# CIRCULAR No. 8

AND

# CIRCULAR No. 9

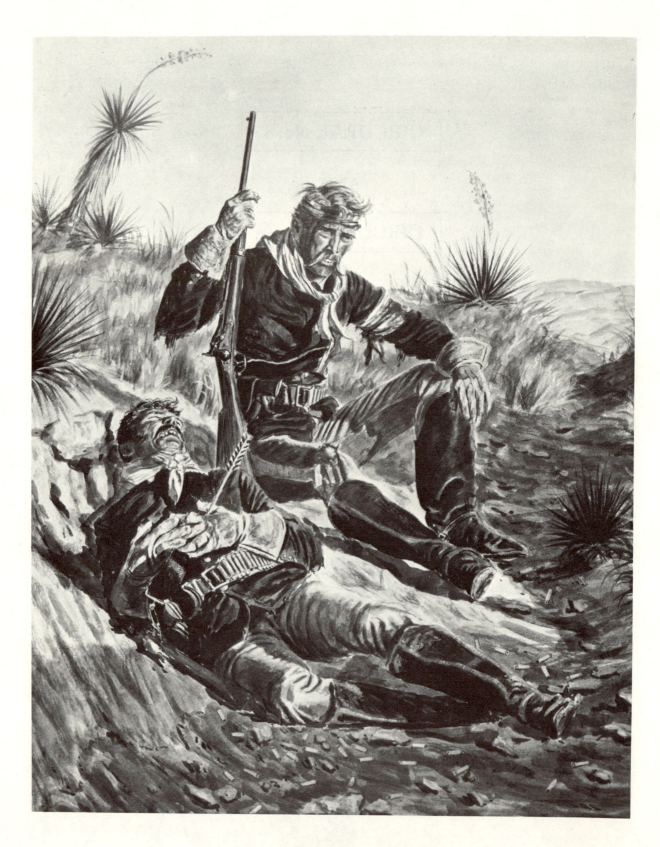

HIS LAST BREATH *by Joe Grandee*

WAR DEPARTMENT
SURGEON GENERAL'S OFFICE

## CIRCULAR No. 8

REPORT ON

# HYGIENE OF THE UNITED STATES ARMY

## WITH DESCRIPTIONS OF MILITARY POSTS

by John S. Billings, Assistant Surgeon, United States Army

AND

## CIRCULAR No. 9

REPORT TO THE SURGEON GENERAL ON THE

TRANSPORT OF SICK AND WOUNDED

BY PACK ANIMALS

by George A. Otis, Assistant Surgeon, United States Army

*With an Introduction by*

Herbert M. Hart

Colonel, United States Marine Corps

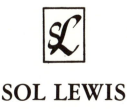

## SOL LEWIS

*New York 1974*

A VOLUME IN THE CUSTERIANA SERIES
John M. Carroll, Editor

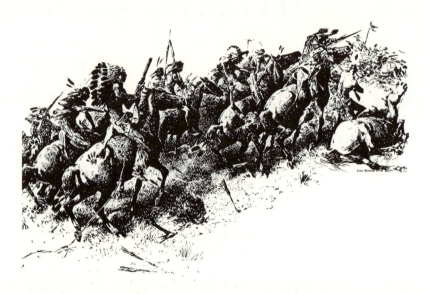

Courtesy: Home Insurance Company

First published by the War Department,
Surgeon General's Office: Circular No. 8,
May 1, 1875; Circular No. 9, March 1, 1877.


Reprinted 1974 in a one-volume Limited
Edition of 500 copies by Sol Lewis.

Library of Congress Catalogue Card Number 72-80857
International Standard Book Number 0-914074-09-1


MANUFACTURED IN THE UNITED STATES OF AMERICA




SOL LEWIS, New York 10003

# PREFACE

The republication of the Surgeon General *Circular #4* and *Circular #8* represents the final fulfillment of an ambition of mine to perpetuate a segment of our western heritage and the role played by the military in its evolution; and it almost did not come about.

Dustin lists *Circular #4* under "Military Posts of the United States Army, with Barracks and Hospitals, Description of . . . 154 Posts described." (Dustin #201) Of it he said: "There is no other publication containing the vast amount of information about frontier posts; contains much natural history." It has always been a difficult publication to obtain and Custer collectors have coveted copies whenever they became available. Fortunately I had a rather good copy in my collection and offered it for reprint purposes so all collectors and students of CUSTER-IANA could share the information it contained. But before the publication got underway I became the possessor of *Circular #8* (not in Dustin) which included the description of an additional 95 posts not in *Circular #4*. Not only did it include most of the information in Circular #4, it addressed itself also to a report on the hygiene of the United States Army, a subject not covered in *Circular #4*. Both circulars are listed in Howes as B-450—indicating their worth.

My perplexity about which edition to reprint was resolved when my good friends, Ruth and Aaron Cohen of Scottsdale, Arizona, insisted both were needed simply because *Circular #8* did not contain everything from *Circular #4*, and *Circular #4* was important because of its listing in Dustin. That settled it! However, I felt uneasy because I feared collectors would be confused about which edition they should own. It was then I hit upon the concept of adding material to each which would make both attractive to the collector.

To *Circular #4* I elected to add that portion of *Circular #3* which addressed itself to the reports of arrow wounds. I opted for this primarily because of the obvious relationship between our western military posts and the ever-present danger of arrow wounds inflicted by Native Americans in the West. The selection of Joe Grandee's great picture, "The Warning," very graphically depicts that real danger.

The addition of *Circular #9* to *Circular #8* makes that one a highly desirable item for any collector because of its immediate association with General Custer. Entitled "Transportation of Sick And Wounded," it contains a section—including drawings—of pack transportation of soldiers from Reno's Hill to Gibbon's Camp. (Dustin #484) A second great painting by Joe Grandee again depicts the potential danger of serving at western posts. Both editions, however, contain a heretofore unpublished picture of Dr. John Shaw Billings, compiler of both circulars on military posts. The picture was discovered by the author of the new Foreward in the process of his research at National Archives in Washington, D. C., and is used here with their permission.

A better choice of author for the new Introduction to these publications than Lieutenant Colonel Herbert M. Hart, USMC. would be difficult to find. Before I made contact with the Colonel I was already certain—in my mind—he would be interested in the project since he was already established as one of the leading authorities in the country on this subject. Fortunately for everyone he was interested. His credentials include *Pioneer Forts of the West, Old Forts of the Far West, Old Forts of the Southwest* and *Old Forts of the Northwest*. To this im-

i

pressive list will soon be added the first of a proposed ten volume series on the same subject; it will be entitled *Guardians Of The Western Frontier* and will be published by Arthur H. Clark Company of Glendale, California.

In addition to his scholarly researched projects, Colonel Hart is Secretary of the Council on Abandoned Military Posts—U.S.A., popularly known as C.A.M.P. Their purpose is to "identify, locate, preserve, and memorialize military installations that no longer serve the roles for which they were originally created." The activities of this worthwhile organization cover the entire North American continent and a very active membership meets annually at which time there are "panel discussions and presentations appropriate to the group and the area [where they are meeting] and visits to the sites of nearby old military posts." They meet at a different location each year. With all these purposeful activities it is astonishing the Colonel finds the necessary time to observe his multiple responsibilities as a marine officer at Quantico, Virginia, but he does. He is presently assigned to the Basic School at the Marine Corps Base there, but is temporarily reassigned from his duties as S-3 to serve full-time on a 9-month panel to study education in the Marine Corps.

Colonel Hart's service tours are equally impressive. He was a platoon leader and executive officer of Company H, 5th Marines in Korea, 1952-53, during which time he was twice awarded the Purple Heart for wounds received, the Navy Commendation Medal with Combat "V" and the Navy Unit Citation. He also served in Korea as a Tactical Air Observer with Marine Observation Squadron Six, receiving five Air Medals and the Presidential Unit citation. He then served in a variety of responsible assignments both in this country and abroad. At the time of the "Lightning War" between Israel and the Arab States in 1967, he was assigned to the U. S. Strike Command at MacDill Air Force Base, Tampa, Florida. From 1967-1969, he was an Arab-Israel-Persian Affairs Plans and Policies Officer in the J-5 (Plans) Directorate of that command's Headquarters of the U. S. Commander-in-Chief, Middle East, Africa South of the Sahara, and Southern Asia, an assignment that took him frequently to the Middle East, including Iran, Kuwait, Saudi Arabia, Lebanon, Bahrain, Jordan, and the Persian Gulf and Red Sea areas. He was awarded the Meritorious Service Medal for this tour of duty. From 1969-70 he was assigned to Southeast Asia, the first six months as commanding officer of Battalion Landing Team, Third Battalion, 9th Marine Regiment, 3d Marine Division, aboard Special Landing Force ships in the South China Sea. The last half of the tour he was the Operations Officer (G-3), 1st Marine Division, based at Danang, Vietnam. For this tour he was awarded The Legion of Merit with combat "V". For his research and publications in the field of military history he was presented the Army Commendation Medal by the Secretary of the Army.

I was grateful to Colonel Hart for accepting my invitation to contribute a new Foreword for these publications, but upon receipt of his insightful and thoroughly researched essay, my gratefulness evolved into deep admiration and respect, for his contribution covers not only all I have said, but it is also a dissertation on the subject which could stand by itself as well.

JOHN M. CARROLL
New Brunswick, New Jersey

# INTRODUCTION

In addition to the research significance of the reprinting of these Surgeon General circulars, the Hart family finds the occasion somewhat sentimental. Having obtained copies through Don Sharp's Roundup Book Company, San Francisco, at the relatively inexpensive prices of ten years ago, I took numbers 4 and 8 with me on my several trips to the sites of about 800 old western forts. Even my children knew what we were talking about when my wife and I referred to "Doctor 4" or "Doctor 8."

As an anesthetist with a master's degree in mental health from Columbia University, New York, my wife was especially interested in the circulars. She assumed the responsibilities of interpreter and custodian for them and on at least one occasion she performed above and beyond the call of duty.

It was during the Memorial Day period, 1962, at Fort Buford, N.D., that this incident occured. I decided to move the station wagon camper slightly in order to get it out of the view for a photograph. Almost immediately I dropped the back wheels into a hidden ditch. From her location in the back of the vehicle my wife could not see what was happening but she decided it would be appropriate to abandon ship. She burst out the side door with her three most valuable posessions in hand: our two-month old baby son and our friends, the "Doctors."

Researching this Introduction also has been a sentimental journey as we visited the National Archives, the Library of Congress, and the National Library of Medicine. Only by going to all of these places were we able to get a good picture of the authors of these circulars, Dr. John Shaw Billings, who was responsible for the larger works, and Dr. George Alexander Otis, who wrote the shorter papers.

Fortunately for our purposes, the records were fairly complete on both officers. Billings, in fact, even had a biographer in the person of Lieutenant Colonel Fielding H. Garrison, Medical Corps, a former Surgeon General's Office associate and the author of "John Shaw Billings: A Memoir" (G. P. Putnam and Sons, 1915). This drew heavily on the journal that Billings kept most of his life.

Billings was born on April 12, 1838, in Switzerland County, Indiana, the son of John Billings and the former Abby Shaw. His English roots were deep: his mother descended from a Mayflower Pilgrim and in later years he made regular trips to England. "Every time I leave England it is more and more like leaving home, so that my affections are about evenly divided," he wrote after a visit in 1889.

Most of Billings' boyhood was spent in Allenville, Indiana, where his father ran a general store, shoemaker shop, and post office "on the road from Rising Sun to Vevay." Money was not plentiful in Billings' younger days and he worked at various occupations during his schooling. Garrison suggests in one writing that many of Billings' adult medical problems, including eight major operations for gallstones or cancer, could be traced to his internship at Miami Medical College, where he subsisted on 75 cents a week, eating mainly eggs and milk.

Entering Miami University in 1852, Billings graduated as class salutatorian in 1857. He entered the Medical College of Ohio (which was combined with the Miami Medical College) in 1858. After receiving his M.D. in 1860, he joined the faculty as demonstrator of anatomy. He held this position until the opening days of the Civil War.

The National Archives has two boxes of Billings' military record, including his letter of application to take the Army Medical Board examination. He faced the examination with a large class and finished first, receiving an appointment as an acting assistant surgeon. He was commissioned an assistant surgeon in the regular Army Medical Corps in April, 1862, with the rank of first lieutenant.

In addition to hospital duties in Pennsylvania and New York, he served in the field with the Army of the Potomac during the "Seven Days Before Richmond" (1862), Chancellorsville (1863), Gettysburg (1863), and Grant's 1864 campaign, including the Wilderness, Todd's Tavern, Spottsylvania, Bloody Angle, North Anna, Cold Harbor, and the Siege of Petersburg.

In April, 1864, Billings was assigned to duty in the Medical Director's Office, Army of the Potomac, in Washington, compiling statistics and data on the medical and surgical activities of that army. This was the start of what would be a major area of interest for the remainder of his Army career and which is reflected in the detailed data presented in Circulars 4 and 8.

Billings was assigned to the Surgeon General's Office in January, 1865, where he was to remain until retirement 30 years later. He spread his talents widely in this duty, with special details to various other government agencies and activities. In 1869 he was loaned to the Secretary of the Treasury for a project which resulted in the reorganization of the Marine Hospital service; he served as professional advisor to the trustees of the Johns Hopkins bequest and designed the hospital of the same name; he collaborated on the design and remodeling of the ventilation of the House of Representatives at the National Capitol; he chaired a committee that modernized the sanitation system of Memphis, Tenn., after a yellow fever epidemic; he was an organizer and an officer of the American Public Health Association and the National Board of Health; and designed the hospital of the University of Pennsylvania, Peter Bent Brigham Hospital in Boston, Mass., and overseas, the Sydney, Australia, City Hospital.

At the time of the 1880 census the War Department was asked to make Billings available as a medical specialist. The statistics involved in this undertaking were a Billings specialty and he compiled the mortality portions for both the tenth and eleventh census, in 1880 and 1890, respectively. His work won high praise, some observers noting that for the first time the census report presented meaningful information. The respect in which he was officially held is suggested by the opening page of the 1890 published result, "Census Report of the 11th Census," part III "Statistics of Deaths" where he is given the title of "Expert Special Agent."

It was in his census work that Billings opened the door for an innovation in statistical compilations by suggesting the use of punched cards and then "sorting them by mechanical means." In 1890, after Herman Hollerith had demonstrated their practical value, punch cards were used in the census. This operation was a forerunner of modern informational retrieval systems now used worldwide.

By the time of the second census project, Billings was nearing the end of his Army career. He had received brevet ranks through lieutenant colonel for his Civil War service but it was not until 1894 that he reached that actual rank.

Although Garrison does not discuss it in his "Memoirs," it appears that in these later years Billings frequently was in the running for the post of Surgeon General. The National Archives' personal file on Billings has a thick packet of letters to Congressmen and the White House from various personages urging that

Billings be made Surgeon General. Almost all the authors suggested that the urging was at their own initiative and without the instigation of Billings. The file also has an anonymous and undated 8-page printed booklet, "Brief Upon the Surgeon Generalship of the Army," which describes Billings' qualifications in glowing terms while those of another officer are deprecated, even to suggesting that the rival already "has been rewarded far beyond his desserts." It is likely that the booklet dates from 1886.

Any chance that Billings had for the surgeon generalship most likely was lost by his specialization in medical literature and statistics rather than active medical field practice. But, as one Medical Corps historian has written, "The work he did was enormously greater than that of any Surgeon General during any period in which he might have been appointed. Let us give thanks."

The two circulars on Army hygiene were not the only products of Billings' research. In 1880 he started to compile the "Index Catalogue," a bibliography of medical writings, of which the first series totaled 16 volumes, when completed 15 years later. From 1879 to 1899 he co-edited the "Index Medicus," a supplement to the "Index Catalogue." He resumed the publication with Carnegie Foundation financing in 1903 and it continues today under the title, "Quarterly Cumulative Index to Current Medical Literature."

In 1885 Billings produced a two-volume "National Medical Dictionary" for a Philadelphia firm, but even his sympathetic biographer, Garrison, had to admit that this was less than impressive. "It contained definitions which did not define and other signs of hasty preparation," Garrison notes in the "Memoir."

Billings represented the United States at numerous medical conventions and received several honorary degrees from both American and European institutions. His work more and more concentrated in the library field: the Surgeon General's Library which he took over in 1865 was increased from 1,800 volumes to 110,000 books and pamphlets by 1880 and today, as the National Library of Medicine, has more than a million and a half holdings and the reputation of being the largest of its kind in the world.

Five years before his retirement and with the concurrence of the Surgeon General, Billings was appointed by the University of Pennsylvania to be the director of its hospital and professor of hygiene. When he retired in 1895 as Deputy Surgeon General and Director of the Army Medical Museum and Library, he moved to active participation on the university faculty. He was not to stay long away from the library field, however.

In 1896 the Board of Trustees of the New York Public Library, newly formed from the merger of three other libraries, elected him superintendent-in-chief for the establishment of the library and construction of the building. In effect the founder of the New York Public Library, he was its director until his death in 1913. He was also the president of the American Library Association in 1902 and, from 1903 until his death, the chairman of the Board of Trustees of the Carnegie Institution of Washington.

Of a more intimate nature are Billings' family and personality. He was married in 1862 to Katharine Mary Stevens, daughter of a former Michigan Congressman. Six children were born of the marriage, one of whom died in infancy. The one son followed his father's lead by becoming a physician in New York City.

Garrison describes Billings as "a man of proud mind and imperious temper, one not given to brooking insults, very much inclined to have his own way, no doubt, yet willing to settle controversy with compromise if he could have peace with honor."

The Dictionary of American Biography expands upon this: "Billings was high-spirited and imperious in temper, and in his later years the recurrent physical pain of which he never spoke added at time an edge to his words. His absorption in matters of large moment interfered with his enduring fools gladly; his Army training developed an innate self-reliance and domination which to some were repellent; his achievements were not such as to split the ears of the ground-lings; and his humor, at times somewhat grim, was not always understood by little men."

Billings' memorials are many. Garrison lists 171 printed works by him but the Dictionary of American Biography notes that this list is incomplete. The entrance to the magnificent National Library of Medicine in Bethesda, Md., bears a plaque crediting Billings with being its founder and further honors him with a John Shaw Billings Collection which is, in turn, housed in a pleasant, deep-carpeted, well-furnished John Shaw Billings Room.

Of greater moment in terms of Billings' memory is the pioneering that he did in turning the primary direction of American medicine from curing the ill to preventing the illness and from caring for the individual patient to caring for community health.

His particular interests which would become his lasting impact on medicine are reflected in the two circulars reprinted in this set. In Circular 4 he devotes an initial 33 pages to the need for proper facilities in barracks, hospitals, messes, guardhouses, and toilets. Today this would be called preventive medicine or sanitation.

A comparison of the so-called "habitability" standards for 1972 military construction reflects considerable progress beyond the minimums prescribed by Billings. Of course the plumbing matters have long out-distanced the methods suggested. Except for recruit-type training and other special situations, the double-deck bunk is a thing of the past.

Billings suggested that barracks have ceilings of at least 12 feet high. The Department of Defense (DOD) "Criteria Manual" of 1972 directs that story heights normally will be nine and a half feet but may go an additional foot if required by a ventilation system. Maximum heights in medical facilities are set at 11 and a half feet.

The Billings standard of 600 cubic feet per man (e.g., a room 6 feet x 10 feet, with a ceiling height of 10 feet) is not too different from the DOD requirement of 72 square feet per recruit with 30 to 60 men per dormitory. With a 10 foot high ceiling this would come out to 720 cubic feet per man, fairly close to Billings' 600 cubic feet, considering the higher number includes common areas and central toilets.

Modern space increases with rank and men in a normal unit supposedly are billeted three to a room of 310 square feet. This would come out to about 1,000 cubic feet per man. Staff noncommissioned officers are to be two to a 310 square foot room, including bathroom; senior staff noncommissioned officers one to a room of the same size.

Even prison cells exceed the 600 minimum. The 1972 standard calls for 300 square feet per prisoner in facilities designed to hold up to 40 prisoners and 250 square feet for larger prisons. Within this space facilities must be included for housing, training, welfare, and advisors so the actual amount per individual probably is reduced by half or two-thirds—but still more than the minimum of 100 years ago.

In Circular 8 Billings takes issue with the diet of the Army and chronicles how the ration was improved, and sometimes reduced, over the years. Although the minimums suggested by Billings may have been sufficient to support a man in 1875, it is unlikely that they would be accepted today.

The soldier of today is larger and requires more intake to keep going. His culture has changed and he is used to more in quantity and in variety. Today's mess halls—called dining rooms by most services—compete for better and bigger salad and dessert bars, choices of several entrees, and a considerable spread of side dishers. Pizzas, tacos, "soul food," curries, sukiyaki now appear on menus. Some services even provide beer machines and all have a wide range of beverages including milk through colas, fruit juices and, of course, the inexhaustible coffee pot.

Investigation of feeding arrangements in the recent conflicts in Korea and Vietnam showed that the diet of the fighting man was close in quality and quantity to that of his stateside counterpart, circumstances permitting, and helicopter missions to deliver ice cream were often the rule rather than the exception. The field combat rations, from canned meat combinations and fruits to the accessories provided as supplements, often were better than the diet which Circular 8 suggests as the standard.

But in these matters pioneers such as Billings took the early steps in improving the lot of the soldier. If Billings' learned prefaces were the only contents of these circulars, they would still be worth reprinting as recognition of their contribution to the future.

The other two circulars in this set were by an associate of Billings, Dr. George Alexander Otis. Equally distinguished in his own right, Otis has not achieved the degree of recognition because of his early death at the age of 51.

Otis was born on November 2, 1830, in Boston, Mass. He was graduated from Princeton with a B.A. in 1850 and M.A. in 1851. Simultaneously he matriculated in the medical department of the University of Pennsylvania and received the M.D. degree in 1851. He was in private practice in Springfield, Mass., at the start of the Civil War and was appointed surgeon of the 28th Massachusetts Volunteers.

Otis served in various duties until 1864 when he resigned from the regiment to accept an appointment as assistant surgeon in the U. S. Volunteers. Assigned to the Surgeon General's Office as assistant to the curator, and then curator, of the Army Medical Museum, he was primarily concerned with the gathering of data for a surgical history of the Civil War.

He wrote several circulars or reports on various wounds and their treatment but his greatest efforts were the three surgical volumes of the "Medical and Surgical History of the War of the Rebellion." He is listed as author and compiler of the first two volumes (1870 and 1875) and was working on the third when he suffered a stroke of paralysis in 1877 and died four years later. He is listed as co-author for this volume.

The two Otis works in this reprint set were first published in 1871 and 1877, respectively. The portion on the treatment of arrow wounds is taken from Circular 3, "A Report of Surgical Cases Treated in the Army of the United States from 1865 to 1871." It is of renewed interest because of its discussion of a wound that became obsolete but now, with conflicts taking place in a guerrilla warfare arena, have become more common again. The entire report consists of 296 pages, covering wounds that range from gunshots to punctures, fractures and dislocations, poisons, burns and frost bite, and operations and amputations.

The arrow wound portion treats 83 cases, 26 of which were fatal, but notes that the discussion is incomplete because reports were not received on at least six major battles of the 1867-70 era. The Fetterman disaster and Custer's Battle of the Washita are two notable omissions.

Otis' second report also has a modern application. "A Report to the Surgeon General on the Transport of Sick and Wounded by Pack Animals" has its own near counterpart on pages 80 and 81 of Army Field manual 8-35, "Transportation of the Sick and Wounded" (Washington, December, 1970). The photographs on these pages show wounded being moved by travois and by litter carried by a pack saddle.

Although helicopter evacuation within minutes may be common in Vietnam, there are exceptions when weather or the absence of suitable landing zone have interfered. Then the wounded had to be man- or animal-packed to safety. Otis vividly describes early practices with an account of the evacuation of 59 wounded from the Battle of the Little Big Horn by travois over 30 dark and rugged miles without "accident or personal inconvenience or discomfort of any sort." It is hard to accept this statement as entirely correct either for the wounded of 1876 or for the wounded in Vietnam who suffered the litter route until faster evacuation means were at hand.

But Otis' main point in Circular 9 is as true today as ever, that it is neither prudent nor economical to confine the matter of transporting the sick to the ingenuity of the troops. He notes that just because makeshift bridges have resulted from battlefield inspiration there is no reason that the engineers should not learn how to build bridges; or quartermasters cease to provide logistical support because foraging has sometimes worked; or ships not to have life boats because crews have devised rafts in emergencies. Otis' lesson has been taken well and today's combat forces are well-equipped for rapid battlefield medical evacuation. From the helicopter to the jeep ambulance, even to the inclusion of animal transport, this area has been given conscientious and effective attention. The Army field manual noted even includes almost 100 pages of drills in the use of litters and stretchers, not leaving that element of the subject to chance.

The bulk of these reprints, and perhaps that which is of the greatest interest and value to the reader, is the discussion of the various posts and stations of the Army in the 1869-74 period. The two circulars describe in varying detail about 250 posts. Some are mere single paragraphs, especially in Circular 8, perhaps included only to satisfy inquiries as to why they were left out of Circular 4. Many of these sites usually were in a caretaker status, or even less than that, and were no longer active. But the addition of these posts meant that considerably more forts are discussed in Circular 8 than in 4. At the same time, because of closings, some forts described in 4 are not in 8 or are greatly condensed. And, throughout, the completeness of a report depended upon submissions from the posts although Billings describes his own efforts along this line in the opening of each circular.

The mission of these posts has long been achieved and few of them are active today. Many of the more prominent or permanent sites are active as parks or museums but many of the lesser known and temporary posts are, at best, memorialized by markers or, at worse, completely lost to memory.

To provide a degree of updating to these circulars and to put the posts in a modern perspective, an attempt has been made to provide a short status comment on each site. In most cases these notes are based on my own personal observations at the sites; in some cases I have been assisted by local sources or fellow members of the Council on Abandoned Military Posts. And in some cases where deadlines or the vagueness of the location dictated, no comment has been possible.

Site location is in terms of 1972 towns and roads but I have not elaborated on directions when those in the original circular still apply. The listing is in the same alphabetical order of the circulars. The numeral after a name indicates that it appears only in that circular, otherwise the post is in both circulars—though sometimes by a different name.

It is with some hesitation that I attempt to pinpoint the location of these sites and thereby draw the attention of treasure hunters, souvenir collectors, and vandals. I ask that anyone visiting a site remember that it is very probably private property and entering without permission is trespassing. Removal of artifacts without permission is stealing. I also ask that the owners of these sites respect their history by not removing or leveling the few evidences that are left and by not permitting others to do so. Let us attempt to retain at least this small portion of our historic past to remind us of the struggles to establish a republic and tame a frontier.

## THE POSTS

*Abercrombie, N.D.,* is a restored, reconstructed state park at Abercrombie. *Abraham Lincoln, N.D.,* (8) Custer's last post, is a state park south of Bismarck in which the building sites are marked and the blockhouses and some other portions of subordinate Ft. McKeen have been reconstructed. *Adams, R.I.,* are massive ruins at the Naval Station, Newport. *Alcatraz Island, Calif.,* has several Army structures surviving the Federal prison and Indian occupation periods but this site is closed and guarded. *Allegheny Arsenal, Penna.,* (8) at 40th and Butler streets, Pittsburgh, is no longer active but some Army buildings are still in use; *Fort Pitt Park* houses the Fort Pitt Museum and the only pre-Revolution building, the original blockhouse, is at 25 Penn avenue, Pittsburgh.

*Andrews, Mass.,* vague site is near the Plymouth Light on Gurnet Point, accessible from Green Harbor down Duxbury Beach, and not to be confused with Fort Andrews (1900-47) on Paddocks Island in Boston Harbor. *Angel Island and Camp Reynolds, Calif.,* are maintained by the State Beaches and Parks Department but the Army buildings, visible from across the bay when fog permits, are closed to general visiting; a ferry makes trips to the island from Tiburon. *Apache, Ariz.,* (8) has many buildings now in use by the Fort Apache Indian Agency whicn encourages visitors at an active resort area. *Augusta Arsenal, Ga.,*

(8) was closed in 1958 and the remaining buildings were turned over to Augusta College.

*Austin, Texas,* post site is shared by a vacant lot and automobile agency at 1214 West 6th street. *Baker, Mont.,* later named Ft. Logan, has several buildings and a blockhouse in private ranch use 20 miles west of White Sulphur Springs. *Barrancas, Fla.,* is preserved and cemented-up on the Pensacola Naval Air Station reservation; visitors are welcome. *Bascom, N.M.* (4) is fully outlined by scattered bricks and mounds on a restricted private ranch north of Tucumcari. *Baton Rouge, La.* has only one Army trace in the Old Arsenal Museum on the state capitol grounds, restored from its earlier days when the Army was here 1810-79 or when the Marines captured it from the Confederates in 1862. *Bayard, N.M.,* has virtually no early appearance after serving as a Veterans Administration hospital and now as a state hospital, north of Bayard.

*Beaver, Utah,* (8) became Ft. Cameron and several building ruins are in a park and race track area 2 miles east of Beaver. *Benicia, Calif.,* (8) was given up by the Army in 1964 and responsibilities for the many historic buildings are shared by several activities.

*Benton, Mont.,* has adobe walls protected by a fence and tin roof, a blockhouse, and an excellent museum next to the town of Ft. Benton. *Bidwell, Calif.,* has several buildings still in use at the Indian agency next to the town of Ft. Bidwell. *Bliss, Tex.,* has several sites in and near El Paso of which the Concordia site noted in both circulars is now Concordia cemetery in the northern part of the city; the present Ft. Bliss has been occupied by the Army since 1894.

*Boise, Idaho,* has several buildings, including quarters, in use at the Veterans Hospital in Boise. *Bowie, Ariz.,* has been stabilized and is now administered by the National Park Service south of the town of Bowie. *Brady, Mich.,* has its original site marked by a plaque at Brady Park drive and Water street, Sault Ste. Marie, while the second site, from which the Army left in 1945, is at South street and Ryan avenue. *Bridger, Wy.,* has restored and reconstructed buildings in Ft. Bridger State Park next to Bridger town. *Brown, Wyo.,* was renamed Ft. Washakie and its buildings 17 miles northwest of Lander still are used by the Indian agency. *Brown, Tex.,* has several buildings in use by Southernmost College and Brownsville city offices.

*Buford, N.D.,* is a state park with several buildings restored or reconstructed south of the town of Buford. *Cady, Calif.,* is a desert swept site 22 miles east of Barstow south of I-15; some buildings are in ranch use. *Canby (or Cape Disappointment), Wash.,* site is shared by a Coast Guard station and abandoned coast artillery foundations at Canby State Park 2.4 miles from Waco. *Carlisle Barracks, Penna.* has several old buildings amidst the modern of the Army War College.

*Carroll, Md.* (8) is in excellent shape because its private island location in Baltimore harbor is inconvenient for vandals to visit. *Caswell, N.C.* (8) has the fortress and other buildings amidst a Coast Guard station at the mouth of the Cape of Fear river 25 miles south of Wilmington. *Charleston, S.C.,* has the Citadel back in educational use on Citadel Square in downtown Charleston. *Chattanooga, Tenn.,* has Grant's 1863 headquarters at 110 East 1st street and the National Cemetery still in use with its main entrance at the south end of National avenue. *Cheyenne Agency, S.D.,* became Ft. Bennett and had three buildings still left when the site 35 miles northwest of Pierre was inundated by the Oahe Reservoir.

*Cheyenne Depot, Wyo.* became Camp Carlin but only a marker is left on the Francis E. Warren Air Force Base near Cheyenne. *Clark, Texas,* has many buildings left, most of them marked and in resort use south of Bracketsville. *Clark's Point, Mass.,* (8), 13 miles south of New Bedford, became Ft. Rodman in 1898 until it was given up in 1947. *Clinch, Fla.,* (8) has been reconstructed as a Florida State Park on Amelia Island 3 miles from Fernandina Beach north of Jacksonville. *Columbia, S.C.* (8) no longer has Army use of the leased quarters noted in the circular but the Army is at nearby Ft. Jackson. *Columbus Arsenal, Ohio,* was designated at Ft. Hayes in 1922 and given up recently; it was at Cleveland avenue and Buckingham streets next to Columbus Depot founded in 1918. *Columbus, N.Y.,* was known by this name 1808-1904 until the original Ft. Jay name was resumed; it became a Coast Guard station in 1966.

*Colorado, Ariz.,* (4) site has been covered by irrigation projects west of Parker, Calif., on the Colorado river. *Colville, Wash.,* has only slight traces left of the military post 3 miles south of Colville city. *Concho, Tex.,* is one of the best restored posts in the country, supported by the San Angelo city council and other organizations as a museum and park in the city. *Constitution, N.H.,* (8) is only a grass-grown ruin east of New Castle 3 miles from Portsmouth. *Craig. N.M.* has adobe ruins that have been so badly vandalized in recent years that the site 30 miles south of Socorro has been fenced and directional signs removed; this is private property.

*Crittenden, Ariz.,* (4) has several adobe ruins on the private Crown C ranch 1 mile west of Sonoita. *Cummings, N.M.,* has elaborate but vandalized adobe ruins on the private Hyatt ranch 20 miles north of Deming. *Date Creek, Ariz.,* (4) site in the circulars was the second of three sites to bear this name; it has scattered rock walls and mounds 80 miles north of Phoenix. *David's Island, N.Y.,* (8) as Ft. Slocum southwest of New Rochelle was in use off and on until given up by the Army in 1966. *Davis Texas,* is an example of careful stabilization, restoration, and reconstruction by the National Park Service next to the town of Ft. Davis. *Delaware, Del.,* is a state park centered on the old fortress on an island accessible only by boat on weekends from Delaware City.

*Detroit Arsenal, Mich.,* (8) should not be confused with present day Detroit Arsenal dating from 1941 and 3 miles from the city limits; the former post was on Morely avenue in Dearborn—once known as Dearbornville—where several buildings are still in public or private use. *Dodge, Kans.,* site is 4 miles east of Dodge City where the old buildings are used by the State Soldiers Home. *Douglas, Utah,* next to Salt Lake City is supposed to be inactive but various military regular and reserve activities, governmental and educational offices occupy the buildings.

*Dutch Island, R.I.,* (8) became Ft. Greble until it was abandoned in 1947. *Drum Barracks, Calif.,* (4) has a single building left,—quarters at 1053 Cary avenue, Wilmington. *Duncan, Tex.,* has many Army buildings preserved in a city park on Adams street south of downtown Eagle Pass. *Ellis, Mont.,* is now the site of the Ft. Ellis Experimental Station east of Bozeman. *Fetterman, Wyo.,* has several buildings in varying stages of restoration as a state park 8 miles northwest of Douglas. *Foote, Md.,* has a man-high 15-inch Rodman gun barrell amidst overgrown brick ruins in the National Park Service's unimproved Ft. Foote Park north of Ft. Washington.

*Frankford Arsenal, Penna.* (8) is still active with 234 buildings covering 112 acres in northeastern Philadelphia. *Frankfort, Ky.,* (8) was a leased site in Frankfort which was given up in 1876. *Gaines, Ala.,* has partly restored ramparts with guns in a park on Dauphin Island in Mobile Bay. *Garland, Colo.,* has been restored or reconstructed as a state museum south of the town. *Gaston, Calif.,* has a few buildings now used by the Hoopa Indian agency at Hoopa. *Gibson, Okla.,* has restored or reconstructed buildings and stockade as a state park of the first Ft. Gibson north of the town; the buildings of the second post are in various stages of repair or use to the east of the park and on the hillside above it. *Gorges, Me.,* (8) has stone ruins on Hog Island in Portland Harbor that seem to rise out of the water without any foundations. *Grand River Agency. S.D.,* (8) site is 5 miles north of Mobridge but inundated by the Missouri river's Oahe Reservoir. *Grant, Ariz.,* has the 1860-72 site of Circular 4 obliterated 40 miles northeast of Tucson but the second site, 1872-1907, is used by the Arizona State Industrial School 25 miles north of Willcox where much of the old officers' row is still in use. *Gratiot, Mich.,* is marked by a plaque at Stone and State streets, Port Huron, but the post was dismantled in 1882.

*Griffin, Tex.,* has numerous ruins amidst rattlesnake-infested grass in Ft. Griffin State Park 15 miles north of Albany. *Griswold, Conn.,* (8) is commemorated by a monument at Fort and Thomas streets, Groton. *Hall, Idaho,* (8) has only rows of trees along the former parade ground at this location 12 miles east of Blackfoot and 25 miles northeast of the inundated site of the Fort Hall trading post. *Halleck, Nev.,* has building excavations and foundation stones on the site 38 miles southeast of Elko. *Hamilton, N.Y.* has the original post and quarters supposedly occupied by Robert E. Lee at this still active installation with the main entrance near 96th street and 7th avenue, Brooklyn.

*Hancock, N.D.* (8) is a single wooden building in use as a museum to Dakota pioneers and Indian tribes at 117 Main avenue, Bismarck. *Harker, Kans.,* has several buildings still in use, one as a museum, in the western edge of Kanopolis. *Harney, Ore.,* has only the cemetery site near the ghost town of Harney City 13 miles north of Burns. *Hartsuff, Nebr.,* (8) is a tribute to Dr. Glen Auble, Ord, who preserved the buildings as best he could until the state finally agreed to accept them as a state park 10 miles from Ord. *Hays, Kans.,* has three buildings at the site in a town park and golf course immediately south of Hays City. *Humboldt, Tenn.,* (8) has not seen the Army since it left in 1876 and now strawberry festivals are the main local activity.

*Independence, Calif.,* has caves of the original post east of the town; the original parade ground is now a meadow; the commanding officer's quarters has been moved to 303 Edwards in town. *Independence, Mass.,* is now a Boston City Park in South Boston where the fortress still is imposing. *Jackson Barracks, La.,* was leased to the state in 1924 and the fortress-like post was remodeled by the WPA for current use by state and federal activities 5 miles from downtown New Orleans at St. Charles and Delery streets. *Ft. Jackson, La.,* (8) is an excellently preserved pentagon 2.5 miles southeast of Triumph on the western bank of the Mississippi. *Jefferson, Fla.,* is now maintained by the National Park Service in the desolate Dry Tortugas islands accessible by boat charter from Key West. *Jefferson Barracks, Mo.*, was inactivated in 1946 and its many buildings are shared by the Veterans Administration, a city park, and the city housing authority, but the National Cemetery is still in use 9 miles south of St. Louis.

*Johnston, N.C.* was abandoned in 1881 and the overgrown site is accessible only by boat south of Wilmington. *Kennebec Arsenal, Me.*, (8) was taken over by the Main State Hospital at the end of Arsenal street when the Army left in 1897. *Kearney, Nebr.*, (4) is a reconstructed stockade and marked building sites in a state park 6 miles southeast of Kearney city. *Key West Barracks, Fla.*, is now in use at the Key West Naval Base. *Klamath, Ore.*, has a museum in a replica of the old guardhouse but there are no other remains, except the cemetery, near the town of Ft. Klamath. *Knox, Me.*, (8) has huge arches and stairways in Ft. Knox State Park at Prospect. *LaPaz, Ariz.*, has only the well left but both post and town have disappeared on the Colorado River Indian Reservation 10 miles north of Ehrenberg. *Lapwai, Idaho*, has many Army buildings still in use at the Lapwai Indian Agency headquarters 1 mile south of the town of Lapwai.

*Laramie, Wyo.*, is one of the most complete National Park Service projects with each building restored or reconstructed to its appearance at its height of activity; the Ft. Laramie National Monument is 2 miles from the town of Ft. Laramie. *Larned, Kans.*, has original buildings around the parade ground on what was the Frizell property but now in National Park Service possession. *Layfayette, N.Y.* (8) never was rebuilt after a fire in 1868, as noted in Circular 8. *Leavenworth, Kans.*, is still active as the location of the Army's Command and General Staff College where many historic buildings still are in use north of the town of Leavenworth.

*Little Rock, Ark.*, has the Army site in a city park at East 9th and Commerce streets with the old armory building as the only structure left. *Livingston, La.*, (8) was not garrisoned after the Civil War and the fort was partly destroyed by a hurricane in 1893; ruins are on the southern point of Grande Terre Island accessible by boat from Grand Isle. *Long Point Batteries, Mass.*, (8) have only a lighthouse across from Provincetown to mark the site. *Lowell, Ariz.*, had two sites with the first one now occupied by the Santa Rita hotel in downtown Tucson and the second—described in the circulars—is a park restored and reconstructed by the Arizona Historical Society east of Tucson.

*Lower Brule Agency, S.D.* (8) had two sites, the 1870 location—usually called Fort Lower Brule—is across the Missouri river from Chamberlain where low hummocks 5 miles north of the Oacoma exit on I-90 are believed to be the site; the post noted in Circular 8 is south of the Big Bend dam's western bank. *Lyon, Colo.*, is now a Veterans Administration hospital with many buildings still in use and an active interest in history by the staff and patients. *Mackinac, Mich.*, is a state park on Mackinac Island with most of the buildings restored or reconstructed.

*Macomb, La.*, (8) is a state monument about 150 yards from the end of Chief Menteur bridge on U. S. 90 about 22 miles northeast of downtown New Orleans. *Macon, N.C.*, is a state park near Atlantic Beach with the fortress restored and reconstructed and housing a museum. *Madison Barracks, N.Y.* was in use until after World War II at the eastern edge of Sackett's Harbor. Its abandoned buildings stand unoccupied. *Marion, Fla.*, (8) was designated a National Monument in

1924 and the historic castillo at St. Augustine (Castillo de San Marcos and nearby Fort Matanzas) had the original name restored in 1942. *McClary, Me.,* (8) is a hexagonal fort now in use as a state park at Kittery. *McDermitt, Nev.,* has several Army buildings left and in use as the Indian agency headquarters 98 miles north of Winnemucca.

*McDowell, Ariz.,* is threatened by reclamation project waters that will inundate the officers' quarters still in use by the Ft. McDowell Indian agency north of Phoenix. The Pioneer Arizona Museum plans to build a replica of the fort as a Bicentennial project. *McHenry, Md.,* is a National Monument in South Baltimore where Marines present a tattoo ceremony every Thursday during the summer months and the Park rangers give tours throughout the year. *McIntosh, Tex.,* was given up by the Army in 1945 but the buildings still are in use by various government agencies, including the Border Patrol and a junior college in Laredo; the original site can still be identified by earthworks north of the main post. *McKavett, Tex.,* has some of Ranald Mackenzie's original buildings still in use as residences in the town of Ft. McKavett about 25 miles from Menard. *McPherson Barracks, Ga.,* (8) no longer has an Army presence at this downtown leased location but modern Ft. McPherson has been located a mile and a quarter to the south since 1889. *McPherson, Nebr.,* has only the cemetery left, as a National Cemetery with the dead of many battles and many Western Forts re-buried there, but there is a monument at the nearby site of the post; all are about 13 miles west of North Platte.

*McRae, N.M.* has stone foundations outlining the entire post in a ravine east of Truth or Consequences and the Elephant Butte Reservoir. *McRae, Fla.,* (8) has vague remains on an islet observable mainly from the air at the western side of Pensacola Bay's channel. *Medicine Bow, Wyo.,* (8) is a vague site about 2 miles south of the town of Medicine Bow. *Mifflin, Penna.* has large ruins next to the runway of Philadelphia International Airport. *Mojave, Ariz.,* has a few traces and the cemetery area left about 90 miles south of Las Vegas, Nev. *Monroe, Va.* is a fortress still in use by the Continental Army Command across Hampton Roads from Norfolk.

*Montgomery, N.Y.* (8) site is on Island Point, an island in Lake Champlain near Rouse's Point and is not to be confused with Revolutionary War Ft. Montgomery 3 miles from Highland Falls. *Morgan, Ala.,* (8) is a fortress in a state park at the end of Alabama 180 at the mouth of Mobile Bay. *Moultrie, S.C.* (8) has maintained ruins of various periods through World War II as part of the National Park Service activities in the Charleston harbor area. *Mount Vernon Barracks, Ala.,* (8) was given up in 1894 and now is the city of Mr. Vernon. *Newport Barracks, Ky.,* was inundated by the Ohio river in 1884 and was re-located 2 miles from the city where it was active as Ft. Thomas until after World War II. *Niagara N.Y.,* is owned and administered by the Old Fort Niagara Association on New York 18 north of Youngstown. *North Platte Station, Nebr.,* has nothing left to mark the site in the 400 block of West Front street.

*Oglethorpe Barracks, Ga.,* (8) has nothing left at this downtown Savannah site, not to be confused with Ft. Oglethorpe (1902-52) 10 miles south of Chattanooga, Tenn. *Omaha Barracks, Nebr.,* is still known as Ft. Omaha but is used by various government activities north of downtown Omaha. *Ontario, N.Y.* has been part of the New York State Park System since 1946 next to Ontario city. *Pem-*

*bina, N.D.* (8) has only the post cemetery site left of the military fort 3 miles south of Pembina city. *Pickens, Fla.,* (8) has massive ruins of defenses into the twentieth century in the Gulf Islands National Seashore on Santa Rosa Island at the eastern side of the Pensacola Bay channel. *Pike, La.,* is a state monument about 32 miles from New Orleans on U. S. 90.

*Pikesville Arsenal, Md.,* (8) was a Confederate Veterans Home for awhile until turned over to Baltimore county in 1932. *Castle Pinckney, S.C.,* has prominent ruins on its island site in Charleston Harbor. *Plattsburg Barracks, N.Y.,* is now Plattsburg Air Force Base. *Point San Jose, Calif.,* has been Ft. Mason for many years but is frequently threatened with the possibility that it, with its historic buildings, will be given up under pressure from commercial interests. *Popham, Me.,* (8) is now a state memorial at Popham Beach. *Porter, N.Y.* was given up at Buffalo when the Army left in 1926. *Portland Head Battery, Me.,* (8) became Ft. Williams but was closed in 1964; the site is at Cape Cottage, 6 miles south of Portland. *Preble, Me.,* (8) was given up in 1947 from its location on Shore road in South Portland.

*Presidio of San Francisco, Calif.,* is still active with a mixture of modern and historic buildings. *Pulaski, Ga.,* is preserved and maintained by the National Park Service. *Quitman, Texas,* has no traces left except for nearby Quitman cemetery but there is a commercial near-replica on I-10 about 18 miles west of Sierra Blanca. *Randall, S.D.,* is now a park below the western end of the Ft. Randall dam west of Pickstown; the chapel and building sites are left. *Ransom, N.D.,* (4) has marked building sites in a state park 1 mile south of town. *Reynolds, Colo.,* (4) has foundation stones that outline most of the buildings on private property 17 miles east of Pueblo.

*Rice, N.D.* The CCC reconstructed much of the stockade and blockhouses at this state park 1 mile east of town. *Richardson, Tex.,* is a park south of Jacksboro with the hospital and other buildings restored. *Riley, Kans.,* is still in active use with many old Army buildings well preserved. *Ringgold Barracks, Texas,* has several Army buildings in use for educational purposes adjacent to Rio Grande City.

*Ripley, Minn.,* was closed in 1880 but the same site north of Little Falls became the 45,000 acre Camp Ripley when the major National Guard post was founded in 1930; it continues in active guard use. *Robinson, Nebr.,* (8) has a museum, resort hotel, camp ground, and marked historic sites at this post which was closed in 1948 about 2 miles west of Crawford. *Rock Island, Ill.,* (8) is on the Mississippi river opposite Davenport, Iowa, as the largest active manufacturing arsenal in the country; its original Ft. Armstrong (1816) has been reconstructed on the post; the John M. Browning Museum has a large collection of firearms and cannon. *D. A. Russell, Wyo.,* is now Francis E. Warren Air Force Base next to Cheyenne and the Army buildings, especially the diamond-shaped quadrangle shown in the circular, are still in use. *St. Augustine, Fla.,* or St. Francis Barracks (8) is known as the State Arsenal, 108 Marine street, and a point of historic interest south of downtown St. Augustine. *St. Louis Arsenal and Barracks, Mo.,* (8) are now part of Jefferson Barracks Historic Park south of St. Louis on the Missisippi; many buildings are preserved.

*St. Philip, La.,* (8) is in primitive condition 2.5 miles south of Triumph on the eastern bank of the Mississippi. *San Antonio, Texas,* has the Alamo museum at

Alamo Plaza in downtown; the old U. S. Arsenal dating from 1858 was at South Flores and Arsenal streets; Gunter Hotel is on the site of the 2-story building used before the Civil War as Army headquarters; the modern Army is at Ft. Sam Houston, founded in 1879 in the northeastern section of the city. *San Carlos, Ariz.,* (8) is beneath the waters of San Carlos Lake behind Coolidge Dam. *Sanders, Wyoming.,* has the guardhouse and magazine ruins in a park south of Laramie city. *Sandy Hook, N.J.* (8) was termed variously as Ft. Hudson and Ft. Lincoln until named Ft. Hancock in 1895; it is still active 15 miles from Red Bank.

*Santa Fe, N.M.* has slight adobe mounds at the site of Ft. Marcy overlooking the plaza, the Governor's Palace is still in state government use as a museum, and other post buildings are in use as residences in the old Army area bounded by Federal, Washington, Palace, and Grant streets north of the Plaza. *Scammel, Me.,* (8) is an abandoned site on House Island in Portland Harbor. *Schuyler, N.Y.* is a fortress that is part of the New York State Maritime Academy reservation. *Winfield Scott, Nev.,* (4) has several original buildings still in private ranch use west of Paradise Valley. *Sedgwick, Colo.,* (4) has only a marker at the site about 3 miles west of Julesburg and across the river.

*Selden, N.M.* is state owned 17 miles north of Las Cruces with a major stabilization program in progress as of spring, 1973, marking and capping the building remnants. *Sewall, Mass.,* (8) was manned until after the Spanish-American War at its site at the northeast end of Front street at the harbor entrance in Marblehead. *Seward, N.D.,* (8) has a cannon and a marker in a town park on a bluff overlooking the city, 2 miles northwest of Jamestown. *Shaw, Mont.,* has almost all of the Army buildings in good condition and in use in the county school system a half mile north of the town of Ft. Shaw. *Sheridan, Nebr.,* (8) has only slight surface traces in a private pasture 14 miles north of Holly Springs.

*Ship Island, Miss.,* (8) and Ft. Massachusetts became part of the Gulf Islands National Seashore in 1970 and the fort is a park. *Sidney Barracks, Nebr.,* (8) has an officers' quarters and a magazine still in use as residences south of U. S. 30 at the eastern edge of Sidney. *Sill, Okla.,* still is in active use with many historic buildings well preserved by the Army and an excellent museum available to visitors. *Sitka, Alaska,* (8) was on the present site of Alaska Pioneers Home built in 1935 and dominating the harbor; the cemetery is still used and annually the Army from other Alaska forts conducts memorial services there.

*Smith, Ark.,* (4) is now Ft. Smith National Historic Site and several Army buildings are preserved. *Snelling, Minn.,* has been the subject of major reconstruction as a state park in St. Paul. *Springfield Armory and Arsenal, Mass.,* (8) is at Armory and Federal streets and, following the Army departure in 1968, is now the location of the General Electric Company's Armament Division. *Stambaugh, Wyo.,* (8) has only a marker and some slight traces of building hollows in open range land about 30 miles southwest of Lander. *Stanton, N.M.,* has numerous buildings in good condition as a state hospital 33 miles west of Roswell. *Fred Steele, Wyo.,* is a collection of collapsing or burned buildings next to a ramshackle cemetery 14 miles east of Rawlins.

*Stevens, Ore.,* is partly owned by the state with some park development plans 13 miles west of Astoria. *Stevenson, N.D.* is now under the waters of the Garrison dam. *Stockton, Texas,* has several quarters and the guardhouse in the southern part of the city of Ft. Stockton, between 5th and 2d streets. *Sullivan, Me.,* has only the magazine left, preserved by the Border Historical Society, Eastport. *Sully, S.D.* has the original site noted by a marker 4 miles east of Pierre; the second site has been inundated by the Oahe Reservoir since 1968 about 30 miles north of Pierre; the hospital building was moved to a farm as a granary and is in Okobojo Creek valley, 17 miles north of Pierre.

*Sumter, S.C.* (8) is managed by the National Park Service as a National Monument in Charleston Harbor, accessible by boat. *Supply, Okla.,* has quarters and other Army buildings still in use at Western State Hospital, 1 mile east of Supply. *Taylor, Fla.,* (8) has remnants of the fortress on the Key West Naval Station. *Thomas Barracks, Ala.,* (8) went through several periods and name changes, including Post at Huntsville, Camp Monte Sano, Camp Wheeler, and Camp Albert G. Forse, until abandoned in 1899. *Three Forks of the Owyhee, Idaho* (4) has a single building left at a desolate site on private range land about 22 miles east southeast of Jordan Valley, Ore. *Totten, N.D.,* is one of the best preserved western forts immediately next to Ft. Totten town in the Devil's Lake area; almost the entire original quadrangle is left.

*Townsend, Wash.,* (8) has only a flagpole, pilings from the wharf, and markers in a state park 5 miles south of Port Townsend city. *Trumbull, Conn.,* has millstone granite fortifications on the Coast Guard Base, East street, New London. *Tulerosa, N.M.* (8) has building sites still obvious and a cemetery on private property immediately northeast of Aragon. *Union, N.M.* is a National Park Service National Monument with stabilized ruins and a fine museum 7 miles from Watrous. *Vancouver, Wash.,* is still used by the National Guard and reserve units but the National Park Service has the adjacent site of the trading post as a National Monument. *Verde, Ariz.,* has several buildings preserved for several years by a citizens' group until accepted as a state park next to the town of Camp Verde.

*Wadsworth, S.D.,* became Ft. Sisseton in 1876, was abandoned in 1890, and its many buildings are now a state park about 40 miles southwest of Sisseton town. *Wadsworth, N.Y.,* is still active at the Staten Island end of Verrazano-Narrows bridge but plans to give it up were discussed by the Army in 1972. *Wallace, Kans.,* cemetery and building indentations are a half mile east of Wallace town. *Walla Walla, Wash.,* (8) has the post cemetery—with the dead of many posts and battles relocated there—and the officers' quarters row still in use at the Veterans Administration Hospital south of Walla Walla. *Warner, Ore.,* (4) had two sites, with the first site (1866-67) now mere indentations and rock piles near the Antelope Blue Sky Hotel atop Hart Mountain 50 miles northeast of Lake View; the stone causeway General Crook built to move to the second site is still visible below the mountain; the second site has several buildings of doubtful lineage in Fremont National Forest, also north of Lake View.

*Warren, Mass.,* is on Georges Island in Boston Harbor where boats from Rowe's Wharf in Boston take visitors to see the ruins, monument, and park. *Washington Arsenal, D.C.* (8) is still active as Ft. McNair and the site of the National War College and the Industrial College of the Armed Forces. Washington, Md., is still a massive fortress maintained by the National Park Service.

*Watertown Arsenal, Mass.,* (8) was recently given up on the north bank of the Charles river, 6 miles east of Boston. *Watervliet Arsenal, N.Y.,* (8) is still active with 82 buildings on 137 acres on South Broadway in Watervliet.

*Wayne Mich.,* is now a museum owned by the city of Detroit at 6301 West Jefferson avenue. *West Point, N.Y.,* is still active in its role as the United States Military Academy. *Whipple, Ariz.,* is a Veterans Administration Hospital 1 mile east of Prescott with many Army buildings, including quarters, still in use. *Whipple, Va.,* is still active as Ft. Myer and the Arlington National Cemetery. *Willet's Point, N.Y.,* was named Ft. Totten in 1898 and many Army buildings are left 15 miles from Manhattan. *Wingate, N.M.,* has some Army structures and the site of the cemetery at the Ft. Wingate Indian School 15 miles from Gallup, but should not be confused with modern Ft. Wingate Army Depot to the west.

*Winthrop, Mass.,* (8) has given way to Boston's Logan International Airport which now occupies this Governors Island site in Boston Harbor. *Wood, N.Y.,* on Bedloe's Island became the location of the Statue of Liberty in 1886. *Wool, Va.,* (8) is an abandoned hulk of concrete coast defenses next to the Norfolk entrance to the Hampton Roads Tunnel between Norfolk and Newport News, Va. The city of Hampton plans to develop its visitor potential. *Wright, Calif.,* (4) has disappeared completely from its location in private pastures west of Covelo in Round Valley. *Yerba Buena Island, Calif.,* is a Naval base below the Oakland Bay Bridge in San Francisco Bay, with many traces of the Army post in evidence. *Yuma, Calif.,* is the headquarters of the Ft. Yuma Indian Reservation at a site where traces of Army buildings and the Army layout are obvious, on the bluff overlooking the Colorado river bridge, north of the highway; *Yuma Depot, Ariz.,* which supported Ft. Yuma, is maintained as a state park at the north end of North 2d avenue in Yuma, Ariz.

HERBERT M. HART
Lieutenant Colonel, U. S. Marine Corps
Quantico, Virginia

CIRCULAR No. 8.

WAR DEPARTMENT,
SURGEON-GENERAL'S OFFICE,
WASHINGTON, MAY 1, 1875.

A REPORT

ON THE

HYGIENE OF THE UNITED STATES ARMY,

WITH

DESCRIPTIONS OF MILITARY POSTS.

WASHINGTON:
GOVERNMENT PRINTING OFFICE.
1875.

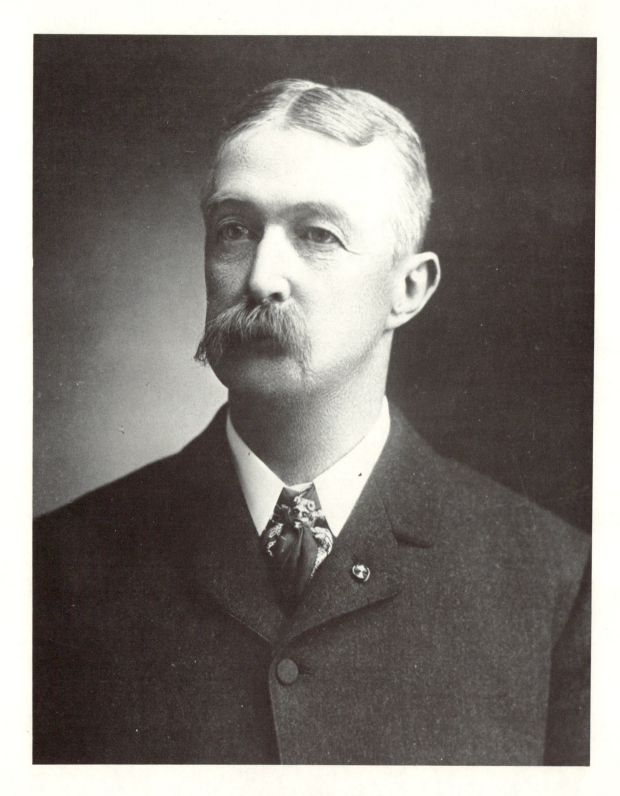

JOHN S. BILLINGS

# CIRCULAR No. 8.

WAR DEPARTMENT, SURGEON-GENERAL'S OFFICE,
*Washington, May* 1, 1875.

The following report on the hygiene of the United States Army, with descriptions of military posts, is published by authority of the Secretary of War, for the information of officers of the Army.

J. K. BARNES,
*Surgeon-General, U. S. Army.*

# REPORT

ON

# THE HYGIENE OF THE UNITED STATES ARMY.

BY JOHN S. BILLINGS, ASSISTANT SURGEON, U. S. A.

SURGEON-GENERAL'S OFFICE,
*Washington, D. C., April* 25, 1875.

GENERAL: In accordance with your directions, I have the honor to submit the following report on the hygiene of the United States Army, with descriptions of military posts, compiled from special and regular sanitary reports made by the medical officers of the Army.

The conditions under which our troops are placed differ greatly, not only from those of civil life, but in many respects from those affecting the military service in other countries, and the problems in sanitation, which are presented to our medical officers, cover nearly the whole field of practical hygiene. Although the medical officers themselves have long recognized that the prevention of disease should be an important part of their duties, and, even at the risk of being considered officious or troublesome, have, from time to time, called the attention of the proper authorities to probable or possible sources of danger to the health of the troops; and although the relations existing between surgeons and commanding officers have usually been such that warnings and recommendations on sanitary matters have been taken in good part and have received proper attention; still, advice volunteered is never welcome; and, in the absence of any law or regulation on the subject, there have always been a few officers who were disposed to resent any suggestion from the surgeon as an attempt at interference, and to look upon any attempt to investigate the sanitary condition of the post as a species of espionage which should be discouraged as much as possible.

Recently, however, the position and duties of the surgeon as a sanitary officer have been defined, while at the same time the general supervision and jurisdiction of commanding officers is fully recognized, by the following General Order:

GENERAL ORDER, }
No. 125. }
WAR DEPARTMENT, ADJUTANT-GENERAL'S OFFICE,
*Washington, November* 17, 1874.

An important part of the duty of a medical officer of the Army is the supervision of the hygiene of the post or command to which he is attached, and the recommendation of such measures as he may deem necessary to prevent or diminish disease among the troops.

For this purpose he shall at least once a month examine and note in the medical history of the post the sanitary condition of the quarters, including all buildings belonging to the post, the character and cooking of the rations, the amount and quality of the water-supply, the drainage, and the clothing and habits of the men, and make a report thereon in writing to the commanding officer, with such recommendations as he may deem proper. If the recommendations be approved and carried out, the medical officer shall note the fact in the medical history of the post. If the action recommended be deemed impracticable or undesirable, the commanding officer shall indorse his objections on the report and forward it to the department commander. A copy of such indorsement shall be furnished to the medical officer, who shall record it in the medical history of the post.

The annual sanitary reports now required from medical officers shall in future be forwarded through their commanding officers, who shall forward them through the regular channels, with such remarks as shall be deemed necessary.

The same course will be taken with the special sanitary reports called for by Circular Orders No. 2, Surgeon-General's Office, October 15, 1874, which, as modified, is as follows:

"Medical officers will forward, with the sanitary reports of December 31, 1874, a special report on the following subjects, to be made as full and be as carefully prepared as possible, as the results are desired for publication:

"I. On the food of the Army, its quantity, quality, and mode of preparation. What is the character of the articles forming the regular ration as furnished to the post? What is the average amount of saving for post fund? What articles of food, and in what amount, are purchased by the post fund, obtained from post garden, or by hunting or fishing? Ice, how obtained and in what quantities furnished? How is the cooking done for the men? Give bill of fare for a week at different seasons. Is the food of the men inspected daily? How often is it inspected by the medical officer? Have any complaints been made by the men about the food, and have any cases of disease occurred which may be attributed to the food or its mode of preparation? If so, specify. Character of kitchen and bakery fixtures. Has any special apparatus, such as the Warren cooker or the felt box, been tried? If so, give results. Character and amount of extra articles furnished by the Commissary Department for officers' use. Diet of the sick, and hospital fund. Remarks, suggestions, and recommendations.

"II. Duties of medical officers in scouting parties and expeditions. Nature and amount of medical supplies required; how carried. Means of transportation for wounded. Remarks.

"III. On military punishments and their effect on the health and morale of the soldier. Give instances, recommendations, &c.

"IV. Personal cleanliness of the men. What are the post regulations, if any, with regard to bathing? What facilities are afforded? How often are the men's blankets washed?

"The above report must be forwarded promptly through the proper channel to the medical director on or before January 1. Medical directors will forward them through the department commanders, with their own observations and comments on the points above referred to."

The medical history of the post shall be kept with the hospital records and shall not be removed therefrom. It shall be open to the examination of the commanding officer, and the attention of inspecting-officers is especially directed to this book, and they will report the manner in which it is kept.

By order of the Secretary of War:

                                                E. D. TOWNSEND,
                                                        *Adjutant-General.*

Under the provisions of this order, it is to be hoped that medical officers will find no obstacles placed in the way of obtaining such information as is needed for sanitary purposes; but they must bear in mind that the majority of the changes and improvements which they recommend cost money; that "les conseillers ne sont pas les payeurs," and should not be surprised or discouraged at the amount of time required to obtain the action desired.

When an epidemic is present, the services of the physician are highly valued, but his efforts to prevent its appearance, which, to be effective, must be made at a time when most people see no special cause for anxiety, and which, therefore, appear to involve unnecessary worry and expense, will be often rated at an inverse ratio to their success. If the expected disease does not appear, the warnings are considered to have been a false alarm, and the precautions taken to have been excessive. The friends of the typhoid fever patient, who will not fail to remember and be grateful for the care and assiduity with which the physician combatted the disease, would very likely have thought him intrusive and meddlesome had he taken one-half the same trouble to see that the possible causes of such affections were removed or destroyed.

In editing the reports descriptive of posts, I have followed the general plan of my previous report (Circular No. 4, Surgeon General's Office, December 5, 1870,) but have condensed or omitted much of the historical data given in that circular, and have in its place given much new material, with the intention of furnishing, as far as possible, such information as would be of interest or value to officers ordered to posts with which they are unacquainted, and to officers of the staff corps.

The medical statistics and the meteorological tables for each post have been compiled under the direction of Assistant Surgeon J. J. Woodward, of this office, and, taken together, covering, as they do, the period of four years for the majority of posts, furnish valuable indications for the medical geography of this country.

Scattered, as our Army is, from Alaska to Florida, its posts give a range of all climates, altitudes, and soils, with the hygienic and endemic influences peculiar to each. Attention is especially invited to the reports from the Departments of the Missouri and the Platte, and more particularly to the remarks of Surgeon Vollum, (Camp Douglas,) and Assistant Surgeons Smart, (Fort Bridger,) Patzki, (Fort Fred. Steele,) Gardner, (Fort Union,) and Happersett, (Fort Garland,) with reference to the effects of high altitudes and mountain climates upon diseases of the lungs.

The opinion of the majority of medical officers is that altitude and a rarified atmosphere are not *per se* beneficial in cases of phthisis, but that it is the dryness of the air, the exercise, and the outdoor life which produce good results in those cases which are "able to stand it."

Owing to the reduction in numbers of the Army, and from other causes, the supply of recruits has exceeded the demand, and recruiting officers have been able to select a physically good class of men for the service. The latest standard for height is fixed as follows:

CIRCULAR.]                  WAR DEPARTMENT, ADJUTANT-GENERAL'S OFFICE,
                                          *Washington, December 14, 1874.*

The standard for recruits will, until further orders, be as follows: For artillery and infantry, five feet four inches, and upward, in height, and weight not less than one hundred and twenty pounds, nor more than one hundred and eighty pounds.

For cavalry, not less than five feet five inches, and not more than five feet ten inches in height, and weight not to exceed one hundred and fifty-five pounds.

\*     \*     \*     \*     \*     \*     \*     \*

By order of the Secretary of War:

E. D. TOWNSEND,
*Adjutant-General.*

The medical examination of recruits is carefully made, and the detailed results, as given in reports on file in this office, afford interesting and valuable data in anthropometry.

It is sufficient for the purposes of this report to say that the standard of health and physical perfection of the enlisted men on entering the service is above the average. These men, thus selected, have their food, habitations, clothing, and occupations prescribed for them, and the result is as follows:

*Table showing ratio per 1,000 of mortality in the United States Army as compared with the mortality of males between twenty and forty years of age in civil life.*

| United States Army. | Mean strength. | Deaths. | | | | | |
|---|---|---|---|---|---|---|---|
| | | From disease. | | From wounds, accidents, and injuries. | | Total. | |
| | | No. | Per 1,000. | No. | Per 1,000. | No. | Per 1,000. |
| WHITE TROOPS: | | | | | | | |
| Year ending June 30, 1871a ........... | 29,365 | 363 | 12 | 156 | 5 | 519 | 17 |
| Year ending June 30, 1872b ........... | 24,101 | 268 | 11 | 99 | 4 | 367 | 15 |
| Year ending June 30, 1873c ........... | 24,844 | 246 | 10 | 166 | 7 | 412 | 17 |
| Year ending June 30, 1874d ........... | 25,647 | 229 | 9 | 112 | 4 | 341 | 13 |
| COLORED TROOPS: | | | | | | | |
| Year ending June 30, 1871a ........... | 2,608 | 28 | 11 | 21 | 8 | 49 | 19 |
| Year ending June 30, 1872b ........... | 2,494 | 44 | 18 | 10 | 4 | 54 | 22 |
| Year ending June 30, 1873c ........... | 2,520 | 46 | 18 | 7 | 3 | 53 | 21 |
| Year ending June 30, 1874d ........... | 2,497 | 25 | 10 | 12 | 5 | 37 | 15 |
| STATES AND TERRITORIES: (*Males between 20 and 40.*) | | | | | | | |
| Arizona ................................ | | | | | | | |
| California ............................. | | | | | | | |
| Colorado .............................. | | | | | | | |
| Dakota ................................ | | | | | | | |
| Kansas ................................ | | | | | | | |
| Minnesota ............................. | | | | | | | |
| Montana ............................... | e564,646 | f3,181 | 5.634 | f895 | 1.585 | f4,076 | 7.219 |
| Nebraska .............................. | | | | | | | |
| New Mexico ........................... | | | | | | | |
| Oregon ................................ | | | | | | | |
| Texas ................................. | | | | | | | |
| Utah .................................. | | | | | | | |
| Washington ........................... | | | | | | | |
| Wyoming .............................. | | | | | | | |
| UNITED STATES ........................ | e5,804,616 | f36,903 | 6.357 | f6,024 | 1.038 | f42,927 | 7.395 |

a Annual Report of the Surgeon-General for 1871.
b Annual Report of the Surgeon-General for 1872.
c Annual Report of the Surgeon-General for 1873.
d Annual Report of the Surgeon-General for 1874.
e Vital Statistics, Ninth Census, Table XXIII.
f Vital Statistics, Ninth Census, Table V.

That is to say, setting aside injuries, to which the soldier is specially liable, the mortality from disease among these picked men is distinctly greater than among men of the same age in civil life under the same conditions of climate.

It is, I think, sufficiently evident, from the above table, that the hygienic conditions under which our troops are placed cannot be considered as satisfactory; and if the descriptions of posts following this report be examined, in connection with the statistics furnished with each, the excessive loss by death and discharge, which preventable excess is probably not less than 100 by death and 200 by discharge, annually, will not seem unaccountable.

For convenience, I propose to comment on the subjects which are related to the health and comfort of the soldier in the following order:

I. Habitations, including barracks, quarters, and guard-houses, with their appendages.

II. The food of the Army, and its preparation.

III. The clothing of the Army.

IV. The hospitals and medical supplies.

## I. HABITATIONS.

The barracks and quarters of the Army have, as a whole, improved within the last five years. The reduction of the Army, and the employment of a large part of it away from the permanent posts, has given a larger air-space, with its accompanying advantages, to those quartered in regular barracks.

It is only necessary, however, to refer to the air-space allowed at many of the posts, to prove that overcrowding still exists.

There is practically no law or regulation in our army as to the amount of air-space which a soldier shall have, nor as to the obtaining the opinions of medical officers in regard to site and plans of habitations for the troops, and the result is that when the defects in such buildings, which are obvious to any one acquainted with the first principles of sanitary architecture, are pointed out, it is usually too late to remedy them.

Since my last report, the board of officers convened to revise the Army Regulations have prepared plans for barracks and quarters, which were issued in a circular from the Quartermaster-General's Office, dated September 14, 1873.

The plan of barrack proposed in this circular is shown in Figure 1: 1, first floor; 2, second floor. A, mess-room, 23 by $46\frac{5}{6}$ feet; B, day-room, 38 by $11\frac{1}{4}$ feet; C, D, non-commissioned officers' rooms, each $20\frac{1}{6}$ by $11\frac{1}{4}$ feet; E, armory, $11\frac{1}{4}$ by 8 feet; F, library, $11\frac{1}{4}$ by $10\frac{1}{2}$ feet; G, wash-room, $11\frac{1}{4}$ by $16\frac{1}{2}$ feet; H, kitchen, 21 by $16\frac{1}{2}$ feet; I, cook's room, 9 by 8 feet; J, room, $16\frac{1}{2}$ by 8 feet; K, L, veranda, 8 feet wide; M, stairway; closet under stairs; Z, dormitory, 133 by 23 feet, to contain 58 beds.

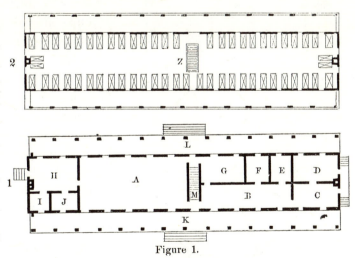

Figure 1.

This plan gives about 500 cubic feet per man, has no arrangements for ventilation, and no provision for bath-rooms. Quarters on this plan have been erected at Camp Douglas, and a detailed description is given in the account of that post. While this is a great improvement on the majority of existing barracks, it cannot be considered perfectly satisfactory; nor will any similar attempts at economy by reducing the air-space in the dormitories prove a success.

M P——II

The plans proposed by the board for officers' quarters are also unsatisfactory, being too small, and lacking the conveniences which should be furnished. The want of bath-rooms in these quarters is especially to be condemned. The providing of conveniences for bathing, both for officers and enlisted men, is too much neglected; and were it not for the fact that the officers and men are very generally aware of the importance of the matter, and hence provide themselves with such makeshifts for bathing conveniences as can be obtained, the results would probably be serious. Next to fresh air and proper food, personal cleanliness is the most important agent in preserving the mind and body in proper working order, and it is not only a duty, but in the highest degree good policy and economy, on the part of the Government, to provide the necessary facilities. A dirty man will, in most cases, be a discontented, disagreeable, and dissolute man; for the condition of his skin has much more to do with a man's morals than is generally supposed.

I would strongly urge that cheap, strong bathing-tubs, or other means of cleansing the whole body, should be as regular a part of the supply of a post as bedsteads. It is by no means sufficient that bathing facilities are good in summer. These should be attended to, for no bath-tub can take the place of a plunge and swimming bath, and there are few posts where the latter cannot be arranged; but winter, as well as summer, should be provided for, and it is to be hoped that no plans for barracks or officers' quarters will be approved in future which do not contain provisions for bathing in cold weather.

The main difficulties in the way of arranging bath-houses for the winter use of the troops arise from deficient water-supply, and from difficulty in heating the room or rooms. Both these obstacles can be overcome, to a considerable extent, and without great expense, by using jets or showers instead of tubs, placing the shower about 5 feet 6 inches from the floor, and using warm water instead of cold. The bathers' stalls need not be large, and can be compactly arranged as shown in Figure 2.

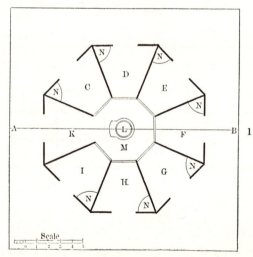

Figure 2.

1, plan; 2, vertical section on line A, B. C, D, E, F, G, H, I, bathing apartments; K, opening to stove; L, stove in central apartment, M, for heating the room and the water in the tank; N, shelves in corner of apartments for wash-basin, soap, &c. The central apartment, M, is 5 feet in diameter. Cells, or bathing apartments, are 4½ feet deep, and 5 feet 3 inches across widest end. There should be eight posts about the central chamber, for the support of the tank between these posts there should be open-work, (slats,) to allow the warm air generated by the stove to pass into the bathing-chambers. Doorways into chambers to be 2 feet wide, and 6 feet 6 inches high. Chambers to be 8 feet high in clear. The floor of the apartments C, D, E, F, G, H, I, should slope downward and inward, (one inch,) and to one point; and at each apartment there should be a drain-pipe, for the waste water to pass off.

The supply of water required is much less than in the ordinary mode, and the central stove can easily be arranged so as to both heat the water and warm the room. Baths upon this principle are in use at Rouen.*

The want of proper means of heating, and an insufficient supply of fuel, are the real reasons for much of the overcrowding and deficient ventilation found at many of our frontier posts, since the present evil of cold will always make that of foul air seem unimportant. I shall consider the subject of heating when speaking of hospitals.

In connection with the subject of ventilation, the following extracts from a special report by Assistant Surgeon Charles Smart, United States Army, on the ventilation of the buildings at Fort Bridger, will be found of interest:

\* \* \* \* \* \* \* \* \*

As the figures relating to the ventilation of the various rooms are deduced from the amount of carbonic acid found by experiment, and as their claim to credit depends on the care and accuracy with which these experiments were performed, it may not be amiss to preface the results by a detail of the steps by which they were attained.

For the standard acid, a solution of oxalic acid was made, containing exactly 2.864 grams in one liter of litmus-tinted water. Pure hydrate of baryta was dissolved in water, and the clear solution transferred to a large bottle, with a blow-tube, containing soda-lime, and an exit-tube, guarded by a strong clip, in its rubber portion. This baryta water was carefully titrated by weight, four experiments agreeing on .987 as the factor to bring the alkaline solution to the strength of the standard acid.

On the afternoon preceding each visit to the quarters, the jars intended for the reception of air were inspected, to determine their perfect dryness, and a corresponding number of two-ounce vials were filled from the baryta reservoir, corked tightly, weighed, and the weight marked on the label of each.

At the visit, the contents of the room were noted, and the walls and windows examined for the discovery of any notable inlets, by which time the jar was conceived to have attained the temperature of its surroundings. The air from on a level with the men's bunks, one and a half to two feet from the floor, was then driven into it, by a large rubber syringe in the absence of a bellows, sixty forcible strokes of the piston being made in each case, to insure the thorough charging of the jar with the air required. The contents of one of the baryta vials were poured in and the jar immediately corked with a tightly-fitting rubber cork, and agitated to diffuse the solution over its sides. The vial was also carefully corked, and the jar and room for which it had been used, together with the temperature, were noted on its label. On two occasions about 10 grams of the baryta solution were retained in the vial and tested with the acid, for the discovery of deterioration.

Eight hours after the visit, the empty baryta vial was weighed, the loss giving the weight of solution transferred to the jar; the number of grams were deducted as cubic centimeters from the capacity of the jar, and the remainder set down as the "quantity of air operated on." The jar was then opened, the baryta transferred to Schuster's alkalimeter, and the weight noted, after which it was permitted to settle. Of the standard acid, 10, 15, or 20 grams were weighed, (according to the clearness or turbidity of the alkaline solution,) and the baryta dropped in through a hole pricked by platinum wire in the parafine which sealed up the nozzle of the alkalimeter. As the excess of acid became diminished, permitting the precipitation of oxalate, the dropping was regulated by the finger admitting or removing atmospheric pressure from the surface of the liquid, until the last

* (Note sur un système d'ablutions pratique à la prison de Rouen, etc., par le Dr. Merry Delabost, Annales d'Hygiène, Janvier, 1875, p. 110.)

drop changed the tint. The alkalimeter was again weighed, the loss giving the weight of baryta equivalent to the grams of acid used, and from this was calculated the weight of acid which would be neutralized by the whole of the baryta solution placed in the jar. The weight so found was deducted from the baryta multiplied by its factor, and the difference in grams called milligrams of carbonic acid. Multiplication by .537042—the volume in cubic centimeters of .001 $CO_2$—transferred weight into volume, and, after correcting the air operated on for temperature, the volume of carbonic acid in 10,000 parts of air was calculated.

There being no barometer at the post, correction for pressure, though desirable, had to be neglected. The "available capacity" of the rooms was found, by deducting so many cubic feet from the total capacity for the more bulky articles contained therein. In this calculation 2.5 was allowed for body bulk and 7 cubic feet for bunk and bedding per man.

The rapid diminution of the carbonic acid in the external air during the period occupied in observation is very noteworthy. Experiments on April 10 and 14, showed the cessation of this diminution, giving 2.6292 and 3.0560 volumes, respectively.

The difference between the carbonic acid found in the external and internal air is set down as "carbonic impurity."

The "ventilation per man" is calculated on the assumption that 4 cubic feet of carbonic acid is evolved hourly by each of the inmates. This quantity diluted with 1,000 cubic feet of air would give to the analyst 4 volumes of carbonic impurity per 10,000, from which the amount of dilution corresponding to a given impurity can be calculated; but, as the air originally in the room takes a part in the dilution, its influence must be deducted to arrive at the ventilation. This is effected by dividing the air-space per man by the number of hours during which the impurity has been accumulating, and subtracting the number of cubic feet so found from the amount of the dilution.

For the purpose of comparison the movement of air through the rooms is expressed in parts of their capacity, as well as by the time required for the entrance of a volume of air equal to their available capacity. It is to be regretted, for the sake of such comparison, that all the experiments were not made in the calm. The wind, however, was noted in each instance. In comparing the ventilation of the guard-house, band-quarters, and C company barracks with that of the other buildings, the great power of the wind as a ventilator must be borne in mind, and the figures diminished proportionately. The three observations in the hospital ward illustrate this power. On April 2 and 8, in the calm the hourly movement was 1.3 and 1.4 times the capacity of the ward; this was raised to 3.5 times on the 4th, by a breeze blowing twenty miles an hour from the southwest.

The excess of moisture was obtained by observation of the dry and wet bulb thermometers and the use of Glaisher's tables.

The organic matter was condensed in one liter of distilled water by means of the rubber bulbs of the local anæsthesia apparatus and a bent glass delivery-tube drawn out to a small orifice. Repeated experiments showed that fifteen times the volume of the rubber bulb were equal to one liter, at 62° Fahrenheit. Permanganate solution, containing one milligram of salt in each gram, was used in the estimation; and, to insure accuracy, an equal volume of distilled water from the same demijohn was treated side by side with that containing the condensed organic matter. Both bottles were immersed in hot water until their temperature reached 140° Fahrenheit; sulphuric acid was added, and the permanganate dropped in until each had a tint which lasted ten minutes. The alkalimeters weighed before and after the operation gave the quantity of permanganate used in each instance. That required for the distilled water and acid was deducted from the other for the weight decolorized by organic matter.

It is noticeable that the results given below differ somewhat on the one hand from those reported by Dr. Hubbard, United States Army, in appendix to Circular No. 4, Surgeon-General's Office, 1870, and on the other very considerably from the experience of Dr. Parkes, as given in his Manual of Hygiene, second edition, page 69; the former reporting the organic matter of 1,000 cubic centimeters of air at 2, 3, and 4 milligrams, and the latter finding that 12 cubic feet of similar air (similar at least in regard to carbonic impurity) were required to destroy .00002 gram of permanganate. For my own part, I conceive this test for organic matter to be useful only in the absence of fires. In the instances reported below, I incline to believe that the permanganate was destroyed more by traces of deoxidizers escaping from the bituminous coal used as fuel than by organic exhalations from the men.

The coincidence in the quantities of permanganate decolorized by the air of the front barracks of B, K, and C companies would seem to give value to these experiments. In each of these rooms were quartered the same number of men, with almost the same air-space; ventilation showing well in these cases its power of dispersing the carbonic acid and its inefficiency with regard to the organic matter; but other experiments recorded throw doubt upon the value of these. Company C's front barrack, for example, with almost the same number of men and ventilation as the rear barrack of the same company, and with two-thirds more space per man, gives double the quantity of test solution destroyed.

At the break-of-day visit the organic odor was perceptible in all the rooms examined, with the exception of the hospital and band-quarters.

In this connection may be mentioned that at inspection on March 31 the odor in the company barracks was quite manifest, to one entering from the fresh air, fully half an hour after the rooms had been vacated by the men, doors opened, and upper window-sashes lowered, through which a light breeze was blowing at the time.

*        *        *        *        *        *        *

*Report on the air and ventilation of sleeping-rooms at Fort Bridger, Wyoming Territory, during March and April, 1874.*

| Barrack. | Date of observation. | Hour of observation. | Available capacity of room in cubic feet. | Number of men. | Air-space per man. | Air operated on in cubic centimeters. | Temperature of room, Fahrenheit. | External temperature. | Wind. | Milligrams $CO_2$ in the air operated on. | Volumes $CO_2$ in 10000 of the air of room at 62° Fahrenheit. | Volumes $CO_2$ in 10000 of external air at 62°. | Carbonic impurity. | Hourly ventilation per man in cubic feet. | Hourly ventilation of room in parts of its capacity. | Ventilation, in minutes, required for admission of a volume of air equal to capacity of room. | Excess of moisture of internal over external air — grains per cubic foot. | Organic matter in grams, permanganate, 6.666 liters of air. |
|---|---|---|---|---|---|---|---|---|---|---|---|---|---|---|---|---|---|---|
| Officers' quarters | March 17 | 4.15 a. m. | 2,777 | 5 | 555 | 7,863 | 56° | 10° | Calm. | 16.6300 | 11.2283 | 4.5011 | 6.7272 | 533 | .959 | 62.5 | | |
| Company B, Fourth Infantry, front barrack | March 24 | 4.45 a. m. | 9,153 | 20 | 458 | 7,994 | 60° | 3° | Calm. | 17.7048 | 11.8497 | 4.0164 | 7.8333 | 454 | .992 | 68.0 | 2.24 | .00140 |
| Company B, Fourth Infantry, rear barrack | March 24 | 5.15 a. m. | 5,280 | 9 | 587 | 7,853 | 56° | 3° | Calm. | 15.4737 | 10.4594 | 4.0164 | 6.4430 | 552 | .941 | 63.7 | 1.64 | .00090 |
| Company K, Fourth Infantry, front barrack | March 26 | 4.45 a. m. | 9,493 | 20 | 475 | 7,850 | 42° | 18° | Calm. | 20.2055 | 13.2931 | 3.7161 | 9.5770 | 359 | .756 | 79.3 | 1.22 | .00130 |
| Company K, Fourth Infantry, rear barrack | March 26 | 5.15 a. m. | 8,565 | 13 | 657 | 7,987 | 49° | 18° | Calm. | 10.6423 | 6.9776 | 3.7161 | 3.2615 | 1,148 | 1.742 | 34.4 | 1.67 | .00030 |
| Company C, Fourth Infantry, front barrack | March 29 | 4.45 a. m. | 9,527 | 20 | 476 | 7,990 | 54° | 23° | N. E.-2 | 10.4470 | 6.9146 | 3.5300 | 3.3846 | 1,122 | 2.355 | 25.4 | 1.42 | .00159 |
| Company C, Fourth Infantry, rear barrack | March 29 | 5.15 a. m. | 5,261 | 19 | 277 | 7,853 | 52° | 23° | N. E.-2 | 10.8420 | 7.2735 | 3.5300 | 3.7435 | 1,035 | 3.738 | 16.1 | 1.58 | .00070 |
| Fourth Infantry band-quarters | March 31 | 4.45 a. m. | 9,780 | 13 | 752 | 7,989 | 37° | 17° | W.-3 | 7.8880 | 5.0485 | 3.2881 | 1.7604 | 2,178 | 2.808 | 20.7 | 1.17 | .00057 |
| Guard-house | March 31 | 5.15 a. m. | 11,290 | 19 | 594 | 7,855 | 56° | 17° | W.-3 | 9.6725 | 6.5373 | 3.2881 | 3.2492 | 1,161 | 1.954 | 30.7 | 1.10 | .00065 |
| Hospital ward No. 1 | April 2 | 5.00 a. m. | 9,444 | 4 | 2,361 | 7,989 | 49° | 15° | Calm. | 6.2721 | 4.1113 | 3.0183 | 1.0930 | 3,398 | 1.440 | 41.7 | 0.95 | .00006 |
| Hospital ward No. 1 | April 4 | 4.00 a. m. | 9,437 | 7 | 1,348 | 7,991 | 42° | 20° | S. W.-4 | 5.3776 | 3.4757 | 2.6560 | 0.8197 | 4,712 | 3.435 | 17.2 | 1.12 | |
| Hospital ward No. 1 | April 8 | 5.00 a. m. | 9,437 | 7 | 1,348 | 7,855 | 59° | 19° | Calm. | 6.9230 | 4.7062 | 2.6033 | 2.1029 | 1,752 | 1.390 | 46.1 | 0.68 | |

All the above quarters, with the exception of those of the band and the guard-house, are shingled log huts, with the crevices between the logs filled in or "chinked" with lime. They are floored, ceiled, and lined internally with lath and plaster or boards.

The officers' quarters have, in addition, a wall-paper over the plaster. These were repaired during the past autumn, being furnished with new floors, roofs, ceilings, doors, &c., as their condition required; but although only a few months have elapsed, the plaster has cracked and fallen off in places, carrying the paper with it, and the doors have warped so as to be anything but air-tight. In the set examined, window-seams were filled with glazier's putty, and door-seams guarded by weather-strips. The set consisted of two rooms, communicating by an open door. Of the inmates two were children, but they are reckoned as adults in the ventilation calculation. From the table may be seen that the air-space and ventilation enjoyed by the officer's family are in no respects superior to the allowance of the enlisted men.

The quarters of Company B, Fourth Infantry, (commanded by senior captain, who has first selection,) were well repaired over a year ago by a previous garrison. Door and window seams at the visit were leaky, but otherwise the two sets were in good condition.

Those of Company K, Fourth Infantry, (commanded by next ranking captain) were repaired during last autumn, and are in good condition. Door and window seams as before, and a broken window-pane in the rear barrack.

Company C's quarters (junior captain) were plastered during the past autumn, but much of it has already fallen. About one-sixteenth of the ceiling of the front barrack is denuded, showing the laths in circular patches, and through these and crevices in the roof above daylight can be seen. The roof of the rear building is in similar condition. At the visit a broken window-pane was found in each room.

The band-quarters, a frame building, shingled and finished inside like the others, was built last autumn. At the visit broken plastering over the doorway admitted a strong current of air.

The guard-house is a solid stone structure, with a prison-room attached behind of heavy logs lined with strong timbers. The two communicate by a grated door. The walls of both are air-tight, but the roof of the former shows daylight through it, and the small windows of the latter, placed near the eaves, have several broken panes.

The hospital excepted, no provision is made for ventilation in any of these buildings, so that the hourly movement of air through them represents their leakiness and the cold draughts to which the men are exposed. There is indeed an appearance of ventilation, for the ceiling of each presents, according to size, one, two, or three openings, which look like the mouths of ventilating-shafts, but they simply communicate with the loft between the ceiling and the roof. I presume it to have been the opinion of the officer who cut them out that they would be sufficient for ventilation, in view of the permeability of the shingled roof. That they are not so is proved by the figures representing the air-movement in the latter sets of quarters. They might have acted as inlets and acted well in former winters when wood was burned in an open fire-place, the chimney of which carried off the foul air; but at present the chimneys are bricked up and coal-burning stoves used, the pipes of which run through the tight-fitting thimbles into the old flues.

The long and severe winters—July and August being the only months during which the temperature does not fall below the freezing point—seem to have made the exclusion of air the great object at this post in the repair of quarters, it having been taken for granted that, no matter how thorough the repair, the building would remain pervious enough to effect proper ventilation. But the impurity in Company K's front and in both of Company B's barracks shows that the log hut can be made so air-tight as to require special ventilation. At the same time, this air-tightness proves that the occupants of some of the other barracks are needlessly exposed to draughts of air through unauthorized crevices.

An investigation of the hospital register was made with the view of detecting any relation between the ventilation and disease. The records for the six months from October, 1873, to March, 1874, inclusive, were examined. Of course accidents and injuries, alcoholism, and such cases as have no bearing on the point at issue, have been omitted. September might have been included but for the fact that Company K was not then in possession of the quarters now occupied by it.

The number of cases registered is small, but the direction in which they point is interesting and practical.

When it is remembered that these commands have the same duties, exposures, water, diet, and cooking arrangements; that the same medical opinion places them on sick-report; that they are filled up from the same detailments of recruits; that in fact they differ only in the matter of quarters and amount of air provided; to this difference must be attributed the difference in the character and amount of disease indicated in the following table as affecting them. I do not think it advancing beyond the facts to entertain the belief that a free supply of air would have reduced the sickness in Company B to Company C's figure, and that a proper distribution of the incoming air would have prevented some of the quinsy cases which form so large a percentage of Company C's sickness.

The cases are as follows: In the band, 7 cases, or 466.6 per thousand; in Company B, 48 cases, or 820.8 per thousand; in Company K, 26 cases, or 448.1 per thousand; in Company C, 24 cases, or 393.4 per thousand.     *     *     *     *     *     *     *

As a contrast to this, take the results of the examination made by Surgeon J. H. Bill, United States Army, of the new barrack at Bedloe's Island, in which each man has over 1,000 cubic feet air-space, and stated by him under date of January 12, 1875, as follows:

      *     *     *     *     *     *     *     *     *

I also examined the dormitory of the new barracks at Bedloe's Island; room 123 feet by 33 feet by 10 feet; thirty-four men present; two stoves; two small louver-ventilators. (open;) a staircase, communicating with lower room, *permanently* open. The time was 1 a. m. Temperature without, 25° F.; within, 49° F. Methods as in previous examination. Carbonic anhydride found in 45.4 liters, (reduced to 0° C., equivalent to 43 liters,) .058 gram, or 6.8 in 10000. Organic impurity, 43 liters (reduced to 0° C.,) taken. Enough organic impurity was found in this to decolorize 0.005 gram of chameleon mineral, corresponding to 0.00199 gram of oxalic acid. This would show one grain in 21,500 cubic inches.

The quantities of organic impurity found were so small that I repeated my experiments, with the solutions of permanganate used at Governor's Island and Bedloe's Island, in a room of the Army headquarters building in this city, after an occupation of two hours by six persons. The room is a small one. In this case I found that 19 liters (reduced to 0° C.) were more than sufficient to decolorize 0.005 gram of chameleon mineral, (I mean some of the same solution used at Governor's Island.) I infer that my results are correct and that the amount of organic matter under question at Governor's and Bedloe's Islands was very small.

I made no examination of the barracks of Governor's Island nor of the casemate quarters of the men; as well make an examination of a pig-stye. They disregard every modern notion of hygiene; they are dark, damp, windy, and cold, and may or may not contain excess of carbonic anhydride, &c. Probably they do not, and hence analytical results would merely mislead.

The following is an extract from a special report made by Surgeon E. Swift, United States Army, stationed at Newport Barracks, Kentucky:

      *     *     *     *     *     *     *     *     *

Companies A and C, permanent party, occupy dormitories in the same building on the second and third stories respectively. These rooms are each about the same size, 57 feet long, 25 feet wide, and 11 feet high, containing 15,675 cubic feet, or 382 cubic feet air-space for each man.

      *     *     *     *     *     *     *     *     *

These dormitories are heated by means of bituminous coal in ordinary cast-iron cylinder stoves; windows and doors afford the only ventilation.

Company E, disposable recruits, occupy the third story of another building, 83 feet long, 25 feet wide, and 11 feet high—22,825 cubic feet. This room has bunks for the accommodation of 120 men, giving 190 cubic feet air-space per man, and is heated in the same manner as the dormitories of companies A and C. It now contains about 100 men, who are, seemingly, comfortable. It is only when more than 200 men are packed into this room, as sometimes necessity demands, covering the floor like red-herrings in a box, that discontent becomes irrepressible and desertion results.

\* \* \* \* \* \* \* \* \*

Company F, unexamined recruits, and the rejected, with those casually at the post, occupy, at the present time and whenever Company E exceeds 120 men, the post-chapel, a small frame building 44 feet long, 27 feet wide, 13½ feet high, and furnished with bunks for 49 men.

\* \* \* \* \* \* \* \* \*

When the strength of the command exceeds the capacity of the garrison, it is not alone that the soldier suffers discomfort on account of the crowded condition of the dormitories, but the absolutely necessary accommodations of the hospital, mess-room, privies, &c., add greatly to his sufferings, morally and physically. He is required to wait patiently his turn to each and every place his poor, frail humanity drives him. It is sad to contemplate the feelings of a young raw recruit, pure as the air upon his native hills, and as verdant as the grass and leaves of his rural home, fresh from clean feather-beds, butter, eggs, and pumpkin-pies, when, having passed his final examination and as an accepted recruit, he is ordered to report to the sergeant in charge of Company E, disposable, and is assigned to little else than standing room in a dormitory and a place in line to wait his turn for a seat in the mess-room, to a pine-table, tin-cups, and everlastingly boiled meat.

\* \* \* \* \* \* \* \* \*

It is sufficiently well established that the evil results of overcrowding and bad ventilation usually are made manifest in an increase of disease of the respiratory organs.

The following table shows that we have reason to think that our barracks are not satisfactory :

| | Mean strength. | Discharges per 1,000 for— | | Deaths per 1,000 from— | | Loss per 1,000 from— | |
|---|---|---|---|---|---|---|---|
| | | Consumption. | Diseases of the respiratory organs. | Consumption. | Diseases of the respiratory organs. | Consumption. | Diseases of the respiratory organs. |
| United States Army, white troops, 1870–'74 ........... | 25,989 | 3.828 | 1.395 | 1.462 | 1.472 | 5.29 | 2.867 |
| United States Army, colored troops, 1870–'74.......... | 2,530 | 2.962 | .296 | 2.47 | 3.162 | 5.432 | 3.478 |
| Arizona................................................. | | | | | | | |
| California............................................. | | | | | | | |
| Colorada............................................... | | | | | | | |
| Dakota................................................. | | | | | | | |
| Kansas................................................. | | | | | | | |
| Minnesota.............................................. | | | | | | | |
| Montana................................................ | 564,646 | ......... | ......... | 1.735 | .953 | 1.735 | .953 |
| Nebraska............................................... | | | | | | | |
| New Mexico............................................. | | | | | | | |
| Oregon................................................. | | | | | | | |
| Texas.................................................. | | | | | | | |
| Utah................................................... | | | | | | | |
| Washington............................................. | | | | | | | |
| Wyoming................................................ | | | | | | | |
| United States.......................................... | 5,804,616 | ......... | ......... | 2.486 | .788 | 2.486 | .788 |

I think it is no exaggeration to say that the service loses by death and discharge on account of overcrowded and badly ventilated barracks and guard-houses, about 100 men every year.

The amount of money appropriated annually for providing quarters for officers and men, even when eked out, as it has been, by employing the labor of troops as much as possible, has been insufficient to meet the legitimate demands made upon it, and no real saving is effected to the Government by expending the health and lives of its employés instead of sufficient money to allow them to have a sufficient supply of fresh air.

I am glad to say that the double and two-story wooden bunks are now very nearly abolished, and that the iron bunks now furnished by the Quartermaster's Department are very satisfactory, with the exception of a few, which are two-story in pattern—that is, an iron frame containing two beds, one four or five feet above the other. Under no circumstances, except for the most temporary emergency, should beds be arranged in this manner. It is connected with deficient air-space, and gives an appearance of room when there is not. Every man should have his sixty square feet of floor space as much as his ration.

But even with the single bunks the supply of bedding is unsatisfactory. No sheets or pillows are furnished, and the men come into direct contact with the blankets, and use their greatcoats for pillows. The blankets are seldom washed, although they are aired and beaten occasionally. The bed-sacks are usually too short, and, as Colonel C. H. Smith, Nineteenth United States Infantry, remarks, "No amount of too short bed can make a man comfortable."

The recommendation of Dr. Patzki, that wire mattresses, hair pillows, and sheets be furnished for the troops, is believed to be a good one, the results of which, in promoting comfort and content among the men, would be a full equivalent for the money it would cost.

The statistics of the prison rooms and cells of the guard-houses of our Army would afford, if they could be collected, some very interesting data as to the effects of cold, damp, and air foul with animal miasms and exhalations upon the human body. Judging from the reports of medical officers, the effects are much less than might be supposed from such guard-houses as those at Camp Apache, Forts Ringgold Barracks McKavitt, Griffin, Stockton, Monroe, Dodge, Craig, and Fetterman.

Among the plans for military buildings submitted by the board above referred to is one for a guard-house, which is shown in Figure 3.

L, sally-port, 18 feet wide; M, guard-room, 38 by 17; N, prison-room, 38 by 28 feet; O, P, Q, banquette; R, officer of the guard, 8 by 10 feet; S, tool-room, 8 by 8 feet; T, U, V, W, X, Y, cells, 5½ by 10 feet.

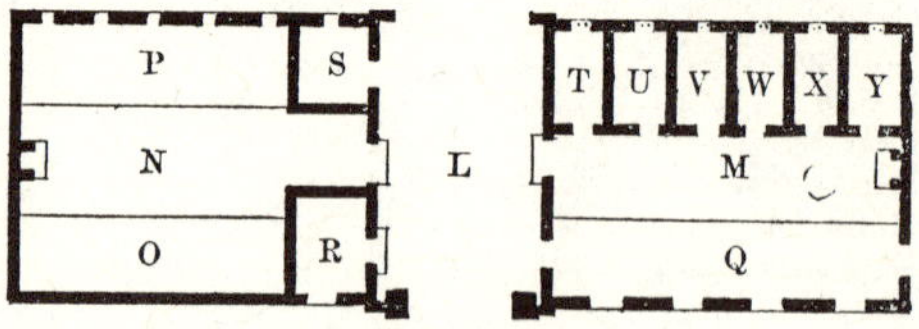

This is intended for ridge ventilation, and if provision is made for the introduction of fresh air in

Figure 3.

such a manner that it can be warmed in winter, may be considered as satisfactory.

Many of the special reports of medical officers contain interesting remarks on the subject of military punishments, and their effects upon the men; but as they report that the present modes of infliction do not specially injure the bodily health of the men, but only tend to damage their morale, for which reason some officers think that this is exclusively a matter of military discipline on which a medical officer has no business to express an opinion, and as my space is too limited to allow of the proper presentation of the subject, I shall not here consider it.

I must remark, however, that the theory advanced in some indorsements, that the observations and comments of a medical officer on the character and effects of the pun-ishments of the soldier, forwarded through the official channels, can be considered as injurious to the service, or subversive of military discipline, is one to which few in the Army, and none out of it, will assent.

In this connection, I give the following extract from a letter addressed to the Hon. Lewis Cass, Secretary of War, dated Headquarters Eastern Department, New York, November 5, 1832, by Maj. Gen. Winfield Scott, United States Army: "I am in the habit, myself, when on duty with troops, of paying great deference, and even of yielding my opinion, on matters deeply affecting health and life, to the advice of the medical staff."

## II. FOOD OF THE ARMY.

The special reports on the food of the Army and its preparation, furnished by medical officers with the sanitary reports of December 31, 1874, are of much interest, and, though presenting various shades of opinion, are remarkably unanimous on many points. As the majority of these reports are long, and space does not permit of printing them in full, and as they necessarily repeat each other to a great extent, I shall give only a summary of the views represented, with extracts.

The following history of the United States Army ration is furnished by Surg. Joseph R. Smith, United States Army :*

\*        \*        \*        \*        \*        \*        \*        \*        \*

---

* The following extracts from the archives, in addition to those given by Dr. Smith, will perhaps be of interest.

[American Archives, fourth series, Vol. IV, 1775-1776. Correspondence, Proceedings, &c., December 24, 1775, pages 307-308. Provincial Council of North Carolina—North Carolina troops.]

The Continental Congress having recommended to the council additional rations for the troops stationed in this province, viz: Three pints of peas or beans per week, or vegetables equivalent, rating the peas or beans at a dollar per bushel; one pint of milk per day, at the rate of $\frac{1}{12}$ of a dollar per pint; half a pint of rice or one pint of Indian meal per man per week; one quart of spruce beer or cider per man, or nine gallons of molasses per company of one hundred men per week; three pounds of candles to one hundred men per week, for guards; twenty-four pounds of soft or eight pounds of hard soap per one hundred men per week.

[American Archives, fourth series, Vol. IV, 1775-1776. Correspondence, Proceedings, &c., December, 1775, p. 457.— General Order—Headquarters Cambridge, December 24, 1775—determined by a board of general officers convened by General Washington, December 23.]

Corned beef and pork, four days in a week. Salt fish one day, and fresh beef two days. As milk cannot be procured during the winter season, the men are to have one pound and a half of beef or eighteen ounces of pork per day. Half pint of rice or a pint of Indian meal per week. One quart of spruce beer per day, or nine gallons of molasses to one hundred men per week. Six pounds of candles to one hundred men per week, for guards. Six ounces of butter or nine ounces of hog's lard per week. Three pints of peas or beans per man per week, or vegetables equivalent, allowing six shillings per bushel for beans or peas, two and eight pence per bushel for onions, one and four pence per bushel for potatoes and turnips. One pound of flour per man, each day; hard bread to be dealt out one day in a week in lieu of flour.

The above allowance is ordered to be issued by the Commissary-General to all the troops of the United Colonies serving in this department, until the honorable the Continental Congress or the commander-in-chief thinks proper to alter it.

[American Archives, fourth series, Vol. IV, 1775-1776. Correspondence, Proceedings, &c., February, 1776, p. 1513.]

Estimate showing the value of different species of provisions to be given in lieu of another, or the value of one species to be given in lieu of the whole species, according to the bill of fare settled by the honorable the Continental Congress, the 9th of November, 1775, viz:

Two pounds of bread or flour and one pound of pork are equal to one ration of all species. One pound of bread or flour, one pound of pork, and two pints of peas are equal to one ration of all species. One pound of bread or flour twelve ounces of pork, and six ounces of butter are equal to one ration of all species. One pound of bread or flour, one and a half pounds of beef, a half pint of rice, or one pint Indian meal, are equal to one ration of all species. One pound of bread or flour, one and a half pounds of beef, one quart of spruce beer or cider, or one gill of rum, are equal to one ration of all species. Five pounds of bread or flour are equal to one ration. Three pounds of beef are equal to one

The first ration of the United States Army of which I find record, is given in the American Archives for 1776, fifth series, vol. 1, p. 865, and as copied from the minutes of the honorable the Continental Congress, is as follows:

Per man per day.

| | |
|---|---|
| Beef | 1 lb.; or |
| Pork | ¾ lb. |
| Bread, or flour | 1 lb.; or |
| Salt fish | 1 lb. |
| Peas, or beans | 3 pints per week; or vegetables equivalent. |
| Milk | 1 pint per day; or at the rate of $\frac{1}{72}$ of a dollar. |
| Rice | ½ pint; or |
| Indian meal | 1 pint per week. |
| Spruce beer, or cider | 1 qt.; or |
| Molasses | 9 gallons per 100 men per week. |
| Candles, (for guards) | 3 lbs. per 100 men per week. |
| Soft-soap | 24 lbs. per 100 men per week; or |
| Hard soap | 8 lbs. per 100 men per week. |

This is less than twenty-five ounces of solid food per day.

The same archives contain a contract for issuing victuals to continental troops in Virginia during the year 1777, in the following amounts:

Per ration.

| | |
|---|---|
| Bacon | 14 oz.; or |
| Beef or pork, either salted or fresh | 1¼ lbs.; or |
| Mutton | 1 lb. |
| Flour | 1¼ lbs.; or |
| Sifted meal | 1½ lbs. |
| Vinegar | ⅐ gill. |
| Salt | ⅐ gill. |

ration. Twenty-eight ounces of pork are equal to one ration. Sixteen ounces of butter are equal to one ration. One gallon and a half pint of peas are equal to one ration. Four pints of rice are equal to one ration. Eight pints of Indian meal are equal to one ration.

[American Archives, fourth series, Vol. V, 1776, p. 578. South Carolina provincial troops.]

Resolution of South Carolina Provincial Congress, February 22, 1776: That the rations of the regular forces be increased to one pound and a half of fresh beef, or to eighteen ounces of salt pork; and that the regiment of rangers' the regiment of riflemen, the two independent companies of artillery, and the militia upon actual service, be allowed rations in like manner with the first and second regiments of foot and the regiment of artillery, and as increased by this establishment.

[American Archives, fourth series, Vol. V, 1776, p. 713. Pennsylvania forces.]

Resolution of Pennsylvania Assembly, April 6, 1776: Upon motion, resolved, that a ration for the Pennsylvania forces shall consist of one pound of beef, or three-quarters of a pound of pork, or one pound of mutton, per man per day. One pound of flour or bread per man per day. Three pints of peas or beans at six shillings per bushel, per man per week, or vegetables equivalent thereto. Half a pint of rice or one pound of Indian meal, per man per week. One pint of milk per man per day. One quart of small beer per man per day, or nine gallons of molasses for one hundred men per week. One gill of vinegar per man per week. Three pounds of candles for one hundred men per week, for guards. Twenty-four pounds of soft or eight pounds of hard soap for one hundred men per week.

[American Archives, fourth series, Vol. V, 1776, p. 1529. Rations for the marines in the service of Maryland.]

Order of Maryland Council of Safety, February 1, 1776: Resolved, that the rations for the marines in the service of this province be according as is expressed in the following table, to wit:

Sunday: 1 pound bread, 1 pound beef, 1 pound turnips, 1 pound potatoes; 1 pound onions per week.

Monday: 1 pound bread, 1 pound pork, ½ pint peas, 4 ounces cheese.

Tuesday: 1 pound bread, 1 pound beef, and pudding.

Wednesday: 1 pound bread, 1 pound pork, ½ pint rice, 2 ounces butter, 4 ounces cheese.

Thursday: 1 pound bread, 1 pound pork, ½ pint peas.

Friday: 1 pound bread, 1 pound beef, and pudding.

Saturday: 1 pound bread, 1 pound pork, ½ pint peas, 4 ounces cheese.

Half a pint of rum per man per day, and discretionary allowance for particular occasions, such as action, extra duty, and the like. Three pints of vinegar for six men per week.

Bacon was to be issued two days per week; salted beef or pork, at least one-half of the former, two days per week; fresh beef or other fresh provisions three days per week.

Instead, or in part, of flour, when demanded by the commanding officer, peas, beans, and potatoes were to be issued three times a week, so long as they could be had, at the rate of two and one-half bushels of peas or beans to one hundred pounds of flour, or one and one-half pounds of potatoes to one ration of flour, or the equivalent in price of vegetables. Butter at eight ounces per ration, and sugar, molasses, rice, coffee, and wine, were to be provided for the sick in lieu of other rations.

\*    \*    \*    \*    \*    \*    \*    \*    \*

Section VIII, article 2, and subsequent, of the original rules and articles of war adopted by Congress September 20, 1776, seems to show that some articles of food were furnished by the Government, and others bought by the men as they needed them, from the sutlers, or other traders. It reads as follows:

All officers, soldiers, and sutlers shall have full liberty to bring into any of the forts or garrisons of the United American [*sic*] States, any quantity or species of provisions, eatable or drinkable, except where any contract or contracts are or shall be entered into by Congress, or by their order, for furnishing such provisions, and with respect only to the species of provisions so contracted for.

ART. 3. All officers commanding in the forts, or barracks, or garrisons of the United States, are hereby required to see that the persons permitted to suttle, shall supply the soldiers with good and wholesome provisions at the market price, as they shall be answerable for their neglect.

Article 4 forbids sutlers to make exorbitant charges, and forbids commanding officers, for their private advantage, to lay any duty or imposition upon, or be interested in, the sale of victuals, &c.

April 14, 1777, Congress changed the above, by the omission of the word "drinkable."

In April, 1785, in the resolution of Congress organizing the troops to be furnished by the several States, it is provided "that the Secretary of War ascertain the necessary clothing and rations proper for the troops, and report the same to Congress."

\*    \*    \*    \*    \*    \*    \*    \*    \*

In the act of April 30, 1790, the ration of the soldier is established as follows:

Beef ..... 1 lb.; or
Pork ..... ¾ lb.
Bread or flour ..... 1 lb.
Rum, brandy, or whisky, or the value thereof ..... ½ gill.

To every hundred rations:

Salt ..... 1 qt.
Vinegar ..... 2 qts.
Soap ..... 2 lbs.
Candles ..... 1 lb.

\*    \*    \*    \*    \*    \*    \*    \*    \*

By the act of March 3, 1775, it was provided, "that to those in the military service who are, or shall be, employed on the western frontier, there shall be allowed, during their term of being so employed, two ounces of flour or bread, and two ounces of beef or pork, in addition to each of their rations, and a half-pint of salt in addition to every hundred of their rations."

\*    \*    \*    \*    \*    \*    \*    \*    \*

In 1799 the ration was again improved, for March 3 of that year Congress established it as follows:

Bread or flour ..... 18 oz.
Rice, (when the above cannot be obtained) ..... 1 qt.; or
Sifted or bolted Indian meal ..... 1½ lbs.
Fresh beef ..... 1¼ lbs.; or
Salted beef ..... 1 lb.; or
Salted pork ..... ¾ lb.

To the hundred rations:

Salt, when fresh meat is issued................................................ 2 qts.
Salt............................................................................ 4 lbs.
Candles........................................................................ 1½ lbs.

\* \* \* \* \* \* \* \* \*

In March, 1802, Congress again legislated for the Army, making, indeed, rather a backward step, and establishing the ration as follows:

Beef.......................................................................... 1¼ lbs.; or
Pork.......................................................................... ¾ lbs.
Bread or flour................................................................ 18 oz.
Rum, whisky, or brandy........................................................ 1 gill.

To the hundred rations:

Salt.......................................................................... 2 qts.
Vinegar....................................................................... 4 qts.
Soap.......................................................................... 4 lbs.
Candles....................................................................... 1½ lbs.

\* \* \* \* \* \* \* \* \*

In 1838 the spirit-ration was abolished, and coffee and sugar substituted therefor, Congress providing that the allowance of sugar and coffee "in lieu of the spirit or whisky component part of the Army ration, now directed by regulation, shall be fixed at six pounds of coffee and twelve pounds of sugar to every hundred rations, to be issued weekly, when it can be done with convenience to the public service, and when not so issued to be paid in money."

\* \* \* \* \* \* \* \* \*

Under the discretionary power granted to the President by the act of 1818, slight modifications were made in the ration, which, as thus modified, was published to the Army in the Regulations of 1841, in these words:

Par. 1102. The component parts of the ration are as follows:

Pork or bacon................................................................. ¾ lb.; or
Fresh or salt beef............................................................ 1¼ lbs.
Bread or flour................................................................ 18 oz.; or
Hard bread.................................................................... 12 oz.; or
Corn-meal..................................................................... 1¼ lbs.

And at the rate of, to the hundred rations—

Soap.......................................................................... 4 lbs.
Candles....................................................................... 1½ lbs.
Salt.......................................................................... 2 qts.
Vinegar....................................................................... 4 qts.

Also, to the hundred rations—

Peas or beans................................................................. 8 qts.; or
In lieu thereof—
Rice.......................................................................... 10 lbs.
Coffee........................................................................ 6 lbs.
Sugar......................................................................... 12 lbs.

On a campaign, or on board of transports at sea and on the lakes, the ration of bread is one pound.

A daily extra issue of one gill of whisky per man was also authorized to men engaged in constant labor of not less than ten days, or a commutation in money for such whisky, at the option of the man.

\* \* \* \* \* \* \* \* \*

In 1857 a new edition of the General Regulations of the Army was published, in which the ration was announced almost the same as in the edition of 1841. The following are the changes:

An equivalent of adamantine or sperm candles was authorized, in lieu of tallow candles. The extra issue of the spirit-ration was no longer authorized, and it was further provided that " when the officers of the Medical Department find antiscorbutics necessary for the health of the troops, the commanding officer may order issues of fresh vegetables, pickled onions, sauerkraut, or molasses, with an extra quantity of rice and vinegar. (Potatoes are usually issued at the rate of one pound per ration, and onions at the rate of three bushels, in lieu of one of beans.) Occasional issues (extra) of molasses are made—two quarts to one hundred rations—and of dried apples of from one to one and a half bushels to one hundred rations. Troops at sea are recommended to draw rice and an extra issue of molasses in lieu of beans."

\* \* \* \* \* \* \* \* \*

In 1860 Congress increased the amounts of coffee and sugar, respectively, to ten and fifteen pounds per hundred rations, and in August, 1861, the war of the rebellion being then under full headway, Congress provided " that the Army ration shall be increased as follows, viz, instead of the present issue,

Bread, or flour...................................................... 22 oz.; or
Hard-bread ........................................................ 1 lb.

"Fresh beef shall be issued as often as the commanding officer of any detachment or regiment shall require it, when practicable, in place of salt meat. Beans, and rice, or hominy, shall be issued in the same ration in the proportions now provided by the regulations; and one pound of potatoes per man shall be issued at least three times a week, if practicable; and when these articles cannot be issued in these proportions, an equivalent in value shall be issued in some other proper food; and a ration of tea may be substituted for a ration of coffee, upon the requisition of the proper officer: *Provided*, That after the present insurrection shall cease, the ration shall be as provided by law and regulation on the 1st day of July, 1861."

\* \* \* \* \* \* \* \* \*

In July, 1862, the Secretary of War was authorized by act of Congress " to commute the Army ration of coffee and sugar, for the extract of coffee, combined with milk and sugar, \* \* if he shall believe it will be conducive to the health and comfort of the Army, and not more expensive to the Government than the present ration, and if it shall be acceptable to the men."

In March, 1863, pepper was added to the ration, in the proportion of four ounces to every hundred rations, and in the 1863 edition of the regulations, the ration, the maximum ration that was ever attained in our Army, was announced in Par. 1190, as follows:

"A ration is the established daily allowance of food for one person. For the United States Army it is composed as follows:

Pork, or bacon ................................................ 12 oz.; or
Salt, or fresh beef............................................ 1 lb. 4 oz.
Soft bread, or flour.......................................... 1 lb. 6 oz.; or
Hard bread.................................................... 1 lb.; or
Corn meal..................................................... 1 lb. 4 oz.

To every one hundred rations—

Beans, or peas................................................ 15 lbs.
Rice, or hominy............................................... 10 lbs.
Green coffee.................................................. 10 lbs.; or
Roasted and ground coffee..................................... 8 lbs.
Tea........................................................... 1 lb. 8 oz.
Sugar......................................................... 15 lbs.
Vinegar....................................................... 4 lbs.
Candles, adamantine, or star.................................. 1 lb. 4 oz.
Soap.......................................................... 4 lbs.
Salt.......................................................... 3 lbs. 12 oz.
Pepper........................................................ 4 oz.
Potatoes, (when practicable).................................. 30 lbs.
Molasses...................................................... 1 qt.

\* \* \* \* \* \* \* \*

Par. 1191 provides that desiccated compressed potatoes, or desiccated compressed mixed vegetables, at the rate of one and a half ounces of the former and one ounce of the latter to the ration, may be substituted for beans, peas, rice, and hominy, or fresh potatoes.

The extra issue of one gill of whisky per man was also authorized in cases of *excessive* fatigue or *severe* exposure.

\*     \*     \*     \*     \*     \*     \*     \*     \*

In March, 1863, Congress enacted "That the officers of the Medical Department shall unite with the line-officers of the Army, under such rules and regulations as shall be prescribed by the Secretary of War, in supervising the cooking within the same, as an important sanitary measure; and the said Medical Department shall promulgate to its officers such regulations and instructions as may tend to insure the proper preparation of the ration of the soldier." Under this act the latter part of the last described directions as to inspections was modified to read as follows:

"The commanding officer of the post, or regiment, attended by the senior medical officer of his command, will make frequent inspections of the kitchens, or messes. The medical officer will submit his suggestions for improving the cooking, in writing, to the commanding officer."

So far as I know, but little attention has ever been paid to this regulation. The regulations and instructions called for by the act of Congress, from the Medical Department, have never been promulgated to this day. It is believed injudicious and impracticable to transfer the charge of inspecting the company messes, and the responsibility for the proper cooking of the food in the company-kitchen, from company to medical officers.

In June, 1864, Congress enacted that "The Army ration shall hereafter be the same as provided by law and the regulations on the first day of July, 1861;" and accordingly General Order 226, Adjutant-General's Office, 1864, publishes the following regulations on the subject, fixing the ration as it exists to the present day, with the one exception of hard bread, now one pound.

\*     \*     \*     \*     \*     \*     \*     \*     \*

In February, 1865, the War Department directed "the issue of a ration of fish, viz: fourteen ounces of dried fish, or eighteen ounces of pickled fish, will be made to the troops once a week, in lieu of the ration of fresh beef." In promulgating this order to officers of his department, the Commissary-General of Subsistence informs them that he is authorized to state that the above order is intended to sanction, but not to require, weekly issues of fish. The frequency of such issues should be controlled by the health and wishes of the troops, economy, &c., as with other articles of food provided by the Government.

\*     \*     \*     \*     \*     \*     \*     \*     \*

In June, 1865, the Secretary of War directed in General Orders that "the whisky ration will no longer be supplied to the troops of the United States by the Subsistence Department. The whisky now on hand will be sold under the orders of the Commissary-General of Subsistence."

In June, 1867, the Secretary of War changed the ration of hard bread from twelve ounces to one pound avoirdupois.

\*     \*     \*     \*     \*     \*     \*     \*     \*

To render complete the history of the ration, it will be proper to mention two other rations issued by order of the War Department during the war.

The first is the ration for prisoners-of-war, which, as announced June 1, 1864, by the Commissary-General of Prisoners, by authority of the Secretary of War, was as follows:

Pork, or bacon, in lieu of fresh beef............................................................. 10  oz.
Fresh beef.............................................................................................. 14  oz.
Flour, or soft bread................................................................................. 16  oz.

    In lieu of flour or soft bread—

Hard bread.............................................................................................. 14  oz.
Corn meal............................................................................................... 16  oz.

    To every one hundred rations—

Beans, or peas........................................................................................ 12½ lbs.; or
Rice, or hominy....................................................................................... 8  lbs.

| | |
|---|---|
| Soap ......................................................................................... | 4 lbs. |
| Vinegar .................................................................................... | 3 qts. |
| Salt ......................................................................................... | 3¾ lbs. |
| Potatoes .................................................................................. | 15 lbs. |

\*    \*    \*    \*    \*    \*    \*    \*    \*

This ration averaged about thirty-two ounces of solid food, the minimum being twenty-eight and a quarter, and the maximum thirty-five ounces, and was abundant for men leading the lazy and idle life of prisoners-of-war, and was only settled on after a long and large experience.

\*    \*    \*    \*    \*    \*    \*    \*    \*

The second was the ration ordered to be issued by the Subsistence Department "to adult refugees, and to adult colored persons, commonly called contrabands, when they are not employed at labor by the Government, and who may have no means of subsisting themselves, viz, ten ounces of pork or bacon, or one pound of fresh beef, one pound of corn-meal five times a week, and one pound of flour or soft bread, or twelve ounces of hard bread, twice a week; and to every one hundred rations ten pounds of beans, peas or hominy, eight pounds of sugar, two quarts of vinegar, eight ounces of adamantine or star candles, two pounds of soap, two pounds of salt, and fifteen pounds of potatoes when practicable. To children under fourteen years of age, half rations will be issued, and to women and children roasted rye-coffee at the rate of ten pounds, or tea at the rate of fifteen ounces, to every one hundred rations.

\*    \*    \*    \*    \*    \*    \*    \*    \*

In order to understand the subject of the food-supply of the soldier, it is necessary to explain its connection with the post, regimental, and company fund, and this can be most briefly effected by quoting the order establishing and regulating these funds, which is as follows:

[General Orders No. 22.]

WAR DEPARTMENT, ADJUTANT-GENERAL'S OFFICE,
*Washington, April 7, 1866.*

The following regulations, which were in force prior to the 1st day of January, 1857, are substituted for paragraphs 198, 199, 200, 201, 202, 203, and 204, Revised Regulations for the Army:

### Post, regimental, and company funds.

When there is a sutler with troops stationed at a post, he shall, for the privilege enjoyèd, be assessed, and held to pay, at the end of every two months or oftener, as may be determined by the council of administration of the post, at a rate not exceeding ten cents a month for every officer and enlisted soldier serving at the post, the monthly average number of such persons to be determined equitably by the said council.

The troops will bake their own bread when practicable; and as the difference between bread and flour is about 33⅓ per cent. in favor of flour, the saving produced thereby will, with the assessment on the sutler as mentioned above, be carried to the credit of, and constitute the—

### Post-fund.

The post-fund shall be under the administration of the post council, and will be collected by and held in the hands of a post-treasurer, who shall be a discreet officer of the post, appointed by the commander. He will also act as the post-librarian.

The post-treasurer shall open an account with the fund, subject to the inspection of the commander of the post and the council and the commander of the regiment; and he will make payments or purchases on the warrants of the commanding officer, which warrants shall only be drawn in pursuance of specific resolves of the council. The commanding officer who approves the appropriations of the council will be held accountable for all expenditures of the fund not made in accordance with the regulations.

M P—IV

The sums received and expended by the post-treasurer, and the balance on hand, shall be reported, after the session of the council of administration, *every four months*, viz, on the last days of April, August, and December, to the Adjutant-General, through the commanding officer of the post, in the manner directed on the blank forms furnished for that purpose. These accounts will be accompanied by a return of property purchased under the authority of the council of administration. When an officer is relieved from the duties of post-treasurer within the period for which accounts are required, he will, in like manner, transmit an account-current for the time during which he was acting as treasurer, a copy of which will be left with his successor.

The following (exclusive of sums transferred to the regimental fund and to companies detached from the post) are the objects to which the post-fund shall be appropriated:

1. Expenses of bake-house.

2. The education at the post school of such uneducated soldiers as may be desirous of improvement, of music boys, and of the children of soldiers.

3. The establishment of a library, and for newspapers—the number of the latter not to exceed *two* for a post garrisoned by a single company, and *one* per company at all other stations.

4. Garden seeds and utensils.

5. Such measures for the moral and religious instruction of the troops at posts which are not allowed chaplains as the state of the funds may allow.

When a post is about to be evacuated, or any company detached permanently, it shall be the duty of the commanding officer of the post to call a council of administration, and direct it to make an equitable distribution among the companies composing the garrison of the post-fund remaining on hand unappropriated, and also of the articles procured by its means—as books, pamphlets, &c.—or of the money-value thereof; and the portion thus determined will be turned over by the post-treasurer to the companies about to leave, invoices and receipts being passed for the same; but on the arrival of any company so detached at the new station, the money and property thus received will be turned over by their captains to the post-treasurer, who will give his receipt therefor. Company commanders who may have received funds, &c., under the provisions of this paragraph, will make returns thereof to the Adjutant-General on the last days of April, August, and December, until the same shall have been turned over. Should the property be held for a less period than four months, the return will be made immediately after the transfer.

*Regimental fund.*

The several councils of administration at posts occupied by companies of the regiment shall, at regular meetings, (on muster-days,) set aside and cause to be paid over to the *regimental treasurer* 50 per cent. (after deducting the expenses of the bakery) of the whole amount accruing to the post-fund during the preceding two months, which amount will be carried by him to the credit of, and will constitute, the regimental fund. Should a post be garrisoned by companies of different regiments, the council will make an equitable division of the sum (50 per cent.) allotted to the regimental fund, and cause it to be paid over to the treasurer of each regiment or corps.

In transmitting sums set aside for regimental funds, the post-treasurer shall name the months for which each sum was appropriated, and the regimental treasurer shall enter each amount, *separately*, upon his own account, naming the posts at which, and the months for which, it was appropriated.

The adjutant shall be treasurer of the fund for his regiment, which he will disburse on warrants drawn by the colonel or commanding officer, under specific resolves of the regimental council of administration. He will render, through the colonel, periodical returns of the state of the fund, and of the property purchased therefrom, in the same manner as prescribed for the post-treasurer, and his accounts will always be open to the inspection of the colonel and regimental council.

The musical instruments, and everything pertaining to the band, shall be kept by the adjutant, and also the regimental library and its appurtenances, for all which he shall be held accountable. The colonel or commanding officer who approves the appropriations of the council will be held accountable for all expenditures of the fund not made in accordance with the regulations.

The following are the objects to which the regimental fund is appropriated exclusively :
1st. The maintenance of a band.
2d. The establishment of a library.

The principles of the foregoing regulations will apply equally in regard to tax on sutler, distribution and accountability of post and regimental funds, when an entire regiment is serving in the field, or as the garrison of a post.

### Company-fund.

The saving arising from an economical use of the rations of the company (excepting the saving of flour from the general baking) will constitute the *company-fund*, which will be kept in the hands of the captain, or other commander of the company, and disbursed by him *exclusively* for the benefit of the enlisted men of the company. An account of the company-fund will be kept by the officer in whose hands it is deposited, which will be subject to the inspection of the commanding officer of the post or regiment; and returns of it will be rendered quarterly (or oftener if required) to the commander of the regiment. After examination at regimental headquarters of these returns, an abstract, showing in detail the receipts and expenditures, will be forwarded to the Adjutant-General of the Army.

The company commander will be held accountable for all expenditures of the fund not made in accordance with the regulations.

Paragraph 1, General Orders No. 58, of April 7, 1865, and all other orders and regulations inconsistent with this order, are rescinded.

By order of the Secretary of War:

E. D. TOWNSEND,
*Assistant Adjutant-General.*

The theories on which these regulations are based are: first, that the ration-allowance is rather more than sufficient for the wants of the men; and second, that the ration is thus made elastic by allowing company officers to use only so much as they please of the regular supplies, and, with the money derived from the sale of that not used, to purchase whatever articles of food are desired. It is manifestly impossible that the same food should be required in Alaska, or Northern Minnesota, and on the Gulf coast, or in the summer and the winter at the same post. But it is supposed that the company commander, through the company fund, can obtain the articles not on the ration that are suited to the climate and station; and some officers find it difficult to understand why the ration can be considered insufficient, seeing that, with all the deductions made from it by the post fund, and purchases from the company fund of other than articles of food, some companies accumulate large funds, are able to buy handsome mess-furniture, &c.

And yet nothing can be more certain, both theoretically and practically, than that the ration *per se*, that is without additions by exchanges and purchase, is insufficient. The following extract from the report of Surgeon Glover Perin, United States Army, medical director, Department of the Missouri, represents clearly and well the views of the majority of medical officers of much experience, and I would call special attention to the statements contained in it. All of the calculations have been verified:

It is believed that it is only necessary to present some of the data recently given by the most eminent chemists and writers upon hygiene, to demonstrate that the present Army ration is not only deficient in quantity, but that it does not contain the elements necessary to preserve the health of the soldier.

The ration, calculated according to tables furnished by Parkes in his work on hygiene, may be shown thus. As usually issued it contains :

| | Albuminates. | Fats. | Carbo-hy-drates. | Salts. | Extracts. |
|---|---|---|---|---|---|
| 20 ounces beef, less ⅕ for bone, 16 ounces, ⅔ of ............... | 1.6 | 0.90 | ......... | 0.17 | ......... |
| 12 ounces bacon, ⅓ of............... | 0.35 | 2.93 | ......... | 0.12 | ......... |
| 18 ounces soft bread ............... | 1.44 | 0.27 | 8.85 | 0.23 | ......... |
| 2.4 ounces beans*............... | 0.54 | 0.05 | 1.20 | 0.06 | ......... |
| 2.4 ounces sugar ............... | ......... | ......... | 2.32 | 0.01 | ......... |
| 0.6 ounce salt............... | ......... | ......... | ......... | 0.60 | ......... |
| 1.6 ounces green, or 1.28 roasted coffee ............... | ......... | ......... | ......... | ......... | 0.26 |
| First total, usually issued ............... | 3.93 | 4.15 | 12.37 | 1.19 | ......... |
| 2.4 ounces beans deducted............... | 0.54 | 0.05 | 1.20 | 0.06 | ......... |
| Total, without beans............... | 3.39 | 4.10 | 11.17 | 1.13 | ......... |
| 1.6 ounces rice added............... | 0.08 | 0.01 | 1.33 | 0.008 | ......... |
| Second total, with rice*............... | 3.47 | 4.11 | 12.50 | 1.14 | ......... |
| Take usual ration............... | 3.93 | 4.15 | 12.37 | 1.19 | ......... |
| Deduct soft bread ............... | 1.44 | 0.27 | 8.85 | 0.23 | ......... |
| Total, without soft bread ............... | 2.49 | 3.88 | 3.52 | 0.96 | ......... |
| Add 16 ounces hard bread............... | 2.50 | 0.21 | 11.74 | 0.27 | ......... |
| Third total with hard bread............... | 4.99 | 4.09 | 15.26 | 1.23 | ......... |
| Deduct ⅔ beef and ⅓ bacon ............... | 1.95 | 3.83 | ......... | 0.29 | ......... |
| Total, with hard bread and without meat............... | 3.04 | 0.26 | 15.26 | 0.94 | ......... |
| Add 12 ounces bacon............... | 1.06 | 8.80 | ......... | 0.35 | ......... |
| Fourth total with hard bread and bacon............... | 4.10 | 9.06 | 15.26 | 1.29 | ......... |

* Cellulose not included.

Expressed as nitrogenous and carbonaceous food, and reduced to grains of nitrogen and carbon, the four methods of issuing the ration compare as follows :

| | Ounces of nitrogenous food. | Ounces of carbonaceous food. | Grains of nitrogen. | Grains of carbon. |
|---|---|---|---|---|
| First, as usually issued............... | 3.93 | 16.52 | 271 | 4,752 |
| Second, with rice instead of beans............... | 3.47 | 16.61 | 239 | 4,655 |
| Third, with hard bread instead of soft bread............... | 4.99 | 19.35 | 344 | 5,539 |
| Fourth, with hard bread and bacon ............... | 4.10 | 24.32 | 283 | 7,049 |

Giving an average of 4.12 ounces of nitrogenous food, 19.2 ounces of carbonaceous food, 284 grains of nitrogen, and 5,474 grains of carbon.

Expressed as water-free food, the

| | |
|---|---|
| First or usual ration gives............... | 21.65 ounces. |
| Second, with rice instead of beans ............... | 21.22 ounces. |
| Third, with hard instead of soft bread............... | 25.57 ounces. |
| Fourth, with hard bread and bacon............... | 29.71 ounces. |
| An average of............... | 24.53 ounces. |
| If coffee is added............... | 0.26 ounce. |
| | 24.79 ounces. |

In estimating the average of anhydrous food, the fourth of the methods of issuing the ration, viz, that where the 12 ounces of bacon and 16 ounces of hard bread are taken, should be excluded, as such a method should be resorted to only when fresh meat cannot be procured. To issue 12 ounces of bacon gives too much carbon and deficiency of nitrogen. Ranke gives as the proportion of nitrogen to carbon in a state of rest as varying between 1 N. to 11 C., and 1 N. to 15 C., average 1 N. to 13 C. Gasparin's calculations give from 1 N. to 21 C. in rest, and 1 N. to 12 C. during activity, mean 1 N. to 16 C. The mean of the observations of both would give 1 N. to 14½ C. The proportion of nitrogen to carbon, when 12 ounces of bacon are issued, would give nearly 1 N. to 25 C.

Excluding, therefore, an improper way of issuing the ration, and taking the mean of the first, second, and third modes of issue, the average anhydrous value would be 22.8 ounces. If the 0.256 ounce of extract of coffee, which by some writers is only estimated as accessory food, be added, the average value will be 23 ounces.

Parkes gives as an average the amount of food taken by man in 24 hours as follows:

When nearly at rest, 18.5 ounces water-free food.

With moderate exercise, 23 ounces water-free food.

When under great exertion, 26 to 30 ounces water-free food.

When under enormous exertion, 30 to 36 or 40 ounces water-free food.

The average of 18.5 : 23 : 26 : 30 and 40 would be 27.5 ounces.

Letheby gives the daily requirements of the body:

During idleness, 2.73 ounces nitrogenous food, 20.6 ounces carbonaceous food. Total, 23.33. ounces.

During routine work, 4.48 ounces nitrogenous food, 26.44 ounces carbonaceous food. Total, 30.92 ounces.

An average of 27.125 ounces water-free food exclusive of salts.

De Lyon Playfair calculates that adults will consume:

With easy work............................................................. 25.01 ounces water-free food.
With active work........................................................... 28.9 ounces water-free food.
With laborious work....................................................... 29 ounces water-free food.

An average of 27.63 ounces water-free food.

Moleschott says the water-free food required for the average laboring-man is 22.866 ounces.

Average requirements of anhydrous food, according to the above writers, is...... 26.28 ounces.
Average of Army ration, first, second, and third issue, is......................... 23 ounces.
Deficiency ....................................................................... 3.28 ounces.

Average Army ration, with the four methods of issue............................. 24.79 ounces.
Deficiency........................................................................ 1.5 ounces

When the best proportions for field service, such as ⅔ beef and ⅓ bacon, with hard bread and coffee, are taken.......................................... 25.8139 ounces.
Deficiency........................................................................ 0.4661 ounce.

Daily average requirements of the body, according to Parkes and Playfair, during activity, is............................................................. 27.45 ounces.
According to Letheby, (without salts) ............................................ 30.92 ounces.
Average during activity.......................................................... 29.185 ounces.

Army ration, when bacon, beans, and hard bread are issued, amounts to......... 29.71 ounces.
Showing apparent excess of........................................................ 0.52 ounce.

above what is the average requirement during activity; but this excess is no benefit, unless its money value is expended in some other food of different form, as will appear by an analysis of the ration when all bacon and hard bread are issued.

That ration consists of 4.10 ounces of albuminates, 9.06 ounces of fat, 15.26 ounces of carbohydrates, and 1.29 ounces of salts. The albuminates are here at least 1.5 ounces deficient for the requirements of men in activity as the soldier is presumed to be when this ration is issued. The fats are about 6 ounces in excess of the average requirements in activity, except in a very cold climate, and the salts 0.41 ounces in excess. Removing, therefore, the excess in fats, and this ration would be equivalent to about 23.7 ounces water-free food; with coffee, 0.256 ounce water-free food, it would amount in real value to but 23.95 ounces water-free food.

It will be seen from the above that the present Army ration does not contain the food required by man during the average state, varying between rest and activity; and taking the mean of what is required during activity, it is far below.

By taking the best combination of the Army ration, viz, two-thirds beef and one-third bacon, hard bread, and beans, with coffee, amounting to 25.82 ounces, it is 3.37 ounces below what is required during activity.

It may be asked how this deficiency is made up in practice. It is accomplished—

1st. By not using all the bacon, sugar, coffee, soap, candles, and vinegar. The savings from the above, and occasionally savings from beans also, are sold or commuted, and flour or other articles purchased instead.

2d. By adding the produce from gardens.

3d. By adding the products from hunting and fishing.

4th. By contributions from the men.

It has been shown that where all the bacon is issued, the ration contains an excess of fats and salts. It is natural, therefore, to expect a saving in what the body does not require. The proceeds from the sale of the savings from bacon constitute the bulk of the company fund; and it may be added also that here is the origin of the exaggerated idea that the Army ration is so abundant that the men cannot consume it.

The savings from sugar and coffee are only justifiable where the albuminates are so low as to require the expenditure of their money value for food containing nitrogenous matter.

The ration of soap is so small that, if reduced, it is only by the sacrifice of means essential to the maintenance of proper cleanliness of clothing and quarters. The whole ration of candles is required to properly illuminate the company quarters.

\*     \*     \*     \*     \*     \*     \*     \*     \*     \*

The necessity for more bread is particularly observable at those posts where gardens cannot be cultivated.

I wish to invite special attention to the fact that much of the company fund is expended for articles of table and kitchen furniture. It is also a fund from whence purchases are made for almost every article of convenience used about the company not furnished by the quartermaster's and commissary departments.

The sanction given to the expenditure of company funds for articles that are not food leads to the gravest abuses. Such an extravagant idea of the value of the ration appears to prevail, that the officer who does not exhibit a large amount of company savings is looked upon as inattentive to his duties. The company commander who has not had much experience undertakes, therefore, to comply with what appears to be expected of him, and the men are often limited to what is barely necessary to supply their wants without causing open murmur.

It requires no argument to prove that this scant and monotonous diet is productive of dissatisfaction with the service, and that it accounts for a large per cent. of desertions.

If the whole of the savings from the ration were expended in food, the diet would be varied more than at present. There is no reason why fresh or canned milk, cheese, fresh or canned vegetables, fresh or canned fruits, or dried fruits should not be purchased to the extent that the fund will admit of.

\*     \*     \*     \*     \*     \*     \*     \*     \*     \*

The ration, besides being deficient in quantity of anhydrous food, is defective in not containing any vegetable element. Troops subsisting entirely upon the present ration, where vegetables cannot be procured, will soon be affected with the scurvy. I observed an instance at Fort McIntosh, Texas, in the year 1851, where, although fresh beef was issued every alternate day, the whole command became more or less scorbutic. After an experience acquired by many years' service with troops, and after patient investigation and discussion of the subject, I unite with Surgeon T. A. McParlin, United States Army, in recommending that the following ration be substituted for the one now established by law: 20 ounces of fresh beef, or other fresh meats, or 20 ounces of salt beef, or 12 ounces of pork or bacon; 22 ounces of flour, or 22 ounces of soft bread, except when on fatigue, and then to have 24 ounces, or 16 ounces of hard bread and 4.8 ounces of flour, or 24 ounces of cornmeal; 2.4 ounces of beans or pease, or the equivalent money value in fresh or canned milk, or cheése; 9.6 ounces of potatoes, whenever practicable, and when not practicable, the equivalent money value in fresh or dried fruits, such as apples, peaches, prunes, and raisins; 1.6 ounces of rice, or the equivalent money value in fresh vegetables, as onions, carrots, parsnips, turnips, cabbage, or fresh or dried fruits; 2.4 ounces of sugar; 1.6 ounces of green coffee, or 1.28 ounces of roasted coffee, or 0.24 ounce of tea.   Candles, soap, vinegar, salt, and pepper to be issued as at present.

The value of the food portion of the above ration is shown by the following table:

|  | Albuminates. | Fats. | Carbo-hy-drates. | Salts. |
|---|---|---|---|---|
| 20 ounces beef, less ⅕ for bone, 16 ounces, ⅔ of | 1.6 | 0.90 | ........ | 0.17 |
| 12 ounces bacon, ⅛ of | 0.35 | 2.93 | ........ | 0.12 |
| 22 ounces soft bread | 1.76 | 0.33 | 10.82 | 0.29 |
| 2.4 ounces beans* | 0.54 | 0.05 | 1.20 | 0.06 |
| 9.6 ounces potatoes | 0.14 | 0.01 | 2.25 | 0.10 |
| 1.6 ounces rice* | 0.08 | 0.01 | 1.33 | 0.008 |
| 2.4 ounces sugar | ........ | ........ | 2.32 | 0.011 |
| 0.6 ounce salt | ........ | ........ | ........ | 0.6 |
| First total, usual issue | 4.47 | 4.23 | 17.92 | 1.36 |
| Deduct 22 ounces soft bread | 1.76 | 0.33 | 10.82 | 0.29 |
| Total, without soft bread | 2.71 | 3.90 | 7.10 | 1.07 |
| Add 16 ounces hard bread | 2.50 | 0.21 | 11.74 | 0.27 |
| Add 4.8 ounces flour | 0.53 | 0.10 | 3.38 | 0.10 |
| Second total, with 16 ounces hard bread and 4.8 ounces flour | 5.74 | 4.21 | 22.22 | 1.44 |
| Deduct ⅔ beef and ⅛ bacon | 1.95 | 3.83 | ........ | 0.29 |
| Total, with hard bread and 4.8 ounces flour, without meat | 3.79 | 0.38 | 22.22 | 1.15 |
| Add 12 ounces bacon | 1.06 | 8.80 | ........ | 0.35 |
| Third total, with hard bread, 4.8 ounces flour, and bacon | 4.85 | 9.18 | 22.22 | 1.50 |

* Cellulose not included.

Expressed as *nitrogenous* and *carbonaceous* food, and reduced to grains of *nitrogen* and *carbon*, the following table is obtained:

|  | Ounces of nitro-genous food. | Ounces of car-bonaceous food. | Grains of nitro-gen. | Grains of car-bon. |
|---|---|---|---|---|
| First issue | 4.47 | 22.15 | 308 | 5,983 |
| Second issue | 5.74 | 26.43 | 396 | 7,107 |
| Third issue | 4.85 | 31.40 | 334 | 8,618 |

Expressed as water-free food, we have:

First issue ................................................................ 27.98 ounces.

Second issue .............................................................. 33.61 ounces.

Third issue ............................................................... 37.75 ounces.

An average of ............................................................ 33.11 ounces.

If coffee is added........................................................ 0.256 ounce.

33.37 ounces.

Excluding the third mode of issue for reasons already stated, the average anhydrous value of the proposed ration would be................................................................... 30.79 ounces.
With coffee ................................................................................ .256 ounce.
                                                                                             —————
                                                                                             31.05 ounces.

\*    \*    \*    \*    \*    \*    \*    \*    \*    \*    \*    \*    \*

The normal state of our soldiers may be fairly considered as one of activity. They are either on guard, drill, daily or extra duty. Their food requirement, therefore, should be rated with those in activity, the average, taken from Parkes, Playfair, and Letheby, being 29.185 in activity. The average proposed ration being 31.05, would show an excess of 1.865 ounces of water-free food.

This excess is purposely made, in order that the necessary variety can be provided.

The articles forming the standard ration are perhaps the cheapest proper food that can be procured. They can be stored or transported with less cost than almost any others. Now, unless the ration is in excess, it is impossible to vary it, for at every attempt to purchase equivalents additional cost will be encountered. The *bacon*, although in excess, as has been shown, of ordinary requirements, has been retained in the same quantity as in the present ration, for it is from the money derived from the sale of the savings of this article that the most of the purchases of other food are to be made.

In regard to the equivalents of the ration of beans or peas, fresh or canned milk or cheese were selected on account of their nutritive value and the facility of procuring them.

The potato was introduced mainly on account of its antiscorbutic value. Whenever it cannot be procured, the dried apples which are furnished by the Commissary Department can.

The evaporated compressed apples, by what is known as the "Alden process," can be furnished at any point desired.

In adding rice, which will only be required for soup, it was designed to furnish in equivalent more vegetables.

No savings are expected on the sugar, coffee, vinegar, and pepper. Neither should any attempt at saving be made on the ration of soap and candles.

Now, unless company commanders are positively prohibited expending any of the money derived from the sale of the savings from the ration for anything but food in some other form, it is useless to increase it.

The evils resulting from attempts at saving from the ration for other purposes than the purchase of food are nowhere more painfully evident than at our recruiting depots. From an experience of five years at Newport Barracks, Ky., I can say that complaints on account of scanty food were most common. On several occasions the men were ready to break into open mutiny. I was member of a board to investigate these complaints, and know that the statements of the men examined were unanimous that the ration was not enough, particularly the bread. The men having just entered the service, did not, as a rule, have money to buy food with, and were thus compelled to subsist on the ration alone. The numerous desertions at that depot were due in great measure, in my opinion, to the deficiency and monotony of the diet. At those depots where men are received into the service everything should be done to attach them to it, by supplying them with personal comforts; and nothing certainly is more productive of contentment than a generous and varied diet.

\*    \*    \*    \*    \*    \*    \*    \*    \*    \*    \*

The question as to the advisability of continuing the present system of post fund is one upon which there is great difference of opinion among officers. Many recommend that it be abolished, on the ground that the objects for which it is expended, although desirable, are no more a proper charge against the soldier's food allowance than against that of his clothing or bedding, and that they should either be provided by direct appropriations or abandoned. On the other hand, to prevent suffering, it is absolutely necessary that the ration be made in excess of what is required where there is a good garden, a skillful administrative officer, and an economical cook; and it is argued that the ration should be made sufficient to supply the wants of the men in all cases, while inducements should be offered for economy and judicious administration, by allowing savings to be made and expended for objects which will benefit the soldier.

Of these two arguments, the first appears to me correct in theory, and the last the most satisfactory in practical results.

So far as the demands of hygiene are concerned, if the flour or bread ration, be made sufficient to meet all emergencies, the question as to what shall be done with the surplus, when such occurs, need not be considered by the Medical Department.

The ration of eighteen ounces of bread is not sufficient, unless it is supplemented by a good supply of the starchy vegetables. The allowance proposed by Surgeon Perin, viz, twenty-two ounces of flour or of soft bread, would be sufficient.

The following recent order effects some improvement, but the allowance is still insufficient:

[General Orders No. 42.]
WAR DEPARTMENT, ADJUTANT-GENERAL'S OFFICE,
*Washington, March 25, 1875.*

I. At posts where fresh vegetables cannot be raised, the ration of bread will be increased, at the discretion of the department commander, from 18 ounces to 22 ounces. Savings on flour will continue to be applied as heretofore.

II. Regimental, post, and company fund accounts will hereafter be transmitted through department headquarters, with a view to the exercise by department commanders of a proper administrative control over the officers charged with their care and disbursement. They will then, as heretofore, be sent to the Adjutant-General for settlement and record.

By order of the Secretary of War:

E. D. TOWNSEND,
*Adjutant-General.*

With regard to the other constituents of the ration it will be most convenient to take them up *seriatim:*

*Beef.*—The testimony is general that, when the quality is good, the quantity is enough; but at many posts, and especially in the winter and spring, or when the grazing is bad, the meat is lean and tough, and there is great excess of bone, amounting from 25 to 35 per cent. of the weight, the proper proportion in good beef being 20 per cent. At Fort Stockton, Texas, the company commanders report that they have to purchase from five to ten ounces for each man to give them enough. A similar statement comes from Fort Richardson. At Fort Buford, at the beginning of winter, enough animals are slaughtered to last from December to March, the meat being packed in ice and snow, to remain frozen until used. This effects a considerable saving to Government in forage, but injures the meat, and a larger quantity should be issued if this course is to be pursued.

The beef is usually baked, or, as the diet-tables phrase it, roasted, and is generally overcooked, as few soldiers will eat rare beef.

The following remarks are made by Surgeon J. R. Smith, United States Army, with regard to the loss in cooking at the post of Fort Monroe. The amount of bone found by him to be present is much less than that reported at the majority of the posts:

Roasting: Thirty-three experiments were made with beef roasted. In these experiments 947 pounds 10 ounces of beef were roasted, averaging a little more than 28 pounds 11 ounces at each cooking, the extremes being 34 and 24 pounds.

M P——V

This beef after roasting weighed 705 pounds 7 ounces; showing a loss of 242 pounds 3 ounces; or 25.55 per cent.

The bone in this beef weighed 155 pounds 5 ounces, or 16.38 per cent., and the amount of beef available as food, after roasting and deducting the bone, was 550 pounds 4 ounces, or 58.06 per cent. of the amount issued.

In these experiments the beef was roasted about three hours, the average time being 2 hours 54 minutes.

This calculation includes only solids by weight, and does not take into account gravies and drippings.

Boiling: Thirty-two experiments were made with beef boiled. In these 865 pounds 11 ounces were cooked, averaging a little over 27 pounds at each cooking, the extremes being 38 and 21 pounds. The weight after boiling was 649 pounds 6 ounces, showing a loss of 216 pounds 5 ounces, or almost exactly 25 per cent. The bone remaining weighed 153 pounds 14 ounces or 17.77 per cent. of the weight of the beef; and the weight of the eatable beef, after cooking and removing bone, was 495 pounds 8 ounces, or 57.23 per cent. of the amount issued.

The average time of boiling in these experiments was 2 hours 55 minutes.

This calculation does not take into account any nutritious matter taken up by the water in which the beef was boiled.

The following tables show concisely the facts:

*Experiments with roasted beef.*

| Letter of company. | Number of experiments made. | Weight of meat, bone and all, before roasting. | Weight after roasting. | Weight of bone. | Per cent. of weight lost during roasting. | Per cent. of bone in meat. | Per cent. of beef, by weight, left after roasting and extracting the bone. | Average weight of beef used in each experiment. |
|---|---|---|---|---|---|---|---|---|
| | | lbs. oz. | lbs. oz. | lbs. oz. | | | | lbs. oz. |
| K | 9 | 253 15 | 174 14 | 45 11 | 31.11 | 17.99 | 50.87 | 28 3¼ |
| C | 6 | 186 3 | 135 6 | 28 8 | 27.29 | 15.10 | 57.40 | 31 00¼ |
| G | 7 | 227 8 | 187 3 | 34 6 | 17.70 | 15.01 | 67.17 | 32 8 |
| A | 11 | 280 00 | 208 00 | 46 12 | 25.71 | 16.69 | 57.58 | 25 7³⁄₁₁ |
| Total | 33 | 947 10 | 705 7 | 155 5 | 25.45 | 16.20 | 58.25 | 29 4⁴⁴⁄₆₆ |

*Experiments with boiled beef.*

| Letter of company. | Number of experiments made. | Weight of beef, bone and all, before boiling. | Weight after boiling. | Weight of bone. | Per cent. of weight lost by boiling. | Per cent. of bone in meat. | Per cent. of beef left after boiling and deducting the bone. | Average weight of beef used in each experiment. |
|---|---|---|---|---|---|---|---|---|
| | | lbs. oz. | lbs. oz. | lbs. oz. | | | | lbs. oz. |
| K | 5 | 136 9 | 95 00 | 25 00 | 30.43 | 18.30 | 51.25 | 27 5 |
| C | 7 | 186 10 | 150 13 | 35 4 | 19.18 | 18.88 | 61.92 | 26 10¾ |
| G | 6 | 192 8 | 157 1 | 28 10 | 18.40 | 14.87 | 65.88 | 32 1¼ |
| A | 14 | 350 00 | 246 8 | 65 00 | 29.57 | 18.57 | 51.85 | 25 00 |
| Total | 32 | 865 11 | 649 6 | 153 14 | 24.99 | 17.77 | 57.23 | 27 12¹¹⁄₆₆ |

*Mutton* is occasionally, but very seldom, issued in place of beef. At a few posts considerable additions are made to the ration by hunting and fishing. In this connection, attention is especially invited to the report of Asst. Surgeon D. Weisel, Fort Johnston, North Carolina.

The reports with regard to the *bacon* and *pork* are somewhat conflicting. Dr. B. F. Pope, at Fort Stockton, reports that the bacon is good, while the pork is more liable to be found damaged than bacon, and is not so good for scouting parties, and on the other hand, that there is a large waste in bacon in hot weather, amounting sometimes to 25 per cent. Dr. De Witt, at Fort Macon, North Carolina, reports the pork mostly sound and of good quality. The medical officers at Saint Augustine and Barrancas, Fla., report that much of the pork is of an inferior quality.

*Flour and bread.*—The flour furnished is usually good. Careful examinations of it have been made by several officers, and in particular by Surgeon J. F. Weeds and Asst. Surgeon Charles Smart, with the following results:

*Examinations by Surgeon J. F. Weeds, United States Army.*—Sample 100 grains. First specimen: Gluten, 12.5 grains; water, $10\frac{4}{5}$ grains. Second specimen: Gluten, 13.5 per cent.; water, 11 per cent. Third specimen: Gluten, 10.25 per cent.; water, 14 per cent.

No attempt was made to determine the quantity of inorganic matter. A microscopical examination showed that the first specimen contained grains of the triticum vulgare, a few fragments of the testa and cellulose of the same plant, the former predominating. No foreign substances were found.

The second specimen was lighter colored, less gritty, more adhesive, and quite free from moldiness, animalculæ or fungi.

The third specimen was inferior in quality to either of the other specimens, darker in color, less adhesive, doughless, spongy, and elastic. No animalculæ or fungi detected.

*Examination by Asst. Surgeon Charles Smart, United States Army.*—Average percentage of three specimens of good flour compared with one specimen of inferior quality:

|  | Inferior. | Good. |
|---|---|---|
| Water | 8.70 | 11.80 |
| Starch | 61.60 | 61.40 |
| Gluten | 14.90 | 13.25 |
| Albumen | 2.00 | 1.15 |
| Dextrin and sugar | 7.20 | 7.00 |
| Ash | 80 | 1.40 |

The bread made in the post-bakeries of the Army is usually of a good quality, and if an inferior article is produced, the attention of the officers is promptly called to it, from the fact that their own bread-supply is obtained from this source. As I have above stated, the supply is insufficient at certain posts. The quality of the bread is always better when potatoes can be obtained for the yeast.

The following extracts from the report of Surgeon E. P. Vollum, at Camp Douglas, are of interest in this connection:

\*        \*        \*        \*        \*        \*        \*        \*        \*

It is very seldom that any complaints are made about the food, excepting as to the quantity of the bread-ration above mentioned, or that any cases of disease may be attributed to its mode of preparation, excepting to sour bread, weak coffee, and insufficiently-cooked beans. Wheat bread made with yeast, the stock of which is allowed to become too old, or when made from flour raised on a sandy soil, or one deficient in the proper amount of lime, unless corrected by the addition of some strengthening agent, makes a weak bread, and though it may rise well enough, when the loaf cools in the sweating-box, it becomes heavy and sour, and when eaten by susceptible cases, produces dyspepsia, diarrhœa, or colic.

\*        \*        \*        \*        \*        \*        \*        \*        \*

Liebig recommended the mixing of this class of flour with lime-water of full strength, and I have often tried it with entire success. A barrel from which the water for mixing the batch is taken is covered on the bottom with about two inches of quicklime, and the barrel filled with water, and stirred up well, and allowed to settle in time for use in the batch, which is mixed with it instead of plain water. As the lime is consumed, more is added to keep up the strength of the water. Liebig assumes that bread made from poor flour in this way simply contains an amount of lime equal to good flour grown on lime soil.

During the war, the great Army bakeries in Washington used the lime-water corrective, at my suggestion, for the various varieties of poor flour that chanced to fall into their hands; and, as far as my observation extended, it was employed with entire satisfaction. It has lately been employed at this post with the same result.

*      *      *      *      *      *      *      *      *

The hard bread is only used on scouts and expeditions, and the men often prefer to draw flour, because, after a few cakes have been taken from a box, the remainder break up from the jolting in transportation. In this connection, Assistant Surgeon Lippincott recommends that yeast-powders be issued for use on scouting parties.

*Beans.*—These are largely used by the troops, to the exclusion of rice, which is seldom drawn. The quality is usually good. At Fort Yuma, the white beans of the ration are often exchanged for the red bean of California and New Mexico, which is preferred by the men.

*Pease.*—These are used only in soup; are of good quality, but not much liked by the men.

*Coffee.*—The article furnished for the use of the troops is "Rio," and is usually of good quality. It is generally badly made, by prolonged boiling, but it would seem that the men prefer strength rather than aroma. Several of the medical officers think that the quantity at present allowed is hardly sufficient, and there is a general disposition to remonstrate against the reduction proposed in the new regulations.

*Tea* is seldom drawn by the men, being used mainly by the laundresses.

The *sugar* is reported as of uniformly good quality. Two or three complaints of insufficient allowance are made, all of which are from colored troops.

Assistant Surgeons Huntington and McElderry recommend that an allowance of about two ounces of cheese be made to the ration, which would certainly be a judicious addition, if it could be preserved.

Dr. Huntington recommends the addition of molasses to the ration. It is much sought for by the men.

At all posts where there are no company gardens, the officers are urgent that vegetables, especially potatoes and onions, be added to the ration.

The want of vegetables is felt in two ways: first, they are required to make good the deficiency in the starchy foods; and second, as antiscorbutics. As there are, and probably will always be, a few posts to which it is impossible to furnish fresh vegetables, it is a question as to the best thing to be done under such circumstances.

The following table shows the localities at which there is a liability to the disease which is caused by a deficient supply of vegetables:

*Table showing, by departments, the number of cases of scurvy, and the posts from which they have been reported, from 1868 to 1874.*

### DEPARTMENT OF TEXAS.

| | 1868. | 1869. | 1870. | 1871. | 1872. | 1873. | 1874. |
|---|---|---|---|---|---|---|---|
| Bliss, Fort | | | | | | 1 | |
| Brazos River | | | | | 1 | | |
| Brownsville | 1 | | | | | | |
| Concordia, Camp | | 2 | | | | | |
| Clark, Fort | 12 | 2 | | 1 | 2 | | 2 |
| Concho, Fort | 4 | 6 | 1 | | 11 | 4 | 4 |
| Davis, Fort | 3 | 8 | 1 | | | | |
| Duncan, Fort | | | | | | 1 | |
| Griffin, Fort | | | | 17 | 4 | 1 | |
| Horse-Head Crossing | | | | | 1 | | |
| Hudson, Camp | | | | | 1 | | |
| Johnson Station | | | | | | | 1 |
| McKavett, Fort | 1 | 11 | | | 1 | | 2 |
| Nueces River, Camp | | | | | 1 | | |
| Quitman, Fort | 2 | 5 | 21 | 1 | 1 | | |
| Ranche San Ignaire | 1 | | | | | | |
| Ranche San Ygnacio | 1 | | | | | | |
| Richardson, Fort | 1 | 2 | | 26 | 16 | | |
| Ringgold Barracks | 3 | | | 1 | | | |
| San Antonio | | 1 | | | | | |
| Stockton, Fort | 15 | 35 | 1 | | 2 | | 1 |
| Verde, Camp | 1 | | | | | | |
| *Miscellaneous.* | | | | | | | |
| In the field | 2 | | | | | | 1 |
| Scouting expedition | | | 6 | | | | |

### DEPARTMENT OF THE MISSOURI.

| | 1868. | 1869. | 1870. | 1871. | 1872. | 1873. | 1874. |
|---|---|---|---|---|---|---|---|
| Arbuckle, Fort, Indian Territory | | 2 | | | | | |
| Bayard, Fort, New Mexico | | | 3 | | | | |
| Beecher, Camp, Kansas | | 2 | | | | | |
| Canadian River, Indian Territory | 1 | | | | 1 | | |
| Craig, Fort, New Mexico | | | 1 | | | | |
| Dodge, Fort, Kansas | *1 | 15 | 1 | 1 | | | 1 |
| Garland, Fort, Colorado | | 1 | 1 | 2 | | | |
| Gibson, Fort, Indian Territory | | | | | | 10 | 5 |
| Harker, Fort, Kansas | | 4 | | | | | |
| Hays, Fort, Kansas | 1 | 2 | | | | | |
| Larned, Fort, Kansas | 1 | | | | | | |
| Lyon, Fort, Colorado | | 2 | 2 | | | 2 | |
| McRae, Fort, New Mexico | 12 | 2 | | | | | |
| Ogallalla Stm., Kansas | 1 | | | | | | |
| Republican River, (near,) Kansas | 3 | | | | | | |
| Sill, Fort, Indian Territory | | 2 | 3 | 7 | 7 | | 2 |
| Supply, Camp, Indian Territory | 1 | 1 | 1 | 2 | 2 | | 1 |
| Sumner, Fort, New Mexico | 1 | | | | | | |
| Union, Fort, New Mexico | | 1 | 2 | 4 | 2 | 5 | |
| Wallace, Fort, Kansas | | 22 | 1 | | | | |
| Willow Springs, Colorado | | | 2 | | | | |
| Wingate, Fort, New Mexico | 1 | 2 | | | | | |
| Witchita, Camp, Indian Territory | | 1 | | | | | |
| *Miscellaneous.* | | | | | | | |
| Field, Indian Territory | 2 | 1 | | | | | |

* Camp near Fort Dodge.

### DEPARTMENT OF THE PLATTE.

| | 1868. | 1869. | 1870. | 1871. | 1872. | 1873. | 1874. |
|---|---|---|---|---|---|---|---|
| Bridger, Fort, Wyoming | | 5 | 2 | | | | 1 |
| Brown, Camp, Wyoming | | | | | | | 1 |
| D. A. Russell, Fort, Wyoming | *2 | | | | | 2 | 1 |
| Fetterman, Fort, Wyoming | 2 | 1 | | | | | |
| Fred. Steele, Fort, Wyoming | | 1 | | | | | |
| Kearney, Fort, Nebraska | | 2 | | | | | |
| Omaha Barracks, Nebraska | | 2 | | 1 | | | |
| Platte River, Camp on, Nebraska | 2 | | | | | | |
| Sanders, Fort, Wyoming | | | | | | 2 | 1 |
| Shell Creek, Camp on, Nebraska | | 2 | | | | | |
| Sidney, Nebraska | | 1 | | | | | |

* Near Fort D. A. Russell.

*Statement showing, by departments, the number of cases of scurvy, &c.*—Continued.

### DEPARTMENT OF DAKOTA.

| | 1868. | 1869. | 1870. | 1871. | 1872. | 1873. | 1874. |
|---|---|---|---|---|---|---|---|
| A. Lincoln, Fort, Dakota | | | | | | 1 | 6 |
| Benton, Fort, Montana | | | 3 | | | | |
| Brulé Agency, Dakota | | | 3 | | | | |
| Buford, Fort, Dakota | | | 1 | | | | |
| C. F. Smith, Fort, Montana | 3 | | | | | | |
| Carroll, Camp, Montana | | | | | | | 1 |
| Cooke, Camp, Montana | | 1 | | | | | |
| Ellis, Fort, Montana | 1 | | | | | 2 | |
| Pembina, Fort, Dakota | | | | | 1 | | |
| Rice, Fort, Dakota | | 2 | 8 | 6 | | 1 | 1 |
| Shaw, Fort, Montana | | | | | 1 | | |
| Stevenson, Fort, Montana | 2 | 5 | | | | | |
| Totten, Fort, Montana | 14 | 4 | 5 | | | | |
| *Miscellaneous.* | | | | | | | |
| Field, Montana | | | 2 | | | | |

### DEPARTMENT OF THE COLUMBIA.

| | 1868. | 1869. | 1870. | 1871. | 1872. | 1873. | 1874. |
|---|---|---|---|---|---|---|---|
| Harney, Camp, Oregon | 1 | 1 | 1 | | | | |
| Sitka, Alaska | | 4 | | | | | |
| Vancouver, Fort, Washington | | | 1 | 2 | | | |
| Warner, Camp, Oregon | 4 | | | 1 | | | |

### DEPARTMENT OF CALIFORNIA.

| | 1868. | 1869. | 1870. | 1871. | 1872. | 1873. | 1874. |
|---|---|---|---|---|---|---|---|
| Benicia Barracks, California | | | | | 1 | | |
| Cady, Camp, California | 1 | | | | | | |
| Churchill Barracks, Nevada | | 2 | | | | | |
| Presidio of San Francisco, California | | | | | | 1 | |

### DEPARTMENT OF ARIZONA.

| | 1868. | 1869. | 1870. | 1871. | 1872. | 1873. | 1874. |
|---|---|---|---|---|---|---|---|
| Apache, Camp | | | | 2 | | | |
| Bowie, Camp | 3 | 3 | 1 | | | 1 | |
| Colorado, Camp | | 6 | | | | | |
| Crittenden, Camp | | 9 | | | | | |
| Date Creek, Camp | | 1 | | 2 | | | |
| Goodwin, Camp | | 3 | | 2 | | | |
| Grant, Camp | 1 | 1 | | 7 | | | |
| Lincoln, Camp | 1 | | | | | | |
| Lowell, Camp | | 6 | 1 | 1 | | | |
| McDowell, Camp | 11 | 1 | 4 | | | | |
| McPherson, Camp | 3 | | | | | | |
| Mojave, Camp | 5 | 1 | 1 | | | | |
| Pinal, Camp | | | | 2 | | | |
| Rawlins, Camp | | | 2 | | | | |
| Toll-Gate, Camp | | | 2 | | | | |
| Verde, Camp | | | | | | | |
| Wallin, Camp | | | | | | 2 | |
| Whipple, Camp | | 2 | | | | | |
| Willow Grove, Camp | 1 | 1 | | | 1 | | |
| Yuma, Fort, (California) | 3 | | | | 5 | | |
| *Miscellaneous.* | | | | | | | |
| Field | | | | | | | 1 |

The remedy for this is, first, to supply the deficiency in carbo-hydrates by an increase in the bread-ration; and, second, to supply the vegetable acids by means of lime-juice or canned tomatoes.

The latter vegetable is especially valuable as an antiscorbutic as I know from practical trial during the late war, far surpassing the potato in this respect, is very cheap, and might easily be furnished in cans at any point.

The canned tomatoes furnished for officers' use by the Subsistence Department contain an excess of water, which might easily be got rid of. A can of tomatoes, obtained from the Washington depot, was examined by Dr. B. F. Craig, with the following results:

A can of tomatoes was found to contain 2.04 pounds avoirdupois, of which, however, only 0.05 pounds (22.75 grams) were solid matter, dried at 212° Fahrenheit. There was, therefore, 97.6 per cent. of water present.

The acid of the tomato I found to be malic, with a trace of citric, the amount of the free malic acid being equivalent to 315 parts in 100,000, or a little over three-tenths of 1 per cent. (Lemon-juice contains about twenty-five times as much free acid.) In tomatoes there is about as much more malic acid in combination with bases.

The amount of vegetable acid—its proportion to the total solid matter—is of itself enough to make tomatoes valuable as antiscorbutics, but it certainly seems desirable, in canning them, to get rid of some of the great excess of water.

Surgeon E. Swift calls attention to the value of the tomato as an article of food, and, if it can be put up in such a way as to dispense with the great amount of water now found in the canned article, it would be an addition to the ration of great value.

At southern posts, the want of ice is strongly felt and expressed, as in the following remarks by the commanding officer at Saint Augustine, Florida, Major John Hamilton, First Artillery:

Greasy, flowing butter and tepid water are just as disagreeable here, where the thermometer is 94°, as they would be North. Give us an ice-house, that our men may put their company fund in ice, and most of it will go that way.

At many of the northern posts a plentiful supply is stored. At Camp Grant, Arizona, compressed snow is brought from the neighboring mountain-tops, with good results. A good ice-machine, suitable for the wants of a one-company post, and at a reasonable price, is much wanted; but, after repeated inquiries, I have not been able to ascertain that such a machine has yet been constructed.

The recommendation is almost unanimous that some change be made in the present regulations with regard to the detail of company cooks, which are that the cooks shall be changed every ten days. This regulation is practically disregarded, as regards the chief cook, at the majority of posts. Were it literally enforced, the results would be very bad, both as regards the health of the men and economy in their provisions. The position of company cook is not a specially desirable one, and it is recommended that extra-duty pay should be allowed to them. Several officers of experience recommend that cooks should be specially enlisted for that duty, and good negro cooks could easily be thus obtained. It is also recommended that at each recruiting depot there should be a school for the training of cooks, as in the English service. The following is an extract from the report of Dr. Vollum:

The plan of detailing cooks for the hospital and companies indiscriminately from the command, with the expectation that because they are detailed and nominated as cooks, they can perform the duty efficiently, faithfully, and economically, is wrong at bottom. It has nothing to recommend it, and should be abolished. It would be as reasonable to expect the like duties to be well done on board of a man-of-war by indiscriminate details among the marines and crew. The cooks in the Army should, in my judgment, form a civil branch of it, uniformed, and subject to military control, and kept recruited up to the wants of the service, as was contemplated by section 10, act of Congress approved March 3, 1863, though the pay therein allowed falls short of the object at this time; but when the act went into operation the pay was enough, and its provisions secured fair cooks, and relieved many men for duty in the ranks.

The following aphorisms of Captain Sanderson should be familiar to all cooks:

*The Cook's Creed.*[1]

Cleanliness is next to godliness, both in persons and kettles. Be ever industrious, then, in scouring your pots. Much elbow-grease, a few ashes, and a little water, are capital aids to the careful cook. Better wear out your pans with scouring than your stomachs with purging; and it is less dangerous to work your elbows than your comrade's bowels. Dirt and grease betray the poor cook, and destroy the poor soldier, while health, content, and good cheer should ever reward him who does his duty and keeps his kettles clean. In military life punctuality is not only a duty, but a necessity, and the cook should always endeavor to be exact in time. Be sparing with sugar and salt, as a deficiency can be better remedied than an overplus.

Remember that beans, badly boiled, kill more than bullets; and fat is more fatal than powder. In cooking, more than in anything else in this world, always make haste slowly. One hour too much is vastly better than five minutes too little, with rare exceptions. A big fire scorches your soup, burns your face, and crisps your temper. Skim, simmer, and scour, are the true secrets of good cooking.

The inspection of the food required by existing laws and regulations is usually made by the company officer, or by the officer of the day. It is inspected by the medical officer from once a week to once a month, and whenever his attention is called to it by the occurrence of disease which may be supposed to be due to its improper quality or preparation.

The mess-furniture of a company is provided from the company fund, and some companies have a very good supply, in which they take much pride. It seems to me, however, that the Government should provide plates and knives and forks, as well as pots and blankets, and relieve the company fund from this source of expense.

The articles kept for sale to officers have been added to and changed, from time to time, and the supply is, as a rule, satisfactory, and is an invaluable addition to the resources of the officer.

At all cavalry or other posts at which a number of horses are kept, a valuable addition to the food-supply can easily be made by the methodical culture of the edible mushroom. This can easily be effected in sheds, cellars, out-houses, &c., and in the open air. The spawn is easily obtained, and crops can be had through the autumn, spring, and winter. I commend to the attention of officers stationed at such posts a small work by W. Robinson, called "Mushroom Culture; its Extension and Improvement;" London, Warne & Co., 1870; in which is given all the information required on this subject.

A comparison of the rations allowed to their armies by different countries is interesting as a comparison of opinions, but affords no data as to comparative value, for the reason that the legal ration never is that which the soldier actually gets to eat. Either by deductions, or exchanges, or additions from the labor or pay of the soldier, the actual bill of fare is usually very different from the ration allowance. I give the following table of different rations, therefore, as of theoretical rather than actual issues:

[1] Camp Fires and Camp Cooking; or, Culinary Hints for the Soldier. By Capt. James M. Sanderson. Washington, Government Printing Office, 1862. Page 4.

*Table showing the daily ration (expressed in grains) of a soldier of the United States Army and of soldiers of different European countries.*

| Ration of— | UNITED STATES. | FRANCE.* | | | | | ENGLAND.† | | | |
|---|---|---|---|---|---|---|---|---|---|---|
| | | Army. | | | Navy. | | Second Battalion Rifle Brigade. | Royal Guard. | First Brigade Artillery. | In war. |
| | | Garrison. | War. | Proposed for war. | On land. | At sea. | | | | |
| Beef, (fresh or salted).........grains | a8,750 | | | | | | | | | |
| Meat, (beef, mutton, &c).........do... | | e4,630 | e4,630 | g7,717 | 3,858 | h4,630 | 5,250 | 5,250 | 5,250 | 7,000 |
| Bread.........do... | b7,875 | 15,434 | f15,434 | f15,434 | 11,576 | i11,576 | 10,500 | 10,500 | 7,000 | 10,480 |
| Flour.........do... | | | | | | | 72.8 | | 1,750 | |
| Barley.........do... | | | | | | | 72.8 | | 437.5 | |
| Beans or peas.........do... | c1,050 | 463 | 926 | 926 | 1,852 | 1,852 | | | | |
| Potatoes.........do... | | | | | | | 8,750 | 8,750 | 7,000 | |
| Mixed vegetables.........do... | | 1,543 | | | | | 765.6 | 875 | 3,500 | |
| Sour-krout.........do... | | | | | | k309 | | | | |
| Butter.........do... | | | | | 231.5 | 231.5 | 93.7 | | | |
| Olive-oil.........do... | | | | | 92.6 | 92.6 | | | | |
| Sugar.........do... | 1,050 | | 324 | 386 | 386 | | 875 | 875 | 1,312.5 | 875 |
| Coffee.........do... | d700 | | 247 | 309 | 309 | | 146 | 146 | 146 | 146 |
| Tea.........do... | | | | | | | 73 | 87.5 | 109 | 73 |
| Milk.........do... | | | | | | | 2 | 2.5 | 2 | |
| Vinegar.........fluid-ounces | 1.28 | | | | | | | | | |
| Wine.........do... | | | | | | 15.55 | | | | |
| Brandy.........do... | | | | | | 2 | | | | |
| Beer.........pints | | | | | | | | | 1 | |

* G. Morache, Hygiène Militaire, Paris, 1874, p. 652 et seq.  
† C. A. Gordon, The Soldier's Manuel of Sanitation, London, 1873.  
a Or 8,750 pork or bacon.  
b Or 7,000 hard bread, or 8,750 corn-meal.  
c Or 700 rice.  
d Or 105 tea.  
e Or 3,704 boned meat.  
f Or 11,576 hard bread.  
g Or 6,174 boned meat.  
h Or 3,087 canned or salt meat, or dry cheese.  
i Or 8,489 hard bread.  
k Or 154 sorrel.

NOTE.—The quantities of salt and other seasonings are omitted.

| *Rations of— | AUSTRO-HUNGARY. | | BAVARIA. | | | BELGIUM. | DENMARK.† | | |
|---|---|---|---|---|---|---|---|---|---|
| | In peace. | In war. | Garrison. | Cantonment. | War. | | Garrison. | Camp and war. | In maritime forts. |
| Beef.........grains | | | | | | 3,858 | | | |
| Meat, (beef, mutton, &c).........do... | 4,322 | 8,643 | 3,858 | 6,945 | 3,858 | | | 3,827 | 4,985 |
| Bread.........do... | 14,817 | 14,817 | 11,576 | 11,576 | 11,576 | 11,885 | ‡11,576 | 11,576 | 11,576 |
| Flour.........do... | 3,473 | 3,473 | | | | | | | |
| Barley, hulled.........do... | | | | | | 15,434 | | 12.5 | 17 |
| Potatoes.........do... | | | Indefinite | Indefinite | 1,482 | | | | |
| Mixed vegetables.........do... | | | | | | 309 | | | |
| Butter.........do... | | | | | | | | | |
| Lard.........do... | | | | | | 154 | | | |
| Coffee, sweetened.........fluid-ounces | | 12.5 | | | | 8.5 | | | |
| Wine.........do... | | 12.5 | | | | | | | |
| Brandy.........do... | | | | | | | | 8.5 | 11.3 |
| Beer.........do... | | | Indefinite | 20 | 20 | | | | |

* G. Morache, pp. 663, 664.  
† On exceptionally severe duty in camp or in the field, the Danish soldier receives a further allowance of 4 fluid ounces of brandy, and from 463 to 3,858 grains of bacon.  
‡ All other articles are procured by the soldier.

M P—VI

*Table showing the daily ration of a soldier of the United States Army &c.—Continued.*

| *Ration of— | HOLLAND. | ITALY. Peace. | ITALY. Camp. | ITALY. War. | PRUSSIA. In peace. Small ration. | PRUSSIA. In peace. Grand ration. | PRUSSIA. In war. Small ration. | PRUSSIA. In war. Grand ration. | RUSSIA. In the Crimea. | RUSSIA. Expedition in Khiva. |
|---|---|---|---|---|---|---|---|---|---|---|
| Beef ........................grains | | | | | | | | | | |
| Meat........................do... | 3,858 | a3,087 | a3,087 | a4,630 | 2,222 | 3,858 | b5,788 | 7,717 | 6,992 | ......... |
| Bacon......................do... | | | 232 | 232 | | | | | | ......... |
| Mutton on the hoof ........do... | | | | | | | | | | 12,656 |
| Bread......................do... | 11,576 | 14,168 | 14,168 | 11,576 | 10,773 | 10,773 | c11,576 | c11,576 | 6,992 | ......... |
| Hard bread.................do... | | | | | | | | | | 12,656 |
| Flour......................do... | | | | | | | | | | 262 |
| Oatmeal....................do... | | | | | | | | | | 3,164 |
| Rice.......................do... | 772 | d2,315 | d2,315 | d1,852 | e1,512 | f1,729 | g1,852 | h2,469 | | ......... |
| Barley.....................do... | | | | | | | | | 7,717 | ......... |
| Beans or peas..............do... | | | | | 3,458 | 4,568 | 3,858 | 4,939 | | 2,160 |
| Potatoes ..................do... | 30,820 | | | | | | | | | ......... |
| Sour-krout.................do... | | | | | | | | | 7,717 | ......... |
| Fresh vegetables ................ | value ½ cent. | value ⅔ cent. | | | | | | | | ......... |
| Lard......................grains | 386 | | | | | | | | | 324 |
| Sugar......................do... | | | | 309 | | | | | | 146 |
| Tea........................do... | | | | | | | | | | 146 |
| Coffee.....................do... | | | | 232 | | | | | | ......... |
| Coffee, roasted............do... | | | | | | 185 | 370 | 370 | | ......... |
| Coffee, sweetened ......fluid-ounces | 8.5 | | | | | | | | | ......... |
| Vinegar....................do... | | | | | | | | | .88 | ......... |
| Wine......................do... | | 8.5 | 8.5 | 8.5 | | | | | | ......... |
| Kwass.....................do... | | | | | | | | | 42 | ......... |
| Brandy....................do... | | | | | | | | | | 6 |

* Morache, p. 666 et seq.
a Fresh.
b Or 2,469 bacon.
c Or 7,717 hard bread.
d Or macaroni.

e Or 1,729 barley, or 3,458 beans or peas, or 6 pints of potatoes.
f Or 3,766 barley, or 4,568 beans or peas, or 8 pints of potatoes.
g Or 1,852 barley, or 3,858 beans or peas, or 23,150 potatoes.
h Or 2,469 barley, or 4,939 beans or peas, or 30,868 potatoes.

| Ration of— | SAXONY. In peace. | SAXONY. In war. | SWEDEN. | SWITZERLAND. Garrison. | SWITZERLAND. In war. | TURKEY. Ordinary times. | TURKEY. During month "Ramadan." |
|---|---|---|---|---|---|---|---|
| Meat, (beef or mutton)............grains | 2,222.5 | 5,788 | ......... | 4,815 | 7,717 | 3,967 | 3,967 |
| Meat, fresh...................do... | | | 2,099 | | | | |
| Meat, salt....................do... | | | 1,404 | | | | |
| Pork, fresh...................do... | | | 386 | | | | |
| Pork, salt....................do... | | | 386 | | | | |
| Codfish......................do... | | | 617 | | | | |
| Herrings.....................do... | | | 1,142 | | | | |
| Bread .......................do... | 10,650 | 11,576 | 13,119 | 11,576 | 11,576 | 14,909 | 14,909 |
| Bread for soup | | | ......... | value 1 cent | value 1 cent | | |
| Flour......................grains | | | 108 | | | | 370 |
| Wheat.......................do... | | | ......... | | | | |
| Barley......................do... | | | 2,300 | | | | |
| Barley, hulled................do... | | | 154 | | | | |
| Rice .......................do... | 1,358 | 1,111 | ......... | | | 1,312 | 5,016 |
| Peas, dried..................do... | | | 1,442 | | | 340 | 340 |
| Peas, green..................do... | | | 2,884 | | | | |
| Potatos .....................do... | | | 11,536 | | | | |
| Vegetables, fresh | | | value 4-5 of cent. | value 2 cts. | value 2 cts. | onions 324 | onions 324 |
| | | | | | | | 200 |
| Cheese, dry ................grains | | | | | | | |
| Butter .....................do... | | | 494 | | | | 146 |
| Sugar ......................do... | | | | | | 146 | 1,142 |
| Coffee......................do... | | 370 | | | | | |
| Coffee, with milk and sugar........fluid-ounces | | | | 25.5 | 25.5 | | |
| Olives....................grains | | | | | | | 200 |
| Preserved fruits..............do... | | | | | | | 200 |
| Wine....................fluid-ounces | | | | 13 | 13 | | |

I append several diet-tables of posts, in different parts of the country, at different times of year. From these it will be seen that the fare of the soldier is rather monotonous, however sufficient and of good quality it may be. But to keep men in good condition, there should be not only abundance but variety, and the want of this is due

partly to the ration itself and partly to the limited knowledge of different modes of preparing food possessed by the cooks.

| Name of post. | Day of week. | Bread. | Coffee. | Beef, roasted. | Beef, boiled. | Beef, roast, cold. | Beefsteak. | Pork, boiled. | Bacon, fried. | Irish stew. | Meat-hash. | Baked beans and bacon. | Bean-soup. | Potatoes. | Vegetable-soup. | Cabbage. | Extra articles. Breakfast. | Dinner. | Supper. |
|---|---|---|---|---|---|---|---|---|---|---|---|---|---|---|---|---|---|---|---|
| Fort Independence, Boston Harbor, Mass. | Sunday | b. d. s. | b. s. | d. | | | | | | | | b. | | d. | | | | Rice soup | |
| | Monday | b. d. s. | b. s. | | | | | | | | | b. | | d. | | | | Fresh pork | |
| | Tuesday | b. d. s. | b. s. | d. | | | | | | | | b. | | | d. | | | | |
| | Wednesday | b. d. s. | b. s. | | d. | | | | | | | b. | | d. | | | | | |
| | Thursday | b. d. s. | b. s. | | | | | d. | | | | b. | | d. | d. | | | | |
| | Friday | b. d. s. | b. s. | d. | | | | | | | | b. | | d. | | | | Rice soup | |
| | Saturday | b. d. s. | b. s. | | | | | | | | | b. | | d. | | | | Turnips and fresh pork. | |
| Fort Mackinac, Mich. | Sunday | b. d. s. | b. d. s. | d. | | | | b. | | | | d. | | | | | | | |
| | Monday | b. d. s. | b. s. | d. | | | | b. | | | | | | d. | d. | | | Beets | |
| | Tuesday | b. d. s. | b. s. | d. | | | | | b. | | | | | | | d. | | Carrots and pea-soup. | |
| | Wednesday | b. d. s. | b. s. | d. | | | | b. | | | | d. | | d. | | | | | |
| | Thursday | b. d. s. | b. s. | d. | | | | b. | | | | | | d. | | | | Pea-soup | |
| | Friday | b d. s. | b. d. s. | d. | | | | d. | b. | | | | | d. | | | | | |
| | Saturday | b. d. s. | b. s. | d. | | | b. | | | | | | | d. | d. | | | Carrots | |
| Saint Augustine, Fla. | Sunday | b. d. s. | b. s. | d. | | | | | | | | b. | | | | | | Sweet potatoes. | Mush and molasses. |
| | Monday | b. d. s. | b. s. | | | | | b. | | | | | | d. | | | | Rice-soup | Stewed beans. |
| | Tuesday | b. d. s. | b. s. | d. | | | | b. | | | | s. | | d. | | | | | |
| | Wednesday | b. d. s. | b. s. | | | | | | | | | b. | | d. | | | | Rice-soup | Mush and molasses. |
| | Thursday | b. d. s. | b. d. s. | | | | b. | s. | | | | d. | | | | | | | |
| | Friday | b. d. s. | b. s. | | | | | b. | | d. | | | | s. | | | | | |
| | Saturday | b. d. s. | b. s. | d. | | | | | | | | b. s. | | d. | | | | | |
| Austin, Tex | Sunday | b. d. s. | b. s. | d. | | s. | | | | | | | | d. | | | | Baked peas and beans. | Rice-pudding |
| | Monday | b. d. s. | b. s. | | d. | | b. | | | | | | | d. | | | | Sweet potatoes. | Fried sausages. |
| | Tuesday | b. d. s. | b. s. | d. | | | | b. | | | | | | d. | d. | | | | Rice and molasses. |
| | Wednesday | b. d. s. | b. s. | d. s. | | | b. | | | | | | | d. | | | Sweet potatoes. | Bread-pudding. | Bread-pudding. |
| | Thursday | b. d. s. | b. s. | | d. | | | | | | | b. | | d. | d. | | | Turnips | Rice and molasses. |
| | Friday | b. d. s. | b. s. | d. | | | b. | d. | | s. | | | | | | | | do | |
| | Saturday | b. d. s. | b. s. | d. | | s. | b. | | | | | | | d. | | | Fried onions | | |
| Fort Sill, Ind. Ter. | Sunday | b. d. s. | b. s. | d. | | | b. | | | | | | | d. | | | | Hominy | Rice and molasses. |
| | Monday | b. d. s. | b. s. | d. | | | b. | | | | | | | d. | | | | | Molasses. |
| | Tuesday | b. d. s. | b. s. | d. | | | b. | | | | | | | d. | | | | Baked beans twice a week. | |
| | Wednesday | b. d. s. | b. | d. | | | b. | | | | | | | d. | | | | | Tea and molasses. |
| | Thursday | b. d. s. | b. s. | d. | | | b. | | | | | | | d. | | | | Hominy | Molasses. |
| | Friday | b. d. s. | b. s. | d. | | | b. | | | | | | | d. | | | | do | |
| | Saturday | b. d. s. | b. s. | d. | | | b. | | | | | | | d. | | | | do | |
| Saint Louis Barracks, Mo. | Sunday | b. d. s. | b. | d. | | | b. | | | | | | | d. | d. | | | | Tea and stewed apples. |
| | Monday | b. d. s. | b. | d. | | | b. | | | | | | | | | | | Pea-soup and hominy. | Tea and fried mush. |
| | Tuesday | b. d. s. | b. | d. | | | | | | | b. | | d. | | | | | Turnips | Tea and stewed apples. |
| | Wednesday | b. d. s. | b. | d. | | | b. | | | | | | | | | | | Baked peas | Do. |
| | Thursday | b. d. s. | b. | d. | | | b. | | | | | | | d. | d. | | | Plum-pudding. | Do. |
| | Friday | b. d. s. | b. | d. | | | | | | | b. | | d. | d. | | | | | Tea and fried mush. |
| | Saturday | b. d. s. | b. | d. | | | | | | | b. | d. | | | | | | | Tea and stewed apples. |
| Fort Randall, Dak. | Sunday | b. d. s. | b. s. | d. | | | | b. | | | | | | d. | | | | Fried onions | |
| | Monday | b. d. s. | b. s. | | | | d. | | b. | | | | d. | d. | | | | | |
| | Tuesday | b. d. s. | b. s. | | d. | | | b. | | | | | | d. | d. | | | | |
| | Wednesday | b. d. s. | b. s. | d. | | | | b. | | | | | | d. | | | | Fried onions | |
| | Thursday | b. d. s. | b. s. | | | | | | | | b. | d. | | | | | | | |
| | Friday | b. d. s. | b. s. | | | | d. | | b. | | | | d. | d. | | | | | |
| | Saturday | b. d. s. | b. s. | | d. | | | | b. | | | | | d. | d. | | | | |
| Fort Ellis, Mont. | Sunday | b. s. | b. s. | d. | | | | b. | | | | | | d. | | | | Plum-pudding. | Pie, cheese, and butter. |
| | Monday | b. d. s. | b. s. | | d. | | b. | | | d. | | | | b. d. | | d. | | | Molasses and head-cheese. |
| | Tuesday | b. d. s. | b. s. | d. | | s. | | | | | b. | | | d. | d. | | | | |
| | Wednesday | b. d. s. | b. s. | d. | | | | | | | b. | | | d. | | | | Plum-pudding. | Head-cheese. |
| | Thursday | b. s. | b. s. | | d. | s. | b. | | | d. | | | | b. d. | | d. | | | Head-cheese. |
| | Friday | b. d. s. | b. s. | d. | | | | | | | b. | | | d. | d. | | | | |
| | Saturday | b. s. | b. d. s. | | | d. | | | | | b. | | | d. | | | | Baked beans | Stewed apples and head-cheese. |

| Name of post. | Day of week. | Bread. | Coffee. | Beef, roasted. | Beef, boiled. | Beef, roast, cold. | Beefsteak. | Pork, boiled. | Bacon, fried. | Irish stew. | Meat-hash. | Baked beans and bacon. | Bean-soup. | Potatoes. | Vegetable-soup. | Cabbage. | Extra article. Breakfast. | Dinner. | Supper. |
|---|---|---|---|---|---|---|---|---|---|---|---|---|---|---|---|---|---|---|---|
| Fort Sanders, Wyo. | Sunday | b. d. s. | b. s. | d. | ... | ... | ... | b. | ... | ... | ... | ... | ... | b. d. | ... | ... | ... | Beets, plum-pudding. | |
| | Monday | b. d. s | b. s. | ... | d. | ... | ... | ... | ... | ... | b. | ... | ... | ... | d. | ... | ... | | |
| | Tuesday | b. s. | b. s. | d. | ... | ... | b. | ... | ... | ... | ... | ... | ... | d. | ... | ... | ... | Vegetables.. | |
| | Wednesday | b. d. s. | b. s. | ... | d. | ... | ... | ... | ... | b. | ... | ... | d. | ... | ... | ... | ... | ...do ... | |
| | Thursday | b. s. | b. s. | d. | ... | ... | ... | ... | ... | ... | b. | ... | ... | ... | ... | ... | ... | ... | |
| | Friday | b. d. s. | b. s. | ... | d. | ... | b. | ... | ... | ... | ... | ... | ... | ... | d. | ... | ... | Turnips and beets. | |
| | Saturday | b. d. s. | b. s. | ... | ... | ... | ... | ... | b. | ... | ... | d. | ... | b. | ... | ... | ... | Vegetables.. | |
| Fort Klamath, Oreg. | Sunday | b. d. s. | b. s. | b. | ... | ... | ... | ... | ... | ... | ... | ... | ... | d. | ... | d. | ... | Fresh pork.. | Butter. |
| | Monday | b. d. s. | b. s. | d. | ... | ... | ... | b. | ... | ... | ... | ... | ... | d. | d. | ... | ... | ... | |
| | Tuesday | b. d. s. | b. s. | ... | ... | ... | ... | d. | ... | ... | b. | ... | ... | d. | ... | d. | ... | ... | |
| | Wednesday | b. d. s. | b. s. | b. d. | ... | ... | ... | ... | ... | ... | ... | d. | ... | ... | ... | ... | ... | ... | |
| | Thursday | b. d. s. | b. s. | ... | d. | ... | ... | ... | ... | ... | b. | ... | ... | d. | ... | ... | ... | ... | |
| | Friday | b. d. s. | b. s. | ... | d. | ... | ... | b. | ... | ... | ... | ... | ... | ... | d. | ... | ... | Turnips ... | |
| | Saturday | b. d. s. | b. s. | b. d. | ... | ... | ... | ... | ... | ... | ... | d. | ... | ... | ... | ... | ... | ... | |
| Benicia Barracks, Cal. | Sunday | b. d. s. | b. s. | d. | ... | ... | ... | ... | ... | ... | b. | ... | d. | d. | ... | ... | ... | ... | |
| | Monday | b. d. s. | b. s. | d. | ... | ... | ... | ... | ... | b. | ... | ... | d. | d. | ... | ... | ... | ... | |
| | Tuesday | b. d. s. | b. s. | d. | ... | ... | ... | ... | ... | ... | b. | ... | ... | d. | d. | ... | ... | ... | Fried mush. |
| | Wednesday | b. d. s. | b. s. | d. | ... | ... | ... | ... | ... | b. | ... | ... | ... | ... | d. | ... | ... | Sweet potatoes. | |
| | Thursday | b. d. s. | b. s. | ... | ... | ... | ... | d. | ... | b. | ... | ... | ... | d. | ... | d. | ... | ... | |
| | Friday | b. d. s. | b. s. | d. | ... | ... | ... | ... | ... | ... | b. | ... | ... | ... | d. | ... | ... | ... | |
| | Saturday | b. d. s. | b. s. | d. | ... | ... | ... | ... | ... | b. | ... | ... | ... | ... | d. | ... | ... | ... | |
| Camp Grant, Ariz. | Sunday | b. d. s. | b. s. | d. | ... | ... | ... | ... | b. | ... | ... | ... | ... | d. | ... | ... | ... | Rice-pudding | |
| | Monday | b. d. s. | b. s. | b. d. | ... | ... | ... | ... | ... | ... | ... | ... | d. | ... | ... | ... | ... | ... | |
| | Tuesday | b. d. s. | b. s. | d. | ... | ... | ... | ... | ... | b. | ... | ... | ... | ... | d. | ... | ... | ... | |
| | Wednesday | b. d. s. | b. d. s. | d. | ... | ... | ... | ... | b. | ... | ... | ... | ... | ... | ... | ... | ... | Baked beans and peas. | |
| | Thursday | b. d. s. | b. s. | b. d. | ... | ... | ... | ... | ... | ... | ... | ... | d. | ... | ... | ... | ... | ... | |
| | Friday | b. d. s. | b. d. s. | d. | ... | ... | ... | ... | ... | ... | b. | ... | ... | d. | ... | ... | ... | ... | |
| | Saturday | b. d. s. | b. s. | b. d. | ... | ... | ... | ... | ... | ... | ... | ... | ... | ... | d. | ... | ... | ... | |

The letters b., d., and s. in the table indicate, respectively, breakfast, dinner, and supper.

The supply of food for the sick of the Army is generally satisfactory, although the commutation value of the ration of the soldier, out of which he is supposed to be fed while in hospital, is not sufficient for that purpose, and, to make it so, an increase of about 25 per cent. on the value of the ration would be necessary. The Medical Department, however, furnishes a considerable quantity of food for the sick, in the shape of the so-called "hospital stores," such as arrowroot, farina, corn-starch, tea, and sugar. With this, and occasional dishes from the table of the medical officer for special cases, it may be said that the sick of the Army are satisfactorily fed. The following table, giving the amounts and principal articles of purchase for the principal posts during the four years ending December 31, 1873, will give an idea of the manner in which the hospital-fund has been managed, and at the same time will give some interesting hints as to the prices of certain articles of food in different sections of the country:

| Post. | Number of rations. | Average cost of ration. | Amount due the hospital. | Value of issues by the commissary. | Milk. Number of gallons. | Milk. Amount expended. | Eggs. Number of dozen. | Eggs. Amount expended. | Butter. Number of pounds. | Butter. Amount expended. | Chickens. Number of chickens. | Chickens. Amount expended. | Amount expended for miscellaneous articles. | Total amount expended. |
|---|---|---|---|---|---|---|---|---|---|---|---|---|---|---|
| | | Cents. | | | | | | | | | | | | |
| Abercrombie, Fort, Dak | 5,168 | 20.92 | $1,081 47 | $952 00 | ...... | ...... | 2½ | $1 00 | 94¼ | $22 39 | 1 | $1 28 | $150 41 | $172 88 |
| Adams, Fort, R. I | 14,835 | 23.70 | 3,518 99 | 2,125 99 | 338⅜ | $118 26 | 132 | 50 49 | 285½ | 121 07 | 58 | 61 48 | 986 82 | 1,352 14 |
| Alcatraz Island, Cal | 19,842 | 20.35 | 4,038 85 | 2,813 63 | 655½ | 300 66 | 101 | 57 65 | 303½ | 155 56 | 4 | 3 45 | 713 79 | 1,220 21 |
| Angel Island, Cal | 19,248 | 20.46 | 3,938 66 | 2,987 77 | 75 | 34 84 | 154¼ | 85 46 | 150 | 73 82 | 91 | 72 25 | 627 51 | 893 88 |
| Austin Tex | 10,081 | 20.93 | 2,110 31 | 1,669 70 | 144⅝ | 72 92 | 153⅓ | 51 28 | 115½ | 46 37 | 48 | 18 95 | 235 58 | 425 10 |
| Apache, Camp, Ariz* | 9,980 | 30.56 | 3,051 12 | 2,280 46 | ...... | ...... | ...... | ...... | 30 | 14 60 | ...... | ...... | 713 09 | 727 69 |
| Baker, Camp, Wyo† | 6,153 | 21.09 | 1,297 84 | 1,005 75 | 11¾ | 6 05 | ...... | ...... | 42 | 24 83 | 4 | 4 00 | 268 87 | 293 70 |
| Barrancas, Fla | 8,036 | 26.78 | 2,146 79 | 1,648 31 | 75¾ | 43 05 | 62 | 30 30 | 72 | 32 70 | 51 | 20 58 | 349 76 | 504 06 |

* From February 1, 1871, to December 31, 1873, inclusive.

† From July 1, 1870, to December 31, 1873, inclusive.

| Post. | Number of rations. | Average cost of ration. | Amount due the hospital. | Value of issues by the commissary. | Milk. | | Eggs. | | Butter. | | Chickens. | | Amount expended for miscellaneous articles. | Total amount expended. |
|---|---|---|---|---|---|---|---|---|---|---|---|---|---|---|
| | | | | | Number of gallons. | Amount expended. | Number of dozen. | Amount expended. | Number of pounds. | Amount expended. | Number of chickens. | Amount expended. | | |
| | | *Cents.* | | | | | | | | | | | | |
| Baton Rouge, La | 19,265 | 19.61 | $3,777 95 | $2,451 39 | 209¾ | $95 52 | 370½ | $138 05 | 150½ | $73 35 | 114 | $49 00 | $969 91 | $1,336 96 |
| Bayard, Fort, N. Mex | 12,518 | 25.30 | 3,167 32 | 2,321 49 | 68½ | 52 40 | 41 | 23 25 | 161 | 70 13 | 48 | 24 00 | 627 06 | 793 25 |
| Benicia Barracks, Cal | 11,916 | 19.02 | 2,267 12 | 1,768 33 | 313½ | 136 92 | 71 | 29 91 | 72 | 32 85 | 103 | 63 25 | 238 55 | 502 00 |
| Benton, Fort, Mont | 7,164 | 21.68 | 1,553 35 | 1,279 96 | 41 1-6 | 30 12 | ...... | ...... | 9 | 3 44 | 12 | 9 00 | 227 62 | 265 68 |
| Bidwell, Camp, Cal | 7,036 | 26.83 | 1,888 31 | 1,564 90 | 96 | 38 40 | 75 | 32 41 | 105 | 48 50 | ...... | ...... | 203 78 | 323 29 |
| Bliss, Fort, Tex | 7,445 | 24.26 | 1,806 12 | 1,679 46 | 86¾ | 34 70 | 20 | 5 50 | ...... | ...... | 2 | 75 | 64 94 | 105 96 |
| Boise, Fort, Idaho | 6,152 | 25.65 | 1,578 13 | 1,413 29 | 42 | 21 00 | 11 | 8 20 | 79 | 58 77 | 4 | 1 00 | 122 91 | 211 88 |
| Bowie, Camp, Ariz | 12,445 | 26.10 | 3,260 18 | 2,610 27 | ...... | ...... | 11½ | 11 50 | 77 | 32 34 | 2 | 2 00 | 605 40 | 651 24 |
| Brady, Fort, Mich | 8,313 | 22.13 | 1,949 85 | 1,535 91 | 130⅞ | 41 80 | 89 | 23 98 | 56 | 19 43 | ...... | ...... | 290 25 | 378 45 |
| Brown, Fort, Tex | 31,333 | 17.23 | 5,501 31 | 4,576 10 | 372¾ | 165 20 | 265 | 79 70 | 53 | 19 20 | 488 | 109 00 | 495 09 | 869 65 |
| Buford, Fort, Dak | 20,199 | 20.28 | 4,097 25 | 2,796 01 | 13½ | 8 10 | 1 | 1 50 | 337 2-16 | 129 15 | ...... | ...... | 1,062 08 | 1,299 21 |
| Bridger, Fort, Wyo | 13,366 | 22.34 | 2,985 60 | 2,701 08 | 30 | 15 00 | 158 | 80 00 | 126 | 59 00 | 3 | 3 00 | 115 35 | 272 35 |
| Charleston, S. C | 11,111 | 21.18 | 2,353 80 | 1,964 10 | 85 5-16 | 31 23 | 46 | 15 27 | 25 | 8 70 | 4 | 2 35 | 322 38 | 369 93 |
| Chattanooga, Tenn | 8,597 | 18.65 | 1,604 16 | 1,206 77 | 43½ | 17 70 | 172 | 32 85 | 466 | 142 30 | 51 | 17 10 | 168 65 | 399 31 |
| Cheyenne agency, Dak* | 10,007 | 18.78 | 1,879 62 | 1,753 55 | ...... | ...... | 5 | 1 75 | 63 | 21 70 | ...... | ...... | 49 70 | 81 69 |
| Clark, Fort, Tex | 23,537 | 10.82 | 4,309 00 | 2,345 29 | 780¼ | 192 40 | 87½ | 41 20 | 149 | 68 90 | 151 | 72 35 | 246 95 | 829 81 |
| Columbia, S. C | 18,477 | 18.64 | 3,437 48 | 2,788 12 | 200 1-6 | 104 35 | 71 | 32 15 | 89 | 35 37 | 25 | 11 40 | 391 89 | 576 36 |
| Columbus, Fort, New York Harbor | 46,059 | 22.82 | 10,513 81 | 7,724 86 | 181½ | 72 60 | 232 | 87 73 | 1,320 | 509 16 | 110 | 79 37 | 2,035 20 | 2,788 95 |
| Colville, Fort, Wash | 4,934 | 21.20 | 1,046 40 | 936 44 | 61 | 24 40 | ...... | ...... | 8 | 4 08 | ...... | ...... | 90 35 | 119 83 |
| Concho, Fort, Tex | 25,946 | 21.42 | 5,559 94 | 4,137 51 | 322½ | 132 20 | 123¾ | 56 72 | 304½ | 134 04 | 204 | 10 80 | 1,012 75 | 1,424 73 |
| Craig, Fort, N. Mex | 9,761 | 23.30 | 2,274 40 | 2,087 40 | 105⅞ | 44 20 | 17½ | 7 00 | 61 | 23 60 | 8 | 4 00 | 171 88 | 258 68 |
| Davis, Fort, Tex | 14,723 | 23.38 | 3,442 92 | 2,906 04 | 53¾ | 21 50 | 47 | 30 00 | 81 | 30 01 | 22 | 12 20 | 392 42 | 485 32 |
| Disappointment Cape. (See Fort Townsend)† | 5,922 | 21.96 | 1,300 98 | 1,195 52 | 17¾ | 8 90 | 27 | 11 85 | 48 | 20 97 | 3 | 1 50 | 72 98 | 127 20 |
| Dodge, Fort, Kans | 21,907 | 21.24 | 4,654 19 | 4,068 94 | 576¼ | 241 05 | 57 | 32 95 | 46 | 17 65 | 9 | 8 50 | 205 05 | 503 74 |
| Douglas, Camp, Utah | 23,624 | 22.26 | 5,260 79 | 3,658 39 | 86¾ | 46 28 | 62 | 20 50 | 382 | 170 15 | 22 | 9 60 | 1,311 72 | 1,547 51 |
| Duncan, Fort, Tex | 19,873 | 18.28 | 3,634 43 | 2,715 11 | 659½ | 162 64 | 169 1-10 | 51 95 | 130 | 42 10 | 378 | 121 56 | 559 96 | 933 61 |
| Ellis, Fort, Mont | 15,153 | 23.63 | 3,581 81 | 2,967 09 | 206¾ | 84 40 | 37 | 18 30 | 89 | 44 30 | 14 | 8 75 | 352 42 | 618 77 |
| Fetterman, Fort, Wyo | 11,981 | 20.89 | 2,403 28 | 1,587 28 | ...... | ...... | 7 | 6 00 | 88½ | 30 04 | 9 | 10 25 | 744 74 | 790 73 |
| Foote, Fort, Md | 8,988 | 22.80 | 2,049 76 | 1,709 82 | 256¼ | 102 60 | 68½ | 19 45 | 20 | 9 30 | 30 | 12 55 | 187 43 | 331 13 |
| Garland, Fort, Colo | 8,909 | 22.85 | 2,036 32 | 1,262 55 | 30 | 3 60 | 66½ | 25 00 | 170 | 78 60 | 6 | 3 00 | 625 32 | 695 62 |
| Gaston, Camp, Cal | 9,606 | 20.11 | 1,931 89 | 1,406 44 | 134 | 54 10 | 61 | 14 14 | 134½ | 34 87 | 69 | 16 56 | 351 27 | 470 73 |
| Gibson, Fort, Ind. Ter‡ | 9,223 | 23.20 | 2,140 15 | 1,634 73 | 237½ | 111 81 | 89 | 51 72 | 136½ | 69 93 | 37 | 25 67 | 211 04 | 456 72 |
| Grant, Camp, Ariz | 12,052 | 28.61 | 3,448 09 | 2,554 73 | 66¼ | 66 25 | 26½ | 29 00 | 112 | 51 63 | 2 | 1 50 | 769 69 | 898 01 |
| Gratiot, Fort, Mich | 8,437 | 19.47 | 1,642 84 | 647 27 | 517½ | 155 73 | 64 5-12 | 15 49 | 189¼ | 61 13 | 28 | 11 28 | 737 67 | 976 30 |
| Griffin, Fort, Tex | 24,149 | 24.76 | 5,980 83 | 5,224 02 | 145⅝ | 53 77 | 202 | 97 90 | 63 | 27 01 | 126 | 62 00 | 524 65 | 746 33 |
| Hall, Fort, Idaho§ | 4,473 | 27.22 | 1,217 87 | 1,068 51 | ...... | ...... | 20½ | 10 05 | 153 | 66 70 | ...... | ...... | 34 11 | 110 86 |
| Halleck, Camp, Nev | 8,347 | 25.58 | 2,135 82 | 1,784 64 | 36½ | 14 94 | 23 | 12 90 | 45¾ | 24 39 | ...... | ...... | 314 45 | 328 70 |
| Hamilton, Fort, New York Harbor | 24,028 | 21.65 | 5,203 89 | 3,336 33 | 912¼ | 358 40 | 206 | 89 74 | 24 | 12 00 | ...... | ...... | 1,425 01 | 1,897 50 |
| Harney, Camp, Oreg | 11,489 | 22.56 | 2,592 75 | 1,919 96 | ...... | ...... | 12 | 12 00 | 80 | 49 76 | 17 | 11 50 | 589 13 | 652 39 |
| Hays, Fort, Kans | 25,153 | 21.46 | 5,399 81 | 4,108 81 | 117 | 60 30 | 48 | 17 10 | 498 | 185 96 | 29 | 16 95 | 1,011 78 | 1,292 88 |
| Humboldt, Tenn | 4,666 | 20.52 | 957 86 | 711 73 | 167⅞ | 64 95 | 82½ | 17 62 | 97¾ | 32 51 | 22 | 5 43 | 170 01 | 282 35 |
| Independence, Fort, Mass | 8,873 | 22.64 | 2,009 44 | 1,189 88 | 468½ | 188 20 | 129¼ | 53 19 | 146 | 63 49 | 4 | 1 08 | 508 57 | 815 43 |
| Indianapolis arsenal | 1,462 | 19.80 | 289 93 | 287 21 | ...... | ...... | 4 | 1 30 | 4 | 1 15 | ...... | ...... | ...... | 2 45 |
| Independence, Camp, Cal | 5,912 | 28.51 | 1,685 83 | 1,497 78 | 3¾ | 1 50 | 18 | 10 50 | 66½ | 35 40 | 18 | 18 00 | 132 61 | 197 01 |
| Jackson Barracks, La | 14,351 | 24.08 | 3,357 74 | 1,789 28 | 378⅞ | 215 20 | 294 | 138 65 | 78 | 32 20 | 186 | 124 65 | 923 97 | 1,433 67 |
| Jackson Barracks, Miss | 14,217 | 20.51 | 2,917 25 | 2,590 45 | 86¾ | 48 05 | 143½ | 52 05 | 85¾ | 39 04 | 81 | 32 15 | 149 64 | 320 93 |
| Jefferson Barracks, Mo | 7,027 | 19.31 | 1,356 77 | 1,077 96 | 2½ | 95 | 22 | 4 70 | 36 | 12 42 | 50 | 15 05 | 248 55 | 281 67 |
| Johnston, Fort, N. C | 6,462 | 21.46 | 1,386 88 | 1,195 53 | 30⅝ | 22 54 | 66¾ | 17 00 | 71 | 32 45 | 23 | 9 55 | 77 86 | 114 36 |
| Key West, Fla | 14,146 | 24.22 | 3,426 90 | 2,643 34 | 45¾ | 14 90 | 136 1-12 | 74 95 | 99 5-6 | 43 60 | 121 | 98 05 | 567 30 | 810 70 |
| Klamath, Fort, Oreg | 16,145 | 22.07 | 3,564 56 | 2,685 47 | 58¾ | 23 50 | 330½ | 128 76 | 52 3-5 | 26 43 | 77 | 35 97 | 616 82 | 840 48 |
| Lapwai, Fort, Idaho | 6,460 | 19.71 | 1,283 53 | 1,166 51 | ...... | ...... | 1 | 50 | 25 | 13 04 | ...... | ...... | 72 42 | 86 16 |
| Laramie, Fort, Wyo | 23,929 | 20.41 | 4,885 33 | 3,553 56 | 137½ | 55 00 | 32¼ | 20 31 | 189 9-16 | 68 76 | 1 | 75 | 1,143 59 | 1,259 37 |
| Larned, Fort, Kans | 11,106 | 21.24 | 2,359 78 | 2,195 88 | 42½ | 17 00 | 38 | 8 21 | 16½ | 6 00 | 19 | 7 75 | 141 54 | 180 50 |
| Leavenworth, Fort, Kans | 44,914 | 18.19 | 8,170 42 | 6,337 51 | 610½ | 244 20 | 1,016 | 246 00 | 1,299¾ | 413 61 | 302 | 67 00 | 823 62 | 1,822 03 |
| Little Rock Barracks, Ark | 9,489 | 20.64 | 1,959 19 | 1,405 80 | 105¼ | 65 87 | 203 | 67 17 | 173½ | 86 22 | 28 | 12 00 | 297 98 | 520 22 |
| Lowell, Camp, Ariz | 16,220 | 24.92 | 4,042 17 | 3,722 14 | 90¼ | 57 32 | 14⅔ | 10 93 | ...... | ...... | 27 | 17 54 | 91 92 | 177 86 |
| Lyon, Fort, Colo | 13,606 | 23.51 | 3,199 47 | 2,228 87 | 338¾ | 135 50 | 47½ | 23 90 | 322 | 140 94 | ...... | ...... | 652 88 | 958 92 |
| McDermit, Camp, Nev | 3,580 | 22.67 | 911 87 | 683 61 | ...... | ...... | 20 | 14 40 | 104 | 44 90 | 2 | 1 70 | 144 57 | 212 88 |
| McDowell, Camp, Ariz | 16,176 | 29.02 | 4,794 42 | 3,625 40 | ...... | ...... | 40⅓ | 50 00 | 89 | 38 98 | 10 | 10 00 | 986 05 | 1,097 03 |
| McHenry, Fort, Md | 24,108 | 21.39 | 5,258 33 | 2,871 07 | 201½ | 83 41 | 328 | 99 96 | 116 | 52 85 | ...... | ...... | 2,136 88 | 2,375 60 |
| McIntosh, Fort, Tex | 8,928 | 18.87 | 1,685 50 | 1,306 78 | 115 22-24 | 42 78 | 18 | 4 49 | ½ | 17 | 12 | 3 15 | 322 16 | 372 75 |
| McKavett, Fort, Tex | 19,976 | 19.22 | 3,839 95 | 2,846 68 | 248¼ | 149 30 | 97½ | 49 55 | 138 | 53 10 | 71 | 44 50 | 455 33 | 751 78 |
| McPherson Barracks, Ga | 21,156 | 19.23 | 4,070 03 | 2,183 83 | 389⅛ | 174 70 | 445½ | 119 30 | 396 1-12 | 186 16 | 144 | 53 30 | 1,225 44 | 1,858 85 |
| McPherson, Fort, Nebr | 24,380 | 18.88 | 4,604 15 | 3,741 16 | ...... | ...... | 69⅓ | 32 38 | 57 | 24 25 | ...... | ...... | 678 25 | 736 68 |
| McRae, Fort, N. Mex | 7,009 | 27.76 | 1,945 93 | 1,733 04 | 10½ | 6 00 | 40 | 20 00 | ...... | ...... | 4 | 2 00 | 381 26 | 413 16 |
| Mackinac, Fort, Mich | 5,172 | 22.46 | 1,161 92 | 870 67 | 129¼ | 41 30 | 54 | 18 17 | 264½ | 83 59 | 12 | 6 65 | 159 25 | 309 06 |
| Macon, Fort, N. C | 19,647 | 11.28 | 2,217 94 | 1,580 93 | 9⅜ | 4 88 | 212 | 39 30 | 127 | 46 66 | 117 | 30 13 | 492 96 | 604 43 |
| Madison Barracks, N. Y | 8,669 | 19.71 | 1,719 80 | 1,200 45 | 608 | 170 66 | 158 | 34 00 | 340½ | 104 41 | 34 | 17 00 | 194 66 | 568 33 |
| Mojave, Camp, Ariz | 8,719 | 25.03 | 2,292 42 | 2,074 23 | 10½ | 10 50 | 12½ | 12 40 | 14 | 2 68 | 3 | 1 80 | 188 91 | 216 27 |
| Monroe, Fort, Va | 20,542 | 22.76 | 4,675 53 | 3,886 33 | 103 | 38 78 | 339 | 81 05 | 23 | 10 00 | 95 | 26 75 | 565 98 | 685 26 |
| Mt. Vernon Barracks, Ala | 14,486 | 20.55 | 2,977 25 | 2,022 46 | 180⅞ | 118 71 | 319 | 112 00 | 302½ | 142 45 | 75 | 51 10 | 534 10 | 957 20 |
| Nashville, Tenn | 20,309 | 18.87 | 3,834 26 | 2,524 41 | 239½ | 69 99 | 269 | 64 68 | 314 | 100 80 | 179 | 51 13 | 959 27 | 1,245 99 |
| Newport Barracks, Ky | 39,577 | 17.83 | 7,068 92 | 4,865 30 | 679½ | 252 60 | 416 | 109 72 | 781 | 293 26 | 631 | 231 65 | 1,209 95 | 2,077 07 |
| Niagara, Fort, N. Y | 5,338 | 24.07 | 1,285 26 | 1,025 72 | 165¼ | 35 08 | 124 | 29 13 | 256 | 72 03 | 4 | 1 40 | 124 36 | 250 35 |
| Oglethorpe Barracks, Ga | 9,336 | 19.42 | 1,813 22 | 1,291 98 | 49¼ | 28 02 | 29 | 10 95 | 86 | 43 20 | 14 | 6 20 | 423 06 | 506 63 |
| Omaha Barracks, Nebr | 30,420 | 19.07 | 5,801 15 | 3,949 40 | 278½ | 80 49 | 515½ | 105 22 | 977 | 293 79 | 60 | 26 25 | 1,335 63 | 1,822 48 |
| Ontario, Fort, N. Y | 6,054 | 20.33 | 1,230 99 | 1,010 17 | 135 5-16 | 39 73 | 57 | 14 96 | 117½ | 35 56 | ...... | ...... | 106 12 | 197 83 |
| Plattsburgh Bar'ks, N. Y | 6,039 | 20.26 | 1,222 85 | 902 13 | 364 | 117 76 | 66 | 15 84 | 32 7-16 | 10 16 | 3 | 45 | 166 28 | 311 29 |
| Point San José, Cal‖ | 1,870 | 20.72 | 388 60 | 340 11 | 8 | 4 00 | 3 | 1 05 | 8 | 4 90 | ...... | ...... | 39 84 | 49 79 |
| Porter, Fort, N. Y | 12,857 | 19.60 | 2,520 42 | 1,998 69 | 413⅛ | 106 41 | 91 | 29 82 | 296⅓ | 111 58 | 15 | 2 78 | 256 00 | 511 38 |
| Preble, Fort, Me | 6,372 | 25.07 | 1,597 87 | 1,599 79 | 482¾ | 147 44 | 228 | 71 65 | 324 | 142 23 | 28 | 16 00 | 409 79 | 797 03 |
| Presidio of San Francisco, Cal | 28,808 | 20.19 | 5,818 10 | 4,127 95 | 539 | 228 80 | 53 | 29 69 | 140 | 75 27 | 56 | 44 15 | 1,294 42 | 1,677 83 |
| Quitman, Fort, Tex | 9,674 | 24.07 | 2,338 68 | 2,064 16 | 62⅜ | 31 18 | 15 | 6 85 | 11 | 7 15 | 33 | 14 15 | 203 87 | 263 20 |
| Raleigh, N. C | 8,681 | 20.73 | 1,797 31 | 1,230 33 | 142⅜ | 52 10 | 112 | 28 83 | 114½ | 45 08 | 34 | 8 50 | 423 96 | 562 47 |
| Randall, Fort, Dak | 14,884 | 18.79 | 2,796 74 | 2,198 58 | 11 | 4 40 | 24 | 13 40 | 116¼ | 40 65 | 27 | 14 90 | 512 42 | 585 50 |

* From August 1, 1870, to December 31, 1873, inclusive.
† From January 1, 1870, to August 31, 1873, inclusive.
‡ Post discontinued from October 31, 1871, to July 1, 1872.
§ From June 1, 1870, to December 31, 1873, inclusive.
‖ From November 1, 1870, to January 31, 1872.

| Post. | Number of rations. | Average cost of ration. | Amount due the hospital. | Value of issues by the commissary. | Milk. | | Eggs. | | Butter. | | Chickens. | | Amount expended for miscellaneous articles. | Total amount expended. |
|---|---|---|---|---|---|---|---|---|---|---|---|---|---|---|
| | | | | | Number of gallons. | Amount expended. | Number of dozen. | Amount expended. | Number of pounds. | Amount expended. | Number of chickens. | Amount expended. | | |
| | | Cents. | | | | | | | | | | | | |
| Rice, Fort, Dak | 20, 840 | 18. 79 | $3, 916 75 | $3, 640 28 | ........ | ...... | 22½ | $13 60 | 11 | $4 00 | 2 | $0 75 | $295 03 | $359 38 |
| Richardson, Fort, Tex | 29, 292 | 23. 43 | 6, 863 65 | 6, 785 57 | 496 | $249 10 | 183½ | 69 85 | 114 | 43 60 | 114 | 48 60 | 344 73 | 758 68 |
| Riley, Fort, Kans | 15, 575 | 20. 46 | 3, 187 32 | 2, 624 45 | 48¾ | 25 70 | 238½ | 85 10 | 180½ | 59 39 | 114 | 43 95 | 281 23 | 496 88 |
| Ringgold Barracks, Tex | 18, 830 | 18. 51 | 3, 497 26 | 2, 738 85 | 220½ | 110 35 | 124 | 36 55 | ........ | ...... | 138 | 42 55 | 375 56 | 577 91 |
| Ripley, Fort, Minn | 8, 857 | 20. 57 | 1, 824 37 | 1, 424 72 | 17¾ | 7 10 | 48 | 14 50 | 43½ | 12 48 | 5 | 2 25 | 361 77 | 398 40 |
| Rock Island Arsenal | 7, 230 | 22. 39 | 1, 619 01 | 964 66 | 170 | 68 00 | 430⅜ | 42 30 | 464 7-15 | 126 61 | 3 | 1 15 | 255 04 | 491 03 |
| Russell, D. A., Fort, Wyo | 33, 002 | 18. 48 | 6, 101 99 | 4, 587 43 | 932½ | 303 54 | 94¾ | 32 22 | 31 | 12 07 | ...... | ...... | 1, 167 24 | 1, 525 34 |
| Saint Louis Barracks, Mo | 22, 458 | 15. 95 | 3, 592 12 | 2, 301 84 | 287⅝ | 89 50 | 329 | 71 30 | 439 | 147 20 | 322 | 130 05 | 762 60 | 1, 186 37 |
| San Juan Island, Cal., (now Fort Townsend) | 6, 982 | 25. 29 | 1, 746 34 | 1, 606 98 | 4 | 2 40 | 5 | 2 72 | 12 | 6 99 | 3 | 1 20 | 122 18 | 135 79 |
| Sanders, Fort, Wyo | 14, 388 | 21. 38 | 3, 078 37 | 2, 040 31 | 89⅞ | 60 03 | 72⅓ | 26 97 | 201 | 73 60 | 1 | 60 | 853 94 | 1, 020 49 |
| Santa Fé, N. Mex | 13, 028 | 21. 34 | 2, 780 84 | 2, 137 79 | ........ | ...... | 178 11-12 | 56 23 | 262 | 118 40 | ...... | ...... | 458 08 | 635 12 |
| Sidney Barracks, Nebr | 6, 316 | 22. 52 | 1, 423 88 | 1, 067 35 | ........ | ...... | 25 | 7 78 | 16⅓ | 5 30 | ...... | ...... | 257 42 | 270 50 |
| Sitka, Alaska | 18, 713 | 25. 29 | 4, 832 91 | 3, 436 63 | 8⅝ | 7 59 | 116½ | 111 88 | 105⅓ | 55 82 | ...... | ...... | 1, 233 80 | 1, 409 09 |
| Selden, Fort, N. Mex | 7, 892 | 24. 01 | 1, 895 44 | 1, 545 33 | 31¾ | 12 80 | 174 | 69 40 | 60 | 31 62 | 23 | 10 20 | 228 35 | 352 27 |
| Shaw, Fort, Mont | 18, 454 | 20. 52 | 3, 786 50 | 3, 681 99 | ........ | ...... | ........ | ...... | ........ | ...... | ...... | ...... | 106 23 | 106 23 |
| Sill, Fort, Indian Ter | 27, 832 | 20. 35 | 5, 665 66 | 3, 360 47 | 227 | 113 38 | 192½ | 84 20 | 410½ | 202 23 | 148 | 74 00 | 1, 667 72 | 2, 142 13 |
| Snelling, Fort, Minn | 13, 919 | 17. 68 | 2, 461 67 | 1, 346 03 | 1, 175 | 363 80 | 453 | 96 60 | 200 | 61 50 | 352 | 100 20 | 502 28 | 1, 121 38 |
| Stanton, Fort, N. Mex | 8, 738 | 21. 97 | 1, 920 66 | 1, 649 56 | ........ | ...... | ........ | ...... | 88 | 34 32 | 21 | 7 00 | 241 88 | 287 01 |
| Steele, Fred., Fort, Wyo | 16, 105 | 20. 42 | 3, 289 93 | 2, 130 96 | 244½ | 106 87 | 29½ | 14 55 | 174⅜ | 61 02 | 15 | 15 00 | 933 07 | 1, 141 48 |
| Stevens, Fort, Oreg | 5, 943 | 22. 01 | 1, 308 29 | 1, 176 54 | 70 | 33 55 | 18 | 5 72 | 50½ | 20 19 | ...... | ...... | 71 64 | 130 90 |
| Stevenson, Fort, Dak | 10, 933 | 18. 73 | 2, 057 53 | 1, 694 35 | ........ | ...... | 15 | 7 50 | 202 | 78 72 | ...... | ...... | 338 80 | 423 33 |
| Stockton, Fort, Tex | 12, 100 | 25. 22 | 3, 052 24 | 2, 522 49 | 106⅞ | 85 50 | 79½ | 51 25 | 78½ | 66 20 | 98 | 98 00 | 184 85 | 508 00 |
| Sully, Fort, Dak | 15, 652 | 18. 07 | 2, 828 78 | 2, 221 47 | ........ | ...... | 11 | 9 50 | 82 | 31 15 | 47 | 44 80 | 537 86 | 593 31 |
| Supply, Camp, Ind. T | 27, 841 | 21. 38 | 5, 953 14 | 5, 244 64 | 337 | 138 00 | 77 | 44 00 | 97 | 55 94 | 14 | 7 00 | 356 29 | 626 89 |
| Thomas Barracks, Huntsville, Ala | 10, 969 | 18. 53 | 2, 032 88 | 1, 464 43 | 436 | 175 43 | 105 | 50 55 | 126 | 41 25 | 104 | 31 20 | 273 58 | 580 01 |
| Totten, Fort, Dak | 11, 425 | 22. 82 | 2, 607 86 | 2, 556 93 | 22 | 8 80 | 2 | 2 00 | 43½ | 22 58 | 29 | 25 75 | 298 11 | 357 12 |
| Trumbull, Fort, Conn | 7, 569 | 21. 63 | 1, 637 54 | 1, 140 33 | 571 | 174 08 | 5 | 170 00 | 95 | 35 88 | ...... | ...... | 299 17 | 506 29 |
| Townsend, Fort, Wash. (See San Juan Island) | ...... | ...... | ........ | ........ | ........ | ...... | ........ | ...... | ........ | ...... | ...... | ...... | ........ | ........ |
| Union, Fort, N. H | 40, 103 | 21. 60 | 8, 662 31 | 7, 347 37 | ........ | ...... | 321 | 92 59 | 352 | 228 19 | 81 | 27 40 | 905 20 | 1, 274 38 |
| Vancouver, Fort, Wash | 16, 789 | 20. 94 | 3, 516 56 | 2, 656 32 | 256⅜ | 139 49 | 285 | 101 74 | 464 | 191 83 | 89 | 35 85 | 438 03 | 914 80 |
| Verde, Camp, Ariz | 10, 731 | 26. 11 | 2, 802 53 | 2, 424 79 | ........ | ...... | 6 | 9 00 | 60 | 30 50 | 8 | 8 00 | 331 63 | 448 52 |
| Wadsworth, Fort, New York Harbor | 10, 158 | 21. 23 | 2, 157 41 | 1, 238 82 | 680⅝ | 221 50 | 105 | 33 80 | 217 | 109 34 | 13 | 5 85 | 520 84 | 904 56 |
| Wadsworth, Fort, Dak | 6, 496 | 23. 26 | 1, 511 40 | 1, 108 89 | ........ | ...... | 65-6 | 5 00 | 131 5-6 | 4 16 | ...... | ...... | 324 87 | 370 97 |
| Wallace, Fort, Kans | 17, 270 | 21. 13 | 3, 649 89 | 3, 011 03 | 42¼ | 15 10 | 47⅓ | 21 93 | 113 | 44 47 | 2 | 1 50 | 532 32 | 625 57 |
| Warner, Camp, Oreg | 13, 931 | 23. 88 | 3, 327 14 | 2, 937 70 | ........ | ...... | 115¾ | 89 37 | 53 | 32 95 | 15 | 11 25 | 292 13 | 425 70 |
| Warren, Fort, Boston Harbor, Mass | 7, 314 | 23. 71 | 1, 734 78 | 1, 308 36 | 31½ | 12 70 | 48 | 17 35 | 148½ | 61 45 | 2 | 1 50 | 357 45 | 455 45 |
| Washington Arsenal | 7, 636 | 23. 79 | 1, 815 98 | 1, 106 51 | 19½ | 9 08 | 135 | 40 87 | 548½ | 213 56 | 2 | 1 25 | 404 52 | 693 73 |
| Watertown Ars'l, Mass* | 2, 289 | 26. 05 | 596 36 | 316 77 | 181¾ | 60 33 | 69 | 25 91 | 194 | 92 26 | ...... | ...... | 101 14 | 279 64 |
| Wayne, Fort, Mich | 10, 550 | 19. 07 | 2, 012 20 | 1, 394 76 | 346¼ | 113 05 | 80½ | 18 54 | 167 | 53 66 | ...... | ...... | 420 70 | 605 45 |
| West Point, N. Y | 10, 170 | 22. 52 | 2, 291 07 | 1, 617 97 | 387 | 149 20 | 50 | 17 74 | 382 | 164 18 | ...... | ...... | 338 70 | 665 53 |
| Whipple, Fort, Ariz | 16, 169 | 25, 77 | 4, 168 40 | 3, 573 74 | 16 | 12 80 | 9 | 14 00 | 91 | 40 34 | 3 | 6 00 | 540 48 | 612 41 |
| Willet's Point, New York Harbor | 19, 194 | 20. 74 | 3, 992 73 | 3, 272 73 | 70 1-25 | 16 79 | 70½ | 30 17 | 198 19-20 | 91 97 | 16 | 12 00 | 504 68 | 655 61 |
| Wingate, Fort, N. Mex | 15, 453 | 23. 93 | 3, 699 02 | 2, 400 67 | 2¼ | 90 | 33 | 18 30 | 248 | 109 27 | 32 | 16 10 | 1, 078 39 | 1, 233 49 |
| Wood, Fort, New York Harbor | 7, 079 | 22. 47 | 1, 589 17 | 989 18 | 163⅓ | 65 27 | 103½ | 41 13 | 142½ | 55 88 | ...... | ...... | 452 85 | 615 13 |
| Wright, Camp, Cal | 7, 288 | 23. 43 | 1, 709 69 | 1, 392 18 | 151¾ | 69 69 | 72 | 26 95 | 37 | 17 08 | 63 | 31 66 | 162 87 | 314 75 |
| Yuma, Fort, Cal | 12, 767 | 22. 36 | 2, 854 67 | 2, 310 63 | 129¼ | 76 87 | 60 7-12 | 68 13 | 114 | 51 72 | 2 | 1 50 | 354 82 | 549 87 |

Total number of rations, 1,937,943; total amount expended, $414,230.35; average cost of ration, 21.37 cents.

* From January 1, 1870, to February 28, 1871.

Recently the mode of management of the hospital fund has been changed by the following order, which is believed to be a simplification and improvement:

[General Orders No. 122.]

WAR DEPARTMENT, ADJUTANT-GENERAL'S OFFICE,
*Washington, November* 6, 1874.

I. The articles named in the second part of paragraph 2 of Circular No. 1, issued from the office of the Commissary-General of Subsistence April 23, 1874, and in paragraph 2 of Circular No. 3, August 20, 1874, from the same office, will be added to the list of articles named in the first part of Circular No. 1, and will be furnished by the Subsistence Department for sale on the same conditions as those articles, *except* that potatoes and onions will be furnished only at posts where they cannot be cultivated or purchased at reasonable rates.

The following articles will also be furnished by the Subsistence Department for sale under paragraph 1229, Army Regulations of 1863: Canned soups, laundry-starch, indigo.

II. The following instructions are substituted for existing regulations and orders in regard to the hospital fund, its management and expenditure, and will go into operation in the month next succeeding the month in which this order is received at any post or station.

*Hospital fund.*

The saving arising from an economical use of the rations of the sick and attendants in a hospital shall constitute the hospital fund.

The rations or parts of rations not drawn shall be paid for by the commissary and taken up by him as purchased, as in the case of company savings. The amount shall be paid to the senior medical officer at the post or station, and shall be expended by him exclusively for the benefit of the men in the hospital, in the purchase of such articles of diet, comfort, or convenience as may be required.

By order of the Secretary of War:

E. D. TOWNSEND,
*Adjutant-General.*

The means of cooking and the mess-furniture of the hospitals are satisfactory. To many of the post-hospitals the Warren cooker, and apparatus for cooking by steam-heat without allowing access of steam to the articles to be cooked, has been sent, and is generally approved. This apparatus has also been tried, to some extent, in the company kitchens, but is not successful, as it is too small. Its great advantage is that a poor cook cannot very well burn or overdo the food when using it.

In concluding this subject, I would respectfully offer the following suggestions with regard to the food-supply of the Army:

1. That the present ration be increased. The allowance suggested by Dr. Perin would give general satisfaction.

2. That the mess-furniture be considered as camp and garrison equipage, to be furnished by the Quartermaster's Department. Galvanized-iron vessels, with covers, for making soup and coffee, should be furnished for cooking in temporary camps or on campaigns.

3. That the company fund shall be used for the purchase of food only.

4. That the chief cook of each company shall be a permanent detail, and shall receive extra-duty pay; that they shall be specially enlisted for that purpose, and that a school for the instruction of cooks be established at the recruiting-depots.

5. That a manual of instructions for Army cooks be prepared and issued by the Subsistence Department, which shall give diet-tables and modes of preparing food suited to the various stations, climates, and seasons.

6. That baking-powders and lime-juice be made a part of the ration for scouts and expeditions, and that canned tomatoes be issued at posts where fresh vegetables cannot be procured.

## III. CLOTHING.

Great improvements have been made in the clothing of the Army, both as to pattern and material, within the last three years, and the articles now being manufactured are more satisfactory than any which have ever been issued to our troops.

I have been permitted to examine the reports made to the Adjutant-General by commanding-officers of posts, in accordance with the following order:

[General Orders No. 6.]

WAR DEPARTMENT, ADJUTANT-GENERAL'S OFFICE,
*Washington, January 29, 1875.*

Commanding-officers of posts will, in consultation with their medical officers, prepare and forward to the Adjutant-General, through the regular channels, by March 15, 1875, or as soon thereafter as practicable, a report on the clothing and accouterments now issued and used by enlisted men of the Army, with regard to their sufficiency, suitability to their purpose, and quantity, and their effects, if any, on the health of the wearers, with remarks and recommendations.

They will also report at the same time on the occupations of the enlisted men, the amount of drill and other military duties, and in general on the character and amount of bodily labor and exercise incurred during the past year, with regard to its effects upon the health of troops.

By order of the Secretary of War:

E. D. TOWNSEND,
*Adjutant-General.*

These reports are almost unanimous in referring to the recent improvement of the clothing, and it may be said that in a hygienic point of view it is satisfactory for temperate climates.

It is probably not possible to devise a uniform which will serve for both Arizona and Minnesota, and accordingly it is found that officers serving in the south recommend the issue of thinner, and those in the north of thicker and warmer articles than those allowed by regulations. Practically, the soldier purchases much clothing from traders, in order to protect himself against extremes of temperature, which cannot be done by the exclusive use of articles furnished by the Government.

Lieut. G. F. Towle, Nineteenth United States Infantry, says: "Many men do not draw their full allowance of clothing, but this does not prove that the allowance is sufficient. Some men want a better article and purchase it; others wish to save money, and effect it by purchasing Government clothing at reduced rates from private dealers."

It would certainly promote health and comfort, and be in accordance with the wishes of the majority of the officers and men, if two distinct kinds of clothing were furnished, one for cold, the other for warm climates, and that each should be of the best quality. This could probably be effected without any material increase of the present allowance considered as money value.

The following is an abstract of the opinions of commanding-officers with regard to some of the articles of clothing and equipment:

*Accoutrements:* The usual statement is that the new patterns are an improvement over the old, but that they are not yet satisfactory.

The recommendation is general that what is known as the prairie or thimble-belt be substituted for the cartridge-box. Complaint is made that the new knapsacks hang too low. On taking the field the knapsacks are not used, the few articles carried being rolled in the blanket and slung round the body from one shoulder to the opposite arm-pit. And if the men be allowed choice in the matter, this mode of carrying their burden would be preferred to any knapsack, except in very warm weather. Probably a simple waterproof-bag is preferable to any form of knapsack.

*Blankets:* The quality of those now furnished is very satisfactory, but complaints are general from posts in northern latitudes that the allowance is insufficient; at least, two are wanted for the first year.

*Blouse:* The plaited blouse is not at all liked by the men; the plaits collect dust, and they are hard to keep clean. The new blouse without plaits is generally approved.

*Boots and Shoes:* The new patterns, cable-screwed, are generally approved and liked when properly made. The new pattern of snow-excluders and the buffalo over-shoes are very satisfactory.

*Canteen:* It is recommended that the canteen-strap shall be made of leather, and wider in the center than elsewhere on account of bearing on the shoulder; also, that the canteen should have two nozzles.

*Drawers:* Complaints are general as to quality and pattern; allowance is considered insufficient. The new pattern proposed by the Quartermaster-General will probably be satisfactory. At least two grades should be furnished.

*Great-coats:* This is the most important article of a soldier's equipment. For northern climates the blanket-lining is not sufficiently warm. It is recommended that a limited number of buffalo or sheep-skin overcoats be issued to northern posts for temporary issue to men on exposed duty. A marked defect in the great-coats is their want of pockets.

*Hats and caps:* The campaign-hat is universally condemned, because of its poor material. It would seem as if the felt had been injured by the dye. A gray hat with a somewhat narrower brim is generally recommended. A light, gray, felt hat, is especially desirable for southern posts. Fur caps with ear-flaps are generally recommended for posts in cold climates. The ear-flaps, especially, are called for by officers in the Departments of Dakota and the Platte, and if not furnished by Government must be purchased by the soldier. The helmet furnished is too heavy, and has too steep a visor; there is a general complaint that it causes headache.

*Mittens:* Those furnished are not suitable for cold climates, and men usually purchase them from dealers. Mittens lined with fur similar to those used by the Canadian troops are recommended.

*Shirts:* Those which have been furnished shrink very much, and are found to irritate the skin. The men purchase many shirts from civilians; the present allowance is insufficient. There should be two qualities, each of flannel, for cold and warm weather.

*Stable-frocks:* There is a general complaint that the allowance is insufficient; two should be furnished the first year.

*Stockings:* There is a general complaint that those which have been furnished are of poor quality, and not properly made. An improvement of the stockings is contemplated by the Quartermaster-General.

In accordance with a request made by the Surgeon-General, a statement has been prepared by the Quartermaster-General with regard to the manufacture of clothing which contains information of interest to all officers of the Army, and is therefore printed in full.

WAR DEPARTMENT, QUARTERMASTER-GENERAL'S OFFICE,
*Washington, D. C., April 24, 1875.*

SIR: In compliance with your request dated February 5, 1875, I have the honor to supply the following statement relative to the selection and manufacture of Army clothing:

On the 27th of July, 1872, the Secretary of War approved the changes in the uniform and

M P——VII

dress of the Army, recommended by a board of officers convened by Special Order No. 260, dated War Department, Adjutant-General's Office, July 3, 1871.

Instructions were given on the 2d of August, 1872, to the officers in charge of the depots at Philadelphia and Jeffersonville to commence the manufacture and purchase of the uniform as described in General Order No. 92, Adjutant-General's Office, 1872.

On the 5th of August, 1872, specifications of the samples of dress-caps and campaign-hats were obtained from the manufacturer, who furnished them to the board referred to, and these specifications were communicated to the depot quartermaster at Philadelphia, with instructions to make the contracts accordingly.

It seems, however, that the campaign-hat does not give satisfaction to the Army, several complaints having been received at this Office of the unsuitableness of this article of head-covering, and the subject is now under investigation. Several practical hatters have examined the hats furnished in connection with the complaints, and have pronounced them to be made in accordance with the specifications. But complaints, mostly of want of durability, continuing to come in, a specimen hat was sent to Col. R. Ingalls, Assistant Quartermaster-General, New York, on the 7th instant, with instructions to submit it to Messrs. Warnock & Co., who made the standard hat upon which the action of the board was based, and obtain their report thereon. When received further action will be taken with a view to securing as durable a hat as possible.

On the 23d of November, 1872, the standard of the forage-cap was adopted and furnished to the officer in charge of the depot at Philadelphia. The quality and make of the cap have since been improved, and on the 9th of November, 1874, a new standard was adopted to be used in making future contracts. It is believed that the new caps will give general satisfaction.

The regulations for the new uniform provide for the issue of mounted overcoats to all arms of the service. On the 26th of May, 1873, the Quarter master-General reported that the supply of mounted great-coats on hand would barely be sufficient for the supply of mounted troops, and recommended that the great-coats, foot, of which there were large quantities on hand, be supplied with a large cape, like that of the new uniform, to be attached to it by buttons under and without removing the old short cape.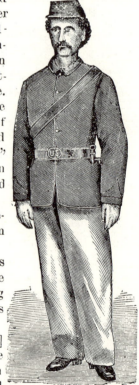

He submitted a sample coat showing the proposed alteration, and the Secretary of War authorized their issue to the enlisted men of all arms of the service. The foot troops have since been furnished with these altered coats, which the Inspector-General pronounces to be " admirable garments." The mounted great-coats will be supplied to all arms of the service as soon as the present stock is exhausted. The large cape can be detached and worn separately in mild weather.

The uniform coats and trousers are now being made after new and revised patterns, and give greater satisfaction as to fit than those made from the old pattern.

The plaited blouse not being satisfactory to the Army, a new one was designed at the Philadelphia clothing depot, which was approved by the Secretary of War on the 27th of February, 1874, and a supply is now being manufactured and issued as fast as the existing stock of the old pattern is exhausted.

[The pattern of the new blouse and of the forage-cap is shown in Fig. 4.]

Owing to the great difficulty in procuring woolen blankets of a suitable quality from the eastern mills, samples were procured from the Mission and Pacific Woolen Mills of San Francisco, which were submitted to a board of officers and adopted as standard by the Secretary of War May 2, 1872, on

Figure 4.

the recommendation of the board. Since that time all purchases have been required to conform to that standard, and the blankets now issued give general satisfaction to officers and enlisted men of the Army.

On the 19th of April, 1872, the Quartermaster-General submitted to the Secretary of War samples of brass-screwed boots and shoes, with a view to improving the standard of these articles, with suggestions that the matter be referred to a board of officers. This was done, and the board recommended that 3,000 pairs of boots and 2,000 pairs of shoes be made for trial in active service, and that reports as to their serviceability be called for with a view to their being adopted as standard, if found satisfactory; which recommendation was approved by the Secretary of War on the 2d of May, 1872. The reports from the officers to whom the shoes and boots were issued being of a favorable nature, the brass-screwed boots and shoes have since been issued to the troops. [Figures 5 and 6 represent the boots and shoes.]

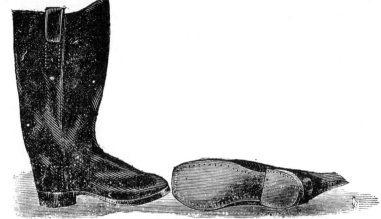

Figure 5.

During the past year several complaints have reached this office from posts in Texas and Kansas that the screws sometimes penetrate the insoles and hurt the feet of the wearers. Immediately upon receipt of these complaints, the chief quartermaster of the military division of the Missouri, the only division from which complaints have been received, was directed to investigate and seek information from local quartermasters relative to defective boots and shoes, and to forward a report to this office.

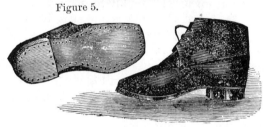

Figure 6.

The reports have been received, and from them it appears that defective boots and shoes have been found at the following posts:

|  | Pairs boots. | Pairs shoes. |
| --- | --- | --- |
| Fort Larned, Kansas | 1 | 2 |
| Fort Lyon, Colorado Territory | 5 | 15 |
| Fort Davis, Texas | 2 | 20 |
| Cheyenne Agency, Dakota Territory | | 26 |
| Fort Leavenworth, Kansas | 5 | 41 |
| Camp Douglas, Utah Territory | 8 | 16 |
| Camp Supply, Indian Territory | 5 | |
| Fort Dodge, Kansas | 1 | |
| Total | 27 | 120 |

All these have been replaced at the cost of the contractor.

Upon investigating the cause of these defects it was ascertained that, owing to the pressing demand for boots and shoes of the new pattern, those of the old patterns having been declared unfit for issue, the screw-cutting machines were run at a high rate of speed, cutting the screw-threads imperfectly, and thus making them liable to penetrate the insoles. Another reason may have been that the boots and shoes were issued to the troops before they were thoroughly seasoned. The Department is now endeavoring to accumulate during each year a small surplus stock, thus avoiding the necessity for issuing boots and shoes immediately after leaving the hands of the manufacturer.

The Quartermaster-General, on the 18th of September, 1874, in order to prevent a recurrence of similar defects, ordered that the factory of the contractor be visited every morning; that the screws be inspected, and a sample be examined with a magnifying-glass, and that, if not perfect, the mahine should not be allowed to work until re-adjusted so as to cut a good screw; a sample of which was furnished to the officer in charge of the Philadelphia depot by this Office. The inspector remains in the factory throughout every day that the machines are on Government work. The following is a detailed statement showing the number of pairs of boots and shoes brass-screwed, purchased and issued to the Army since 1869:

|  | Boots. | Shoes. |
|---|---|---|
| Purchased | 109,990 | 175,403 |
| On hand March 31, 1875 | 15,974 | 39,417 |
| Total issued to Army | 94,016 | 135,986 |

Taking these figures into consideration, it will be seen that the number of pairs found defective is very small compared with the number issued; and it is belived that the precautions now taken will hereafter prevent any defective boots and shoes from reaching the Army from this Department.

The quantity of stockings has also been improved, but is not yet what is desired. The agent of the Mission and Pacific Woolen Mills, of San Francisco, is now having manufactured a few pairs of improved quality, with a view to making a new standard. This will probably be done in time for procuring a supply for next fiscal year.

The old stock of shirts and some of the sizes of drawers being about exhausted, the patterns of these articles have been improved. A new standard shirt was adopted on the 5th of August last, and a sample of the improved drawer is now ready to be submitted to the Secretary of War for his approval. [The new patterns are represented in Figure 7.]

New and higher standards of dark-blue cloth and sky-blue kersey were adopted by the Secretary of War on the 12th of November, 1874, upon the recommendation of a board of officers convened under the provisions of Special Order No. 241, paragraph 2, Adjutant-General's Office, 1874. Materials purchased under these specifications will be used in the manufacture of coats and trousers next year.

The specifications for sky-blue kersey are as follows:

To be 6-4 wide; to be of pure, long-staple American fleece wool, free from shoddy or flocks, and dyed with pure indigo to color of standard sample; the nap to be slightly raised; to weigh not less than twenty-two ounces per linear yard; to have thirty-four threads of filling and forty threads of chain in each square inch; the breaking-strain to be not less than fifty-five (55) pounds to one inch width of warp in the piece, and forty-five (45) pounds to one inch width of filling in the piece.

The specifications for the dark-blue cloth are as follows:

To be 6-4 wide; to be of pure, long-staple American fleece wool, dyed with pure indigo to color of standard sample; to be free from shoddy or flocks, and the nap to be very slightly raised; to have fifty-six threads of filling and sixty threads of chain in each square inch; to weigh not less than twenty-one ounces per linear yard; the breaking-strain to be not less than sixty-eight (68) pounds to one inch width of warp, and fifty (50) pounds to one inch width of filling in the piece. All cloth to be of the standard strength here given, with an allowance of three pounds for variation in samples; but no cloth breaking under a strain four pounds less than the standard will be accepted from contractors.

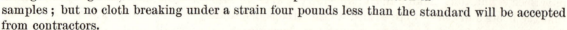

Figure 7.

On the 3d of February, 1871, the Quartermaster-General recommended to the Secretary of War that, at posts north of the forty-second degree of north latitude, an overcoat lined with blanket be issued, according to the present allowance; also that one pair of buffalo overshoes be issued the first and third year, and two pairs of woolen mittens in each year of enlistment. This was authorized and published to the Army in General Order No. 9, Adjutant-General's Office, 1871. Issues of these articles are now being made to troops, regardless of station, upon the approval of the department commander, as authorized by the Secretary of War, and communicated to the Army in General Order No. 10, Adjutant-General's Office, 1875.

Standards for buffalo overshoes were adopted on the 6th of June, 1873, and for woolen mittens on the 3d of July, 1873.

The stock of inferior blankets used for the purpose of lining great-coats is now nearly exhausted, and hereafter such coats will be lined with dark-blue cloth or sky-blue kersey, similar to that used for the manufacture of coats and trousers.

Arctic overshoes, called the "buckle-gaiter" and "snow-excluder," have been purchased and issued for trial during the last year, and have given such satisfaction that now the buffalo overshoes are seldom called for, and it is supposed that the arctics will soon replace them. They are as good in cold, dry weather as the buffalo overshoes, and are much better in wet weather.

[The arctic overshoes are represented by Figure 8; *a*, the "buckle-gaiter;" *b*, "the snow-excluder."]

The practice of this Department is to thoroughly investigate all complaints relative to the character of clothing and equipage, and, *(b.)* when well founded, to improve the quality and correct errors of manufacture.

A change was made on the 29th of September, 1874, in the wall-tent. Heretofore they were so made that when pitched the small pins *(a.)* were outside the tent, and interfered with the sod-cloth; now the pins are inside the tent and the sod-cloth outside, forming a valve to keep out the wind.

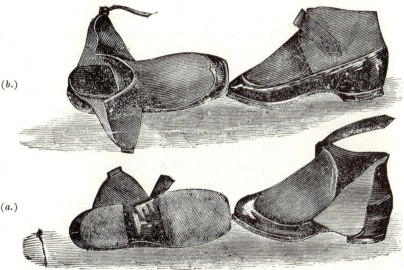

Figure 8.

When covered with sods or earth, it does not interfere with or cover up the pins. Stay-pieces have also been stitched inside the corners, at the junction of the wall and roof, and a few have been manufactured with stay-pieces, four inches wide, extending from the junction of the wall and roof across the back of the tent, and sent out for trial.

\*    \*    \*    \*    \*    \*    \*    \*    \*    \*    \*    \*

Very respectfully, your obedient servant,

M. C. MEIGS,
*Quartermaster-General,*
*Brevet Major-General U. S. A.*

The SURGEON-GENERAL OF THE ARMY.

## IV. HOSPITALS.

The hospitals of the Army are all post hospitals, and, as a rule, are barrack or temporary structures intended to contain twelve or twenty-four beds. The regulations governing their construction, with plans and specifications, are given in Circular No. 2, dated Surgeon-General's Office, July 27, 1871.

Previous to June 6, 1872, no specific sum was appropriated for hospital construction and repair, the wording of the law being—

For hire of quarters for officers on military duty, hire of quarters for troops, of store-houses for the safe-keeping of military stores, and of grounds for summer cantonments; for the construction of temporary huts, hospitals, and stables; and for repairing public buildings at established posts —— dollars.

Since that date a specific appropriation has been made annually for the construction and repair of hospitals, the amount allowed being $100,000 per annum, a plan which is much more satisfactory than the old one, the only difficulty being the same which applies to all appropriations for housing troops, viz, its insufficiency.

Under the present system the responsibility for the proper construction and good repair of the hospital rests primarily on the medical officer. It is his duty to report at the beginning of each fiscal year (July 1) as to what is needed in the way of hospital construction or repair at his post. That he made a similar report or request the year before, or a few months before, without success, is no reason why he should not repeat the process *de novo*, if, in his opinion, it is necessary for the interests of the sick; and it will be found best to make each report, estimate, or request on this subject complete in itself; that is, there should be no references to previous reports for estimates or information, as it may not be possible for the reviewing officer to have access to the paper referred to. This repetition of papers is necessary, for the reason that each fiscal year has its own specific appropriation, which can only be used in that year; and as the amount allowed is only about two-thirds what it should be, a certain number of applications, no matter how meritorious they may appear, must be rejected.

As it requires about a month, under the present system, to obtain the action of all the reviewing officers who must supervise each request for hospital construction and repair; and as in many localities but a small part of the year is available for transportation and labor, it has happened that the fiscal year has expired with a hospital unfinished, when the unspent balance which had been reserved for it must be turned into the Treasury, and, of course, a fresh request must be made to obtain funds from the succeeding appropriation.

There are about one hundred and forty post hospitals to be kept up, and the average cost of each is about $7,000. The average duration of one of these hospitals is intended to be about ten years, during which time it will probably cost about $3,000 for repairs.

In one of our 12-bed hospitals the office and dispensary, kitchen, dining-room, bathroom, and steward's quarters, require nearly as much room as they would for thirty-six beds, and thus such small hospitals are disproportionately expensive. So long, however, as our Army is cut up into detachments of one or two companies, it will probably be found difficult to properly care for the sick and be ready for emergencies with smaller buildings than are now used.

Two permanent and rather expensive hospitals are in process of construction in connection with the Army, each presenting certain peculiarities.

One of these is the new hospital for cadets at West Point, for description and plan of which see page 91 in the description of that post. The other is the Barnes Hospital, at the Soldiers' Home near Washington, and, as an attempt has been made in its construction to solve some of the problems of hospital construction as presented in civil life, a reference to these is necessary.

The question, "What is the best plan for a hospital?" is often asked, as if but one set of conditions were possible. The fact is, that hardly any two hospitals can or should be alike. The "pavilion plan," which for a time was supposed to be a perfect panacea against all evil, has been found, by sad experience, to furnish no security against the

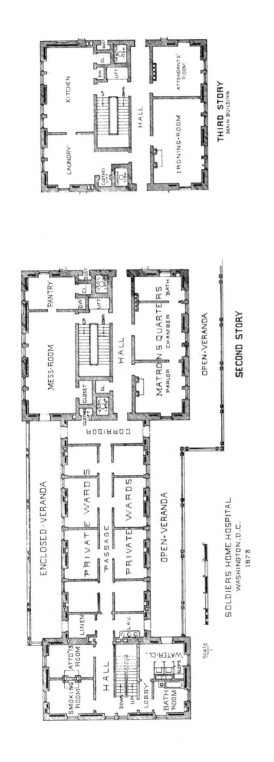

THIRD STORY
MAIN BUILDING

SECOND STORY

SOLDIERS HOME HOSPITAL
WASHINGTON. D.C.
1873

Scale

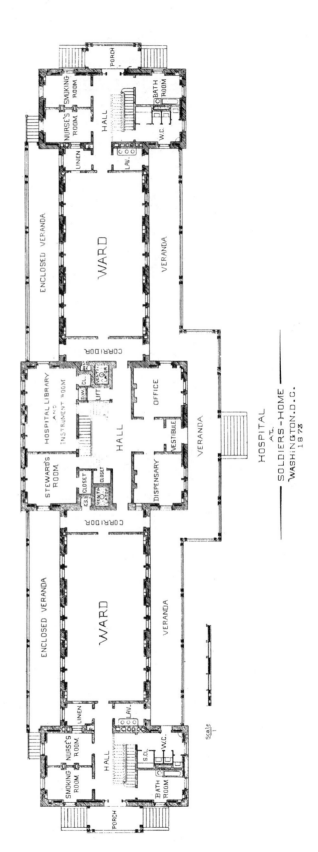

HOSPITAL
AT
SOLDIERS-HOME
WASHINGTON.D.C.
1873

Scale

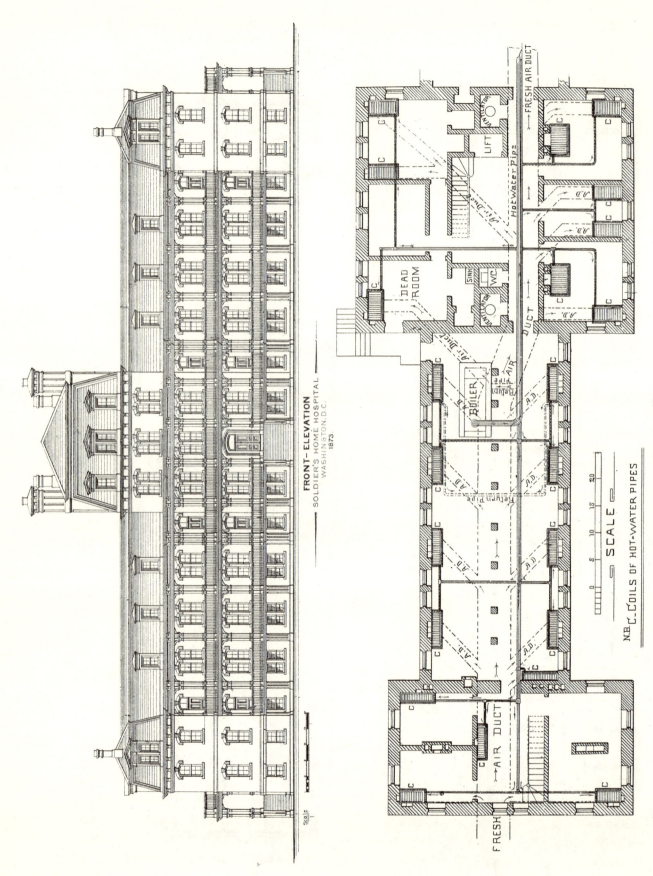

FRONT-ELEVATION

SOLDIER'S HOME HOSPITAL
WASHINGTON. D.C.
1873

PLAN OF BASEMENT

— WITH FRESH-AIR DUCTS AND HEATING APPARATUS —

N.B. C. COILS OF HOT-WATER PIPES

SCALE

0   5   10   15   20

DEAD ROOM

BOILER

LIFT

WC

SINK

FRESH AIR DUCT

FRESH AIR DUCT

Hot Water Pipe

Return Pipe

Air Duct

A.D.

evils summed up in the word "hospitalism;" and the results of practical trial in recent wars, both in this country and in Europe, have led to the recommendation of the so-called "barrack hospitals;" that is, temporary wooden structures, intended to last but ten or twelve years; in fact, such as are now used in the Army.

But to obtain the benefit of the barrack plan, the buildings must not be crowded or superimposed; and, especially, no ward or room for patients should have another room over it. Our large city hospitals are usually connected with medical schools, and it is considered necessary to place them near the city, where space is limited and costly. What, then, is the best plan for the construction within a limited space, and, therefore, of several stories, of a building which shall be satisfactory for hospital purposes?

The hospital at the Soldiers' Home is a 50-bed hospital, built of brick, and consists of a central or executive building, two wings or pavilions for wards, and towers at the distal ends of the pavilions for ward offices. The general arrangement is shown in the plates opposite. The kitchen and laundry are placed in the third story of the executive building, thus avoiding back or out-buildings, and contributing to ventilation.

The building is heated in accordance with the following specifications:

Set in complete working order a hot-water apparatus, whose maximum temperature at the boilers shall not exceed 210° Fahrenheit, sufficient for heating, during the coldest weather, all the rooms, halls, and corridors of the first, second, and third floors of the two pavilions and two end towers, and all the space on the first, second, and third floors, and the hall of the fourth floor of the center building, the kitchen and laundry excepted.

"The coils under the pavilions must be capable of heating for each ward 60,000 cubic feet of air per hour, from zero to 85° Fahrenheit.

The apparatus to consist of two wrought-iron horizontal tubular boilers, 42 inches in diameter; 9 feet long, containing 80 3-inch by 9-foot flues. * * * These boilers to be located adjoining the ventilating-stacks; where marked on plan, * * * the smoke-flues from each boiler to be connected with main smoke-flue in ventilating-stack; these connections to be fitted with perfectly tight dampers to allow fire to be used in the summer furnaces constructed at base of main smoke-flues. * * * The radiating surface to consist of coils of 3-inch cast-iron pipe having an average depth of 50 inches. * * * * * *

The fresh-air supply is provided by a bricked duct, six feet square, running from the fan—about one hundred and fifty yards away—under the building, and giving off a branch to each coil. Ventilation for the pavilions is effected by two chimneys, six feet square and one hundred feet high, in the center of which, from base to top, runs a smoke-flue of boiler-iron two feet in diameter. Into these iron tubes open the boiler smoke-flues, as above provided for: the smoke-flue from the engine, and, in the third story, the flues from the kitchen and laundry furnaces. These smoke-flues have also extra grates at the base.

Into the aspirating space in these chimneys open the foul-air flues, which are tubes four feet wide by twelve inches deep, running from end to end beneath the floor under the center of each ward. These flues or boxes have registers opening into the ward above through the floor, and into the ward below through the ceiling. These registers close air-tight, so that the air from any ward can be taken out either above or below. The fresh-air flues for the lower wards are double, one opening near the floor, the other near the ceiling, and can be controlled by registers, so that the air can be introduced at top or bottom. This arrangement is intended for experimental purposes, and will be modified in accordance with the results obtained by trial.

The clothes lift, the main lift, and the dumb-waiter open above into the main ventilating stacks. The ventilation of the center building is by a large Emerson ventilator over the central hall and staircase, and by fire-places in the rooms. The end towers, containing the ward offices, have independent ventilation by aspirating chimneys heated by furnaces in the basement which supply hot water to the lavatories and bath-rooms. The water-closets are ventilated downward through the seats, except in one set, where the Jennings closet is placed for purposes of comparison. The gas-jets contribute to the ventilation, having flues over them which connect with the foul-air ducts. One end of the building is finished in Parian, the other in ordinary hard finish, so arranged that it can easily be removed and replaced. All re-entering angles are rounded.

The hospital fronts the south, and is surrounded by piazzas, those on the north side being arranged with sashes, removable in summer.

The difficulty in properly ventilating a ward is in direct proportion to the number of beds it contains, and to the variety of ailments of the patients. The smaller the wards, and the nearer to isolation that can be obtained for grave cases, provided that an allowance of about one cubic foot of fresh air per second per man is furnished, the more satisfactory the results. Even in our most roomy and best ventilated barrack-hospitals, during the war, the use of tents was often resorted to on account of the appearance of hospital diseases.

All systems of ventilation in practical use act on the theory of diluting the vitiated air, by securing the introduction and proper diffusion of a large amount of fresh supply.

As regards deleterious gases, this will do very well; but the real danger of hospitalism arises from solid particles, probably living, and the results of attempting to dilute these have been, and will probably continue to be, very much like those obtained by Chauveau and Sanderson in diluting vaccine—the probability of infection for one exposure may be diminished, but when the small particle does happen to be present, its effects will be the same as though no dilution had been attempted.

These organic poisons are necessarily more dangerous to others than to the one who produces them, and who may therefore be supposed to be more or less saturated by them; and it seems probable that they increase in virulence by successive transmissions. Their prompt and complete removal as fast as formed is the only certain way of preventing their peculiar zymotic effects, and I do not believe that any system of hospital construction or ventilation will prevent hospitalism which does not allow of a much more minute classification of cases than is now practiced, and in which ample provision is not made for the isolation of cases when needed.

In our small hospitals, with few grave cases and no risk of puerperal contamination, these considerations need not often be taken into account; but it is well to remember that even in a twelve or six bed ward, the presence of a case of erysipelas or septic disease, or of extensive suppuration, is a special source of danger to the other inmates of that room, and if contagion be conveyed it will, in most cases, not be necessary to refer to saturation of walls and floors with organic poison to account for it, but rather to look to baize screens, woolen clothing of attendants, upholstered furniture, and dressings as the probable sources of the trouble.

A mode of obtaining a local low temperature in cases of hyperpyrexia has been employed by Assistant Surgeon A. H. Hoff, in the hospital at Sitka, and again in that at Governor's Island, New York Harbor, which is worth remembering. It consists in cutting a hole about one foot square in the floor immediately under a bed, the opening communicating with the outer air, and then covering this with a latticed box in such a way as to break up the incoming current of cold fresh air, and to cause it to envelop the bed. In cold weather, and using a thin mattress, Dr. Hoff has in this way obtained a local reduction of temperature of the air of 35° Fahrenheit, and has treated cases of typhoid fever in such a bed with good effect.

In my previous report I recommended, as a means of heating the wards of our post hospitals, a ventilating fire-place, consisting of two fire-places placed back to back, with a space between, through which fresh air could be introduced and warmed, being a modification of the Galton fire-place.

About a dozen such fire-places were constructed and sent out for trial, and reports with regard to their efficiency have been rather contradictory. Owing to defects of construction, a part of them were entirely deficient in heating-power. Those set up in the twelve-bed wards of the hospitals at Fort Whipple and at Fort McHenry worked very well, ventilating the rooms at the rate of about 36,000 cubic feet per hour, and giving sufficient warmth, except when the temperature fell to zero. But they need improvement in mode of construction, especially as regards facility of transportation, and they will not give sufficient heat, except with anthracite as fuel, when the temperature is below freezing-point.

For these reasons their issue has been stopped, and the majority of the hospitals are now heated with sheet-iron cylinder-stoves. If the fresh-air box be brought under the ward to open under one of these stoves, and then the stove be encased with a sheet-iron cylinder about 18 inches greater in diameter than itself, and open at the top, the difficulties attending the introduction of fresh air are in a large measure obviated.

It is not possible, in a barrack-hospital, to obtain both satisfactory heating and ventilation, with the temperature of the external air near zero, by any stove or fire-place placed in the ward itself, and therefore ventilation must be to some extent sacrificed. It is impossible to warm the fresh entering air, and at the same time introduce it at any point except at the stove itself, while the foul air must either be taken out at the ceiling or by the stove or fire-place. It is evident that the air surrounding the beds cannot be directly changed in this way, as there is no provision for mixing it with the fresh incoming air. In our hospitals this is a matter of very little practical importance, and I allude to it only because many persons seem to think that there are no difficulties in ventilating a one-story barrack-building.

To obtain satisfactory heating and ventilation, with the outside temperature at or below the freezing-point, in any room occupied by a number of men, whether it be hospital or barrack, is not possible unless the heating apparatus be placed below the room to be heated, and arranged in such a way that if the fresh, warmed air is delivered at the center it can be taken out at the sides near the floor, and *vice versa*.

By way of comparison, I quote from the Report of the Sanitary Commissioner for Bombay, 1866, Appendix II, page 33, the following:

*Principles of construction of hospitals for European and native troops, by Lieutenant-Colonel Crommelin, Royal Engineers.*

PROPOSAL No. III.—That all regimental or detachment hospitals, which may hereafter be constructed in the plains of India, shall be double-storied buildings, in which the whole of the wards for the sick, together with a certain necessary amount of subsidiary accommodation, shall be arranged in the upper floors, and the day-room administrative offices, quarters for medical subordinates, &c., shall be provided in the lower stories; further, that the kitchen, guard-room, dead-house, shed for ambulance-carts, privy, and lavatory for general use, shall be in out-buildings.

*Conclusion of the government of India.*—Looking to the great expense that is involved in the future provision of hospital accommodation throughout India, to the excess of space for auxiliary purposes, in the lower floors, that will be the consequence of the construction of buildings unnecessarily large, to the fact that the proportion of sick only exceeds 7 and 8 per cent. of strength for a period during each year, and, lastly, to the positive advantage there may be in having accommodation in the lower floor for a small number of certain classes of patients, the government of India considers that it is not necessary to provide accommodation in the upper floor for more than three-fourths of the total complement of patients, the remaining one-fourth being arranged for in well-raised and well-ventilated lower floors. By such an arrangement the actual necessity of placing patients in the lower floor will rarely occur.

\*    \*    \*    \*    \*    \*    \*    \*    \*

PROPOSAL No. VI.—That the subdivision of a hospital into a number of small buildings is objectionable, because it tends to unnecessary expense, to the occupation of too great space, and to the overtaxing of the powers of the establishments; and further, that it is not necessary in military hospitals, which are rarely fully occupied, in which the generality of cases treated are not of a serious character, and in which the whole of the sick have liberal accommodation provided for them in upper floors.

*Conclusion of the government of India.*—The government of India approves of the proposal, and the subdivision of a hospital into a number of very small buildings is objectionable on sanitary, administrative, and financial grounds.

\*    \*    \*    \*    \*    \*    \*    \*    \*

PROPOSAL No. IX.—That the component parts of every military hospital shall consist of—
1. Wards for the sick and convalescents.
2. Ward-offices, viz: Superintendent's rooms, sculleries, privies, and urinaries, bath and ablution rooms.
3. Day-rooms for sick and convalescents.
4. Quarters for medical subordinates.
5. Quarters for hospital-sergeant.
6. Quarters for hospital-orderlies.
7. Store-rooms.
8. Surgery.
9. Receiving-room.
10. Outdoor kitchen.
11. Outdoor lavatory, (with shower-bath.)
12. Outdoor privy.
13. Guard-room.
14. Shed for ambulance-carts, hearse, &c.
15. Dead-house.
16. Inclosure-wall or railing.

*Conclusion of the government of India.*—The government of India considers that a separate dispensary is unnecessary, and that one room will suffice for a combined surgery and dispensary. The following, however, should be added to the above list:
1. Houses for native establishment.

2. Laundry.

3. A small detached building for contagious diseases.

\*   \*   \*   \*   \*   \*   \*   \*   \*

PROPOSAL No. XII.—That the following is a suitable distribution of beds in the wards of the several hospitals:

*Infantry male hospital.*

Beds.

4 wards of 24 beds each..................................................... 96

1 ward of 12 beds........................................................ 12

2 wards of 2 beds each................................................... 4

                            —————

Total ................................................................ 112

\*   \*   \*   \*   \*   \*   \*   \*   \*

PROPOSAL No. XIV.—That all large wards be 26 feet in width, and 21 feet in height to wall-plate, and that the wall space per bed in them be 10 feet, thus giving an area of 130 superficial feet per bed; that the wall space per bed in wards for convalescents be $7\frac{1}{2}$ feet only, which length will give an area of $97\frac{1}{2}$ superficial feet per bed; and that in small wards the area per bed may average from 150 to 180 superficial feet per bed.

*Conclusion of the government of India.*—The government of India considers that the space in the main wards should be as follows:

In the plains: 10 running feet per bed; 24 running feet width of ward; 20 running feet height of wards from floor to wall-plate.

These dimensions give 120 superficial feet and 2,400 cubic feet per bed.

When the lower floor is not intended to be occupied by patients, the height from floor to wall-plate to be 16 feet.

In hill stations: $8\frac{1}{2}$ running feet per bed; 24 running feet width of ward; height of wards 16 to 18 feet, according to the altitude of the station.

These dimensions give 102 superficial feet, and 1,632, or 1,836 cubic feet per bed.

The space in the small wards should average, as proposed, from 150 to 180 superficial feet per bed; but $7\frac{1}{2}$ running feet, and 90 superficial feet per bed, will suffice for the large convalescent wards of regiments.

In view of the theories which have been advanced as to hospital walls becoming contaminated and a source of disease, I have endeavored to obtain some data as to the influence of adobe barracks and hospitals, and other buildings, and especially those which have been long in use, upon the health of their occupants. I have been unable, however, to obtain any satisfactory information as to the relative healthfulness of such structures. A few medical officers report that they consider adobe houses as conducive to rheumatic affections; but the majority appear to be of the opinion that they are as healthful as any other class of habitation. A very satisfactory mode of constructing hospitals for warm climates is to line them with canvas instead of plaster, and white-wash directly upon the canvas. This has been tried in several cases, and with good results. Taken as a whole, I have great pleasure in reporting that the condition of the Army hospitals, including their furniture, supplies, and means of caring for the sick and wounded, are very satisfactory, and are so considered by the medical officers of the Army.

Very respectfully, your obedient servant,

JOHN S. BILLINGS,

*Assistant Surgeon, United States Army.*

General J. K. BARNES,

  *Surgeon-General United States Army,*

# DESCRIPTIONS OF MILITARY POSTS.

# MILITARY DIVISION OF THE ATLANTIC.

(Embracing the States of Maine, New Hampshire, Vermont, Massachusetts, Rhode Island, Connecticut, New York, New Jersey, Pennsylvania, Delaware, Maryland, Virginia, West Virginia, Ohio, Indiana, Michigan, and Wisconsin.)

## POSTS.

Adams, Fort, R. I.
Allegheny Arsenal, Pa.
Andrew, Fort, Mass.
Brady, Fort, Mich.
Carlisle Barracks, Pa.
Carroll, Fort, Md.
Clark's Point, fort at, Mass.
Columbus Arsenal, Ohio.
Columbus, Fort, N. Y.
Constitution, Fort, N. H.
Davids Island, N. Y.
Delaware, Fort, Del.
Detroit Arsenal, Mich.
Dutch Island, fort on, R. I.
Finn's Point, battery at, N. J.
Foote, Fort, Md.
Frankford Arsenal, Pa.
Gerrish's Island, battery on, Me.
Gorges, Fort, Me.
Gratiot, Fort, Mich.
Griswold, Fort, Conn.
Hamilton, Fort, N. Y.
Independence, Fort, Mass.
Indianapolis Arsenal, Ind.

Jerry's Point, battery on, N. H.
Kennebec Arsenal, Me.
Knox, Fort, Me.
Lafayette, Fort, N. Y.
Lazaretto Point, fort at, Md.
Lee, Fort, Mass.
Long Island Head, battery at, Mass.
Long Point Batteries, Mass.
McClary, Fort, Me.
McHenry, Fort, Md.
Mackinac, Fort, Mich.
Madison Barracks, N. Y.
Mifflin, Fort, Pa.
Monroe, Fort, Va.
Montgomery, Fort, N. Y.
Niagara, Fort, N. Y.
Ontario, Fort, N. Y.
Phœnix, Fort, Mass.
Pikesville Arsenal, Md.
Plattsburgh Barracks, N. Y.
Popham, Fort, Me.
Porter, Fort, N. Y.
Portland Head Battery, Me.
Preble, Fort, Me.

Sandy Hook, fort at, N. J.
Scammel, Fort, Me.
Schuyler, Fort, N. Y.
Sewall, Fort, Mass.
Springfield Armory and Arsenal, Mass.
Standish, Fort, Mass.
Sullivan, Fort, Me.
Trumbull, Fort, Conn.
Wadsworth, Fort, New York Harbor.
Warren, Fort, Mass.
Washington Arsenal, D. C.
Washington, Fort, Md.
Watertown Arsenal, Mass.
Watervliet Arsenal, N. Y.
Wayne, Fort, Mich.
West Point Military Academy, N. Y.
Whipple, Fort, Va.
Willett's Point, N. Y.
Winthrop, Fort, Mass.
Wolcott, Fort, R. I.
Wood, Fort, N. Y.
Wool, Fort, Va.

## FORT ADAMS, RHODE ISLAND.

REPORTS OF SURGEONS J. F. HEAD AND JOHN CAMPBELL, UNITED STATES ARMY.

Fort Adams is situated upon Brenton's Point, the southern boundary of the entrance to the harbor of Newport, R. I., about three miles from the mouth of Narraganset Bay. Latitude, 41° 28′ north; longitude, 5° 4′ east.

It is distant from Newport one mile by water and three miles by land.

The underlying rock upon which the post is built is a stratified slate, inclosing two thick beds of compact variegated limestone, which, with the slate, are traversed by veins of quartz. The reservation includes 138½ acres, of which the fort proper covers 21½. The parade is about 30 feet above low-water mark and includes about 6¼ acres, most of which is turfed.

The quarters for officers and men are in casemates, arched with brick and covered with sheet-lead, the valleys between the arches being filled with earth surmounted by a thin layer of concrete, and a brick pavement over all.   The defects of this arrangement are shown in the following extract from a communication from General G. K. Warren, United States Engineers, dated September 16, 1874:

The weight of the covering above the lead pressed the hard parts, (like pebbles,) and probably ice aided, through it, so as to allow the water to reach the arches.   The escape-pipes in the scarp will sometimes become stopped up, and notably so on the north and west sides, by filling with ice in the winter.   The valleys thus filled with water, and this kept up a continual supply for percolation through the concrete and arch.

In the year 1863 the covering was removed from the two casemates in the flank north of the east sally-port because of their extensively leaky condition.   Then was first apparent the injury to the lead covering above alluded to.

The injured lead was taken up from the concrete (and from the side of the vertical walls, against which the arch covering abutted, which was also covered with lead) and an asphaltum coating put on in its place.   The earth and brick pavement were then replaced.   No complaint has since been made of the leaks in these casemates, but there is a danger of cracks forming in the concrete where the arch covering joins the vertical walls, and in that case the leaking would begin again.

At the same time (in 1868) the coverings were removed from two casemates on the west front, and these were regarded as the most leaky casemates in the work.

I do not know the month they were uncovered, but the valleys were found filled with ice, showing that the cold weather was sufficient to close the drain-pipes.   The lead was pierced with holes, and in the winter icicles formed by the percolation on the outside of the casemate roof.

These were covered up with asphaltum as the others had been.   In addition, drain-pipes were placed so as to prevent the earth filling from becoming saturated.   The earth was put back, finished with a top layer of concrete 6 inches thick, and upon this the usual tar pavement was laid, with sufficient slope toward the parade wall to carry off the surface water.   This alone should be security against leakage, but being liable to injury should not be solely relied upon.   The covering was put on in the autumn of 1870, and no leaks have since occurred, as far as known.

Many, if not all, of the casemates leak somewhat, and this seems to occur to the greatest extent along the line of junction of the terre-plein and parade-wall, so as to run down the windows and doors of the quarters, in some places in streams during heavy rains.

*     *     *     *     *     *     *     *     *     *     *     *     *

It is believed that proper construction would wholly prevent leakage, but nothing can ever be done to make them proper dwellings as permanent quarters in time of peace.

The exterior walls are strong masonry, with either narrow vertical slits or loop-holes for small-arms, or an occasional embrasure for a cannon.   The parapets above being designed to support cannon *en barbette*, the arches have to be supported by piers of masonry, (which piers serve as partitions to quarters,) and the whole requiring to be bomb-proof in war necessitates a very thick covering.

Unlike a cave, (which in many features they resemble,) they do not preserve the uniform mean temperature of the latitude, but in winter become often thoroughly chilled through, (as shown by the ice in the valleys between the arches in summer.)   This temperature they retain during a large part of the warm season, losing it but gradually ; and while thus much below the temperature of the atmosphere, they receive the moist warm air and fogs from the ocean, so that heavy condensation is unavoidable without fires to dispel it.

Quarters built in this way, practically *cellars*, are, of course, except in winter, excessively damp; more than ordinarily so in this climate, which is a peculiarly humid one.   Fires are necessary during a part of almost every day, even in midsummer, to make the quarters at all habitable.   Arms and instruments rust, and clothing and equipments decay rapidly.   It is needless to say that such dwelling-places are unhealthy.

The dormitories for enlisted men measure 54 by 18 or 19 feet, with an average height of 11 feet, affording, during the year 1873, an average air-space of 560 feet per man.   The allowance has at times been not more than half so much; and were the estimated full garrison for this fort ever packed into it the result would certainly be a pestilence.

Three circular apertures, each 20 inches in diameter, in the roof of each dormitory, open into a space between the arched roof and the flat ceiling, from the outer end of which space is a communication with the external air by the smoke-hole, 5 by 1½ feet, the shaft opening on the parapet 12 feet above the ceiling.

A few years ago a deficiency in extent of quarters caused the erection of three temporary wooden buildings as officers' quarters, one as quarters for two captains, each of the others as quarters for two lieutenants.   These buildings, although badly planned and slightly built, are much more suitable than the casemates as quarters.

An elegant residence, two stories and L, with Mansard roof, was completed in June, 1873, for the commanding officer. It is located about 50 yards south of the redoubt, on high ground, which was formerly a part of the post garden, contains fourteen rooms, and is provided with the usual modern appliances for distributing heat and hot and cold water throughout the building.

The cells for prisoners are four in number; average dimensions 7½ by 6 feet, and 9 feet 5 inches high; ventilation by two loop-holes, 3½ by 20 inches.

In these cells, and a hall in front, giving a total cubic space of less than 5,000 cubic feet, thirty prisoners have been confined at one time, giving each man about 170 cubic feet.

The hospital stands on the crest of land between Brenton's Cove and Narraganset Bay, a dry and airy site, and is upon the plan given in Circular No. 2, Surgeon General's Office, April 27, 1867, for a hospital of twenty-four beds, with the addition of a porch at each end.

The wards allow space for twelve beds in each, with superficial area of 94¾ square feet, and air space of 1,421¼ cubic feet per bed. But one ward is in use, with an average occupancy of one attendant and three patients. It is warmed by a ventilating fire-place.

The light is sufficient, and the ventilation ample and satisfactory. The water-closets, one to each ward, contain but one seat each and one urinal. There is no stench-trap, and no separate ventilating-shaft for the closets. Each bath-room has a good planished copper fixed tub and two basins, supplied with hot and cold water.

The bath-tubs, sinks, fixed basins, water-closets, &c., are fed by a tank in the attic, with capacity of 580 gallons, filled by a force-pump in the kitchen.

The hospital has been much improved within the past three years. The main building has been entirely surrounded by a veranda; a spacious yard inclosed by a substantial fence; the plot in front sodded and planted with young pines; and the space in the rear converted into a garden. Two cisterns have been constructed to receive the water from the roof, and a small stable built for the hospital cow. It has also received new flooring, cooking-range, storm-doors, and windows, and repainting within and without.

The natural supply of water is sufficient, and the well water of reasonably good quality, though rather hard. There are in use one well within the main work, and seven outside. The best water is that of a spring near Brenton's Cove. It is soft, and is used by the laundresses. In addition to the wells several large cisterns afford a supply of rain-water.

The men have no lavatories. For sea-bathing during the warm months the facilities are very good.

Earth-closets have been in constant use at this post and have proved thoroughly successful. The casemate occupied by the apparatus is conveniently near the men's quarters. Sufficient light and air is admitted through three embrasures. The furnace and drying-pans are in the same apartment. Only one-half of the closets are used at a time, which use continues for two weeks, when the other half is brought into play. The caissons or drawers of the vacated half are then removed, emptied, aired, and deodorized. The contents are shot out of one of the embrasures into carts. This work is done without causing offensive odor. Two soldiers are detailed to keep in order the casemate and closets—to prepare the earth, &c. The urine is carried from the trough by tubes running through the scarp-wall into the sewer in the ditch. The earth-closet, as now in use by the soldiers at this post, is a most thorough success. It obviates, as nearly as possible, all the objections to be urged against most other species of privy. It insures convenience, cleanliness, and safety from unhealthy emanations. Further improvements in the closets will perhaps secure still more entire suitableness. The necessity of a detail of men to keep the closets in working order may be urged as an objection to them; but it is more than probable that any other system of sinks would necessitate at least as great an amount of labor in the course of a year and a greater outlay of money.

The climate of the southern part of this island is in some respects an exception to that of the region in which it is classed. Its peculiarities, which, with the facilities for sea-bathing, have made Newport a favorite summer resort, are due to its insular position, its general slope toward the south, and doubtless to the nearness of the western edge of the Gulf Stream. The winter temperature is much milder than that of Providence, and the summers are remarkably cool and equable. The same cause, however, which produces these results, occasions in spring and early summer the heavy fogs for which this vicinity is famous. The influence of the dampness upon the health of the inhabitants is less unfavorable than might reasonably be expected.

*Meteorological report, Fort Adams, R. I., 1870–'74.*

| Month. | 1870–'71. Temperature. Mean. | Max. | Min. | Rain-fall in inches. | 1871–'72. Temperature. Mean. | Max. | Min. | Rain-fall in inches. | 1872–'73. Temperature. Mean. | Max. | Min. | Rain-fall in inches. | 1873–'74. Temperature. Mean. | Max. | Min. | Rain-fall in inches. |
|---|---|---|---|---|---|---|---|---|---|---|---|---|---|---|---|---|
| | ° | ° | ° | | ° | ° | ° | | ° | ° | ° | | ° | ° | ° | |
| July | 68.95 | 88 | 56 | 2.96 | 68.27 | 92* | 53* | 1.91 | 71.68 | 88* | 57* | 5.83 | 69.38 | 90* | 57* | 1.41 |
| August | 70.22 | 81 | 56 | 1.93 | 69.37 | 86* | 54* | 8.16 | 70.39 | 83* | 47* | 3.70 | 68.50 | 86* | 54* | 4.00 |
| September | 63.26 | 76* | 45* | 1.52 | 59.17 | 74* | 40* | 1.39 | 62.62 | 87* | 46* | 3.89 | 61.78 | 80* | 44* | 2.48 |
| October | 54.91 | 75* | 22* | 5.22 | 53.85 | 66* | 31* | 5.83 | 51.71 | 68* | 38* | 4.06 | 53.95 | 69* | 36* | 4.92 |
| November | 43.89 | 62* | 27* | 2.07 | 38.42 | 59* | 8* | 4.15 | 40.58 | 56* | 15* | 3.62 | 36.22 | 61* | 14* | 4.89 |
| December | 32.42 | 61* | 8* | 1.37 | 28.94 | 46* | 0* | 1.79 | 25.49 | 46* | 0* | 1.46 | 34.63 | 53* | 14′ | 4.24 |
| January | 26.38 | 48* | −13* | 1.97 | 27.61 | 43* | 2* | 2.07 | 26.09 | 49* | −11* | 5.79 | 32.61 | 51* | 7* | 3.20 |
| February | 27.41 | 50* | −5* | 2.19 | 27.69 | 45* | 3* | 1.06 | 26.70 | 43* | −15* | 2.43 | 28.58 | 49* | 8* | 2.77 |
| March | 39.24 | 58* | 25* | 4.07 | 26.00 | 44* | −6* | 2.10 | 32.81 | 49* | 14* | 1.84 | 33.80 | 52* | 13* | 1.41 |
| April | 45.44 | 67* | 29* | 2.27 | 42.14 | 69* | 26* | 1.52 | 42.11 | 61* | 34* | 4.09 | 37.57 | 56* | 18* | 6.99 |
| May | 53.41 | 73* | 36* | 2.82 | 54.21 | 81* | 33* | 3.23 | 51.66 | 76* | 33* | 3.85 | 51.66 | 73* | 35* | 3.99 |
| June | 61.82 | 82* | 50* | 3.15 | 63.81 | 84* | 47* | 1.48 | 61.99 | 88* | 46* | 0.58 | 62.17 | 83* | 48* | 3.71 |
| For the year | 48.95 | 88 | −13* | 31.54 | 48.29 | 92* | −6* | 34.69 | 47.00 | 88* | −15* | 41.14 | 47.57 | 90* | 7* | 44.01 |

* These observations are made with self-registering thermometers. The mean is from the standard thermometer.

*Consolidated sick-report, Fort Adams, R. I., 1870–'74.*

| Year | | 1870–'71. | | 1871–'72. | | 1872–'73. | | 1873–'74. | |
|---|---|---|---|---|---|---|---|---|---|
| Mean strength { Officers | | 18 | | 18 | | 15 | | 15 | |
| { Enlisted men | | 325 | | 222 | | 230 | | 243 | |
| Diseases. | | Cases. | Deaths. | Cases. | De | Cases. | Deaths. | Cases. | Deaths. |
| GENERAL DISEASES, A. | | | | | | | | | |
| Typhoid fever | | | | 3 | | | | | |
| Remittent fever | | 2 | | 4 | | 2 | | | |
| Intermittent fever | | 31 | | 7 | | 15 | | 7 | |
| Diphtheria | | | | | | | | 1 | |
| Other diseases of this group | | 105 | | 12 | | 26 | | 12 | |
| GENERAL DISEASES, B. | | | | | | | | | |
| Rheumatism | | 44 | | 24 | | 31 | | 46 | |
| Syphilis | | 11 | | | | 6 | | 5 | |
| Consumption | | | | 1 | 1 | | | 2 | |
| Other diseases of this group | | 1 | | | | | | 2 | |
| LOCAL DISEASES. | | | | | | | | | |
| Catarrh and bronchitis | | 44 | 1 | 50 | | 48 | | 73 | |
| Pneumonia | | 4 | | | | 3 | 1 | | |
| Pleurisy | | 1 | | | | 1 | | 1 | |
| Diarrhœa and dysentery | | 71 | | 30 | 1 | 49 | | 29 | |
| Hernia | | 4 | | 3 | | | | | |
| Gonorrhœa | | 12 | | 3 | | 5 | | 4 | |
| Other local diseases | | 167 | 1 | 161 | 2 | 167 | | 131 | 1 |
| Alcoholism | | 4 | | 4 | | 10 | 1 | 32 | |
| Total | | 501 | 2 | 302 | 4 | 366 | 2 | 345 | 1 |
| VIOLENT DISEASES AND DEATHS. | | | | | | | | | |
| Accidents and injuries | | 109 | | 70 | | 56 | | 98 | |
| Suicide | | | | | 1 | | | | |
| Total violence | | 109 | | 70 | 1 | 56 | | 98 | |

# ALLEGHENY ARSENAL, PENNSYLVANIA.

## REPORT OF ACTING ASSISTANT SURGEON JAMES ROBISON, UNITED STATES ARMY.

This arsenal is located within the limits of the city of Pittsburgh, on the left bank of the Allegheny River, three miles from its mouth. Latitude, 40° 32′ north; longitude, 3° 2′ west; altitude, 704 feet.

The reservation was purchased in 1814, and contains about thirty-eight acres.

The mean annual temperature is about 50°; maximum, 98°, minimum, —6°; rain-fall about 34 inches.

The barracks are two brick buildings, each 125 by 25 feet, two stories high, with slate roofs. One is divided into 18 rooms, and is at present occupied by married soldiers and their families. The other barrack is in part occupied by the detachment of ordnance. Half of the first floor is used as a mess-hall and kitchen. The mess-hall is 22 by 40 by 10 feet, and the kitchen 13 by 16 by 8 feet. Both are well supplied with the appropriate furniture and utensils. The second floor is divided into four rooms, two of which are dormitories, each 40 by 22 by 8 feet. The air-space per bed is about 586 cubic feet. There are two small rooms partitioned off at each end of each dormitory. One is occupied by the first sergeant, and the other by the hospital steward and his family. The dormitories are warmed by coal-stoves, lighted at night by gas, and ventilated by means of the doors and windows.

The officers' quarters are four buildings, divided into five sets of quarters, two of which are built of stone, with attached wings of brick. These quarters are all two stories high, are very large and commodious, and are fitted up with all the modern improvements.

The guard-house is a brick building 53 by 17 feet, and contains three rooms, one room for the use of the guard, a prison room with three cells attached, seldom used, and a small store-room over the passage-way. The guard and prison rooms are warmed by coal-stoves, lighted by gas, and ventilated by doors and windows.

The hospital occupies five rooms in the barrack already described. The space is considered ample, and the general arrangement satisfactory.

The sinks of the detachment are about 100 feet from the barrack, and are frequently disinfected in warm weather. The natural drainage of the post is excellent, the grounds sloping to the river, and the artificial drainage is all that could be desired. All drains and gutters connect with two large underground sewers terminating at the Allegheny River. All the slops, offal, and rubbish of the post are thrown into the river.

Pure soft-water is brought in iron pipes from a never-failing spring, about half a mile east of the arsenal, to two brick reservoirs, and from them distributed through a system of pipes.

The men bathe in the Allegheny River in summer, and use a bath-tub and basins in winter.

*Consolidated sick-report, Allegheny Arsenal, Pa., 1870–'74.*

| Year | | 1870-'71. | | 1871-'72. | | 1872-'73. | | 1873-'74. | |
|---|---|---|---|---|---|---|---|---|---|
| Mean strength { Officers | | 3 | | 3 | | 3 | | 3 | |
| { Enlisted men | | 48 | | 30 | | 28 | | 30 | |
| Diseases. | | Cases. | Deaths. | Cases. | Deaths. | Cases. | Deaths. | Cases. | Deaths. |
| GENERAL DISEASES, A. | | | | | | | | | |
| Small-pox and varioloid | | | | 1 | | | | | |
| Remittent fever | | 4 | | | | 1 | | | |
| Intermittent fever | | | | | | 1 | | | |
| Other diseases of this group | | 1 | | 1 | | | | | |
| GENERAL DISEASES, B. | | | | | | | | | |
| Rheumatism | | 6 | | 3 | | 2 | | | |
| Syphilis | | 4 | | 1 | | 3 | | | |
| Other diseases of this group | | | | | | 1 | | | |
| LOCAL DISEASES. | | | | | | | | | |
| Catarrh and bronchitis | | 7 | | 3 | | 2 | | 8 | |
| Pneumonia | | 1 | | | | | | | |
| Diarrhœa and dysentery | | 2 | | 4 | | 3 | | 6 | |
| Gonorrhœa | | 1 | | | | | | | |
| Other local diseases | | 25 | | 8 | | 8 | 1 | 8 | |
| Alcoholism | | 3 | | 2 | | | | 3 | |
| Total | | 54 | | 23 | | 21 | 1 | 25 | |
| VIOLENT DISEASES AND DEATHS. | | | | | | | | | |
| Accidents and injuries | | 13 | | 7 | | 6 | | 3 | |
| Total violence | | 13 | | 7 | | 6 | | 3 | |

## FORT ANDREW, MASSACHUSETTS.

Established in 1863 on Gwinet Point, north side of the entrance to Plymouth Harbor, in latitude 42° north, longitude 6° 23′ east. The fort is distant nine miles by water and twenty-four by land from the city of Plymouth.

Water is supplied by a well within the fort.

The works are in charge of an ordnance-sergeant.

---

## FORT BRADY, MICHIGAN.

REPORTS OF ASSISTANT SURGEONS M. K. TAYLOR AND J. H. T. KING, UNITED STATES ARMY.

Fort Brady is on the south bank of the Sault Ste. Marie, Mich., six miles from Lake Superior; latitude, 46° 30′ north; longitude, 7° 46′ west; altitude, 600 feet.

For early history and plate of this post see Circular 4, Surgeon General's Office, 1870, page 124.

The eastern portion of the garrison grounds slopes gently to the river, but that between the commanding officer's quarters and the river forms an abrupt bluff of about 26 feet in height. To the rear of the garrison inclosure, at a distance of 400 feet, there is a bowlder ridge ranging from 30 to 34 feet above the surface of the river in front, which is the dividing elevation between the river slope on the one hand and the watershed to the creek in the swamp on the other. This bowlder ridge extends from the head of the rapids to Hay Lake, a distance of four miles, and constitutes what may be called the second terrace. Back of this ridge, ranging from a third of a mile wide at the head of the rapids to a mile and a half at the head of Hay Lake, there is a slight depression of three to five feet, the surface of which is wet and known as the "Swamp," through which runs a small stream most of the year. In dry weather in summer, and when the lake above is at low water, this stream may be dry, but in high water of Lake Superior, with strong winds from the north or northwest, water will flow from Ashman's Bay at the head of the rapids through this little stream to Hay Lake, probably falling about 22 feet in four miles. Back of this swamp are the highlands, at an elevation of from 100 to 150 feet above Lake Superior. On the Canadian shore, at a distance of from six to ten miles, there are high lands ranging from 400 to 600 feet above Lake Superior, and on Sugar Island, in Saint Mary's River, the elevation in the central portion attains to 300 or 400 feet.

All the swamp land situated between the hills on the river, from the head of the Portage, as it is called, to Hay Lake is susceptible of cultivation if properly drained, and would unquestionably be very productive; but as it is now the line of cultivation does not extend beyond the bowlder ridge except for a short distance along the Mackinac road. The swamp is densely covered with *coniferæ* and thick beds of moss, which hold water like a sponge, almost from one year to another.

The Saint Mary's River properly commences at "Pointe aux Pins," six miles above the falls, where the river leaves the lake at a right angle with the general trend of its shores. From its commencement to the head of the rapids its current is moderate, but gradually accelerating until reaching the falls, the waters plunge tumultuously over the rocks on a declivity of 18 feet in three-quarters of a mile.

The special geology of the immediate vicinity of the post has some interesting features in a sanitary point of view. Sandstones crop out on the rapids and appear on the surface about 500 feet on the American side, barely covered by a light soil. This occurs to the west of the garrison inclosure about 1,500 feet, and can be traced to the hills in the rear. It forms the barrier to the drainage of the great lake above, and has resisted for ages the combined disintegrating action of water, ice, and frost in maintaining the general level of that vast inland sea. Superimposed on this are the clay hills forming the table-lands between this and Mackinac, which are stratified in the following order from the surface downward, as appears by a dry well sunk about two miles from the river, viz: first, soil and clay, 20 feet; second, clay marls, 5 feet; third, bowlders, 10 feet; fourth, gravel, 10 feet; fifth, sandrock, 10 feet—total, 55 feet. The rock in this instance is dense and very hard, light-colored, and of the same color as that on the rapids. The superficial strata of these rocks are light-colored, compact, with matted patches colored with oxide of iron, very hard to work, and withstand the weather most excellently. Beneath these it readily splits into thin layers, and there is more oxide of iron mixed with its constituents, so that on exposure it readily disintegrates and crumbles into a dark-red sand. Below it becomes hard again, has a dark brown color, and is more compact. Within the fort limits these several strata appear as follows, from the surface downward:

First. Soil, fine sand, infiltrated with a little clay from one to one and a half feet thick.

Second. A hard, compact ferruginous stratum, consisting of sand with clay and iron cement almost impervious to water, and difficult to disturb, except with a pick; depth, three inches to one foot. This almost totally prevents the water from percolating through to the loose lake sands of variable depths beneath, and hence wherever it is thickest, water stands until removed by evaporation, unless drained off by surface ditches.

Third. White sand, loose, pervious to water. In the lower parts of the garrison water may be obtained in it by sinking shallow wells, except during the drier seasons of the year. It appears to be the natural under-drainage of the swamp. Southwest of the officers' quarters, near the angle of the inclosure, and also along the Portage road in several places where the side ditches cut the dense stratum above, water comes to the surface; depth from two to three feet.

Fourth. A second dense stratum, consisting of white sand and clay and a little lime, moderately pervious to water, and rather hard to disturb with a spade simply; depth variable, from a few inches to one and a half feet.

Fifth. Lake sand of variable depth, extending down to the bowlders.

Sixth. Bowlders, infiltrated with sand and gravel to variable depths, extending down to the sandrock in places.

The inclination of the several strata is toward the river, but where the same have been cut away by the river at a former higher level, the bowlders appear very profusely on the surface. These bowlders are quite peculiar in their character; they consist of large granite, gneiss, greenstone, porphyritic trap, and other azoic water-worn masses, weighing in many instances more than 30 tons, with smaller rocks closely intervening, and the interstices filled with loose sand and gravel. Their general lithological characters would indicate that they had been transported from the north shore of Lake Superior, by glacial action, and that they had been subjected to very great attrition.

The shores of the lake and river exhibit terraces corresponding to the different water-levels of past periods. There are four of these on the river below the rapids and three above, which correspond with the terraces on the lake shore. The business part of the village of Sault Ste. Marie is built on the first, counting from the river. Fort Brady stands on the second river terrace, with an elevation above the first of from 10 to 12 feet. The bowlder ridge constitutes the second lake or third river terrace. All along the clay bluffs the last in the series may be distinctly seen. Those terraces may be traced nearly the whole length of the river, and, according to Messrs. Foster and Whitney, constitute one of the characteristic features of the Lake Superior shore.

Water is furnished to the garrison by water-carts. It is obtained from the river below the landing, where the slope of the river is such as to allow the carts to be driven into the stream about 150 feet, near the verge of the channel. The supply thus obtained is excellent. What is needed, however, is a more abundant supply, kept in reservoirs near the places where it is to be used for cooking and police purposes, and where, in the event of fires breaking out, it can be made available in their extinguishment. As the matter now stands, there is no adequate means of saving the garrison from a general conflagration if any one of the permanent buildings should take fire when the wind is in a favorable direction for the spreading of the flames. Lake water can be obtained and conducted to all the garrison grounds by a conduit not exceeding 4,300 feet in length; the fall

2 M P

would be approximately between two and three feet; and with suitable reservoirs the garrison could be abundantly supplied with pure water for all purposes at a moderate expense. With force-pumps or water-rams it could then be made available for any emergency. This subject needs special attention, for in four instances, within a short time, the post has been in danger of being burned out from causes arising within the military limits; and, in addition to this, the garrison is so near the middle of the village of Sault Ste. Marie, which is built in a shabby manner and with none but the simplest means of arresting fires, that it is at all times in danger of a general conflagration.

The barrack is a two-story building, 120 by 24 feet; has been recently refloored and repaired. Each man has a separate iron bedstead and about 280 cubic feet air-space. The ventilation is very defective.

The building is surrounded on all sides by a veranda 6 feet wide, and extending to the roof. Back of the main building, at a distance of 10 feet from the veranda, are the company kitchens, the two being connected by a covered passage-way, 6 feet wide. At a distance of 12 feet from the rear of the kitchens the company store and commissary rooms are located, being temporary structures of frame-work, weather-boarded. Still farther to the rear is the bakery, an old building erected in 1822 for a guard-house, constructed of hewn logs and weather-boarded. It is in a dilapidated condition, and should be replaced by a suitable structure, planned so as to be convenient and cleanly, and located where it will not endanger the other buildings in case of fire.

The guard-house is a small building one story high, situated to the west of the barracks, at a distance of 160 feet. It is divided into four apartments, the front half being in one room, and occupied by the guard, and the rear being divided into a prison-room and two small cells. It was erected in 1867; size 24½ by 20½ feet, with a porch, 4 feet wide, in front. During the winter months this porch is boarded up and three small windows introduced at the respective sides and ends, so as to shield the sentinel from the cold, and yet allow a watchful care of the grounds and buildings.

The commanding officer's quarters is a building 32 by 42¾ feet on the ground, and one and a half stories high, and contains four rooms, a hall, and two closets; having a porch, 6 feet wide, extending along the front and half of the north end. The second or attic story has but two rooms. To the rear, at a distance of 10 feet, is the kitchen, 12 by 20 feet, one story high. The building is situated near the bluff at the northwest part of the inclosure, and has a beautiful view of the river and Canadian shore.

South of the commanding officer's quarters, at a distance of 88 feet, is the building for the line and staff officers' quarters. It consists of a one and a half story building, 52 by 56 feet on the ground, with a porch, 6 feet wide, on the front.

It is divided through the middle, from front to rear, by a partition, extending from the ground floor to the attic, whereby the house is separated into two distinct parts, and on either side of which is a long hall, extending the whole length. The first floor of each side is divided into three rooms. To the rear, at a distance of 12 feet, is a covered passage-way leading to the kitchens, the latter being one story high and 15 by 15 feet, each, and under one roof, but separated by a hall, 4 feet wide, leading to the water-closet in the rear. The building was intended to accommodate two families. There are cellars under the kitchens only. The foundations of the main part are sunk but little below the surface of the ground, and hence during the winter months the buildings, more especially the line officers' quarters, are subject to being raised by the upheaval of the earth by the frost, whereby they are more or less damaged every season. They were erected in 1866, but the walls are now badly damaged, and will soon have to be repaired to make them habitable and look decent. Already the south end of the porch of the officers' quarters has become detached from the main building by the frost and considerably injured. In consequence of the drifting of the snow, the foundations receive but very little protection during the winter, and hence are subject to the direct action of the frost.

New officers' quarters, consisting of a two-story frame house, located south of and in a line with the other officers' quarters, have been recently completed and occupied. This structure, which constitutes two sets of quarters, is 44½ by 50½ feet, with a hall extending through the center from front to rear. Each set comprises a hall and six rooms, each about 15 feet square, and a pantry; coal-sheds, with water-closets, are attached in the rear. A veranda extends along the whole front. These quarters are lathed, plastered, and ceiled, weather-boarded, and have shingle roofs. Large cellars are underneath, but, owing to defective drainage, are half filled with water, rendering them useless.

The sinks of the officers' buildings, hospital, and barracks are all in bad condition for want of proper drainage and ventilation. In the spring they are nearly filled with water, which, as the warm weather comes on, drains away until the contents of the vaults become in some degree inspissated.

The garrison grounds are very inadequately drained. Nowhere within the Government reservation, except in the immediate vicinity of the commanding officer's quarters, can a cellar be excavated to the depth of three feet without having water stand in it more than two-thirds of the year. The cellar of the officers' quarters has not been dry for months, although it purports to be drained by a small conduit about two inches square, in sections, put in at the erection of the building, three years since. The garrison fields to the rear of the cemetery were cultivated in vegetables the past season, and, although an unusually dry one for this region, when the fall-rains commenced it was found difficult to secure the crop because of the grounds being covered with water.

At the Baptist Mission a well has been dug to the depth of twelve feet, with an unfailing supply of water, coming to within nine feet of the surface, or about two feet above the grounds in front of the officers' quarters. This indicates about the height of the surface-water of the swamp. Last spring the water stood to the depth of two feet for two months on the surface between the officers' quarters and the corner of the inclosure containing the springs. Underneath the hospital a cellar has been excavated to the depth of three feet, yet it is practically useless, for, in the first place, it is not deep enough to be of any service, and, in the next place, it is always wet.

Heretofore the slops from the company kitchens have been drained by an open ditch, less than two feet deep, round by the rear of the hospital toward the river, and those from the hospital take the same direction. In warm weather the stench arising from this ditch is intolerable, and in more southern localities would be productive of the greatest harm.

What is required, therefore, is a proper system of drainage, and it seems strange that a Government post like this should be occupied so long without any attention being given to this very important matter. A large sewer, sufficient to carry off all the kitchen slops of the barracks, the hospital, and the water falling from the roofs of the buildings and surface-water, as well as to drain the garrison privies, seems imperatively demanded.

The building used as a post-hospital being more than fifty years old, and very dilapidated, a new hospital was commenced June 10, 1874, and at the date of latest advices was expected to be ready for occupancy by the first of November.

The building is to be of wood, upon a stone foundation, one story in height, and 12 feet from floor to ceiling throughout. It is to contain one ward, for eight beds, 30 by 24 feet; dispensary and mess room, each 16 by 12 feet; isolation-ward, store-room, and matron's room, each 12 by 9 feet; and steward's room, 12 by 15 feet. A veranda, 8 feet wide, is to run along the entire front and the end of the ward. The outside of the building is to be boarded up and down, and lined within with tar-paper; the entire inside to be lathed and plastered. The windows are to be 18 inches above the floor, and those of the ward double. Those of the ward and front of the building are to be furnished with venetian shutters, painted green. The entire wood-work, outside and inside, is to be well painted with white lead.

Communication with Fort Brady is by water during the period of lake navigation; that is, from the first of May to the end of November. During the rest of the year it is overland, upon snow-shoes and dog-sledges. The mails are very irregular the year round, seldom arriving oftener than twice a week in the summer, and in winter New York papers are often three weeks old when they arrive. Accidents to the mails are not unfrequent. In September, 1873, the Western Union Telegraph Company established lines of communication from the village of Sault Ste. Marie with Marquette and Detroit.

*Meteorological report, Fort Brady, Mich., 1870–'74.*

| Month. | 1870–'71. | | | | 1871–'72. | | | | 1872–'73. | | | | 1873–'74. | | | |
|---|---|---|---|---|---|---|---|---|---|---|---|---|---|---|---|---|
| | Temperature. | | | Rain-fall in inches. | Temperature. | | | Rain-fall in inches. | Temperature. | | | Rain-fall in inches. | Temperature. | | | Rain-fall in inches. |
| | Mean. | Max. | Min. | | Mean. | Max. | Min. | | Mean. | Max. | Min. | | Mean. | Max. | Min. | |
| | ° | ° | ° | | ° | ° | ° | | ° | ° | ° | | ° | ° | ° | |
| July | | | | | | | | | 64.92 | 90* | 38* | 2.06 | 62.70 | 85* | 35* | 2.50 |
| August | | | | | | | | | 65.64 | 90* | 43* | 1.62 | 63.65 | 91* | 42* | 1.72 |
| September | | | | | | | | | 56.13 | 85* | 30* | 6.28 | 51.15 | 82* | 29* | 6.88 |
| October | 49.30 | 68 | 30 | ? | | | | | 44.05 | 68* | 28* | ? | 39.74 | 67* | 16* | 3.74 |
| November | 37.54 | 56 | 10 | ? | | | | | 28.77 | 54* | – 7* | ? | 23.89 | 44* | – 7* | 0.92 |
| December | 23.27 | 46 | –10 | 1.80 | | | | | 10.06 | 36* | –41* | ? | 26.31 | 45* | – 8* | 2.32 |
| January | 11.74 | 36 | –27 | ? | | | | | 7.54 | 36* | –42* | ? | 17.78 | 46* | –34* | 2.76 |
| February | 16.71 | 44 | –28 | ? | | | | | 7.51 | 32* | –47* | ? | 13.54 | 40* | –41* | 1.30 |
| March | 29.95 | 46 | 8 | 2.54 | | | | | 18.92 | 36* | –24* | ? | 20.73 | 53* | –15* | 1.32 |
| April | 38.70 | 55 | 24 | 1.78 | | | | | 37.13 | 65* | 18* | ? | 27.56 | 63* | –14* | 0.68 |
| May | 52.86 | 90 | 37 | 0.72 | | | | | 48.01 | 76* | 28* | 2.24 | 49.99 | 89* | 23* | 2.14 |
| June | | | | | | | | | 58.95 | 86* | 31* | 2.76 | 59.47 | 89* | 30* | 3.58 |
| For the year | | | | | | | | | 37.22 | 90* | –47* | ? | 38.04 | 91* | –41* | 29.86 |

* These observations are made with self-registering thermometers. The mean is from the standard thermometer.

*Consolidated sick-report, Fort Brady, Mich., 1870–'74.*

| Year | 1870–'71. | | 1871–'72. | | 1872–'73. | | 1873–'74. | |
|---|---|---|---|---|---|---|---|---|
| Mean strength { Officers | 6 | | 6 | | 4 | | 5 | |
| { Enlisted men | 73 | | 75 | | 82 | | 73 | |
| Diseases. | Cases. | Deaths. | Cases. | Deaths. | Cases. | Deaths. | Cases. | Deaths. |
| GENERAL DISEASES, A. | | | | | | | | |
| Typhoid fever | 2 | | | | | | | |
| Intermittent fever | 10 | | 12 | | 6 | | | |
| Other diseases of this group | 3 | | 1 | | 6 | | 2 | |
| GENERAL DISEASES, B. | | | | | | | | |
| Rheumatism | | | 8 | | 9 | | 4 | |
| Syphilis | 6 | | 1 | | 1 | | | |
| Consumption | | | 1 | | 3 | | | 1 |
| Other diseases of this group | | | 1 | | | | | |
| LOCAL DISEASES. | | | | | | | | |
| Catarrh and bronchitis | 13 | | 7 | | 17 | | 20 | |
| Pneumonia | | | | | 1 | | | |
| Pleurisy | 2 | | | | | | | |
| Diarrhœa and dysentery | 2 | | 4 | | 8 | | 2 | |
| Hernia | | | | | | | 1 | |
| Gonorrhœa | 3 | | 1 | | | | | |
| Other local diseases | 26 | | 30 | | 33 | | 23 | 1 |
| Alcoholism | 18 | | 10 | | 5 | | 3 | |
| Total diseases | 85 | | 76 | | 89 | | 55 | 2 |
| VIOLENT DISEASES AND DEATHS. | | | | | | | | |
| Drowning | | | | | | | | 2 |
| Other accidents and injuries | 14 | | 15 | | 14 | | 15 | 1 |
| Total violence | 14 | | 15 | | 14 | | 15 | 3 |

# CARLISLE BARRACKS, PENNSYLVANIA.

Carlisle Barracks is situated near the center of the Cumberland Valley, about midway between the north and south mountain spurs of the Allegheny range, which are at this point ten miles apart. Latitude, 40° 12′ north; longitude, 7′ west; height above the sea, 500 feet. The post is exposed to the northwest wind, coming from the mountains about five miles distant; but its other aspects are in some degree protected by woods and by the town of Carlisle, situated on a slight eminence, half a mile off.

The underlying rock of the vicinity is carboniferous limestone, which crops out at short and irregular intervals all over the eastern portion of the valley. All the cellars of the garrison are dug out of this solid rock.

The quarters for enlisted men consist of three brick buildings. Two of these are respectively 271 by 24 feet, and 251 by 24 feet, and two stories high. The third is a three-story building, including the basement; its first and second floors designed for married soldiers and their families, the remaining portion for armory and shops.

The officers' quarters consist of two-story brick buildings, in good condition, with kitchens and quarters for servants; also convenient yards in the rear. A commodious veranda for both stories extends along the whole front of the buildings. Ten sets of quarters consist each of parlor, dining-room, two bed-rooms, kitchen, servants' room, and a bath-room. These quarters are liberally supplied with hydrants.

The commandant's residence, a two-story brick building, with wings attached, is appropriately located, and, with the exception of gas, contains all modern improvements and appurtenances.

The guard-house, about 70 by 30 feet, was originally built for a powder-magazine; it is a brick vault, 6 feet thick; the summit of the arch is about 20 feet high in the clear.

Carlisle has been occupied as a military station almost continuously since the colonial period, yet was never provided with a separate hospital until 1864, when the present temporary structure was erected. It is badly located, on the edge of a marsh, and was not designed with any special adaptation to its use as a hospital.

The post of Carlisle Barracks was discontinued as a depot of recruits June 20, 1871, since which time it has been occupied only by a small detachment, as a guard. No repairs having been made for three years, the buildings, &c., are rapidly deteriorating.

*Meteorological report, Carlisle Barracks, Pa., 1870–'74.*

| Month. | 1870–'71. Temperature. | | | 1870–'71. Rain-fall in inches. | 1871–'72. Temperature. | | | 1871–'72. Rain-fall in inches. | 1872–'73. Temperature. | | | 1872–'73. Rain-fall in inches. | 1873–'74. Temperature. | | | 1873–'74. Rain-fall in inches. |
|---|---|---|---|---|---|---|---|---|---|---|---|---|---|---|---|---|
| | Mean. | Max. | Min. | | Mean. | Max. | Min. | | Mean. | Max. | Min. | | Mean. | Max. | Min. | |
| July | 76.61 | 96 | 57 | 8.70 | 73.83 | 90 | 56 | 4.76 | 79.16 | 97 | 68 | 6.88 | 78.16 | 96* | 50* | 4.70 |
| August | 72.71 | 91 | 55 | 4.64 | 75.05 | 97 | 56 | 8.92 | 77.72 | 94 | 60 | 3.12 | 71.99 | 95* | 51* | 8.91 |
| September | 65.01 | 88 | 40 | 5.90 | 58.67 | 79 | 34 | 2.54 | 67.26 | 97 | 44 | 2.81 | 64.73 | 91* | 35* | 2.81 |
| October | 52.48 | 75 | 32 | 4.44 | 52.53 | 76 | 28 | 3.44 | 50.92 | 80 | 28 | 4.88 | 50.32 | 70* | 17* | 5.40 |
| November | 40.37 | 66 | 21 | 1.76 | 38.17 | 62 | 20 | 4.32 | 36.59 | 56 | 14 | 3.84 | 34.68 | 56* | 14* | 2.16 |
| December | 30.78 | 58 | 3 | 3.40 | 26.44 | 44 | — 4 | 1.06 | 24.28 | 46 | —14 | 4.26 | 35.91 | 68* | 15* | 2.44 |
| January | 26.84 | 58 | 5 | 3.96 | 27.25 | 48 | 0 | 1.01 | 22.94 | 45 | —28 | 2.36 | 32.36 | 66* | 0* | 3.44 |
| February | 28.51 | 52 | — 1 | 4.35 | 27.62 | 50 | 0 | 1.34 | 26.29 | 50 | — 6 | 3.25 | 29.86 | 63* | — 6* | 2.80 |
| March | 43.44 | 64 | 29 | 4.76 | 31.57 | 61 | 8 | 1.65 | 33.48 | 53 | — 6 | 3.88 | 37.79 | 64* | 14* | 2.30 |
| April | 52.57 | 82 | 35 | 2.63 | 51.70 | 88 | 32 | 3.14 | 48.66 | 67^ | 28* | 4.54 | 42.62 | 67* | 23* | 4.08 |
| May | 62.49 | 92 | 39 | 3.49 | 65.53 | 92 | 46 | 3.10 | 59.99 | 90* | 38* | 4.18 | 60.72 | 91* | 38* | 2.60 |
| June | 70.93 | 92 | 58 | 3.40 | 73.64 | 94 | 52 | 4.50 | 72.64 | 95* | 45* | 2.43 | 75.21 | 100* | 45* | 1.80 |
| For the year | 51.87 | 96 | — 1 | 51.43 | 50.17 | 97 | — 4 | 39.78 | 49.99 | 97 | —28 | 46.43 | 51.19 | 100* | — 6* | 43.44 |

* These observations are made with self-registering thermometers. The mean is from the standard thermometer.

*Consolidated sick-report, Carlisle Barracks, Pa., 1870–'74.*

| Year | | 1870–'71. | | 1871–'72.* | | 1872–'73.† | | 1873–'74.‡ | |
|---|---|---|---|---|---|---|---|---|---|
| Mean strength { Officers | | 7 | | 5 | | ............ | | 1 | |
| { Enlisted men | | 222 | | 60 | | ............ | | 6 | |
| Diseases. | | Cases. | Deaths. | Cases. | Deaths. | Cases. | Deaths. | Cases. | Deaths. |
| GENERAL DISEASES, A. | | | | | | | | | |
| Typhoid fever | | 1 | | | | | | | |
| Intermittent fever | | 58 | | | 1 | | | | |
| Other diseases of this group | | 18 | | | | | | 1 | |
| GENERAL DISEASES, B. | | | | | | | | | |
| Rheumatism | | 22 | | | | | | | |
| Syphilis | | 12 | | | | | | | |
| Consumption | | 3 | | | 1 | | | | |

* July, 1871, only.     † No reports.     ‡ March and April, 1874, only.

*Consolidated sick-report, Carlisle Barracks, Pa., 1870–'74—Continued.*

| Year | 1870–'71. | | 1871–'72.* | | 1872–'73.† | | 1873–'74.‡ | |
|---|---|---|---|---|---|---|---|---|
| Mean strength { Officers | 7 | | 5 | | ......... | | 1 | |
| { Enlisted men | 222 | | 60 | | ......... | | 6 | |
| Diseases. | Cases. | Deaths. | Cases. | Deaths. | Cases. | Deaths. | Cases. | Deaths. |
| LOCAL DISEASES. | | | | | | | | |
| Catarrh and bronchitis | 32 | ..... | ..... | ..... | ..... | ..... | ..... | ..... |
| Pneumonia | 7 | 1 | ..... | ..... | ..... | ..... | ..... | ..... |
| Diarrhœa and dysentery | 82 | ..... | 12 | ..... | ..... | ..... | ..... | ..... |
| Gonorrhœa | 28 | ..... | 1 | ..... | ..... | ..... | ..... | ..... |
| Other local diseases | 110 | ..... | 3 | ..... | ..... | ..... | ..... | ..... |
| Alcoholism | 3 | 1 | 1 | ..... | ..... | ..... | ..... | ..... |
| Total disease | 376 | 3 | 18 | ..... | ..... | ..... | 1 | ..... |
| VIOLENT DISEASES AND DEATHS. | | | | | | | | |
| Gunshot wounds | 2 | ..... | ..... | ..... | ..... | ..... | ..... | ..... |
| Other accidents and injuries | 88 | ..... | 2 | ..... | ..... | ..... | 1 | ..... |
| Total violence | 90 | ..... | 2 | ..... | ..... | ..... | 1 | ..... |

*July, 1871, only.      † No reports.      ‡ March and April, 1874, only.

## FORT CARROLL, MARYLAND.

Fort Carroll was commenced in 1850, on Sollers's Point Flats, in the Patapsco River, eight miles below the city of Baltimore, in latitude 39° 15′ north, longitude 28′ east.

The works are in charge of an ordnance-sergeant.

---

## CLARK'S POINT, MASSACHUSETTS.

A fort was commenced in 1857 on Clark's Point, about three miles south of the city of New Bedford, latitude 41° 35′ north, longitude 6° 10′ east.

The reservation comprises sixty acres, and has a bountiful supply of water furnished by wells.

The principal buildings are, officers' quarters, of wood, one and a half stories high, 50 by 25 feet, containing five rooms, with kitchen and dining-room; one barrack, built of wood, without lath or plaster, 100 by 25 feet, one and a half stories high, with mess-room attached, much out of repair; hospital, of wood, two stories high, 28 by 22 feet, and guard-house, constructed of wood, 30 by 18 feet, one and a half stories high, both much out of repair.

---

## COLUMBUS ARSENAL, OHIO.

An arsenal of construction was established in 1863 in the northeastern suburbs of the city of Columbus. The extent of ground inclosed with the arsenal is seventy-seven and three-fourths acres.

The quarters of the commanding officer are of brick, 73 by 40 feet, two stories in height, and are divided into ten rooms.

The ordnance store-keeper's quarters are of brick, two stories high, 65 by 48 feet, containing eight rooms.

The barracks for enlisted men are of brick, two stories in height, 73 by 32 feet, divided into eleven rooms, of which two, 18 by 32 feet, are used as a hospital.

The guard-house is a one-story brick building, 25 by 22 feet, containing one room and three cells.

*Consolidated sick-report, Columbus Arsenal, Ohio, 1870–'74.*

| | 1870–'71. | | 1871–'72. | | 1872–'73. | | 1873–'74. | |
|---|---|---|---|---|---|---|---|---|
| Year | Cases. | Deaths. | Cases. | Deaths. | Cases. | Deaths. | Cases. | Deaths. |
| Mean strength { Officers | 2 | | 2 | | 1 | | 1 | |
| { Enlisted men | 24 | | 13 | | 13 | | 13 | |
| **GENERAL DISEASES, A.** | | | | | | | | |
| Small-pox and varioloid | | | 1 | | | | | |
| Remittent fever | | | 1 | | | | | |
| Intermittent fever | 5 | | 3 | | 1 | | 6 | |
| Diphtheria | | | 1 | | | | | |
| Other diseases of this group | 1 | | | | 1 | | 1 | |
| **GENERAL DISEASES, B.** | | | | | | | | |
| Rheumatism | | | 1 | | 1 | | | |
| Syphilis | 1 | | | 1 | | | | |
| Consumption | | 1 | 1 | 1 | | | | |
| **LOCAL DISEASES.** | | | | | | | | |
| Catarrh and bronchitis | 7 | | | | | | 1 | |
| Pneumonia | | | | | | | 1 | |
| Gonorrhœa | 2 | | | | | | | |
| Other local diseases | 7 | | | | 3 | | 2 | |
| Alcoholism | 1 | | | | | | | |
| Total disease | 24 | 1 | 8 | 2 | 6 | | 11 | |
| **VIOLENT DISEASES AND DEATHS.** | | | | | | | | |
| Accidents and injuries | 7 | | | | 1 | | 3 | |
| Total violence | 7 | | | | 1 | | 3 | |

# FORT COLUMBUS, GOVERNOR'S ISLAND, NEW YORK HARBOR.

## REPORT OF SURGEON J. J. MILHAU, UNITED STATES ARMY.

Governor's Island is situated in the upper bay of New York Harbor, at the entrance of the East River, about 1,000 yards south of the Battery, New York, and 6 miles north by east of the Narrows; latitude 40° 41' 5'' north; longitude 3° 2' 45'' east. Buttermilk Channel, a quarter of a mile wide, with sufficient water for the largest vessels, separates it on the south and southeast from the Atlantic docks, Brooklyn. A full account of the early settlement of the island by the Dutch, and its subsequent history, is given in Circular No. 4, Surgeon General's Office, December 5, 1870.

The island contains nearly 65 acres, has a circumference of about one mile and a quarter, with a mean elevation of 20 feet above the highest tides; in general contour it is somewhat egg-shaped, with the point looking to the northwest. The surface is covered by a luxuriant growth of grass with a good sod. While the eastern portion is level and shaded by fine trees, the western is without tree or bush, and is diversified only by the slopes of the glacis.

The soil is fertile, consisting of a clayey loam two feet in depth, with an underlying stratum of sand of about ten feet; below this the drift deposit entirely covers the basis rock to the depth of one hundred feet in some places.

The whole of Governor's Island is reserved by the United States for military purposes. The northern part is fenced off and occupied by the Ordnance Department as the " New York Arsenal." All the rest is embraced within the limits of the post of Fort Columbus, at present the principal depot of the general recruiting service.

Fort Columbus, a permanent stone work near the center of the island, contains four large buildings, constructed of stone and brick, with two stories and basements, and roofed with slate; a broad portico shelters the whole front of each building. The building on the west side of the parade is intended for officers' quarters, and divided into eight sets of two rooms and kitchen each. The rooms are from 14 to 15 by 19½ feet, with two windows in each. The two rooms of a set communicate by a door, only one of the rooms opening on the hall-way. The eight kitchens are in the basement, are dark, and very badly ventilated. There is but one hall-way and one stairway in common for four sets of quarters.

The other three buildings are for enlisted men.  Each is intended to quarter two small companies.  They are at present occupied by companies "A" and "C," permanent party, and "B," music boys.  The dormitories or squad rooms, orderly rooms, and company offices are on the first and second floors, are well lighted, and pretty well ventilated by doors and windows.  The larger dormitories contain either 16 or 18 single bunks, with an average allowance for each of 46 superficial feet and an air-space of nearly 450 cubic feet.  As one-quarter or more of the men are generally absent from their bunks by reason of being on guard, in hospital, or on leave, the air-space is materially increased for those remaining.  The mess-rooms, store-rooms, and kitchens, two sets in each building, are in the basements, and are dark and very badly ventilated.

Light iron stairways and balconies on the portico serve for communication between different parts of the building.

At each angle of the parade are two small pentagonal buildings two stories high.  Company tailors and married soldiers occupy the upper stories, while the ground floors are used, one for the bakery, one for the barber-shop, three for sculleries, and three for privies.

Castle William, completed in 1811, is prominently located on the northwest point of the island, and is a stone work with three tiers of casemates inclosing five-sixths of a circle, the rear being open.  This is the only structure at the post available as quarters for recruits and transient troops, but is ill adapted to the purpose on account of dampness and the difficulty of properly heating it and regulating the ventilation.

In the third tier the casemates are separated by thick walls which support the arched ceiling.  The rear of each is inclosed by a wooden partition with a door and two windows, and window-sashes are fitted into the embrasures.  The air-space in each is about 5,000 cubic feet, with sufficient floor-space for 16 single bunks, the number usually placed therein.  The prisoners and their guard occupy five of these casemates, while the others serve as quarters for recruits.  In the two lower tiers the casemates communicate by archways forming continuous galleries around the castle ; the lower one is paved, and a portion of it is used for messing when occasion requires.  The second tier, though occupied by guns, has frequently accommodated large numbers of men, the bedding being spread on the floor around the gun-carriages.  A frame building, 60 by 30 feet, in the interior court is fitted up with a large range, and serves as kitchen and mess-hall for the occupants of the castle.

The South Battery, a well-known land-mark, is a small triangular work, situated on the southerly point of the island.  The rear is inclosed by a two-story brick building, which is at present occupied by non-commissioned officers and their families, one room in it being reserved for the post-school and occasionally used as a Catholic chapel.

The band quarters are in a one-story frame building, with basement, located 25 yards east of the South Battery.  The dormitory, a single room, occupies the whole floor, and is 19 by 54 feet, and 11 feet high, and contains 20 single bunks.  The mess-room, 42 by 18½ feet, and the kitchen, with a cooking-range, are in the basement.

At the northeast corner of the post and near the wharf is located a two-story brick building, with front and rear piazzas and basement.  On the first and second floors are the offices of the commanding officer, adjutant, and clerks.  The basement is occupied as the guard-room for the main guard, and opens on a terrace which commands the landing and its approaches.  Prisoners are confined in Castle William.  Those sentenced to solitary confinement are placed in dark cells in the basement of one of the buildings in Fort Columbus.

Besides the quarters described as inside of the fort, the officers occupy three buildings facing to the west, and situated on the eastern part of the island.  The principal one, the commanding officer's quarters, 130 feet south of the adjutant's office, is a large double house, built of brick, with two stories, attic, and basement.  High and broad piazzas protect the front and rear.  There are four large rooms on the first floor, five on the second, and two in the attic, with kitchen and laundry in the basement.  The house is fitted up with bath-rooms, water-closets, furnace, and range.  The grounds attached contain fruit-trees and a good vegetable-garden.

The other two buildings are 50 feet south of the commanding officer's house, with a space of fifty feet between them.  They are frame cottages, 46 feet front by 36 feet deep, with two stories, attic, and basement, and piazzas front and rear. Each building is divided into two dwellings, with separate entrances, halls, and stairways. In each dwelling are, on the first floor, two rooms; on the second, two assignable rooms and two hall-rooms, and two finished rooms in the attic. The kitchen and store-rooms are in the basement. In the rear of each house a plot of ground, reaching nearly to the water, is fenced in for the cultivation of fruits and vegetables.

The post hospital and the grounds, inclosed by a picket-fence, occupy about five-sixths of an acre on the southeastern part of the island. (Figure 1.)

A, front entrance to main building; B, dispensary, 19 by 20 feet; C, surgeon's office, 12 by 20 feet; D, attendant's room, 12 by 20 feet; E, mess-room, 24 by 20 feet; F, pantry, 9 by 10 feet; G, kitchen, 19 by 20 feet; H, hall; I, east ward-building, 90 by 24 feet; J, west ward-building, 90 by 24 feet; K, court-yard, 100 by 42 feet; L, nurse's room, 9 by 12½ feet; M, vestibule, 11 by 13 feet, with small closet adjoining; N, smoking-room, 9 by 9 feet, with small closet adjoining; O, nurse's-room, 9 by 12½ feet; P, covered way, 5 feet wide; Q R S, veranda, 7 feet wide; T T T, wells and cisterns; U V, water-closets, 8 by 9 feet; W, dead-house; X, sea-wall; Y and Z, underground drains.

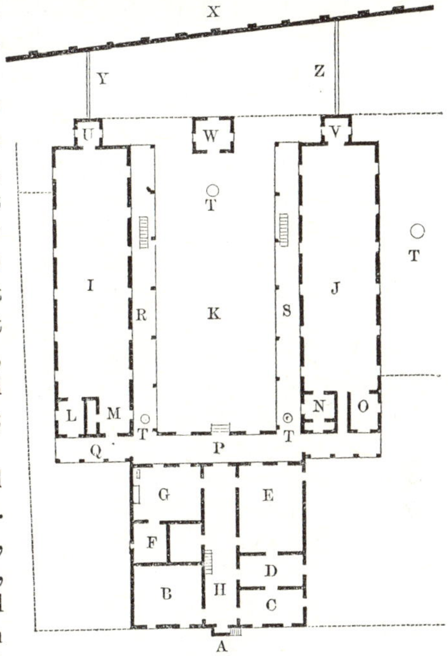

The administration-building, built in 1840, is constructed of brick, with two stories and basement, and roofed with tin. A high granite stoop in front gives access to the first floor, which is divided by a hall, 9 feet wide, into two large rooms, 48 by 20½ feet each. These rooms were originally intended as wards for patients, but for want of proper ventilation are not adapted to the purpose. They are at present used

Figure 1.

for the examination of recruits, and occasionally for entertainments, such as balls, concerts, &c. The second floor is divided off into five rooms, which are used as wards for the treatment of special cases, store-rooms, and occasionally as quarters for medical officers and hospital-stewards temporarily at the post. The largest room has a bath-room and a water-closet attached. The basement is reached by descending a flight of four steps under the front stoop. A hall, 9 feet wide, divides it through the center. On the right is the surgeon's office, supplied with desk, tables, and book-case, an attendant's room, and the mess-hall. On the left, the dispensary, very fully fitted up, and the kitchen, with cooking-range boiler, sink, pump, &c. In the rear of the basement an inclosed covered way communicates with the front of the two wards, enabling patients to reach the mess-hall without unnecessary exposure.

The wards are two frame pavilions, built in 1874 from the material obtained by taking down the general hospital described in Circular No. 4 of 1870. They are located in rear of the administrative building, on ground sloping toward the water. Each pavilion is 90 by 24 feet, with a ceiling of 12 feet, and a veranda, 7 feet wide, on front and inner side. The walls are filled in with brick, lathed and plastered on the inside, and the floor is deadened. Thirteen feet at the northern end of the building is partitioned off and divided into a vestibule or hall-way, an attendant's room, and a knapsack-closet. In the west ward there is, in addition, a smoking-room. The ward proper is 77 by 24 feet, with twelve full-sized windows, admitting favorable location for twenty-four beds; but it is the intention to limit the number of patients to twenty, so that each may enjoy an air-space of over 1,100 cubic feet, and an area of 92 superficial feet. Each ward is heated by two stoves, with the pipes running up through metal-shaft ventilators. Additional ventilation is secured by large openings in the ceiling, communicating directly with the outer air through open boxes placed along the ridge of the roof. The water-closets and lavatories are in a projection of 9 by 8 feet at the southern end. Under the southern end of each building there is a basement, 30 by 24 feet, which, owing to the grade, is almost entirely out of ground. Under the west ward the basement contains, first, the laundry, supplied with range, boiler, pump, and stationary tubs;

second, a bath-room, with hot and cold water; and, third, a small store-room. That under the east ward contains a store-room and the coal-bins. In the basement of the projections are the privies for the convalescents.

The dead-house, located at the foot of the court, is on the same level with the basements of the wards, and hence does not intercept the view or the breezes; it is lighted by skylights. Quarters for the steward and for the two matrons have been very comfortably fitted up in a building which formed a part of the old general hospital.

The hospital barn and stable is outside of the inclosure near the water; it contains stalls for four animals and a hay-mow. All the frame buildings of the hospital are covered with gravel roofing. Drain-pipes connect the water-closets and privies with tide-water. The reconstruction of the hospital buildings and the laying out of the grounds have involved a great deal of labor, which, the plumbing and roofing excepted, was performed entirely by soldiers under the immediate super-vision of Assistant Surgeon A. H. Hoff, United States Army, to whom should be accorded the full credit of having successfully completed the work.

The post library, the court-martial room, and the billiard-room are contained in a low brick building, 100 by 25 feet, situated next to the adjutant's office.

The commissary and quartermaster's storehouse is a brick building, 50 by 40 feet, situated between the adjutant's office and the commanding officer's house.

The blacksmith-shop, the carpenter-shop, the paint-shop, and the quartermaster's stables are frame buildings situated on the southeastern part of the island near the water. The post bakery occupies one of the pentagonal buildings within the fort, and is supplied with two ovens, with an aggregate capacity of 800 rations.

Laundress quarters, a long frame building of one story and attic, with piazzas front and rear, was put up in 1871 near the South Battery and to the west of it. The building is divided off into 16 sets of neat and comfortable quarters, each set having two rooms 12 by 12 feet on the first floor and two similar ones in the attic.

The chapel, a neat gothic frame structure, is situated in a grove 25 yards north of the South Battery; it is capable of seating about 150 persons. On the southwestern part of the island half an acre of ground, inclosed by an iron fence, has long served as the resting-place of the remains of those dying on the island. Within the last year further interments in it have been interdicted, and the bodies of soldiers are now escorted to New York and placed in charge of the undertaker for burial in the Cypress Hill National Cemetery, Long Island.

Privies for the men are placed over the water at several points along the shore, and the excreta carried off by the tides. The privies in rear of the officers' cottages are over small hopper-shaped pits, from the bottom of which drain-pipes run to the water. Within the fort are three sinks, two of them attached to the officers' quarters; they require to be emptied every two or three years by nightmen from the city, and, though disinfected daily with copperas, and but little used, they are frequently very offensive. A recommendation has been made to have a large sewer constructed from the interior of the fort to the water, through which all foul matters might be carried off directly into the bay.

The rain-fall is collected from nearly all the buildings, and stored in cisterns located near them. When, for want of sufficient rain, these cisterns become empty, which happens frequently during the year, they are thoroughly cleansed and fumigated, and then filled up with Croton water brought over in the tanks of the quartermaster's steamer. There are several wells on the island; the water from all of them is quite hard, containing an undue amount of magnesia and lime-salts. The per-manganate test shows the presence of but a small percentage of organic matter. While the water from two of the wells is pleasant to the taste, that from the others is more or less brackish. The water from any of the wells produces, in some persons, gastric derangement, and there is reason to believe that its use during the prevalence of diseases affecting the bowels is decidedly injurious. It is to be hoped that the day is not far distant when the importance of having an abundant sup-ply of good water on the island will be fully recognized. A submarine tube connecting with the mains of either New York or Brooklyn would effect the object.

Owing to the peculiar location of the island, each tide washes up on its shores carcases, offal, and floating *débris* of every description, including mattresses, matting, and a variety of articles thrown overboard from the shipping in the harbor. Although this material is daily disposed of by burning or burying, it is evident that a portable disease can thus be communicated to the occupants of the island through *fomites* coming directly from an infected vessel. Were the island entirely surrounded by a sea-wall, built near the low-water line, the danger of having diseases introduced in this manner would be averted. Some portions of the island are already protected by a permanent sea-wall of granite, and it is the intention of the engineers to continue the work as soon as they can obtain appropriations for the purpose. The proximity of populous cities calls for the early completion of this protection against the introduction of diseases liable to become epidemic.

The boat-houses afford limited facilities for salt-water bathing. During the summer the men bathe on the west beach after sundown, generally twice a week. For recruits a bathing-room, with hot and cold water, is attached to the castle.

The police of the post is generally very good. The slops and garbage are kept in barrels, which are emptied into the bay twice a day. The beach is regularly policed once or twice daily. A liberal use of copperas in solution is made daily in all places requiring disinfection.

By means of a stationary-engine on the dock, and a hose, all silt-basins, sewers, and drains are frequently flushed out with salt-water, at least once a week in summer.

Communication with New York is frequent and easy, though occasionally interrupted by ice or by fogs. Besides the post barge and the quartermaster's steamer, which make several trips a day, a small steam propeller, owned by private parties, runs regularly every hour during the day till sundown from the barge-office in New York.

Since 1870 a number of sanitary improvements have been made, including the removal of old dilapidated buildings, and filling up and closing of cesspools, laying of drains, &c.

*Meteorological report, Fort Columbus, New York Harbor, 1870-'74.*

| Month. | 1870-'71. Temperature. Mean. | Max. | Min. | Rain-fall in inches. | 1871-'72. Temperature. Mean. | Max. | Min. | Rain-fall in inches. | 1872-'73. Temperature. Mean. | Max. | Min. | Rain-fall in inches. | 1873-'74. Temperature. Mean. | Max. | Min. | Rain-fall in inches. |
|---|---|---|---|---|---|---|---|---|---|---|---|---|---|---|---|---|
| July | 76.03 | 93 | 60 | 3.93 | 72.16 | 87 | 60 | 4.22 | 77.27 | 97* | 62* | 8.35 | 76.06 | 94* | 58* | 3.64 |
| August | 74.96 | 90 | 62 | 3.98 | 73.91 | 87 | 63 | 7.60 | 75.56 | 93* | 54* | 7.68 | 73.28 | 88* | 51* | 8.28 |
| September | 68.16 | 82 | 56 | 1.79 | 62.22 | 81* | 39* | 2.30 | 66.22 | 92* | 49* | 2.57 | 67.10 | 87 | 45* | 2.73 |
| October | 57.53 | 74 | 37 | 5.88 | 56.20 | 73* | 31* | 6.44 | 53.33 | 74* | 35* | 1.76 | 57.51 | 78* | 30* | 2.32 |
| November | 45.14 | 63 | 30 | 2.97 | 40.45 | 62* | 17* | 3.88 | 40.88 | 59* | 15* | 3.83 | 38.76 | 60* | 20* | 4.32 |
| December | 34.67 | 56 | 10 | 1.97 | 29.92 | 54* | −3* | 2.24 | 28.10 | 47* | 3* | 3.77 | 36.84 | 64* | 19* | 4.81 |
| January | 28.41 | 49 | 4 | 2.76 | 29.87 | 49* | 7* | 2.03 | 27.12 | 49* | 0* | 6.32 | 34.95 | 59* | 11* | 3.28 |
| February | 29.43 | 50 | −3 | 3.95 | 30.68 | 54* | 13* | 2.16 | 28.48 | 46* | −2* | 4.00 | 31.20 | 66* | 7* | 2.01 |
| March | 42.74 | 65 | 32 | 5.39 | 31.09 | 58* | 2* | 4.53 | 35.72 | 52* | 12* | 2.33 | 38.58 | 58* | 13* | 7.92 |
| April | 51.80 | 77 | 35 | 2.66 | 49.94 | 78* | 28* | 2.29 | 46.12 | 68* | 35* | 4.78 | 42.29 | 62* | 19* | 2.06 |
| May | 59.78 | 87 | 45 | 3.83 | 62.30 | 90* | 40* | 2.77 | 58.20 | 83* | 40* | 4.40 | 58.13 | 88* | 31* | 3.15 |
| June | 68.31 | 87 | 58 | 6.25 | 70.82 | 94* | 54* | 2.60 | 70.80 | 95* | 51* | 1.12 | 70.92 | 94* | 50* | |
| For the year | 52.58 | 93 | −3 | 45.36 | 50.79 | 94* | −3* | 43.06 | 50.65 | 97* | −2* | 50.91 | 52.13 | 94* | 7* | 47.43 |

* These observations are made with self-registering thermometers. The mean is from the standard thermometer.

*Consolidated sick-report, (white troops,) Fort Columbus, New York Harbor, 1870-'74.*

| Year | 1870-'71. Cases. | Deaths. | 1871-'72. Cases. | Deaths. | 1872-'73. Cases. | Deaths. | 1873-'74. Cases. | Deaths. |
|---|---|---|---|---|---|---|---|---|
| Mean strength { Officers / Enlisted men | 8 / 627 | | 7 / 589 | | 8 / 529 | | 10 / 439 | |
| **GENERAL DISEASES, A.** | | | | | | | | |
| Small-pox and varioloid | 3 | 1 | 5 | 2 | | | | |
| Cerebro-spinal fever | | | 2 | 1 | | | | |
| Typhoid fever | 2 | 1 | 3 | | 6 | | 1 | |
| Remittent fever | | | 2 | | 8 | | 3 | |
| Intermittent fever | 71 | | 68 | | 96 | | 80 | |
| Yellow fever | 105 | 43 | | | | | | |
| Other diseases of this group | 144 | 1 | 45 | | 96 | | 42 | |

*Consolidated sick-report, (white troops,) Fort Columbus, New York Harbor, 1870–'74.—Continued.*

| Year | 1870–'71. | | 1871–'72. | | 1872–'73. | | 1873–'74. | |
|---|---|---|---|---|---|---|---|---|
| Mean strength   { Officers | 8 | | 7 | | 8 | | 10 | |
|           { Enlisted men | 627 | | 589 | | 529 | | 439 | |
| Disease. | Cases. | Deaths. | Cases. | Deaths. | Cases. | Deaths. | Cases. | Deaths. |
| GENERAL DISEASES, B. | | | | | | | | |
| Rheumatism | 27 | | 24 | | 54 | | 59 | |
| Syphilis | 34 | | 17 | | 37 | | 31 | |
| Consumption | 1 | 3 | 5 | 2 | 7 | 1 | 3 | |
| Other diseases of this group | 3 | | 2 | 2 | 5 | | 4 | |
| LOCAL DISEASES. | | | | | | | | |
| Catarrh and bronchitis | 256 | | 103 | | 267 | | 158 | |
| Pneumonia | 2 | | 6 | 1 | 1 | | 3 | 1 |
| Pleurisy | | | 3 | | | | 1 | |
| Diarrhœa and dysentery | 494 | | 96 | 1 | 255 | | 264 | |
| Hernia | | | 6 | | 2 | | | |
| Gonorrhœa | 59 | | 8 | | 68 | | 62 | |
| Other local diseases | 381 | 2 | 167 | 1 | 432 | 3 | 321 | 2 |
| Alcoholism | 34 | | 20 | | 29 | | 25 | |
| Total disease | 1,616 | 51 | 582 | 10 | 1,363 | 4 | 1,057 | 3 |
| VIOLENT DISEASES AND DEATHS. | | | | | | | | |
| Gunshot wounds | 1 | 1 | 1 | | | | | |
| Drowning | | 1 | | | | | | |
| Other accidents and injuries | 118 | | 67 | 1 | 122 | | 74 | 1 |
| Total violence | 119 | 2 | 68 | 1 | 122 | | 74 | 1 |

*Consolidated sick-reports, (colored troops,) Fort Columbus, New York Harbor, 1870–'74.*

| Year | 1870–'71.* | | 1871–'72.† | | 1872–'73. | | 1873–'74.† | |
|---|---|---|---|---|---|---|---|---|
| Mean strength   Enlisted men | 21 | | 18 | | 7 | | 8 | |
| Diseases. | Cases. | Deaths. | Cases. | Deaths. | Cases. | Deaths. | Cases. | Deaths. |
| GENERAL DISEASES, A. | | | | | | | | |
| Small-pox and varioloid | 1 | | 1 | | | | | |
| Typhoid fever | 1 | | | | | | | |
| Intermittent fever | 1 | | 2 | | 1 | | | |
| Other diseases of this group | 4 | 1 | | | 3 | | 1 | |
| GENERAL DISEASES, B. | | | | | | | | |
| Rheumatism | 2 | | | | 1 | | | |
| Syphilis | 4 | | 1 | | 1 | | | |
| Consumption | | | 1 | | 2 | | | |
| Other diseases of this group | 1 | | 1 | | | | | |
| LOCAL DISEASES. | | | | | | | | |
| Catarrh and bronchitis | 17 | | 6 | | 5 | | 2 | |
| Diarrhœa and dysentery | 6 | | 6 | | 5 | | 2 | |
| Gonorrhœa | 6 | | 1 | | 1 | | 2 | |
| Other local diseases | 16 | | 8 | | 8 | | 6 | |
| Unclassified | 1 | | | | | | | |
| Total disease | 59 | 1 | 27 | | 27 | | 13 | |
| VIOLENT DISEASES AND DEATHS. | | | | | | | | |
| Accidents and injuries | 4 | | 4 | | 2 | | 2 | |
| Total violence | 4 | | 4 | | 2 | | 2 | |

*10 months only.        †11 months only.

# FORT CONSTITUTION, NEW HAMPSHIRE.

This post was established in 1808, on a peninsula of Great Island, forming the most eastern point of New Hampshire, at the entrance to the harbor of Portsmouth, from which city it is distant about three miles. The reservation is a rocky ledge of about six acres, within 300 yards of the main channel of entrance.   United States troops were first stationed here in 1806, in an old earthwork erected by the English government, and named William and Mary.   The fort stands in latitude 43° 4′ north, longitude 6° 14′ east.

The quarters, hospital, &c., are wooden buildings, most of which are old and out of repair. Good water is obtained from two wells, dug to the depth of 12 and 20 feet.

The post is in charge of an ordnance-sergeant.

----

## DAVIDS ISLAND, NEW YORK.

Davids Island is situated at the southwestern extremity of Long Island Sound, latitude 40° 54′ north, longitude 3° 20′ east, distant twenty-seven miles from the Battery, and one and a half miles southwest of New Rochelle, in the State of New York.   It was first established as a hospital-station in 1861, and extensive buildings of a temporary character were put up—frame structures, with roofs of felt and gravel—which are now all more or less out of repair.   The island having been purchased by the United States, was, in 1869, made a sub-depot for the reception of recruits.   It has been abandoned and re-occupied several times, and was last discontinued as a post October 1, 1874.

The buildings are old and in bad condition; but as a site for a recruiting depot, a military prison, or a hospital, this island presents special advantages.

*Consolidated sick-report, Davids Island, New York Harbor, 1870–'74.*

| Year | | 1870–'71. | | 1871–'72. | | 1872–'73. | | 1873–'74. | |
|---|---|---|---|---|---|---|---|---|---|
| Mean strength | { Officers | 30 | | 27 | | 7 | | 8 | |
| | { Enlisted men | 670* | | 376 | | 94† | | 79 | |
| Diseases. | | Cases. | Deaths. | Cases. | Deaths. | Cases. | Deaths. | Cases. | Deaths. |
| GENERAL DISEASES, A. | | | | | | | | | |
| Small-pox and varioloid | | 3 | | | | | | | |
| Typhoid fever | | | | | 1 | | | | |
| Typho-malarial fever | | | | | 1 | | | | |
| Remittent fever | | 31 | | 20 | | | | | |
| Intermittent fever | | 154 | | 79 | | 19 | | 4 | |
| Other diseases of this group | | 89 | 1 | 52 | | 2 | | 2 | |
| GENERAL DISEASES, B. | | | | | | | | | |
| Rheumatism | | 83 | | 84 | | 15 | | 18 | |
| Syphilis | | 90 | | 27 | | 4 | | 4 | |
| Consumption | | 1 | 1 | | 2 | 1 | | | |
| Other diseases of this group | | 18 | 1 | 1 | | | | | |
| LOCAL DISEASES. | | | | | | | | | |
| Catarrh and bronchitis | | 376 | | 193 | | 79 | | 26 | |
| Pneumonia | | 4 | | 1 | 1 | | | | |
| Pleurisy | | 28 | | 18 | | | | | |
| Diarrhœa and dysentery | | 234 | 1 | 234 | | 25 | | 16 | |
| Hernia | | | | 6 | | | | | |
| Gonorrhœa | | 41 | | 23 | | 4 | | 4 | |
| Other local diseases | | 469 | | 311 | 1 | 39 | | 42 | |
| Alcoholism | | 49 | | 24 | | | | 1 | |
| Unclassified diseases | | 24 | | | | | | | |
| Total disease | | 1,694 | 4 | 1,073 | 6 | 188 | | 117 | |
| VIOLENT DISEASES AND DEATHS. | | | | | | | | | |
| Gunshot wounds | | 3 | | | | | | | |
| Drowning | | | | | | | | | 1 |
| Other accidents and injuries | | 146 | | 140 | | 15 | | 14 | |
| Total violence | | 149 | | 140 | | 15 | | 14 | 1 |

* No reports July, August, September, 1870; post not open.
† Discontinued July 5, 1872; no reports for July, August, September, October, 1872.

## FORT DELAWARE, DELAWARE.

Fort Delaware is situated on Pea-Patch Island, in the Delaware River, one and one-eighth miles distant from the Delaware shore, one mile from the New Jersey shore, and forty-two miles below the city of Philadelphia.  Latitude 39° 35′ 18″ north, longitude 1° 28′ 29″ east.

The island is a flat mud-bank, irregularly oval in form, and has an area of eighty acres.  Its average level is 3 feet 4 inches, and its highest point 9 feet 8 inches above mean low water.  It is surrounded by an embankment, faced with broken stone, 10 feet 10 inches above mean low water, and is drained by means of a net-work of ditches, through which the tide, which has an average of 6½ feet, is permitted to flood and ebb, under the control of two sluice-gates.  These ditches vary in width from 3 to 30 feet, and in depth from 8 inches below to 1 foot above mean low water.

Fort Delaware is placed midway between the center and the southern extremity of the island, and is a bastioned work of granite, lined with concrete brick.  Within the fortification are three brick buildings, three stories in height, and provided with painted iron roofs.  Their third floors are nearly on a level with the terre-plein, and communicate directly with it.

The largest of these buildings, constituting the barracks proper, is 279 feet long, 66 feet 6 inches wide, and 51 feet 6 inches high, from the parade to the crest of the roof.  The sally-port is in the center of this building.  The ground floor is divided into fifteen rooms, which are severally designed as subsistence store-rooms, mess-rooms, prison-rooms, kitchen and laundresses' quarters. The third floor has sixteen rooms, for quartermaster store-rooms, company offices, and laundresses' quarters.  The height of the first floor in the clear is 12 feet 6 inches; of the second, 12 feet 9 inches; and of the third, 13 feet 9 inches.  The kitchens, two in number, measure, respectively, 20 feet 6 inches by 19 feet 6 inches.  The mess-rooms are also two in number.  They are 39 feet long by 30 feet broad, and are immediately adjacent to the kitchens.  The floors of all the rooms on the first story are flagged.  There are four squad-rooms or dormitories, each 57 feet 6 inches long by 30 feet broad.  They are all furnished with ventilators, wash-sinks, pumps, &c.

One guard-room and three prison-rooms are situated in the second story of the barracks, above the sally-port.  The former measures 19 feet 9 inches by 13 feet; the latter, respectively, 13 feet by 8 feet 6 inches, 19 feet 9 inches by 10 feet, and 29 feet by 17 feet 9 inches.  In addition to these, there are two cells on the ground floor, one on each side of the main gate, each 6 feet 6 inches long, 5 feet 11 inches broad, and 10 feet high, and a prison-room 24 feet 6 inches by 14 feet 9 inches.  A bastion-room on the lower tier is set apart for the post bakery.

The two remaining buildings are designed for officers' quarters and for offices.  They are each 95 feet in length, 70 feet in depth, and 53 feet 6 inches in height, from the parade to the crest of the roof.  The height of the first floors in the clear is 13 feet; of the second, 13 feet; and of the third, 14 feet.  The ground floor of each building is divided into eight rooms, for offices and kitchens.  The second floor contains nine rooms, and the third eight, set apart for officers and their families.

The water-supply of the fort is principally derived from the fall of rain on the terre-plein.  The water from this source passes successively through six inches of sand, two feet of earth, nine inches of gravel, and several layers of brick, the vertical joints of which are open, to an arched brick gutter, whose bottom is covered with asphaltum.  From this gutter it runs through conduits, made in part of iron and in part of earthen-ware crocks, to filters placed, with the cistern to which each is attached, under the floor of the first tier of casemates.

The cisterns, twenty-two in number, are of various sizes.  Their aggregate capacity is 543,710⅔ gallons; and it has been estimated that the water-shed is sufficient to fill them three times annually.  They are built wholly of brick, lined throughout with hydraulic cement.

The rain that falls on the buildings inside the fort is conveyed to iron tanks placed a short distance under every roof.  The dimensions of these tanks are 12 feet by 8 feet by 4 feet.  There are six in the barracks and three in each of the other buildings. The water derived from those in the officers' quarters is used in the privies. The water from those in the barracks is conveyed to wash sinks situated in the second and in the third stories, and is chiefly used by the laundresses. The number of privies in the barracks is sixteen, equally divided between the first and the second floors. They communicate with the moat by means of a perpendicular well, 4 by 3 feet, which extends from the second story to the grillage of the foundation. In each of the other buildings there are three privies on the first and three on the second story, constructed on the same plan, but in addition having a supply of water from the tanks. The excrement from these privies passes into the moat through sixteen openings, each 4 feet long and 3 feet 8 inches high, and placed 2 feet above the bottom of the well. The drainage of the interior of the fort is secured by a large brick culvert, which discharges into the moat, and by tributary side-drains.

There are also a number of cottages outside the works for the use of officers and their families, married soldiers, and the employés of the Quartermaster's and Engineer Departments.

The hospital is situated 350 yards from the sally-port; is a wooden structure, placed upon brick piers, 3 feet 4 inches high, on the plan promulgated in Circular No. 4, Surgeon General's Office, 1867.

The post was evacuated in October, 1870, and turned over to the Engineer Department. For further description see Circular No. 4, Surgeon General's Office, 1870.

---

# DETROIT ARSENAL, MICHIGAN.

This arsenal was established in 1832, at Dearbornville, 10 miles west of the city of Detroit, in latitude 42° 20' north, longitude 6° 7' west, (approximately.) The reservation comprises 230 acres.

The quarters for officers are two buildings, constructed substantially of brick, two stories and basement in height, with slate roofs, and piazza, 10 feet wide, on three sides. They each contain 12 rooms, averaging 16 by 18 feet, and three attic-rooms, averaging 10 by 12 feet. For enlisted men there is one substantial brick building, 75 by 28 feet, two stories and basement in height, with slate roof, capable of accommodating 100 men.

The hospital is built of wood, 44 by 29 feet, one and a half stories high, and contains three rooms besides the dispensary. The guard-house is 35 by 18 feet, built of brick, one story high, with slate roof. It is used as an office.

*Consolidated sick-report, Detroit Arsenal, Mich., 1870-'74.*

| Year | | 1870-'71. | | 1871-'72. | | 1872-'73. | | 1873-'74. | |
|---|---|---|---|---|---|---|---|---|---|
| Mean strength | Officers | 1 | | 1 | | 1 | | 1 | |
| | Enlisted men | 15 | | 9 | | 8 | | 8 | |
| Diseases. | | Cases. | Deaths. | Cases. | Deaths. | Cases. | Deaths. | Cases. | Deaths. |
| GENERAL DISEASES, A. | | | | | | | | | |
| Typho-malarial fever | | 2 | | | | | | | |
| Remittent fever | | 19 | | 7 | | 5 | | | |
| Intermittent fever | | 7 | | 9 | | 5 | | 4 | |
| Other diseases of this group | | | | 1 | | 4 | | | |
| LOCAL DISEASES. | | | | | | | | | |
| Catarrh and bronchitis | | 2 | | 1 | | 1 | | 1 | |
| Pneumonia | | | | | | | | 3 | |
| Diarrhœa and dysentery | | 14 | | 2 | | 2 | | 4 | |
| Other local diseases | | 1 | | 1 | | | | 2 | |
| Total disease | | 45 | | 21 | | 17 | | 14 | |
| VIOLENT DISEASES AND DEATHS. | | | | | | | | | |
| Accidents and injuries | | 3 | 1 | 1 | | 1 | | | |
| Total violence | | 3 | 1 | 1 | | 1 | | | |

## DUTCH ISLAND, RHODE ISLAND.

Dutch Island was purchased for defensive purposes in 1863. It is situated in the western entrance to Narraganset Bay, between Conanicut Island and the western shore of the bay, latitude 41° 29′, longitude 5° 44′ east, 4½ miles west of Newport and 26 miles south from Providence.

The reservation includes the whole island, about 75 acres. There are no permanent buildings for quarters or hospital.

## FINN'S POINT, NEW JERSEY.

A battery was commenced in 1872 on Finn's Point, in the Delaware River, and is now in course of construction.

## FORT FOOTE, MARYLAND.

Fort Foote is situated on the Maryland side of the Potomac River, 8 miles below Washington and 3 miles below Alexandria, with both of which there is daily communication by steamboat. The post occupies an elevation of about 100 feet above tide-water, and commands the river for several miles in both directions, as the channel here runs close to the shore.

With the interior of the country there is communication by a road connecting with the main road leading across the Eastern Branch of the Potomac to Washington. During severe winters the garrison is frequently provisioned by stores sent over this route.

In the rear of the fort is an extensive ravine running in a northerly direction until it gets within about 500 yards of the river, when it flattens out into a large morass, loaded with all kinds of organic matter in every stage of decomposition, giving forth exhalations most prejudicial to the health of the garrison. Along the shore of the river this place assumes somewhat the form of a cove, acting as a receptacle for all the filth floating down the stream, which, being driven over the marsh by the tide, remains until destroyed by time. This piece of ground is overflowed by every high tide, leaving in all directions stagnant pools. It is believed that the malarial diseases prevailing at the post are largely due to the action of the sun's rays upon this large surface of decomposing organic matter. It has been thought by persons who have examined the locality that a moderate outlay would drain and protect this marshy tract, and transform it from a source of disease to a most valuable post-garden.

In the rear of the officers and company quarters there is a quite extensive forest, consisting principally of red and black oak, chestnut, beech, hickory, and maple. Many of the trees are old and hollow, affording comfortable homes for large numbers of gray squirrels, while their tops are the favorite resort of eagles, for the purpose of building their nests.

About a mile and a quarter below Fort Foote lies a flat and marshy piece of land of about two hundred acres, known as Broad Creek, where malaria, frequently of a most virulent character, prevails, not uncommonly making its appearance in a congestive form, sometimes of a very fatal character. Fortunately, between the fort and the marsh there intervenes an extensive belt of woods, which, in a great measure, protects the post.

The water-supply at this post is sufficient in quantity, but is rather defective in quality, containing a large proportion of organic and inorganic matter. The best water naturally at the post is a large spring, but in consequence of its proximity to the stables it is little used, except for police purposes. If the water used for cooking and drinking could be thoroughly filtered through some suitable apparatus, it would greatly mitigate the obstinate bowel complaints that prevail here during the hot season. Water for cleansing purposes is obtained from cisterns, and that used for drinking from a well 60 feet deep.

The original fortifications were of a temporary character, and are fast falling into decay. The work has been commenced to replace them by substantial works of masonry.

The buildings at the post consist of the officers' quarters, barracks, married soldiers' quarters, guard-house, hospital, storehouses, bake-house, and stables. These, with the exception of the stables, are all new and in good condition, built on a uniform plan, and containing all the modern arrangements for perfect ventilation. They are built of wood, painted of a warm brown color, with doors and windows white, which adds much to their appearance and durability.

The officers' quarters consist of two one-story buildings, each containing two sets of quarters. Each set of quarters contains one parlor 14 by 16 feet, one kitchen 17 by 10 feet, a dining-room same size as the parlor, and a bed-room. Under each kitchen is a cellar. The buildings are first class, and quite ornamental in appearance. Immediately around them are flower-gardens, while in front is a fine lawn, wide gravel-walks, some large trees, and a fine view of the river.

Distant from the officers' quarters about seventy yards, and on a parallel line, but a little farther back, are the company quarters, a two story building, 163 feet long, with verandas in front and rear. The upper floor is occupied by the dormitory, 162 by 23 feet, built for two companies, and affording more than sufficient air-space for one. During the past winter it was sufficiently heated by two coal-stoves. The first floor of the barracks contains the kitchen, 27 by 13 feet, with cook's room, 12 by 9, and store-room, 15 by 9, attached, a large dining-room, 48 by 23 feet, a reading-room, 49 by 11 feet, back of which is the wash-room, 22 by 11 feet, shoemaker-shop, 19 by 11 feet, and baker-shop, 12 by 11 feet. The southeast end of the first floor contains the company office and store-room, each 24 by 11 feet. All these rooms are 8¾ feet high. Under the building is a large cellar.

The quarters for married soldiers consist of five sets of quarters, each set containing two rooms, 20 by 14 by 9 feet, and 14 by 8 by 9 feet, respectively.

The guard-house consists of a guard-room, 18¼ by 15 feet, a prison-room of the same dimensions, and four cells, 7 by 4½ feet. It is badly lighted, and, in consequence of the thickness of the walls, insufficiently heated. The number of the prisoners, however, is generally small.

The hospital is a substantial, new, and well-ventilated building. The ward is well lighted and aired. Its internal dimensions are 32½ by 23½ and 12 feet high. The ceiling is lathed and plastered, with the exception of a strip 3 feet wide, which is latticed, and communicates with the roof ventilation. The flooring of the ward, and of the hospital generally, is very inferior, being made of green lumber, which has shrunk and left crevices in all directions, rendering it very difficult to keep properly warm in cold weather.

A good deal of attention is given to the post garden, but the soil, being a tenacious clay, is unsuited to the cultivation of many vegetables.

The site of the old cemetery having been selected for the erection of a battery, a new location has been chosen on the slope directly north of the officers' quarters. The ground has been cleared, and is to be inclosed and ornamented with suitable trees.

*Meteorological report, Fort Foote, Md., 1870–'74.*

| Month. | 1870–'71.† | | | | 1871–'72. | | | | 1872–'73. | | | | 1873–'74. | | | |
|---|---|---|---|---|---|---|---|---|---|---|---|---|---|---|---|---|
| | Temperature. | | | Rain-fall in inches. | Temperature. | | | Rain-fall in inches. | Temperature. | | | Rain-fall in inches. | Temperature. | | | Rain-fall in inches. |
| | Mean. | Max. | Min. | | Mean. | Max. | Min. | | Mean. | Max. | Min. | | Mean. | Max. | Min. | |
| | ° | ° | ° | | ° | ° | ° | | ° | ° | ° | | ° | ° | ° | |
| July | | | | | 72.72 | 90 | 55 | 3.37 | 81.12 | 100* | 70 | 0.86 | 77.94 | 94* | 58* | 4.93 |
| August | | | | | 75.39 | 91 | 62 | 2.38 | 78.98 | 95* | 56* | 5.88 | 73.86 | 92* | 55* | 8.37 |
| September | | | | | 58.63 | 91* | 37* | 2.50 | 67.85 | 94* | 47* | 4.34 | 66.52 | 89* | 43* | 1.63 |
| October | | | | | 52.04 | 73* | 31* | 3.00 | 54.83 | 76* | 32* | 4.15 | 53.31 | 78* | 26* | 3.52 |
| November | | | | | 42.03 | 67* | 22* | 3.22 | 39.95 | 59* | 15* | 2.37 | 39.29 | 63* | 21* | 2.40 |
| December | | | | | 30.43 | 61* | −2* | 1.19 | 28.00 | 53* | 4* | 2.33 | 38.61 | 67* | 18* | 0.76 |
| January | | | | | 29.91 | 59* | −2* | 0.70 | 29.38 | 65* | −5* | 3.31 | 37.90 | 68* | 8* | 1.60 |
| February | | | | | 31.78 | 60* | −2* | 0.98 | 32.79 | 58* | 4* | 4.36 | 35.30 | 72* | 16* | 0.95 |
| March | | | | | 34.49 | 69* | 4 | 5.34 | 39.34 | 66* | 5* | 0.87 | 43.56 | 68* | 22* | 1.93 |
| April | | | | | 54.60 | 87* | 29 | 2.13 | 52.19 | 84* | 38* | 2.33 | 46.31 | 67* | 23* | 5.75 |
| May | | | | | 67.04 | 90* | 47 | 2.21 | 62.23 | 88* | 44* | 4.34 | 63.03 | 86* | 38* | 2.44 |
| June | | | | | 74.78 | 95* | 58 | 3.42 | 73.54 | 93* | 44* | 1.86 | 75.65 | 97* | 50* | 1.81 |
| For the year | | | | | 51.99 | 95* | −2* | 30.44 | 53.35 | 100* | −5* | 37.00 | 54.27 | 97* | 8* | 36.09 |

* These observations are made with self-registering thermometers. The mean is from the standard thermometer.
† Not on file for this year.

*Consolidated sick-report, Fort Foote, Md., 1870–'74.*

| Year | | 1870–'71. | | 1871–'72. | | 1872–'73. | | 1873–'74. | |
|---|---|---|---|---|---|---|---|---|---|
| Mean strength | { Officers ........... | 3 | | 3 | | 2 | | 4 | |
| | { Enlisted men ...... | 59 | | 52 | | 49 | | 57 | |
| Diseases. | | Cases. | Deaths. | Cases. | Deaths. | Cases. | Deaths. | Cases. | Deaths. |
| GENERAL DISEASES, A. | | | | | | | | | |
| Remittent fever .................... | | 17 | ...... | 12 | ...... | ...... | ...... | 7 | ...... |
| Intermittent fever .................... | | 118 | ...... | 134 | ...... | 45 | ...... | 99 | ...... |
| Other diseases of this group .................... | | 1 | ...... | ...... | ...... | 7 | ...... | 1 | ...... |
| GENERAL DISEASES, B. | | | | | | | | | |
| Rheumatism .................... | | 8 | ...... | 6 | ...... | 14 | ...... | 27 | ...... |
| Syphilis .................... | | 11 | ...... | 3 | ...... | 9 | ...... | 4 | ...... |
| Consumption .................... | | ...... | 1 | 1 | ...... | ...... | ...... | ...... | ...... |
| Other diseases of this group .................... | | 3 | ...... | ...... | ...... | ...... | ...... | ...... | ...... |
| LOCAL DISEASES. | | | | | | | | | |
| Catarrh and bronchitis .................... | | 7 | ...... | 2 | ...... | 1 | ...... | 13 | ...... |
| Pleurisy ....... | | ...... | ...... | 1 | ...... | ...... | ...... | ...... | ...... |
| Diarrhœa and dysentery .................... | | 22 | 1 | 9 | ...... | 16 | ...... | 22 | ...... |
| Gonorrhœa .................... | | 4 | ...... | 1 | ...... | 3 | ...... | 1 | ...... |
| Other local diseases .................... | | 32 | ...... | 16 | ...... | 18 | 1 | 32 | ...... |
| Alcoholism .................... | | 8 | ...... | 4 | ...... | 17 | ...... | 32 | ...... |
| Total disease .................... | | 231 | 2 | 189 | ...... | 130 | 1 | 238 | ...... |
| VIOLENT DISEASES AND DEATHS. | | | | | | | | | |
| Gunshot wounds .................... | | 1 | ...... | ...... | ...... | ...... | ...... | ...... | ...... |
| Other accidents and injuries .................... | | 27 | ...... | 21 | ...... | 22 | ...... | 13 | ...... |
| Total violence .... .................... | | 28 | ...... | 21 | ...... | 22 | ...... | 13 | ...... |

# FRANKFORD ARSENAL, PENNSYLVANIA.

This is an arsenal of construction established in 1816. It is located in the twenty-third ward of the city of Philadelphia, at the confluence of the Frankford Creek and Delaware River, having a front on each.

The quarters consist of three two-story brick houses, with capacity for four officers in all. The barracks are a two-story brick building, capable of accommodating one hundred single men, and two buildings occupied by twelve enlisted men and their families.

The building used as a hospital has four beds, a dispensary, and quarters for a matron. There is a guard-house, built of brick, containing a guard-room and four cells for prisoners, all well lighted and aired.

*Consolidated sick-report, Frankford Arsenal, Pa., 1870–'74.*

| Year | | 1870–'71. | | 1871–'72. | | 1872–'73. | | 1873–'74. | |
|---|---|---|---|---|---|---|---|---|---|
| Mean strength | { Officers ........... | 4 | | 4 | | 4 | | 4 | |
| | { Enlisted men ...... | 49 | | 30 | | 30 | | 31 | |
| Diseases. | | Cases. | Deaths. | Cases. | Deaths. | Cases. | Deaths. | Cases. | Deaths. |
| GENERAL DISEASES, A. | | | | | | | | | |
| Remittent fever .................... | | | | | | | | 1 | ...... |
| Intermittent fever .................... | | 8 | ...... | 2 | ...... | 5 | ...... | 9 | ...... |
| Other diseases of this group .................... | | 6 | ...... | 1 | ...... | 1 | ...... | ...... | ...... |
| GENERAL DISEASES, B. | | | | | | | | | |
| Rheumatism .................... | | 3 | ...... | ...... | ...... | ...... | ...... | ...... | ...... |
| Syphilis .................... | | 2 | ...... | 1 | ...... | ...... | ...... | ...... | ...... |
| LOCAL DISEASES. | | | | | | | | | |
| Catarrh and bronchitis .................... | | 13 | ...... | 5 | ...... | 2 | ...... | 3 | ...... |
| Pneumonia .................... | | 8 | ...... | ...... | ...... | ...... | ...... | ...... | ...... |
| Pleurisy .................... | | ...... | ...... | ...... | ...... | ...... | ...... | 1 | ...... |
| Diarrhœa and dysentery .................... | | 7 | ...... | 3 | ...... | 3 | ...... | 2 | ...... |

*Consolidated sick-report, Frankford Arsenal, Pa., 1870-'74—Continued.*

| Year | | 1870-'71. | | 1871-'72. | | 1872-'73. | | 1873-'74. | |
|---|---|---|---|---|---|---|---|---|---|
| Mean strength | Officers | 4 | | 4 | | 4 | | 4 | |
| | Enlisted men | 49 | | 30 | | 30 | | 31 | |
| Diseases. | | Cases. | Deaths. | Cases. | Deaths. | Cases. | Deaths. | Cases. | Deaths. |
| LOCAL DISEASES—Continued. | | | | | | | | | |
| Gonorrhœa | | 3 | ...... | ...... | ...... | ...... | ...... | ...... | ...... |
| Other local diseases | | 61 | ...... | 18 | 1 | 22 | ...... | 16 | 1 |
| Alcoholism | | 1 | ...... | ...... | ...... | 2 | ...... | ...... | ...... |
| Total disease | | 112 | ...... | 30 | 1 | 35 | ...... | 32 | 1 |
| VIOLENT DISEASES AND DEATHS. | | | | | | | | | |
| Accidents and injuries | | 6 | ...... | 6 | ...... | 4 | ...... | 11 | ...... |
| Total violence | | 6 | ...... | 6 | ...... | 4 | ...... | 11 | ...... |

# GERRISH'S ISLAND, MAINE.

A battery was commenced in June, 1873, on Gerrish's Island, Me., in the harbor of Portsmouth, N. H.

---

# FORT GORGES, MAINE.

This fort, commenced in 1857, is located on Hog Island Ledge, in Portland Harbor, latitude 43° 39' north, longitude 6° 43' east. The works are undergoing extensive modifications.

---

# FORT GRATIOT, PORT HURON, MICHIGAN.

REPORTS OF ASSISTANT SURGEONS M. K. TAYLOR AND W. M. NOTSON, UNITED STATES ARMY.

Fort Gratiot is situated on the west bank of the Saint Clair River, about 1,300 feet south of the forty-third parallel, in longitude 5° 21' west. The distance from the fort to the light-house, at the foot of Lake Huron, is three-quarters of a mile, and the general direction north-northeast. Elevation above the sea 598 and above the lake 20 feet. North of the post, and adjoining the reservation, is the village of Gratiot, containing about 500 inhabitants. In the report made for Circular No. 4, Port Huron was stated to be one mile distant. At this writing, September, 1874, Port Huron, a city of 10,000 inhabitants, is built up to the grounds adjoining the post and rapidly progressing. New streets have been opened and two street-railways now in operation connect the city with the village of Gratiot, one company running immediately in front of the fort and the other along the west line of its inclosure. The Detroit branch of the Grand Trunk Railroad passes in the vicinity of the post. For history of the post see Circular No. 4, page 120.

All the wells sunk in the vicinity pass through the following formations from above downward: 1. Soil and yellow sand, 8 to 12 feet; 2. Compact blue clay, 85 to 100 feet; 3. Vein of coarse sand and gravel, 1 to 10 feet; 4. Limestone shale, intercalated with thin veins of sand and gravel, 875 feet; making a total depth of 1,000 feet. Immediately beneath the strata of blue clay immense quantities of gas have escaped in many places, and continued to do so even after the lapse of twenty-five years; and, at the depth of two or three feet in the limestone shales, pure water has always been obtained, which has risen in the wells about to the level of Lake Huron, or within ten to twenty feet of the surface of the earth. At the depth of about 500 feet salt-water veins were struck, with a supply and strength quite sufficient to warrant investments for the manufacture of that commodity. The soil is mostly a sandy loam, and the proportion of marsh is small. Most of the surrounding country is covered with forest.

The physical peculiarities of the Saint Clair and Black Rivers, which form the peninsula upon which the post is situated, are noteworthy in many respects. The latter is formed chiefly by the superficial drainage of the bottom-lands situated to the west and northwest, the smaller tributaries constituting its origin arising in the upland districts of the interior portions of the State. Its course through the low districts is tortuous, the current sluggish, the water highly colored with de- composing vegetable matter, to the extent of suggesting its appropriate appellation.

The officers' quarters and barracks are so situated as to inclose a parallelogram 100 feet wide and 191 feet long, which is used for the parade-ground. To the rear of the buildings is a pasture- field, and to the south, between the buildings and the railroad, is the post-garden. The field south of the railroad is the drill-ground.

For several years (since the fall of 1870) this post has been garrisoned by but a single company. The one barrack-building on the north, 100 by 30 feet, and 10 feet between floor and ceiling, affords ample accommodation, allowing 604 cubic feet per man for the average occupants. Kitchen and mess-room are well arranged, and of sufficient size to meet all present requirements. One objec- tionable feature of the barrack-room is the retention of the old wooden bunks or lockers, afford- ing receptacles for hidden filth and fostering vermin.

The married soldiers' quarters have met with the condemnation of every medical officer whose reports are available to the writer. They consist of rotten, leaky huts, and are discreditable to the service. One new one has recently been erected, partly by private expenditure, and is occupied by the commissary-sergeant.

The officers' quarters are all old buildings, and in severe weather leaky and continually damp,

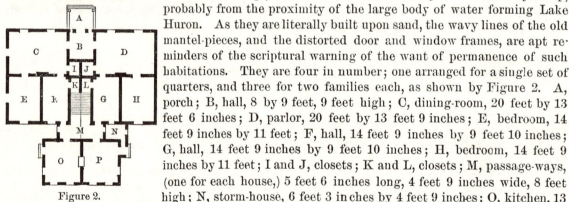

Figure 2.

probably from the proximity of the large body of water forming Lake Huron. As they are literally built upon sand, the wavy lines of the old mantel-pieces, and the distorted door and window frames, are apt re- minders of the scriptural warning of the want of permanence of such habitations. They are four in number; one arranged for a single set of quarters, and three for two families each, as shown by Figure 2. A, porch; B, hall, 8 by 9 feet, 9 feet high; C, dining-room, 20 feet by 13 feet 6 inches; D, parlor, 20 feet by 13 feet 9 inches; E, bedroom, 14 feet 9 inches by 11 feet; F, hall, 14 feet 9 inches by 9 feet 10 inches; G, hall, 14 feet 9 inches by 9 feet 10 inches; H, bedroom, 14 feet 9 inches by 11 feet; I and J, closets; K and L, closets; M, passage-ways, (one for each house,) 5 feet 6 inches long, 4 feet 9 inches wide, 8 feet high; N, storm-house, 6 feet 3 inches by 4 feet 9 inches; O, kitchen, 13 feet 9 inches by 12 feet; P, office, 13 feet 9 inches by 12 feet. They possess much similarity of external appearance. The rooms have about the same height, varying an inch above or below 9 feet, with windows 5 feet 4 inches by 3 feet, with base-sill about 30 inches above the floor, varying slightly, depending upon the distortion before referred to.

The guard-house consists of a frame building, divided into two rooms, one for the guard and one for the prisoners. The prison-room is lighted and ventilated by two small windows with grating. Adjoining there are two cells, built of brick. The average occupancy of the guard-house under the present command is 1.6; average air-space for prisoners, 4,200 cubic feet; minimum under present garrison, 1,167 cubic feet per man.

The hospital is a one-story frame building with attic, clapboarded outside and plastered within, erected about 1828. The building was designed for officers' quarters, and has at times been occu- pied as a dwelling by Grand Trunk Railway employés. In 1867 it was removed to its present site, to the rear of the post, some changes made in its interior, and the back-building erected, and has since that time been used for hospital purposes. Figure 3 shows general arrangement, &c. A, veranda; B, ward, 20 feet 6 inches by 28 feet 8 inches; C, office and dispensary, 14 by 13 feet; D, steward's and matron's room, 14 by 12 feet; E, store-room, 14 by 8 feet; F, steward's and matron's room, 14 by 8 feet; G, wash-room, 10 feet 6 inches by 8 feet; H, bath-room, 5 feet 6 inches by 8 feet; I, front hall, 28 feet long, 8 feet wide, and 8 feet 10 inches high; J, back hall, connecting with kitchen, 10 feet long, 7 feet wide, and 8 feet high; K, kitchen, 17 feet 6 inches by 12 feet 8 inches; L, steward's pantry, 11 feet by 7 feet 6 inches; M, kitchen pantry, 7 feet 6 inches by 6 feet; N, wood-room, 14 by 6 feet. The ward usually contains six beds, allowing 908 cubic feet of air-space to each. Five windows afford ample ventilation, as there are seldom more than two beds occupied. The bath-room contains a zinc tub, one 20-gallon caldron, and three fixed porcelain wash-bowls. A dead-house has recently been erected.

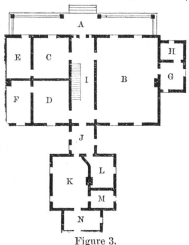

Figure 3.

The barracks, hospital, officers' quarters, and most of the offices, are heated by coal-stoves; the pattern used is styled "the American Base-Burner." The stoves are large, having a central reservoir opening from the top, with a capacity of about half a bushel. This reservoir is closed by a sliding-plate, the base of an urn, which moves on a pivot. With an ordinary fire the action upon the supply of fuel is precisely like that of a retort in a gas-factory. The imperfect joint of the cover allows large quantities of impure carburetted hydrogen to escape into the rooms, and at times, when through damp and dirty coal the reservoir is rendered impervious to the gas, the gas, by sudden combustion, causes the atmospheric pressure to burst in the mica windows with a loud report. This mephitic gas permeates every sleeping and living room of the garrison. The post surgeon has not deemed it necessary to prove the existence of the gas by chemical tests, it being so evident to the ordinary senses. He has proved it dangerous to animal life by carefully supplying every other favorable hygienic condition to gold-fish, and finding them dead on four different occasions, after exposure for six hours in the ordinary living-room of his own quarters. Probably the same stoves, desirable in other respects, if fitted with a water-joint for the reservoir bonnet, like that used for some of the inodorous vessels issued by the Medical Department, and a gas-conducting tube, made to connect by a perforated plate with about one-third of the surface of the reservoir, and emptying at some distance from the stove into the pipe, would remedy the defect, but at present it is prejudicial to health if not dangerous to life.

Shallow wells have been sunk on the reservation, and are readily filled with surface water to within four or five feet of the top, and afford a moderate supply of very inferior quality. One well has been sunk in the rear of the adjutant's office. The water in this is used for general police purposes and for Government horses. This is the only well of any real use to the garrison. At the foot of the bluff there are several places where small springs appear. A wind-mill, with force-pump and water-tank, has been procured, and pipes have been laid connecting each building with the tank, with two open taps upon the parade-ground. The water is pumped from the Saint Clair River, and promises to be abundant enough for the ordinary uses of the garrison, but will be of little service in case of fire. The cistern water at most of the officers' quarters is suitable for police purposes only, as it is generally colored either by the dropping foliage of the surrounding trees, or by collections on the roofs of the buildings of soot, dirt, or other matters thrown out by the passing locomotives. The total amount of all the water supply would be soon exhausted in the event of a conflagration of any magnitude breaking out in the garrison. The drainage of the post and of the surrounding country is bad. After heavy rains the water remains in pools.

In March, 1874, one set of officers' quarters was entirely burned down. Although a steam fire-engine from Port Huron was early on the ground, the difficulty of running it through the tracks of the railroad-yard was so great that the building was destroyed before it could get into operation.

As the Port Huron water-works, on the Holly force-pump plan, are in active operation within half a mile of the fort, and the gas-pipes have been laid to within even less distance, it is hoped that at an early day the garrison may be furnished with both water and gas from those sources.

The proximity of the Grand Trunk Railway, of Canada, and the disregard shown by that corporation for the health and comfort of the post, exercise an unfavorable influence on the hygiene of the locality. In addition to the unavoidable sources of annoyance, such as noise and jarring, it would seem as if the employés of the company deliberately made things as unpleasant as possible. Cars with dead animals and offal are left standing in front of the post, the right of the inmates to a free entrance has been denied, the water-supply is interfered with, and no regard has been paid to protests or complaints.

The views upon Lake Huron from the fort, the natural and unsurpassed magnificence of the Saint Clair River, with the busy and ever-varying scene presented by the passage through one narrow channel of less than three hundred yards width of all the commerce of the great lakes, and it within one hundred yards of the quarters, are attractions beyond description. Facilities for boating in all its forms are present, while duck, snipe, woodcock, and the wild pigeon reward and tempt the sportsman. There are no drives in the vicinity; the soil being loose and sandy, is dusty in dry weather, muddy in wet, and too rough for light vehicles in cold. A covering of snow, however, hides all defects, and sleighing is practicable during the greater part of the winter.

*Consolidated sick-report, Fort Gratiot, Mich., 1870–'74.*

| Year | 1870–'71. | | 1871–'72. | | 1872–'73. | | 1873–'74. | |
|---|---|---|---|---|---|---|---|---|
| Mean strength { Officers | 4 | | 4 | | 4 | | 3 | |
| { Enlisted men | 79 | | 48 | | 46 | | 48 | |
| Diseases. | Cases. | Deaths. | Cases. | Deaths. | Cases. | Deaths. | Cases. | Deaths. |
| GENERAL DISEASES, A. | | | | | | | | |
| Small-pox and varioloid | 1 | | | | | | | |
| Typhoid fever | | | | | 1 | | | |
| Typho-malarial fever | | | | | 1 | | | |
| Remittent fever | 1 | | | | | | | |
| Intermittent fever | 36 | | 3 | | 8 | | 11 | |
| Other diseases of this group | 9 | | 1 | | 2 | | | |
| GENERAL DISEASES, B. | | | | | | | | |
| Rheumatism | 6 | | 2 | | 4 | | | |
| Syphilis | 6 | | 1 | | | | 3 | |
| Consumption | | | 1 | | 2 | 1 | 1 | 1 |
| Other diseases of this group | 1 | | | | | | | |
| LOCAL DISEASES. | | | | | | | | |
| Catarrh and bronchitis | 13 | | 2 | | 2 | | 10 | |
| Pneumonia | 2 | | | | | | | |
| Pleurisy | | | 2 | 1 | | | | |
| Diarrhœa and dysentery | 17 | | 1 | | 4 | | 13 | |
| Gonorrhœa | 1 | | | | | | | |
| Other local diseases | 19 | | 10 | | 21 | | 22 | |
| Alcoholism | 3 | | | | 2 | | 8 | |
| Total disease | 115 | | 23 | 1 | 47 | 1 | 68 | |
| VIOLENT DISEASES AND DEATHS. | | | | | | | | |
| Drowning | | 1 | | | | | | |
| Other accidents and injuries | 20 | | 9 | | 9 | | 7 | |
| Total violence | 20 | 1 | 9 | | 9 | | 7 | |

# FORT GRISWOLD, CONNECTICUT.

Fort Griswold was originally established in 1778, on the east bank of the Thames River, on the heights of Groton, directly opposite to the city and overlooking the harbor of New London, in latitude 41° 22′ north, longitude 4° 54′ east. After the war of 1812 the original work was abandoned, until the construction of the present battery was commenced in 1842. The extent of the reservation is fourteen acres. Water is supplied by wells. There are no quarters other than the small frame dwelling occupied by the ordnance-sergeant.

# FORT HAMILTON, NEW YORK.

INFORMATION FURNISHED BY SURGEONS H. R. WIRTZ, R. H. ALEXANDER, AND C. E. GODDARD, U. S. A.

Fort Hamilton is situated on the southwest shore of Long Island, in latitude 40° 37′ 28″ north, longitude 3° 1′ 15″ east, and 5½ statute miles due south of the city of New York. At this point the shores of Long Island and Staten Island approach within a mile of each other, and form the strait known as the "Narrows," by which the inner bay of New York communicates with the outer or maritime bay. Fort Hamilton, in conjunction with Fort Wadsworth, on Staten Island, commands the Narrows; and Fort Lafayette, erected on an artificial island, lies off Fort Hamilton to the east of the main ship-channel. Nothing separates Fort Hamilton on the southeast from the Atlantic but a narrow strip of sand, called "Coney Island."

The name Fort Hamilton is applied not only to the military work but also to the village that has sprung up in its neighborhood. The fort is really situated in the town of New Utrecht, Kings County, New York.

The features of the country to the north and east of the fort are peculiar. Along the shore the banks are precipitous, and the fort itself stands on an elevation of about forty-seven feet above low water. Back from the shore the land becomes rolling, and exhibits a series of elevations and depressions till we arrive at Flatlands and Flatbush, names which sufficiently express the character of the surface.

This peculiar feature is the most important element, next to its insular position, in the topography of the post, the soil being alluvial, consisting for the most part of clay on top, then sand, pebbles, &c., and frequently a second stratum of clay, and the rolling character of the surface, producing numerous depressions, some round, some oblong, varying in size from thirty feet in diameter to as many yards. The result is that the whole country is dotted over with ponds from the surface-drainage. Some of these ponds are clear, with a gravelly or clayey bottom and grassy borders; others are surrounded with trees, and filled up with bushes and rank grasses, and covered in summer with a green slime. It has been calculated that within a radius of a mile about Fort Hamilton there are at least sixty of these ponds. East of the fort, near the new battery, is a marsh of considerable extent, formed by the drainage of the higher land, and imperfectly separated by a bank of sand from tide-water.

The reservation contains about 96 acres, and exhibits all the peculiar features of the surrounding country. There is scarcely a level spot on it; it is a series of ridges and round elevations, with depressions of every conceivable shape between them. Its general direction is northeast and southwest. The highest part is the northeast corner, which is sixty-six feet above sea-level. The hospital is built on an elevation of forty-two feet; back of it the land rises to fifty-three feet.

The soil, where it is not stony, consists of a clayey loam, with rich muck and peat beds in places, and a substratum of sand. Bowlders of all sizes are scattered over the surface, and patches of pebbles and gravel crop out here and there on the sides of the declivities. The bowlders and blocks are principally of granite, red sandstone, greenstone, &c. Trees of various kinds are sparsely scattered over the reserve, the principal collection being a grove of oak, poplar, maple, dogwood, &c., near the northeast extremity. There is no running water, and there are no springs. The climate is variable.

The quarters for the men are stone casemates, each 44 by 14 by 12 feet, badly ventilated, damp, and leaky, and totally unfit for quarters. The air-space per man is about 175 cubic feet. The majority of the enlisted men sleep upon bedsteads composed of board slats, an inch thick, supported by iron trestles, and well adapted for the purpose. There are no bath-rooms or lavatories, the men performing their ordinary ablutions at the wells and cisterns near their quarters. During the summer months they bathe frequently in the bay near the fort. The water-closet is built upon the fort dock, over the water, and the excreta removed by the tide. Several earth-closets have been placed near the casemates for use at night.

The kitchens are in casemates adjoining the quarters; they are in good condition and of sufficient capacity.

The quarters of the laundresses and married soldiers are two sets of weather-boarded frame buildings, built on the northeastern portion of the reserve, near the hospital, on a slight elevation. One set occupied by the non-commissioned staff, 75 by 26 feet, containing four rooms 12 by 18 feet, two on the ground floor and two in the attic, with doors intervening and piazzas in front and rear; ventilation excellent. The other set, occupied by laundresses, is 116½ by 43 feet, constructed similar to that occupied by the non-commissioned staff, with the exception that there are no doors communicating between the front and rear rooms, thereby preventing the proper amount of ventilation, and making the quarters so excessively warm during the summer season as to be almost insupportable.

Ten of the casemates are occupied by officers, eight by bachelors, and two by officers with their families. These quarters are even more unhealthy than those of the men, as they are intersected by numerous partitions, and have no ventilation. Earth-closets are used in them, and give entire satisfaction. There are also three sets of one-story frame buildings, filled in with brick, and with Mansard roofs, consisting of one set of colonel's quarters, occupied by the commanding officer, one double set captains', and one set major's. They are heated by coal, in grates and stoves, during the winter months, and supplied with water from wells and cisterns. The casemates are dark and damp. The frame buildings were put up in the cheapest manner, without closets or other conveniences. One of them, occupied by the post surgeon, is on the edge of a peat-bog, which must always render it an unhealthy residence. It was built there in opposition to the advice of the surgeon of the post. The water-closets for the frame buildings consist of the ordinary privy vaults.

The building occupied formerly as the post hospital is divided into two sets of captain's quarters. It has been recently painted inside, and is in fair condition.

The post hospital is a "temporary hospital," built of frame, in 1869, and partly lathed and plastered inside and weather-boarded outside, with ridge ventilation in the wards. It it situated near the upper northeast end of the reserve, on a moderate eminence, about 130 yards back from the State road, fronting to the northwest, its greater length being northeast and southwest. It consists of the administration building, two wards, and a kitchen. The original materials and workmanship were so inferior that a constantly increasing expenditure will be necessary to keep the buildings in repair.

The administration building is two stories high, 36 by 25 feet, shingle roof, weather-boarded outside, and lathed and plastered inside. A passage-way runs through from front to rear, and a flight of steps leads thence to the second story. There are four rooms on each floor, two on each side the entry-way about 10 by 12 feet, each lighted by four windows. The ground-floor rooms on the left of the entrance are used as surgeon's office and dispensary. These communicate, and the dispensary has a sliding window opening into the entry for the delivery of prescriptions. The two rooms on the right of the entrance are used as store-rooms, one for medical supplies, and the other for bedding, furniture, &c. Three of the upper rooms are occupied by the hospital steward and his family, and the remaining room is applied to the purposes of dissection and chemical and microscopical investigation. The two wards, one on each side of the administrative building, are on a line with its rear, and are 88 feet long by 25 feet wide; height of wall to the eaves, 12 feet; to the peak of the roof, 18 feet. The walls are plastered inside, but not ceiled above, being open to the roof, where a ridge ventilator with shutters extends the whole length. The northwest ward forms one large, beautiful room, with two small apartments boarded off at the far end, one for nurses the other for wash and bath-room.

The southwest ward is divided into two rooms by a passage-way through the building from front to rear. The farther room is used as a ward, and has two small apartments boarded off, as in the large ward. The other room has never been occupied by sick, but could be applied to that purpose if needed. It has, however, served for examining recruits, as a sort of sitting-room for convalescents, &c. The wards are well lighted by windows on all sides, two at each end and seven front and seven rear, with space between each window for two beds. A porch, 6 feet wide, runs the whole length of each ward on the side facing the northwest. The superficial area of the large ward is 2,200 square feet; of the small one, 1,075 square feet; total, 3,275 square feet, now applied to hospital purposes, and furnishing in cubic space 47,487 cubic feet, or about 1,180 cubic feet of air-space per bed. At the end of each ward is a door opening upon a platform, leading to a small water-closet, from which a urinal and drain convey the water to a cess-pool, and in which provision is made for the reception of the discharges of patients who are too sick to resort to the privy. Each little house, about the size of a sentry's box, is separated from the ward, so that a current of air passes between them.

The kitchen is a one-story structure, forty feet to the rear of the administrative building. The walls are plastered, but the ceiling is open to the roof. It is divided into two rooms. The kitchen proper is 14 by 24 feet, and the mess-room 10 by 24 feet. A small apartment for a pantry is boarded off from one end of the kitchen, and a snug little cellar, bricked all around, with entrance from the outside, is built under it.

The above-described buildings are all connected by means of a covered corridor, 40 by 50 feet, and 4 feet wide, in the shape of a cross, which makes a convenient passage-way between the administrative building, the wards, and the kitchen.

The large ward contains thirty iron bedsteads, with chairs and bedside tables; the small ward contains twelve iron bedsteads. The hospital is warmed by stoves, two in the large ward and one in the small one, and one in each of the other rooms when required. The water is furnished by two cisterns, 14 feet deep by 12 diameter, bricked and cemented and arched above. One cistern supplies water to the kitchen, the other is fitted with a pump in the open air. The large and clean surface of the shingle roofs affords an unfailing supply of good water. Two cess-pools, with drains of vitrified pipe, are connected, one with the wash-room and water-closet of the northeast ward, the other with the southwest ward and kitchen. They are 8 feet deep by 7 feet in diameter, of open brick-work.

The hospital grounds embrace about two acres, and are surrounded with a good picket fence. The larger portion lies in front of the hospital, between it and the State road, and has vated as a garden. The grounds in the rear of the buildings are still in grass. The privy is situated here, about fifty yards back of the kitchen; it contains eight seats, separated from each other by partitions shoulder high. A good root-house has been built; it is 20 feet square and 6 feet deep, covered with earth and sod, and further protected from the rains by a shingle roof. It is boarded inside, is perfectly dry, and maintains a temperature never below 40° F., even in the coldest part of winter.

Water is supplied from wells and cisterns; it is abundant and of good quality, except that supplied from cisterns, which occasionally becomes foul from earthy deposits.

The natural drainage is bad; the ground being hilly, the water collects in the hollows, forming ponds, that have become filled with rank vegetation, the depth of water continually varying, being filled during the winter and spring by rain and snow, and in the summer and autumn becoming so nearly dry as to expose almost the entire beds to the direct solar rays.

The artificial drainage consists of a large sewer, built in connection with the ditch in the permanent fortification, and into which the superficial drains and water-pipes lead, discharging into the bay. Slops, offal, and excreta are thrown into the bay and removed by the tide.

*Meteorological report, Fort Hamilton, New York Harbor, 1870-'74.*

| Month. | 1870-'71. | | | | 1871-'72. | | | | 1872-'73. | | | | 1873-'74. | | | |
|---|---|---|---|---|---|---|---|---|---|---|---|---|---|---|---|---|
| | Temperature. | | | Rain-fall in inches. | Temperature. | | | Rain-fall in inches. | Temperature. | | | Rain-fall in inches. | Temperature. | | | Rain-fall in inches. |
| | Mean. | Max. | Min. | | Mean. | Max. | Min. | | Mean. | Max. | Min. | | Mean. | Max. | Min. | |
| | ° | ° | ° | | ° | ° | ° | | ° | ° | ° | | ° | ° | ° | |
| July | 75.55 | 94 | 61* | 2.72 | 72.61 | 87 | 47* | 4.78 | 77.27 | 96* | 62* | 8.04 | 74.27 | 89* | 59* | 4.12 |
| August | 73.91 | 78 | 58* | 2.96 | 74.30 | 88 | 55* | 9.10 | 74.78 | 91* | 54* | 8.34 | 71.14 | 89* | 55* | 7.11 |
| September | 67.03 | 82 | 54* | 1.70 | 61.59 | 78 | 41* | 2.26 | 66.12 | 89* | 46* | 3.89 | 64.02 | 86* | 44* | 2.23 |
| October | 57.02 | 79 | 29* | 5.20 | 56.28 | 75* | 32* | 5.36 | 54.13 | 72* | 35* | 2.69 | 54.81 | 71* | 30* | 1.30 |
| November | 43.84 | 65 | 27* | 1.40 | 38.70 | 53* | 16* | 3.47 | 40.31 | 58* | 13* | 3.88 | 37.41 | 58* | 20* | 1.95 |
| December | 34.64 | 54 | 10* | 1.52 | 29.95 | 45* | −2* | 1.62 | 27.09 | 48* | 3* | 2.05 | 36.07 | 62* | 17* | 1.24 |
| January | 28.20 | 47 | 4* | 1.85 | 28.69 | 44 | 8 | 1.50 | 26.75 | 48* | −4* | 4.52 | 34.16 | 57* | 12* | 3.29 |
| February | 30.38 | 53 | 2* | 2.15 | 29.57 | 51 | 11 | 1.11 | 26.04 | 48* | −2* | 3.06 | 29.78 | 70* | 5* | 1.27 |
| March | 43.83 | 62 | 28* | 4.90 | 29.66 | 60 | 0* | 2.21 | 33.35 | 52* | 9* | 1.88 | 37.07 | 63* | 10* | 1.18 |
| April | 52.35 | 84 | 30* | 3.12 | 48.66 | 82* | 25* | 1.47 | 44.29 | 60* | 33* | 3.05 | 40.83 | 62* | 21* | 6.63 |
| May | 60.87 | 91 | 37* | 3.90 | 61.24 | 90* | 40* | 2.03 | 57.16 | 81* | 38* | 2.62 | 57.77 | 87* | 34* | 1.50 |
| June | 69.31 | 86 | 40* | 5.94 | 70.57 | 92* | 41* | 1.91 | 68.73 | 92* | 51* | 1.19 | 69.64 | 91* | 49* | 1.53 |
| For the year | 53.08 | 94 | 2* | 37.36 | 50.15 | 92* | −2* | 36.82 | 49.67 | 96' | −4* | 45.21 | 50.58 | 91* | 5* | 33.35 |

* These observations are made with self-registering thermometers. The mean is from the standard thermometer.

5 M P

*Consolidated sick-report, Fort Hamilton, New York Harbor, 1870–'74.*

| Year | | 1870–'71. | | 1871–'72. | | 1872–'73. | | 1873–'74. | |
|---|---|---|---|---|---|---|---|---|---|
| Mean strength { Officers<br>{ Enlisted men | | 15<br>242 | | 17<br>233 | | 17<br>231 | | 19<br>238 | |
| Diseases. | | Cases. | Deaths. | Cases. | Deaths. | Cases. | Deaths. | Cases. | Deaths. |
| GENERAL DISEASES, A. | | | | | | | | | |
| Remittent fever | | 6 | 1 | ...... | ...... | 2 | ...... | 3 | ...... |
| Intermittent fever | | 197 | ...... | 292 | ...... | 140 | ...... | 66 | ...... |
| Other diseases of this group | | | | 6 | ...... | 24 | 1 | 10 | ...... |
| GENERAL DISEASES, B. | | | | | | | | | |
| Rheumatism | | 16 | ...... | 16 | ...... | 15 | ...... | 16 | ...... |
| Syphilis | | 24 | ...... | 28 | ...... | 28 | ...... | 16 | ...... |
| Consumption | | 3 | 1 | 3 | 3 | 2 | ...... | 1 | ...... |
| Other diseases of this group | | 1 | 1 | 1 | ...... | 1 | ...... | | |
| LOCAL DISEASES. | | | | | | | | | |
| Catarrh and bronchitis | | 68 | | 32 | ...... | 42 | ...... | 44 | ...... |
| Pneumonia | | ...... | ...... | 1 | 1 | ...... | | | |
| Diarrhœa and dysentery | | 45 | 1 | 71 | ...... | 90 | ...... | 65 | ...... |
| Hernia | | | | | | 1 | ...... | 2 | ...... |
| Gonorrhœa | | 23 | ...... | 24 | ...... | 24 | ...... | 10 | ...... |
| Other local diseases | | 86 | 1 | 72 | ...... | 140 | 1 | 201 | ...... |
| Alcoholism | | 1 | ...... | | | 13 | | 24 | |
| Total disease | | 470 | 5 | 546 | 4 | 522 | 2 | 458 | ...... |
| VIOLENT DISEASES AND DEATHS. | | | | | | | | | |
| Gunshot wounds | | 2 | ...... | | | | | | |
| Drowning | | | | | | | | | 1 |
| Other accidents and injuries | | 69 | ...... | 66 | ...... | 85 | ...... | 68 | ...... |
| Total violence | | 71 | ...... | 66 | ...... | 85 | ...... | 68 | 1 |

# FORT INDEPENDENCE, BOSTON HARBOR, MASSACHUSETTS.

## INFORMATION FURNISHED BY ASSISTANT SURGEONS J. W. BREWER AND C. E. MUNN, U. S. A.

Fort Independence is situated on Castle Island, in Boston Harbor, in latitude 42° 20′ north; longitude 6° 2′ 3″ east. From India wharf, in a southeast direction, it is distant two miles and three furlongs; from City Point (Rochester Point) it is distant about 900 yards; and from Governor's Island, (Fort Winthrop,) from which it is separated by the main channel, 1,160 yards. The surface will measure, perhaps, twelve acres at high water. The southern extremity of the island is a level plain, but a few feet above water-mark. For history of the post see Circular No. 4, Surgeon-General's Office, December 5, 1870.

The fort is a pentagonal, five-bastioned fortification, occupying the northern portion of the island. The casemates contain the squad-rooms and dormitories, the dining-room and kitchen of the men, the married soldiers' quarters, laundresses' quarters, store-houses, bakery, &c. These casemates are all about the same size, averaging 21 feet long, 17 feet broad, and 11 feet high, floored with jointed pine flooring, and the walls and ceilings plastered. Each room looks out on the parade-ground, and, externally, is separated by a wooden partition from the general gun-gallery and outer walls. Six of these casemate-rooms are assigned as squad-rooms and dormitories of the men, containing from ten to thirteen men each, giving about 300 cubic feet air-space per man—hardly one-third enough if there were any proper ventilation; but no ventilation is provided for save by a movable transom over the door, which, opening over the beds of those farthest from the stove, is diligently kept closed by them. Each room is heated by one cast-iron coal-stove, placed in the corner farthest from the door, and alternately heated to redness by those who sleep farthest from it, or allowed to go out entirely by those whose beds are nearest to it. The air in these rooms is always foul and offensive, and is rendered still more hurtful by dampness and moisture, the walls and ceiling being constantly wet, sometimes dripping, from the water that soaks through from the terre-plein above. The married soldiers and laundresses have each one of these casemates, similar to the squad-rooms, and to them the same remarks will apply, save that they are not so overcrowded. All of these casemates are damp, ill ventilated, badly lighted, and worse heated. They are a constant and prolific source of catarrh, bronchitis, rheumatism, and neuralgia, and probably increase the sick-report from ten to fifteen per cent. The furniture of these squad-rooms is little besides the stove, bunks and bedding, the clothing, arms, and accouterments of the men. The bunks are single, each composed of two iron tressels connected by slats, and furnished with a bed-sack filled with hay or straw, and two or three blankets.

The officers' quarters are situated without the walls, on the south of the fortification, and consist of three almost similar double houses, and one isolated set of quarters immediately west of the southwest bastion; the isolated set of quarters is but one story high; it has seven rooms on the lower floor, and a basement, and is occupied by the commanding officer. The other sets of quarters are each one story and a half high; they have each three rooms on the lower floor and too low attic rooms on the upper. All the officers' quarters are well finished, and are each provided with a range in the kitchen and grates for coal in the other lower rooms; they are all supplied with water from a tank filled by a forcing-pump from the general cistern. The rooms are 15 feet square.

Two adjoining casemate rooms in the southwest bastion are now occupied by the post-guard and prisoners. The larger room, 33 by 18 by 9 feet, is the guard-room. Ten feet of its length is separated by an open fence, and provided with bunks for garrison prisoners. The room is floored and its walls cased with pine boards. It is warmed by a cast-iron coal-stove and ventilated by a door and four windows. The average occupancy is six members of the guard and four prisoners, leaving an average air-space of 534 cubic feet, and, on rare occasions of crowding, 334 feet.

The other apartment is 31 by 18 by 14 feet, and was formerly a gun-room. It contains an air-space of about 5,500 cubic feet; is furnished with a coal-stove, bunks, and bedding; is ventilated by a grated door, two embrasures, 2½ feet square, and three loop-holes, 6 by 32 inches. Pine boards are laid upon its concrete floor, but the bare granite walls and arched roof are always cold and wet. This cheerless place is occupied exclusively by prisoners sentenced by general courts-martial to long terms of confinement. Their number at present is 15, sent from differents posts in this Military Division. At one time a ventilating-shaft was conducted from the roof of this room, but in adapting new works upon the terre-plein it was unavoidably closed. Both rooms are carefully policed while the prisoners are at work out of doors. By careful supervision a degree of comfort is maintained; but after the above description it seems unnecessary to say that either apartment is totally unfit for prolonged occupancy by human beings.

On the extreme southern point of the island is the post hospital, a brick building, fronting the north, and consisting of a central administration building, and two wards arranged as wings, in conformity with Circular No. 4, Surgeon-General's Office, series of 1867.

The central or main building is two stories high and 36 feet square; the wings or wards are each one story high, and 45 feet long by 25½ feet broad. All the roofs are of slate and all the walls are of brick, those of the main building and wings being double, with air-chambers between the inner and outer courses; but from some cause, either from having no substance inlaid near the ground course to prevent the dampness from rising, or from the improper manner in which the inner and outer walls are bound together, the inner walls are continually wet and the white-wash constantly discolored. The flooring is of good, well-matched yellow pine, but the baseboards have so shrunk away from the floor that a current of air enters so forcibly in many places as to extinguish a candle. Ridge elevation is provided for in the wards, and in all the other rooms there are ventilators connecting with the air-chamber between the walls. Bath-rooms and latrines are supplied with water from the common tank, the waste water and sewerage being carried off by a drain emptying in the bay. There is at the post hospital a library, consisting of two hundred selected volumes, for the use of patients, with the addition of a set of Chambers' Cyclopædia.

There are six wells and an equal number of cisterns on the island. Four of the cisterns are connected with the officers' quarters in the casemates, one cistern connected with the commanding officer's quarters, and one with the hospital. Water for culinary purposes is obtained from two wells. The water from the well but a few yards from the sea-wall contains a larger quantity of saline impurities than the other wells, the principal salts being chloride of sodium, chloride and bromide of magnesium, with traces of chloride of potassium and sulphate of lime. This well is doubtless subject to tidal impregnations. The water of the well near the soldiers' barracks is not so strongly impregnated with earthy and alkaline salts as the former. Two quarts of water from this well gave, on evaporation, five grains of solid residue, one and a half grains of which was combustible organic matter and the remainder earthy and alkaline salts, principally chloride of sodium and carbonate of lime. During the extreme heat of summer the wells become quite low, necessitating economy in the use of water, but at the other seasons the supply is more than suffi-cient for all ordinary purposes. The expediency and practicability of obtaining the water supply of the post from the city water-works, by laying pipes from South Boston to the island, has been discussed. The pipes would necessarily be exposed every twelve hours, and thus be subject to injury from the frost.

The insular position of the fort makes drainage simple and easily effected. The sink or latrine of the enlisted men is a deep pit or vault under the northeast bastion ; it is connected by a covered-way or large drain with the bay. Earth-closets having been tried at one time, and found to require much care to keep them in proper order, were considered unsatisfactory and abandoned. The cottages occupied by officers are furnished with water-closets which are faulty, because the discharge-pipes have no traps.

During the summer the men bathe in the sea. The only other bathing facilities are in the hospital.

The prevailing diseases are those incident to the insular situation of the post and the damp and unhealthy quarters.

Fort Independence is doubtless as free from such conditions and influences as are prejudicial to health as any spot in the United States. The surface in the vicinity of the post is flooded at stated intervals by the tide, and sewerage is thus thoroughly removed.

*Meteorological report, Fort Independence, Mass., 1870–'74.*

| Month. | 1870–'71. Temperature. Mean. | Max. | Min. | Rain-fall in inches. | 1871–'72. Temperature. Mean. | Max. | Min. | Rain-fall in inches. | 1872–'73. Temperature. Mean. | Max. | Min. | Rain-fall in inches. | 1873–'74. Temperature. Mean. | Max. | Min. | Rain-fall in inches. |
|---|---|---|---|---|---|---|---|---|---|---|---|---|---|---|---|---|
| | ° | ° | ° | | ° | ° | ° | | ° | ° | ° | | ° | ° | ° | |
| July.................. | 71. 55 | 91 | 35* | 2. 46 | 69. 43 | 86 | 51* | 2. 18 | 73. 37* | 98* | 52* | 6. 49 | 69. 51* | 94* | 54* | 3. 95 |
| August.............. | 70. 02 | 91 | 41* | 1. 15 | 70. 26 | 83* | 55* | 3. 78 | 71. 53* | 90* | 49* | 6. 40 | 67. 09* | 90* | 49* | 5. 17 |
| September........... | 63. 46 | 83 | 36* | 0. 54 | 58. 08 | 81* | 41* | 1. 04 | 61. 65* | 89* | 43* | 5. 85 | 60. 46* | 87* | 36* | 2. 01 |
| October ............. | 54. 74 | 75* | 31* | 4. 28 | 52. 33 | 73* | 31* | 6. 04 | 51. 40* | 72* | 34* | 4. 80 | 48. 72* | 70* | 30* | 2. 18 |
| November ........... | 42. 78 | 62 | 28* | 2. 84 | 37. 09 | 61* | 7* | 1. 98 | 40. 16* | 58* | 13* | 4. 51 | 31. 43* | 55* | 5* | 6. 02 |
| December ........... | 31. 66 | 49 | 2* | 1. 78 | 27. 11 | 50* | — 2* | 3. 67 | 22. 77* | 43* | —10* | 3. 95 | 29. 61* | 58* | 8* | 4. 55 |
| January ............ | 24. 66 | 49 | — 8* | 1. 32 | 27. 29 | 44* | — 5* | 1. 76 | 25. 12* | 52* | — 3* | 5. 29 | 26. 42* | 52* | — 3* | 2. 94 |
| February ........... | 27. 73 | 54 | —10* | 2. 55 | 25. 94 | 48* | — 4* | 1. 30 | 22. 17* | 46* | —10* | 2. 70 | 22. 19* | 50* | 0* | 2. 08 |
| March .............. | 41. 63 | 62 | 25* | 2. 78 | 18. 42 | 34* | — 6* | 7. 68 | 28. 67* | 52* | — 3* | 3. 30 | 28. 19* | 58* | 5* | 3. 09 |
| April ............... | 45. 87 | 82 | 28* | 2. 50 | 39. 48* | 82* | 20* | 1. 75 | 41. 80* | 59* | 29* | 2. 15 | 32. 66* | 55* | 20* | 6. 85 |
| May ................ | 56 32 | 90 | 37* | 3. 30 | 55. 02* | 72* | 34* | 3. 95 | 53. 51* | 82* | 34* | 2. 74 | 51. 36* | 82* | 31* | 3. 45 |
| June ................ | 64. 90 | 80 | 49* | 4. 73 | 65. 08* | 99* | 35* | 3. 95 | 66. 27* | 89* | 44* | 1. 54 | 63. 66* | 96* | 40* | 1. 80 |
| For the year....... | 49. 61 | 91 | —10* | 30. 24 | 45. 45 | 99* | — 6* | 39. 08 | 46. 53 | 98* | —10* | 49. 73 | 44. 27 | 96* | — 3* | 44. 09 |

* These observations are made with self-registering thermometers. The mean is from the standard thermometer.

NOTE.—The monthly means have been computed from the registering-thermometers since April, 1872, there being no standard-thermome-ter at post.

*Consolidated sick-report, Fort Independence, Mass., 1870–'74.*

| Year ................................................................ | 1870–'71. | 1871–'72. | 1872–'73. | 1873–'74. |
|---|---|---|---|---|
| Mean strength ................................................ { Officers ........... { Enlisted men ..... | 5 59 | 6 49 | 5 51 | 6 68 |

| Diseases. | Cases. | Deaths. | Cases. | Deaths. | Cases. | Deaths. | Cases. | Deaths. |
|---|---|---|---|---|---|---|---|---|
| GENERAL DISEASES, A. | | | | | | | | |
| Small-pox and varioloid................................... | | | | | 5 | | | |
| Typhoid fever............................................ | 1 | | | | | | | |
| Intermittent fever....................................... | 4 | | | | 6 | | 6 | |
| Other diseases of this group............................. | 12 | | 5 | | 4 | | 24 | |
| GENERAL DISEASES, B. | | | | | | | | |
| Rheumatism ............................................. | 16 | | 16 | | 10 | | 23 | |
| Syphilis ................................................. | 2 | | 1 | | | | | |
| Consumption ............................................. | | | 4 | | 1 | | 2 | |
| Other diseases of this group............................. | 2 | | 1 | | | | | |

*Consolidated sick-report, Fort Independence, Mass., 1870-'74.—Continued.*

| ear | | 1870-'71. | | 1871-'72. | | 1872-'73. | | 1873-'74. | |
|---|---|---|---|---|---|---|---|---|---|
| Mean strength { Officers........... Enlisted men.... | | 5 59 | | 6 49 | | 5 51 | | 6 68 | |
| Diseases. | | Cases. | Deaths. | Cases. | Deaths. | Cases. | Deaths. | Cases. | Deaths. |
| LOCAL DISEASES. | | | | | | | | | |
| Catarrh and bronchitis | | 23 | ...... | 20 | ...... | 28 | ...... | 37 | ...... |
| Pneumonia | | 2 | 1 | ...... | ...... | ...... | ...... | ...... | ...... |
| Pleurisy | | 2 | ...... | ...... | ...... | ...... | ...... | 1 | ...... |
| Diarrhœa and dysentery | | 15 | ...... | 17 | ...... | 10 | ...... | 32 | ...... |
| Gonorrhœa | | 4 | ...... | 7 | ...... | 3 | ...... | 1 | ...... |
| Other local diseases | | 44 | ...... | 17 | ...... | 32 | ...... | 4 | ...... |
| Alcoholism | | 8 | ...... | 14 | ...... | 11 | ...... | 17 | ...... |
| Total disease | | 135 | 1 | 102 | ...... | 110 | ...... | 190 | ...... |
| VIOLENT DISEASES AND DEATHS. | | | | | | | | | |
| Gunshot wounds | | ...... | ...... | ...... | ...... | 1 | ...... | ...... | ...... |
| Drowning | | ...... | ...... | ...... | ...... | ...... | ...... | ...... | 1 |
| Other accidents and injuries | | 22 | ...... | 20 | ...... | 13 | ...... | 22 | ...... |
| Total violence | | 22 | ...... | 20 | ...... | 14 | ...... | 22 | 1 |

# INDIANAPOLIS ARSENAL, INDIANA.

This arsenal, established as an arsenal of construction, occupies an area of seventy-five acres within the limits of the city of Indianapolis, latitude, 39° 46′ north; longitude, 9° 2′ west. There are quarters for two officers and fifty enlisted men, built of brick and stone, and in good condition. Two rooms in the barracks are used as a hospital.

*Consolidated-sick report, Indianapolis Arsenal, Ind., 1870-'74.*

| Year | | 1870-'71. | | 1871-'72. | | 1872-'73. | | 1873-'74. | |
|---|---|---|---|---|---|---|---|---|---|
| Mean strength { Officers........... Enlisted men ..... | | 1 22 | | 1 13 | | 1 13 | | 1 16 | |
| Diseases. | | Cases. | Deaths. | Cases. | Deaths. | Cases. | Deaths. | Cases. | Deaths. |
| GENERAL DISEASES, A. | | | | | | | | | |
| Typhoid fever | | ...... | ...... | ...... | ...... | ...... | ...... | 1 | ...... |
| Remittent fever | | ...... | ...... | 1 | ...... | ...... | ...... | 2 | ...... |
| Intermittent fever | | 21 | ...... | 5 | ...... | 13 | ...... | 14 | ...... |
| Other diseases of this group | | 5 | ...... | 5 | ...... | 4 | ...... | 3 | ...... |
| GENERAL DISEASES, B. | | | | | | | | | |
| Rheumatism | | ...... | ...... | 2 | ...... | 3 | ...... | 1 | ...... |
| Syphilis | | ...... | ...... | ...... | ...... | ...... | ...... | 1 | ...... |
| LOCAL DISEASES. | | | | | | | | | |
| Diarrhœa and dysentery | | ...... | ...... | 2 | ...... | ...... | ...... | 3 | ...... |
| Gonorrhœa | | ...... | ...... | ...... | ...... | 1 | ...... | ...... | ...... |
| Other local diseases | | ...... | ...... | 3 | ...... | 3 | ...... | 2 | ...... |
| Total disease | | 26 | ...... | 18 | ...... | 24 | ...... | 27 | ...... |
| VIOLENT DISEASES AND DEATHS. | | | | | | | | | |
| Accidents and injuries | | ...... | ...... | 1 | ...... | 1 | ...... | 2 | ...... |
| Total violence | | ...... | ...... | 1 | ...... | 1 | ...... | 2 | ...... |

# JERRY'S POINT, NEW HAMPSHIRE.

Battery commenced in June, 1873, on Jerry's Point, the southern extremity of Great Island, in Portsmouth Harbor.

## KENNEBEC ARSENAL, AUGUSTA, MAINE.

The arsenal is situated on the east side of the Kennebec River, in latitude 44° 19′ north; longitude 7° 13′ east, in the city of Augusta, with the business part of which it is connected by a covered bridge.

The reservation is in the form of a parallelogram, and contains thirty-nine and seven-eighths acres. The ground rises gradually from the bank of the river until it attains a height of 200 feet. The buildings, with the exception of the hospital and a barn, are of granite, covered with slate. The quarters of the commanding officer and military store-keeper are large, commodious residences, furnished with the usual modern conveniences. The enlisted men and their families are quartered in two large barracks, a separate kitchen and bed-room, and in some cases a sitting-room, being assigned to each family.

The hospital is a room 20 by 20 feet, furnished with 10 beds, 5 of which are kept ready for use. There is little sickness at the post, and the enlisted men, most of whom have families, are treated in quarters.

An abundance of excellent water is supplied by springs, and distributed to all the buildings by means of a reservoir and pipes. The sewerage is perfect, consisting of a system of covered drains, terminating at the river.

*Consolidated sick-report, Kennebec Arsenal, Me., 1870–'74.*

| Year | | 1870–'71. | | 1871–'72. | | 1872–'73. | | 1873–'74. | |
|---|---|---|---|---|---|---|---|---|---|
| Mean strength { Officers | | 1 | | 1 | | 1 | | 1 | |
| { Enlisted men | | 17 | | 9 | | 9 | | 9 | |
| Diseases. | | Cases. | Deaths. | Cases. | Deaths. | Cases. | Deaths. | Cases. | Deaths. |
| GENERAL DISEASES, A. | | | | | | | | | |
| Typhoid fever | | | | 1 | | | | | |
| Other diseases of this group | | 7 | | 1 | | 3 | | | |
| GENERAL DISEASES, B. | | | | | | | | | |
| Rheumatism | | 2 | | 2 | | 1 | | 4 | |
| LOCAL DISEASES. | | | | | | | | | |
| Catarrh and bronchitis | | 1 | | 2 | | | | 2 | |
| Pneumonia | | 2 | | | | | | | |
| Pleurisy | | | | | | 1 | | 1 | |
| Diarrhœa and dysentery | | 12 | | 3 | | | | 1 | |
| Hernia | | | | | | | | 1 | |
| Gonorrhœa | | 1 | | | | | | | |
| Other local diseases | | 5 | | 3 | | 1 | | 1 | |
| Total disease | | 30 | | 12 | | 6 | | 10 | |
| VIOLENT DISEASES AND DEATHS. | | | | | | | | | |
| Accidents and injuries | | 1 | | | | | | | |
| Total violence | | 1 | | | | | | | |

## FORT KNOX, MAINE.

This fort is on the western bank of the Penobscot River, about 50 miles from its mouth, in latitude 44° 35′ north; longitude 8° 13′ east, three-fourths of a mile from Bucksport, in Hancock County, the nearest town. The reservation is one hundred and fifty acres, a part of which is woodland. The construction of the fort was begun in 1844. The officers' quarters consist of two buildings, four rooms in all, each 50 by 20 feet, unfinished. There is also a frame building outside the main works, measuring 40 by 20 feet, containing five small rooms.

The men's quarters in the main works are bomb-proof, and divided into eight rooms, about 30 by 15 feet. There is also a frame building outside the main works 100 by 20 feet. There are several workshops and barns at the post, but no building specially designed for hospital or guard-house.

Water is supplied by springs and cisterns.

The post is in charge of an ordnance-sergeant.

# FORT LAFAYETTE, NEW YORK.

This fort, originally called Fort Diamond, was commenced in 1812, upon an artificial island, in that part of New York Harbor called the "Narrows," to the east of the main ship-channel, and directly west of Fort Hamilton. It was first garrisoned in September, 1822, and in the following year the name was changed to Fort Lafayette.

The fort was partially destroyed by fire on the first day of December, 1868. The outer walls, the magazines, and the quarters for officers and men remain intact. The works have not been restored, and the remaining buildings are now chiefly used for the storage of ordnance supplies.

# LAZARETTO POINT, MARYLAND.

Fortifications were commenced in 1872 at Lazaretto Point, in Baltimore Harbor, opposite Fort McHenry. The works are in course of construction.

# FORT LEE, MASSACHUSETTS.

Fort Lee was rebuilt in 1862, on the site of an old revolutionary work, in the center of Salem Neck, commanding the entrance to Salem and Beverly Harbors; latitude, 42° 31′ north; longitude, 6° 10′ east.

In charge of an ordnance-sergeant.

# LONG ISLAND HEAD, MASSACHUSETTS.

These works, commenced in 1871, at the entrance into Boston Harbor through Broad Sound, are still in course of construction.

# LONG POINT BATTERIES, MASSACHUSETTS.

These works were commenced in 1863, at the south entrance into Provincetown Harbor, Cape Cod, in latitude 41° 57′ north; longitude 7° 3′ east. Communication is by water, except at low tide, when Provincetown can be reached by land.

The officers' quarters are a frame building, 42 by 24 feet, containing four rooms and a kitchen. The quarters for the men are a frame building, 82 by 24 feet, intended to accommodate 100 men. Water is obtained from cisterns.

In charge of an ordnance-sergeant.

# FORT McCLARY, KITTERY, MAINE.

This was originally established as a military post in 1812, on Kittery Point, opposite Fort Constitution, in Portsmouth Harbor, latitude, 43° 5′ north; longitude, 6° 18′ east. The present works were commenced in 1841. The fort, which stands upon a rocky eminence, was partly torn down, and new works, still incomplete, commenced in 1863.

There are no officers' quarters at the post, but a barrack, chapel, hospital, and guard-house, all unimportant, unoccupied, and out of repair. The reservation contains fifteen acres.

The works are in charge of an ordnance-sergeant.

# FORT McHENRY, BALTIMORE, MARYLAND.

## REPORTS OF SURGEONS J. SIMPSON AND D. BACHE, UNITED STATES ARMY.

Fort McHenry is situated on Whetstone Point, a peninsula formed by the junction of the northwest branch of the Patapsco with the main river, latitude, 39° 15′ 44″ north; longitude, 28′ 32″ east. It is about three miles southeast from the center of the city of Baltimore.

This site was first occupied for military purposes in 1775, at which time a water-battery was constructed here in connection with obstructions in the river, consisting of three massive wrought-iron chains and some sunken vessels. In 1794 the fort was repaired, the star fort of brick-work added, and the whole was ceded to the United States and received its present name. It was named after James McHenry, a secretary to General Washington during the revolutionary war, and Secretary of War in 1798.

The military reservation covers an area of about forty-nine and one-half acres, of which about four and one-fourth is occupied by the fort and water-battery. The surrounding country is comparatively low and level, and subject to occasional inundations.

The formation of the land upon which the fort is located, as shown by the borings of the artesian well at the post, consists of yellow sand, clay, with bowlders, iron ore, &c., in layers varying from 1 to 33 feet in thickness, until, at the depth of 140 feet, water of an excellent quality is found in abundance.

The fort occupies the whole of the extremity of the peninsula. The parade ground is $31\frac{1}{3}$ feet above low-water mark.

The men's barracks inside the fort, as originally built and intended to accommodate two companies, are two substantial brick buildings occupying two adjacent sides of a pentagon. They are each $97\frac{2}{12}$ feet by $21\frac{2}{3}$ feet, and two stories high, with a covered porch, 10 feet wide, to each floor, extending the entire length of the west or front side. Each story contains three rooms of equal size. In the lower are the kitchen, mess-room, orderly and store rooms. In the upper are three squad-rooms as quarters, each $30\frac{1}{2}$ by $21\frac{2}{3}$ by 10 feet, plastered and ceiled, giving to each man about 330 cubic feet of air-space. In these rooms the men live almost entirely, there being no separate provision for lounging, smoking, reading, &c. Iron bedsteads of the new pattern are furnished. The number of soldiers in each dormitory is seldom less than twenty, and the ventilation is very insufficient, especially in winter.

The barracks situated outside of the fort are on the northeastern part of the sea-wall, built of brick, and, unlike those described above, are large and commodious. They consist of two stories, the lower used for mess-hall, office, kitchen, &c.; the upper as dormitories. In these rooms iron bedsteads are used, which contribute greatly to the comfort of the men and neatness of the barracks. Upon the roofs of these buildings are placed two large ventilators, and there being a sufficient number of windows, the air is kept tolerably sweet and pure. The principal objection to these rooms is the lowness of ceiling, the air-space for each man being 520 cubic feet; at night the air in all the sleeping-rooms is very impure. Another objection to the sea-wall barracks is the location near the water. It has been found by observation that in the spring, summer, and fall, the sick-list of the companies occupying these quarters is twice as large as that of the companies garrisoned within the fort. All the barrack buildings are heated by stoves, and the windows are ranged on opposite sides.

The men's sinks, four in number, are located on the sea-wall, but are not built sufficiently far out to secure removal of the excreta by the tide. A kitchen and mess-room are attached to each company quarters. The laundresses' quarters, situated on the northeast side of the main entrance to the fort, are three one-story frame battened buildings, originally put up for confederate prisoners, but used for quarters by troops, and subsequently divided into rooms, and occupied by laundresses. In these buildings too many persons are crowded.

The quarters for officers having been built at different periods in the history of the post, and to meet varying conditions in the size of the command, are much scattered and not uniform. Some of the buildings are good, others decidedly objectionable, being much out of repair, damp, and located on low and badly drained ground. That occupied by the commanding officer is situated near the chapel, between the two roads leading to the wharf. It is an old brick building two and one-half stories high, formerly used as a hospital. Recently a two-story frame wing, containing kitchen, bath-room, &c., has been added, increasing its convenience and comfort. Opposite to these are two frame houses used as officers' quarters. That nearest to the fort is one and one-half stories high; the other, consisting of two buildings joined at right angles, is partly one and partly two stories high. In addition to these quarters there are situated on the main road leading to the fort one single and three double frame cottages. The single cottage contains three rooms, a kitchen, and four attic rooms. The double cottages are divided into two single sets, each of two rooms, a kitchen, and two attic rooms. These buildings are well located, and for the most part comfortable, though presenting obvious faults of construction.

The guard-house is situated at the entrance of the fort, and occupies the fifth side of a pentagon. It is a substantial brick building, the archway or sally-port passing through it, on one side of which are two rooms, one 21 feet 5 inches by 14 feet 2 inches; the other, 12 feet 10 inches by 12 feet 2 inches, used for the confinement of prisoners. These rooms are deemed too small for the strength of the garrison. The guard-room, 21 feet 5 inches by 14 feet 2 inches, is on the other side of the archway, and communicates, by means of a door of iron bars, with three cells, each about 10 by 4 feet, intended for solitary confinement. The guard-house is warmed by stoves, ventilation is rather imperfect, and the building is believed to be decidedly unhealthy. Its average occupancy is about ten prisoners, giving to each about 265 cubic feet of air-space.

The hospital building proper is a substantial brick structure, located within the fort limits, upon elevated ground, and fronts to the southeast. It was erected about thirty-five years ago. Its dimensions are 53½ by 27 feet, and two stories high. Covered porches, 10 feet wide, extend around the building on its lower and upper floors. The first floor being raised from the ground about four feet, is reached by stairs at the front and rear porches. The building is warmed by means of stoves.

Kerosene oil is used for artificial illumination at night. Large windows secure natural lighting and ventilation. The plan of this building is shown in Figure 4. 1, lower floor; 2, upper floor; A A, wards; B, bath and wash-room; D, dispensary; H H, halls; O, office; W, water-closets.

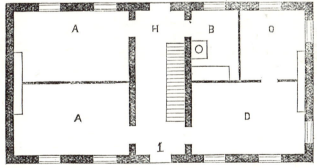

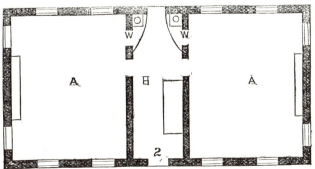

Figure 4.—Scale 16 feet to 1 inch.

The wards on the upper floor measure 23 feet 10 inches by 19 feet 4 inches, and are 12 feet 10 inches high. These wards contain six beds, giving to each 979 cubic feet of air-space. Each room has a water-closet attached, which, on account of their improper construction, rendering disinfection imperfect, are no longer used. (The earth-closet has been sent to this hospital.) The bath-room is on the first floor, adjoining the office. The basement story extends only under one-half of the building, and contains the kitchen, which is low and dark, and at present not in use. Water is supplied from the main tank inside the fort, and conveyed in pipes to the first floor of the hospital. A fine spring is located near the building, but cannot be used on account of the proximity of the hospital privy.

During the recent war it became necessary to provide additional hospital accommodations, and a frame building 150 by 30$\frac{5}{12}$ feet was erected, adjoining the hospital on the southwest side, by an addition 60½ by 25¼ feet, extending from the center of each. The connecting building contains the mess-room, store-room, and linen-room. The frame building was originally one large ward, but latterly a portion of it has been partitioned off sufficient to contain twenty beds, with an air-space of 1,200 cubic feet to each. The principal objection to this ward is its defective ventilation; the windows are sufficient in number, but too high from the floor. The upper part of the ward is thoroughly purified by the windows and ridge-vents, while on the floor and five feet above the air is never fresh.

The post bakery, located near the wharf, is a very old frame building, one story high, and contains two large ovens, with a respective capacity for 200 and 300 loaves per day.

The chapel, situated west of the commanding officer's residence, is a two-storied building, the first floor being used as a library and school-room. On the second floor is the auditory, which will comfortably seat 200 persons. This building was erected some twenty-four years ago by the Methodists of Baltimore.

The post and regimental libraries contain over 1,000 volumes of standard literature, and are being constantly increased.

The principal supply of water is furnished by an artesian well sunk in the center of the parade-ground. The well is 142 feet in depth, 12 inches in diameter 92 feet down, 88 feet of 8-inch pipe extending to 138 feet, double pipe 46 feet. The water is forced, by means of a steam-engine of 8 horse-power, from a depth of 30 feet, into an iron tank of a capacity of 3,322 gallons, and from thence distributed through iron pipes to the following hydrants, viz: one in the center of the fort; one in the center of the road leading from the sally-port to the wharf, located between the commanding officer's and officers' quarters; one to each cook-house of the barracks; one near the southwest corner of the laundresses' quarters; one in the hospital yard; one in the dispensary; one in the hospital kitchen; one in the second story of the brick hospital; one in every kitchen of the officers' quarters, and one at a convenient distance from each row of laundresses' quarters.

The post is also supplied by means of pumps from wells located as follows, viz: one in the southeast corner of the fort; one in the southwest corner of the yard, in rear of the commanding officer's quarters; one between the stable and bakery, and one in the hospital grounds. Means of subduing fire are water-buckets, a force-pump, and ladders; in addition to which there should be a steam fire-engine.

The drainage is naturally good, the whole of the reservation having a gradual slope to the water. The ground outside of the fort is drained by stone and brick gutters, following the natural slope and emptying into the river. The fort is drained by a sewer extending from the southeast side. The marshy piece of ground, spoken of in reference to a portion of the officers' quarters, and which fronts northeast on the Patapsco, should be filled in, or some means devised to prevent the overflow it is subject to, as it is a fruitful source of disease.

The hospital garden consists of three patches of ground within the hospital reservation proper, and is cultivated by convalescents; it is not only ornamental, but useful, a sufficiency of vegetables having been raised to supply all the wants of the hospital.

*Meteorological report, Fort McHenry, Md., 1870–'74.*

| Month. | 1870–'71. | | | | 1871–'72. | | | | 1872–'73. | | | | 1873–'74. | | | |
|---|---|---|---|---|---|---|---|---|---|---|---|---|---|---|---|---|
| | Temperature. | | | Rain-fall in inches. | Temperature. | | | Rain-fall in inches. | Temperature. | | | Rain-fall in inches. | Temperature. | | | Rain-fall in inches. |
| | Mean. | Max. | Min. | | Mean. | Max. | Min. | | Mean. | Max. | Min. | | Mean. | Max. | Min. | |
| July | 82.44 | 95 | 65 | 0.35 | 75.97 | 88 | 62 | 5.65 | 81.92 | 100* | 69* | 1.10 | 78.66 | 91* | 62* | 2.77 |
| August | 79.64 | 93 | 68 | 1.68 | 78.17 | 89 | 64 | 2.04 | 78.79 | 97* | 55* | 6.12 | 74.07 | 91* | 62* | 9.37 |
| September | 70.77 | 85 | 42 | 1.76 | 64.72 | 83 | 47 | 1.76 | 68.31 | 92* | 50* | 6.09 | 67.70 | 88* | 48* | 4.50 |
| October | 59.77 | 79 | 44 | 3.00 | 60.77 | 78 | 42 | 3.98 | 56.98 | 80* | 38* | 4.02 | 55.51 | 73* | 30* | 6.30 |
| November | 47.42 | 66 | 32 | 0.28 | 42.89 | 59 | 28 | 4.44 | 41.70 | 66* | 11* | 4.08 | 40.18 | 61* | 22* | 2.74 |
| December | 35.89 | 60 | 12 | 1.04 | 32.15 | 54* | 0* | 2.01 | 27.56 | 54* | — 1* | 1.46 | 40.17 | 73* | 10* | ? |
| January | 32.33 | 50 | 12 | 2.20 | 31.38 | 50* | 0* | 1.22 | 29.28 | 57* | —15* | 1.50 | 36.50 | 66* | 7* | 1.24 |
| February | 36.16 | 60 | 15 | 2.92 | 31.90 | 56* | 6* | 1.48 | 30.98 | 52* | — 3* | 2.70 | 36.41 | 74* | 9* | 1.56 |
| March | 50.60 | 66 | 39 | 3.38 | 32.36 | 48* | 6* | 5.04 | 41.88 | 65* | 0* | 2.83 | 42.53 | 70* | 15* | 0.56 |
| April | 59.76 | 74 | 42 | 1.88 | 53.38 | 85* | 30* | 3.50 | 51.89 | 72* | 37* | 2.18 | 45.27 | 64* | 20* | 3.56 |
| May | 64.58 | 84 | 51 | 2.19 | 69.36 | 87* | 44* | 1.68 | 62.75 | 84* | 44* | 5.51 | 60.86 | 84* | 31* | 1.81 |
| June | 74.01 | 89 | 64 | 2.96 | 77.93 | 96* | 58* | 4.46 | 73.18 | 93* | 50* | 0.85 | 76.66 | 96* | 57* | 1.07 |
| For the year | 57.78 | 95 | 12 | 23.64 | 54.25 | 96* | 0* | 37.26 | 53.77 | 100* | —15* | 38.44 | 54.54 | 96* | 7* | ........ |

* These observations are made with self-registering thermometers. The mean is from the standard thermometer.

NOTE.—Monthly means from June, 1872, to June, 1874, are derived from registering thermometers, there being no standard thermometer at post.

*Consolidated sick-report, Fort McHenry, Md., 1870–'74.*

| Year | 1870–'71. | | 1871–'72. | | 1872–'73. | | 1873–'74. | |
|---|---|---|---|---|---|---|---|---|
| Mean strength { Officers / Enlisted men | 10 / 196 | | 12 / 168 | | 11 / 173 | | 12 / 221 | |
| Diseases. | Cases. | Deaths. | Cases. | Deaths. | Cases. | Deaths. | Cases. | Deaths. |
| GENERAL DISEASES, A. | | | | | | | | |
| Small-pox and varioloid | | | | | 2 | | 1 | |
| Typhoid fever | 1 | | | 1 | | | 1 | |
| Remittent fever | 6 | | 3 | | 1 | | 1 | |
| Intermittent fever | 75 | | 86 | | 41 | | 45 | |
| Other diseases of this group | 41 | | 18 | | 12 | | 10 | |
| GENERAL DISEASES, B. | | | | | | | | |
| Rheumatism | 27 | | 24 | | 9 | | 19 | |
| Syphilis | 14 | | 9 | | 28 | | 18 | |
| Consumption | 2 | | | 1 | 1 | | 1 | |
| Other diseases of this group | | | 4 | | 1 | 1 | 1 | |
| LOCAL DISEASES. | | | | | | | | |
| Catarrh and bronchitis | 30 | | 23 | | 23 | | 13 | |
| Pneumonia | 1 | | 3 | 1 | | | 2 | |
| Pleurisy | 2 | | | | 1 | | | |
| Diarrhœa and dysentery | 55 | | 47 | 1 | 49 | | 63 | |
| Hernia | | | | | 1 | | 1 | |
| Gonorrhœa | 14 | | 19 | | 4 | | 6 | |
| Other local diseases | 80 | | 47 | 1 | 56 | | 67 | |
| Alcoholism | 32 | | 25 | 1 | 18 | | 22 | |
| Unclassified | | | | | 1 | | 1 | |
| Total disease | 380 | | 308 | 6 | 248 | 1 | 271 | |
| VIOLENT DISEASES AND DEATHS. | | | | | | | | |
| Gunshot wounds | 1 | | | | | | | |
| Drowning | | 1 | | | | 1 | | 2 |
| Other accidents and injuries | 65 | | 38 | | 52 | | 64 | |
| Total violence | 66 | 1 | 38 | | 52 | 1 | 64 | 2 |

# FORT MACKINAC, MACKINAC, MICHIGAN.

REPORT OF ACTING ASSISTANT SURGEON H. R. MILLS AND OF ASSISTANT SURGEON C. CARVALLO, UNITED STATES ARMY.

Fort Mackinac is situated on a bluff on the southeastern portion of the island of Mackinac, near the straits of the same name which connect Lakes Huron and Michigan, latitude, 45° 51′ 22″ north; longitude, 7° 38′ 22″ west. Height above the lake, 155 feet; above the sea, 728 feet. The nearest post is Fort Brady, 60 miles to the northeast. The only town of importance near the post is Sheboygan, on the mainland, 18 miles south. Its population is about 2,000. The nearest railroad station is at Saginaw, 150 miles distant. The island was first occupied by the English as a military post, soon after the destruction of old Fort Mackinac and its garrison on the mainland by the French in 1763, on account of its security from attacks from Indians. About 1795 it was turned over to the United States Government by treaty, as a part of the result of the revolutionary war, but in 1812 it was again occupied by the English. The island is about nine miles in circumference, and rises on its eastern and southern shore in abrupt rocky cliffs, the highest point being 250 feet above the water, Fort Mackinac being situated on the south side, near the lake. Situated on the highest point of the island, and about half a mile to the rear of the fort, is "Fort Holmes," which was built by the English during their occupancy of the island in 1812–'13–'14, and called by them "Fort George." It was upon this point that the United States forces were making an attack when Major Holmes, of the United States Army, was killed, which circumstance subsequently gave the present name to the work.

The timber on the island is mostly small, probably owing to its having been cut down at not a very remote period. It is composed of beech, maple, oak, and poplar, principally, with a liberal supply of the *coniferæ*, viz: pine, spruce, hemlock, cedar, tamarack, &c. *Conium maculatum* is found in abundance.

The reservation contains a little over two square miles. The surface is regular, but there is very little soil covering the underlying rock.

The fort consists of stone and earthworks, inclosing about half an acre of ground.

The barrack is a two-story frame building, 112 by 29 feet, with a porch on the south-southeast side, fronting the parade. The dormitories are 11 feet 5 inches high; are fitted with single iron bedsteads, and give an air-space of 496 and 749 cubic feet per man, respectively.

The kitchen, mess-room, and wash-room are in a one-story frame building; capacity, one company.

The officers' quarters are in two buildings; one of stone, built in 1780–'83, 103 by 40 feet, divided into two sets of quarters, each of four rooms, with a basement; the other, a one and a half story frame building, 52 by 48 feet, containing two sets of quarters.

The guard-house is a one-story frame building, 30 by 20 feet. The prison-cell is a dark ill-ventilated room, 16 feet 11 inches by 11 feet 10 inches and 8 feet 3 inches high. Fourteen prisoners have been confined in this cell for one night.

The commissary storehouse is a one-story frame building, 49 by 30 feet. The quartermaster's storehouse is 46 by 20 feet.

The hospital was built in 1860. It is a two and a half story frame building, with shingle roof, with three wards, giving room for ten beds, with an air-space of from 600 to 800 cubic feet to each. It has no bath-room.

The water-supply of the post is from the lake, by water-carts, and from cisterns.

The natural drainage is good, and the post is a healthy one.

*Consolidated sick-report, Fort Mackinac, Mich, 1870–'74.*

| Year | | 1870–'71. | | 1871–'72. | | 1872–'73. | | 1873–'74. | |
|---|---|---|---|---|---|---|---|---|---|
| Mean strength { Officers | | 3 | | 4 | | 4 | | 4 | |
| { Enlisted men | | 35 | | 43 | | 39 | | 41 | |
| Diseases. | | Cases. | Deaths. | Cases. | Deaths. | Cases. | Deaths. | Cases. | Deaths. |
| GENERAL DISEASES, A. | | | | | | | | | |
| Typhoid fever | | | | | | | | 2 | 1 |
| Remittent fever | | 1 | | | | | | 4 | |
| Intermittent fever | | | | 2 | | 18 | | 3 | |
| Other diseases of this group | | | | | | | | 1 | |
| GENERAL DISEASES, B. | | | | | | | | | |
| Rheumatism | | 2 | | 1 | | 8 | | 1 | |
| Syphilis | | 3 | | 3 | | 2 | | 2 | |
| Consumption | | 2 | | 2 | | 4 | 1 | | |
| LOCAL DISEASES. | | | | | | | | | |
| Catarrh and bronchitis | | | | | | 29 | | 2 | |
| Pleurisy | | | | 1 | | 5 | | | |
| Diarrhœa and dysentery | | 3 | | 4 | | 14 | | 20 | |
| Hernia | | 1 | | 3 | | 1 | | | |
| Gonorrhœa | | | | | | 1 | | | |
| Other local diseases | | 16 | | 11 | | 30 | 1 | 28 | |
| Alcoholism | | 1 | | 1 | | | | 1 | |
| Total disease | | 29 | | 28 | | 112 | 2 | 64 | 1 |
| VIOLENT DISEASES AND DEATHS. | | | | | | | | | |
| Gunshot wounds | | | 1 | | | 1 | | | |
| Other accidents and injuries | | 8 | | 8 | | 8 | | 9 | |
| Total violence | | 8 | 1 | 8 | | 9 | | 9 | |

# MADISON BARRACKS, SACKETT'S HARBOR, NEW YORK.

## REPORTS OF SURGEONS E. P. VOLLUM AND L. A. EDWARDS, UNITED STATES ARMY.

Madison Barracks is situated at Sackett's Harbor, New York, on the south shore of Black River Bay, about ten miles from Lake Ontario, latitude, 43° 57′ north; longitude, 0° 48′ east; height, 262 feet above the sea. Black River, a stream of considerable size and importance as an unfailing water-power, falls into the head of Black River Bay, eight miles east of the post, at the town of Dexter, a manufacturing place; and the mouth of Mill Creek bounds the reservation in the same direction. The land in the neighborhood is free from marsh, but at the head of Black River Bay there are some marshy places, which, however, do not produce any appreciable bad effects. The surface of the surrounding country is gently undulating, and the soil, originally rich, is now somewhat worn out by careless cultivation. The timber is mostly cleared off, and the country is thickly settled.

The site of the post is about thirty feet above the water, and, excepting a short space in front of the parade, overlooks it by a perpendicular bluff of limestone.

The soil of the reservation is chiefly a dark loam, resting on a stratum of fossiliferous limestone, which lies from one to four feet below the surface. A large part of the surface, especially the cultivated portion, is flat, and difficult to drain in a thorough manner. The reservation contains thirty-nine and one-fourth acres, purchased in parcels at different dates. The whole is inclosed by a substantial cedar stockade.

The roads about the post are partly covered with broken stones, with a covering of sifted hard-coal ashes about an inch deep, thrown on, wetted, and packed down by a horse-roller. The result has been a smooth and quite durable light carriage-road and foot-path, which can be easily and cheaply repaired.

All of the buildings, except the ordnance-sergeant's quarters, stables, ice-house, and engine-house, are constructed of limestone, used in pieces of various sizes and shapes, and neatly fitted together, making the walls about 19 inches thick, and sufficiently durable to stand for centuries to come.

The roofs of all the buildings are shingled, except the quartermaster's and commissary storehouses and guard-house, which are covered with tin, painted. The parade is a smooth grassy surface, 552 by 452 feet, bounded on three sides by officers' and men's quarters, and open on the water side, allowing a beautiful and extended view of the bay and opposite country. The officers' quarters face the northwest, and consist of two rows of buildings on the same line, raised about two feet above the ground and separated by the sally-port, which is 30 feet wide. Each row is 217 feet by 33 feet, and consists of five double sets of quarters, protected in front by a continuous portico, six feet wide. The first set of quarters on each side of the sally-port is two stories high. In the quarters on the right of the sally-port there are two rooms on each side of the hall on both stories, and a kitchen in a wooden extension in rear. The ceilings on both stories are 10 feet high. The lower rooms on the right, in front, measure 15 feet by 16 feet 7 inches; in rear, 14 feet 3 inches by 15 feet 6 inches; up stairs, same side, in front, 14 feet 7 inches by 15 feet 6 inches; in rear, 11 feet 8 inches by 15 feet 3 inches; left of hall, lower story, front, 13 feet by 15 feet; rear, 12 feet 6 inches by 15 feet 1 inch; up stairs, front, 13 feet 2 inches by 14 feet 4 inches; rear, 13 feet 3 inches by 14 feet 5 inches; kitchen, 23 feet 8 inches by 11 feet 10 inches, by 10 feet high, with a sky-light. Inclosing the yard, which is 25 by 30 feet, are a carriage-house and stable for two horses, water-closets, wood-shed, and coal-bin, constructed of wood, and a root-house constructed of stone and covered with earth and sod. The walls of the quarters are hard-finished. In the front of the second-story hall is a bath-room, 6 by 16 feet, the water for which is carried up by hand. There are plenty of closets and cupboards. The first set of quarters, on the left of the sally-port, is the same as the above in every particular, excepting the bath-room and out-houses. The kitchen is a wooden extension in rear, 11 feet 9 inches by 11 feet 4 inches, by 10 feet high; the water-closet is an ordinary wooden structure in the yard. The remainder of the officers' quarters are all one story and an attic high. Each set consists of a front and rear room on the first floor, a front and rear attic room, and a kitchen; a hall and stairway are in common for the two sets, a very objectionable arrangement for domestic comfort and privacy. The height of all the ceilings on the first story measures 9 feet 2 inches, and the height of the attics is 8 feet 4 inches in the middle, 5 feet 2 inches at the side, with a slope of 8 feet. The front rooms on the first story are 13 feet by 14 feet 6 inches; rear rooms 13 feet by 15 feet. The end set of the right-hand row is divided up on the lower story into three rooms; the front one is 34 feet 6 inches by 15 feet 6 inches, with five windows, and is used as a post-library, reading-room, and school; the two rear ones are respectively 13 feet 2 inches by 21 feet 6 inches, and 12 feet 4 inches by 13 feet 2 inches, and are used as court-martial rooms. The attic is thrown into one apartment, 34 feet 6 inches by 29 feet 3 inches, with four dormer windows on each side, and is used as a ball-room and chapel. The end set on the left is partitioned off the same as the above, except the attic, which is divided into four sleeping-rooms, averaging each 12 feet by 12 feet 6 inches. The large room on the lower story has five windows, and is used as an officers' mess-room. A board fence, 7 feet high, extends along the rear of each row of quarters, and separates the yards which, excepting the first set described, are 60 feet by 60 feet. A ditch for drainage runs underneath each row along the middle. The heating of the officers' quarters is effected at present partly by coal-stoves and partly by grates. The ventilation in the rooms having grates is found to be sufficient. In front of the portico is a grassed terrace, 10 feet wide and the length of each row, with a stone path and steps leading from each front door to the carriage-road. This road describes a circle at each end of the line of quarters and in the middle at the sally-port, and the parade-ground and the circles are protected by rows of cedar posts turned in the form of cannon and connected by chains. The circles are sodded and raised about two feet, and surmounted by brass field-pieces for ornament.

The men's quarters consist of two buildings, one story and an attic high, constructed of lime-stone, each 452 feet by 23 feet. These buildings face each other from the opposite sides of the parade, and run perpendicularly to the water-front. A portico extends along the front of each. The windows of the western barracks are, as formerly, all in the face looking upon the parade, excepting two in the kitchens, but in the eastern barracks, in addition to these, three windows have been cut in the blind wall into each squad-room. Owing to the slope of the ground toward the water, the buildings at that end are considerably higher than at the other, allowing in one space enough below the squad-rooms for mess and store rooms, in the other for coal-cellars. The ceilings of all the rooms on the lower story are 9 feet high. Each building is subdivided into four squad-rooms, 64 feet by 20 feet, two mess-rooms, 30 feet by 20 feet, two kitchens, 20 feet by 19 feet 9 inches, two wash-rooms, 20 feet by 7 feet 9 inches, two sergeants' rooms, 20 feet by 10 feet 9 inches, and two store-rooms, 19 feet by 10 feet 9 inches.

Each squad-room is thoroughly fitted up with gun-racks, lockers for the clothing and effects of the men, tables, chairs, shelves, and clothes-hooks. Each man has an iron bedstead, of the hospital pattern, to himself, and his locker and shelf are painted with his name and company number. The ventilation of the squad-rooms is effected by wooden shafts, 16 inches square, reaching from the ceiling at each end of the squad-room to latticed ventilators in the roof. The lower openings of the shafts are covered by ornamental iron registers for controlling the passage of air, and in the attics an aperture is cut into the shaft for the ventilation of those apartments. The heating is effected by one coal-stove in each squad-room, which is found to be sufficient for ordinary winter weather.

In the eastern barracks there are nine windows in the squad-rooms, six in the dining-rooms, and three in the kitchens; and in the western barracks, six in the squad-rooms, four in the dining-rooms, and four in the kitchens.

The wash-rooms open out of the squad-rooms, and each is provided with a trough on each side, with holes for basins, and a barrel of water with a faucet. Every man has a tin basin, which has its appropriate hook and number. In summer a half hogshead is placed in the room for the use of such men as do not bathe in the bay.

The men's sinks are wooden structures, set over deep pits, walled up, and situated sixty paces to the rear of each barrack building. They are emptied in the winter season by chopping out the soil in frozen blocks and depositing them on the ice about half a mile out from shore.

The guard-house, situated near the south gate, on the main road to the sally-port, is a very durable, fine-looking stone structure, 54 feet by 39 feet, roofed with tin, painted. The portico, supported by five wooden columns, is 39 feet by 10 feet. All the ceilings are 9 feet 6 inches high. It is partitioned off into a room for the officer of the day, 14 feet 11 inches by 13 feet; a guard-room, 20 feet by 18 feet; a prisoners' room, 30 feet by 20 feet; six cells, each 8 feet 11 inches by 4 feet; and a passage in front of the cells, 34 feet by 5 feet. The officer of the day's room and guard-room are well lighted by two windows each. The building is well ventilated, except the prisoners' room, into which pure air can only enter by the windows, which are seldom opened in cold weather, and by a grated opening a foot square in the door leading into the guard-room. The cells have no ventilation whatever, and there is no light, except a narrow spot that appears at an aperture near the ceiling, 12 inches by 3 inches in size. They are dark, cold, damp, and gloomy, and in them a prisoner is smothered and punished in a chilly, stony den, in a style worthy of the dark ages. The exhalations of a man in a single night accumulate in sufficient quantity to nearly extinguish a lighted candle set on the floor. In them a man is not only deprived of his liberty, light, and his life's breath, but his own effluvia turn upon him as a poison. Happily they are seldom occupied. The heating is effected by coal-stoves, and is sufficient. The guard-room and prisoners' room are furnished with the customary board platforms used in the Army guard-houses to sleep upon. Whatever may be said as to the propriety of the prisoners being compelled, as part of their punishment, to sleep in that uncomfortable way, there is no good reason why the members of the guard should be forced to catch the little sleep and rest allowed them between their hours of guard on hard boards in the same manner. The members of the guard, the *élite* for the time, always charged with the most important duties known to army life, should be lodged in time of peace as comfortably as when they are in quarters, and when off post their inducements for sleep should be as good as may be—a straw mattress at least. The sink is a wooden structure, set over a deep pit, walled up, and is situated 20 feet in rear. It is reached by a covered way, opening into the passage in front of the cells, from which it is separated by two doors. The object of the covered way is to protect the prisoners from the weather, and to prevent their escape at night.

The storehouse, formerly used by the quartermaster and subsistence departments, was destroyed by fire in the winter of 1871–'72, and has not been rebuilt.

The wharf is a wooden crib, filled with stone, 75 feet long, L-shaped, 61 feet front. Upon it are a boat-house and a force-pump housed in. The bakery, situated at the water's edge near the quartermaster and commissary storehouse, is a stone structure, divided into two rooms. The oven, recently rebuilt of brick, is capacious enough for a regiment.

The ice-house is a wooden structure, situated near the water, 32 feet by 16 feet by 10 feet to the eaves. It rests on a stone foundation 2 feet high, on a gentle slope favoring the drainage, which is allowed to sink into the ground. The floor is made of inch boards, not tongued and grooved, and the outer and inner walls, of the same stuff tongued and grooved, are separated 5 inches and filled with coarse sawdust. An aperture in each end, 3 inches wide, runs across nearly to the eaves and communicates with the space above the eaves inside. There is a single door, 4 feet square, on the north side, 5 feet above the ground. The roof is shingled, and projects 3 feet over the sides, which are whitewashed. It is calculated for 150 tons.

There is a fire-engine, a hose-cart, and 600 feet of rubber hose. Besides these, each barrack-building, store-house, the hospital, and the guard-house, are well supplied with ladders, hooks, axes, and fire-buckets, which are always kept filled with water and standing in convenient places. The water-supply for this purpose is from the bay and from a well in rear of the eastern barracks, and another in the rear of the officers' quarters. In case of fire, the bay would be too far off for some of the buildings, and the wells, if used, would soon give out.

The water-supply for drinking and cooking, as taken from the bay, is a mixture of the waters of Black River and Lake Ontario. At times it is clear from the lake, at others it is the brownish water from the river, according as the winds drive the waters about the bay and mix them together. Formerly the Black River water was regarded as unwholesome, but this has been proved to be a mistake by the experience of Watertown, a place ten miles off, of some twelve thousand inhabitants, where, for a number of years past, this water has been used exclusively, without any bad effects whatever. The water is forced up by a hand-pump, situated on the end of the wharf, where it is taken from a place 12 feet deep, free from much current and the effects of surface drainage. From thence it is conveyed by a rubber hose to barrels placed on an army wagon, and thus distributed about the post. This arrangement occupies five men and two horses for most of the day, with a decided damage to the health of the men, especially in winter, and a considerable expenditure for forage and wear and tear of wagon and harness. An estimate of cost shows that this work could be done cheaper by a steam-pump and reservoir, with a great saving to the health of the command.

The post-garden comprises about ten acres within the stockade.

Shade-trees have been set out from time to time in various places about the post, but with little success, owing, doubtless, to the shallowness of the soil and the prevalence of strong winds that disturb the tender roots of the young trees.

The drainage is effected by ditches leading to the bay. In a few level spots the ditches have to be cleaned out occasionally.

The hospital is situated at the eastern limits of the reservation, about 50 feet from the water. The site is sandy, and elevated about 15 feet above the bay, and the grounds, which are well sodded, slope off in every direction from the building, making the drainage excellent. It commands a beautiful and extensive view of the harbor and islands toward the lake; but the situation is exceedingly bleak in winter. The building is square, with wings on either side, and constructed of cut limestone, with a hipped roof, shingled and painted. The main building has two stories, and measures 56 feet 5 inches by 53 feet 6 inches, by 35 feet high; and the wings have one story, 18 feet 2 inches by 15 feet 3 inches, by 20 feet 5 inches high. The basement is dry, and is lighted by windows above ground. The building is entered by stone steps, 12 feet wide, front and rear, and by basement doors under the steps. The basement is 8 feet 4 inches high. For plan of division of the basement and second floor, see Figure 5.

1. *Basement.*—K, kitchen; M, dining-room; X, pantries; H, hall; S, store-room; T, closet; V, matron's quarters.

2. *Second floor.*—A, wards; S, lavatories; T, closet; W, water-closet.

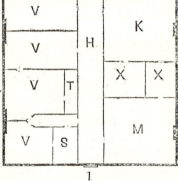

The kitchen is provided with a boiler and pipes for sending hot water to the bath on the first story, and a force-pump for sending water from a rain-water cistern to a tank on the second story. The pantries are well fitted up with shelves and cupboards.

There are two wards opening into each side of the halls on both stories, making eight in all, and all of the front and rear wards communicate by passages 8 feet 4 inches by 4 feet 6 inches; from each side of which open closet-rooms, eight in all, appropriated to uses to be mentioned below. The four wards on the first story measure 20 feet by 19 feet 9 inches, by 12 feet 9 inches high each, and those on the second story measure the same, except in the height, which is 3 inches less. Two wards on each story on the south side are generally the only ones in use, and are occupied by from four to six beds each. When there are four patients in a ward, omitting fractions, each has 1,290 cubic feet of air and 101 superficial feet of area; when there are six, each has 860 cubic feet of air and 67 superficial feet of area. On the right of the passage, between the lower wards on the south side, is a bath-room, 7 feet 2 inches by 8 feet, by 12 feet 9 inches high, in which is a water-closet; the bath is furnished with hot and cold water. Opposite the bath-room is a lavatory, 7 feet 3 inches by 8 feet, by 12 feet 9 inches high, furnished with ordinary tin basins and towels. Opening from the passage between the wards, on the north side of the same story, are two medical store-rooms, each 7 feet 3 inches

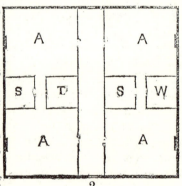

Figure 5.

by 8 feet, by 12 feet 9 inches high, furnished with shelves and double locks. The second story is reached by a stairway, 4 feet 2 inches wide, in the hall leading from the front, the steps of which are only 6 inches high, for ease of ascent for the sick. Opening from the right of the passage between the wards on the south side of this story is a room, 7 feet 7 inches by 7 feet 2 inches, by 12 feet 6 inches high, containing a water-closet and a water-tank for supplying the bath and water-closets; opposite this is a lavatory, 7 feet 7 inches by 7 feet 2 inches, by 12 feet 6 inches high. Opening from the passage between the wards on the opposite side are a lavatory and closet of the same size. A skylight in the apex of the roof, with a wooden railing about it, admits abundance of light upon the halls and stairway. Iron balconies project from the front and rear windows in the hall of the second story. The uses of all the rooms are indicated by tin signs over the doors; the wards are lettered.

The wing rooms on each side open out of the front wards, 16 feet by 11 feet 2 inches, by 12 feet 9 inches high, and each has a rear door and stone stairway to the ground. The one on the south side is used as a surgery, the other as a *post-mortem* room. Both are grained in imitation of oak. Under each of the wings is a stone masonry rain-water cistern, arranged with a filter. The one on the north side is not in use, for want of water-pipes from the roof, which seem never to have been put up; the other is in good order, and is fed from the roof by copper pipes. Except in winter, when all the water is hauled, this cistern supplies about half the quantity required. The lighting is ample. The windows on the first and second stories and wings are furnished with double sash for winter weather. The heating is sufficient, and is effected by base-burner hard-coal stoves, except in one ward, where there is a wood fireplace, for the accommodation of a special class of patients. The ventilation is effected by fireplaces in each room, which are kept partly open, by the draught of the stoves, and by letting down the tops of the window-sash when required. The drainage from the bath, water-closets, and kitchen, passes off by a main into the ground under the hospital. Occasionally the water-closets taint the air, as is usual when they are built indoors, but they are only used when the weather is too severe for the patients to go to the sink in the yard. The sink, situated 50 feet in the rear, is built of limestone, and measures 10 feet by 20 feet, by 9 feet high, and is divided into three apartments. The pit, the area of the building, is very deep, and walled up with stone, and seems to drain into the ground, as it always keeps the same level. A substantial picket-fence incloses the grounds; foot-paths describing ornamental figures have been laid out, and hundreds of trees, bushes, shrubs, and plants have been set out; but, unfortunately, owing to the light, sandy character of the soil, but few of these have survived, except some 430 feet of lilac hedging along the edge of the bluff, a few rose-bushes and Missouri currants, a few Lombardy poplars, set out especially to embellish the effect of the building, and a number of plum-trees.

*Meteorological report, Madison Barracks, N. Y., 1870-'74.*

| Month. | 1870-'71. Temperature. Mean. | Max. | Min. | Rain-fall in inches. | 1871-'72. Temperature. Mean. | Max. | Min. | Rain-fall in inches. | 1872-'73. Temperature. Mean. | Max. | Min. | Rain-fall in inches. | 1873-'74. Temperature. Mean. | Max. | Min. | Rain-fall in inches. |
|---|---|---|---|---|---|---|---|---|---|---|---|---|---|---|---|---|
| July | 72.44 | 88 | 56 | 1.46 | 68.71 | 94 | 52 | 2.17 | 71.94 | 92* | 60* | 1.55 | 70.66 | 75 | 45* | 1.96 |
| August | 73.59 | 92 | 58 | 1.61 | 69.42 | 90 | 50 | 6.14 | 71.36 | 95* | 58* | 3.64 | 68.45 | 81 | 47* | 2.70 |
| September | 63.87 | 80 | 40 | 4.55 | 58.07 | 90* | 28* | 1.40 | 62.44 | 87* | 36* | 3.85 | 60.98 | 85 | 30* | 2.20 |
| October | 49.82 | 70 | 26 | 2.05 | 52.51 | 75* | 23* | 1.55 | 46.87 | 80* | 22* | 5.20 | 50.13 | 70 | 18* | 5.25 |
| November | 38.15 | 60 | 17 | 1.27 | 30.43 | 62* | − 4* | 3.68 | 35.52 | 53 | 8* | 2.39 | 27.56 | 52 | − 6* | 1.55 |
| December | 23.44 | 42 | −15 | 1.60 | 17.76 | 50* | −44* | 1.98 | 19.42 | 40 | −36* | 1.39 | 28.63 | 47 | −12* | 1.05 |
| January | 13.17 | 55 | −24 | 1.60 | 18.52 | 42* | −16* | 2.00 | 14.83 | 52 | −25 | 1.90 | 23.89 | 65 | −25* | 4.71 |
| February | 20.13 | 52 | −20 | 1.05 | 15.82 | 52* | −15* | 2.00 | 18.49 | 42 | −16* | 0.30 | 17.72 | 48 | −30ᴬ | 2.24 |
| March | 35.91 | 66 | 20 | 2.36 | 15.23 | 40* | −36* | 1.54 | 24.59 | 50 | −13* | 5.60 | 28.45 | 60 | − 5* | 2.07 |
| April | 44.66 | 75 | 26 | 2.15 | 40.61 | 79* | 12* | 1.60 | 38.66 | 60 | 22* | 2.72 | 34.11 | 54 | 7* | 0.97 |
| May | 53.83 | 85 | 35 | 1.58 | 53.06 | 80* | 35* | 2.14 | 54.54 | 86 | 25* | 0.92 | 54.63 | 78 | 21* | 0.92 |
| June | 64.99 | 90 | 50 | 1.38 | 65.35 | 85* | 40* | 2.90 | 67.27 | 90 | 42* | 3.80 | 63.80 | 86 | 40* | 1.84 |
| For the year | 46.17 | 92 | −24 | 22.67 | 42.12 | 94 | −44* | 29.10 | 43.83 | 95* | −36* | 33.26 | 44.09 | 86 | −30* | 27.46 |

* These observations are made with self-registering thermometers. The mean is from the standard thermometer.

*Consolidated sick-report, Madison Barracks, Sackett's Harbor, N. Y., 1870-'74.*

| Year | | 1870-'71. | | 1871-'72. | | 1872-'73. | | 1873-'74. | |
|---|---|---|---|---|---|---|---|---|---|
| Mean strength { Officers | | 6 | | 6 | | 5 | | 7 | |
| { Enlisted men | | 95 | | 90 | | 77 | | 110 | |
| Diseases. | | Cases. | Deaths. | Cases. | Deaths. | Cases. | Deaths. | Cases. | Deaths. |
| GENERAL DISEASES, A. | | | | | | | | | |
| Typhoid fever | | 1 | 1 | | | | | | |
| Typho-malarial fever | | | | | | | | 1 | |
| Remittent fever | | | | 5 | | | | | |
| Intermittent fever | | 26 | | 16 | | 3 | | 4 | |
| Other diseases of this group | | 21 | | 26 | | 16 | | 75 | |

7 M P

*Consolidated sick-report, Madison Barracks, Sackett's Harbor, N. Y., 1870–'74—Continued.*

| Year | | 1870–'71. | | 1871–'72. | | 1872–'73. | | 1873–'74. | |
|---|---|---|---|---|---|---|---|---|---|
| Mean strength { Officers | | 6 | | 6 | | 5 | | 7 | |
| { Enlisted men | | 95 | | 90 | | 77 | | 110 | |
| Diseases. | | Cases. | Deaths. | Cases. | Deaths. | Cases. | Deaths. | Cases. | Deaths. |
| GENERAL DISEASES, B. | | | | | | | | | |
| Rheumatism | | 21 | ...... | 12 | ...... | 14 | ...... | 10 | ...... |
| Syphilis | | | ...... | 3 | ...... | | ...... | 2 | ...... |
| Consumption | | | ...... | 1 | ...... | | ...... | | ...... |
| LOCAL DISEASES. | | | | | | | | | |
| Catarrh and bronchitis | | 51 | ...... | 40 | ...... | 9 | ...... | 7 | ...... |
| Pneumonia | | 1 | ...... | | ...... | 1 | ...... | | ...... |
| Pleurisy | | 2 | ...... | 1 | ...... | | ...... | | ...... |
| Diarrhœa and dysentery | | 34 | ...... | 28 | ...... | 10 | ...... | 14 | ...... |
| Hernia | | 2 | ...... | 5 | ...... | | ...... | | ...... |
| Gonorrhœa | | | ...... | | ...... | 2 | ...... | 7 | ...... |
| Other local diseases | | 65 | ...... | 80 | ...... | 46 | ...... | 46 | ...... |
| Alcoholism | | 10 | ...... | 10 | ...... | 10 | ...... | 19 | ...... |
| Total disease | | 234 | 1 | 227 | ...... | 110 | ...... | 185. | ...... |
| VIOLENT DISEASES AND DEATHS. | | | | | | | | | |
| Gunshot wounds | | 1 | ...... | 1 | ...... | | ...... | | ...... |
| Other accidents and injuries | | 27 | ...... | 14 | ...... | 17 | ...... | 25 | 1 |
| Suicide | | | ...... | | ...... | | 1 | | ...... |
| Total violence | | 28 | ...... | 15 | ...... | 17 | 1 | 25 | 1 |

## FORT MIFFLIN, PENNSYLVANIA.

Fort Mifflin is situated on Mud Island, in the Delaware River, one mile below the mouth of the Schuylkill and seven miles below Philadelphia City proper. The site was occupied for military purposes during, and perhaps before, the Revolution. The present works were commenced in 1798. The reservation contains about three hundred and seventeen acres.

The quarters consist of commanding officers' quarters, one and a half stories, brick, rough-coated, with tin roof, 70 feet by 34½ feet; subalterns' quarters, two stories, 80 feet by 20½ feet, brick, with slate roof, kitchen attached, 14½ feet by 12½ feet; company quarters for one company of artillery, one and a half stories high, 117½ feet by 28 feet, brick, with slate roof, divided into three squad-rooms, one mess-room, kitchen, one orderly-room, and a small room for sutler's store on the first floor, and six rooms for company laundresses and one company store-room on the second floor.

The guard-house is of wood, with tin roof, divided into a guard-room and a prison-room, 30½ feet by 16 feet.

The hospital, which is outside of the fort, is a wooden building, with shingle roof, 51 feet by 20 feet, and two stories high. There are also separate adjoining buildings for hospital kitchen, wash-house, storehouse, and ice-house.

Water is taken exclusively from the Delaware River, there being no well at the post fit for use.

The post is in charge of an ordnance-sergeant.

---

## FORT MONROE, VIRGINIA.

### REPORTS OF SURGEONS G. E. COOPER AND J. E. SUMMERS, UNITED STATES ARMY.

Fort Monroe is situated on Old Point Comfort, a peninsula at the south end of the west shore of Chesapeake Bay; latitude, 37° 2' north; longitude, 51' east. The peninsula is connected to the mainland by a strip of beach about four hundred yards wide, over which, during heavy easterly storms, with a full spring tide, the sea washes; and by a bridge over Mill Creek.

The fort is built at the extremity of the peninsula, and commands the entrance to Hampton

Roads, into which empty the waters of the James, Elizabeth, and Nansemond Rivers. The waters on all sides of the fort are salt. The land upon which the fort is built is some four feet above mean high-water mark. Salt marshes are on the north and northwest of the fort, but these seem to have but little, if any, effect upon its sanitary condition.

The geological formation of the peninsula upon which the fort is built is ocean sand, resting upon marl-impregnated clay. Boring to the depth of 850 feet, within the inclosure of the fort, has shown nothing but sand, lying upon marl-impregnated clay, with here and there small veins of sharp bluish sand of fine grain, admirably adapted for polishing and grinding metals. The country on the mainland is flat, and there are no hills within a radius of eight or ten miles. The soil to the north of Mill Creek, which bounds the reservation in that direction, is aluminous and quite productive, giving, under favorable circumstances, abundant yields of wheat, corn, oats, and potatoes, as well as of all the market vegetables. There are no rocks of any description in the neighborhood.

The whole country to the north and northwest of the fort is underlaid by extensive beds of marl, at depths varying from 20 feet to 50 feet. The water procurable on the mainland, from wells, is, in consequence, quite unpalatable, and, to many persons, acts as a strong cathartic, while to others it has the effect of causing discharges of bloody urine. All, previous to the war of secession, who had the means, erected cisterns to collect rain-water for drinking purposes.

The soil inside the fort, which incloses over eighty acres, is artificial, and has been brought from the mainland. By careful cultivation and an artificial supply of water during the dry seasons vegetables for kitchen use and flowers for ornament can be raised. The live-oak is found within the inclosure of the work, having been undisturbed when the clearing was made to build the fort.

On the Chesapeake Bay beach, distant some 2,000 yards to the north, are heavy sand hills, and on and around these are found numerous live-oaks, as well as the southern pine. This is said to be the most northern position in the United States at which the live-oak is to be met with.

In the gardens of the fort are to be found numerous fig trees, which flourish, though the late frosts of spring often destroy the fruit.

The waters surrounding the fort are well stocked with fish, principally rock, sheephead, bay mackerel, trout, white perch, sun, spot, hog, chub, green, flounders, moss-bunkers, and toad. Porpoises are quite numerous, and white shark not scarce. Crabs, both hard and soft, are abundant. Oysters cover the banks where the tide runs not too fast and the bottom is not sand; they are the quality highest prized in all the markets.

The climate of Old Point Comfort is comparatively mild. The winters are open, and the thermometer, except in extremely rare instances, does not fall below 12° F. The duration of the cold periods seldom passes seventy-two hours, when the cold snaps give way and the mercury indicates an increase of temperature. The cold is, however, felt more perceptibly than in those regions where it is continuous, and the system is far more susceptible to the influence of a decrease of temperature than it is in the more northern latitudes.

Within the walls of the fort the heat is much more oppressive than without, as they serve to obstruct, in a great measure, the free range of the breeze which may be blowing. At night, however, the reverse holds, as a damp, murky atmosphere arises from the ground, imparting a chilly sensation, with a feeling of moisture. There is, at night, a difference of two or three degrees in the temperature inside and outside the fort.

The prevailing winds of spring and summer are southeast and southwest; those of fall and winter east, northeast, and northwest. The easterly winds are the most severe in February and March, and with them come diseases of the throat and lungs to both adults and infants. With the latter croup is most common in February and early March, when the winds, chilled by the icebergs on the banks, continue blowing from the northeast for several successive days.

The fort is a massive work, built of granite, surrounded by a moat filled with water, which is fed by a tide-gate opening into Mill Creek. The depth of water in the moat is 8 feet. Bridges, five in number, crossing the moat, furnish the means of entrance into the fort. The officers and men composing the garrison are quartered within the walls of the work.

The quarters for officers are, respectively, brick buildings, frame buildings, and casemates. The brick buildings are large, roomy, and well ventilated, though badly arranged for household conveniences. They all have basement stories, which are really untenable, in consequence of their excessive humidity, caused principally by large fresh-water cisterns being built in contact with one of the walls, one side of which they form. In the winter time this excessive dampness is overcome by the large fires kept in the basements. During the summer time all articles kept in the basement stories are soon covered with a greenish-white mold. The same objection, as far as humidity is concerned, is applicable to the casemates. They are very damp and poorly ventilated. Even in the warmest days of summer it is necessary to have large fires in them to overcome the humidity and render them tenantable. The use of them as dwellings is very conducive to rheumatic affections, as well as to diseases of the pulmonary organs. Persons suffering from intermittent fevers find that it is almost impossible to have them broken up as long as they reside in the casemates without having them dried by constant fires.

The quarters for the enlisted men are temporary frame structures, erected on the northern side of the parade, seven in number, each 120 feet by 25 feet. The houses are built some 40 feet distant from each other. These buildings are not sufficiently roomy, nor are they built of the proper material, being made of green, unseasoned lumber. Kitchens of the same materials are built to the rear of each set of company quarters, separated from them by a street some 25 feet in width.

The company quarters are one-story structures, raised from the ground 5 feet, and rest on piles. The ventilation is by means of windows and doors, as well as by ventilating orifices in the ceiling, which can be opened or closed as are shutters. These orifices connect with roof-ventilators. The air-space for each man is 251 cubic feet. In consequence of the shrinking of the green lumber and the opening of the joints there is more than a sufficiency of fresh air admitted.

In the winter time there is great difficulty experienced in keeping the quarters sufficiently warm by two large 18-inch cylinder stoves kept burning night and day. Near to the stoves the heat is too oppressive, and distant from them the cold is much too perceptible. There is all the light that could be required. The men sleep in the main room of the company quarters, the same which is occupied by them during the day, and in which, too, are kept their boxes, extra clothing, apparatus for cleaning arms, accouterments, &c. The bunks used in the company quarters are similar to those which were made for the hospital department during the war, being iron frames with wooden slats. The troops have a sufficiency of blankets and covering. The accommodations furnished the soldiery to assist them in the way of personal cleanliness are of the most limited character. The company wash-rooms are too contracted, being but 12 feet by 5 feet, and are built to the outside of the company kitchens.

There is not a sufficiency of fresh water for general use, and there are no means of washing the whole person afforded the men, save during the summer time, when salt-water bathing can be indulged in. The greater part of the command do not wash their whole persons from November till June. A bath-house attached to each company quarters, with the means of heating water during the winter, would be a great desideratum in a sanitary point of view. With the exception of small shelves at the head of the bunks, a few benches, and two or three large tables, there is no furniture in the company quarters. The company kitchens are rather contracted in size, but answer the purpose quite well. To each company kitchen a large-sized range has been furnished, and by means of it cooking of the finest kind can be done for even a greater number of men than a full company. The company mess-rooms, which are 24 feet by 24 feet, are all too contracted for the accommodation of a full company.

The quarters of the married soldiery and laundresses are badly built and worse arranged. They are two-story buildings of battened frame, with porches on the south sides, by means of which porches access to the second story is gained by stairs running from the lower to the upper porch, and by no other way. In each of these are fourteen sets of quarters, seven on the lower and seven on the upper floor. The quarters on the upper floor are, in the summer time, rendered almost uninhabitable, in consequence of the pipes from the cooking-stoves on the lower floor coming up through the ceiling and floor of the second stories. There are fourteen stoves, doing the cooking of the same number of families, in a frame building 87 feet long by 30 feet deep. These quarters were constructed partly of green lumber and partly of old lumber taken from the laundresses' quarters, which were torn down in 1867. The green, yellow-pine lumber, in drying and shrinking, has, to all intents, opened the rooms adjoining to each other, for the joints of the ceilings and partition walls have so much opened as to allow what occurs in one room to be seen in the next set of quarters. The quarters are built most disadvantageously in case of fire, for, should it occur in the lower story, there would be but little chance of escape for those occupying the upper one, the only stairs being those joining the porches, and there is no fire-escape.

To partially isolate a case of contagious disease, or an infectious one, in these quarters, is a matter of impossibility, and to have even a moderate share of quiet is impracticable. Should any disease, contagious or infectious in its nature, make its appearance in these buildings, it will go through the whole of them as if it were a single room.

There are no regular storehouses in the fort. Unoccupied casemates are made use of to store supplies.

The stables for public horses are some quarter of a mile distant from the fort, on the road leading to the Mill Creek bridge. Near the stables are the store-houses of the quartermaster's depot, large frame buildings, containing supplies collected at the closing of the war.

Inside of the fort there are no sinks, in the general acceptation of the term. Officers residing in the casemates make use of the officers' commode in the flagstaff bastion, which is now a series of six earth-closets, which are admirably adapted for the purpose, and fulfill every indication required of them. They are a great improvement on the copper tank on wheels. The families in the casemates who have not furnished themselves with earth commodes must use chamber utensils, and throw their contents into the waters of the moat. The water-closets of officers not residing in casemates are furnished with small boxes, which are removed at intervals, and are sprinkled with crude lime, or its chloride, at the option of the men who have charge of them. The same arrangement exists in the hospital yard, with the exception of the use of the disinfectant, which is regulated by order of the surgeon on duty.

The sinks for the men are large copper tanks, mounted on wheels, which are run under the closets, and changed every twenty-four hours, summer and winter. They are used only during the night by the men, whose main sink is at the north side of the fort, outside of the work, and covers a portion of Mill Creek below low-water mark. The night-soil tanks are drawn out of the fort and emptied into the Roads to the northwest of the work, and the filth is carried off by the tide, sooner or later. At times, during midsummer, the excrement is not carried off sufficiently promptly to prevent it from giving off unpleasant smells, perceptible to persons passing in the vicinity.

There is no drainage or sewerage. The rains, when heavy, collect on the parade-ground, and there remain till soaked up by the soil or evaporated by the sun.

The troops are supplied with vegetables and other articles needed by means of their company fund. As a general thing the troops are well fed, and with a sufficient variety of food to keep them healthy and in good condition.

There are neither company nor post gardens belonging to the fort, consequently everything not issued by the subsistence department must be procured by purchase. Fish and oysters are abundant in season, and are to be purchased at reasonable rates. Did the companies own seines, the men could catch more fish than they could possibly make use of; as it is, they, by means of hooks and lines, procure quite a number, and thus are enabled to change their diet at will.

The general police of the garrison is excellent.

The guard-houses of the fort are situated to the right and left of the main entrance, and are casemates appropriated for that purpose. The prison-rooms are two, and to one of these is attached a cell-room for solitary confinement. The main prison-room includes both the casemated room and the gun-room; is 44 feet long and 17 feet wide; has a large door and two large windows in front and an embrasure in the rear. Both the windows and the embrasure are shielded by immovable blinds, which prevent the ingress of sunlight and interfere greatly with the wind. The only ventilation to this room, which often has from twenty to forty men confined in it, is furnished through the small embrasure, not more than 3 by 4 feet wide, which is greatly interfered with by the crossed bars built into it and by the screen outside. Into this prison-room sunlight scarcely ever enters and never warms. During the winter the room is heated by stoves, which keep it comparatively dry and comfortably warm. In the summer time, however, it is always damp, and the water condenses in large drops on the walls and trickles thence to the floor. The prison-rooms are well floored, and they are made as tenantable as circumstances will permit, but at night, when the doors are closed, they are unendurable in consequence of the very imperfect ventilation. The smaller of the prison-rooms is worse, in point of ventilation, than the larger, as it has not even the embrasure to allow a current of air to pass through. The cells are much worse, in a sanitary point of view, than either of the prison-rooms. They are contracted, ill-ventilated, never warmed, and the light of the sun never enters them. They are always cold, damp, most disagreeable, and really unfit to confine men in.

The hospital building is near to the main entrance of the fort and faces the parade-ground. (Figures 6 and 7.)

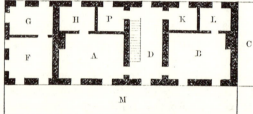

Figure 6, (1st story.)

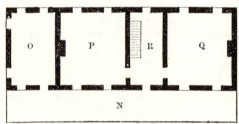

Figure 7, (2d story.)

A, office, 22 feet 3 inches by 15 feet 2 inches; B, dispensary, 22 feet 3 inches by 16 feet; C, cistern, 25 feet by 10 feet and 7 feet 6 inches above ground; D, hall and staircase, (hall, 11 feet 6 inches wide, staircase, 3 feet 6 inches wide;) F, hospital-steward's quarters, 15 feet by 14 feet 9 inches; G, hospital-steward's quarters, 10 feet by 14 feet 9 inches; (F and G, new part;) H, store-room for medical supplies, 12 feet 4 inches by 8 feet 4 inches; I, commissary-room, 9 feet 2 inches by 8 feet 4 inches; K, store-room for bedding, 10 feet 8 inches by 7 feet 6 inches; L, store-room for medicines, 11 feet 4 inches by 7 feet 6 inches; M, veranda, 80 feet long, 10 feet 8 inches wide; N, veranda, same size as first story; O, isolation-ward, (new part,) 23 feet 6 inches by 14 feet 9 inches; P, ward, 23 feet 3 inches by 25 feet; Q, ward, 23 feet 3 inches by 25 feet; R, hall and staircase, (hall, 11 feet 6 inches by 25 feet.) Rooms F and G and ward O, above them, is an addition to the building.

It is a structure of three stories, with garrets, which are used as store-rooms for bedding, and as a small ward for isolating contagious diseases. On the front of the building, on the first and second stories, there is a large porch much used by the convalescents. The wards, four in number, are large airy rooms in the second and third stories of the building, measuring 23 feet 7 inches by 24 feet 9 inches, and accommodating in each ten beds. The ventilation of the wards is afforded by a door opening into a spacious hall and by four windows, the sash of which raise and lower from above and below. The wards are heated by stoves burning anthracite coal, and are kept most comfortably warm by them during the coldest days of winter. The first floor of the building is occupied as a dispensary, steward's room, and two small store-rooms, which are much too contracted to accommodate the supplies requiring storage.

The hospital kitchen and mess-room are in a small brick building in the hospital yard, immediately to the west of the main building. (Figure 8.)

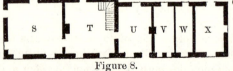

Figure 8.

S, dining-room, 19 inches by 17 feet 3 inches; T, kitchen, 17 feet by 17 feet 3 inches; U, special diet and hospital-steward's kitchen, 11 feet 6 inches by 16 feet 1 inch; V, bath-room, 7 feet 6 inches by 16 feet 1 inch; W, store-room for the Tompkins wheeled litters, 6 feet 6 inches by 16 feet 1 inch; X, shed for fuel, open in front, 10 feet 2 inches by 16 feet 1 inch.

This is sufficiently large, and is well adapted to the purpose. It has a second story which is used as a dormitory for the cook and as a store-room for kitchen utensils. Attached to the hospital, in the yard, is a two-story frame building, which was erected during the war of secession, and is now used as quarters for the hospital matron. (Figure 9.)

O, hospital matron's room, 14 feet 3 inches by 15 feet 6 inches; P, laundry-room, 15 feet 2 inches by 15 feet 6 inches; Q, *post-mortem* room, 8 feet 9 inches by 15 feet 6 inches; R, hall and staircase, (hall, 7 feet 6 inches wide and 15 feet 6 inches long, stair, 3 feet wide;) S, hall and staircase, (same width as below;) T, matron's room, 14 feet 3 inches by 15 feet 6 inches; U, matron's room, 14 feet 2 inches by 15 feet 6 inches; V, matron's room, 9 feet 9 inches by 15 feet 6 inches.

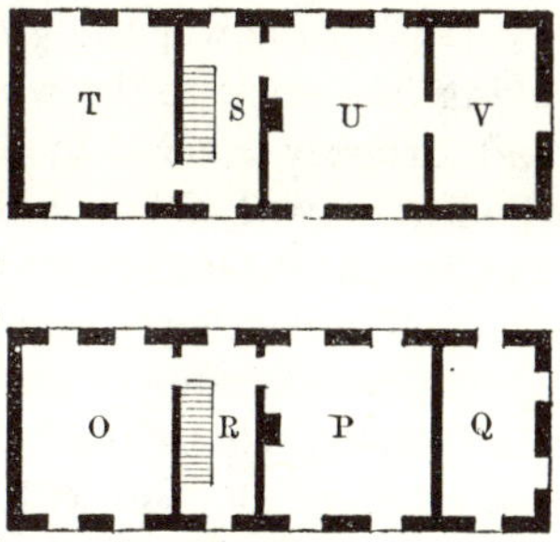

The close stools used in the wards are earth commodes, and they are infinitely superior to anything of the kind ever before furnished for the purpose. It is impossible to discover the slightest disagreeable smell arising from them, no matter how freely they may be used.

The water used for drinking purposes, as well as for cooking in the hospital, is procured from the large cistern attached to it. The roofing

Figure 9.

of the building being of slate furnishes perfectly pure water, and it is as good as can be procured anywhere. It is generally believed by persons residing in this country that those who use rain-water for drinking are not as subject to malarial fevers as are those who are in the habit of having the water they drink furnished by wells or springs. The water used in the garrison is either rain-water or that produced by condensation from sea-water. There is in the fort a large condensing apparatus, and much of the water used by the troops for drinking and culinary purposes is thus procured. Water, too, is collected from the roofs of the barracks, and carried to cisterns, which is used for drinking. This is somewhat unpalatable in consequence of having run over the shingles, and when warm it is somewhat nauseating. The condensed water is very disagreeable to most palates, and produces, when first used, considerable irritation of the intestinal canal, which, however, passes away in the course of a few days.

Prior to the war of secession there was but little if any malarial disease, originating at Old Point Comfort proper, met with, and Fort Monroe was regarded as one of the few places in the tide-water region of Virginia exempt from its influence. So highly was its sanitary condition regarded that it became the great watering-place of the Southern States. Pleasure-seekers, in great numbers, congregated here during the summer months to enjoy the salt-water bathing, and many invalids who had been suffering from the effects of malarial cachexia came to Old Point Comfort to recuperate their health by the tonic sea-breezes, and, at the same time, remove themselves from the depressing influences of the fever poison to which, at their homes, they had been subjected. Now, however, the sanitary status has changed, and malarial disease is quite common here. There is no doubt of its being contracted not only on the Point, but within the walls of the fort. Formerly the few cases of malarial fever reported occurred in men who had been on picket-guard at Mill Creek Bridge, or in those who, going on leave, would get drunk and, sleeping out during the night, expose themselves to the malarial exhalations on the mainland. To what this great change may be attributable is not certain. Two hypotheses are, with claims of reason, advanced. Before the war occurred, the lands under cultivation were well drained and well cared for. They had been worked for a long time, and could not be regarded as fresh soil, the upturning of which is always productive of malarial disease in the Southern States; much of the country, too, was covered with virgin forests of pine, oak, and hickory, extending from a short distance north and west of Mill Creek to Back River, thus intercepting, to a great extent, the winds impregnated with malarial exhalations which came from over the swamp-lands in its vicinity. This Back River is the receptacle of the waters of the many small streams and creeks which head in the swamp-lands, and find their way through it into Chesapeake Bay at a distance of about a league to the north of the fort. The lands proximate to these creeks are swampy for the greater part, the waters upon them being only brackish. These swamps, when the tides are low and the rains heavy, as is often the case in late summer and early autumn, become stagnant fresh-water marshes, and furnish all the material necessary for the production of southern autumnal fevers. On the banks of, and in all the country near to Back River, malarial fevers have full sway during the greater portion of the year, and in the autumn, when not promptly and skillfully treated, are very destructive to life, as in many cases they assume the malignant type here called congestive-remittent, corresponding to the disease so admirably described by Professor George B. Wood, in his work on the Practice of Medicine, under the name of pernicious fever. There has been no case of this type of disease at Fort Monroe in 1866, '67, '68, or '69, though several have occurred immediately over Mill Creek, a distance of no more than a mile from the fort.

During the war the greater part of the forest to the northwest of the fort was cut down, thus giving free scope to the winds blowing over the marshes of Back River. Much, too, of the virgin land formerly covered by forest has been turned up for cultivation. The cultivated land, too, which was lying fallow during the five years of the war, is once more being worked, poorly it is true, for the drains are all filled up or choked, and the owners, wanting as they are in labor or the means of procuring it, cannot put them in proper order. The result of this want of proper drainage is that the rains collect upon the low-lands, to be removed only by solar evaporation.

Immediately to the north of Mill Creek many large excavations have been made for the purpose of procuring soil with which to erect military works and repair defective ones. These large holes, never yet filled up, collect the rain-water in considerable quantities, and form ponds, which, exposed to the hot sun of summer, furnish fruitful sources of malarial poison.

The other hypothesis—more probably the correct one as far as the production of malarial disease inside the fort is concerned—is " that large quantities of clay and soil have been brought into and around the fort for the purpose of repairing and filling up the roads inside and outside of the same, as well as for repairing portions of the work." This clay and soil were procured at and brought from the western side of Mill Creek, in the locality where malarial fevers are most common. Prior to the spreading of this clay upon the roads there were few, if any, fevers of a malarial type originating in the fort, but in a very short time afterward they presented themselves for medical treatment. Previous to this the young children who went not outside of the walls in the night, or in the early morning, did not suffer from malarial disease, but since then children who seldom go outside the fort, and never off the point, are attacked with both remittent and intermittent fever. In addition to fevers of a malarial origin, diarrhœas and dysenteries are frequently met with, caused either by irritating ingesta or showing symptoms and complications of malarial disease; indeed, there is scarcely any disease of importance presented for treatment which does not in its course give indications of malarial complications, and which does not require for its treatment anti-periodics of some kind or other. In early summer, which is generally hot and humid, there is much derangement of the hepatic secretions, at times excessive, producing diarrhœas, at others diminished, running oftentimes into jaundice. These conditions, if not promptly relieved, seem to be but the precursors of remittent fever, more or less severe. The locality is unfavorable to those affected with diseases of the lungs.

*Meteorological report, Fort Monroe, Va., 1870-'74.*

| Month. | 1870-'71. | | | | 1871-'72. | | | | 1872-'73. | | | | 1873-'74. | | | |
|---|---|---|---|---|---|---|---|---|---|---|---|---|---|---|---|---|
| | Temperature. | | | Rain-fall in inches. | Temperature. | | | Rain-fall in inches. | Temperature. | | | Rain-fall in inches. | Temperature. | | | Rain-fall in inches. |
| | Mean. | Max. | Min. | | Mean. | Max. | Min. | | Mean. | Max. | Min. | | Mean. | Max. | Min. | |
| | ° | ° | ° | | ° | ° | ° | | ° | ° | ° | | ° | ° | ° | |
| July | 80.97 | 98* | 67* | 0.89 | 75.56 | 95* | 61* | 5.97 | 80.42 | 97* | 68* | 4.54 | 78.36 | 95* | 64* | 1.70 |
| August | 78.15 | 96* | 66* | 2.31 | 78.58 | 93* | 68* | 4.11 | 78.93 | 92* | 58* | 1.30 | 76.37 | 92* | 60* | 4.72 |
| September | 72.61 | 90* | 64* | 2.66 | 68.71 | 82* | 48* | 2.80 | 72.07 | 89* | 55* | 3.73 | 70.83 | 89* | 53* | 5.88 |
| October | 63.71 | 80* | 49* | 2.74 | 62.25 | 78* | 42* | 4.46 | 59.69 | 78* | 48* | 8.70 | 58.37 | 79* | 35* | 2.74 |
| November | 51.27 | 72* | 34* | 2.27 | 48.89 | 72* | 25* | 4.15 | 47.02 | 69* | 15* | 4.02 | 47.18 | 65* | 26* | 3.12 |
| December | 39.63 | 61* | 9* | 1.82 | 39.51 | 64* | 7* | 1.83 | 35.27 | 60* | 13* | 5.40 | 44.71 | 67* | 20* | 3.82 |
| January | 38.45 | 65* | 18* | 2.40 | 36.25 | 60* | 17* | 1.66 | 38.61 | 65* | 17* | 3.67 | 44.64 | 71* | 14* | 2.32 |
| February | 42.69 | 70* | 20 | 3.68 | 37.29 | 61* | 10* | 5.79 | 39.16 | 57* | 10* | 6.12 | 42.03 | 68* | 27* | 3.70 |
| March | 53.34 | 77* | 35 | 7.05 | 39.07 | 68* | 14* | 4.66 | 43.93 | 64* | 13* | 0.66 | 47.08 | 67* | 21* | 3.48 |
| April | 61.30 | 86* | 44* | 3.40 | 56.29 | 82* | 35* | 2.01 | 53.95 | 82* | 37* | 1.08 | 51.38 | 75* | 33* | 5.38 |
| May | 66.20 | 90* | 50* | 3.53 | 68.29 | 87* | 45* | 3.63 | 62.15 | 87* | 47* | 4.89 | 62.53 | 83* | 43* | 3.69 |
| June | 75.11 | 91* | 66* | 2.96 | 74.31 | 89* | 57* | 2.38 | 73.60 | 94* | 50* | 3.00 | 76.55 | 97* | 58* | 1.84 |
| For the year | 60.28 | 98* | 9* | 35.71 | 57.08 | 95* | 7* | 43.45 | 57.06 | 97* | 10* | 47.11 | 58.33 | 97* | 14* | 42.39 |

* These observations are made with self-registering thermometers. The mean is from the standard thermometer.

*Consolidated sick-report, Fort Monroe, Va., 1870–'74.*

| Year | 1870–'71. | | 1871–'72. | | 1872–'73. | | 1873–'74. | |
|---|---|---|---|---|---|---|---|---|
| Mean strength { Officers | 32 | | 37 | | 33 | | 34 | |
| { Enlisted men | 380 | | 302 | | 297 | | 382 | |
| **Diseases.** | Cases. | Deaths. | Cases. | Deaths. | Cases. | Deaths. | Cases. | Deaths. |
| GENERAL DISEASES, A. | | | | | | | | |
| Cerebro-spinal fever | | | 1 | | 1 | | | |
| Typho-malarial fever | | | | | | | 1 | |
| Remittent fever | 11 | | 7 | | 7 | | 25 | 1 |
| Intermittent fever | 148 | | 51 | | 12 | | 19 | |
| Diphtheria | 2 | | | | 2 | | | |
| Other diseases of this group | 17 | | 6 | | 6 | | 17 | |
| GENERAL DISEASES, B. | | | | | | | | |
| Rheumatism | 24 | | 26 | | 26 | | 26 | |
| Syphilis | 41 | | 7 | | 10 | | 7 | |
| Consumption | 7 | | 2 | | 2 | 1 | 5 | 2 |
| Other diseases of this group | 7 | | 7 | | 5 | | 1 | |
| LOCAL DISEASES. | | | | | | | | |
| Catarrh and bronchitis | 45 | | 31 | | 33 | | 67 | |
| Pneumonia | 1 | 1 | | | 1 | | 6 | 2 |
| Pleurisy | | | | | 1 | | 2 | |
| Diarrhœa and dysentery | 88 | | 35 | 1 | 69 | | 114 | |
| Hernia | | | | | 2 | | 1 | |
| Gonorrhœa | 43 | | 20 | | 7 | | 12 | |
| Other local diseases | 169 | 1 | 108 | 1 | 84 | | 105 | 2 |
| Alcoholism | 17 | | 5 | | 14 | 1 | 18 | |
| Unclassified | 1 | | | | | | | |
| Total disease | 621 | 2 | 306 | 2 | 283 | 2 | 426 | 7 |
| VIOLENT DISEASES AND DEATHS. | | | | | | | | |
| Gunshot wounds | 2 | 1 | 1 | | | | 2 | |
| Drowning | | 2 | | | | | | |
| Other accidents and injuries | 147 | | 63 | | 57 | | 91 | |
| Homicide | | | | | | 1 | | |
| Total violence | 149 | 3 | 64 | | 57 | 1 | 93 | |

# FORT MONTGOMERY, NEW YORK.

Fort Montgomery, commenced in 1841, is located at Rouse's Point, near the outlet of Lake Champlain, in latitude 45° north; longitude, 3° 43' east. The extent of the reservation is six hundred acres. The officers' quarters are built of limestone and bluestone, with arches of brick. They comprise forty-one rooms, 18 feet by 20 feet. The quarters for enlisted men are of the same material, and number twenty-three rooms.

Water is obtained from the lake. The locality is healthy, but the climate is severe in winter.

---

# FORT NIAGARA, NEW YORK.

INFORMATION FURNISHED BY ASSISTANT SURGEONS C. K. WINNE AND G. P. JAQUETT, UNITED STATES ARMY.

Fort Niagara is situated on a point of land at the junction of Lake Ontario and the Niagara River, latitude, 43° 15' north; longitude, 2° 5' west. Elevation above the sea, about 271 feet. The nearest town and post-office is Youngstown, on the bank of the river, one mile south; it contains about 800 inhabitants. Lewistown, six miles farther south, also on the bank of the river, is the terminus of a branch railroad from Suspension Bridge, and of a steamboat line from Toronto. The land near the river is low and sandy, being but a few feet above high-water mark. Immediately east of this the bank rises about 20 feet to a level plateau, on which the fort is built. The underlying rocks are limestone and sandstone. For history of the post see Circular No. 4, Surgeon-General's Office, December 5, 1870.

8 M P

The old barrack is a stone building within the fort, 134 by 24 feet. The walls are but 8 feet high, and as it is situated very near the western wall the ventilation is very deficient. The barrack now occupied is outside the fort, in an open and airy situation, and was erected in 1868–'69 It is a two-story brick building, the lower floor being divided into kitchen, mess-room, and wash-room, the latter supplied with hot and cold water, and furnished with a trough for the reception of basins. The wash-room is also used as a bath-room in winter—half-barrels serving for bath-tubs. The second floor contains two dormitories, each 52 by 22 by 10 feet, giving 476 cubic feet air-space per man. They are heated by stoves, and lighted and ventilated by sixteen windows each. The bunks are iron bedsteads. New sinks have recently been built near the barrack. The kitchen is well furnished, containing a range and apparatus for hot water; and the mess-room is commodious and well lighted.

Laundresses' quarters are contained in a new frame building situated 200 yards south of the fort; they comprise six rooms, and are in good condition and well ventilated.

The officers' quarters consist of three frame houses—two double and one single, making five sets of quarters—completed in 1871. They stand near the edge of the river-bluff, about 600 yards south of the fort. The one occupied by the commanding officer is 40 feet square and two stories high, the second story being in the Mansard roof. It contains eight rooms, two on each side of the hall in each story. The first story is 10 feet; the second, 8½ feet high. The kitchen is furnished with a range. The other rooms are provided with grates, and are well lighted. Each double house is divided by a partition from front to rear, making two sets of quarters, each consisting of two rooms and a kitchen, besides an attic of three low and dark rooms. The front room in each set is 15¾ by 17¾ feet; the next room, 15¾ by 19½ feet, and 10 feet high, and the kitchen is 13¼ by 14¼ feet. To avoid contiguity, the entrances are on opposite sides of the buildings. The main door of each opens into a small hall communicating with the two rooms and a stairway leading to the attic. The rooms are furnished with grates; three of the kitchens with stoves, and the remaining one with a range. None of the officers' quarters have cellars.

The guard-house, erected in 1869, is a two-story frame building, 32 by 26½ feet. The first floor contains two rooms for the guard and six cells, the latter divided by a hall measuring 13 feet 8 inches by 10 feet 5 inches. The cells measure 7 feet by 4 feet 4 inches, and are ventilated by small windows opening exteriorly, and openings over the door into the hall between them. The windows are 2½ feet long and 1 foot wide, and the openings 1½ feet long and 6 inches wide, with a board sliding over it. There is no ridge ventilation, except for the halls and space between the ceiling and roof; this is 2 feet square. The second story is divided into three rooms and a hall, each 10 feet high, and ventilated by windows. These rooms measure, respectively, 14 by 24½ feet, 6 by 10 feet, 9 by 24½ feet. The room designed as court-martial room is now used as a billiard-room for both officers and men. Fresh and foul air are exchanged through the same openings. The whole building is ventilated by windows.

The hospital, located near the river, about 400 yards south of the fort, is a temporary wooden structure, ill adapted for the purpose. For the general arrangement of the building see Figure 10.

A, ward, 23 by 40 feet; B, steward's room, 9 by 17 feet; C, surgery, 9 by 17 feet; D, attendant's room, 10 by 15 feet; E, store-room, 10 by 15 feet; F, wash-room; H, commissary store-room; K, kitchen, 24 by 17 feet; L, coal-shed.

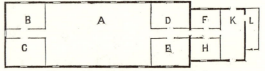

Figure 10.—Scale, 37 feet to 1 inch.

Its location, on the high bank of the Niagara River, insures all the air necessary, and sometimes more than is comfortable. The rooms are ventilated by windows opening at the top, aided by small openings near the floor, the latter communicating by flues with the attic above. Stoves are used for heating, and kerosene-oil for the artificial illumination of the building. The ward contains nine beds, giving to each 1,431 cubic feet of air-space. The water-closets are situated to the right and rear of the hospital. They are two compartments in a small wooden building, and conveniently arranged. The dead-house is a small frame structure, situated 70 yards to the north of the hospital. The water-supply for the hospital is from the Niagara River. The water at times is unpleasant, and at all times unsuitable for hospital purposes, owing in part to the great number of dead animals which are thrown into the river and find their way to its mouth, or are stranded along its shores in various stages of decomposition. The most unpleasant water is obtained after a severe storm of rain and wind. Besides the washings from an extended surface, the bottom of the river is made to yield largely of a deposit, which, when diffused, does not add to the pleasant character of the water. There have been, however, no cases of disease traced to its impurities, nor any unpleasant effect produced by its use.

The laundresses are mostly supplied with river water, which is furnished by police parties, in a cart duly constructed for the purpose. Buckets filled with water, and hooks and ladders are conveniently placed in and about the various buildings of the post, to be used in case of fire.

The country lying back of the fort, though generally level, is sufficiently undulating to afford perfect drainage. The cleared portions of the public lands mostly discharge their waters into the Niagara River by natural surface-drainage. The portion still covered by timber has its drainage eastward, and through a small creek enters Lake Ontario. The hospital grounds are especially well provided with natural drainage. Slops and offal from the kitchens are consumed by swine, and the excreta either buried or used as a fertilizer.

There are about fifteen acres under cultivation near the post, known as the company garden. This amount of land produces sufficient for the use of the entire garrison.

*Meteorological report, Fort Niagara, N. Y., 1873-'74.*

| Month. | 1870-'71. | | | | 1871-'72. | | | | 1872-'73. | | | | 1873-'74. | | | |
|---|---|---|---|---|---|---|---|---|---|---|---|---|---|---|---|---|
| | Temperature. | | | Rain-fall in inches. | Temperature. | | | Rain-fall in inches. | Temperature. | | | Rain-fall in inches. | Temperature. | | | Rain-fall in inches. |
| | Mean. | Max. | Min. | | Mean. | Max. | Min. | | Mean. | Max. | Min. | | Mean. | Max. | Min. | |
| | ° | ° | ° | | ° | ° | ° | | ° | ° | ° | | ° | ° | ° | |
| July | | | | | | | | | | | | | 71.72 | 86 | 60 | 4.22 |
| August | | | | | | | | | | | | | 69.53 | 85 | 56 | 2.17 |
| September | | | | | | | | | | | | | 61.57 | 84 | 44 | 2.48 |
| October | | | | | | | | | | | | | 49.28 | 70 | 31 | 4.03 |
| November | | | | | | | | | | | | | 31.54 | 48 | 17 | 2.27 |
| December | | | | | | | | | | | | | 31.52 | 55 | 15 | 3.08 |
| January | | | | | | | | | | | | | 26.42 | 65 | 8 | 4.45 |
| February | | | | | | | | | | | | | 24.97 | 48 | 2 | 3.06 |
| March | | | | | | | | | | | | | 31.69 | 54 | 10 | 1.57 |
| April | | | | | | | | | | | | | 35.57 | 59 | 17 | 3.31 |
| May | | | | | | | | | | | | | 53.82 | 83 | 35 | 2.10 |
| June | | | | | | | | | 66.50 | 86 | 51 | 1.74 | 64.99 | 90 | 53 | 2.46 |
| For the year | | | | | | | | | | | | | 46.05 | 90 | 2 | 35.20 |

*Consolidated sick-report, Fort Niagara, N. Y., 1870-'74.*

| Year | | 1870-'71. | | 1871-'72. | | 1872-'73. | | 1873-'74. | |
|---|---|---|---|---|---|---|---|---|---|
| Mean strength { Officers | | 5 | | 3 | | 3 | | 3 | |
| { Enlisted men | | 51 | | 41 | | 40 | | 48 | |
| Diseases. | | Cases. | Deaths. | Cases. | Deaths. | Cases. | Deaths. | Cases. | Deaths. |
| GENERAL DISEASES, A. | | | | | | | | | |
| Remittent fever | | | | | | 3 | | | |
| Intermittent fever | | 1 | | 4 | | 9 | | 2 | |
| Other diseases of this group | | 1 | | 3 | | 1 | | | |
| GENERAL DISEASES, B. | | | | | | | | | |
| Rheumatism | | 3 | | 4 | | 1 | | 1 | |
| Syphilis | | | | 1 | | | | 5 | |
| Other diseases of this group | | | | 1 | | | | | |
| LOCAL DISEASES. | | | | | | | | | |
| Catarrh and bronchitis | | 1 | | 4 | | 4 | | 11 | |
| Diarrhœa and dysentery | | 12 | | 13 | | 18 | | 4 | |
| Other local diseases | | 18 | | 21 | | 12 | | 12 | |
| Alcoholism | | | | 2 | | 2 | | | |
| Total disease | | 36 | | 53 | | 50 | | 35 | |
| VIOLENT DISEASES AND DEATHS. | | | | | | | | | |
| Drowning | | | 8 | | | | | | |
| Other accidents and injuries | | 18 | | 8 | | 6 | | 9 | |
| Homicide | | | | | | | 1 | | |
| Total violence | | 18 | 8 | 8 | 1 | 6 | | 9 | |

# FORT ONTARIO, OSWEGO, NEW YORK.

### REPORT OF ASSISTANT SURGEON H. E. BROWN, UNITED STATES ARMY.

Fort Ontario is situated in latitude 43° 27′ 30″ north, longitude 30′ east, and is 282 feet above the level of the ocean and 49 feet above the level of Lake Ontario. It is on the right bank of the Oswego River, at its junction with Lake Ontario, and faces the lake. The city of Oswego, a flourishing town of about 26,000 inhabitants, is in the immediate vicinity.

For history of the post see Circular No. 4, Surgeon General's Office, December 5, 1870, page 103.

The reservation embraces about seventy-five acres, extending from the river on the west to Ninth street, in Oswego, on the east, and from the lake on the north to Schuyler street.

There are no springs or ponds of water on the reservation. The ground is boggy, and saturated with water in some places, being merely the drainage toward the lake from the higher ground behind the town. Several wells have been dug in the fort, which obtain their water in this way, at a depth of 25 or 30 feet. One was bored to a depth of 280 feet without striking a spring.

The soldiers' barrack is a two-story building, constructed in 1842, of limestone quarried on the lake shore, about 30 miles from Oswego. The building is 62 feet front by 39 feet deep, and 24 feet from floor to eaves, and contains on the first floor a mess-room and kitchen, 35 feet by 27 feet 9 inches, and 10 feet 2 inches from floor to ceiling, and a reading-room of the same dimensions. The second story contains two squad-rooms, each 35 by 28 feet, and 12 feet from floor to ceiling, each having a small non-commissioned officers' room partitioned off in one corner, giving, with the present command, about 550 cubic feet of air per man. They are warmed in winter by sheet-iron coal-stoves, and lighted and ventilated by the ordinary windows and doors. The building has a piazza, 10 feet broad, in front, and at either end of the piazza, on the ground floor are a urinal and wash-room, supplied by pipes from the city water-works. The men's sinks are in the ditch of the fort, outside the main work.

The quarters for married soldiers and laundresses consist of four small wooden buildings and one of stone, (the latter the old post hospital,) situated on the reservation outside the work. Each wooden cottage contains three rooms, and is well adapted for the purpose. The officers' quarters are two two-story limestone buildings, each intended for two sets of quarters. Each set of quarters contains, on the ground floor, one dining-room, 15 feet 6 inches by 14 feet 10 inches, and a kitchen of nearly the same dimensions, with a closet opening in each room. The second story contains a parlor, 15 feet 10 inches by 14 feet, and a bed-room, 15 feet 6 inches by 14 feet. There is also a small hall bed-room, 7 feet 8 inches by 9 feet 6 inches.

In the attics are two good rooms, on either side, measuring, one 16 feet by 13 feet, and the other nearly the same. There is a large closet in every room. The quarters are comfortable, well built, well lighted and ventilated, the only objection to them being the common passage-way for two families. There are no arrangements for bathing purposes. The water-closets or sinks are in out-houses, detached from the main building, and are very defective in their arrangement. At one end of each out-house is a cistern, and at the other the sink, only separated by a stone wall, and so constructed that there is always great danger of the contamination of water in the cistern. The water-closets consist merely of a well, communicating with the main drain of the fort by a small drain, which, instead of leading from the bottom of the sink-well, opens some two feet above it, thus causing the drainage to be always incomplete. The sinks can be flushed with water by means of hose attached to the fire-plug on the parade, and this, to some extent, obviates the defective drainage. There is one other two-story building inside the work; the upper story, containing two rooms, used for ordnance and commissary store-rooms, and the lower story being in temporary use for a guard-house. The room for the guard is 16 by 13 feet, and 9 feet 10 inches from floor to ceiling. Behind this are two prison-rooms, one 12 feet 6 inches by 6 feet, and the other 12 feet 6 inches by 9 feet. Through the center of the building runs a hall, 26 feet by 6 feet, and on the other side of the hall is a tool-room and three cells, each 8 feet long by 3 feet 6 inches broad, and 9 feet 5 inches from floor to ceiling. These cells hold but 264 cubic feet of air, and are utterly without ventilation, except a small grated aperture over the door, six inches square. Fortunately they are but very seldom used. The guard-room is warmed by a coal-stove in winter, but the prison-rooms, behind, are never supplied with stoves, and are very imperfectly heated, being entirely dependent on what heat comes from the front room through an open door and a small grated window. The permanent guard-houses are on either side of the sally-port, and are now used for adjutant's office and first sergeant's quarters.

The hospital is situated on the reservation, outside the fort, about 275 yards from the sally-port. It is built on the plan indicated in Circular No. 4, Surgeon General's Office, April 27th, 1867; there being a central executive building, two stories high, with two wings, each one story, and accommodations for twenty patients. The whole built of wood, lathed and plastered. The wings are each 44 feet long by 24 feet broad, and are divided into a ward, 33 feet by 23 feet 6 inches, a water-closet and bath-room, 11 feet by 8 feet 6 inches, and an attendant's room of the same dimensions. Between these small rooms is a passage-way, 11 by 6 feet. The hospital is warmed by coal-stoves, lighted at night by oil-lamps and candles, and ventilated by the ridge system. The water-closets and baths are arranged with a pull connecting with the water-pipes, so as to keep a constant stream of water flowing in them. There is no dead-house, an unoccupied room in the hospital being so used when required. The hospital is too far from the garrison; is on the lowest ground of the reservation, and very much exposed to cold winds.

The post bakery has a capacity of 100 loaves per day.

There is no laundry, chapel, or school-house at the post. A room in the soldiers' barracks is fitted up as a reading-room, where the soldiers receive occasional instruction from the commanding officer. There is no post library. The officers and soldiers have access to the Gerritt Smith Free Library and the City School Library of Oswego, two excellent collections, embracing over 10,000 volumes. The post is supplied with water by the City Water Company, obtaining its water from the Oswego River, about three miles above the city. The supply is unlimited, and of good quality. There are also four wells inside the work, the water of which is more or less impregnated with lime, and of ordinary quality, and a cistern of small dimensions attached to each officer's quarters, the water of which, on account of its contiguity to the privies, is unfit for general use. The means of extinguishing fire are ample, by hose attached to the hydrants of the water company. Fire-buckets, constantly filled, are also kept for immediate use in the hospital. The post is drained by means of sewers of masonry work, there being one main sewer encircling the parade, and having subdrains connecting with each building. The main sewer discharges into the lake just below the fort. The system is good, but the construction of some of the drains is bad, and some of them are out of repair. The troops have unlimited opportunity for bathing in the lake in the summer season. In winter there are no facilities for that purpose.

The post garden contains about two and one-half acres of land, and is cultivated by details from the post.

Mails are received and depart morning and evening to all points. It requires twenty-four hours for a letter to go to department headquarters at New York City, and forty-eight to Washington. There are no ambulances at the post.

*Meteorological report, Fort Ontario, N. Y., 1870–'74.*

| Year. | 1870-'71. | | | | 1871-'72. | | | | 1872-'73. | | | | 1873-'74. | | | |
| | Temperature. | | | Rain-fall in inches. | Temperature. | | | Rain-fall in inches. | Temperature. | | | Rain-fall in inches. | Temperature. | | | Rain-fall in inches. |
| | Mean. | Max. | Min. | | Mean. | Max. | Min. | | Mean. | Max. | Min. | | Mean. | Max. | Min. | |
| July | 73.91 | 94 | 60 | 4.34 | 69.41 | 90 | 58 | 2.38 | 72.26 | 93* | 55* | 1.75 | 70.37 | 90* | 45* | 1.95 |
| August | 73.06 | 98 | 53 | 2.54 | 71.77 | 89 | 57 | 5.83 | 73.37 | 96* | 50* | 0.64 | 67.19 | 84* | 41* | 1.56 |
| September | 65.72 | 90 | 47 | 4.23 | 58.78 | 93 | 35 | 0.91 | 63.92 | 96* | 40* | 2.20 | 61.12 | 88* | 31* | 2.95 |
| October | 53.90 | 81 | 33 | 2.59 | 52.26 | 82* | 26* | 1.40 | 49.39 | 76* | 26* | 4.92 | 50.23 | 78* | 28* | 5.42 |
| November | 41.27 | 73 | 27 | 1.93 | 33.40 | 60* | 1* | 2.76 | 36.61 | 52* | 8* | 1.97 | 31.04 | 53* | 10* | 1.97 |
| December | 28.76 | 49 | 4 | 3.45 | 24.05 | 50* | −15* | 3.69 | 21.02 | 40* | −20* | 2.49 | 31.31 | 67* | 9* | 3.12 |
| January | 23.15 | 62 | −16 | 2.46 | 23.03 | 42* | − 7* | 3.04 | 19.97 | 44* | −20* | 1.72 | 28.56 | 64* | −10* | 5.32 |
| February | 26.03 | 51 | − 8 | 2.21 | 22.08 | 51* | − 9* | 2.12 | 22.27 | 48* | − 5* | 2.16 | 25.12 | 45* | −15* | 1.72 |
| March | 39.98 | 70 | 28 | 2.87 | 21.94 | 42* | −21* | 1.35 | 28.02 | 49* | −10* | 5.65 | 33.39 | 60* | 1* | 1.55 |
| April | 46.19 | 80 | 27 | 2.67 | 42.90 | 76* | 19* | 1.14 | 39.80 | 57* | 25* | 2.38 | 35.44 | 59* | 12* | 1.96 |
| May | 55.86 | 89 | 40 | 0.82 | 52.34 | 81* | 33* | 2.27 | 55.58 | 85* | 33* | 1.63 | 53.03 | 86* | 26* | 2.45 |
| June | 65.55 | 92 | 50 | 2.00 | 63.92 | 90* | 35* | 3.72 | 65.78 | 89* | 45* | 0.95 | 62.99 | 91* | 42* | 3.28 |
| For the year | 49.45 | 98 | −16 | 32.11 | 44.66 | 93 | −21* | 30.61 | 45.67 | 96* | −20* | 28.46 | 45.82 | 91* | −15* | 33.25 |

* These observations are made with self-registering thermometers. The mean is from the standard thermometer.

*Consolidated sick-report, Fort Ontario, N. Y., 1870–'74.*

| Year | | 1870–'71. | | 1871–'72. | | 1872–'73. | | 1873–'74. | |
|---|---|---|---|---|---|---|---|---|---|
| Mean strength { Officers | | 4 | | 3 | | 3 | | 4 | |
|             { Enlisted men | | 54 | | 43 | | 35 | | 46 | |
| Diseases. | | Cases. | Deaths. | Cases. | Deaths. | Cases. | Deaths. | Cases. | Deaths. |
| GENERAL DISEASES, A. | | | | | | | | | |
| Remittent fever | | 1 | | | | | | | |
| Intermittent fever | | 5 | | | | 4 | | | |
| Other diseases of this group | | 34 | | 10 | | 9 | | 8 | |
| GENERAL DISEASES, B. | | | | | | | | | |
| Rheumatism | | 3 | | 5 | | 3 | | 5 | |
| Syphilis | | 3 | | | | | | | |
| Consumption | | 2 | | | | | | | |
| Other diseases of this group | | 2 | | | | | | 1 | |
| LOCAL DISEASES. | | | | | | | | | |
| Catarrh and bronchitis | | 95 | | 37 | | 32 | | 33 | |
| Pleurisy | | | | | | | | 2 | |
| Diarrhœa and dysentery | | 25 | | 19 | | 18 | | 28 | |
| Hernia | | | | | | 1 | | | |
| Gonorrhœa | | 6 | | 1 | | 1 | | | |
| Other local diseases | | 81 | | 46 | | 34 | | 23 | |
| Alcoholism | | 7 | | 7 | | 4 | 1 | 2 | |
| Unclassified diseases | | | | | | | | 1 | |
| Total disease | | 264 | | 125 | | 106 | 1 | 103 | |
| VIOLENT DISEASES AND DEATHS. | | | | | | | | | |
| Accidents and injuries | | 46 | | 14 | | 20 | | 17 | |
| Total violence | | 46 | | 14 | | 20 | | 17 | |

# FORT PHŒNIX, MASSACHUSETTS.

Construction commenced in 1841 on Fort Point, on the east side of the entrance to the harbor of New Bedford, one mile south of the village of Fairhaven, in latitude 41° 38′ north ; longitude, 6° 8′ east.

The reservation is two acres. There is no hospital or guard-house; the quarters for officers and men are small and decayed. The post is in charge of an ordnance-sergeant.

# PIKESVILLE ARSENAL, MARYLAND.

Pikesville Arsenal was established in 1819, at Pikesville, Md., latitude, 39° 18′ north ; longitude, 26′ east. The reservation includes fifteen acres, and is on the Reisterstown road, eight miles north of Baltimore.

The quarters for officers and men are built of pressed brick, and are in good condition. The officers' quarters are one two-story building, 71 by 38 feet, containing eight rooms. The quarters for the men are one building, two stories, 80 by 27 feet, containing ten rooms.

The guard-house, also of pressed brick, is 50 by 21 feet.

There is no hospital at the arsenal.

# PLATTSBURGH BARRACKS, NEW YORK.

INFORMATION FURNISHED BY ASSISTANT SURGEONS S. M. HORTON AND L. Y. LORING, U. S. A., AND ACTING ASSISTANT SURGEON J. P. FOOTE, U. S. A.

This post is situated on the west side of Lake Champlain, about one mile from the village of Plattsburgh, New York, latitude, 44° 41′ north; longitude, 3° 38′ east; and 186 feet above the sea. The Saranac, a small river rising in a range of lakes forty miles southwest, enters the lake at this point. This vicinity was first occupied by United States troops in 1812. Troops were stationed here from 1814 to 1825, from 1840 to 1846, from 1848 to 1852, from 1859 to 1861, and from 1865 to the present. The post was established in June, 1838.

The geology of the vicinity may be briefly presented as follows, the strata being given from above downward:

1. Drift of sand and gravel, depth 25 to 30 feet. 2. Trenton limestone, 400 feet. This is the surface rock of Plattsburgh and Lumberland Head, and includes two varieties—one black and close-grained, taking a fine polish; the other gray and crystalline. 3. Birdseye limestone, 50 feet. 4. Chazy limestone, 130 feet. 5. Calciferous sandstone, from 250 to 300 feet.

The soil of the vicinity is sandy, and not productive unless fertilizers are used extensively.

The post is situated on a sandy plain 25 rods from the lake and 90 feet above its level, the buildings being arranged around a square parade of 200 feet each side. The principal buildings are substantially constructed of uncut limestone.

The barracks for the enlisted men were erected in 1838–'40, and consist of a building two and a half stories high, 200 feet long by 26 feet wide, containing eighteen rooms. On the second floor are three large and commodious sleeping-rooms for each company. They are warmed by stoves, well lighted and ventilated by windows, and contain 420 cubic feet of air-space per man. Each bunk is arranged for two occupants. A camp privy for each company and one for the hospital are located 100 feet distant from the barracks. A capacious company kitchen adjoins each mess-room and occupies a portion of the first floor of the building. In the eastern end of this building, four rooms on the lower floor are set apart for the use of the hospital department, and are occupied as office, dispensary, ward-room, and kitchen. The arrangement of the barracks and hospital is shown in Figure 11.

1, first story; 2, second story; A, hospital kitchen; B, ward; C, office; D, dispensary; E, company kitchen; F, mess-room; H, sergeants' room; I, company office; M, hospital bath-room; K, storm-shed; P, piazza; L L, dormitories. Height of rooms on first floor, 10 feet; on second floor, 10 feet 6 inches.

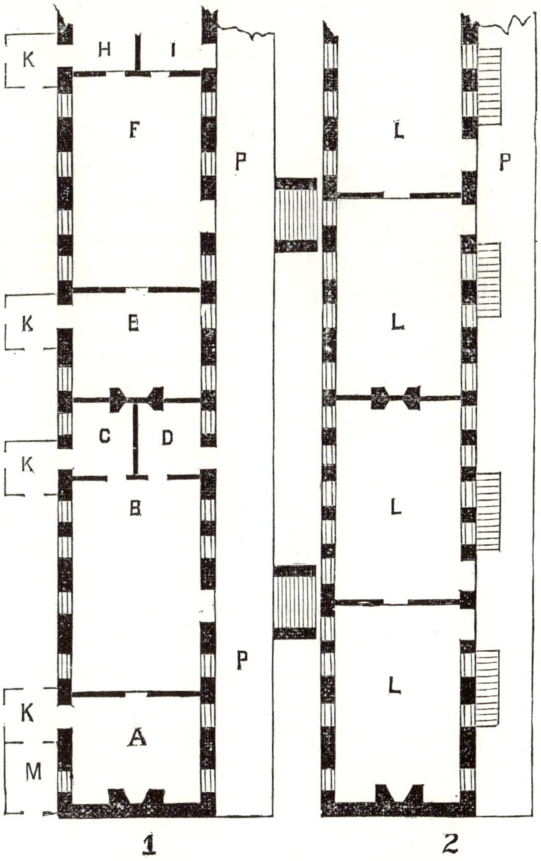

Figure 11.—Scale, 32 feet to 1 inch.

The quarters of the non-commissioned staff and also the quarters of the company laundresses, located outside of the inclosure of the post, are three old wooden buildings, each one and a half stories high. The first of these buildings is divided into three rooms, one 20 by 12 feet and two 12 by 12 feet, and occupied by the non-commissioned staff, hospital-steward, and matron. The other buildings toward the north, containing two rooms and two attics each, are occupied by laundresses. A new wooden building, 80 by 28 feet, has been erected on the south side of the barracks, and 20 feet distant from the inclosure. This is occupied by four families, affording to each two rooms 16 by 14 feet, with air-space of 1,568 cubic feet.

The building assigned to the use of commissioned officers is composed of the same materials as the main building, and is 70 feet long, 25 feet wide, two and a half stories high, and contains 16 rooms. The building is erected at right angles with the main building, and 20 feet distant. In its rear is an open veranda. It is intended for eight sets of quarters.

The headquarters of the post is a small one-story building 24 by 18 feet, a portion of which is set apart for the purpose of a library and reading-room for the use of the command.

The commissary storehouse is a two and a half story wooden building, 40 feet long and 18 feet wide, divided into two store-rooms and an office.

On the east side is a one-story building, 60 by 16 feet, used for a carpenter's shop, with the exception of a small portion on the western end, which is set apart for a sutler's store.

The guard-house is a wooden building, 50 by 15 feet, and divided into three rooms and two cells. The front room, 13 by 12 feet, is used as a guard-room; adjoining are the cells designated for prisoners sentenced to solitary confinement. The cells are 4½ feet wide and 10 feet long, with a grated window, 1 foot square, near the top of the wall, and a similar grating in the door for ventilation. A small opening from the top of the cell serves to allow a part of the foul air to escape. These cells are found to be unsuitable for the purpose by reason of defective ventilation and bad arrangement for warming the rooms in cold weather. Adjoining the guard-room is a room 27 by 14 feet, used as a "lock-up" for prisoners. This apartment could be improved by more ample ventilation.

The hospital is in the building occupied as soldiers' barracks, the men's quarters being immediately over the sick-ward, as shown in Figure 11. Though rather inconvenient, this arrangement will answer the purpose for a command of two companies. The hospital is warmed by coal-stoves and well ventilated. Two rooms, each 10 by 10 feet, are used for office and dispensary.

The ward contains eight beds; superficial area, 792 feet; air-space per bed, 990 cubic feet. A room for bathing and lavatory purposes has been erected in rear of the building and adjoining the ward. The hospital sink is 100 feet distant, and kept in good condition. This privy is constructed on the system of earth-closets, the result proving quite satisfactory. The substance used as an absorbent is dry coal-ashes, (sifted,) which is regularly applied to each deposit in a sufficient quantity, and is found to be a good deodorizer.

The school-house is an old one-story building, situated at the northeast corner of the post.

The ice-house is a wooden building, 10 by 12 feet, with a stone wall 10 feet deep below ground, and frame building 8 feet high above the surface. An ample supply of ice is obtained from Lake Champlain during the months of January and February, and is found to be of an excellent quality.

The library contains a good supply of the most desirable of the daily and weekly journals; stationery and materials for writing are supplied gratis to members of the command.

The supply of water is obtained from two deep wells in close vicinity to the buildings; the quality of this water is excellent for drinking and cooking, and it is perfectly free from impurities. Rain-water is chiefly used for cleansing clothes and habitations.

The post is well drained by reason of being located on elevated ground and the alluvial nature of the soil.

The close proximity of Lake Champlain affords good facilities in summer for bathing purposes; and in winter a bath-room is used, which is well supplied with tubs and hot and cold water.

Fronting the western entrance to the post is a square plot of ground, inclosed with fence, containing about two acres. This ground is supposed to have been originally designed for a park or parade-ground, but has recently been converted into a vegetable garden, and cultivated for the benefit of the officers of the post.

The company gardens are located about half a mile northwest from the barracks, and consist of about five acres of fertile soil, under a good state of cultivation. The hospital garden is located about the same distance east of the post, and near the bank of the river. It is about half an acre in extent, and is cultivated by the hospital attendants.

*Meteorological report, Plattsburgh Barracks, N. Y., 1870–'74.*

| Month. | 1870–'71. | | | | 1871–'72. | | | | 1872–'73. | | | | 1873–'74. | | | |
|---|---|---|---|---|---|---|---|---|---|---|---|---|---|---|---|---|
| | Temperature. | | | Rain-fall in inches. | Temperature. | | | Rain-fall in inches. | Temperature. | | | Rain-fall in inches. | Temperature. | | | Rain-fall in inches. |
| | Mean. | Max. | Min. | | Mean. | Max. | Min. | | Mean. | Max. | Min. | | Mean. | Max. | Min. | |
| July | 73.75 | 95 | 50 | 1.91 | 69.19 | 84 | 51 | 4.65 | 72.59 | 97 | 59 | 4.72 | 70.22 | 86 | 48* | 4.90 |
| August | 70.40 | 87 | 46 | 1.31 | 69.20 | 85 | 54 | 3.48 | 71.29 | 86 | 53 | 5.86 | 66.51 | 85 | 45* | 2.02 |
| September | 61.42 | 80 | 45 | 2.54 | 55.64 | 79 | 34 | 1.15 | 61.35 | 80 | 45 | 3.27 | 58.27 | 75 | 29* | 1.95 |
| October | 49.86 | 67 | 29 | 2.70 | 49.56 | 72 | 28 | 1.95 | 46.74 | 68 | 28 | 3.40 | 48.20 | 67 | 22* | 5.15 |
| November | 38.02 | 57 | 22 | 1.29 | 30.27 | 52 | — 5 | 1.09 | 36.02 | 50 | 10* | 2.16 | 25.32 | 46 | —10* | 3.94 |
| December | 25.35 | 47 | — 5 | 1.26 | 19.34 | 40 | —21 | 2.32 | 14.35 | 37 | —26* | 1.59 | 24.07 | 48* | —14* | 1.86 |
| January | 14.62 | 46 | —21 | 1.13 | 18.98 | 39 | —12 | 0.68 | 15.51 | 40 | —28* | 3.26 | 24.19 | 49 | —16* | 3.69 |
| February | 19.58 | 45 | —21 | 1.09 | 17.95 | 43 | — 8 | 1.42 | 16.99 | 47 | —24* | 0.36 | 17.72 | 50 | —29* | 1.96 |
| March | 34.99 | 57 | 21 | 3.63 | 19.67 | 38 | —18 | 1.17 | 26.84 | 42 | — 2* | 3.68 | 27.22 | 50 | — 2* | 1.83 |
| April | 44.69 | 59 | 25 | 3.98 | 42.46 | 82 | 26 | 1.66 | 40.71 | 60 | 25 | 2.00 | 33.63 | 54 | 4* | 3.60 |
| May | 56.14 | 84 | 41 | 1.73 | 56.58 | 83 | 43 | 2.37 | 54.18 | 78 | 30* | 1.26 | 53.73 | 77 | 28* | 3.89 |
| June | 66.01 | 85 | 53 | 1.34 | 68.82 | 88 | 48 | 2.85 | 66.57 | 86* | 42* | 2.01 | 64.12 | 83 | 44* | 2.40 |
| For the year | 46.23 | 95 | —21 | 23.91 | 43.14 | 88 | —21 | 24.79 | 43.60 | 97 | —28* | 33.57 | 42.77 | 86 | —29* | 37.19 |

* These observations are made with self-registering thermometers. The mean is from the standard thermometer.

*Consolidated sick-report, Plattsburgh Barracks, N. Y., 1870–'74.*

| Year | 1870–'71. | | 1871–'72. | | 1872–'73. | | 1873–'74. | |
|---|---|---|---|---|---|---|---|---|
| Mean strength { Officers | 5 | | 7 | | 4 | | 5 | |
| { Enlisted men | 74 | | 94 | | 63 | | 52 | |
| Diseases. | Cases. | Deaths. | Cases. | Deaths. | Cases. | Deaths. | Cases. | Deaths. |
| GENERAL DISEASES, A. | | | | | | | | |
| Intermittent fever | 25 | | 16 | | | | | |
| Other diseases of this group | 33 | | 63 | | 4 | | 4 | |
| GENERAL DISEASES, B. | | | | | | | | |
| Rheumatism | 14 | | 9 | | 4 | | 1 | |
| Syphilis | 3 | | | | 2 | | 2 | |
| Consumption | 2 | | | | 2 | | | |
| Other diseases of this group | | | | | 1 | | 1 | |
| LOCAL DISEASES. | | | | | | | | |
| Catarrh and bronchitis | 3 | | 3 | | 29 | | 19 | |
| Pneumonia | | | 1 | | | | | |
| Pleurisy | 3 | | 1 | | 1 | | | |
| Diarrhœa and dysentery | 12 | | 34 | | 35 | | 13 | |
| Gonorrhœa | | | | | 1 | | 2 | |
| Other local diseases | 92 | | 115 | | 48 | | 23 | |
| Alcoholism | 7 | | 16 | | 3 | | 1 | |
| Total disease | 194 | | 258 | | 130 | | 66 | |
| VIOLENT DISEASES AND DEATHS. | | | | | | | | |
| Gunshot wounds | | | | | 1 | | | |
| Other accidents and injuries | 36 | | 63 | | 33 | | 22 | |
| Suicide | | | | 1 | | | | |
| Total violence | 36 | | 63 | 1 | 34 | | 22 | |

# FORT POPHAM, MAINE.

This fort was commenced in 1857 on Hunniwell's Point, on the west bank and near the mouth of the Kennebec River; latitude, 43° 50′ north; longitude, 7° 8′ east. It is distant from Bath, the nearest town, ten miles, and two and a half miles by water from the little village of Parker's Head, which is the nearest post-office.

The reservation comprises two and a half acres of unimproved land. The works, which are incomplete, are designed for one company, and are in charge of an ordnance-sergeant.

9 M P

# FORT PORTER, BUFFALO, NEW YORK.

## REPORT OF SURGEON A. F. MECHEM, UNITED STATES ARMY.

This post is pleasantly located within the city limits of Buffalo, on the right bank of the Niagara River, about half a mile from where Lake Erie empties into that stream. Latitude, 42° 53' north; longitude, 1° 52' west; altitude, 660 feet.

The post grounds at present in use are about 200 yards from the river, and 60 feet above its level. A part of the ground was ceded to the United States by the State of New York in 1844, and other lots have since been purchased, making the reservation at present about twenty-eight acres, one-half of which is used for the purposes of the post.

There are at the post one set of commandant's quarters, one set of surgeon's quarters, two sets of captain's quarters, and eight sets of lieutenant's quarters. The quarters of the commandant are of stone; all the others are of wood. There are also quarters for two companies of infantry, with complement of laundresses. The company quarters can each accommodate comfortably 70 men; have mess-rooms, kitchens, wash-room, office, and store-rooms for each company, and are built of wood. Their condition is serviceable, but they are not of quality suitable for a permanent post.

The hospital is an L-shaped frame building. One wing, 63 feet long by 23 feet wide, and one and a half stories high, contains the offices, kitchens, &c. The other wing, 80 by 27 feet, and one story high, contains the hospital ward, 41 by 26 feet, and 12 feet high. The ward is warmed by stoves, and ventilated by an air-shaft of ingress one foot square, which conveys the air underneath the ward and opens under one of the stoves, which is partially surrounded by a zinc sheathing. The vitiated and heated air is carried off by a shaft passing with the stove-pipe through the roof. The bath-room, water-closets, attendant's room, and mess-room are also in this wing.

The quartermaster's and commissary's storehouse is a frame building, 56 feet 10 inches long by 20 feet wide. It is one story and a half high, and contains an office and two store-rooms on the lower floor. On the upper floor are two rooms, one used as quartermaster's and the other as subsistence store-room. A good cellar extends about one-half the length of the building.

The guard-house is a stone building, one story and a half high, converted from a stable to its present use. On the first floor are the guard-room, 17 by 19 feet, and cell-room, 15 by 19 feet, containing eight cells, four on each side of a corridor opening into the guard-room. The prison-room, 16 by 17 feet, is on the second floor, and is tolerably well lighted and ventilated.

The subsoil drainage of the parade and other grounds about the fort is by means of tile-drains emptying into the larger earthen-pipe drains, which carry off the drainage and sewage from the barracks and some of the officers' quarters. All the contents of the sewers and drains of this part of the post are discharged into the Erie Canal, at least 50 feet below the lowest part of the post grounds now used, and 100 yards from the stable, which is the building nearest the mouth of the sewer. The drainage and sewage from the hospital and the officers' quarters, which are on the higher ground, are carried off by means of earthen-pipe drains connecting with the city sewer.

The post is supplied with good water by means of iron pipes extending from the Buffalo City reservoir to the fort. The reservoir, two squares distant from the fort, is filled with water pumped from the Niagara River. In winter the supply is insufficient, as it is necessary to allow the water to run from the hydrants in very cold weather to prevent it from freezing in the pipes, the feed-pipe not being large enough. The supply fails in some of the officers' quarters and at the hospital, which is on higher ground, and the last point that the water reaches. Independent of this supply, the officers' quarters have large cisterns, which are filled with rain-water from the roofs of the buildings.

Seven acres of ground are cultivated by the enlisted men as a post-garden. A garden is also cultivated by the hospital attendants, and in favorable seasons furnishes a good summer supply of vegetables.

There is a well-selected post library of about 200 volumes.

*Meteorological report, Fort Porter, N. Y., 1870–'74.*

| Year. | 1870–'71. | | | | 1871–'72. | | | | 1872–'73. | | | | 1873–'74, | | | |
|---|---|---|---|---|---|---|---|---|---|---|---|---|---|---|---|---|
| | Temperature. | | | Rain-fall in inches. | Temperature. | | | Rain-fall in inches. | Temperature. | | | Rain-fall in inches. | Temperature. | | | Rain-fall in inches. |
| | Mean. | Max. | Min. | | Mean. | Max. | Min. | | Mean. | Max. | Min. | | Mean. | Max. | Min. | |
| July | 71.24 | 84 | 53 | 3.63 | 68.29 | 87 | 48* | 3.31 | 74.42 | 98 | 46* | 1.10 | 70.88 | 93* | 48* | 6.27 |
| August | 69.86 | 87 | 44* | 0.48 | 71.00 | 92 | 46* | 4.10 | 74.71 | 98 | 48* | 1.64 | 68.82 | 83* | 43* | 2.20 |
| September | 65.81 | 83 | 42* | 4.28 | 57.83 | 77 | 31* | 0.93 | 65.51 | 89 | 40* | 2.71 | 60.12 | 79* | 32* | 2.04 |
| October | 53.72 | 73 | 34* | 3.06 | 53.46 | 73 | 28* | 1.12 | 48.83 | 79 | 20* | 2.22 | 48.74 | 73* | 27* | 4.35 |
| November | 40.23 | 67 | 20* | 2.34 | 33.99 | 65 | −15* | 3.10 | 36.43 | 60 | 0* | 2.43 | 30.74 | 50* | 10* | 2.83 |
| December | 29.30 | 50 | 5* | 2.69 | 25.43 | 56 | −18* | 1.50 | 23.02 | 48 | −18* | 1.82 | 31.35 | 57* | 3* | 4.03 |
| January | 25.08 | 53 | −3* | 1.08 | 22.64 | 48 | −16* | 0.83 | 21.28 | 50 | −22* | 2.52 | 27.48 | 62* | 0* | 5.40 |
| February | 26.83 | 49 | −4* | 0.97 | 21.68 | 52 | − 7* | 0.53 | 24.31 | 49 | −15* | 1.15 | 25.50 | 54* | −3* | 3.37 |
| March | 38.56 | 65 | 22* | 3.31 | 24.61 | 50 | −17* | 0.56 | 28.96 | 54 | −10* | 5.46 | 30.55 | 55* | 8* | 1.50 |
| April | 47.23 | 70 | 26* | 1.44 | 42.89 | 86 | 7* | 1.18 | 39.60 | 60 | 22* | 3.52 | 35.05 | 60* | 12* | 2.38 |
| May | 55.36 | 81 | 31* | 1.49 | 53.43 | 74 | 24* | 2.58 | 53.28 | 90* | 30* | 2.00 | 53.64 | 83* | 26* | 2.58 |
| June | 65.72 | 86 | 42* | 2.03 | 68.08 | 89 | 49* | 2.41 | 67.55 | 92* | 44* | 1.53 | 65.29 | 87* | 38* | 2.04 |
| For the year | 49.08 | 87 | −4* | 26.80 | 45.28 | 92 | −18* | 22.15 | 46.49 | 98 | −22* | 28.10 | 45.68 | .93* | −3* | 38.99 |

\* These observations are made with self-registering thermometers. The mean is from the standard thermometer.

*Consolidated sick-report, Fort Porter, N. Y., 1870–'74.*

| Year | 1870–'71. | | 1871–'72. | | 1872–'73. | | 1873–'74. | |
|---|---|---|---|---|---|---|---|---|
| Mean strength { Officers | 8 | | 7 | | 6 | | 6 | |
| { Enlisted men | 165 | | 102 | | 99 | | 101 | |
| **Diseases.** | Cases. | Deaths. | Cases. | Deaths. | Cases. | Deaths. | Cases. | Deaths. |
| GENERAL DISEASES, A. | | | | | | | | |
| Typhoid fever | 2 | | 2 | 1 | 1 | | | |
| Intermittent fever | 35 | | 2 | | 3 | | 14 | |
| Other diseases of this group | 32 | | 18 | | 5 | | 2 | |
| GENERAL DISEASES, B. | | | | | | | | |
| Rheumatism | 33 | | 9 | | 3 | | 1 | |
| Syphilis | 52 | | 29 | | 5 | | 11 | |
| Consumption | 1 | | | | 1 | | | |
| Other diseases of this group | 4 | | 1 | | | | 3 | |
| LOCAL DISEASES. | | | | | | | | |
| Catarrh and bronchitis | 79 | | 48 | | 7 | | 3 | |
| Pneumonia | 1 | 1 | 3 | 1 | 1 | 1 | 1 | |
| Pleurisy | 9 | | 2 | | 1 | | 1 | |
| Diarrhœa and dysentery | 99 | | 71 | | 17 | | 13 | |
| Hernia | 4 | | 1 | | | | | |
| Gonorrhœa | 10 | | 5 | | | | 1 | |
| Other local diseases | 149 | 1 | 68 | | 17 | | 22 | 1 |
| Alcoholism | 79 | | 34 | | 8 | | 2 | |
| Total disease | 589 | 2 | 295 | 2 | 69 | 1 | 74 | 1 |
| VIOLENT DISEASES AND DEATHS. | | | | | | | | |
| Gunshot wounds | 1 | | | | | | | |
| Other accidents and injuries | 102 | | 33 | | 16 | | 6 | |
| Total violence | 103 | | 33 | | 16 | | 6 | |

# PORTLAND HEAD BATTERY, MAINE.

Was commenced June 1, 1873, on Portland Head, in Portland Harbor.

---

# FORT PREBLE, MAINE.

Fort Preble is situated on Spring Point, the northern extremity of Cape Elizabeth, on the south side of Portland Harbor, latitude, 43° 38′; longitude, 6° 50′ east. It is distant about a mile from the city, which may be reached either by land or water. The reservation contains about twenty-four acres, a considerable addition having been made by purchase in 1871. The rock on which the fort stands is talcose schist, whose highest points are about 38 feet above the sea. The soil is gravelly and thin; the drainage is perfect; the water, supplied from a spring and two wells, is of bad quality and insufficient, especially in case of fire. A stationary hand-engine has been placed upon one of the wells, which is conveniently located on the parade.

The barracks for troops are four two-story wooden buildings with basement, each 52 by 37½ feet. The basements are used for post bakery, furnace-rooms, coal-rooms, &c. On the first floor are four rooms—mess-room, 33 by 17 feet; dormitory, 34 by 17 feet; and two office rooms. On the second floor are three dormitories, two measuring 33 by 17 feet, and the third 34 by 17 feet. The height of rooms on the first floor is 10 feet 10 inches; on the second floor, 9 feet 8 inches. Each dormitory is lighted by three windows, and is intended to contain twelve beds, which would give an average of 475 cubic feet air-space per man.

These barracks are placed contiguous to each other, leaving interspaces of 10 feet, on the west side of the parade. One is used for dormitories, in another is the company kitchen, mess-room, and reading-room; a third serves as a storehouse, and the fourth is occupied temporarily as a hospital, the hospital building having been taken down in 1871 by the Engineer Department in extending the earth-works.

The barracks are warmed by furnaces. In each of the upper dormitories an opening, 8 by 12 inches and 7 feet from the floor, communicating with an air-shaft in the chimney, furnishes the only special means of ventilation. The beds are low single bunks formed of boards on movable iron supports. A small room in one of the barracks is used as a bath-room, having two bath-tubs and a large caldron for heating water.

The sinks for the men are built over tide-water, and are arranged in stalls, each for one man, and, instead of having a seat or bar, an opening is cut in the floor 20 inches long, 5 inches wide behind, and 2 inches wide in front. This form of water-closet has proved very satisfactory. The quarters for married soldiers are one convenient frame cottage, in excellent repair, for the ordnance-sergeant, and three small frame houses adjoining the garrison rented for laundresses. Authority has been given for their purchase.

The guard-house is a one-story wooden building, 43 by 31 feet, and contains the guard-room, 17 by 15 feet; two prison-rooms, 14 feet 10 inches by 15 feet, and 18 feet 4 inches by 7 feet 4 inches; and five cells, each 7 feet 10 inches by 3 feet 10 inches. The height of all these rooms is 12 feet. There are two windows, 4 feet 4 inches by 2 feet 6 inches, in each of the prison-rooms and in the guard-room; none in the cells, and no special means of ventilation. Cubic air-space per cell is about 370 feet.

The officers' quarters are four frame cottages of one story, with cellars and attics, and with verandas in front. They are heated by stoves, lighted by lamps or candles, and have no bath-rooms. Each building contains four rooms, with two small rooms for kitchens, &c.

The hospital is a two-story frame building, 62 by 40½ feet, with basement and attic. The kitchen and laundry are in the basement. On the first floor are two wards, each 25½ by 19 feet, and 11⅔ feet high. The second floor contains four wards, 25½ by 19 and 7⅔ feet. There is one small ventilator in each upper ward only, opening in the outer wall; it is 10 inches in diameter and communicates by a tin flue with the outer air. The capacity of the wards is reckoned at eight beds each, giving 706½ cubic feet per man. Only one ward is usually used, containing four beds. There are wash and bath-rooms and water-closets for both first and second floors.

There are no gardens at the post, fresh vegetables being obtained by purchase.

The post library contains about three hundred and fifty volumes, and receives the principal periodicals.

Interments are made in a private burial ground adjacent to the reservation. Its purchase is desirable for the use of the garrison.

*Meteorological report, Fort Preble, Me., 1870–'74.*

| Month. | 1870–'71. | | | | 1871–'72. | | | | 1872–'73. | | | | 1873–'74. | | | |
| --- | --- | --- | --- | --- | --- | --- | --- | --- | --- | --- | --- | --- | --- | --- | --- | --- |
| | Temperature. | | | Rain-fall in inches. | Temperature. | | | Rain-fall in inches. | Temperature. | | | Rain-fall in inches. | Temperature. | | | Rain-fall in inches. |
| | Mean. | Max. | Min. | | Mean. | Max. | Min. | | Mean. | Max. | Min. | | Mean. | Max. | Min. | |
| July | 69.25 | 90* | 52* | 2.63 | 67.81 | 86* | 46* | 2.70 | 70.81 | 90* | 50* | 2.58 | 66.91 | 87* | 52* | 1.80 |
| August | 66.53 | 86* | 48* | 4.02 | 68.14 | 84* | 49* | 4.50 | 69.08 | 87* | 45* | 8.20 | 67.64 | 83* | 51* | 2.38 |
| September | 58.62 | 81* | 41* | 2.11 | 60.44 | 80* | 35* | 2.36 | 61.78 | 87* | 40* | 2.46 | 58.85 | 84* | 44* | 1.41 |
| October | 50.40 | 71* | 29* | 6.01 | 56.02 | 73 | 29* | 5.07 | 50.71 | 67 | 28* | 2.94 | ....... | ....... | ....... | 3.09 |
| November | 39.14 | 56* | 26* | 4.19 | 36.33 | 60* | 7* | 5.57 | 39.73 | 70* | 11* | 4.81 | 30.58 | 54* | 1* | 1.72 |
| December | 27.97 | 47* | 1* | 3.94 | 23.16 | 45* | — 5* | 2.60 | 28.05 | 46* | —10* | 3.91 | 27.14 | 50* | 5* | 2.80 |
| January | 18.65 | 41* | —11 | 2.58 | 21.92 | 40* | 1* | 1.69 | 19.86 | 47* | —12* | 4.46 | 25.59 | 47* | — 2* | 2.52 |
| February | 23.86 | 48 | —11 | 2.23 | 22.87 | 42* | — 3* | 1.20 | 21.83 | 43* | — 3* | 1.62 | 24.51 | 48* | — 7* | 1.10 |
| March | 36.56 | 52* | 25* | 4.10 | 22.41 | 45* | — 5* | 2.10 | 29.63 | 44* | 7* | 3.54 | 32.18 | 49* | 8* | 3.38 |
| April | 41.83 | 63 | 26* | 2.88 | 41.90 | 75* | 25* | 1.32 | 39.82 | 56* | 32* | 3.37 | 36.21 | 58* | 13* | 4.00 |
| May | 52.69 | 82* | 35* | 3.47 | 53.44 | 70 | 38* | 2.74 | 50.15 | 75* | 34* | 3.30 | 51.56 | 74* | 36* | 1.82 |
| June | 61.89 | 82* | 45* | 2.00 | 64.16 | 83* | 44* | 4.88 | 61.62 | 83* | 44* | 1.26 | 60.69 | 82* | 49* | |
| For the year | 45.60 | 90* | —11 | 30.76 | 44.88 | 86* | — 5* | 36.73 | 45.26 | 90* | —12* | 42.45 | ....... | 87* | — 7* | ....... |

* These observations are made with self-registering thermometers. The mean is from the standard thermometer.

NOTE.—No observations made in October, 1873, on account of the absence of the observer.

*Consolidated sick-report, Fort Preble, Me., 1870–'74.*

| Year | 1870–'71. | | 1871–'72. | | 1872–'73. | | 1873–'74. | |
| --- | --- | --- | --- | --- | --- | --- | --- | --- |
| Mean strength — Officers | 5 | | 6 | | 5 | | 3 | |
| Enlisted men | 52 | | 36 | | 43 | | 39 | |
| Diseases. | Cases. | Deaths. | Cases. | Deaths. | Cases. | Deaths. | Cases. | Deaths. |
| GENERAL DISEASES, A. | | | | | | | | |
| Small-pox | | | 1 | | | | | |
| Remittent fever | | | | | | | 1 | |
| Intermittent fever | 1 | | 5 | | 3 | | 5 | |
| Other diseases of this group | 3 | | 2 | | 1 | | 1 | |
| GENERAL DISEASES, B. | | | | | | | | |
| Rheumatism | 3 | | 1 | | 3 | | 2 | |
| Consumption | | | | | 2 | | | |
| LOCAL DISEASES. | | | | | | | | |
| Catarrh and bronchitis | 15 | | 9 | | 20 | | 8 | |
| Pneumonia | | | | | | | 1 | |
| Pleurisy | 1 | | 1 | | | | | |
| Diarrhœa and dysentery | 16 | | 4 | | 6 | | 4 | |
| Gonorrhœa | 3 | | 3 | | | | | |
| Other local diseases | 42 | | 15 | | 20 | | 11 | |
| Alcoholism | | | 1 | | 3 | | | |
| Total disease | 84 | | 42 | | 58 | | 33 | |
| VIOLENT DISEASES AND DEATHS. | | | | | | | | |
| Drowning | | 1 | | | | | | 1 |
| Other accidents and injuries | 25 | | 9 | | 23 | | 15 | |
| Suicide | | | | | | 1 | | |
| Total violence | 25 | 1 | 9 | 1 | 23 | | 15 | 1 |

## SANDY HOOK, NEW JERSEY.

A fort was commenced in 1857 on the northern end of Sandy Hook, at the entrance to the lower harbor of New York, in latitude 40° 28′ north, longitude 3° 3′ east. The works were first occupied April 3, 1863. The soil is an accumulation of sand, partially grown over with coarse grass and shrubs, together with cedar timber of good growth. Communication is by water in the summer season; but the post is seldom accessible in winter on account of the ice. Water is obtained anywhere by sinking wells in the sand.

The quarters, store-houses, &c., are unimportant, and occupied only by the ordnance-sergeant in charge.

## FORT SCAMMEL, MAINE.

This fort was begun in 1841 on House Island, Portland Harbor, latitude, 43° 39′ north; longitude, 6° 43′ east. Undergoing extensive changes.

## FORT SCHUYLER, NEW YORK.

### REPORT OF ASSISTANT-SURGEON C. B. WHITE, UNITED STATES ARMY.

Fort Schuyler is situated upon Throgg's Point, a narrow projection of Westchester County, New York, at the junction of the East River with Long Island Sound, latitude, 40° 48′ 45″ north; longitude, 3° 16′ east. Distant from the City Hall, New York City, 17 miles, from Long Island shore about one mile, and 3 miles from Westchester, the post-office of the fort. There is daily communication with New York City by steamer; and the city can be reached by rail at any time in about two hours.

The reservation was purchased in 1826, work was begun on the fort in 1833, and it was first garrisoned in January, 1861. The neck of the peninsula was the site of the McDougall general hospital during the late war. The peninsula is a narrow strip of ground nearly half a mile in length, with an average elevation above the water of 25 feet, and including an area of fifty-two acres.

The fort is on the outer end of the peninsula, and is a regular casemated structure of gneiss.

The quarters for the troops are casemates upon the land side of the fort; eight in number, and in two tiers. The lower rooms measure 47 feet 6 inches by 18 feet, and the upper ones 48 feet by 18 feet 6 inches, the height of each averaging about 13 feet. Each room has two large fire-places, but to warm them properly in severe winter weather it has been found necessary to resort to stoves. Each room has three windows in the rear, two windows and a door in front, and at the end of the room, over the windows and doors, an opening for ventilation 2 by 1½ feet, closing with a shutter.

Within 30 feet of the quarters is a shed over a well and pump, fitted up as a wash-room for the use of enlisted men. There is no bath-room connected with the quarters. The privies for the men's use are in a flagged yard inclosed from the parade, in front of and about 35 feet from the quarters. The kitchens and mess-rooms are wooden buildings, outside the fort.

The larger portion of the rooms available at this post for officers' quarters are in the land-side line of casemates south of the main entrance. These casemates, similar in size to those occupied by the men, have been plastered, and divided by halls and partitions into rooms averaging 16½ by 18½ feet. A wide veranda, communicating with the lower floor by iron stairways, runs along the front of the second story. The lower floors are damp in summer. In front the courtyard is laid out in garden plots, with greensward and some trees. The sinks are in the front yard, like those of the enlisted men.

There are no bath-rooms connected with the officers' quarters, and their water-supply is by water-cart and barrels.

The guard-house is in a casemate by the sally-port. The guard-room measures 8 by 36 feet; the prison-room 28½ by 24½ feet; the height of each being 12 feet. Each room has a ventilating tube passing through the masonry of the ceiling, and they are sufficiently lighted and dry.

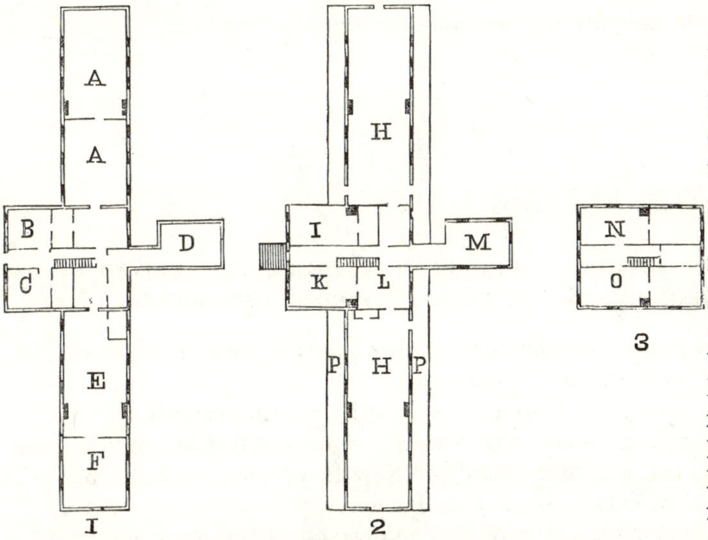

Figure 12.

The hospital is a frame building 171 feet in length, 22 feet wide in the wings, and 32 feet wide in the center buildings. It was originally a part of the general hospital above referred to, and is situated at the foot of the glacis.

The plan of the building is given in Fig. 12: 1 designating the basement, 2 the first floor, and 3 the second floor of the central part of the building; A A, store-rooms; B, laundry; C, linen-room; D, pump-room; E, kitchen; F, mess-room; H H, ward; I, dispensary; K, office; L, bath-room; M, water-closets; N, matron's room; O, steward's quarters; PP, verandas.

Each ward is 63 by 21 feet and 15 feet in height, and has ridge ventilation.

The water-supply of the post is from wells; the quantity is ample, and the quality usually good. The natural drainage is excellent. A sewer underlies the fort, connected with a large reservoir, which is filled at high tide, from which the water can be let off as required to flush the sinks, &c.

The garrison was withdrawn October 5, 1870.

## FORT SEWALL, MASSACHUSETTS.

A very old work, commenced about the close of the last century, situated on the west point of Marblehead, adjoining the town, in latitude 42° 30' north; longitude 6° 13' east.

In charge of an ordnance-sergeant.

## SPRINGFIELD ARMORY AND ARSENAL, MASSACHUSETTS.

The arsenal of construction at Springfield, Mass., (latitude, 42° 6' north; longitude, 4° 27' east,) was established in 1794. The reservation comprises between 200 and 300 acres.

In addition to the workshops and storehouses, the principal buildings are: commanding officer's quarters, of brick, two stories high, thirteen rooms; officers' double quarters, brick, two stories high, ten rooms in each; for ordnance store-keeper and paymaster, one two-story brick, seventeen rooms; for master-armorer, one two-story brick, eleven rooms; for clerks, four two-story bricks, eleven rooms in each; for foreman of laborers, one one-story wooden house, containing nine rooms. All of these are in good condition.

## FORT STANDISH, MASSACHUSETTS.

Commenced in 1863 on Saquish Head, northern entrance to Plymouth Harbor, in latitude 41° 57' north; longitude 6° 23' east. The fort is distant 4 miles by water and 24 miles by land from the city of Plymouth.

The quarters, hospital, guard-house, &c., are unimportant and require repairs.

In charge of an ordnance-sergeant.

## FORT SULLIVAN, MAINE.

INFORMATION FURNISHED BY ACTING ASSISTANT SURGEON H. C. FESSENDEN, UNITED STATES ARMY, AND ASSISTANT SURGEON J. W. WILLIAMS, UNITED STATES ARMY.

Fort Sullivan is located on Moose Island, Passamaquoddy Bay, in the town of Eastport, Me., in latitude 44° 54' north, longitude 9° 59' east from Washington.

The island is a sterile mass of trap-rock, about four miles long by two in breadth.

The fort is an eminence on the southeastern side of the island, about 150 feet above tide-water, and overlooks the village, the harbor, the adjacent islands of New Brunswick, and the mouth of the Saint Croix River. The amount of reservation is about nine acres.

The buildings are of wood and for the most part old. The barrack is one story and an attic, 94 by 21 feet, and 10 feet from floor to ceiling. The hospital, built in 1808, is 55 by 20 feet, and two stories high. The second story contains two large rooms, one for the use of the steward, and the other a ward for six beds, giving 624 cubic feet per man. The guard-house is 30 by 25 by 10 feet, divided into one room for the guard and four cells. The guard-room is 29 by 16 by 10 feet; cubic capacity, 4,640 feet; has two windows, 5 by 3 feet each. The large cell is 18 by 9 by 10 feet; cubic capacity, 1,620 feet; ventilated by a grated window, 2 by 2 feet. The small cells, three in number, are 3 by 7 by 10 feet each; cubic capacity, 210 feet; ventilated by a small grating, one foot square, in the door.

There are two buildings, of a plain, cheap character, for officers' quarters, one of one story for the commandant; the other of two stories, divided into four tenements. These quarters have no water-closets or bath-rooms.

The drainage is perfect. An abundance of excellent water is obtained from wells.

During the winter weekly communication is had by steamboat with Portland, Me., and Boston, Mass.; during the summer there is tri-weekly communication with the same cities by boat. The nearest railroad station is Calais on the river Saint Croix, 30 miles north of Fort Sullivan. Steamboats communicate between the port and Calais during the summer months and until the Saint Croix is closed by ice, after which time daily stages take the place of boats. There is a daily mail by land and one by every steamboat.

The troops were withdrawn September 30, 1873.

For further particulars see Circular No. 4, Surgeon-General's Office, December 5, 1870.

*Meteorological report, Fort Sullivan, Me., 1870–'74.*

| Month. | 1870–'71. | | | | 1871–'72. | | | | 1872–'73. | | | | 1873–'74. | | | |
|---|---|---|---|---|---|---|---|---|---|---|---|---|---|---|---|---|
| | Temperature. | | | Rain-fall in inches. | Temperature. | | | Rain-fall in inches. | Temperature. | | | Rain-fall in inches. | Temperature. | | | Rain-fall in inches. |
| | Mean. | Max. | Min. | | Mean. | Max. | Min. | | Mean. | Max. | Min. | | Mean. | Max. | Min. | |
| July | 64.05 | 85 | 48 | 1.46 | 63.03 | 80 | 46 | 2.88 | 63.37 | 92* | 46* | 4.52 | 63.42 | 89* | 44* | 4.82 |
| August | 65.10 | 81 | 51 | 1.12 | 62.52 | 78 | 50 | 5.68 | 61.27 | 82* | 46* | 5.94 | 61.63 | 85* | 45* | 1.94 |
| September | 59.14 | 68 | 49 | 2.72 | 54.33 | 77 | 35 | 2.96 | 57.62 | 81* | 44* | 6.06 | 54.21 | 75* | 37* | 3.82 |
| October | 48.06 | 68 | 24 | 5.22 | 48.89 | 63 | 26 | 5.96 | 47.22 | 65 | 27* | 7.22 | ...... | ...... | ...... | ...... |
| November | 39.37 | 56 | 23 | 5.14 | 30.06 | 50 | − 5* | 2.14 | 36.00 | 52 | 12* | 6.92 | ...... | ...... | ...... | ...... |
| December | 27.71 | 48 | − 5 | 3.14 | 22.92 | 42 | −14* | 1.96 | 16.14 | 40 | −20* | 3.66 | ...... | ...... | ...... | ...... |
| January | 18.55 | 54 | −20 | 2.00 | 21.82 | 40 | −11* | 3.30 | 21.43 | 48 | − 8* | 3.84 | ...... | ...... | ...... | ...... |
| February | 21.07 | 40 | −18 | 1.52 | 23.47 | 39 | − 6* | 1.46 | 21.03 | 37 | −11* | 2.82 | ...... | ...... | ...... | ...... |
| March | 31.65 | 55 | 19 | 1.32 | 21.55 | 48 | −15* | 4.64 | 26.84 | 40 | 9* | 3.20 | ...... | ...... | ...... | ...... |
| April | 42.29 | 59 | 23 | 2.38 | 38.23 | 67 | 22* | 1.14 | 36.52 | 50 | 24* | 2.52 | ...... | ...... | ...... | ...... |
| May | 49.17 | 88 | 31 | 2.58 | 47.17 | 58 | 33* | 7.76 | 49.03 | 68 | 30* | 2.32 | ...... | ...... | ...... | ...... |
| June | 57.94 | 76 | 36 | 2.16 | 56.58 | 87* | 35* | 5.98 | 60.39 | 81* | 40* | 3.64 | ...... | ...... | ...... | ...... |
| For the year | 43.67 | 88 | −20 | 30.76 | 40.88 | 87* | −15* | 45.86 | 41.40 | 92* | −20* | 52.66 | ...... | ...... | ...... | ...... |

* These observations are made with self-registering thermometers. The mean is from the standard thermometer.

*Consolidated sick-report, Fort Sullivan, 1870–'74.*

| Year | | 1870–'71. | | 1871–'72. | | 1872–'73. | | 1873–'74. | |
|---|---|---|---|---|---|---|---|---|---|
| Mean strength { Officers | | 5 | | 6 | | 5. | | 3 | |
| { Enlisted men | | 66 | | 45 | | 50 | | 53* | |
| Diseases. | | Cases. | Deaths. | Cases. | Deaths. | Cases. | Deaths. | Cases. | Deaths. |
| GENERAL DISEASES, A. | | | | | | | | | |
| Remittent fever | | ...... | ...... | ...... | ...... | 5 | ...... | ...... | ...... |
| Intermittent fever | | ...... | ...... | ...... | ...... | 17 | ...... | ...... | ...... |
| Other diseases of this group | | 7 | ...... | 2 | ...... | 3 | ...... | ...... | ...... |
| GENERAL DISEASES. B. | | | | | | | | | |
| Rheumatism | | 2 | ...... | 9 | ...... | 17 | ...... | ...... | ...... |
| Syphilis | | ...... | ...... | ...... | ...... | 2 | ...... | ...... | ...... |
| Consumption | | 1 | ...... | ...... | 1 | 3 | ...... | ...... | ...... |
| LOCAL DISEASES. | | | | | | | | | |
| Catarrh and bronchitis | | 3 | ...... | 1 | ...... | 13 | ...... | ...... | ...... |
| Pneumonia | | 3 | ...... | ...... | ...... | ...... | ...... | ...... | ...... |
| Pleurisy | | ...... | ...... | ...... | ...... | 1 | ...... | ...... | ...... |
| Diarrhœa and dysentery | | ...... | ...... | 2 | ...... | 9 | ...... | ...... | ...... |
| Gonorrhœa | | 1 | ...... | ...... | ...... | 1 | ...... | ...... | ...... |
| Other local diseases | | 8 | ...... | 15 | ...... | 12 | ...... | 2 | ...... |
| Alcoholism | | 1 | ...... | 2 | ...... | 6 | ...... | ...... | ...... |
| Total disease | | 26 | ...... | 32 | 1 | 89 | ...... | 2 | ...... |
| VIOLENT DISEASES AND DEATHS. | | | | | | | | | |
| Accidents and injuries | | 10 | ...... | 7 | ...... | 20 | ...... | 2 | ...... |
| Total violence | | 10 | ...... | 7 | ...... | 20 | ...... | 2 | ...... |

* Three months only.

---

# FORT TRUMBULL, NEW LONDON, CONNECTICUT.

## REPORT OF SURGEON JOHN CAMPBELL, UNITED STATES ARMY.

Fort Trumbull lies in latitude 41° 20′ 33″ north; longitude 5° 2′ 52″ east. It occupies the extreme southeast point of a peninsula or neck, formerly called "Mamacock," now Fort Neck, which projects into the harbor of New London. It is half a mile below the city, and a mile and a half above the mouth of the river Thames. The Government grounds are of a very limited

10 M P

extent, embracing but a small portion of the "Neck," and the buildings are crowded into very uncomfortable proximity to each other. (For history of the post see Circular No. 4, Surgeon General's Office, December 5, 1870.)

A few of the officers occupy very comfortable casemates in the fort. The remainder of the garrison occupy quarters outside the fort.

In parallel lines at a short distance from the sally-port, and running west therefrom, lie the officers' quarters, the men's barracks, and the hospital, a space of not more than 50 feet separating the buildings. The officers' quarters consist of a block of four two-story buildings of granite, comfortable, and in good repair. The soldiers' quarters consist of one building of granite, one story, with kitchen and offices underneath, and one frame building, continuous with the other. One company occupies each of the buildings. To the rear of these lies the hospital. Its main building, erected many years before the present fort, is a one-story granite building, with a central hall, on one side of which is the surgery, on the other, a ward; beneath are a kitchen and mess-room, the fall of the ground making two clear stories in the rear. Toward the end of the war two frame wings were affixed to the hospital, the eastern one of which is now used as a ward, while the western one has been converted into a quartermaster's and commissary's storehouse.

Four detached cottages are occupied by married soldiers and laundresses; and in the summer of 1873 an old barrack was converted into quarters for the same purpose, and a substantial house of 8 rooms built.

The garrison is supplied with water from four wells sunk into the granite which underlies the whole tract. The water is pure, pleasant, and wholesome. It is carried by hand by the police party to the quarters, hospital, &c. The river Thames runs directly southward past the fort and opens upon Long Island Sound. The harbor is one of the finest on the coast. The garrison has always enjoyed extraordinary exemption from severe disease and epidemics. A large proportion of the inhabitants of the neighboring country reach a great age, and the climate seems remarkably favorable to the rearing of children. Wounded patients sent here during the war recovered with great rapidity.

Fish of every variety and excellent quality are found in the river and in the sound—shad, cod, bass, blue-fish, mackerel, eels, flat-fish, black-fish, tautog, with oysters, clams, muscles, crabs, &c. In fact, this is reputed one of the finest fish markets and harbors in the country, and is the headquarters for the sporting yachts in the blue-fish and mackerel season.

*Meteorological report, Fort Trumbull, Conn., 1870-'74.*

| Month. | 1870-71. | | | | 1871-72. | | | | 1872-73. | | | | 1873-74. | | | |
|---|---|---|---|---|---|---|---|---|---|---|---|---|---|---|---|---|
| | Temperature. | | | Rain-fall in inches. | Temperature. | | | Rain-fall in inches. | Temperature. | | | Rain-fall in inches. | Temperature. | | | Rain-fall in inches. |
| | Mean. | Max. | Min. | | Mean. | Max. | Min. | | Mean. | Max. | Min. | | Mean. | Max. | Min. | |
| July | 73.94 | 92 | 53* | 2.09 | 71.02 | 89 | 51* | 1.76 | 77.81 | 98* | 58* | 5.02 | 73.20 | 96* | 56* | 1.10 |
| August | 73.87 | 87 | 52* | 1.84 | 71.51 | 87 | 53* | 3.80 | 72.68 | 94* | 48* | 6.56 | 70.19 | 93* | 52* | 5.16 |
| September | 64.77 | 83 | 43 | 1.38 | 59.26 | 87* | 36* | 1.36 | 63.59 | 90* | 41* | 6.26 | 62.92 | 85* | 39* | 2.82 |
| October | 57.59 | 73 | 28* | 4.67 | 55.27 | 73* | 28* | 7.62 | 52.08 | 74* | 32* | 3.32 | 53.57 | 74* | 30* | 5.02 |
| November | 44.37 | 63 | 25* | 2.66 | 37.36 | 65* | 11* | 4.90 | 41.14 | 59* | 14* | 5.56 | 34.56 | 61* | 17* | 4.76 |
| December | 34.27 | 59 | 0* | 2.53 | 29.84 | 52* | —2* | 2.76 | 26.21 | 49* | —3* | 3.50 | 33.06 | 58* | 10* | 5.68 |
| January | 27.34 | 48 | —4* | 2.28 | 28.61 | 49* | 5* | 2.42 | 26.30 | 50* | —7* | 6.46 | 31.50 | 52* | 3* | 3.96 |
| February | 29.02 | 53 | —6* | 3.41 | 28.43 | 51* | 5* | 2.74 | 26.45 | 46* | —1* | 4.18 | 28.42 | 56* | 4* | 2.70 |
| March | 41.24 | 59 | 25 | 6.09 | 27.75 | 57* | —3* | 5.22 | 33.02 | 53* | 9* | 1.50 | 33.50 | 58* | 10* | 2.14 |
| April | 48.16 | 71 | 27* | 3.49 | 44.57 | 80* | 28* | 1.78 | 43.26 | 61* | 30* | 3.28 | 38.44 | 57* | 15* | 8.20 |
| May | 57.06 | 80 | 34* | 2.82 | 58.06 | 92* | 30* | 3.29 | 55.07 | 83* | 32* | 5.92 | 55.52 | 85* | 25* | 4.64 |
| June | 66.36 | 87 | 42* | 4.58 | 67.79 | 90* | 43* | 3.46 | 66.80 | 92* | 45* | 0.60 | 66.64 | 92* | 45* | 2.98 |
| For the year | 51.49 | 92 | —6* | 37.84 | 48.29 | 92* | —3* | 41.11 | 48.70 | 98* | —7* | 52.12 | 48.46 | 96* | 3* | 49.16 |

* These observations are marked with self-registering thermometers. The mean is from the standard thermometer.

*Consolidated sick-report, Fort Trumbull, Conn., 1870–'74.*

| Year | 1870–'71. | | 1871–'72. | | 1872–'73. | | 1873–'74. | |
|---|---|---|---|---|---|---|---|---|
| Mean strength { Officers............. { Enlisted men...... | 9 102 | | 7 79 | | 7 77 | | 7 79 | |
| Disease. | Cases. | Deaths. | Cases. | Deaths. | Cases. | Deaths. | Cases. | Deaths. |
| GENERAL DISEASES, A. | | | | | | | | |
| Remittent fever ........................ | ...... | ...... | ...... | ...... | 1 | ...... | ...... | ...... |
| Intermittent fever........................ | 1 | ...... | ...... | ...... | ...... | ...... | ...... | ...... |
| Other diseases of this group............ | 16 | ...... | 14 | ...... | 10 | ...... | 9 | ...... |
| GENERAL DISEASES, B. | | | | | | | | |
| Rheumatism ............................ | 26 | ...... | ...... | ...... | 5 | ...... | 7 | ...... |
| Syphilis ................................ | 4 | ...... | 9 | ...... | 1 | ...... | ...... | ...... |
| Consumption ............................ | ...... | ...... | ...... | 1 | 1 | ...... | ...... | ...... |
| Other diseases of this group............ | ...... | ...... | 1 | ...... | 1 | ...... | ...... | ...... |
| LOCAL DISEASES. | | | | | | | | |
| Catarrh and bronchitis................. | 25 | ...... | 17 | ...... | 20 | ...... | 43 | ...... |
| Pneumonia............................. | 1 | ...... | ...... | ...... | ...... | ...... | 1 | ...... |
| Diarrhœa and dysentery ............... | 22 | ...... | 12 | ...... | 31 | ...... | 12 | ...... |
| Gonorrhœa............................. | 5 | ...... | 1 | ...... | ...... | ...... | ...... | ...... |
| Other local diseases................... | 69 | ...... | 65 | ...... | 67 | ...... | 39 | ...... |
| Alcoholism............................. | 9 | ...... | 3 | ...... | 14 | ...... | 13 | ...... |
| Total disease ..................... | 178 | ...... | 122 | 1 | 150 | ...... | 124 | ...... |
| VIOLENT DISEASES AND DEATHS. | | | | | | | | |
| Gunshot wounds ....................... | 1 | ...... | ...... | ...... | ...... | ...... | ...... | ...... |
| Drowning ........ | ...... | 1 | ...... | ...... | ...... | 1 | ...... | ...... |
| Other accidents and injuries............ | 47 | ...... | 31 | ...... | 21 | ...... | 20 | ...... |
| Total violence................... | 48 | 1 | 31 | ...... | 21 | 1 | 20 | ...... |

# FORT WADSWORTH, STATEN ISLAND, NEW YORK HARBOR.

### REPORTS OF SURGEON J. COOPER M'KEE AND ASSISTANT SURGEON H. R. TILTON, UNITED STATES ARMY.

The fortifications and government reserve on Staten Island, west of the Narrows, commanding the entrance on that side of New York Harbor, are known by the name of Fort Wadsworth. They are in latitude 40° 35' 50'' north, longitude 3° east; distant from Fort Hamilton, one mile; and are named in honor of General Wadsworth, a distinguished soldier who fell in the late civil war. It was formerly known by the name of Fort Richmond, being placed in the county of that name, State of New York. The fortification on the top of the hill, the commanding point on the reserve, is known by the name of Fort Tompkins, and commands the work of Fort Wadsworth, a triple casemate of granite, as well as Battery Hudson, and the other continuous water-batteries which defend the passage. It lies 140 feet above the level of the sea.

The reserve contains about 100 acres; surface very broken and rugged; its slopes and declivities are steep and rapid.

The hills on the island surround many deep hollows or basins, some of which are in the limits of the reservation, exercising an important influence on its hygiene. The soil is very spongy and porous, and absorbs a large quantity of water. During the warm weather great atmospheric humidity is maintained from the rapid evaporation arising from the surface of the earth, which is said to be hardly ever dry, and when exposed or denuded of vegetation, is never free from fungi. Having no outlets, and receiving the drainage from the surrounding surface, the valleys already mentioned usually contain ponds or swamps, which, during the summer and autumn, emit great quantities of vapor, in connection with the diffusible products of organic decomposition.

The men occupy for dormitories casemates in Fort Tompkins, averaging ten men and beds in each. The casemates are comfortably warmed by a large anthracite coal-stove in each, lighted by candles at night, ventilated and lighted by two windows in the rear, 5 feet high and 8 inches wide, two in front 6 feet 6 inches high and 3 feet wide, and a transom over the door 3 feet by 2. Air-space ample; each occupant has five hundred cubic feet. These casemates have recently been improved by lining them with brick, leaving an air-space between the lining and wall, and covering the floors and ceilings with boards. Bedsteads are of iron, single, made with a hinge in the middle so as to fold up in day-time. One casemate is used for bathing and washing; basins are supplied; water is furnished in sufficient quantity from a large hogshead on a platform. In winter, bathing once a week is required, in tubs in a compartment fitted up in a casemate; in summer men bathe in the ocean. The dining-room and kitchen are adjoining casemates, and are well furnished and in good condition.

There is one large brick water-closet or sink on the slope facing the sea, in addition to several temporary sinks, which are pits dug in the ground, and removed and rebuilt as required.

Four sets of quarters for married soldiers and laundresses, and a cottage for the ordnance sergeant, were erected in 1873 near the barracks south of the fort. A fine large oven was constructed in the same year in the frame building formerly used as a library.

The officers' quarters are situated at the northern end of the reservation, and comprise the commanding officer's quarters, a one-story and attic frame building, erected in the latter part of 1869; three frame buildings, erected in 1871, two of which contain each two sets of captains' quarters, and the other four sets of quarters for subaltern officers. All these quarters are furnished with cisterns, and the three sets first mentioned with supplies of hot and cold water. The temporary buildings erected for officers' quarters during the war have been removed, with the exception of one, now used for offices for commanding officer, adjutant, quartermaster, and commissary of subsistence.

The guard-house is placed in two casemates in the western wing; one is occupied by the guard and the other by the prisoners. The guard-house for the prisoners is divided into six cells, each 7 feet long, 4 feet broad, and 6 feet 10 inches in height. The top is secured and guarded by heavy plank lattice, so as to secure the equable ventilation of each cell with the air in the casemate. Prisoners are locked in cells at bed-time; are furnished with bedsacks and straw; have the same diet as the company; and are supplied from company kitchen. They use the company sink, and are required to bathe once a week. The average occupation during the past year was four.

The post hospital is a frame building, constructed in September and October, 1869, in accordance with plan of "Circular No. 4, Surgeon General's Office, Washington, April 27, 1867," and consists of an administration building two stories high, back building (kitchen) one story high, and one wing (ward) one story high, and has a capacity of twelve beds; it is well built, and properly and neatly furnished. It has recently been improved by the addition of a porch, and of boilers, tanks, and force-pumps for the distribution of hot water. The building is, however, inconveniently located; has no isolation ward for the treatment of contagious diseases, and would be found inadequate in the event of any considerable increase of the garrison, or the breaking out of an epidemic.

There is no chapel, school, general laundry, or bakery at the post. Flour is exchanged with a village baker for bread, which is of good quality.

The water-supply is by means of a large cistern of about 2,000 gallons capacity, and is of good quality. Water is hauled to the officers' quarters, hospital, &c., from a well near the light-house, in a water-wagon, the quantity daily being about 200 gallons; about 40 gallons of this go to the hospital.

There is no effective fire-apparatus at the fort. The drainage, which is partly natural and partly artificial, has heretofore been insufficient; but a drain 10 inches in diameter has recently been laid in the rear of the hospital and officers' quarters, and will be an important sanitary improvement.

A post garden of one and a quarter acres is inclosed, in which all the usual garden vegetables are cultivated with success.

*Meteorological report, Fort Wadsworth, N. Y., 1873–'74.*

| Month. | 1870–'71. | | | | 1871–'72. | | | | 1872–'73. | | | | 1873–'74. | | | |
|---|---|---|---|---|---|---|---|---|---|---|---|---|---|---|---|---|
| | Temperature. | | | Rain-fall in inches. | Temperature. | | | Rain-fall in inches. | Temperature. | | | Rain-fall in inches. | Temperature. | | | Rain-fall in inches. |
| | Mean. | Max. | Min. | | Mean. | Max. | Min. | | Mean. | Max. | Min. | | Mean. | Max. | Min. | |
| | ° | ° | ° | | ° | ° | ° | | ° | ° | ° | | ° | ° | ° | |
| July | | | | | | | | | | | | | 73.35 | 94 | 54 | 3.10 |
| August | | | | | | | | | | | | | 70.71 | 86 | 52 | 5.41 |
| September | | | | | | | | | | | | | 63.69 | 88 | 38 | 2.25 |
| October | | | | | | | | | | | | | 52.24 | 73 | 24 | 2.25 |
| November | | | | | | | | | | | | | 33.11 | 59 | 16 | 4.90 |
| December | | | | | | | | | | | | | 31.99 | 63 | 11 | 3.83 |
| January | | | | | | | | | | | | | 30.19 | 65 | − 3 | 3.50 |
| February | | | | | | | | | | | | | 26.57 | 74 | 0 | 1.32 |
| March | | | | | | | | | | | | | 34.06 | 65 | 9 | 0.75 |
| April | | | | | | | | | | | | | 33.70 | 66 | 14 | 3.10 |
| May | | | | | | | | | | | | | 56.71 | 90 | 30 | 2.80 |
| June | | | | | | | | | 68.40 | 96 | 48 | 1.04 | 68.81 | 92 | 48 | 2.15 |
| For the year | | | | | | | | | | | | | 47.93 | 94 | − 3 | 35.36 |

NOTE.—All observations are made with self-registering thermometers.

*Consolidated sick-report, Fort Wadsworth, N. Y., 1870–'74.*

| Year | | 1870–'71. | | 1871–'72. | | 1872–'73. | | 1873–'74. | |
|---|---|---|---|---|---|---|---|---|---|
| Mean strength { Officers | | 6 | | 5 | | 5 | | 5 | |
| { Enlisted men | | 62 | | 48 | | 44 | | 54 | |
| Diseases. | | Cases. | Deaths. | Cases. | Deaths. | Cases. | Deaths. | Cases. | Deaths. |
| GENERAL DISEASES, A. | | | | | | | | | |
| Typho-malarial fever | | 5 | | 9 | | 1 | | | |
| Remittent fever | | 194 | | 133 | | 1 | | 54 | |
| Intermittent fever | | 2 | | 2 | | 54 | | 5 | |
| Other diseases of this group | | | | | | 2 | | | |
| GENERAL DISEASES, B. | | | | | | | | | |
| Rheumatism | | 9 | | | | 2 | | 29 | |
| Syphilis | | 4 | | | | 1 | | 3 | |
| Consumption | | 1 | 1 | 1 | | 1 | | | |
| LOCAL DISEASES. | | | | | | | | | |
| Catarrh and bronchitis | | 26 | | 14 | | 10 | | 35 | |
| Pneumonia | | 1 | | | | | | 1 | |
| Pleurisy | | | | | | | | | |
| Diarrhœa and dysentery | | 15 | | 10 | | 18 | | 71 | |
| Hernia | | | | 1 | | 1 | | 1 | |
| Gonorrhœa | | 2 | | | | | | | |
| Other local diseases | | 48 | | 21 | | 28 | | 48 | |
| Alcoholism | | 25 | | 15 | | 6 | | 3 | |
| Total disease | | 332 | 1 | 206 | | 125 | | 250 | |
| VIOLENT DISEASES AND DEATHS. | | | | | | | | | |
| Accidents and injuries | | 23 | | 14 | | 22 | | 34 | |
| Total violence | | 23 | | 14 | | 22 | | 34 | |

# FORT WARREN, BOSTON HARBOR, MASSACHUSETTS.

REPORTS OF ASSISTANT SURGEONS J. H. KINSMAN AND J. W. BREWER, UNITED STATES ARMY

Fort Warren is situated at the mouth of Boston Harbor, Mass., in latitude 42° 19' 30'' north; longitude 6° 4' east, on George's Island, seven and one-quarter miles east-southeast of Boston; five miles east-southeast of Fort Independence and Fort Winthrop. The height of the parade above the sea is 38 feet.

The island is an irregular oval, 1,800 by 1,200 feet, and contains about 28 acres. It originally consisted of two hills, which were leveled for the building of the fort, and the only land at present not thus occupied is a few acres on the northwest and southwest points of the island. This space is used as a post garden, and for the accommodation of the engineer building, laundresses' quarters, and stables.

Although the prevailing winds of summer are westerly, the heat is much mitigated by the frequent occurrence of winds from the east, which often spring up early in the afternoon, and last, unaccompanied by rain, for five or six hours.

The east and northeast winds bring with them violent storms of snow in winter and rain in summer, which have a general duration of two or three days. A true north wind is comparatively rare.

The fort is built of granite, and contains about 18 acres. The casemates are used as quarters, averaging in dimension 30 by 18 by 15 feet, with hard-finished walls and floors of concrete, covered with hard pine, accommodating nine men to each. The casemates are warmed by stoves, and lighted and ventilated by three embrasures looking outward and two windows looking upon the parade.

The beds are single iron bunks, with the usual bedding. A water-closet for winter use is within the fort—the excreta passing into the main sewer running under the ditch. It requires to be flushed with water every day, and is inadequate to the wants of the command, the arrangement being very imperfect, and it is only used when the weather is too inclement to make use of the summer water-closet, which is a wooden building outside the fort upon the sea-wall, overhanging the water.

Three of the casemates are used as kitchens and mess-rooms combined; they are well furnished and adapted for the purpose.

The quarters for laundresses and married soldiers consist of three wooden buildings outside the

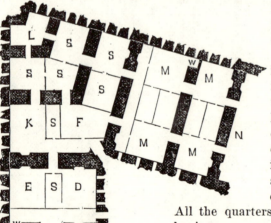

fort. They are one story high, 175 feet long, 25 feet broad, and divided into five sets of quarters, each containing about four rooms.

The officers' quarters are the casemates forming the northwest side of the fort. They are hard-finished, with plain white walls, and comprise twelve sets of one story, with basements below the level of the parade, and two sets of one story without basements. The number of rooms to a set is either four or six. The average size of the rooms is 16 by 18 feet. The two sets without basements are single sets, and contain each four rooms. Two of the sets contain six rooms, including basements. All the quarters with basements, except one set, are double sets, having a common entrance, but separated by a wall running from front to back. They are heated by grates, and lighted by embrasures on one side and by windows looking upon the parade on the other, which also afford ventilation. Water is supplied from a pump in the kitchen, leading to a cistern below each set of quarters. A water-closet and bath-room is in common for each double set of quarters, and is situated at the end of the hall which separates the quarters. The two single quarters have water-closets, but no bath-rooms.

The offices and storehouses are in casemates, principally in the north bastion of the fort.

The guard-house is of stone, at the entrance of the road leading to the sally-port, between the cover-face and the wall of the fort.

Figure 13.

It is one story high, 40 by 18 feet, and contains two rooms and a hall. The building is warmed by stoves, and ventilated principally by windows. It is not any too large for the exclusive use of the guard, and it ought not to contain prisoners.

The hospital is situated in casemates on the western side of the fort, and is contained in a space of 202 by 39 feet. The walls are hard-finished, and the floor is of hard pine. The rooms are warmed by grates and stoves, and ventilated by windows and embrasures and by tubes passing up from the ceilings. The arrangement and division of the space are shown in Fig. 13. The massive lines represent stone; the fine lines, wooden partitions. A, wards, 39 by 25 feet; B, bath and wash-room; D, dispensary; E, steward's room; F, clothing-room; K, kitchen; L, cook's room; M, surgeon's quarters; N, commanding-officer's quarters; O, well; S, store-rooms; W, water-closet.

The ward is intended to contain thirty beds, giving to each a cubic air-space of 1,226 feet. The bath-room contains a large sink with pump, and three bath-tubs. Hot water is furnished by a small perpendicular boiler in the coal-room. The ceiling of the hospital is arched, the height from the floor to the center being 16 feet 4 inches.

The post bakery is a casemate containing two ovens, situated in the north bastion. It is commodious, and well adapted for that purpose.

On the eastern side of the fort is a casemate used as a chapel and furnished with plain wooden benches. Adjoining the chapel is the school-room—also a casemate—and furnished with benches and blackboards.

The library is contained in a casemate on the east side of the fort, near the chapel. It comprises about 1,900 volumes of all branches of literature. Changes now in progress will have the effect of rendering a part of the casemates no longer available as quarters.

The fort is abundantly supplied with water from wells and cisterns. Although the water contains a considerable amount of lime and soda salts, the quality is good. In case of fire at the post, the only available means of water-supply would be the pumps.

The drainage of the fort is entirely artificial, effected by drains and sewers, which run beneath the parade, and, extending under the ditch, discharge into the sea.

In summer the men bathe in the sea, but there are no special arrangements providing bathing accommodations for them within the fort.

The post garden contains about one and a half acres of ground, which is cultivated by a detail from the command.

The means of communication with Boston is a steam-tug belonging to the Engineer Department, but under orders to call at the fort three times a week. It is regular in summer, but liable to occasional interruptions in winter from ice and violent storms.

*Meteorological report, Fort Warren, Mass., 1870–'74.*

| Month. | 1870–'71. | | | | 1871–'72. | | | | 1872–'73. | | | | 1873–'74. | | | |
|---|---|---|---|---|---|---|---|---|---|---|---|---|---|---|---|---|
| | Temperature. | | | Rain-fall in inches. | Temperature. | | | Rain-fall in inches. | Temperature. | | | Rain-fall in inches. | Temperature. | | | Rain-fall in inches. |
| | Mean. | Max. | Min. | | Mean. | Max. | Min. | | Mean. | Max. | Min. | | Mean. | Max. | Min. | |
| | ° | ° | ° | | ° | ° | ° | | ° | ° | ° | | ° | ° | ° | |
| July ............... | 73.34 | 94 | 60 | 1.00 | 70.99 | 90 | 60 | 1.82 | 72.71 | 100* | 55* | 3.70 | 69.57 | 92* | 50* | 3.30 |
| August ............. | 73.01 | 95 | 60 | 1.60 | 72.43 | 92 | 62 | 3.45 | 72.62 | 95* | 59* | 8.20 | 68.02 | 87* | 50* | 5.44 |
| September ......... | 63.42 | 85 | 49 | 1.10 | 60.52 | 80 | 45 | 0.70 | 65.00 | 100* | 45* | 4.00 | 62.66 | 86* | 45* | 1.27 |
| October ............ | 55.46 | 72 | 35 | 3.31 | 53.44 | 73* | 32* | 5.29 | 50.78 | 73* | 36* | 5.70 | 53.84 | 69* | 35* | 3.69 |
| November ........... | 43.69 | 62 | 31 | 2.34 | 36.83 | 60* | 9* | 2.49 | 40.22 | 60* | 17* | 2.55 | 34.43 | 60* | 10* | 1.90 |
| December ........... | 31.75 | 49 | 8 | 1.34 | 27.64 | 48* | 0* | 3.52 | 23.51 | 44* | — 8* | (13.?91) | 32.32 | 58* | 5* | 1.35 |
| January ............ | 24.66 | 52 | — 9 | 0.82 | 27.22 | 44* | 6* | 1.65 | 25.58 | 52* | —10* | 7.25 | 39.99 | 56* | 2* | 2.80 |
| February ........... | 28.08 | 52 | — 5 | 1.07 | 27.75 | 54* | 2* | 1.57 | 25.76 | 46* | — 8* | (14.?00) | 27.39 | 56* | 0* | 3.20 |
| March .............. | 41.82 | 61 | 31 | 2.75 | 27.14 | 53* | — 2* | 2.80 | 33.64 | 55* | 12* | (11.?20) | 34.13 | 56* | 5* | 1.98 |
| April .............. | 47.14 | 76 | 34 | 2.05 | 45.23 | 73* | 30* | 1.25 | 43.03 | 63* | 28* | (8.?15) | 37.49 | 64* | 16* | 9.85 |
| May................. | 57.73 | 94 | 42 | 1.75 | 57.31 | 74* | 41* | 7.00 | 54.88 | 80* | 35* | 7.00 | 53.88 | 80* | 35* | 3.30 |
| June ............... | 66.49 | 86 | 53 | 3.60 | 66.37 | 92* | 46* | 3.30 | 64.89 | 90* | 45* | 1.75 | 63.33 | 92* | 39* | 3.93 |
| For the year..... | 50.55 | 95 | — 9 | 22.73 | 47.74 | 92* | — 2* | 34.84 | 47.72 | 100* | —10* | (?) | 48.88 | 92* | 0* | 42.01 |

* These observations are made with self-registering thermometers. The mean is from the standard thermometer.

*Consolidated sick-report, Fort Warren, Mass., 1870–'74.*

| Year | 1870–'71. | | 1871–'72. | | 1872–'73. | | 1873–'74. | |
|---|---|---|---|---|---|---|---|---|
| Mean strength { Officers / Enlisted men | 6 / 75 | | 6 / 47 | | 5 / 46 | | 6 / 50 | |
| Diseases. | Cases. | Deaths. | Cases. | Deaths. | Cases. | Deaths. | Cases. | Deaths. |
| GENERAL DISEASES, A. | | | | | | | | |
| Typhoid fever | | | | | 1 | 1 | | |
| Intermittent fever | | | 2 | | 6 | | 1 | |
| Other diseases of this group | 5 | | 2 | | 5 | | 14 | |
| GENERAL DISEASES, B. | | | | | | | | |
| Rheumatism | 15 | | 2 | | 3 | | 4 | |
| Syphilis | 3 | | | | | | 4 | |
| LOCAL DISEASES. | | | | | | | | |
| Catarrh and bronchitis | 13 | | 7 | | 11 | | 13 | |
| Pneumonia | | | | | 1 | | 1 | |
| Pleurisy | | | | | 1 | | | |
| Diarrhœa and dysentery | 8 | | 1 | | 9 | | 9 | |
| Gonorrhœa | 1 | | 2 | | | | 1 | |
| Other local diseases | 33 | | 23 | | 19 | | 18 | |
| Alcoholism | 4 | | 2 | | 2 | | 3 | |
| Total disease | 82 | | 41 | | 58 | 1 | 68 | |
| VIOLENT DISEASES AND DEATHS. | | | | | | | | |
| Accidents and injuries | 20 | | 15 | | 12 | | 9 | |
| Total violence | 20 | | 15 | | 12 | | 9 | |

# WASHINGTON ARSENAL, DISTRICT OF COLUMBIA.

### REPORT OF ACTING ASSISTANT SURGEON J. R. REILY, UNITED STATES ARMY.

The arsenal at Washington occupies the most southern point of the city, known as Greenleaf Point, at the extremity of Four-and-a-half street west, and at the confluence of the Anacostia or Eastern Branch with the Potomac River. Government workshops appear to have been erected here at a very early period in the history of the city, but the post is said to have been first officially established as an arsenal in 1816.

The ground at present occupied is 69 acres.

Four buildings are in use as officers' quarters. They are plain brick buildings, two stories high, 63 feet by 30, containing each eight rooms. The average dimensions of the rooms are 20 by 15 feet, and 12 feet high. One entire building is allowed to each officer. They are heated by stoves, lighted by gas, and ventilated by the ordinary windows. Each house contains a water-closet and bath-room, and has hot and cold water throughout. The residence of the commanding officer, completed in the winter of 1873–'74, is a brick building, three stories and basement in height, possessing all the modern improvements. The eastern front is plastered in imitation of Connecticut freestone. The height of the different stories is as follows: basement, 7 feet; first story, $13\frac{1}{2}$ feet; second story, 12 feet; and third story, 11 feet. The average dimensions of the rooms are 21 by 18 feet. The parlor is 40 by 18 feet.

One brick building is used as barracks. It is two stories and basement in height, 84 by $20\frac{1}{2}$ feet, and contains 8 rooms used as dormitories, besides a mess-room, kitchen, and bath-room in the basement. The dormitories are warmed by coal-stoves, lighted by candles, and ventilated by windows front and rear. The average air-space per man is 910 cubic feet. The bunks are of iron. One room in the basement of the barrack is used as bath and wash room, to which the men have access daily. It contains two bath-rooms, a large iron tank, communicating with the boiler in the kitchen, from which hot water is obtained, and a shower-bath. The kitchen is 22 by 19 feet, and 8 feet in height. It contains one large range, capable of cooking for 150 men, and the necessary utensils. The mess-room is 40 by 22 feet, and 9 feet in height. It contains 6 tables and 6 benches, with a capacity for seating 100 men.

There are 14 sets of quarters for married soldiers and laundresses. Three sets are in wooden cottages, one story each in height, and each containing three rooms. The others are in two-story and basement brick buildings, each containing 6 rooms, which are distributed among three families, allowing two rooms for each.

The guard-house, built of brick and one story in height, is 30 by 25 feet, and 14 feet high. On the northern end is an extension 12 by 29 feet, in which are contained the cells, two in number. These cells are each 12 feet square and 10 feet high, with a passage 4 feet wide between them. They are damp within, in consequence of the floors resting immediately upon the ground. They are ventilated by skylights in the roof, but have no provision for heating. The guard-room, which occupies the entire main building, is warmed by a coal-stove, and ventilated by four windows.

The building in which is the hospital is of brick, two stories in height, 76 by 25 feet. It contains 12 rooms, 6 of which are used by the hospital department, and the rest by the hospital matron and married soldiers. The hospital is heated by stoves, lighted by gas, and ventilated by windows. There are two wards with five beds in each, the hospital cook and nurse occupying beds in one of the wards. The air-space per man is 748 cubic feet. There is no bath or wash room. The bath-tub is placed in a small closet, 3 by 10 feet, in the basement. The water-closet is about 40 feet west of the hospital, and is drained into the river. There is no dead-house at the post; and in case of a death the body awaits burial in one of the hospital wards.

The bakery is a small brick building, with a capacity for baking for 200 men.

There is no laundry, chapel, or school-house at the post. The post library, kept in the office building, contains about 500 volumes of miscellaneous works.

The water-supply is abundant and good, being derived from the city water-pipes. The pressure is sufficient to throw a stream through 100 feet of hose to the top of the highest buildings. The fire-plugs are distributed liberally about the post, and there is in addition a well-organized fire company provided with fire-engine, hose-carts, ladders, &c.

*Consolidated sick-report, Washington Arsenal, D. C., 1870–'74.*

| Year | | 1870–'71. | | 1871–'72. | | 1872–'73. | | 1873–'74. | |
|---|---|---|---|---|---|---|---|---|---|
| Mean strength { Officers | | 5 | | 5 | | 5 | | 5 | |
| { Enlisted men | | 80 | | 43 | | 45 | | 45 | |
| Diseases. | | Cases. | Deaths. | Cases. | Deaths. | Cases. | Deaths. | Cases. | Deaths. |
| GENERAL DISEASES, A. | | | | | | | | | |
| Remittent fever | | 1 | | | | | | 2 | |
| Intermittent fever | | 52 | | 65 | | 39 | | 36 | |
| Diphtheria | | 1 | | | | | | | |
| Other diseases of this group | | 5 | | 1 | | 2 | | | |
| GENERAL DISEASES, B. | | | | | | | | | |
| Rheumatism | | 7 | | | | 5 | | 6 | |
| Consumption | | 1 | | | | | | | |
| Other diseases of this group | | 1 | | | | 1 | | | |
| LOCAL DISEASES. | | | | | | | | | |
| Catarrh and bronchitis | | 18 | | 9 | | 13 | | 7 | |
| Pneumonia | | 1 | | | | 1 | 1 | | |
| Pleurisy | | 5 | | 3 | | 1 | | | |
| Diarrhoea and dysentery | | 11 | | 4 | | 13 | | 13 | |
| Gonorrhoea | | 2 | | | | | | | |
| Other local diseases | | 30 | | 8 | 1 | 17 | 2 | 20 | 1 |
| Alcoholism | | 12 | | 7 | | 8 | | 7 | |
| Total disease | | 147 | | 97 | 1 | 105 | 3 | 91 | 1 |
| VIOLENT DISEASES AND DEATHS. | | | | | | | | | |
| Accidents and injuries | | 16 | | 4 | | 8 | | 2 | |
| Total violence | | 16 | | 4 | | 8 | | 2 | |

# FORT WASHINGTON, MARYLAND.

## REPORT OF ASSISTANT SURGEON J. C. G. HAPPERSETT, UNITED STATES ARMY.

Fort Washington, in latitude 38° 41' north, longitude 3' west, stands on a high ridge, at the confluence of Piscataway Creek with the Potomac River, 14 miles below Washington City. This ridge extends from Swan Creek, (a short, wide arm of the river, half a mile north of the post,) nearly parallel with the river, and terminates in a narrow promontory below the fort. Behind is a deep ravine, 300 feet wide at the top, with sides sloping precipitously about 80 feet, terminating in a narrow plain about 100 feet wide; this ravine opens on Piscataway Creek, a small portion of which, near the creek, is marshy and covered with swamp willow. The sides of the ravine were formerly heavily timbered, but this was cut away during the late war, and they are now covered by a thick undergrowth, principally chestnut and locust. The river at this point is about 1,300 yards wide; the channel, however, is not more than 500, and entirely on the fort or Maryland side of the river. The shore is gradually sloping, sandy, and hard; the Virginia side being flat and muddy, both sides covered in summer by the ordinary river grass, which is exposed at low tide, the rise and fall of which is between five and six feet. The shores of the creeks are muddy.

This site was early occupied as a military post, and the small work which formerly stood here, (near where the water battery now is,) known as Fort Warburton, was blown up in 1814, by order of the officer in command, to prevent its probable capture by the English fleet. The present structure, laid out in 1815, is an irregular bastioned fortification of stone and brick. The parade of the main work is 115 feet above high-water mark. The entire government reservation contains between 40 and 50 acres.

The buildings originally constructed are one brick building designed as quarters for four officers; one brick building for barracks for one company, (both inside the fort,) and one brick building outside the fort, intended as quarters for the commanding officer. In the winter of 1867–'68, three small double cottages, intended as officers' quarters, and one large building for barracks, all frame buildings, were erected outside the fort, and in the winter of 1868–'69 one long frame building for laundresses, and a small house for the hospital steward. The old or brick barrack is intended to accommodate 60 men. It is without means for proper ventilation, is two stories high, with piazza facing the west. The upper story is divided into two rooms for dormitories; the lower story has three rooms, kitchen, mess-room, and one sleeping-room.

The frame barrack is a two-story building, standing near the edge of the ravine on the eastern side of the reservation. It is intended to accommodate 100 men with an allowance of 460 cubic feet of air per man. The lower story is divided into kitchen, mess-room, wash-room, store-room, and company offices. The walls and ceilings of this story are all plastered; of the upper story, only the sides. Two wide piazzas extend the entire length of the building, front and rear.

The officers' quarters consist of one brick building inside the fort, intended for four officers, the set at each end of the building consisting of two rooms and a basement kitchen; the others of similar rooms, but without the kitchen. One brick building outside the fort, for the commanding officer, has four rooms, with a basement and attic. To accommodate officers, three small frame cottages, each for two sets of quarters, have been erected. Two of these cottages (four sets of quarters) have two rooms and a small kitchen on the ground floor, with low attic above; the other cottage is smaller and without the kitchen.

The hospital, erected in 1863, is a frame building, 192 by 24 feet, and 16 feet high, with a small kitchen, connected with the main building by a covered porch. This building is badly arranged, and has never been finished. The ground on which it stands is fast crumbling away.

The water-supply is obtained from cisterns, and when these fail, in dry weather, by hauling from the river.

The post was evacuated in September, 1872, and turned over to the Engineer Department for repair and modification.

# WATERTOWN ARSENAL, MASSACHUSETTS.

The arsenal was established in 1816 at Watertown, Mass., about six miles west of Boston. The grounds, 100 acres in extent, are bounded on the south by the Charles River.

The quarters at the arsenal are, one set for commanding officer 64 by 46, with a wing 47 by 30, two and a half stories high, completed in 1866, (brick;) two sets of officers' quarters, two stories, each 30 by 40, with wing, (brick;) one set officers' quarters, two stories, 27 by 62, (brick;) one set officers' quarters, two stories, 43 by 33, (wood;) one barrack, two stories, 65 by 25, (brick;) two barracks, one story, 68 by 21, (brick;) one mess-hall, one story, 38 by 19, (brick;) and two wooden cottages for married men.

There is no hospital-building. The shops and storehouses are numerous and extensive.

Water is obtained from wells and cisterns, and in emergencies from the Charles River.

*Consolidated sick-report, Watertown Arsenal, Mass., 1870–'74.*

| Year | 1870-'71. | | 1871-'72. | | 1872-'73. | | 1873-'74. | |
|---|---|---|---|---|---|---|---|---|
| Mean strength { Officers / Enlisted men | 5 / 47 | | 4 / 29 | | 4 / 28 | | 4 / 32 | |
| Diseases. | Cases. | Deaths. | Cases. | Deaths. | Cases. | Deaths. | Cases. | Deaths. |
| GENERAL DISEASES, A. | | | | | | | | |
| Intermittent fever | 4 | | 1 | | 1 | | 1 | |
| Other diseases of this group | 7 | | | | 1 | | 2 | |
| GENERAL DISEASES, B. | | | | | | | | |
| Rheumatism | 7 | | 1 | | 9 | | | |
| Syphilis | 2 | | 1 | | 1 | | 1 | |
| Consumption | | 1 | | | | | | |
| Other diseases of this group | 1 | | | | 1 | | | |
| LOCAL DISEASES. | | | | | | | | |
| Catarrh and bronchitis | 5 | | 4 | | 1 | | 12 | |
| Pneumonia | 6 | | 2 | | | | 2 | |
| Diarrhœa and dysentery | 6 | | 1 | | 1 | | 1 | |
| Gonorrhœa | 3 | | 1 | | | | | |
| Other local diseases | 75 | | 40 | | 16 | | 21 | 1 |
| Alcoholism | 5 | | 2 | | 2 | | 3 | |
| Total disease | 121 | 1 | 53 | | 33 | | 43 | 1 |
| VIOLENT DISEASES AND DEATHS. | | | | | | | | |
| Accidents and injuries | 6 | | 7 | | 7 | | 5 | |
| Total violence | 6 | | 7 | | 7 | | 5 | |

# WATERVLIET ARSENAL, NEW YORK.

This is an arsenal of construction, established in 1814 at West Troy, N. Y.; latitude, 42° 44′ north; longitude 3° 23′ east. The reservation includes 106 acres. The officers' quarters are two stone buildings of two stories each, one for the commanding officer and the other for two subalterns and their families; one two-story brick building for one family, and quarters of unmarried officers. The men's quarters consist of one set of barracks of stone, two stories and basement, and brick cottages for married soldiers. These are sufficient to accommodate 100 men and 14 families.

The guard-house and hospital are two-story brick structures, the latter having a basement in addition.

The extremes of temperature observed in a number of years are 100° and —22°.

*Consolidated sick-reports, Watervliet Arsenal, N. Y., 1870–'74.*

| Year. | | 1870–'71. | | 1871–'72. | | 1872–'73. | | 1873–'74. | |
|---|---|---|---|---|---|---|---|---|---|
| Mean strength { Officers | | 6 | | 4 | | 4 | | 4 | |
| Enlisted men | | 48 | | 34 | | 35 | | 35 | |
| Diseases. | | Cases. | Deaths. | Cases. | Deaths. | Cases. | Deaths. | Cases. | Deaths. |
| GENERAL DISEASES, A. | | | | | | | | | |
| Typhoid fever | | | | | | | | | |
| Remittent fever | | | | 1 | | 2 | | | |
| Intermittent fever | | 5 | | 4 | | 1 | | | |
| Diphtheria | | | | 2 | | 2 | | 3 | |
| Other diseases of this group | | 13 | | 4 | | 3 | | 3 | 1 |
| GENERAL DISEASES, B. | | | | | | | | | |
| Rheumatism | | 10 | | 3 | | 1 | | 2 | |
| Syphilis | | | | 1 | | 1 | | | |
| LOCAL DISEASES. | | | | | | | | | |
| Catarrh and bronchitis | | 9 | | 2 | | 7 | | 6 | |
| Pneumonia | | 1 | | 1 | | 1 | | | |
| Diarrhœa and dysentery | | 14 | | 4 | | 10 | | 5 | |
| Gonorrhœa | | 1 | | | | | | | |
| Other local diseases | | 18 | | 15 | 1 | 19 | | 14 | |
| Alcoholism | | 1 | | 5 | | 2 | | | |
| Total disease | | 72 | | 42 | 1 | 49 | | 31 | |
| VIOLENT DISEASES AND DEATHS. | | | | | | | | | |
| Gunshot wounds | | | | 1 | | | | | |
| Other accidents and injuries | | 7 | | 4 | | 6 | | 3 | |
| Total violence | | 7 | | 5 | | 6 | | 3 | |

# FORT WAYNE, MICHIGAN.

## REPORTS OF SURGEONS B. J. D. IRWIN AND J. R. SMITH, UNITED STATES ARMY.

Fort Wayne is situated on the right bank of the Detroit River, 2½ miles from the city of Detroit. Latitude, 42° 23′ north; longitude, 5° 55′ west. Height above sea-level, 580 feet. The reservation lies parallel with and fronting the river, and contains about 63 acres. The country in the vicinity is level, and at many points marshy.

The fort is constructed of brick and stone with earth-works, with a square parade in the center containing 84,759 square yards.

The barracks are of stone, three and a half stories high, 186 feet long, and 36 feet 6 inches wide. The rear of the building has solidly-constructed balconies, 10 feet in depth on the second and third stories, extending the whole length of the structure.

The quarters were evidently designed and finished for the accommodation of a battalion of five small companies. The building is divided into five equal divisions, which are in turn subdivided into halls, dormitories, dining-rooms, &c. The halls are 33½ feet long, 6 feet wide, and 11½ feet high. Cast-iron stairways lead from the ground-floor to the several stories of each set of quarters. The facilities for heating the quarters consist of large open fireplaces in the dining-rooms and dormitories. Wood-stoves, placed in the center of the sleeping-apartments, are used in preference to fireplaces. The walls of the building on each floor are perforated with ventilators. The amount of cubic space allowed to each occupant of the sleeping-apartments is seldom in excess of 300 feet. The quarters are furnished with iron bedsteads. The dormitories connect with ablution-rooms and the balconies previously described. These quarters are good and well adapted for troops serving in this latitude, and are every way superior to the wooden or frame quarters at the post. The sinks are badly arranged and constructed, being nothing more than a temporary shed over an open trench, which latter is shifted as often as it becomes filled. The kitchens, store-rooms, and mess-rooms occupy the first floor of the barracks, which are divided into five equal sections, allowing one to a company.

On the grounds outside, and to the south of the fortifications, a number of wooden buildings have been erected. The officers' quarters, hospital, guard-house, quarters for the post band, non-commissioned officers, married soldiers, and laundresses; the storehouse, bakery, sutler's store, artillery stables, quartermaster's stables, ice-house, workshop, and corrals are irregularly scattered over the grounds, covering an area of some 300 yards from east to west, and 500 yards from north to south. Excepting the officers' quarters, the buildings are one-story frame structures, of a frail and very imperfect character, and appear to have been constructed with a view to meeting the temporary wants of the garrison until such time as casemate quarters and other buildings suitable for a permanent stronghold could be furnished. The quarters occupied by laundresses and married soldiers are well-constructed pavilion barracks, divided into twenty-four sets, which are excellent and ample for the wants of the command.

The officers' quarters are two-story frame cottages. The house for the commanding officer is unexceptionable, while the remainder of the officers' quarters are miserably constructed, badly arranged, and unsuitable, owing to a variety of defects. The rooms are all under the regulation size, varying from 10 feet to 14 feet square. The lighting is sufficient. The quarters are built to face the east and the river, to which they are parallel. There are three double buildings, with common entrances to halls which lead to four sets of quarters. Owing to the frail nature of the material used in their construction, and to the fact that the buildings are raised about two feet above the ground, they are cold and uncomfortable during the winter season. Their position is bad, and they are necessarily crowded, both as to location and in their subdivision into so many sets of quarters. The privies are inconveniently situated within a few feet of the dining-room doors. Bath-rooms have been constructed for the quarters on the lower floors, but, owing to the difficulty of obtaining a supply of water, they are seldom used for their legitimate purpose.

The artillery stables have been occupied temporarily as commissary and quartermaster's store-rooms since the battery was dismounted. They are properly fitted up for the purpose, and in good condition.

The guard-house is a strongly constructed frame building, 54 feet by 30 feet. It is divided into the guard-room, 30 feet by 26 feet by 12 feet, two prison-rooms, and seven small cells. The ventilation is by twelve windows and two doors and a chimney. The windows in the cells and prison-rooms are heavily barred with close iron gratings. The heating is afforded by one large No. 10 wood-stove, placed in the center of the guard-room. There are no stoves or fireplaces in the cells or prison-rooms.

The hospital is a wooden building of one story, with a detached building one and a half stories high. The ward contains 20 beds, with 1,133 cubic feet of space and $83\frac{1}{2}$ superficial feet to each.

The plan of the hospital is shown in Figure 14.

A, ward, 73 by 23 feet; B, bath-room; D, dispensary; E E, steward's quarters; L, lavatory; K, kitchen; M, mess-room; O, office; R, reading-room; S S, store-rooms. Height of ward, 13 feet 6 inches. It is heated by the necessary number of wood and coal stoves. On the west side and at right angles to the end of the pavilion are two buildings, each containing one and a half stories, constructed over brick cellars, 7 feet deep. They are 12 feet distant from the main structure, allowing the porch to extend, without interruption, around the main building, thereby affording a full and unimpeded circulation of air. The detachment on the north end is 24 feet by 16 feet, and is subdivided above and below into two compartments, which are set apart for and used as quarters by the hospital steward on duty at the post. Parallel with this, on the corresponding end, a new structure, 36 feet by 18 feet, has been erected, the main floor of which is divided equally into a spacious kitchen and dining-room. The upper or half story is intended for an extra ward, to be used in case of necessity.

The building has recently been painted and repaired, and is in good condition.

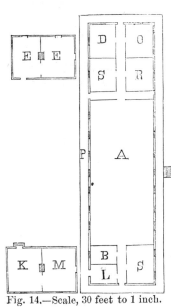

Fig. 14.—Scale, 30 feet to 1 inch.

The post bakery is a suitable frame building, 30 feet by 18, with brick ovens capable of baking for one thousand men. The building is divided into a capacious, well-ventilated work-room, store-room, and a sleeping-apartment for the baker.

There is no general laundry at the post, the washing of the command being done by the laundresses at their quarters.

The post chapel consists of a frame structure, 44 feet long by 24 feet wide, by 15 feet high, with a gabled roof, a vestry-room, 10 feet by 10, and a vestibule or entrance, 10 by 8 feet, which is carried up above the main building, forming a contracted steeple.

The stables consist of a strongly constructed frame building one and a half stories high, 250 feet long by 26 feet wide. One half thereof is subdivided into quartermasters' and commissary's store-rooms, and the remainder into stables for officers' private horses and those pertaining to the transportation of the post. It is built of heavy, rough plank, and is well ventilated.

The post library is a room 15 feet square, and adjoins and opens into the school-room. There are some 200 volumes of miscellaneous light reading. It is under the charge of the post treasurer, supervised by the post council.

The supply of water is furnished from the Detroit River; that for the use of the troops quartered within the fort is hauled in barrels from the dock, which extends into the river 75 or 100 yards.

The level nature of the ground in the vicinity causes the drainage to be defective in an extreme degree. A system of sewerage is connected with the interior of the fort, but it is frequently choked or disarranged. The sewer from the officers' quarters draining the privies empties into the river about 50 feet *above* the mouth of the pipe which carries water from the river for the use of those quartered outside the main work.

During the summer and autumn the men of the command are ordered to bathe daily, and are conducted to the river at dusk by the first sergeants of the companies. In winter there are no facilities afforded, nor is there any disposition on the part of the men to indulge in general ablution.

The cemetery is located near the extreme southwest angle of the reserve, and is surrounded by a neat picket-fence. The area inclosed is 150 by 75 feet.

Instead of a post garden the troops at this station cultivate company gardens. The amount cultivated consists of a piece of rich, loamy soil, measuring 1,100 by 140 feet. The hospital garden contains 250 feet by 100 feet. That set apart as an officers' garden has an area of 400 feet by 100 feet. They are cultivated by details from the command, and yield an abundance of almost all varieties of table vegetables.

The rations procured through the post commissary have been abundant, and are generally of good quality. Eggs, milk, butter, chickens, and all varieties of fruits and vegetables are abundant in the vicinity of the post.

The medical supplies are obtained from the purveying depot in New York City, and are received in good condition.

From the physical and geological peculiarities of the military reserve and the neighboring country, it will be readily inferred that fevers of a malarial type usually constitute a large proportion of the sickness prevalent among the troops at this station.

The great defect of the post in a hygienic point of view is the want of proper drainage and sewerage and of pure-water supply. This last might be remedied by connecting with the pipes of the Detroit water-works, and the cost of doing this would be well repaid by the improvement in the health and comfort of the garrison which it would produce.

*Meteorological reports, Fort Wayne, Mich., 1873–'74.*

| Month. | 1870–'71. | | | | 1871–'72. | | | | 1872–'73. | | | | 1873–'74. | | | |
|---|---|---|---|---|---|---|---|---|---|---|---|---|---|---|---|---|
| | Temperature. | | | Rain-fall in inches. | Temperature. | | | Rain-fall in inches. | Temperature. | | | Rain-fall in inches. | Temperature. | | | Rain-fall in inches. |
| | Mean. | Max. | Min. | | Mean. | Max. | Min. | | Mean. | Max. | Min. | | Mean. | Max. | Min. | |
| July.................... | ...... | ...... | ...... | ...... | ...... | ...... | ...... | ...... | ...... | ...... | ...... | ...... | 71.54 | 90 | 57 | 4.31 |
| August................. | ...... | ...... | ...... | ...... | ...... | ...... | ...... | ...... | ...... | ...... | ...... | ...... | 70.38 | 85 | 58 | 0.48 |
| September ........... | ...... | ...... | ...... | ...... | ...... | ...... | ...... | ...... | ...... | ...... | ...... | ...... | 59.76 | 85 | 37 | 2.29 |
| October .............. | ...... | ...... | ...... | ...... | ...... | ...... | ...... | ...... | ...... | ...... | ...... | ...... | 46.24 | 70 | 22 | 1.83 |
| November ........... | ...... | ...... | ...... | ...... | ...... | ...... | ...... | ...... | ...... | ...... | ...... | ...... | 31.37 | 49 | 9 | 1.52 |
| December ........... | ...... | ...... | ...... | ...... | ...... | ...... | ...... | ...... | ...... | ...... | ...... | ...... | 30.72 | 46 | 12 | 3.05 |
| January .............. | ...... | ...... | ...... | ...... | ...... | ...... | ...... | ...... | ...... | ...... | ...... | ...... | 27.84 | 53 | 4 | 3.54 |
| February ............. | ...... | ...... | ...... | ...... | ...... | ...... | ...... | ...... | ...... | ...... | ...... | ...... | 26.20 | 44 | 8 | 1.54 |
| March ................ | ...... | ...... | ...... | ...... | ...... | ...... | ...... | ...... | ...... | ...... | ...... | ...... | 33.74 | 61 | 14 | 1.04 |
| April ................. | ...... | ...... | ...... | ...... | ...... | ...... | ...... | ...... | ...... | ...... | ...... | ...... | 36.74 | 69 | 11 | 1.14 |
| May .................. | ...... | ...... | ...... | ...... | ...... | ...... | ...... | ...... | ...... | ...... | ...... | ...... | 58.90 | 88 | 34 | 1.83 |
| June .................. | ...... | ...... | ...... | ...... | ...... | ...... | ...... | ...... | ...... | ...... | ...... | ...... | 71.49 | 93 | 50 | 3.71 |
| For the year ........ | ...... | ...... | ...... | ...... | ...... | ...... | ...... | ...... | ...... | ...... | ...... | ...... | 47.08 | 93 | 4 | 26.28 |

*Consolidated sick-report, Fort Wayne, Mich., 1870–'74.*

| Year ........................................................................ | 1870–'71. | | 1871–'72. | | 1872–'73. | | 1873–'74. | |
|---|---|---|---|---|---|---|---|---|
| Mean strength ............... { Officers............ / Enlisted men...... | 12 / 178 | | 11 / 168 | | 11 / 173 | | 10 / 191 | |
| Diseases. | Cases. | Deaths. | Cases. | Deaths. | Cases. | Deaths. | Cases. | Deaths. |
| GENERAL DISEASES, A. | | | | | | | | |
| Typhoid fever ......................................... | 3 | ...... | 1 | ...... | 3 | 1 | 1 | ...... |
| Remittent fever ...................................... | ...... | ...... | 1 | ...... | ...... | ...... | 1 | ...... |
| Intermittent fever.................................... | 214 | ...... | 58 | ...... | 62 | ...... | 32 | ...... |
| Other diseases of this group........................ | 23 | ...... | 2 | ...... | 6 | ...... | ...... | 1 |
| GENERAL DISEASES, B. | | | | | | | | |
| Rheumatism........................................... | 18 | ...... | 4 | ...... | 10 | ...... | 6 | ...... |
| Syphilis............................................... | 15 | ...... | 5 | ...... | 6 | ...... | 2 | ...... |
| Other diseases of this group ....................... | ...... | ...... | 1 | ...... | ...... | ...... | ...... | ...... |
| LOCAL DISEASES. | | | | | | | | |
| Catarrh and bronchitis............................... | 16 | ...... | 3 | ...... | 3 | ...... | 13 | ...... |
| Pneumonia............................................ | ...... | ...... | 1 | ...... | 2 | ...... | 3 | ...... |
| Pleurisy............................................... | ...... | ...... | 1 | ...... | ...... | ...... | 1 | ...... |
| Diarrhœa and dysentery ............................. | 36 | ...... | 11 | ...... | 1 | ...... | 4 | ...... |
| Gonorrhœa............................................ | 9 | ...... | 1 | ...... | ...... | ...... | 1 | ...... |
| Other local diseases ................................. | 49 | ...... | 23 | ...... | 19 | ...... | 20 | 2 |
| Alcoholism............................................ | 10 | 1 | 15 | ...... | 12 | ...... | 2 | ...... |
| Unclassified........................................... | ...... | ...... | 1 | ...... | 1 | ...... | ...... | ...... |
| Total disease....................................... | 393 | 1 | 128 | ...... | 125 | 1 | 85 | 3 |
| VIOLENT DISEASES AND DEATHS. | | | | | | | | |
| Gunshot wounds ..................................... | ...... | ...... | 1 | 1 | ...... | 1 | 1 | ...... |
| Drowning ............................................. | ...... | 2 | ...... | ...... | ...... | 1 | ...... | ...... |
| Other accidents and injuries......................... | 39 | 2 | 16 | ...... | 11 | 1 | 13 | ...... |
| Total violence..................................... | 39 | 4 | 17 | 1 | 11 | 3 | 14 | ...... |

# UNITED STATES MILITARY ACADEMY, WEST POINT, NEW YORK.

## REPORT OF SURGEON B. J. D. IRWIN, UNITED STATES ARMY.

West Point is situated on the right bank of the Hudson River, fifty-one miles above New York City, in the midst of a range of the Alleghany Mountains known as the Highlands, latitude, 41° 23′ north; longitude, 3° 3′ east.

The river at this point takes two abrupt bends, and on the peninsula thus formed, containing about 100 acres, is located the National Military Academy, with its appurtenances. This is the only portion of the public lands (2,105 acres) now used for military purposes. The remainder consists of rugged cliffs and hills, rising precipitously to the west, which were occupied during the war of the Revolution by forts and redoubts. At the foot of these hills, and 157 feet above the river, is a level plateau, a large part of which serves as a parade-ground and plain for military evolutions, and on which are situated the cadets' barrack, mess-hall, and hospital, the academic buildings, administration offices, hotel, and residences of professors and officers.

The north side of the plateau, sloping quite steeply toward the river, and irregularly terraced, is occupied by soldiers' barracks and hospital, cottages of married soldiers, residences of employés, ordnance laboratory, gas-works, equipment-sheds and storehouses, sutler's store, school-house, and workshops. The riding-hall and stable are on the south side of the plain.

The geological formation is primary stratified rock—gneiss—covered with deposits of drift. The soil is gravelly, and, except on the plain, of little depth. The slope is sufficient to allow of easy and complete drainage to the river. Access of air is unobstructed.

Besides numerous unfailing springs and wells scattered about the post, water is supplied by three reservoirs, each having an independent source. Two of them are fed by mountain brooks, the other by springs at the bottom, and by rills from the mountain side. Pipes from these three reservoirs convey the water to a common tank or water-house, whence it is distributed, by a main seven inches in diameter at its exit, to nearly all parts of the post. This tank is 15 feet deep, and its bottom 62 feet above the level of the plain. The supply from this source is estimated at 60,000 gallons per diem.

Numerous hydrants are placed at convenient distances about the post for use in case of fire.

The cadets' barrack, mess-hall, and academic buildings are drained by a sewer, in height, 3 feet; width, 2 feet; fall, 1 foot in 40 for the first 150 feet, after which it is much greater. This sewer opens on the bank of the river nearly a hundred yards from the water's edge, and its contents are conveyed to the river through an open conduit of masonry, and discharged near the southern entrance of the tunnel through which the West Side Railway passes under the plain. The noxious gases from it are carried up the bank under certain conditions of the atmosphere, much to the disgust of the inhabitants on the crest of the hill.

The several sets of officers' quarters south of the cadets' mess-hall are now having drains made from them which connect with this main sewer. The new cadet hospital will have a separate sewer so as to avoid the evils that might arise from connection with the other sewers.

There is another sewer discharging into the river at the soldiers' hospital. Except during the winter months this is constantly supplied with water from the overflow of a spring in front of the hospital. This also has the defect of opening on the river bank, and of being unprovided with traps. With the exception of these two sewers, the means of getting rid of excrementitious and refuse matter are as follows:

1. *Close cesspits*, at some distance from the houses, into which excreta are conveyed through a pipe by water from the water-closets, and whence the soluble portions sink into the soil. The sides and tops of these cesspits are of masonry, the top being about three feet from the surface of the ground; the bottom of the chamber is simply the loose, gravelly soil. The pipe in its passage is bent so as to contain water, forming a valve to prevent the reflux of gases. But one of these cesspits has been opened for years; its condition is said to have been by no means offensive, only a few inches deep of soil remaining in the bottom of the vault. This arrangement prevails at the cadets' hospital and at the residences of some of the professors and officers.

2. *Open cesspits or vaults.* The hotel, band barracks, most of the quarters of officers and professors, and all the cottages of soldiers, are provided with these. There is one also at the encampment-ground of cadets. The pits are of varying size, and, when of sufficient depth and frequented but by few persons, seem not to be offensive. Excepting the ones at the hotel and camp-grounds, they are seldom or never cleaned. In some cases old ones have been filled up and new ones constructed. As the area over which they are scattered is very large, they are far from being the nuisance that they would be in a densely-populated village. At the same time it must be remembered that the soil is thin and underlaid by ledges, which serve to a great extent either as an impervious receptacle for this filth, or as a shed to convey it to the surface at a lower level.

## ACADEMIC BUILDINGS.

The observatory and library on the southeast corner of the plain was erected in 1841. It is a stone structure, 160 feet front and 78 feet in depth, castellated and corniced with red sandstone in the Elizabethan style. The east wing contains the library, 46 feet square and 31 feet high; it contains 25,000 volumes, besides unbound serials, maps, &c.

A new building was completed in 1870 for the administrative offices. It is fire-proof, with rooms for records, archives, and for offices of the superintendent, adjutant, quartermaster, and the treasurer of the academy. The building is constructed of hewn gneiss, (obtained in the vicinity,) trimmed with Kingston blue-stone, having arched floors and iron beams, with the party walls of brick. The location is on the south side of the chapel, and east of the academic building.

The chapel, a stone structure west of the library, 83 by 54 feet, was built in 1836.

The academy fronting east and situated directly west of the chapel was erected in 1838. It is a stone edifice, with red sandstone pilasters, 275 by 75 feet, and three stories high. This building is occupied by laboratories, lecture and recitation rooms, model rooms, and cabinets.

The ordnance and artillery laboratory, on the north side of the plain, was erected in 1840, and consists of three two-story stone buildings used for fabrication of ammunition, repairing, &c., all within a stone-inclosed yard, containing, besides, shelter for field batteries. Near the cavalry stables, on the east slope of the plain, stands the riding-hall, 218 by 78 feet, built of stone in 1855.

### THE RESIDENCES OF PROFESSORS AND OFFICERS

Are substantial and commodious structures, built, with few exceptions, of stone or brick, and provided, for the most part, with bathing-rooms and water-closets. Some of the officers occupy quarters in the west angle of the cadet barrack.

The hotel, built in 1829, is a stone building, stuccoed, 50 by 60 feet, and contains sixty-four rooms. A wing three stories, 62 by 29 feet, of brick, has since been added.

The cadets' barrack, on the south side of the plain, fronting north, was built in 1851. It is of stone, four stories high, with fire-proof rooms, castellated and corniced in the Elizabethan style of architecture. It is 360 by 60 feet, with a wing extending in rear of the west tower, 100 by 60 feet. It contains one hundred and seventy-six rooms, of which one hundred and thirty-six are cadets' quarters, arranged in eight divisions without interior communications. The basement contains bathing-rooms and quarters of employés.

The arrangement of the rooms is shown in Fig. 15: K, cadets' rooms; O, officers' rooms; A, partition between beds.

Each room is occupied by two cadets—is 22 by 14 by 9½ feet. It has a window 6½ by 3½ feet; a door 7⅙ by 3 feet, a glazed transom over the door; a transom 12 by 18 inches, provided with lattice and shutter, opening into the hall near the inner end of the room; a fireplace flue 9 by 30 inches, and a ventilating flue near the ceiling, with a circular aperture 7 inches in diameter. Two alcoves are formed by a wall projecting from the center of the rear end of the room.

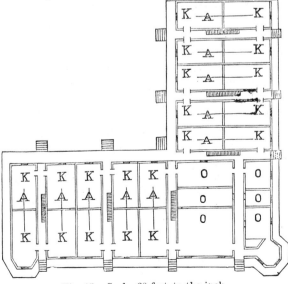

Fig. 15.—Scale, 60 feet to the inch.
12 M P

The dimensions of the room, 22 by 14 by 9½, give 2,926 cubic feet. Deduct chimney, furniture, occupants, &c., 186 cubic feet, and there remain 2,740 cubic feet, or 1,370 cubic feet of air to each occupant—an ample supply, provided its renewal is sufficiently accomplished. The means of ventilation mentioned above are adequate to effect this result.

Bathing facilities are extensive, but there are none for swimming. The privies and urinals are sufficiently commodious and well arranged; they discharge by a sewer into the river.

The engineer barrack, built in 1858, is a brick

building of two stories and a basement, 103 by 43 feet. It fronts north, having an eligible site, with free access of air, on an open terrace about 300 yards from the river. The basement contains the kitchen, dining-room, and store-rooms. The first floor has two sergeant's rooms, each 14 by 14 feet, and three squad-rooms, each 30 by 18 feet, and 12 feet high. Each squad-room is fitted up with double bunks in two tiers for twelve men, giving 530 cubic feet air-space to each. The ventilation is by doors and windows. For the general arrangement of the engineer barrack see Fig. 16.

     1. *Basement.*—B, bath-room; H, hall; K, kitchen; M, dining-room; S, store-rooms.
     2. *First floor.*—A, squad-rooms; C, sergeant's room; S, store-room; H, hall; O, officers' quarters.

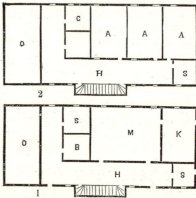

Fig. 16.—Scale, 50 feet to 1 inch.

The cavalry barrack, 57 by 41 feet, two stories high, of brick, with a stone basement, was erected in 1857. The artillery barrack, 46 by 30 feet, was built soon after, on a similar plan. The kitchens, mess-rooms, and store-rooms of both barracks are large and convenient.

The squad-rooms of the cavalry barrack have single bunks for 84 men, giving to each 371 cubic feet and $35\frac{1}{2}$ superficial feet of space.

The artillery barrack has single bunks for 58 men, giving to each 434 cubic feet and 39 superficial feet. The means of ventilation in both are doors and windows.

A commodious set of barracks for the military band was completed in 1873. The structure is of brick, two stories, with basement and attic, built on the site of the old band quarters. It is arranged so as to allow a room to each member of the band, and from two to four rooms to each of the non-commissioned officers and married men of the organization. The water-closets are outside the quarters, and are drained by a sewer that discharges into the river to the right of and a short distance from the front of the hospital for enlisted men.

Accommodations for some twenty-four laundresses, or married soldiers, have lately been added, which will have the effect of relieving the hitherto crowded quarters known as "Logtown." The buildings are two-story frame structures, with stone basements, and afford two rooms for each set of quarters, 12 by 14 by 9 feet; are well lighted and ventilated, and lathed and plastered inside. Five of them are situated on high ground, near the road leading north and west of the cemetery.

The other building is a two-story brick, with slate roof, situated near the engineer barracks, and is intended for the laundress of the engineer company.

A neat and substantial brick building, of two stories and basement, is in course of construction for the leader of the Academy band.

The hospital for cadets, built in 1830, 131 by 40 feet, is a stone building, fronting east and overlooking the river, of two stories and a basement. The two wings are used as quarters of medical officers. The central portion contains twelve rooms, two being used as quarters for the steward, two for dispensary, one as an office, and the remaining seven as wards for the sick. Two of the latter are 32 by $14\frac{1}{2}$ by 10 feet, one $28\frac{1}{2}$ by $14\frac{1}{2}$ by 10 feet, and the other five 16 by $14\frac{1}{2}$ by 10 feet. The two largest wards are partially divided by partition walls. For general arrangement of the hospital see Fig. 17.

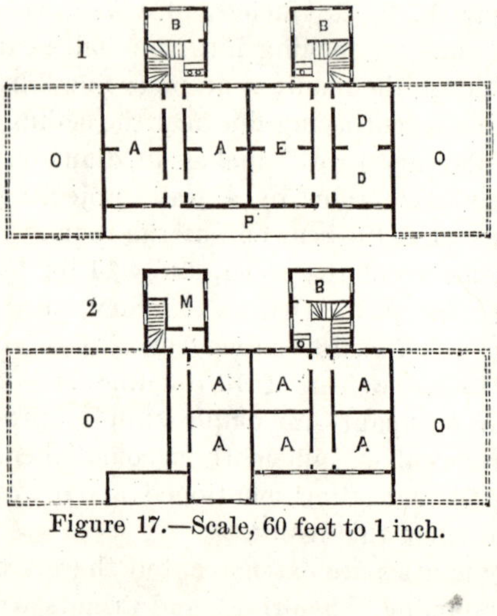

1 represents the first floor, 2 the second floor of the build-

Figure 17.—Scale, 60 feet to 1 inch.

ing; A, wards; B, bath-rooms; D, dispensary; E, steward's quarters; P, veranda; O, medical officers' quarters; M, dining-room.

A new hospital for cadets is now being built on a knoll between the old hospital and the mess-hall. The material is granite quarried on the Government lands, and it is to consist of a center building of three stories and two wings each two stories in height. The general arrangement is shown in Figures 18, 19, 20, and 21, which represent, respectively, the basement, ground floor, second story, and the third story of the main building.*

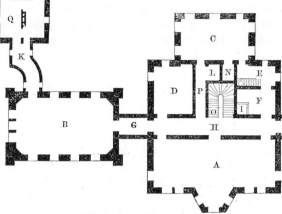

Figure 18.  (Basement.)

main building to ward building; H, hall (main building;) 

Fig. 18. A, examining room; B, cellar under the ward; C, store-room for kitchen supplies; D, boiler-room; E, back entrance and stairs; F, dark store-room and passage; G, passage from main building to ward building; H, hall (main building;) I, ventilating shaft; K, passage from ward-building to out-building, Q; L, lift; N, strong closet or dumb-waiter; O, main stair-case; P, passage; Q, foundation for out-building.

Fig. 19. A, reception hall; B, library; C, dispensary; D, store-room; E, back entrance and stairs and water-closet for surgeon; F, passage-way and closets; G, corridor; H, main hall; I, ventilating-shaft; K, passage between ward and out-building; L, lift; M, mess-room for servants; N, dumb-waiter; O, main stair-case; P, passage; Q, water-closet; R, lavatory; S, bath-room; W, ward.

The mess-room is divided by a partition, affording a dormitory for attendants.

Figure 19.  (Ground floor.)

Fig. 20. A, convalescents' parlor and reading-room; B, dormitory for matron; C, pantry; D, water-closet and urinal for attendants; E, back entry and stairs; F, linen-room; G, corridor; H, main hall; I, ventilating-shaft; L, lift; M, mess-room for patients; N, dumb-waiter; O, main stair-case; P, passage from front to rear; Q, water-closets; R, lavatory; S, bath-room.

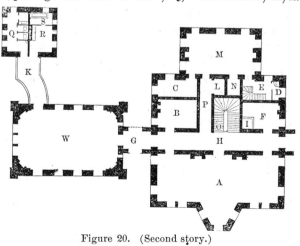

Figure 20.  (Second story.)

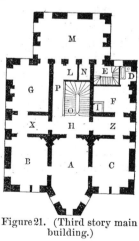

Figure 21. (Third story main building.)

---

* But one wing is at present being constructed, namely, the north; the diagram erroneously represents the south wing.

Fig. 21. A, room for sick officer; B, isolation ward; C, steward's room; D, bath-room; E, back stair-case; F, steward's room; G, laundry; H, hall; I, ventilating shaft; L, lift; M, kitchen; N, dumb-waiter; O, main stair-case; P, passage; X, attendant's room; Z, steward's room.

Each room in the building is provided with a separate air-chamber in the basement, to which the fresh air is admitted by a capacious duct, and where it is heated by a coil of steam-pipes. Flues one foot square conduct the heated air to the rooms, where it is admitted at the ceiling, provision being made to admit it also at the bottom of the room if desired.

The coils are calculated to heat 100 cubic feet of air per minute for each person from 0° to 70° F.; each coil is arranged in three equal sections, any one of which can be thrown out of use at any time to enable the heat to be readily moderated without reducing the quantity of fresh air admitted.

A foul-air duct, one foot square, leads from the bottom of each room down through the outer walls under the basement-floor to the ventilation-shaft. The latter extends from the ground up through the roof; it is 4 feet square, and about 60 feet high. To increase its draught the smoke-stack from the boiler-room is carried up through its axis. The smoke-stack is of iron. Provision is made for keeping a small fire in it during the summer when the steam-apparatus is not in use.

Fireplaces are constructed in the rooms for occasional use in the early or late summer, arrangements being made to shut off the ventilating-apparatus at such times, since the two will not work together.

### SOLDIERS' HOSPITAL.

This hospital, built in 1851, is of brick, 50 by 28 feet, having two stories and a basement. The height of the first story is 12 feet; of the second, 10½ feet; and of the basement, 9 feet. It is situated near the foot of a wooded hill, with a steep northern slope, the ground being as high as the eaves of the hospital at a distance of 100 feet, horizontally, in front. Air and sunshine have, consequently, an imperfect access to the southern or front windows, and the only other windows opening into the wards are on the north. These defects give it the twofold disadvantage of being very hot in summer and very cold in winter. There are accommodations for twelve patients. This allowance, with two additional beds in the wards for attendants, gives to each bed 982 cubic feet and 94 superficial feet of space. Doors, windows, and transoms (one over each door) furnish the only means of ventilation. Only one ward has a privy attached. The bathing-room is inconvenient, opening, as it does, from the dispensary.

The mode of heating is by coal-stoves. An abundance of water is supplied from the reservoir, except during the coldest weather, when, owing to freezing of the pipes, it has to be obtained from a spring in front of the hospital.

### GUARD-HOUSE.

This is a one-story brick building with stone basement. It has a guard-room and six cells for prisoners. Four of the six cells are in the basement, and have no facilities for heating, two of them being dark and badly ventilated. One end of the building is occupied by soldiers' families.

The quartermaster's stables occupy a commanding bluff looking north from the cavalry and artillery barracks, and fronting them, on the Hudson River, opposite Constitution Island. Its dimensions are 146½ by 39 feet, and three stories high. The basement is of stone, containing stalls for 50 animals. The second floor is of frame, for storage of wagons, &c., having, also, a grain-bin capable of holding 7,000 bushels of oats. On the third floor there is storage-room for 250 tons of hay.

The buildings are lighted by coal-gas manufactured at the station. A new building, tank, &c., has recently been completed, furnishing an abundance of illuminating gas at $2 per 1,000 feet.

*Meteorological report, United States Military Academy, West Point, N. Y., 1870–'74.*

| Month. | 1870–'71. | | | | 1871–'72. | | | | 1872–'73. | | | | 1873–'74. | | | |
|---|---|---|---|---|---|---|---|---|---|---|---|---|---|---|---|---|
| | Temperature. | | | Rain-fall in inches. | Temperature. | | | Rain-fall in inches. | Temperature. | | | Rain-fall in inches. | Temperature. | | | Rain-fall in inches. |
| | Mean. | Max. | Min. | | Mean. | Max. | Min. | | Mean. | Max. | Min. | | Mean. | Max. | Min. | |
| July | 78.95 | 98* | 59* | 2.53 | 73.62 | 89* | 58* | 8.55 | 77.32 | 96* | 62* | 1.10 | 74.73 | 97* | 56* | 2.46 |
| August | 77.97 | 93* | 60* | 2.95 | 75.42 | 91* | 50* | 6.60 | 77.93 | 98* | 56* | 4.57 | 70.79 | 87* | 54* | 5.11 |
| September | 70.39 | 88* | 52* | 2.40 | 63.31 | 89* | 36* | 1.03 | 68.14 | 99* | 48* | 2.78 | 63.75 | 88* | 38* | 3.52 |
| October | 58.39 | 80* | 34* | 3.52 | 58.90 | 87* | 33* | 4.96 | 52.30 | 70* | 30* | 2.18 | 52.20 | 71* | 30* | 5.75 |
| November | 47.06 | 64* | 29* | 1.11 | 40.64 | 68* | 9* | 4.40 | 39.32 | 58* | 11* | 4.73 | 33.79 | 54 | 14* | 2.77 |
| December | 35.69 | 55* | 6* | 2.00 | 27.23 | 60* | – 7* | 2.73 | 24.56 | 48* | – 3* | 2.89 | 32.12 | 61* | 12 | 5.00 |
| January | 28.71 | 60* | – 6* | 1.48 | 28.53 | 58* | 4* | 1.70 | 22.90 | 47* | –30* | 4.81 | 29.87 | 61* | 9 | ? |
| February | 29.40 | 83* | – 6* | 2.77 | 30.12 | 65* | 5* | 1.00 | 25.97 | 46* | – 6* | 4.60 | 26.31 | 48* | – 6 | 1.56 |
| March | 45.53 | 65* | 30* | 5.24 | 29.87 | 60* | 0* | 2.40 | 32.36 | 51* | – 6* | 2.79 | 35.41 | 64* | 10* | 1.68 |
| April | 54.40 | 82* | 31* | 3.97 | 52.23 | 89* | 28* | 1.70 | 45.48 | 64* | 33* | 3.82 | 39.54 | 75* | 18* | 6.49 |
| May | 63.79 | 92* | 42* | 3.85 | 65.06 | 92* | 41* | 2.41 | 57.74 | 85* | 29* | 3.46 | 59.79 | 93* | 32* | 2.15 |
| June | 70.78 | 90* | 56* | 7.36 | 73.16 | 92* | 53* | 3.18 | 70.14 | 93* | 45* | 0.76 | 71.51 | 99* | 48* | 2.17 |
| For the year | 55.09 | 98* | – 6* | 39.18 | 51.51 | 92* | – 7* | 40.66 | 49.48 | 99* | –30* | 38.49 | 49.15 | 99* | – 6 | ........ |

* These observations are made with self-registering thermometers. The mean is from the standard thermometer.

*Consolidated sick-report, United States Military Academy, West Point, N. Y., 1870–'74.*

| Year | 1870–'71. | | 1871–'72. | | 1872–'73. | | 1873–'74. | |
|---|---|---|---|---|---|---|---|---|
| Mean strength, officers and cadets | 259 | | 262 | | 262 | | 292 | |
| Diseases. | Cases. | Deaths. | Cases. | Deaths. | Cases. | Deaths. | Cases. | Deaths. |
| **GENERAL DISEASES, A.** | | | | | | | | |
| Typhoid fever | 23 | ...... | 2 | ...... | 176 | ...... | 127 | ...... |
| Intermittent fever | 50 | ...... | 74 | ...... | 64 | ...... | 71 | ...... |
| Other diseases of this group | | | 59 | | | | | |
| **GENERAL DISEASES, B.** | | | | | | | | |
| Rheumatism | 12 | ...... | 6 | ...... | 22 | ...... | 14 | ...... |
| Syphilis | 1 | | 1 | | 5 | | | |
| Consumption | | | 1 | 1 | | | 1 | |
| Other diseases of this group | | | | | | | | |
| **LOCAL DISEASES.** | | | | | | | | |
| Catarrh and bronchitis | 172 | ...... | 139 | ...... | 234 | ...... | 66 | ...... |
| Pneumonia | 80 | ...... | 39 | ...... | 144 | ...... | 1 | |
| Diarrhœa and dysentery | | | | | 8 | | 62 | |
| Hernia | 4 | ...... | 4 | ...... | 1 | | | |
| Gonorrhœa | 473 | 1 | 539 | 1 | 499 | ...... | 295 | ...... |
| Other local diseases | | | | | | | | |
| Total disease | 815 | 1 | 864 | 2 | 1,153 | ...... | 637 | ...... |
| **VIOLENT DISEASES AND DEATHS.** | | | | | | | | |
| Gunshot wounds | 1 | ...... | 3 | ...... | | | | |
| Other accidents and injuries | 229 | ...... | 236 | ...... | 252 | ...... | 77 | ...... |
| Drowning | | | | | 1 | | | |
| Total violence | 230 | ...... | 239 | 1 | 252 | ...... | 77 | ...... |

*Consolidated sick-report, United States Military Academy, West Point, N. Y., 1870–'74.*

| Year | 1870–'71. | | 1871–'72. | | 1872–'73. | | 1873–'74. | |
|---|---|---|---|---|---|---|---|---|
| Mean strength, enlisted men | 320 | | 302 | | 307 | | 281 | |
| Diseases. | Cases. | Deaths. | Cases. | Deaths. | Cases. | Deaths. | Cases. | Deaths. |
| **GENERAL DISEASES, A.** | | | | | | | | |
| Remittent fever | 18 | ...... | 62 | ...... | 64 | ...... | 1 | 1 |
| Intermittent fever | 25 | ...... | 17 | ...... | 21 | ...... | 50 | ...... |
| Other diseases of this group | | | | | | | 13 | |

*Consolidated sick-report, United States Military Academy, West Point, N. Y., 1870–'74—Continued.*

| Year | 1870–'71. | | 1871–'72. | | 1872–'73. | | 1873–'74. | |
|---|---|---|---|---|---|---|---|---|
| Mean strength, enlisted men | 320 | | 302 | | 307 | | 281 | |
| Diseases. | Cases. | Deaths. | Cases. | Deaths. | Cases. | Deaths. | Cases. | Deaths. |
| GENERAL DISEASES, B. | | | | | | | | |
| Rheumatism | 19 | ...... | 20 | ...... | 17 | ...... | 14 | ...... |
| Syphilis | ...... | ...... | ...... | ...... | 5 | ...... | 1 | ...... |
| Consumption | 5 | ...... | 2 | ...... | 4 | ...... | 2 | ...... |
| LOCAL DISEASES. | | | | | | | | |
| Catarrh and bronchitis | 140 | ...... | 83 | ...... | 42 | ...... | 25 | ...... |
| Pneumonia | 1 | 1 | 2 | ...... | | | 2 | ...... |
| Diarrhœa and dysentery | 109 | ...... | 52 | ...... | 62 | ...... | 45 | ...... |
| Hernia | 1 | ...... | 9 | ...... | 1 | ...... | 2 | ...... |
| Gonorrhœa | 3 | ...... | 6 | ...... | | | 1 | ...... |
| Other local diseases | 220 | ...... | 170 | ...... | 180 | 2 | 110 | ...... |
| Alcoholism | ...... | ...... | ...... | ...... | ...... | ...... | 1 | ...... |
| Total disease | 541 | 1 | 423 | ...... | 396 | 2 | 267 | 1 |
| VIOLENT DISEASES AND DEATHS. | | | | | | | | |
| Accidents and injuries | 97 | 1 | 94 | ...... | 139 | ...... | 67 | ...... |
| Total violence | 97 | 1 | 94 | ...... | 139 | ...... | 67 | ...... |

# FORT WHIPPLE, VIRGINIA.

### REPORT OF ACTING ASSISTANT SURGEON L. W. RITCHIE, UNITED STATES ARMY.

Fort Whipple is situated on the Arlington Heights, about one mile from Georgetown, D. C. The ground rises rapidly from the Potomac until it attains a height of 200 feet. It is one of the cordon of forts erected for the defense of Washington, and was considered the strongest. So completely, however, has it yielded to the encroachments of time that it is now difficult to find any vestige of its former embankments. It commands an admirable view of the Potomac River, of the cities of Washington and Georgetown, and the country to the south and east.

The garrison consists of 140 men, embracing Signal-Service detachment and sergeants of division of telegrams and reports for the benefit of commerce and agriculture.

The buildings at the post are nearly all of recent construction, and are so placed as to inclose the four sides of the parade-ground. The barrack is a building on the west side of the parade-ground, consisting of a central portion and two wings, the whole length being 250 feet, allowing an occupancy of 200 men, and a cubic capacity of 360 feet to each occupant. Fresh air is admitted by ridge ventilation, by doors and windows. Heat is supplied by coal-stoves, and light by windows and candles. The headquarters of the post are located in the instruction building, which contains twelve rooms, all occupied and used for the instruction of enlisted men previous to their being sent to stations for the observation and report of storms. The company kitchen and mess-hall, situated 175 feet north of the company barracks, are ample and commodious. The bakery has a capacity of 1,000 loaves per day. The quarters for married soldiers consist of two buildings, intended for the accommodation of eight families, and well adapted to their purpose. Two sets of officers' quarters recently built, are comfortable and well arranged. Two unmarried officers are compelled to occupy the old building, and have but limited accommodation. The guard-house, situated south of the company barracks, is well adapted to its purpose.

The hospital was erected in November, 1871, in accordance with plans contained in Circular No. 2, Surgeon-General's Office, July 27, 1871, being the regulation two-story hospital for 12 beds, and is sufficient for the requirements of the command. The grounds have been enlarged and cleared up, and trees planted at intervals. An acre of ground has been set apart for a hospital-garden, and when put in proper cultivation will yield sufficient vegetables for the use of the hospital during the summer and fall.

The post garden consists of 15 acres under cultivation.

The sinks are situated in a ravine northwest of, and 100 yards from, company barracks, and are sufficient for the requirements of the command.

Excellent water is obtained from a spring. The construction of a reservoir and of a steam force-pump and water-main is contemplated in order to secure an abundant supply, and diminish the labor now required to supply the garrison. Five cisterns are also in process of construction, with a capacity of 1,500 gallons each; two for the officers' quarters, two for the barracks, and one for the post stables.

An ice-house has been constructed at the post, but has not yet been filled.

The means of subduing fire are four fire-extinguishers, twelve hand force-pumps, improved pattern, and a good supply of rubber and water buckets.

*Consolidated sick-report, Fort Whipple, Va., 1870–'74.*

| Year | 1870–'71. | | 1871–'72. | | 1872–'73. | | 1873–'74. | |
|---|---|---|---|---|---|---|---|---|
| Mean strength { Officers / Enlisted men | 3 / 71* | | 5 / 88 | | 5 / 104 | | 5 / 143 | |
| Diseases. | Cases. | Deaths. | Cases. | Deaths. | Cases. | Deaths. | Cases. | Deaths. |
| GENERAL DISEASES, A. | | | | | | | | |
| Small-pox and varioloid | | | 1 | | | | | |
| Typhoid fever | 1 | | | | | | | |
| Typho-malarial fever | 1 | | | | | | 3 | |
| Remittent fever | 4 | | 3 | | | | 2 | |
| Intermittent fever | 95 | | 90 | | 38 | | 27 | |
| Other diseases of this group | 3 | | | | 9 | | 11 | |
| GENERAL DISEASES, B. | | | | | | | | |
| Rheumatism | | | 4 | | 5 | | 14 | |
| Syphilis | 3 | | 4 | | 5 | | 10 | |
| Consumption | | | | | | | 1 | 1 |
| Other diseases of this group | | | 1 | | 1 | | 1 | |
| LOCAL DISEASES. | | | | | | | | |
| Catarrh and bronchitis | 14 | | 12 | | 14 | | 20 | |
| Diarrhœa and dysentery | 23 | | 26 | | 40 | | 59 | |
| Gonorrhœa | 2 | | 2 | | 5 | | 1 | |
| Other local diseases | 29 | | 29 | | 45 | | 68 | |
| Alcoholism | 10 | | 3 | | 3 | | 7 | |
| Total disease | 185 | | 175 | | 165 | | 224 | 1 |
| VIOLENT DISEASES AND DEATHS. | | | | | | | | |
| Accidents and injuries | 11 | | 14 | | 10 | | 22 | |
| Total violence | 11 | | 14 | | 10 | | 22 | |

* Ten months only, September, 1870, first report.

---

# WILLET'S POINT, NEW YORK.

INFORMATION FURNISHED BY SURGEON C. C. BYRNE, AND ASSISTANT SURGEONS C. DEWITT, J. H. JANEWAY, AND C. B. BYRNE, UNITED STATES ARMY.

This point is a part of Long Island, situated on the south bank of the East River, seventeen miles from New York City, and opposite Fort Schuyler, in latitude 40° 48′ north; longitude 3° 16′ east. The construction of the works was commenced in September, 1862, an area of 136 acres being obtained by purchase.

In 1864 the Grant General Hospital was established on the point, consisting of thirty-seven wards, with a capacity of 1,410 beds. This hospital was in existence for one year. After the close of the war the post was made a depot for engineer stores and material, headquarters of battalion of engineers, and has since that time been garrisoned by three companies of the engineer battalion.

Willet's Point is an irregular, oval, undulating tract of land, the long axis running from the northwest to southeast, the highest point being the extreme northwest portion, which is 80 feet above low water. Communication with the mainland is made by a narrow strip of land on the southwest. On the north, northeast, and southeast it is bounded by Great and Little Bays; on the northwest by the East River and Little Bay, and on the south and southwest by a salt marsh and the narrow strip of land above referred to. The shores are washed by tide-water, the average rise of which is 8 feet; the spring tides overflow the salt marsh.

The quarters for enlisted men, erected in 1870, are comprised in one frame building, the walls being filled in with brick, upon foundations of stone or concrete, one story high, 180 feet long by 24 feet wide, with a rear projection 90 by 24 feet. The main floor is divided into three rooms, each 90 by 24 feet, and designed for one company. Beneath the rear projection is a basement of the same extent, and 9 feet high, containing carpenter, tailor, and shoemaker shops, lavatories and bath-rooms, vegetable, coal, and wood cellars.

The residence of the commanding officer is a two-story double house with finished attic and basement, the first floor containing four, and the second six rooms. Convenient out-buildings are attached, and in the rear there is a large garden; it is well finished and arranged, having all the modern improvements.

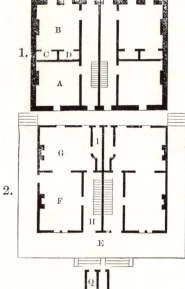

The quarters for married officers are two wooden buildings lined with brick, of two stories and basements, with finished attics, containing each two sets of quarters, as shown by Figure 22. 1, basement; 2, first story; 3, second story; A, cellar; B, kitchen; C and D, closets; E, veranda; F, parlor, 15 by 20 feet; G, dining-room, 18 feet 3 inches by 14 feet 10 inches; H, hall; I, pantry, with dumb-waiter in recess; K, chamber, 15 by 17 feet; L, chamber, 13 feet 9 inches by 14 feet 2 inches; M, bed-room, 8 feet by 9 feet 8 inches; N and O, closets; P, passage; Q, bath-room. Each room is heated separately, all are well lighted and ventilated; but some of the modern and desirable improvements could not be introduced for want of funds.

A separate building was erected in 1871, as quarters for unmarried officers. It is 35 feet 4 inches by 40 feet, its height being two stories and basement. The basement is of concrete, the remainder of the walls of wood. The height of basement and first and second stories is 7 feet 4 inches and 10 feet respectively. Each story contains four rooms, 15 by 17 feet, intended for two officers. There is also an attic for servants, 18 by 15 feet. Two sets of quarters for married officers were built in 1873. They form one building, 46 by 36⅓ feet, the first and second stories 10 feet in height, the basement and attic each 7½ feet. Of each set the basement contains a kitchen and cellar, each 15½ by 15 feet; the first floor, two rooms and one closet; the second floor, three rooms, two closets, and bath-room; the attic, three rooms, store-room, and two closets.

During the year 1873 four separate cottages were erected for the depot ordnance-sergeants and sergeant-major of battalion of engineers.

Figure 22.

The guard-house was erected in 1867. The basement is of granite, with thick concrete floor, divided into one large cell 30 by 18 feet, and 10 feet high, one light cell 8 by 9 feet, and one dark cell 5 by 9 feet, each of the latter being 10 feet high. The large cell is lighted by three long, narrow iron-barred windows, and ventilated by these and two air-shafts.   Each of the other cells has a similar ventilating-shaft.   The arrangement of the building is shown in Figure 23.

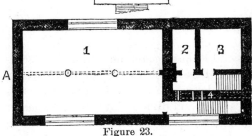

A, basement; 1, general prison; 2, dark cell; 3, light cell; 4, ventilating-box.

B, first floor; 1, non-commissioned officers' room; 2, guard-room; 3, trap to dungeons; 4, stove; 5, lights to dungeon.

The erection of a hospital was commenced in 1867, and in April, 1869, although not completed, the sick were moved into it.

The building is 75 feet 6 inches long by 31 feet 6 inches wide, and 50 feet high, surmounted by an oblong cupola, (arranged to increase the ventilation,) 26 feet long, 7 feet wide, and 5 feet 6 inches high from the top of the ridge.   The basement has walls of concrete 2 feet 3 inches thick and 8 feet 6 inches high, and is divided into six rooms.   The kitchen is 25 feet by 13 feet 5 inches, furnished with a large range capable of cooking full and special diet for at least one hundred

Figure 23.

men, with a good though narrow closet, a sink for washing dishes, &c., and a dumb-waiter leading to the first and second floors.   The mess-hall is 28 feet 10 inches by 13 feet 5 inches, well lighted by three large windows, and having a pantry, 13 feet 5 inches by 2 feet 9 inches, attached.   Two rooms are used as store-rooms, one is occupied by the cook and his assistant as a sleeping apartment, and another is to be fitted up as a library, museum, and reading-room for the convalescents and attendants of the hospital.

Outside the basement walls is an area of 8 feet wide laid in concrete 6 inches thick, with a gutter of the same material, from which on two sides and a part of the third of the building the ground slopes up at an angle of forty-five degrees to the level of the garden, and is well sodded. The gutter leads to an open drain on the southeast of the building, carrying off all the water that falls.   The walls of the rest of the building are of brick cased on the outside with boards; on the inside they are lathed, plastered, and hard-finished.   The first floor is approached by two sets of steps—one at the main entrance, and one at the office.

The plan of the upper floors of this hospital is shown in Figure 24.

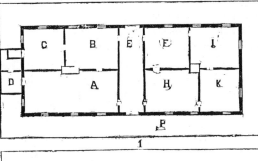

1. *First Floor.*—A, ward for isolation of contagious diseases, 74 by 30 feet; B, keeper's room, 17 feet 8 inches by 12 feet 8 inches; C, prison-room, 15 feet by 12 feet 8 inches; D, bath-room; E, hall; F, inspection-room, 14 feet 1 inch by 14 feet 2 inches; H, dispensary, 18 feet 6 inches by 14 feet 2 inches; I, steward's room, 18 feet 3 inches by 14 feet 2 inches; K, office, 14 feet 2 inches by 14 feet 3 inches; P, veranda.

2. *Second Floor.*—A, main ward, 74 feet by 30 feet; L, wardrobe; M, chimneys.

The height of the rooms on the first floor is 9 feet 8 inches; of the main ward on the second floor, 12 feet 6 inches.   The ward A, on the first floor, has floor and eave ventilation.

The windows and door of the prison-room are heavily ironed.   This room is used for sick prisoners undergoing sentence of court-martial, or for cases of delirium tremens.   It has a water-closet attached.

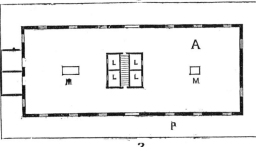

Figure 24.

The ventilation of the main ward on the second floor is excellent. There are eight openings at the floor, and the same number at the top of the walls, each being 3 feet 6 inches long by 6 inches high, and fitted with doors. In addition to this there is the ridge ventilation in connection with the cupola.

In a projection at the north end of the building is a tank holding sufficient water to supply the bath-rooms and water-closets.

In the center of the ward the stairway leading from the first floor is cased, and includes three small closets: one for the clothing of the patients entering the hospital, one for dressings, and one used as a dressing-room; and also the dumb-waiter for the kitchen.

At present only sixteen beds, of which six are usually occupied, are furnished in this ward, giving 1,734 cubic feet of air to each bed. On the two floors a piazza, 8 feet wide, extends around the three sides of the building and a part of the fourth.

The ground allotted to the hospital contains a little more than two and a half acres, of which about half an acre is inclosed by a picket-fence.

The ground in front and on the south side of the hospital is neatly laid out and cultivated as a vegetable and flower garden. Close to the rear fence, and 61 feet from the hospital, are placed the chicken-house, wood, coal, and cow house, each 12 feet long by 8 feet wide, and also a sink, used by the convalescents and attendants, 13 feet 6 inches long, and divided into two apartments.

A post bakery was erected during the summer of 1867. The ovens have a capacity of six hundred rations.

A large two-story frame building was erected in 1873 as post headquarters, containing offices, library, printing-office, clerks' rooms, &c.

The building formerly occupied as a hospital, having been remodeled, is used as a chapel and school-house.

The post library is large and well selected, containing 2,350 volumes, besides periodicals and newspapers. The men have a literary and dramatic club, a billiard-room containing two tables, a bowling-alley, and are allowed to use a part of the old mess-hall for dancing purposes.

The water-supply for the post is derived from sixteen wells, and a large cistern, (oval, 50 feet by 30 feet broad and 7 feet deep) receiving its supply of rain-water from the adjacent buildings. Thus far the supply has proved to be ample, and, with but one exception, has been found to be good.

The buildings of the post, being constructed of wood, are constantly liable to catch fire, especially in winter, when, to keep the majority of them warm, it is necessary to maintain large fires in the stoves. To provide against the same there is an organized fire-company, under the command of a sergeant, and provided with a large hand-fire-engine. In addition to the engine, six force-pumps of great power have been placed at different parts of the post.

The natural drainage of the post is very fine, as the land slopes in all directions toward the water. There is but little artificial drainage, the greater portion being superficial, and used to carry off water from the laundresses' quarters and barracks. One large sewer extends from the kitchen to tide-water; another, from the married officers' quarters and mess-hall to the swamp on the southeast part of the post, has recently been built, and is well adapted for the purpose.

Each company barrack is furnished with three iron bath-tubs; cold water is supplied from cisterns, and hot water from caldrons adjacent to the bath-rooms.

The burial place for the soldiers is situated near the salt marsh, southwest of the post, on ground slightly elevated, at good distance from any building; is 180 by 100 feet, and is inclosed by a neat fence.

There are two gardens at the post, the post and hospital. The post garden is located on the northwest half of the point, contains nine acres, and is under charge of a sergeant. The garden attached to the hospital contains about two and a half acres, and is under charge of the hospital steward. It is cultivated by the hospital attendants and convalescents. Its yield is very large, supplying an abundance of vegetables for summer and fall use.

The post stable is located on the southeastern shore, at some distance from the occupied barracks, is large, well built and ventilated, and excellently arranged for the health and comfort of its inmates; all the water that drains from or around it is led by superficial drains into the tide.

A number of chickens and one cow are kept for the use of the post hospital, which more than repay all outlay.

*Meteorological report, Willet's Point, N. Y., 1870–'74.*

| Month. | 1870–'71. Mean. | Max. | Min. | Rain-fall in inches. | 1871–'72. Mean. | Max. | Min. | Rain-fall in inches. | 1872–'73. Mean. | Max. | Min. | Rain-fall in inches. | 1873–'74. Mean. | Max. | Min. | Rain-fall in inches. |
|---|---|---|---|---|---|---|---|---|---|---|---|---|---|---|---|---|
| July | 75.57 | 94 | 58 | 2.49 | 71.42 | 88 | 60 | 5.58 | 76.76 | 99* | 60* | 6.28 | 73.94 | 91 | 56* | 2.62 |
| August | 75.31 | 92 | 58 | 3.37 | 73.42 | 90 | 65 | 7.16 | 74.84 | 98* | 52* | 8.68 | 71.95 | 91 | 55* | 5.66 |
| September | 68.47 | 95 | 54 | 1.48 | 61.32 | 88* | 41* | 1.74 | 65.88 | 95* | 45* | 3.62 | 69.94 | 88 | 43* | 2.22 |
| October | 58.15 | 80 | 37 | 4.52 | 58.52 | 76* | 33* | 4.00 | 53.03 | 77* | 34* | 1.80 | 54.51 | 74 | 30^ | 3.00 |
| November | 42.27 | 62 | 28 | 1.32 | 38.85 | 65* | 12* | 4.06 | 39.84 | 58* | 11* | 4.36 | 36.74 | 61 | 15* | 2.52 |
| December | 32.29 | 53 | 8 | 1.22 | 28.67 | 58* | 5* | 1.50 | 25.97 | 49* | — 3* | 2.54 | 32.87 | 61 | 6* | 5.42 |
| January | 26.70 | 50 | 5 | 1.68 | 28.34 | 49* | 4* | 2.98 | 25.26 | 48* | —15* | 4.08 | 28.70 | 49 | 2* | 1.66 |
| February | 27.12 | 47 | — 1* | 0.48 | 28.48 | 55* | 5* | 2.12 | 26.86 | 51* | — 7* | 2.20 | 36.32 | 63 | 11* | 1.88 |
| March | 32.77 | 60 | 26* | 2.66 | 28.99 | 60* | — 3* | 2.94 | 34.23 | 49 | 3* | 1.62 | 33.93 | 64 | 17* | 8.14 |
| April | 52.06 | 85 | 32* | 1.98 | 48.61 | 82* | 27* | 1.22 | 44.63 | 62 | 30* | 2.38 | 58.34 | 89 | 30* | 1.90 |
| May | 59.86 | 93 | 39* | 2.98 | 61.19 | 94* | 40* | 2.84 | 57.16 | 86 | 35* | 2.72 | | | | |
| June | 70.14 | 89 | 52 | 5.40 | 70.15 | 104* | 52* | 3.40 | 69.11 | 95 | 41* | 2.94 | 70.13 | 96 | 48* | 2.50 |
| For the year | 51.73 | 94 | — 1* | 29.58 | 49.83 | 104* | — 3* | 39.64 | 49.46 | 99* | —15* | 43.22 | 50.84 | 96 | 2* | 41.55 |

*These observations are made with self-regulating thermometers. The mean is from the standard thermometer.

*Consolidated sick-report, Willet's Point, N. Y., 1870–'74.*

| Year | 1870–'71. Cases. | Deaths. | 1871–'72. Cases. | Deaths. | 1872–'73. Cases. | Deaths. | 1873–'74. Cases. | Deaths. |
|---|---|---|---|---|---|---|---|---|
| Mean strength { Officers | 10 | | 11 | | 10 | | 12 | |
| Mean strength { Enlisted men | 271 | | 223 | | 220 | | 248 | |
| **GENERAL DISEASES, A.** | | | | | | | | |
| Small-pox and varioloid | 2 | 2 | | | | | | |
| Typho-malarial fever | | 1 | | | | | | |
| Remittent fever | | | 1 | | 3 | | 8 | |
| Intermittent fever | 214 | | 89 | | 56 | | 57 | |
| Other diseases of this group | 3 | | 9 | | 5 | | | |
| **GENERAL DISEASES, B.** | | | | | | | | |
| Rheumatism | 40 | | 16 | | 17 | | 18 | |
| Syphilis | 15 | | 21 | | 9 | | 9 | |
| Consumption | 1 | 1 | | | 2 | | 3 | 1 |
| Other diseases of this group | 1 | | | | | | | |
| **LOCAL DISEASES.** | | | | | | | | |
| Catarrh and bronchitis | 68 | | 21 | | 26 | | 14 | |
| Pneumonia | | | 6 | | | | 1 | |
| Diarrhœa and dysentery | 169 | 1 | 44 | | 26 | | 28 | |
| Gonorrhœa | 7 | | 10 | | 3 | | 8 | |
| Other local diseases | 143 | | 87 | | 91 | | 102 | |
| Alcoholism | 45 | | 38 | | 19 | | 35 | |
| Total disease | 708 | 5 | 342 | | 257 | | 283 | 1 |
| **VIOLENT DISEASES AND DEATHS.** | | | | | | | | |
| Gunshot wounds | | | | | | | 1 | 1 |
| Other accidents and injuries | 125 | 1 | 105 | | 83 | 1 | 62 | |
| Total violence | 125 | 1 | 105 | | 83 | 1 | 63 | 1 |

# FORT WINTHROP, MASSACHUSETTS.

This post was established as a military station in 1798, on the site of old Fort Warren on Governor's Island, Boston Harbor. It is in latitude 42° 21′ north; longitude, 6° 2′ 30″ east, two miles east of Boston City, and 760 yards from Fort Independence, from which it is separated by the main channel of entrance to Boston Harbor.

The tower, or citadel, is a new granite building, 100 feet square, 45 feet high, with casemate quarters inside.

The officers' quarters consist of two frame buildings, one 60 by 25 by 15 feet, having two kitchens; the other is 40 by 25 by 15 feet, with one kitchen adjoining. The men's quarters consist of one frame building, 95 by 25 by 18 feet. The laundress's quarters consist of a frame building 50 by 20 by 10 feet. There is no hospital.

Good water is supplied by four wells and a cistern. The post is in charge of an ordnance-sergeant.

## FORT WOLCOTT, RHODE ISLAND.

Fort Wolcott, established by the English before the revolutionary war, was rebuilt as an earthwork by the American Government in 1798–1800. It is located on Goat Island, in the center of Newport Harbor, a half mile west of the city, in latitude 41° 30' north; longitude, 5° 43' east.

The buildings at the post are unimportant, out of repair, and occupied only by an ordnance-sergeant.

## FORT WOOD, NEW YORK HARBOR.

### REPORT OF ACTING ASSISTANT SURGEON H. C. YARROW, UNITED STATES ARMY.

Bedloe's Island, upon which is situated Fort Wood, is a small island of about twelve acres in extent, situated in Upper New York Bay, about twenty statute miles from Sandy Hook, one and a half miles from Jersey City, and 2,950 yards from the Battery, New York City. (For history see Circular, No. 4, Surgeon-General's Office, December 5, 1870.)

Fort Wood is a star-shaped fort, built of Quincy granite. According to a stone which is inserted in one of the garrison buildings, the date of its commencement was the year 1814. The men's barracks within the quadrangle of the fort are sufficiently capacious to hold about two hundred men, allowing an air-space of about 600 cubic feet to each; and there are also comfortable accommodations for eight or ten officers. The barracks are two stories, built of brick, and their dimensions are as follows: Upper room, 53 feet long by 20 feet wide; lower room, 56 feet long by 20 feet wide. In addition to the men's quarters in the brick buildings spoken of above, there are the following rooms: Men's kitchen, 54 feet long by 18 feet wide; wash-room, 19 feet long by 18 feet wide; bake-house, 19 feet long by 15 feet wide; six rooms for officers' mess house and quarters of ordnance-sergeant, besides officers' quarters, guard-house, office, &c., making in all forty-four rooms.

The garrison is supplied with water by four large cisterns, holding in all about 400,000 gallons. These cisterns are filled with Croton water, brought over in the tanks of the quartermaster's steamers. Outside the garrison there are seven small cisterns, holding about 15,707 gallons, which are supplied in the same way as those within the garrison.

During the late war of the rebellion Bedloe's Island was chosen as a general hospital, and a number of temporary barracks of wood were erected. At present there are nine of these barracks or wards occupied as men's quarters, beside others used as storehouses, offices, ordnance store-rooms, laundress's quarters, &c. These buildings were constructed substantially of boards, but are now out of repair, difficult to warm and ventilate properly, and should be replaced by new ones.

The post hospital at Fort Wood, built in 1851–'52, consists of a three-story brick building, situated at the northwest extremity of Bedloe's Island, 50 feet long by 42 feet wide, and 60 feet high. Its front or principal entrance faces to the southeast. The building is placed directly upon the ground, has no basement or cellar beneath it, and the ground floor has been found by experience to be very damp. The ground floor is divided into the following rooms: To the right of the passage a small room, 19 feet long by 8 feet wide, used as an office; next, a small room, 18 feet long by 8 feet wide, used as a furnace, lamp, and porter's room; next, a small room, 7 feet long by 6 feet wide, in which the cook sleeps; and finally, the dining-room, 18½ feet long by 18 feet wide, communicating by a small passage with the kitchen, which is 17½ feet long by 8 feet wide. It will be plainly seen that space has not been economized in the arrangements of the first story, and it is a matter of regret that no better place exists for the keeping of the hospital food. The ceilings on the first floor are 8 feet high. On the second floor there are four wards, two on each side of the passage, and a bath-room and water-closet. The wards are 18 feet long by 18 feet wide, and are separated from each other by small doors. The arrangements of the third floor are even worse than that of the ground floor, as it is divided into no less than nine rooms, occupied as steward's room, bath-room and water-closet; tank-room, knapsack-room, linen-room, store-room, &c.

The supply of water for the hospital is from a cistern containing about 10,000 gallons. The water, which is from the Croton aqueduct, is brought to the island by means of water-boats. With the hospital cistern there is connected a powerful force-pump, worked by hand, and placed in the kitchen. This pump throws the water into a tank placed in the third story of the building. Constant care is taken to keep the cistern and tank clean and sweet, and where it is suspected that organic matter is present, permanganate of potassa is added sufficient to render innocuous any deleterious substances.

Of the water-closets in the building (two in number) too much cannot be said of their evil arrangements. They are connected, by means of pipes, with a cistern in the yard, which, it should be stated, is not more than 6 or 8 feet from the drinking-water cistern. The drain from the privy passes under the sea-wall upon the beach. The objection to this system of drainage is as follows: In case the drain between the foul-water cistern and the privy becomes choked up, it becomes necessary to remove the stone slabs which cover it and remove the cause of stoppage. If care be not taken to dig out the drain from the privy to the beach every day, the constant action of the tide fills up the passage-way. Last, though not least, the close proximity of the drinking-water cistern to the foul-water cistern must certainly be considered as dangerous to the well-being of the patients who use the water. Large quantities of various and approved disinfectants have been used to sweeten the foul-water cistern, but without effect, and the stench arising therefrom at times is intolerable. The only means by which it can be kept in any way approaching to cleanliness has been to force water from the bay into it, by means of a fire-engine, and allow it to rush through the drain, thus carrying off the accumulated filth.

The heating of the hospital building is accomplished by means of a large furnace and numerous grates, and the consumption of coal in winter averages 16,000 pounds monthly.

The ventilation of the hospital is bad.

The necessity of frequent bathing for the enlisted men at this post as a sanitary agent in promoting their health has been fully recognized. Each company quarters has a bath-room containing a portable bath-tub, and a stove and boiler for heating water, and the men bathe twice a week.

*Burials.*—In the event of the death of an enlisted man at this post, the Government undertaker is notified, and the body sent to New York City in charge of a guard of honor; thence it is removed to Cypress Hills Cemetery.

The bunks are the iron ones now generally in use, consisting of iron end-pieces connected by wooden slats.

*Consolidated sick-report, Fort Wood, N. Y., 1870-'74.*

| Year | | 1870-'71. | | 1871-'72. | | 1872-'73. | | 1873-'74. | |
|---|---|---|---|---|---|---|---|---|---|
| Mean strength | Officers.......... | 7 | | 7 | | 5 | | 5 | |
| | Enlisted men...... | 82 | | 99 | | 55 | | 47 | |
| Diseases. | | Cases. | Deaths. | Cases. | Deaths. | Cases. | Deaths. | Cases. | Deaths. |
| GENERAL DISEASES, A. | | | | | | | | | |
| Typhoid fever | | | | | | | | 1 | |
| Typo-malarial fever | | | | | | 1 | | | |
| Remittent fever | | 5 | | | | | | 2 | |
| Intermittent fever | | 9 | | 8 | | 5 | | 2 | |
| Diphtheria | | | | | | | | 2 | |
| Other diseases of this group | | 6 | | 26 | | 6 | | 3 | |

*Consolidated sick-report, Fort Wood, N. Y., 1870-'74—Continued.*

| Year | 1870–'71. | | 1871–'72. | | 1872–'73. | | 1873–'74. | |
|---|---|---|---|---|---|---|---|---|
| Mean strength { Officers............ \\ Enlisted men...... | 7 82 | | 7 99 | | 5 55 | | 5 47 | |
| Diseases. | Cases. | Deaths. | Cases. | Deaths. | Cases. | Deaths. | Cases. | Deaths. |
| GENERAL DISEASES, B. | | | | | | | | |
| Rheumatism.............. | 7 | ...... | 9 | ...... | 6 | ...... | 2 | ...... |
| Syphilis................. | 7 | ...... | 1 | ...... | 3 | ...... | 2 | ...... |
| Consumption............. | ...... | ...... | ...... | 1 | ...... | ...... | ...... | ...... |
| Other diseases of this group ...... | ...... | ...... | 1 | ...... | ...... | ...... | ...... | ...... |
| LOCAL DISEASES. | | | | | | | | |
| Catarrh and bronchitis............ | 11 | ...... | 6 | ...... | 2 | ...... | 4 | ...... |
| Pneumonia...................... | ...... | ...... | 1 | ...... | ...... | ...... | ...... | ...... |
| Diarrhœa and dysentery........... | 9 | ...... | 13 | ...... | 10 | ...... | 9 | ...... |
| Hernia.......................... | 1 | ...... | ...... | ...... | 3 | ...... | ...... | ...... |
| Gonorrhœa...................... | 4 | ...... | 6 | ...... | 2 | ...... | 1 | ...... |
| Other local diseases............. | 42 | 1 | 34 | 1 | 18 | ...... | 20 | ...... |
| Alcoholism..................... | 14 | ...... | 11 | ...... | 2 | ...... | 5 | ...... |
| Total disease............. | 115 | 1 | 116 | 2 | 58 | ...... | 53 | ...... |
| VIOLENT DISEASES AND DEATHS. | | | | | | | | |
| Gunshot wounds.............. | ...... | ...... | 2 | ...... | ...... | ...... | ...... | ...... |
| Other accidents and injuries......... | 26 | ...... | 20 | ...... | 11 | ...... | 14 | ...... |
| Total violence............. | 26 | ...... | 22 | ...... | 11 | ...... | 14 | ...... |

# FORT WOOL, VIRGINIA.

This fort is located on the Rip Raps in Hampton Roads, opposite Fort Monroe, in latitude 37° 2' north; longitude, 51' east. The construction of the work, under the name of Fort Calhoun, was commenced in 1818. The name was changed to Fort Wool March 18, 1862.

# MILITARY DIVISION OF THE SOUTH.

# DEPARTMENTS OF THE SOUTH AND OF THE GULF.

(Embracing the States of North Carolina, South Carolina, Georgia, Florida, Alabama, Kentucky, Tennessee, Louisiana Arkansas, and Mississippi.)

## POSTS.

| | | |
|---|---|---|
| Atlanta, Ga. | Jackson, Fort, and Fort Saint Philip, La. | Nashville, Tenn. |
| Augusta Arsenal, Ga. | | Newberry, S. C. |
| Barrancas, Fort, Fla. | Jefferson, Fort, Fla. | Newport Barracks, Ky. |
| Baton Rouge Barracks, La. | Johnston, Fort, N. C. | Pickens, Fort, Fla. |
| Battery Bienvenue, La. | Key West Barracks, Fla. | Pike, Fort, La. |
| Caswell, Fort, N. C. | Lancaster, Ky. | Pinckney, Castle, S. C. |
| Charleston, S. C. | Lebanon, Ky. | Pulaski, Fort, Ga. |
| Chattanooga, Tenn. | Little Rock, Ark. | Raleigh, N. C. |
| Clinch, Fort, Fla. | Livingston, Fort, La. | Savannah, Ga. |
| Columbia, S. C. | Macomb, Fort, La. | Saint Augustine, Fla. |
| Dupre's Tower, La. | Macon, Fort, N. C. | Saint Philip, Fort, (see Fort Jackson,) La. |
| Frankfort, Ky. | Marion, Fort, Fla. | |
| Gaines, Fort, Ala. | McRea, Fort, Fla. | Ship Island, Miss. |
| Humboldt, Tenn. | Mobile, Ala. | Sumter, Fort, S. C. |
| Huntsville, Ala. | Morgan, Fort, Ala. | Taylor, Fort, Fla. |
| Jackson, Miss. | Moultrie, Fort, S. C. | Yorkville, S. C. |
| Jackson Barracks, La. | Mount Vernon Barracks, Ala. | |

## NOTES ON THE DEPARTMENT OF THE SOUTH, BY SURGEON W. J. SLOAN, U. S. A., MEDICAL DIRECTOR.

The Department of the South was constituted in July, 1868, by the consolidation of the second and third military districts. In June, 1870, the Department of the Cumberland was discontinued, and the States of Kentucky, Tennessee, and Mississippi, of which it was composed in part, attached to the Department of the South. Further changes were made in November, 1871, by which the State of Mississippi was detached, together with the Gulf posts, not including those in Mobile Bay. The military posts then occupied were Fort Taylor, at Key West; Fort Jefferson, at Dry Tortugas; and Fort Barrancas, Pensacola Harbor.

As now constituted, the department includes the States of North Carolina, South Carolina, Georgia, Florida, Alabama, Tennessee, and Kentucky, with the exception of the Gulf posts above recited.

The military posts in the department may, very properly, be classified as permanent and temporary. The fortifications on the Atlantic sea-board, which were garrisoned for years previous to the war, have not all been re-occupied. No troops are quartered in the forts in Charleston Harbor, but occupy the citadel in that city. Fort Pulaski, at the mouth of the Savannah River, was evacuated on the 25th of October, 1873, and transferred to the Engineer Corps for repair, alteration, and reconstruction.

14 M P

Forts Macon and Johnston, N. C.; Oglethorpe Barracks, Ga.; Saint Augustine Barracks, Fla.; and Mount Vernon Barracks, Ala., are the only permanent forts or barracks now occupied by troops.

The temporary posts in the interior of the department, constituted after the war, during the reconstruction of the Southern States, are of a two-fold character, those which have been established for a long period, and those established for temporary purposes, from causes connected with the condition of civil affairs, and which are abandoned when there no longer exists any necessity for their continuance. The continued occupancy of many of the temporary posts is no doubt due to the fact that after the war, barracks were built by the Government on lands leased for a term of years, and in those sections of the country where the presence of troops was most important. These barracks furnished comparatively comfortable accommodations for the men at that time. Time and climate have caused rapid decay and dilapidation, and constant repairs are necessary to render them at all tenable. The posts of Columbia, S. C.; Raleigh, N. C.; Atlanta, Ga.; Chattanooga, Nashville, and Humboldt, Tenn.; Huntsville, Ala.; and Lebanon, Lancaster, and Frankfort, Ky., are of this character. From these points of concentration detachments are sent whenever demanded by the nature of the service.

The troops stationed at other temporary posts in the interior, and placed there on account of sudden emergencies of service, have generally been quartered in buildings hired for the purpose, and made habitable. Many posts of this character were scattered in that section of South Carolina denominated the Ku-Klux district, and were all abandoned some time since, except those at Yorkville and Newberry.

Recent events in the South, which are familiar to all, have changed the aspect of affairs, and a portion of the troops stationed at the various posts above described have been re-distributed throughout the States of North Carolina, South Carolina, Alabama, and Tennessee, to twenty-four localities, viz: Marion, N. C.; Unionville, Spartanburgh, Edgefield, Abbeville, Barnwell, Marion, Laurens, and Hamburgh, S. C.; Livingston, Eufaula, Carrolton, Butler, Demopolis, Mobile, Tuscaloosa, Eutaw, Greensborough, Tuskegee, Opelika, and Greenville, Ala.; and Somerville and Memphis, Tenn.

The whole number of troops in the department, distributed as above stated, is about two thousand one hundred and thirteen, and the headquarters at Louisville, Ky. The number of posts is forty-three, including one arsenal; and the number of medical officers, thirty-two; while eleven of the posts recently occupied for temporary purposes have not yet been supplied with medical attendance. The medical service is performed by four surgeons United States Army, (two of them now on sick-leave,) twelve assistant surgeons United States Army, twelve contract physicians, transferable, and six local physicians, who are permanently located in the vicinity and are under contract to give the necessary medical attendance and medicines, but are not transferable or subject to orders.

The contract system, though unsatisfactory in many respects, has given us many able, reliable medical officers, who, after having become fully acquainted with their duties, and trained by observation and experience, have given great satisfaction; have secured the confidence of those under their professional charge; have become attached to the service, and discharged their various duties with a conscientious regard for the public interest. These observations apply especially to those who have served continuously for a long period; a status, the natural result of faithful and efficient service, and "the survival of the fittest."

The employment of local physicians without contract will soon become a necessity, under the law of Congress limiting the number of contract physicians to seventy-five after January 1, 1875. The effect of this action cannot yet be estimated, but it is very certain that in the management of hospitals, the expenditure of medical and other supplies, and all the varied duties of the medical officer, efficiency and responsibility will be lessened. Looseness of administration will naturally follow the absence of binding terms and military accountability. The only guarantee for a perfect system of medical administration is the commission, and the duties and privileges entailed thereby.

The department, extending from the Ohio River to the Gulf of Mexico, possesses a varied climate. On the sea-board the fervid heat of summer is tempered by the breezes from the Atlantic. The posts in the uplands of North and South Carolina, as Raleigh, Columbia, &c., on the foot-hills of the Appalachian chain, as Atlanta on the spurs of the mountains, as Chattanooga and Huntsville, are comparatively free from the severer forms of malaria—hot in summer but pleasant and desirable in winter; while those in Middle Tennessee and the interior of Kentucky have a climate more assimilated to the true temperate zone. All the posts are convenient to railroads and very accessible. The comforts and necessaries of life are attainable; most of the inconveniences and drawbacks result from the dilapidated condition of the quarters and the want of genial society. In this latter respect there is a marked difference between this and other departments, which time alone will correct. At some of the posts gardens have been cultivated, and wherever this has been done successfully a greater degree of contentment has been the result. There is no better way of relieving the dullness and monotony of these small posts than this limited cultivation of the soil, which, while giving employment to mind and body, adds so much to the material comfort and health of the whole command.

The medical supplies for the hospitals in the department are received from the medical purveyors in New York and Saint Louis, Mo. They have always been of good quality, and ample for every emergency. Troops on detached service are supplied from the larger posts. The temporary posts are not so amply furnished with medical books, furniture, and miscellaneous property as those more permanently established.

The health of the troops has been satisfactory. Although liable to all the diseases peculiar to the climate, and the influence of malaria in all its protean forms, the command has not suffered to any unusual extent. It cannot be doubted, however, that long-continued service in this portion of our country is followed by more or less physical prostration and constitutional derangement.

The medical officers have been active in the enforcement of stringent hygienic measures for the prevention of disease; and commanding and other officers cheerfully carry out their recommendations in almost all cases. A livelier interest in this subject is manifested from year to year, and disinfectants have been purchased and judiciously expended so far as the limited appropriation of funds would admit.

It is much to be regretted that the military posts have scarcely any improved systems of latrines, sewerage, or means of ablution; and that from the want of such system, generally from deficiency in funds, we maintain the old-fashioned cess-pits, and have advanced but little beyond the ancient Jewish civilization. It is to be hoped that with the increasing interest in sanitary science, these matters will be as thoroughly considered and acted upon as their great importance demands.

Epidemic yellow fever has occasionally prevailed on the Atlantic and Gulf coasts. The spread of the disease among the troops at those posts exposed to it has been prevented by a prompt removal of the command a few miles to non-infected and healthy camps. This policy, adopted and stringently enforced, has been productive of the most salutary results, and entire immunity from attack. The appearance of the first case in Charleston, Mobile, or any other locality liable to the inroads of the pestilence, has always been promptly reported to department headquarters. The post commander in some instances had instructions to assume the responsibility of removing the garrison; or, if not, those instructions were transmitted without delay. This policy of removal and subsequent quarantine being enforced, the advent of the disease is not dreaded.

The same course was pursued during the prevalence of epidemic cholera in many of the Southern States during the summer of 1873, and in towns where our troops were in barracks. In those instances where the transfer of the command to a healthy camp in the vicinity was made immediately after the appearance of the disease in the city or town, and camp quarantine enforced, every one escaped. In other cases where the removal was not effected until after cases and deaths occurred in the command, one or two deaths resulted subsequent to the occupation of the new camp, and no more.

Without theorizing upon these subjects it has been fully demonstrated that this policy, in yellow fever and cholera, has been successful; and to it we are indebted for the comparative immunity of the troops in the department from their destructive ravages.

# ATLANTA, GEORGIA. (McPHERSON BARRACKS.)

### REPORT OF ASSISTANT SURGEON A. A. WOODHULL, UNITED STATES ARMY.

Atlanta, Ga., became a military post shortly after the close of the war, but the exact date of its occupation is now unknown.

The earliest retained post-return is that for March, 1866, and represents five companies of the Thirteenth Connecticut Volunteers.

The central and healthy location of Atlanta rendered it a desirable rendezvous for detachments doing duty in the department, and, owing to the presence of department headquarters in the town several years after the barracks were built, troops were kept in camp there, while the present post also was occupied. The buildings constituting McPherson Barracks were erected in 1867 and 1868. The first order now in the adjutant's office from the present post bears date of 31st May, 1868. The hospital was occupied 1st May of that year. The post is situated in the southwestern part of the city of Atlanta, the limits of the corporation passing through it. It is about 33° 54′ north and 7° 28′ west, and the flagstaff enters the ground at an elevation of 1,078.5 feet above the sea. It is said to be on the divide of the water-shed separating the waters which enter the Gulf of Mexico through the Chattahoochee, here distant eight miles, from those which find the Atlantic through Proctor's Creek, the South and Ocmulgee Rivers. The Blue Ridge terminates about fifty miles to the northeast, and bifurcating from it westward are Sweet's Mountain, the Allatoona Range, Great and Little Kenesaw and Lost Mountains.

Stone Mountain, an isolated peak of granite about eight hundred feet high, is sixteen miles southeast of Atlanta. The surrounding country is very rolling, affording good surface-drainage, and there are no swamps near. It has once been covered with pine, oak, chestnut, and gum trees, of which there is a large second growth, and is now imperfectly cultivated.

The post is between fifty-three and fifty-four acres in area, is ellipsoidal in outline, and irregular in surface, occupying two small knolls and an intervening ravine, is inclosed by a high board fence, and is distant from the center of the city one and a half miles.

The grounds are leased by the Government for a term of years. For the general arrangement of the post, see plate in Circular No. 4, page 145.

All the buildings, except the bakery and magazine, which are brick, are of pine lumber.

The company barracks are ten in number, built on the pavilion plan, elevated on brick piers from 2 to 15 feet, according to the slope of the ground, and each is surrounded by a veranda. The space between the verandas of adjacent buildings is 60 feet. Each pavilion is 158 by 27 by 13 feet, interior measurement.

Deducting four small rooms for offices and store-rooms, the barrack contains 47,736 cubic feet. At the date of the erection of these buildings, the strength allowed an infantry company was 119 enlisted men. This would give an air-space to each man of 401.14 cubic feet. With the present maximum strength of 60 men, if all were present, each would have about 795.6 feet, and in practice, counting out the absentees, the air-space to each soldier is about 918 cubic feet.

Ventilation is secured by thirty-two windows, both sashes being movable, four doors, and three openings in the ceiling, each 4 by 2 feet. These latter are closed by movable slats, like Venetian blinds, and communicate with as many hooded, louvered openings in the roof. They are warmed by wood-stoves, and are imperfectly lighted at night by candles and fixed oil. Each man has an iron bunk with wooden slats and a tick for straw. Over the head of his bed is a shelf, and a gun-rack fixed against the wall. The barracks are wainscoted for the height of 3 feet and 8 inches, and are well built. No wash or bath rooms are provided, but the barrack-floors are elevated sufficiently to allow of washing on long platforms or troughs underneath the buildings.

When the garrison is small some of the companies make use of vacant kitchens for bath-rooms, having the water constantly renewed in ordinary wash-tubs by fatigue details. When, as at present, the garrison is full, some of the companies have tents pitched on the rear veranda for bath-rooms. But in the plan of the post opportunities for bathing were not provided.

The company kitchens are five cruciform cottages, 60 feet in rear of the line of barracks. Each contains four rooms, a kitchen and a mess-room for two companies. There are ten buildings for laundresses' quarters, each 36 feet square, surrounded by a veranda, and divided into four rooms. These buildings are raised on piers in common with all that are inhabited at this station.

It will be observed that, although McPherson Barracks were built for a ten-company or regimental post, there is no provision for band-quarters or for quarters for the non-commissioned staff. At present, with eight companies, one barrack is divided between the band and the quartermaster's store-room, and the vacant one is being fitted up for a chapel, hop-room, and place for musical and other entertainments for the men.

There is a well in rear of each kitchen-building, and there is also one well to every two laundresses' buildings, between them and the rear. The company sinks are 50 feet in rear of the laundresses' quarters, and the only provision of this nature for the women and children is by one end of each sink being partitioned off for them. There appears to be no available remedy for this very objectionable condition.

The wood-yard, stables for ninety-two animals, granaries, and work-shops are still farther in rear of the laundresses' quarters. There is a well with a copious supply of water near the stable. The headquarters building is two stories high, with four rooms in each story. It has two wings, each 50 by 28 by 14 feet, used for store houses by the quartermaster and subsistence officers.

The bakery is of brick, 18 by 45 feet.

Thirty-three sets of officers' quarters are contained in nineteen frame buildings, each, excepting the commanding officer's, fifty-five by thirty-five and a half feet, a story and a half high, elevated on piers and having a veranda in front. The commanding officer's house is in the center of the southwesterly line, and contains four rooms to the floor, each 18 by 20 feet. The four houses to the right of this, on the same line, are designed for field-officers, and have three rooms to the story. These rooms are two on one side of the hall, each fifteen by eighteen feet, and one on the other side, eighteen by twenty-five and a half feet. Those on the second story are of corresponding superficies. They are twelve feet high down-stairs and eight feet above. The stairs ascend in rear of the large room, and are not in sight from the front door. The hall is six feet wide. The kitchen is a detached single room, sixteen feet square, and is connected with the house by an opened covered way, fourteen feet long. The company officers' quarters are arranged in double houses, as shown in the accompanying plan. Each set of quarters contains two rooms down-stairs and two up-stairs of the same size as the smaller ones in field officers' houses. The hall is wider and the stairway ascends from near the front door. The kitchens for the captains are single rooms, side by side, connected with the main houses, as already described. The lieutenants' quarters do not differ from the captains', except as to the kitchens. These are singularly arranged, and it is not at all clear what was the design of the constructing officer. The buildings that contain the lieutenants' quarters are arranged in sets of twos, requiring four subalterns to live near each other. Between the two houses and to the rear of them is a detached T-shaped house of two rooms. Tradition has it that the constructing quartermaster (who was a field-officer in rank) designed the rear room for a kitchen and the front room for messing-purposes, expecting the four officers concerned to provide a common table. This may be an error, but there is no more reasonable hypothesis on which to account for their disposition. They are entirely unconnected with the main houses. None of the quarters have any rooms especially designed for servants. Every room, including the kitchens, has four windows and a fire-place for burning wood. There are no shutters to the windows, except when occasionally provided by private means. There are no gutters to conduct the rain-water, which, in wet seasons, falls in considerable quantities from the eaves, except along the commanding officer's veranda. There are no cellars. All of the sets of quarters are not identical in the minor details of internal arrangement, but in the most of them the two similar rooms communicate by single doors, and there is a large closet in the wall in nearly every room.

It has never been permitted to paint the exterior of any building at the station, and as a consequence their weather-beaten aspect is gloomy and desolate in the extreme. As a further and more important consequence the officers' quarters under heavy rains leaked badly, defacing the walls and in some cases damaging the furniture, as well as making residence very unpleasant. In the autumn of 1873 the quartermaster was authorized to make certain repairs, and the worst leaks were accordingly patched over. The quarters are not yet entirely sound, however, and severe rains demand vigilance from the occupants in order to avoid injury to their personal property. The doors and windows have shrunk considerably, or were originally ill-fitting, and admit much cold air during the severe weather that occasionally occurs in the winter. The officers' quarters are very scantily supplied with plain tables and fire-place furniture. There are enough heating-stoves to give one or two to a house. The most of the officers are obliged to supply their own cooking-stoves. An application made to the chief-quartermaster for enough for all the officers' families, in the fall of 1873, was rejected on the ground that as the kitchens had fire-places, cooking-stoves could not be allowed. The front yards are neatly sodded, and a picket-fence separates them from the road. The back yards are large, but on the easterly side are not arranged so as to give a separate one to each subaltern. In like manner some of the privies, which are about fifty yards in the rear, are on that row common to two families.

The guard-house is elevated on piers, and consists of a main building, 33 by 46 feet, one story high, and a wing, 44 by 8 feet 5 inches. The main portion contains two rooms, 20 feet 5 inches by 14 by 10 feet 7 inches, and 12 feet 5 inches by 14 by 10 feet 7 inches, for the guard; a jail-room, 17 by 32 feet by 10 feet 7 inches, and five cells, each 6 feet 5 inches by 10 by 10 feet 7 inches. The jail-room has a cubic air-space of 5,757 feet, and each cell of 679 feet. The wing is divided into ten cells, 4 by 8 feet 5 inches by 9 feet 3 inches, having a cubic air-space of 303 feet each. Ventilation is effected by six grated windows in the jail-room, and by one in each of the cells 2 by 2 feet 3 inches. In the cells of the wing the doors contain in addition a grated aperture 3 by 6 inches. A sink is attached by an inclosed covered-way. The guard-room is warmed by a stove, but there is no provision for heating the prisoners' apartments.

The hospital consists of a main building 36 feet square, with two lateral wings forward and an L in rear for kitchen. It is elevated on piers, and, except the kitchen, is surrounded by a broad veranda. The main building contains on the first floor three rooms, each 14 feet square, (including a chimney in each,) used as office, dispensary, and store-room for medicines, and a fourth room, 14 by 20 feet, used as a mess-room. This last must be traversed to reach the kitchen, which opens into it. A strong closet for liquors has been built under the stairway. The second story of the main building is divided into five rooms, two, each 14 feet square, in front, and three, 11 by 14 feet, behind. The front rooms are used as sleeping apartments for attendants, and the rear rooms for storing hospital property. These last are insufficient, and are not well adapted for the purpose. Some additional shelving has been put up within the past six months, and a rack for mattresses has been erected in the upper hall. The two wards are each 65 feet 6 inches by 24 by 14 feet 6 inches internal measurement. There are also two rooms at the outer extremity of each ward, each 11 feet 3 inches by 8 feet 6 inches, used for general purposes of convenience. Allowing 24 beds, there would be 949.3 cubic feet to each, or 18 beds would have 1,266 cubic feet to each. At present but one ward is used, and but 20 beds are set up. (As two stewards are on duty at the hospital, the nurses and cook are obliged to sleep in the ward, leaving but 15 beds for patients.) As it is very seldom that all are occupied, each inmate has in practice a much greater air-space. The wards have ridge ventilation, reached by eight slatted openings each 4 by 2 feet, operated like Venetian blinds in each ceiling. There are two similar openings in the hall between the adjacent small rooms. There is but one chimney-shaft to each ward. Heretofore the wards have been heated by a stove at each end, the pipes being carried to the center shaft. An improved ventilating double fire-place was set up in the autumn of 1873, and up to the date of writing this report (late in January,) it heated the ward fairly, and ventilated it excellently. The chief difficulty was from its occasionally smoking, under certain atmospheric conditions. Each ward has twelve windows, six on a side, 3 by 6 feet 5 inches each, and four doors, two of which are half glass. The hospital kitchen is reached from the interior of the building through a door in the mess-room, and from the exterior through a door from the veranda, each opening close to each other. The kitchen is small, 14 by 12 feet, with a closet 6 by 8 feet, which is the only place for keeping rations and utensils. There is a fire-place in the kitchen, but the cooking is done upon a range of the "Union" pattern, set up in a room. There is, and can be, no cellar. It has not been necessary to use more than one ward at a time for the sick, and the other, therefore, has been used as a place for storing the more bulky articles.

The sick are transferred from one ward to another, according to the season. The well is near and just north of the kitchen. The hospital grounds are inclosed by a neat picket fence, and include a garden of nearly an acre in extent. The privy is about forty yards in rear of the building. It has no vault, but is provided with drawers, which are emptied nightly, and are disinfected with dry earth. An earth-closet and close-stools are kept in one of the small rooms adjoining the ward. A bath-tub is kept in another adjacent small room, which is also provided with basins for washing. There is a one-roomed frame dead-house, 15 by 14 feet, with a chimney and fire-place near and behind the easterly part of the hospital.

The privies throughout the garrison are situated as already described, and the most of them are provided with sliding boxes that are taken out nightly and the contents removed by a scaven- ger to pits about three-quarters of a mile distant. They are deodorized by fresh earth, and are kept in very good condition. A few of the officers' privies have shallow brick vaults, which are frequently cleaned out and deodorized like the others.

There are twenty-six wells located as already detailed. These average nearly thirty feet in depth and four and a third feet in diameter. The water they furnish is soft and desirable for drinking and washing purposes, but the supply has not been very abundant. In December, 1873, they were cleaned out and the most of them deepened, to their great improvement. There are two large underground cisterns in the parade, with a capacity of 45,000 and 90,000 gallons respectively. They are supplied by the rain-fall from the roofs of some of the buildings. They may also be filled by forcing water with the post steam fire-engine, and its attached 2,000 feet of hose, from a small creek several hundred yards away. There are also several portable fire-extinguishers of the "American" pattern. There is an abundance of fire-ladders, each building being supplied with several, and all the public buildings have a number of fire-buckets kept constantly filled. But, curiously, there is no building that has any scuttle or trap in the roof. As the lumber is pine, saturated with turpentine, and as the walls are not filled in between the inner plastering and the weather-boarding, an accidental fire that gained any headway would almost surely result in at least the destruction of the building where it originated.

The post library, containing several hundred volumes of good general reading, is kept in the headquarters building. A school for children, taught by an enlisted man, is held in one of the vacant quarters.

There is no sewerage and no artificial drainage, except the pipes conveying the water to the cisterns, as already mentioned, and shallow brick gutters around the hospital and barracks. Nor is any needed for general purposes, the natural slope of the ground conveying the surplus water beyond the post. Gutters to the eaves of the officers' houses would, however, prevent occasional dampness under these houses, which now occurs.

A post garden has once or twice been cultivated by details on ground outside of the post. None has been kept up for a year or two, however, the men being supplied with vegetables by purchase from the company funds. Small gardens are cultivated by some officers in their back yards. The neighboring citizens expend very little intelligent labor on their gardens, and but few of the finer vegetables are brought into market.

A line of street cars makes access to the business part of Atlanta from the barracks very easy.

Staple dry-goods and furniture in fair variety may be purchased in the town at prices more reasonable than in most southern cities, and at such rates that it is cheaper to buy here than to purchase new articles elsewhere and transport them here. The markets are not very good, the most of the supplies coming from Tennessee. Fish, oysters, oranges, and lemons are plentiful in season from the South.   The best cuts of beef sell for fifteen cents, dressed poultry from 12½ to 20 cents a pound, eggs from 20 to 35 cents a dozen.   Good vegetables are scarce and comparatively high.   Manufactured ice of good quality is retailed at a cent and a half a pound.   The town of Atlanta, whose population approaches 30,000, is considered healthy, although sickness among young children in the hot weather is said to be excessive.

The locality is said to be an unfortunate one for persons with the rheumatic diathesis.   The post is certainly a healthy one for the latitude, and appears to have no local causes of disease. Most of the troops in garrison have been stationed elsewhere in miasmatic districts, and they show occasionally the effect of previous malarial influence, but serious sickness is rare.   During 1873 there was from disease but one death among the families at the post—a young child of a newly-arrived soldier.   In the same period among the men there were four deaths from disease, viz, one each from consumption following typhoid fever, debility and general paralysis of old age, Bright's disease, and consumption.   The prevalent complaints are mild malarial fevers, intestinal and venereal diseases.

Several springs in this vicinity contain iron in sufficient quantity to render their waters available for medicinal purposes.  Chief among these is the "Atlanta Mineral Spring," situated near the Macon and Western Railroad Depot, in the city of Atlanta.

The iron of this water is said to be in the form of a carbonate of the protoxide, by Prof. A. Means, of the Atlanta Medical College, whose complete analysis, based upon one gallon imperial measure, is appended:

Specific gravity, (distilled water being 1)............................ 1.0005
Temperature................................................................ 66° F.
Quantity per hour.......................................................... 32⅓ gallons.

### GASEOUS CONTENTS.

Carbonic acid ............................................................. 9.96 cubic inches.
Hydrosulphuric acid ...................................................... 2.33 cubic inches.
Atmospheric air...............................................about      1½ per cent.

### SOLID CONTENTS.

Iron as a protocarbonate, suspended in carbonic-acid gas .......... 13.34 grains.
Sulphate of magnesia................................................... 11.84 grains.
Carbonate of magnesia ................................................ 4.15 grains.
Magnesia as base in both.............................................. 6.01 grains.
Sulphate of soda ...................................................... 8.82 grains.
Chloride of sodium .................................................... 16.06 grains.
Lime .................................................................. a trace.
Silica.................................................................not estimated.
Entire solid contents................................................. 55.11 grains.

This analysis was made some years ago.   The quantity yielded per hour in 1870 was from sixty to seventy gallons.

There is another spring, situated in the suburb called West End, and known as the West End Mineral Spring, which has a considerable local reputation.

The following analysis, bearing date of April 24, 1873, was made by Mr. W. J. Land, a chemist of Atlanta:

### ONE UNITED STATES STANDARD GALLON.

Sulphureted-hydrogen gas ............................................. 0.1720 grains.
Protocarbonate of iron ............................................... 2.0350 grains.
Sesquicarbonate of iron............................................... .3520 grains.
Protocarbonate of manganese.......................................... .0050 grains.
Carbonate of magnesia................................................ .0520 grains.
Carbonate of lime..................................................... .2130 grains.
Sulphate of lime ..................................................... .3020 grains.
Chloride of calcium .................................................. .1190 grains.

Chloride of sodium . . . . . . . . . . . . . . . . . . . . . . . . . . . . . . . . . . . . . . . . . . . . . . . . . . . . . . . . . . .   .1310 grains.
Silicates of soda and lime . . . . . . . . . . . . . . . . . . . . . . . . . . . . . . . . . . . . . . . . . . . . . . . . . .   .4300 grains·
Crenic and apocrenic acids . . . . . . . . . . . . . . . . . . . . . . . . . . . . . . . . . . . . . . . . . . . . . . . . .   .0180 grains.
Free carbonic acid . . . . . . . . . . . . . . . . . . . . . . . . . . . . . . . . . . . . . . . . . . . . . . . . . . . . . . . . . .   1.0370 grains.

      Total . . . . . . . . . . . . . . . . . . . . . . . . . . . . . . . . . . . . . . . . . . . . . . . . . . . . . . . . . . . . . . . . . . .   4.8660 grains.
      Total solid matter, dried at 212° F., = . . . . . . . . . . . . . . . . . . . . . . . . . . . . . . . . . . . . . .   3.5324 grains.

The flow of this spring is more copious at some seasons than at others.

There is another spring in Atlanta, styled Ponce de Leon, of the same general character.

### Meteorological report, McPherson Barracks, Atlanta, Ga., 1870–'74.

| Month. | 1870–'71. Temperature. | | | 1870–'71. Rain-fall in inches. | 1871–'72. Temperature. | | | 1871–'72. Rain-fall in inches. | 1872–'73. Temperature. | | | 1872–'73. Rain-fall in inches. | 1873–'74. Temperature. | | | 1873–'74. Rain-fall in inches. |
|---|---|---|---|---|---|---|---|---|---|---|---|---|---|---|---|---|
| | Mean. | Max. | Min. | | Mean. | Max. | Min. | | Mean. | Max. | Min. | | Mean. | Max. | Min. | |
| | ° | ° | ° | | ° | ° | ° | | ° | ° | ° | | ° | ° | ° | |
| July | 81.44 | 94 | 73 | 2.25 | 79.93 | 93 | 65 | 1.12 | 80.56 | 96* | 69* | 3.91 | 79.64 | 93* | 65* | 3.87 |
| August | 80.84 | 94 | 72 | 4.69 | 80.87 | 96 | 68 | 6.49 | 80.13 | 95* | 61* | 5.84 | 78.20 | 97* | 56* | 2.08 |
| September | 74.14 | 91 | 64 | 9.40 | 71.34 | 89 | 46 | 4.44 | 75.21 | 96* | 54* | 2.26 | 72.44 | 96* | 52* | 5.40 |
| October | 67.06 | 91 | 41 | 0.67 | 66.34 | 92* | 31* | 2.09 | 64.79 | 88* | 42* | 0.74 | 59.85 | 86* | 21* | 1.23 |
| November | 53.86 | 81 | 30 | 5.42 | 56.33 | 80* | 25* | 3.41 | 50.35 | 74* | 10* | 2.12 | 49.71 | 75* | 10* | 3.15 |
| December | 43.08 | 78 | 7 | 3.74 | 44.48 | 71* | 6* | 3.36 | 42.82 | 77* | 10* | 4.48 | 45.12 | 73* | 15* | 2.41 |
| January | 48.06 | 72 | 24 | 2.03 | 39.53 | 63* | 8* | 2.94 | 42.77 | 71* | 3* | 3.36 | 45.24 | 69* | 12* | 3.14 |
| February | 50.91 | 70 | 32 | 6.20 | 46.51 | 70* | 15* | 5.28 | 49.44 | 75* | 15* | 12.04 | 46.63 | 74* | 22* | 6.86 |
| March | 57.67 | 79 | 37 | 6.01 | 49.83 | 76* | 23* | 7.66 | 50.83 | 77* | 12* | 2.58 | 53.97 | 78* | 27* | 7.38 |
| April | 65.18 | 84 | 39 | 5.20 | 64.69 | 89* | 33* | 3.09 | 62.42 | 89* | 36* | 1.96 | 59.20 | 79* | 34* | 10.42 |
| May | 68.39 | 86 | 44 | 7.77 | 72.43 | 90* | 44* | 3.75 | 70.87 | 89* | 47* | 6.05 | 71.24 | 94* | 46* | 3.00 |
| June | 78.52 | 92 | 67 | 5.97 | 77.82 | 92* | 60* | 1.82 | 76.17 | 90* | 63* | 7.06 | 78.19 | 95* | 59* | 7.71 |
| For the year | 64.09 | 94 | 7 | 59.35 | 63.51 | 96 | 6* | 45.45 | 62.20 | 96* | 3* | 52.40 | 61.62 | 97* | 10* | 56.65 |

ᐟ These observations are made with self-registering thermometers.   The mean is from the standard thermometer.

### Consolidated sick-report, McPherson Barracks, Atlanta, Ga., 1870–'74.

| Year | | 1870–'71. | | 1871–'72. | | 1872–'73. | | 1873–'74. | |
|---|---|---|---|---|---|---|---|---|---|
| Mean strength { Officers | | 20 | | 11 | | 13 | | 19 | |
| { Enlisted men | | 420 | | 195 | | 189 | | 363 | |
| Diseases. | | Cases. | Deaths. | Cases. | Deaths. | Cases. | Deaths. | Cases. | Deaths. |
| **GENERAL DISEASES, A.** | | | | | | | | | |
| Small-pox and varioloid | | | | 1 | | | | | |
| Typhoid fever | | 8 | 3 | 11 | 2 | 2 | | 3 | 1 |
| Typho-malarial fever | | 1 | | | | | | | |
| Remittent fever | | 5 | | 2 | 1 | | | 24 | |
| Intermittent fever | | 137 | | 114 | | 66 | | 29 | |
| Other diseases of this group | | 41 | | 10 | | 9 | | 8 | |
| **GENERAL DISEASES, B.** | | | | | | | | | |
| Rheumatism | | 43 | | 22 | | 39 | | 22 | |
| Syphilis | | 44 | | 34 | | 24 | | 37 | |
| Consumption | | 1 | 1 | 2 | | 3 | 2 | 2 | |
| Other diseases of this group | | | | | | 3 | | | |
| **LOCAL DISEASES.** | | | | | | | | | |
| Catarrh and bronchitis | | 31 | | 34 | | 36 | | 36 | |
| Pneumonia | | 3 | 1 | 1 | | | | 1 | |
| Pleurisy | | 4 | | | | | | 2 | 1 |
| Diarrhœa and dysentery | | 206 | 2 | 63 | | 79 | | 91 | |
| Hernia | | 3 | | 1 | | 1 | | 2 | |
| Gonorrhœa | | | | 2 | | 8 | | 33 | |
| Other local diseases | | 242 | 2 | 116 | | 106 | 2 | 136 | |
| Alcoholism | | 9 | | 6 | | 10 | | 9 | |
| Unclassified | | | | | | | | 1 | |
| Total disease | | 778 | 9 | 419 | 3 | 386 | 4 | 436 | 2 |
| **VIOLENT DISEASES AND DEATHS.** | | | | | | | | | |
| Gunshot wounds | | 6 | | 3 | | 1 | | 4 | |
| Other accidents and injuries | | 82 | | 38 | | 40 | 2 | 82 | |
| Suicide | | | 1 | | | | | | |
| Total violence | | 88 | 1 | 41 | | 41 | 2 | 86 | |

## AUGUSTA ARSENAL, GEORGIA.

This is an " arsenal of construction," established in 1816, about three miles from the city of Augusta, Ga., and three miles from the Savannah River, in latitude 33° 28′ north, longitude 4° 51′ west. It is situated in what is known as the Sand Hill region of Georgia, the soil of which is white sand covered with a scanty growth of small yellow pine, black-jack, and scrub-oak. There are two sets of officers' quarters, and a brick barrack for thirty-five men, all in good repair. The hospital consists of a ward, 20 by 22 feet, and dispensary, 20 by 8 feet, in an old brick building, in fair condition. The guard-house is a new brick building, 18 by 24 feet, in good order. Water is obtained from a well 170 feet deep, and from cisterns.

*Meteorological report, Augusta Arsenal, Ga., 1870–'74.*

| Month. | 1870–'71. Mean. | Max. | Min. | Rain-fall in inches. | 1871–'72. Mean. | Max. | Min. | Rain-fall in inches. | 1872–'73. Mean. | Max. | Min. | Rain-fall in inches. | 1873–'74. Mean. | Max. | Min. | Rain-fall in inches. |
|---|---|---|---|---|---|---|---|---|---|---|---|---|---|---|---|---|
| July | 81.81 | 96 | 71 | 3.78 | 81.29 | 96 | 66 | 5.20 | 81.02 | 98* | 69* | 7.74 | 81.30 | 99* | 68* | 2 07 |
| August | 80.87 | 96 | 73 | 3.23 | 79.41 | 100 | 64 | 5.67 | 79.37 | 96* | 64* | 4.86 | 78.96 | 96* | 66* | 5.41 |
| September | 75.50 | 90 | 64 | 1.25 | 71.83 | 91* | 49* | 8.00 | 75.91 | 94* | 59* | 0.38 | 74.52 | 95* | 59* | 2.93 |
| October | 67.57 | 87 | 43 | 5.29 | 67.76 | 85* | 46* | 2.07 | 64.79 | 91* | 35* | 0.96 | 63.12 | 87* | 28* | 2.09 |
| November | 56.46 | 79 | 33 | 1.84 | 55.46 | 76* | 31* | 6.92 | 50.28 | 72* | 11* | 3.87 | 52.51 | 73* | 16ᴬ | 7.99 |
| December | 44.07 | 75 | 10 | 4.27 | 47.53 | 76* | 14* | 5.84 | 42.66 | 67* | 15* | 2.70 | 47.27 | 74* | 16* | 3.44 |
| January | 49.64 | 71 | 29 | 1.26 | 41.65 | 72* | 15* | 4.22 | 45.16 | 75* | 8* | 4.37 | 47.82 | 73* | 18* | 3.55 |
| February | 59.23 | 79 | 33 | 9.41 | 45.95 | 75* | 17* | 6.25 | 51.88 | 76* | 22* | 4.38 | 49.85 | 81* | 28* | 6.07 |
| March | 61.08 | 84 | 40 | 3 64 | 50.80 | 77* | 27ᵗ | 9.11 | 52.45 | 82* | 15* | 3.24 | 58.29 | 85* | 35* | 9.77 |
| April | 66.86 | 89 | 45 | 4.44 | 66.37 | 89* | 41* | 2.80 | 63.92 | 90* | 38* | 4.04 | 63.94 | 82* | 37* | 9.98 |
| May | 70.28 | 87 | 46 | 7.42 | 73.00 | 89* | 54* | 5.77 | 71.83 | 91* | 48* | 8.57 | 73.31 | 96* | 50* | 4.49 |
| June | 78.79 | 93 | 69 | 3.70 | 78.14 | 92* | 67* | 3.61 | 78.10 | 92* | 57* | 2.77 | 83.20 | 99* | 67* | 2.68 |
| For the year | 66.04 | 96 | 10 | 49.53 | 63.27 | 100 | 14* | 65.46 | 63.11 | 98* | 8ᵃ | 47.88 | 64.51 | 99* | 16* | 60.47 |

\* These observations are made with self-registering thermometers. The mean is from the standard thermometer.

*Consolidated sick-report, Augusta Arsenal, Ga., 1870–'74.*

| Year | 1870–'71. Cases. | Deaths. | 1871–'72. Cases. | Deaths. | 1872–'73. Cases. | Deaths. | 1873–'74. Cases. | Deaths. |
|---|---|---|---|---|---|---|---|---|
| Mean strength { Officers | 2 | | 2 | | 2 | | 2 | |
| { Enlisted men | 35 | | 20 | | 20 | | 23 | |
| **GENERAL DISEASES, A.** | | | | | | | | |
| Remittent fever | | | 1 | | 1 | | | |
| Intermittent fever | 7 | | 7 | | 5 | | 9 | 1 |
| Other diseases of this group | | | 1 | | | | | |
| **GENERAL DISEASES, B.** | | | | | | | | |
| Rheumatism | 3 | | | | 1 | | | |
| Syphilis | 5 | | 1 | | 1 | | 2 | |
| Consumption | | | | | 1 | | | |
| Other diseases of this group | | | | | | | 1 | |
| **LOCAL DISEASES.** | | | | | | | | |
| Catarrh and bronchitis | 11 | | 7 | | 2 | | 5 | |
| Pleurisy | | | | | 1 | | | |
| Diarrhœa and dysentery | 6 | | 5 | | 5 | | 5 | |
| Gonorrhœa | 2 | | 2 | | 1 | | 2 | |
| Other local diseases | 28 | | 19 | | 24 | | 18 | |
| Alcoholism | 1 | | 1 | | 3 | | | |
| Total disease | 63 | | 44 | | 45 | | 42 | 1 |
| **VIOLENT DISEASES AND DEATHS.** | | | | | | | | |
| Accidents and injuries | 17 | | 2 | | 4 | | 2 | |
| Total violence | 17 | | 2 | | 4 | | 2 | |

# FORT BARRANCAS, FLORIDA.

REPORT OF ASSISTANT SURGEON GEORGE M. STERNBERG, UNITED STATES ARMY.

Fort Barrancas, Fla., is situated in latitude 30° 19' north, and longitude 10° 13' west. The military reservation is 1,667.37 acres in extent, and is located on a peninsula, bounded by the bay of Pensacola on the south, and the Grand Bayou (an arm of the bay) on the north. The naval reservation, upon which is located the Pensacola navy-yard, occupies the extremity of the peninsula, and bounds the military reservation on the east.

On the opposite side of the bay, at the extremity of Santa Rosa Island, and 2,300 yards distant from Fort Barrancas, is Fort Pickens. In a southeasterly direction, on a peninsula of the mainland formed by the lagoon, (an arm of the bay,) are the ruins of Fort McRea.

The city of Pensacola is nine miles distant, in a northeasterly direction. The ordinary means of communication with it are by the post-yacht, by the steam-tug Rose, belonging to the Navy Department, or by a land conveyance. The land-route leads through the villages of Warrington and Woolsey, across the Grand Bayou and the Little Bayou by bridges, and through the " piney woods" along the shores of the bay. A railroad from Pensacola connects with the Mobile and Montgomery Railroad at Pollard Junction. The steamers Lizzie and Reliance ply between Pensacola and New Orleans, landing freight or passengers at the Barrancas wharf when desired.

Warrington is a small village on the naval reserve, inhabited mainly by employés of the navy-yard and pilots.

Woolsey is on the north and east of the navy-yard, and is a continuation of Warrington.

Upon the naval reserve are also located a national cemetery, the ruins of the Pensacola naval hospital, and the ruins of the marine barracks. These buildings were destroyed during the late war.

Fort Barrancas proper is a brick-work with a glacis on the land side, and with counterscarp and flank defense. It has no casemates or quarters for troops. Immediately in front of it, and connected with it by a covered way, is the old Spanish fort, Fort San Carlos de Barrancas. This is a small semicircular work, which was constructed by the Spaniards, and was the only fort for the protection of the harbor when Florida was ceded to the United States, October 24, 1820.

The garrison of Fort Barrancas occupies Barrancas barracks, a three-story brick building, situated on a sand plateau, which has an elevation of about 30 feet from the level of the sea, overlooking the bay of Pensacola, Santa Rosa Island, and the Gulf of Mexico, and distant from the fort 470 yards. The building is 186 feet long and 36 feet wide. It contains fifteen rooms, each 32 by 26 by 16 feet, and several smaller rooms, occupied as store-rooms and company offices. Four of the five rooms on the ground-floor are used as kitchens and mess-rooms. The remaining rooms are distributed among the four companies as quarters for men. There is a veranda for each story in the rear of the building, but none in front, where it is most needed. The rooms are well lighted and ventilated by windows in front and rear. Each one has an open fire-place. The air-space per man, with the present garrison, June 15, 1874, is 1,030 cubic feet. The bunks are single iron frame with wooden slats.

Immediately in rear of the barracks are four detached two-story buildings. Three of these have heretofore been used as quarters for laundresses and married soldiers. They were, however, poorly adapted for this purpose, and new quarters for laundresses have recently been completed, and are now occupied. It is proposed to give the companies rooms in these buildings for lavatories and reading-rooms. The lower story of the fourth building is used as a guard-house, the upper story as a billiard-room for enlisted men. The men's sink is new and good.

The commanding officer's house contains nine rooms. It faces the bay, is shaded by large live-oak trees, and has a veranda 12 feet wide in front and at the sides. There is a detached building in rear of it containing a kitchen and laundry. Three houses were built by contract in 1871. They are elevated from 3 to 6 feet above the ground, and have a veranda 12 feet wide running all around them. The lower story contains two rooms, 16 by 22 feet each, and is without hallway or closet. An outside stairway on the back veranda leads to the two rooms in the second story, each 22 by 28 feet, and destitute of closets. A detached building, 10 feet in rear of the main building, and having two rooms, 12 by 10 feet each, is intended as kitchen and servant's room.

Two buildings have recently been repaired and remodeled to serve as officers' quarters. There are seven rooms in one, all on one floor. In the other there are two rooms and a detached kitchen on the ground-floor, and two good attic-rooms above.

The officers' quarters are all inclosed with rough picket-fences, and most of them have some improvements in the way of fruit and shade trees, grape-vines, and flower-beds.

There is an elevated cistern of cypress-wood, having a capacity of 5,000 gallons for each set of quarters, except the last described.

The new building, erected as quarters for laundresses, is 200 feet long, and has a veranda 8 feet 6 inches wide in front and rear. It contains twelve sets of quarters, each of two rooms, 14 by 16 by 10 feet. Each set of quarters has a yard in rear, 50 by 16 feet, surrounded by a high board fence. There is a sink in the rear of each yard. For every two sets of quarters there is a cistern having a capacity of 4,500 gallons.

The ground-floor of a detached brick building in rear of the barracks is occupied as a guard-house. It has recently been greatly improved and remodeled. The prisoners' room is 38 by 20 by 10 feet, and has six windows and one fire-place for ventilation. There are four dark cells, 7 by 4 by 9 feet, ventilated by a grating over the door, which opens into the main prison-room. The room for the guard is 38 by 20 by 10 feet, and is well ventilated by a fire-place, five windows, and two doors.

The adjutant's and quartermaster's offices are two rooms, each 14 by 16 feet, in a small building located 100 yards south of the barracks. There is an ample parade-ground in front, and to the left of the barracks, which is in great part covered with a good sod of Bermuda grass.

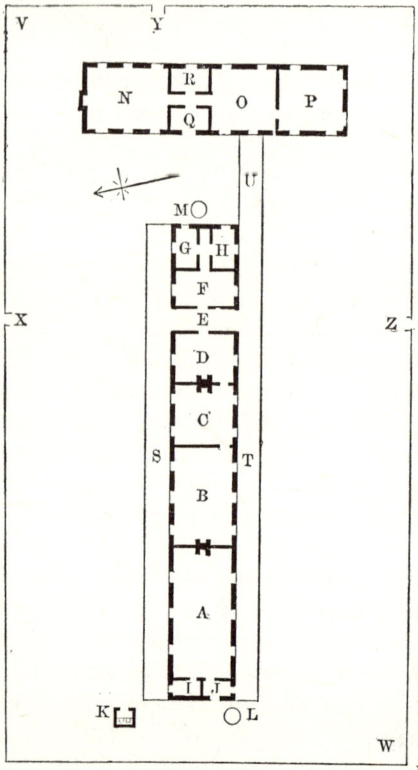

Figure 25.

The post hospital is located 370 yards west of the barracks. It is a one-story frame building elevated 4 feet from the ground, and having a veranda 8 feet wide in front and rear of the main building. It is situated near the edge of the elevated sand plateau on which the fort is built, and has an unobstructed outlook over the bay and Gulf, receiving the full benefit of the prevailing summer winds, which are from the southwest. It has recently been improved by the addition of a bath-room, wardmaster's room, cistern, and new dispensary fixtures. It is now in excellent order, and is well adapted to the climate and the requirements of the post. It is inclosed by a substantial picket-fence, and the grounds are embellished by fruit and shade trees, and flowering shrubs and vines. The capacity of the hospital is for thirty beds, with 1,000 cubic feet of air-space for each. The ventilation is excellent by doors, windows, open fire-places, and special ridge-ventilators. The ground-plan of the hospital is shown in Figure 25.

A, ward, 45 by 22 feet, twelve beds; B, ward, 33 by 22 feet, eight beds; C, ward, 20 by 22 feet, six beds; D, steward's room, 18 by 22 feet; E, hall-way, 8 by 22 feet; F, dispensary, 12 by 22 feet; G, store-room; H, linen-room; I, closet; J, bath-room; K, sink; L and M, cisterns; N, kitchen, 30 by 22 feet; O, mess-room, 22 by 22 feet; P, ward, 24 by 22 feet, four beds; Q, store-room; R, cook's room; S and T, veranda, 160 feet long, 8 feet wide; U, covered way, 30 feet long, 8 feet wide; V and W, picket-fence, inclosing hospital grounds; X, Y, and Z, gate-ways; arrow points to the north.

The dead-house is located 100 yards north of the hospital. It has a single room 10 by 12 by 14 feet, is well ventilated, and contains a post-mortem table.

The buildings already mentioned are inclosed by a new and substantial picket-fence, which includes 40 acres. Outside of this inclosure are the following buildings:

The commissary and quartermaster's storehouse, 100 feet long and 50 feet wide, (recently repaired.)

The carpenter's shop, 20 by 32 feet.

The forage-shed, 30 by 50 feet, (new.)

Forage store-house, (old.)

The wharf and wharf boat-house, (new.)

The stable, 40 by 40 feet; has stalls for ten horses; (old, but serviceable.)

Wagon-shed, 20 by 95 feet, (new.)

Bake-house, 58 by 31 feet; has recently been repaired, and has three ovens, with a capacity for 1,500 loaves of bread.

The post garden is located 1,050 yards north of the barracks. It has recently been enlarged by the clearing of 8 acres of land on the north side of the old garden, and now contains 11 acres, inclosed by a new and substantial board fence. The soil is a sandy loam. By careful cultivation, and the liberal use of manure, it produces excellent crops of sweet potatoes, corn, okra, melons, tomatoes, &c. Cabbage, turnips, and lettuce may be grown with ease during the winter and spring months. Peas, beans, beets, and other garden-vegetables do well during the early spring.

The water-supply for the post is obtained from nineteen cisterns, distributed as follows: Two at the post hospital; three at the barracks; six at the laundresses' quarters, and eight at the officers' quarters. The total capacity of these cisterns is about 80,000 gallons. Five more cisterns, with a capacity of 25,000 gallons, are in process of erection in rear of the barracks. Prior to August 1, 1873, the garrison depended for water upon eight wells, which are distributed about the post. The supply was ample, but inconvenient to obtain, and in the opinion of the post-surgeon the water was very objectionable for drinking purposes. This opinion was founded upon the fact that several of the wells most used had old privy-vaults in their immediate vicinity; that diarrhœa prevailed among the men to a considerable extent, and that, during the summer of 1873, a number of cases of typhoid fever occurred. Since cisterns have been obtained, and the use of water from the wells prohibited by order, there has not been a case of typhoid fever at the post, and the number of cases of diarrhœa has notably diminished. (Cases of diarrhœa during the first six months of 1873, when well-water was used exclusively, 64; cases during the first six months of 1874, when cistern-water was used exclusively, 32. Mean strength of the command during the first period, 109; during the second period, 144.)

The natural drainage of the post is good, as the pervious, sandy soil quickly absorbs any liquid falling upon it. No artificial drains or sewers are required. Slops and refuse from the kitchens are deposited in barrels and daily removed to sink-holes several hundred yards in rear of post.

The enlisted men of the command are marched down to the beach, immediately after retreat, thrice a week from May 2d, to October 1st, for the purpose of bathing. The gently-sloping beach is of pure white sand, and the water is clear and of pleasant temperature.

The climate of this part of Florida may be pronounced pleasant and healthful, although it is subject to somewhat sudden variations in winter, and at times is uncomfortably warm in summer. The prevailing winds in summer are southerly and westerly. In winter east, northeast, and southwest, with occasionally a severe "norther." During the hottest part of the summer there is commonly a refreshing breeze from the Gulf, and when sheltered from the direct rays of the sun, and properly clothed, one may most always be comfortable. In rooms facing the sea, and with open windows, the temperature at night is mild and agreeable throughout the summer.

The prevailing diseases are, in winter, catarrhal affections; in spring and autumn, mild forms of malarial fevers, and throughout the year acute diarrhœa.

Yellow fever has prevailed at Fort Barrancas as a more or less severe epidemic three times since the post was first occupied, viz., in 1822, 1853, and 1873. It was, without doubt, in every instance introduced from abroad. There are no local causes of disease to add to its malignancy. Pure air, pure water, and well-ventilated quarters leave nothing to be desired, so far as favorable sanitary conditions are concerned. The proximity of the village of Warrington, however, makes it almost impossible to maintain an effective quarantine when the disease is prevailing there or in Pensacola It therefore becomes necessary in such a case to remove the command into camp in some more isolated position. Last year (1873) yellow fever prevailed in New Orleans and Pensacola. From one of these cities, without doubt, it was introduced to Barrancas, and 12 cases and 3 deaths occurred among the enlisted men of the command. The prompt removal of the main part of the command into camp on Santa Rosa Island, and the enforcement of rigid quarantine regulations, proved effectual in protecting from the disease all those who were so removed.

The soil of the Barrancas reservation and vicinity is, first, extending back from the waters of the bay for a distance of 100 to 1,000 yards, sand of a dazzling snowy whiteness; then a bluff, 30 feet high, forming the margin of a plateau of yellow sand. The white sand supports in places a scanty growth of sage-bushes, (*Calamintha canascens*,) golden-rod, (*Solidago tortifolia*,) holly, (*Ilex glaber*,) &c.

The waters of the bay and gulf abound in fish. The most valuable for the table are the following: Pompino, Spanish mackerel, red snapper, bluefish, redfish, sheep's head, trout, flounder, mullet. Sharks are plentiful, and attain a great size. Of reptiles, the gopher, a land terrapin, is the only one valuable as food. Snakes are numerous, but mostly harmless. Alligators abound.

Subsistence supplies are obtained from the post commissary, the grocers of Warrington, and to a small extent from the settlers in the vicinity.

The native cattle furnish beef of an inferior quality, and western or Texas beef is scarce. The contract-price for the former ranges from 6 to 10 cents per pound; of the latter, from 10 to 15 cents per pound. The standard price for butter is 50 cents per pound; milk, 20 cents per quart; eggs, 50 cents per dozen. Vegetables are scarce, and command extravagant prices.

There are a few settlers along the Grand Bayou, the Lagoon, and their branches, who obtain a precarious subsistence by raising sweet-potatoes and other vegetables for market, and by fishing.

*Meteorological report, Fort Barrancas, Fla., 1873–'74.*

| Month. | 1870–'71. | | | | 1871–'72. | | | | 1872–'73. | | | | 1873–'74. | | | |
|---|---|---|---|---|---|---|---|---|---|---|---|---|---|---|---|---|
| | Temperature. | | | Rain-fall in inches. | Temperature. | | | Rain-fall in inches. | Temperature. | | | Rain-fall in inches. | Temperature. | | | Rain-fall in inches. |
| | Mean. | Max. | Min. | | Mean. | Max. | Min. | | Mean. | Max. | Min. | | Mean. | Max. | Min. | |
| | ° | ° | ° | | ° | ° | ° | | ° | ° | ° | | ° | ° | ° | |
| July.......... | | | | | | | | | | | | | 84.76 | 100 | 70 | 6.65 |
| August........ | | | | | | | | | | | | | 84.99 | 96 | 78 | 7.59 |
| September...... | | | | | | | | | | | | | 81.99 | 98 | 70 | 11.15 |
| October....... | | | | | | | | | | | | | 71.38 | 92 | 28 | 2.22 |
| November...... | | | | | | | | | | | | | 62.68 | 86 | 19* | 2.58 |
| December...... | | | | | | | | | | | | | 57.84 | 87 | 15* | 0.24 |
| January....... | | | | | | | | | 48.66 | 75 | 15 | 4.80 | 56.27 | 78 | 21* | 1.58 |
| February...... | | | | | | | | | 56.52 | 71 | 34 | 2.70 | 59.31 | 76 | 25* | 3.04 |
| March......... | | | | | | | | | 59.61 | 75 | 32 | 2.73 | 65.25 | 80 | 33* | 3.02 |
| April......... | | | | | | | | | 66.49 | 84 | 48 | 1.63 | 65.21 | 82 | 30* | 10.11 |
| May........... | | | | | | | | | 75.15 | 89 | 58 | 5.69 | 73.81 | 93 | 36* | 0.24 |
| June.......... | | | | | | | | | 81.21 | 93 | 67 | 7.70 | 79.56 | 92 | 51* | 12.80 |
| For the year..... | | | | | | | | | | | | | 70.25 | 100 | 15* | 61.23 |

* These observations are made with self-registering thermometers. The mean is from the standard thermometer.

*Consolidated sick-report, Fort Barrancas, Fla., 1870–'74.*

| | 1870–'71. | | 1871–'72. | | 1872–'73. | | 1873–'74. | |
|---|---|---|---|---|---|---|---|---|
| Year | | | | | | | | |
| Mean strength { Officers | 4 | | 3 | | 5 | | 6 | |
| { Enlisted men | 82 | | 50 | | 95 | | 124 | |
| **Diseases.** | Cases. | Deaths. | Cases. | Deaths. | Cases. | Deaths. | Cases. | Deaths. |
| GENERAL DISEASES, A. | | | | | | | | |
| Typhoid fever | | | | | | | 4 | 1 |
| Remittent fever | 4 | | | | 3 | | 5 | |
| Intermittent fever | 32 | | 21 | | 36 | | 7 | |
| Yellow fever | | | | | | | 12 | 3 |
| Other diseases of this group | 4 | | 1 | | 5 | | 1 | |
| GENERAL DISEASES, B. | | | | | | | | |
| Rheumatism | 2 | | 6 | | 8 | | 4 | |
| Syphilis | 8 | | 4 | | | | 3 | |
| Consumption | | | | | | | | |
| Other diseases of this group | | | | | 4 | | 4 | |
| LOCAL DISEASES. | | | | | | | | |
| Catarrh and bronchitis | 5 | | | | 40 | | 26 | |
| Pleurisy | | | | | 1 | | | |
| Diarrhœa and dysentery | 79 | | 33 | | 138 | | 80 | |
| Gonorrhœa | 3 | | 2 | | 3 | | 8 | |
| Other local diseases | 87 | | 31 | | 104 | | 133 | |
| Alcoholism | 12 | | | | 5 | | 13 | |
| Total diseases | 236 | | 98 | | 347 | | 300 | 4 |
| VIOLENT DISEASES AND DEATHS. | | | | | | | | |
| Gunshot wounds | 2 | | | | 2 | | | |
| Drowning | | | | | | | | 1 |
| Other accidents and injuries | 36 | | 22 | | 68 | | 39 | |
| Total violence | 38 | | 22 | | 70 | | 39 | 1 |

# BATON ROUGE BARRACKS, LOUISIANA.

## REPORT OF ASSISTANT SURGEON C. EWEN, UNITED STATES ARMY.

Baton Rouge is situated on the east bank of the Mississippi River, in latitude 30° 26′ north ; longitude, 14° 6′ west, on the first high land or bluff found in ascending the river. This bluff is about 22 feet above high water in the river, and 60 feet above the level of the Gulf. The ground here occupied by the Government is 210¾ acres, within the limits of the city of Baton Rouge. The surface is undulating, and has good natural drainage. On the north is a bayou, which empties into the river about 200 yards above the barracks. The post is supposed to have been first occupied in 1820. Baton Rouge Arsenal, discontinued June 15, 1871, formerly occupied a portion of these grounds. The arsenal buildings became a part of the present military post.

The barracks consisted originally of five nearly uniform brick buildings, two stories in height, disposed in a pentagon near the bank of the river ; but the one nearest the water was removed many years ago. Of those that remain, the two nearest the river are each 184 by 34 feet, with 12-feet verandas running along the front and rear, and outside staircases leading to both galleries. The other two are similar, except that their dimensions are 182 by 24 feet. The two larger barracks are similar in their arrangements. Each is divided in the middle into quarters for two companies. Each set of quarters has in the basement a store-room, 31 by 24 ; kitchen, 19 by 31 ; and mess-room, 39 by 31 feet. The mess-rooms are furnished with tables and benches. The second floor of each set is divided into two squad-rooms, 30 by 31 feet, and 44 by 31 feet ; a first-sergeant's room, and store-room, each 15 by 14 feet. These rooms are furnished with single iron bunks. A third building, situated about 250 feet northeast from the original pentagon, and formerly belonging to the arsenal, is now used as quarters for two companies. It is a three-story brick building, 40 feet high to the eaves, 120 feet long by 38 feet wide. The basement is divided by wooden bulkheads into two kitchens and two mess-rooms, each apartment being 28½ by 33 feet. The second floor is reached by outside staircases at both ends, and contains a dormitory 102 by 33 feet, a first-sergeant's room 17 by 14 feet, and a small space under the staircase which leads to the third story. The dormitory in the third story is of the same dimensions as the other, except that two small rooms are partitioned off at the east end for a first sergeant's room, and store-room. The furniture is similar to that in the other company-quarters. All are warmed by stoves.

The two smaller buildings of the pentagon are occupied as officers' quarters. The upper story of each contains nine rooms of the average size of 19 by 21 feet. Each room has two average-sized windows, and a door opening front, and the same in the rear. The doors and windows are provided with outside blinds. The walls are plastered, except of three center rooms which are partitioned and ceiled with boards. Most of the rooms communicate by inside doors. There are no inside stairs. The basements are divided into kitchens and dining-rooms, and are damp and unfit to live in. The windows have iron gratings and board shutters. The rooms are warmed by open fire-places.

There are also four detached buildings for officers' quarters. The quarters of the commanding officer front the parade, and are 300 feet east from the buildings last described. The building is of brick, two stories high, 36 by 34 feet, very nicely finished inside. The second story is surrounded by a veranda, 12 feet wide. The upper story contains one large room, 30 by 15 feet, occupying the south side of the building, and two on the north side, 15 by 14½ feet, the whole surrounded by a veranda, 12 feet wide. Under the veranda is a small bath-room. The ground floor has the same arrangement as the upper story. The rooms are hard-finished and have marble mantels. Each of the large rooms has two doors and six windows; each of the smaller, one door and four windows. The doors and windows have outside blinds. In the rear is a two-story brick building containing kitchen, servants' room, and water-tank. There are also in the yard two small frame buildings for servants' quarters, storage of tools, &c., and a cistern covered with a shed.

The second of these detached dwellings is a two-story brick cottage, 60 by 30 feet, with slate roof. It contains an entrance-hall, 18 by 10 feet, a large room at each end, 18 by 27 feet—each room with five windows cut down to the floor—a room back of the hall, 18 by 17 feet, with one window, and, in an adjoining wing, (a frame structure,) a dining-room, 15 by 13 feet, and a kitchen 13 feet square. The walls are hard-finished, the ceilings of wood, and the doors and windows furnished with blinds. The third is a brick cottage of one story, 60 by 26 feet, with slate roof, and contains two sets of officers' quarters. There is a veranda, 9 feet wide, running along the front. Each set comprises one large room, 22 by 18 feet, and a smaller, 22 by 10 feet, with kitchen and dining-room in detached frame building reached by a covered gallery. The finish of this building is similar to that of the other. They are warmed by open grates. The fourth is a brick building with slate roof, two stories and basement in height, 78 by 30 feet. The two upper stories have a gallery, 9 feet in width, running the length of the building, front and rear. The building is divided into four sets of quarters, two on each of the main floors. The several stories communicate by a central hall and stairway, and granite steps lead from the ground, front and rear, to the entrance of the first floor above the basement. The basement contains two kitchens. The rooms are heated by open fire-places.

The hospital is a frame building, plastered within, built after the plan prescribed in Circular No. 4, Surgeon-General's Office, April 27, 1867, for twenty-four beds, with administration building and two wings. A veranda, 12 feet wide, extends around the whole building. The administration building is warmed by open fire-places, except the office and dispensary, which have grates. The wards are warmed by stoves. Each ward contains twelve beds, with an air-space of 1,200 feet to each. Ventilating-shafts are used in winter and ridge ventilation in summer. There is a bath-room and water-closet at the end of each ward, containing bath-tubs, basins, and inodorous chambers. The room opposite the bath-room is used for the storage of the baggage of patients. The dead-house, laundry, and sink are in a small frame building, 28 by 10 feet, standing about 200 feet in rear of the hospital. The sink consists of a deep vault. There is a flower and vegetable garden in the rear of the hospital, which is cultivated by the attendants, and furnishes a sufficient supply of vegetables for the hospital.

A closed sally-port in the center of one of the barracks first above described has been used for several years past as a guard-house. This is about to be superseded by a new building now in progress. The new building is of brick, two stories in height, 60 by 27 feet outside measurement. The lower floor contains the guard-room, 29 by 24 feet, lighted by four windows, and divided off by wooden bulk-heads from the apartments for the confinement of general military convicts of the Department of the Gulf. There are three apartments for this purpose—one 28½ by 13 feet, lighted by two windows; the others 14 by 11 and 13 by 11 feet, each lighted by one window. The second floor is for the confinement of the garrison prisoners, and contains one large room, 43 by 24 feet, and a smaller, 27 by 13½ feet, designed for a mess-room. The building is surrounded by a plank stockade, 14 feet high, with a parapet at top for the sentry and sentry-boxes at the angles. There is a detached kitchen in one corner of the inclosure, 18 by 16 feet.

In the vicinity of the guard-house, which is located near the river, are two small frame houses, consisting each of one room and a shed, occupied as laundresses' quarters. A one-story frame building, directly north of the hospital, 128 by 23 feet, is divided into laundresses' quarters. Each room has a door and window front and rear.

The extensive grounds of the post are pleasantly shaded with live and water oaks, pecan and China trees.

The natural drainage is very good.

The officers' sinks are furnished with boxes, which are emptied every day; those of the men are benches placed in sheds over deep pits, difficult to disinfect or clean.

The malarial diseases prevailing at the post are immediately due in great part to the tract of swamp bordering the northern edge of the reservation, and the continuance of winds from that quarter is accompanied by a marked increase in the number and gravity of the cases.

*Meteorological report, Baton Rouge, La., 1873–'74.*

| Month. | 1870–'71. Temperature. | | | Rain-fall in inches. | 1871–'72. Temperature. | | | Rain-fall in inches. | 1872–'73. Temperature. | | | Rain-fall in inches. | 1873–'74. Temperature. | | | Rain-fall in inches. |
|---|---|---|---|---|---|---|---|---|---|---|---|---|---|---|---|---|
| | Mean. | Max. | Min. | | Mean. | Max. | Min. | | Mean. | Max. | Min. | | Mean. | Max. | Min. | |
| July | | | | | | | | | | | | | 80.61 | 95 | 72 | 7.42 |
| August | | | | | | | | | | | | | 79.97 | 94 | 71 | 5.02 |
| September | | | | | | | | | | | | | 76.62 | 93 | 60 | 5.92 |
| October | | | | | | | | | | | | | 64.44 | 91 | 33 | 1.40 |
| November | | | | | | | | | | | | | 58.59 | 82 | 27 | 6.65 |
| December | | | | | | | | | | | | | 58.39 | 80 | 23 | 3.06 |
| January | | | | | | | | | | | | | 53.82 | 79 | 28 | 3.88 |
| February | | | | | | | | | | | | | 56.29 | 80 | 33 | 4.93 |
| March | | | | | | | | | | | | | 65.05 | 84 | 47 | 6.87 |
| April | | | | | | | | | | | | | 63.74 | 81 | 43 | 14.18 |
| May | | | | | | | | | | | | | 75.33 | 95 | 60 | 0.23 |
| June | | | | | | | | | | 80.97 | 93 | 72 | 5.76 | 81.02 | 95 | 71 | 6.31 |
| For the year | | | | | | | | | | | | | 67.82 | 95 | 23 | 65.87 |

*Consolidated sick-report, Baton Rouge, La., 1870–'74.*

| Year | | 1870–'71. | | 1871–'72. | | 1872–'73. | | 1873–'74. | |
|---|---|---|---|---|---|---|---|---|---|
| Mean strength | { Officers<br>{ Enlisted men | 7<br>117 | | 14<br>255 | | 9<br>144 | | 7<br>134 | |
| Diseases. | | Cases. | Deaths. | Cases. | Deaths. | Cases. | Deaths. | Cases. | Deaths. |
| GENERAL DISEASES, A. | | | | | | | | | |
| Typho-malarial fever | | 2 | 2 | | | 2 | 1 | 1 | 1 |
| Remittent fever | | 6 | 1 | 8 | 1 | 6 | | 66 | |
| Intermittent fever | | 181 | | 673 | | 139 | | 150 | 1 |
| Other diseases of this group | | 1 | | 6 | | 15 | | 4 | |
| GENERAL DISEASES, B. | | | | | | | | | |
| Rheumatism | | 12 | | 37 | | 20 | | 5 | |
| Syphilis | | 11 | | 14 | | 6 | | 22 | |
| Consumption | | 1 | | 1 | 1 | 2 | 2 | 2 | 1 |
| Other diseases of this group | | 4 | | 9 | | 4 | | | |

16 M P

*Consolidated sick-report, Baton Rouge, La., 1870–'74—Continued.*

| Year | 1870–'71. | | 1871–'72. | | 1872–'73. | | 1873–'74. | |
|---|---|---|---|---|---|---|---|---|
| Mean strength { Officers / Enlisted men | 7 / 117 | | 14 / 255 | | 9 / 144 | | 7 / 134 | |
| Diseases. | Cases. | Deaths. | Cases. | Deaths. | Cases. | Deaths. | Cases. | Deaths. |
| LOCAL DISEASES. | | | | | | | | |
| Catarrh and bronchitis | 10 | ...... | 67 | ...... | 32 | ...... | 12 | ...... |
| Pneumonia | 1 | ...... | 1 | ...... | 1 | ...... | 3 | ...... |
| Pleurisy | 1 | ...... | | | 1 | ...... | 1 | ...... |
| Diarrhœa and dysentery | 56 | ...... | 145 | ...... | 51 | 1 | 79 | ...... |
| Hernia | 1 | ...... | 1 | ...... | | | | |
| Gonorrhœa | 4 | ...... | 12 | ...... | 11 | ...... | 21 | ...... |
| Other local diseases | 105 | 3 | 168 | ...... | 108 | 1 | 89 | 1 |
| Alcoholism | 17 | ...... | 27 | 1 | 33 | ...... | 43 | ...... |
| Total disease | 413 | 6 | 1,169 | 3 | 431 | 5 | 498 | 4 |
| VIOLENT DISEASES AND DEATHS. | | | | | | | | |
| Gun-shot wounds | | ...... | 1 | 1 | 1 | ...... | 1 | ...... |
| Drowning | | ...... | | | 1 | 1 | | 1 |
| Other accidents and injuries | 33 | ...... | 45 | ...... | 37 | ...... | 52 | ...... |
| Homicide | | ...... | | 1 | | | | |
| Suicide | | ...... | | | 1 | 1 | | |
| Total violence | 33 | ...... | 46 | 4 | 38 | 2 | 53 | 1 |

*Baton Rouge, La., (military convicts.)*

| Year | 1873–'74. | |
|---|---|---|
| Mean strength ... Enlisted men | *21 | |
| Diseases. | Cases. | Deaths. |
| GENERAL DISEASES, A. | | |
| Remittent fever | 19 | ...... |
| Intermittent fever | 32 | ...... |
| GENERAL DISEASES, B. | | |
| Rheumatism | 2 | ...... |
| Syphilis | 1 | ...... |
| Other diseases of this group | 1 | ...... |
| LOCAL DISEASES. | | |
| Catarrh and bronchitis | 8 | ...... |
| Pleurisy | 1 | ...... |
| Diarrhœa and dysentery | 13 | ...... |
| Hernia | 2 | ...... |
| Other local diseases | 22 | ...... |
| Total diseases | 101 | ...... |
| VIOLENT DISEASES AND DEATHS. | | |
| Accidents and injuries | 5 | ...... |
| Total violence | 5 | ...... |

\* Eleven months only.

# BATTERY BIENVENUE, LOUISIANA.

Construction commenced in 1826, on the right bank of Bayou Bienvenue, near New Orleans, in latitude 29° 58′ north, longitude 12° 47′ west. Not now occupied.

# FORT CASWELL, NORTH CAROLINA.

The construction of Fort Caswell was commenced in 1825, on Oak Island, on the right bank of Cape Fear River, at the mouth of the river, in latitude 34° north, longitude 57′ west. It is two miles south of Smithville, N. C., which is the nearest post-office.

The reservation consists of a peninsula, containing between four and five hundred acres, on the eastern extremity of which the fort stands.

Inside the fort the brick walls of barracks are standing, all the wood-work having been burned out, it is believed, by the confederate forces when they evacuated the place after the fall of Fort Fisher, which is eight miles above, at the mouth of New Inlet. Outside the fort are two or three small frame shanties, one of which is occupied by the ordnance-sergeant in charge of the post. The water-supply is obtained from a well inside the fort. Communication is by a small boat furnished the ordnance-sergeant by the quartermaster at Fort Johnston.

---

# CHARLESTON, SOUTH CAROLINA.

INFORMATION FURNISHED BY ASSISTANT SURGEON J. R. GIBSON AND ACTING ASSISTANT SURGEON T. C. SKRINE, UNITED STATES ARMY.

The military post of Charleston consists of the citadel of Charleston, and the barracks—formerly Charleston Arsenal.

The city of Charleston is situated in latitude 32° 46′ north, longitude 2° 54′ west, on a neck of land between the Cooper and Ashley Rivers, and now includes an area of three miles in length by two in breadth at the widest part. The soil is alluvium, and a large part of the present city was formerly subject to inundation, and was cultivated as rice-fields. The neighboring country is low and swampy, and is prolific in malaria. The climate is mild. The temperature in summer seldom exceeds 90° or falls below 76°, the average being about 83° from May to October. The range of temperature in winter is between 68° and 35°.

The citadel was originally built for a State military academy, and also, probably, for defense in case of servile insurrection. The central portion was completed in 1827, the wings two or three years later. The western wing was destroyed by fire in October, 1869

It was first occupied by the United States in 1865. It forms a hollow parallelogram, constructed of brick and stone, two stories and a basement in height, for the general plan of which see Figure 26.

1, basement; 2, first floor; 3, second floor.

A, quarters of enlisted men; B, gate

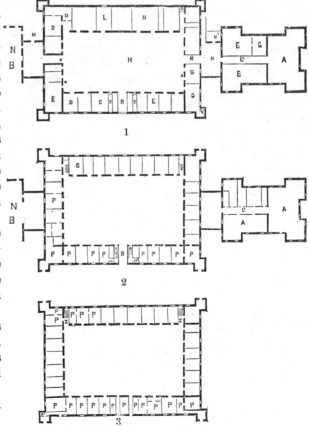

Figure 26.—Scale 120 feet to 1 inch.

and sally-port; C, guard-room; D, guard-house; E, dining-room; G, kitchen; H, yard; L, engine-house; M, privies; N, commissary; P, quarters of officers; L, hall; S, dispensary.

There are no special arrangements for ventilation in any of the rooms.

The dormitories are fitted up with double bunks in two tiers, and allow about 850 cubic feet of air-space per man.

The water-supply of the building is from cisterns, and is sufficient in quantity and of good quality. A room in the basement is fitted up as a bath-room for the enlisted men.

The present hospital, a plain wooden pavilion, is situated about 80 yards from the citadel, and was formerly the eastern ward of the Tradd Street Hospital, now occupied by the quartermaster's department. It measures 90 by 25 feet, has a capacity of fourteen beds, allowing 1,243 cubic feet air-space to each, is well lighted, and has ridge ventilation. It has no water-closet or bath-room and no piazzas, and is not well adapted to its purpose.

The drainage of the post is good, being connected with the city system of sewerage.

The general sanitary condition of the post is good, and few of the cases of disease are supposed to be due to local causes.

The garrison was transferred to Summerville, S. C., October 26, 1874, on account of the prevalence of yellow fever in the city.

Charleston Barracks, formerly Charleston Arsenal, is situated within the corporate limits of the city, near the left bank of the Ashley River. The extent of the grounds is 11¼ acres, surrounded by a wall. In addition to the store-houses and dismantled work-shops there is one brick building, for barracks, two stories high, 78 by 28½ feet, containing seven rooms, with kitchen and bakery attached; also, one brick building for officers' quarters, 125 by 40 feet. There is no hospital or guard-house at the barracks.

### Consolidated sick-report, Charleston, S. C., 1870–'74.

| Year | | 1870–'71. | | 1871–'72. | | 1872–'73. | | 1873–'74. | |
|---|---|---|---|---|---|---|---|---|---|
| Mean strength { Officers | | 9 | | *12 | | 12 | | 12 | |
| { Enlisted men | | 125 | | *132 | | 157 | | 187 | |
| Diseases. | | Cases. | Deaths. | Cases. | Deaths. | Cases. | Deaths. | Cases. | Deaths. |
| GENERAL DISEASES, A. | | | | | | | | | |
| Typhoid fever | | 2 | ...... | 1 | 1 | ...... | ...... | ...... | ...... |
| Remittent fever | | 7 | ...... | 1 | ...... | ...... | ...... | 1 | ...... |
| Intermittent fever | | 40 | ...... | 24 | 1 | 21 | ...... | 42 | ...... |
| Other diseases of this group | | 3 | ...... | 2 | ...... | 2 | ...... | 3 | ...... |
| GENERAL DISEASES, B. | | | | | | | | | |
| Rheumatism | | 25 | ...... | 33 | ...... | 9 | ...... | 11 | ...... |
| Syphilis | | 8 | ...... | 18 | ...... | 17 | ...... | 21 | ...... |
| Consumption | | 2 | ...... | ...... | ...... | 1 | 1 | 2 | 1 |
| Other diseases of this group | | 9 | ...... | ...... | ...... | ...... | ...... | ...... | ...... |
| LOCAL DISEASES. | | | | | | | | | |
| Catarrh and bronchitis | | 4 | ...... | 27 | ...... | 21 | ...... | 29 | ...... |
| Pneumonia | | 1 | ...... | 2 | ...... | ...... | ...... | 1 | 1 |
| Diarrhœa and dysentery | | 42 | ...... | 25 | ...... | 28 | ...... | 42 | ...... |
| Hernia | | 1 | ...... | ...... | ...... | 1 | ...... | ...... | ...... |
| Gonorrhœa | | 5 | ...... | 9 | ...... | 12 | ...... | 10 | ...... |
| Other local diseases | | 73 | ...... | 68 | ...... | 61 | ...... | 86 | 1 |
| Alcoholism | | 14 | ...... | 24 | ...... | 6 | ...... | 6 | ...... |
| Total disease | | 236 | ...... | 234 | 2 | 179 | 1 | 254 | 3 |
| VIOLENT DISEASES AND DEATHS. | | | | | | | | | |
| Gunshot wounds | | ...... | ...... | ...... | ...... | ...... | ...... | 1 | ...... |
| Other accidents and injuries | | 34 | ...... | 35 | ...... | 30 | ...... | 40 | ...... |
| Total violence | | 34 | ...... | 35 | ...... | 30 | ...... | 41 | ...... |

\* Nine months only.

# CHATTANOOGA, TENNESSEE.

### REPORT OF ASSISTANT SURGEON CHARLES STYER, UNITED STATES ARMY.

This post is about 1½ miles from the center of the city of Chattanooga, near the national cemetery, on the left or southern bank of the Tennessee River, which is about 1¾ miles distant. Troops have been stationed in this vicinity since the occupation of the town by General Rosecranz, in September, 1863, but barracks were not constructed until the fall of 1867. The tract of land purchased by the Government contains about 125 acres, 75 acres of which are inclosed by a good stone wall, and form the cemetery proper.

Chattanooga is a manufacturing and railroad center, and has about 10,000 inhabitants.

The site of the post is not good, being too low, and the buildings are in bad condition. They are mostly built of undressed lumber, with shingle roofs.

The post is intended for two companies.

The barrack is a two-story frame building, 88 by 24 feet, the dormitories giving with present strength about 790 cubic feet per man. If occupied by two companies this would be reduced to about 360 cubic feet per man.

Two buildings in rear, each 50 by 24 feet, contain the kitchens and mess-rooms.

The officers' quarters are small frame cottages. The hospital is a frame building 44 by 17 feet, and 10 feet from floor to ceiling. The ward contains six beds, with an air-space per man of 678 cubic feet. It has no bath-room.

The quartermaster's and commissary store-houses are frame buildings, the latter 61 by 16, the former 45 by 17 feet.

The guard-house is a frame building divided into four small rooms.

The water-supply is hauled from a spring three-fourths of a mile distant. In hot weather it is also obtained from a well at the residence of the cemetery superintendent.

*Consolidated sick-report, Chattanooga, Tenn., 1870–'74.*

| Year | | 1870–'71. | | 1871–'72. | | 1872–'73. | | 1873–'74. | |
|---|---|---|---|---|---|---|---|---|---|
| Mean strength { Officers | | 4 | | 4 | | 4 | | 4 | |
| { Enlisted men | | 79 | | 90 | | 56 | | 45 | |
| Diseases. | | Cases. | Deaths. | Cases. | Deaths. | Cases. | Deaths. | Cases. | Deaths. |
| GENERAL DISEASES, A. | | | | | | | | | |
| Small-pox and varioloid | | | | 1 | | | | | |
| Typhoid fever | | 1 | | | | | | | |
| Remittent fever | | 13 | | 1 | | | | | |
| Intermittent fever | | 33 | | 105 | | 16 | | 10 | |
| Cholera | | | | | | 1 | 1 | | |
| Other diseases of this group | | | | 5 | | 2 | | 1 | |
| GENERAL DISEASES, B. | | | | | | | | | |
| Rheumatism | | 3 | | 3 | | 1 | | 4 | |
| Syphilis | | 7 | | 22 | | 13 | | 6 | |
| Consumption | | 1 | | 2 | 1 | | | 1 | |
| Other diseases of this group | | | | 1 | | | | | |
| LOCAL DISEASES. | | | | | | | | | |
| Catarrh and bronchitis | | 7 | | 12 | | 3 | | 9 | |
| Pneumonia | | 1 | | 2 | | | | 1 | |
| Pleurisy | | | | 1 | | | | | |
| Diarrhœa and dysentery | | 17 | | 18 | | 8 | | 11 | |
| Gonorrhœa | | 4 | | | | 1 | | | |
| Other local diseases | | 24 | | 26 | | 15 | | 8 | |
| Alcoholism | | | | | | 7 | | 2 | |
| Total disease | | 111 | | 199 | 1 | 67 | 1 | 53 | |
| VIOLENT DISEASES AND DEATHS. | | | | | | | | | |
| Gunshot wounds | | 2 | | 1 | | | | | |
| Other accidents and injuries | | 18 | | 15 | 1 | 10 | | 3 | |
| Total violence | | 20 | | 16 | 1 | 10 | | 3 | |

# FORT CLINCH, FLORIDA.

The construction of this fort was commenced in 1847, on Amelia Island, at the mouth of Saint Mary's River, near Fernandina, in latitude 30° 41' north, longitude 4° 25' west. The reservation was declared February 9, 1842, and enlarged in 1849 and 1850. Now in charge of an ordnance-sergeant

---

# COLUMBIA, SOUTH CAROLINA.

### REPORT OF ASSISTANT SURGEON J. H. FRANTZ, UNITED STATES ARMY.

This post is within the limits and near the southern boundary of the city of Columbia, which is on the left bank of the Congaree River; latitude, 34° north : longitude, 4° 4' west; altitude above the sea, about 300 feet. The city is on a granite formation, which forms an isolated outcrop between the older formations of the upper part of the State and the tertiary deposits of the lower country. The granite is of a uniform, fine-grained texture, resists well the action of the elements, contains few seams, and therefore possesses all the requisites of good building-material. The State-house is built of granite quarried in the vicinity of the city.

The rock immediately beneath the city is covered to a considerable, but varying, depth with an alluvium composed of sand mixed with ferruginous clay. The principal element of the soil being quartz sand, it is quite porous. Surface water sinks in rapidly. The porous soil forms an excellent filter, so that wells and springs of pure water are numerous. As the alluvium is cut through, circumscribed layers are struck containing a larger per cent. of clay than the average. These layers crop out at certain points along the river, and are made use of to manufacture an inferior article of brick.

With the exception of malarious fevers, which are endemic, the place is remarkably healthful. During the prevalence of epidemics of yellow fever in Charleston this has always been a favorite resort for fugitives from that place. Physicians of this place, conversant with the facts, inform me that though cases have occurred, and ended fatally among such fugitives, in *no case* has it been known to become epidemic, or even be communicated to residents who visited or were in attendance upon the sick. The same, in effect, is averred by physicians with regard to cholera. The profession do not believe either of these diseases could prevail as an epidemic. To some extent this belief is grounded on the geological character of the locality. Whether this theory would hold good in a general application or not, it seems borne out by the facts in this special instance.

Though the city has a population of nearly 10,000 the houses are much scattered. No part of it is compactly built up, and dwelling-houses usually have large yards around them. The scattered dwellings and wide streets, and the fact that dwellings are constructed with a view to comfort in hot weather, elevated on piers, with high ceilings and good ventilation, must also be considered in accounting for the city's immunity from the diseases referred to. In this connection I may mention that typhoid fever is of very rare occurrence. No case has occurred in the command within the last two years.

Cotton is the principal product of the surrounding country. Its production, however, has decreased very materially. Little attention is paid to the cultivation of fruit. The best the markets afford is brought from States north, and hence commands very high prices. Meats are reasonable in price, but of inferior quality. Especially is this true of beef. Vegetables command good prices, and merchandise generally is about 25 per cent. in advance of New York prices.

Colored servants are plentiful, but, as a rule, indifferent, an aggravation to housekeepers. In short, the cost of living, for an inland town, is high.

Game is not abundant, but deer and wild turkeys are still found in the woods, and quail and other small game in the open fields and along the marshes, in sufficient numbers to attract sportsmen.

The grounds occupied by the barracks, store-houses, and other public buildings connected with the post are rented or leased by the Government.

The parade-ground is about 900 by 400 feet—that is, two squares and the width of a street front and one square deep. While it is comparatively level, there is sufficient declination toward the south to drain off superfluous water. Toward the eastern end of the southern edge of the parade-ground the earth declines suddenly and rapidly, forming a sharp hill, at whose foot is a damp valley, traversed by a slow stream, distant nearly a quarter of a mile. Near this edge and overlooking the valley are barracks occupied by four companies. I cannot but regard the position of these barracks as bad, from a sanitary point of view. The valley extends in a south westerly direction, widens into quite a swamp, and, again narrowing, terminates in a comparatively stagnant mill-pond, distant about a mile from the barracks. No obstacles intervene between the low grounds and these barracks to arrest the marsh poison in its march up the hill-side, and certainly all the conditions—heat, moisture, and vegetable decay—which we are taught are the main factors in the production of malaria, obtain in this valley during the autumn months. Much of the space intervening between this valley and the other two barracks is occupied by dwelling-houses, and they impede the miasm in its progress, so that its influence is not felt to so great a degree as in the sites of the barracks first alluded to. Graduation of the intensity of the miasm in its progress through this portion of the city is quite apparent.

The barracks are four frame buildings, and the floor of each, except the one on the eastern side of parade-ground, is elevated from 3 to 5 feet above the ground, on piers. The floor of the excepted barrack is only a few inches from the ground. I have noticed no evil effects from this fault in construction.

The dimensions of these barracks are 145 by 25, 160 by 30, 240 by 25, and 240 by 28 feet. The last of these has three lateral extensions in the rear, used for kitchens and mess-rooms.

Each dormitory is heated by means of two large stoves, in which wood is burned, and is furnished with neat, strong, iron bedsteads, rough tables, and benches. The mess-rooms have ordinary tables and benches manufactured at the post, and generally good mess-furniture. Kitchens have wrought-iron ranges of sufficient capacity to do the required cooking, and the necessary cooking utensils.

Each company has a sink at a proper site. The sinks are deep trenches covered with a movable wooden building. They are disinfected with lime and fresh earth. When necessary, the buildings are removed and placed over new trenches, and the old trenches filled to their surface with earth.

The guard-house is sufficiently lighted and ventilated, but is entirely too small for the present command, the dimensions of the building being 25 by 40 feet. It is divided into a guard-room, 25 by 12 feet; a prison-room, 17 by 28 feet; a passage, 3½ by 28 feet, and six cells. The average occupancy during the year 1873 was 19 prisoners; the maximum, 47.

There is one frame building, 50 by 100 feet, occupied as store-room for quartermaster supplies, and as offices for officer of the day, post quartermaster, and post commissary.

A stable for public animals, forage-house, granary, post bakery, a carpenter and smith shop, constitute, with the barracks described above, the Government buildings at the post.

The basement of a large building hired by the Government is used as a store-room by the subsistence department.

There are no public quarters for officers, company laundresses, and hospital matron. Quarters for them are hired by the quartermaster department at various and at as eligible points relative to the post as can be obtained in the city.

The building used as the post hospital is a frame dwelling-house, containing 18 large, well-ventilated rooms, which will accommodate 16 patients, giving to each an air-space of 1,318 cubic feet. It is leased by the Government by the year. Being private property no detailed description is deemed necessary.

It is located on one of the most elevated points in the city, and in regard to healthfulness the site is entirely satisfactory. It is, however, an inconvenient distance (more than half a mile) from the post.

The city, however, affords no more suitable building and location for the purpose.

Medical supplies are received from the medical purveyor at New York.

Malarious fevers are the prevailing diseases at this post. They may be said to be endemic through the country at large. Cases at this place are generally of a mild type. Though met with occasionally, congestive fever is rare.

*Meteorological report, Columbia, S. C., 1872–'74.*

| Month. | 1870–'71. | | | | 1871–'72. | | | | 1872–'73. | | | | 1873–'74. | | | |
|---|---|---|---|---|---|---|---|---|---|---|---|---|---|---|---|---|
| | Temperature. | | | Rain-fall in inches. | Temperature. | | | Rain-fall in inches. | Temperature. | | | Rain-fall in inches. | Temperature. | | | Rain-fall in inches. |
| | Mean. | Max. | Min. | | Mean. | Max. | Min. | | Mean. | Max. | Min. | | Mean. | Max. | Min. | |
| | ° | ° | ° | ° | ° | ° | ° | ° | ° | ° | ° | | ° | ° | ° | |
| July | | | | | | | | | 82.71 | 99 | 74 | 6.65 | 81.37 | 96 | 72 | 7.50 |
| August | | | | | | | | | 80.49 | 97 | 65 | 5.05 | 79.69 | 96 | 71 | 9.74 |
| September | | | | | | | | | 76.90 | 97 | 57 | 0.60 | 74.65 | 93 | 60 | 9.70 |
| October | | | | | | | | | 62.65 | 88 | 36 | 2.51 | 61.78 | 84 | 34 | 0.80 |
| November | | | | | | | | | 49.22 | 70 | 18 | 3.80 | 51.77 | 73 | 26 | 4.63 |
| December | | | | | | | | | 41.93 | 66 | 18 | 3.30 | 48.44 | 74 | 22 | 2.62 |
| January | | | | | | | | | 45.46 | 72 | 17 | 3.85 | 50.23 | 72 | 25 | 4.29 |
| February | | | | | | | | | 51.47 | 72 | 32 | 4.60 | 49.70 | 77 | 32 | 5.54 |
| March | | | | | | | | | 53.09 | 80 | 20 | 2.21 | 58.68 | 85 | 36 | 4.28 |
| April | | | | | | | | | 65.80 | 92 | 43 | 1.85 | 63.51 | 83 | 44 | 7.41 |
| May | | | | | | | | | 73.34 | 91 | 58 | 1.09 | 72.99 | 96 | 53 | 2.10 |
| June | | | | | | | | | 79.08 | 93 | 58 | 5.66 | 82.79 | 98 | 68 | 6.24 |
| For the year | | | | | | | | | 63.51 | 99 | 17 | 41.17 | 64.61 | 98 | 22 | 64.85 |

*Consolidated sick-report, Columbia, S. C., 1870–'74.*

| Year | | 1870–'71. | | 1871–'72. | | 1872–'73. | | 1873–'74. | |
|---|---|---|---|---|---|---|---|---|---|
| Mean strength | { Officers<br>{ Enlisted men | 9<br>171 | | 13<br>194 | | 14<br>213 | | 19<br>307 | |
| Diseases. | | Cases. | Deaths. | Cases. | Deaths. | Cases. | Deaths. | Cases. | Deaths. |
| GENERAL DISEASES, A. | | | | | | | | | |
| Typhoid fever | | | | 1 | | | | 1 | 1 |
| Typho-malarial fever | | 2 | | 5 | 1 | | | | |
| Remittent fever | | 4 | | 18 | | 35 | | 42 | |
| Intermittent fever | | 48 | | 104 | 2 | 149 | | 188 | |
| Other diseases of this group | | 9 | | 8 | | 17 | | 11 | 1 |
| GENERAL DISEASES, B. | | | | | | | | | |
| Rheumatism | | 15 | | 21 | | 29 | | 26 | |
| Syphilis | | 47 | | 33 | | 26 | | 18 | |
| Consumption | | 3 | | 2 | | 1 | 1 | 2 | 1 |
| Other diseases of this group | | 1 | | | | 8 | | | |
| LOCAL DISEASES. | | | | | | | | | |
| Catarrh and bronchitis | | 20 | | 21 | | 54 | | 4 | |
| Pneumonia | | | 1 | 1 | | 3 | 1 | | |
| Pleurisy | | | | 1 | | | | | |
| Diarrhœa and dysentery | | 55 | 1 | 29 | | 57 | | 80 | |
| Hernia | | | | | | 1 | | | |
| Gonorrhœa | | 15 | | 10 | | 11 | | 16 | |
| Other local diseases | | 82 | 1 | 65 | 1 | 131 | | 168 | 1 |
| Alcoholism | | 7 | | 6 | | 7 | | 9 | |
| Total disease | | 303 | 3 | 325 | 4 | 529 | 2 | 565 | 4 |
| VIOLENT DISEASES AND DEATHS. | | | | | | | | | |
| Gunshot wounds | | 1 | | 1 | | | | 1 | |
| Drowning | | | | | | | | | 1 |
| Other accidents and injuries | | 64 | | 57 | | 34 | 1 | 48 | |
| Total violence | | 65 | | 58 | | 34 | 1 | 49 | 1 |

# DUPRE'S TOWER, LOUISIANA.

Construction commenced in 1829 on the right bank of Bayou Dupre, Lake Borgne, near New Orleans, in latitude 29° 55' north, longitude 12° 37' west, approximately. Not now occupied.

# FRANKFORT, KENTUCKY.

REPORT OF ASSISTANT SURGEON P. MIDDLETON, UNITED STATES ARMY.

The city of Frankfort, the capital of Kentucky, is a handsome town situated on the right (or N. E.) bank of Kentucky River, in latitude 38° 14′ north, longitude 7° 37′ west, 24 miles W. N. W. of Lexington and 53 miles E. of Louisville. A military post was established in April, 1871, at the base of one of the hills that surround the city on the land side. The ground was leased from a private citizen, who erected the necessary buildings. The principal of these are four brick buildings designed for barracks, although only one is now required for that purpose. The one now occupied by the troops is 116 by 32 feet and allows an air-space of 650 feet per man. One building, 100 by 32 feet, is used for offices and store-rooms; and another, of the same dimensions, is partitioned off into rooms 16 feet square for laundresses' quarters. The remaining barrack, 116 by 32 feet, is now fitted up as a post hospital. The dormitories are well lighted and ventilated by windows opposite, and heated by stoves. Single iron bedsteads are used.

The officers reside in the city of Frankfort, no quarters having been provided for them.

The hospital ward is 52 by 32 feet, ceiled, but not plastered. It is well lighted and ventilated by opposite windows and warmed by stoves; contains 8 beds, with an air-space of 9,000 feet. Adjoining is a store-room, 28 by 32 feet. At one end of the building the dispensary and steward's room are partitioned off, and at the other the kitchen and mess-room.

The guard-house consists of two rooms, each 16 feet square, one for the guard and one for prisoners. They are in the basement underneath the laundresses' quarters. They are well lighted and ventilated by windows.

An abundant supply of water is obtained from a spring on the grounds. It is, however, rather strongly impregnated with salts of lime.

# FORT GAINES, ALABAMA.

The present works were commenced in 1848, on the site of old Fort Tombigbee, on Dauphin Island, in Mobile Bay; latitude, 30° 13′ north; longitude, 10° 56′ west. The fort is in charge of an ordnance sergeant.

# HUMBOLDT, TENNESSEE, SWAYNE BARRACKS.

REPORT OF ASSISTANT SERGEON B. F. POPE, UNITED STATES ARMY.

The post of Humboldt, or Swayne Barracks, as it was formerly called, is one-half mile north of the town of Humboldt; latitude, 35° 47′ 28″ north; longitude, 10° 50′ 41″ west; elevation above the sea, 368 feet.

The town of Humboldt is at the junction of the Louisville and Memphis and the Mobile and Ohio Railroads, and contains about 2,300 inhabitants. The surrounding country is undulating; the staple crops are cotton and corn. The principal duties of the garrison have been to furnish detachments to assist civil officers in the discharge of their duties. The reservation of about 10 acres is leased by the Government. It is a knoll or hill giving good natural drainage. The geological formation of this part of the country is, for the most part, the Orange sand, or La Grange

17 M P

Group, belonging to the tertiary. The ferruginous sands, of which this is composed, give rise to chalybeate springs.

The barrack is a one-story wooden building 269 by 30 feet, with an L at each end 30 by 30. It is boxed on a balloon frame, weather-stripped and shingled, and raised on posts at one end from 7 to 9 feet.

The dormitories are furnished with single iron bedsteads; allow about 790 cubic feet space per man; are badly ventilated; cannot be well heated in cold weather, and are in bad condition. This building also contains laundresses' quarters, kitchen, mess-room, office, store-room, &c.

The officers' quarters are in a frame building 96 by 32 feet, with a veranda 8 feet wide on the north and east. It contains 12 rooms, each 16 by 16 feet, plastered, ceiled, and painted. At one end the building is elevated on posts about 6 feet from the ground, giving a desirable sub-floor ventilation in summer, but making it almost impossible to keep warm in winter. The kitchens are in a detached building, 20 by 16 feet, in rear of the quarters. These building are in bad condition.

The hospital is a frame building 52 by 20 feet, and about 9 feet high. The ward is 25 feet 11 inches by 19 feet 3 inches, and contains 5 beds, giving to each 723 cubic feet. The hospital has no bath-room, mess-room, nor closets.

The guard-house is 24 by 16 feet, divided into a guard-room, 16 by 13 feet, and two cells, 11 by 11 and 11 by 15 feet.

The cells are close boxes, with auger-holes in ceilings, floors, and sides. They are not lighted. During the still, hot nights of summer the sufferings of the prisoners are very great. As many as thirteen suffocating wretches have been locked at once into these sweat-boxes, which are entirely unfit for their purpose.

The military store-house is 50 by 30 feet, and in better repair than any other building at the post.

The water-supply is from three wells, is sufficient, and of fair quality. It contains about 60 grains of solid matter to the gallon, chiefly sand and clay. In this vicinity there is a belief in water filtered through a non-calcareous alluvium, as a protective against epidemic cholera. The exemption of this locality from the disease is certainly remarkable.

*Meteorological report, Humboldt, Tenn., 1870–'74.*

| Month. | 1870–'71. | | | | 1871–'72. | | | | 1872–'73. | | | | 1873–'74. | | | |
|---|---|---|---|---|---|---|---|---|---|---|---|---|---|---|---|---|
| | Temperature. | | | Rain-fall in inches. | Temperature. | | | Rain-fall in inches. | Temperature. | | | Rain-fall in inches. | Temperature. | | | Rain-fall in inches. |
| | Mean. | Max. | Min. | | Mean. | Max. | Min. | | Mean. | Max. | Min. | | Mean. | Max. | Min. | |
| July ............... | 83.66 | 98 | 69 | 1.70 | 81.80 | 98 | 67 | 3.00 | 81.03 | 98* | 61* | 4.88 | 80.82 | 95* | 58* | 3.75 |
| August............. | 81.77 | 96 | 63 | 5.80 | 80.85 | 104 | 61 | 4.40 | 80.23 | 101* | 50* | 1.09 | 78.88 | 97* | 52* | 3.46 |
| September.......... | 77.63 | 91 | 54 | 1.75 | 71.04 | 89 | 44* | 0.80 | 71.67 | 96* | 40* | 1.87 | 71.64 | 97* | 42* | 2.56 |
| October ........... | 62.92 | 84 | 41 | 5.50 | 63.50 | 80* | 44* | 6.06 | 58.13 | 88* | 30* | 2.66 | 55.07 | 85* | 20* | 5.19 |
| November.......... | 50.30 | 74 | 28 | 1.62 | 50.06 | 75* | 27* | 10.57 | 42.47 | 69* | 9* | 1.97 | 48.57 | 71* | 14* | 3.48 |
| December .......... | 37.16 | 68 | 4 | 4.75 | 39.13 | 72* | 7* | 2.72 | 29.47 | 62* | — 3* | 5.92 | 44.22 | 72* | 18* | 5.48 |
| January............ | 43.85 | 68 | 18 | 5.00 | 34.14 | 70* | 2* | 2.07 | 33.76 | 65* | — 8* | 14.55 | 42.65 | 66* | 9* | 4.73 |
| February........... | 50.58 | 77 | 29 | 5.35 | 41.99 | 72* | 16* | 2.30 | 42.76 | 70* | 11* | 10.26 | 44.70 | 72* | 20* | 4.82 |
| March............. | 56.90 | 79 | 29 | 8.60 | 45.44 | 74* | 16* | 2.30 | 48.56 | 73* | 11* | 5.06 | 52.75 | 82* | 27* | 6.36 |
| April.............. | 66.94 | 84 | 40 | 2.60 | 63.25 | 89* | 31* | 7.79 | 59.23 | 88* | 29* | 1.54 | 55.84 | 82* | 31* | 9.20 |
| May .............. | 72.14 | 92 | 52 | 3.50 | 69.94 | 89* | 39* | 4.46 | 69.56 | 91* | 45* | 9.56 | 73.10 | 98* | 41* | 0.82 |
| June .............. | 81.75 | 99 | 65 | 4.80 | 76.25 | 95* | 55* | 4.15 | 78.87 | 95* | 62* | 6.04 | 83.10 | 104* | 54* | 2.42 |
| For the year..... | 63.80 | 99 | 4 | 50.97 | 59.78 | 104 | 2* | 50.62 | 57.98 | 101* | — 8* | 65.40 | 60.94 | 104* | 9* | 52.2 |

* These observations are made with self-registering thermometers. The mean is from the standard thermometer.

*Consolidated-sick report, Humboldt, Tenn., 1870–'74.*

| Year | | 1870-'71. | | 1871-'72. | | 1872-'73. | | 1873-'74. | |
|---|---|---|---|---|---|---|---|---|---|
| Mean strength { Officers | | 2 | | 3 | | 3 | | 4 | |
| { Enlisted men | | 48 | | 47 | | 48 | | 52 | |
| **Diseases.** | | Cases. | Deaths. | Cases. | Deaths. | Cases. | Deaths. | Cases. | Deaths. |
| GENERAL DISEASES, A. | | | | | | | | | |
| Typhoid fever | | | | 1 | 1 | | | | |
| Typho-malarial fever | | 2 | | | | | | | |
| Remittent fever | | 6 | | | | 2 | | 8 | |
| Intermittent fever | | 12 | | 35 | | 69 | | 43 | |
| Other diseases of this group | | 1 | | 3 | | 1 | | 2 | |
| GENERAL DISEASES, B. | | | | | | | | | |
| Rheumatism | | 3 | | 9 | | 11 | | 9 | |
| Syphilis | | | | 13 | | 5 | | 2 | |
| Consumption | | 4 | | | | | | | |
| Other diseases of this group | | 3 | | | | | | | |
| LOCAL DISEASES. | | | | | | | | | |
| Catarrh and bronchitis | | 1 | | 13 | | 5 | | 7 | |
| Pneumonia | | 1 | | 2 | | | | | |
| Pleurisy | | | | 3 | | | | | |
| Diarrhœa and dysentery | | 8 | | 16 | | 24 | | 25 | |
| Gonorrhœa | | 4 | | 7 | | 3 | | | |
| Other local diseases | | 23 | | 27 | | 49 | | 26 | |
| Alcoholism | | 1 | | 3 | | 5 | | 13 | |
| Total disease | | 69 | | 132 | 1 | 174 | | 135 | |
| VIOLENT DISEASES AND DEATHS. | | | | | | | | | |
| Gunshot wounds | | | | 1 | | | | 1 | |
| Other accidents and injuries | | 5 | 1 | 6 | | 15 | 1 | 13 | |
| Homicide | | | | | | | | | 1 |
| Total violence | | 5 | 1 | 7 | | 15 | 1 | 14 | 1 |

# HUNTSVILLE, ALABAMA, THOMAS BARRACKS.

### REPORT OF ASSISTANT SURGEON C. R. GREENLEAF, UNITED STATES ARMY.

This post is about two miles northeast of the city of Huntsville, Alabama; latitude, 34° 45′ north; longitude, 9° 44′ west; 600 feet above the sea, and 75 feet above the valley of Huntsville.

The barracks are two frame buildings, designed to quarter one company each. When the post was built all the quarters and store-houses were put together in a very inferior manner, and upon insufficient foundations, so much so that they were constantly settling, warping joints and timbers out of place, and necessitating frequent repairs to make them safe for habitation. Upon one occasion the company quarters had fallen so much out of plumb that they had to be replaced by block and tackle, and extensively braced.

Owing to the slope of the hill the company quarters are built on brick piers 10 feet high. The large space thus left beneath made them very cold. Recently this has been boarded up under the west set, and a new wash-room made under the kitchen and store-room. The company quarters are ceiled inside, and divided into the following rooms, viz: first sergeant's quarters, 12 by 13 feet; quarters for the men, 114 by 20 feet; dining-room, 20 by 23 feet; kitchen, 20 by 16 feet; store-room, 12¼ by 6¾ feet; height of all, 11 feet. Covered porches 12 by 8 feet have quite recently been built over the doors on the west side of the west set of quarters, and on the front of each set is a porch running the whole length of the building. They are warmed by two stoves burning coal, lighted by six windows on opposite sides of the building, and ventilated by three ventilators in the roofs. The rooms are open from the floor to the roof. The air-space for each company of 50 men is 507 feet per man. The quarters are supplied with single iron bedsteads. Privies are located 300 feet south of the barracks, built over sinks 8 feet deep, well calculated for the purpose. The seats have self-closing covers, and the vaults are ventilated. The buildings were erected on the recommendation of the post surgeon.

The laundresses' quarters are 12 rooms 12 by 14 feet, built of wood, like the barracks, without interior ceiling or plastering, although authority has lately been received for ceiling them. Over the doors of the west set, on the south side, covered porches have been built. One set is now in temporary use as a carpenter's shop, and another as guard-house.

The officers' quarters are four frame buildings, three double, and one single, which has been used by the medical officer. They are built of wood, one story high, a very plain finish inside, and undressed weather-boarding. The lumber was unseasoned when put up, and, as a result, the panels have nearly shrunken out of the doors, and all the interior wood-work shrunken equally. The double houses are divided through the middle by parallel halls 5½ feet wide. The suites of quarters for captains consist of three rooms, namely, a front room, 15 by 16 feet, and 10½ feet high, middle room of same size, and a dining-room or kitchen, 10 by 12 feet and 9½ feet high. The subalterns' quarters consist of two rooms, the same size and arrangements as those in the captains' quarters. The set of single quarters consist of a single building divided into three rooms of the same size and arrangements as those of the captains' quarters, and one hall 32 feet long, 6 feet wide. The halls in all the double buildings are without light, except when the doors are open. Heating is by stoves and small fire-places burning wood. The fire-places were wholly inadequate for the purpose during the cold weather. In rear of the quarters small temporary sheds have been built for kitchen purposes. Drinking-water is obtained from a large tank a few feet in rear of the quarters, and washing-water from a cistern close by, which is supplied with a chain-pump. The privies are built 75 feet in rear of the quarters, over deep sinks; they are really the best constructed buildings about the post.

The offices and store-rooms are in a large frame building on the south front of the post, 45 by 46 feet, divided by a hall 7 feet wide, on each side of which are four rooms, 18 by 20 feet, used as headquarters, adjutant's office, quartermaster and commissary officers; a wing on each side of the main building, 50 by 28 feet, is used as quartermaster and commissary store-rooms.

There is no guard-house at the post; a set of laundresses' quarters is temporarily used, but is not suited for the purpose; the rooms are, however, well ventilated, but indifferently heated; average occupancy, 2.

The hospital is a frame building, 35 by 35 feet, two stories high, with a ward 24 by 32 feet, built on the east end to accommodate twelve beds, giving an air-space per man of 975 feet. On the east end of the ward are the bath and wash rooms, 9½ by 10½ feet, each separated by a hall 5 feet wide. The lower floor of the main building is divided by a hall, 5 by 15 feet, on each side of which are four rooms, 15 by 15 feet, used respectively as dispensary, office, attendants' and dining room. At the end of the hall is the kitchen, 15 by 15 feet. A hall, 5 by 15 feet, cuts the main hall at right angles, and affords passage from the ward to the stairway leading to the second story. All the rooms in the hospital are warmed by stoves and lighted naturally by windows and artificially by lard-oil lamps. The second story is divided by a passage-way, 5 by 35 feet, on each side of which are three rooms used as store-rooms and quarters for the steward. The privies are in rear of the hospital, and, like those in other parts of the post, well adapted for the purpose for which they were built. Upon the recommendation of the post-surgeon a veranda, 8 feet wide, was built all around the hospital, and the building, which was very much out of repair and badly settled, was put in as complete order as possible. Opposite the kitchen a large tank is built, capable of holding 1,500 gallons, which supplies the hospital with rain-water for cooking and washing purposes.

The post bakery, 15 by 38 feet, is made of old lumber set upright, ceiled inside, and has a moderately good oven. There is no laundry, chapel, or school-house, the orderly room, in vacant quarters, being used for latter purposes.

The post library consists of about one hundred volumes of a miscellaneous character. Several magazines and newspapers are taken.

The water supply is excellent, and is obtained from a spring in hill in rear and above the garrison; it contains, however, a considerable percentage of lime. The water is carried into the post through wooden pipes laid under ground for a distance of 500 feet from the spring to the edge of a ravine in rear of the officers' quarters, and thence over a trestle-work 550 feet in length and 27 feet high, to a tank on the north line of the garrison; thence 534 feet, through pipes laid under ground, to a tank on the south line of the garrison; thence, about 50 feet under ground, to the stables, from which the wastage runs into the valley below. The capacity of the tank in rear of the officers quarters is 3,200 gallons, which furnishes an ample supply to the officers and their families, and also means of extinguishing fires in the quarters through a fire-play attachment at its base. The tank on the south line has a capacity of 1,600 gallons and furnishes water to the men, laundresses, and hospital through a wooden spigot. Between the two tanks, and in the center of the parade, the main-pipe is tapped by a small service-pipe and a very pretty fountain of water is constantly playing. The entire length of piping from the spring to the outflow is a little over 1,600 feet. The tanks can be emptied and cleaned at any time, and are washed out as often as occasion requires to keep them perfectly clean, and furnish a supply of pure water at all times.

In addition to this supply of spring water there are three large cisterns, one in rear of each set of company quarters, and one in rear of the officers' quarters; rain-water is supplied to them from the roofs through tin gutters and pipes, and is drawn by chain-pumps.

A garden of about 4 acres is cultivated by detail from the command, and an abundance of vegetables of all kinds raised for the use of the entire command, the post-garden supplying the officers and their families and the hospital.

The natural drainage is excellent. No artificial drainage.

The rations are of good quality and ample quantity. There is a fair market in Huntsville. Milk costs 10 cents per quart; butter, 25 to 50 cents per pound; eggs, 15 to 40 cents per dozen; chickens, 20 to 40 cents each; turkeys, 75 cents to $1 each; potatoes, 75 cents to $1.50 per bushel; sweet-potatoes, 75 cents to $1; apples raised in this section, $1.50 per bushel; those from the North, $6 per barrel.

Communication with Huntsville, the nearest railroad station, is by means of a spring-wagon; mails arrive and depart once daily; length of time to reach department headquarters by letter, two days; Washington, three days.

During warm weather dysentery, diarrhœa, and intermittent fevers prevail, and during the winter months influenza, catarrh, intermittents, and a mild form of muscular rheumatism of a malarial origin, and a few cases of diseases of the pulmonary organs.

The climate is particularly healthy, and the beautiful location of the garrison ought to make this one of the most salubrious stations in the country.

The geological formation belongs to the carboniferous period; the blue limestone rocks, sometimes designated as the cavernous limestone of this region, crop out within, above, and below the garrison inclosure. The soil is clay, thoroughly impregnated with iron, and has the intensely red color of this mountainous region.

Deer, foxes, raccoons, rabbits, squirrels, wild-turkeys, quails, pigeons, &c., abound in the neighboring mountains.

*Consolidated sick-report, Thomas Barracks, Ala., 1870–'74.*

| Year | | 1870–'71. | | 1871–'72. | | 1872–'73. | | 1873–'74. | |
|---|---|---|---|---|---|---|---|---|---|
| Mean strength | Officers | 8 | | 4 | | 4 | | 4 | |
| | Enlisted men | 157 | | 63 | | 54 | | 53 | |
| Diseases. | | Cases. | Deaths. | Cases. | Deaths. | Cases. | Deaths. | Cases. | Deaths. |
| GENERAL DISEASES, A. | | | | | | | | | |
| Remittent fever | | 1 | | | | | | | |
| Intermittent fever | | 93 | | 17 | | 24 | | 8 | |
| Other diseases of this group | | 40 | | 7 | | 10 | | 3 | |
| GENERAL DISEASES, B. | | | | | | | | | |
| Rheumatism | | 24 | | 6 | | 10 | | 4 | |
| Syphilis | | 8 | | 4 | | 2 | | 5 | |
| Other diseases of this group | | 1 | | | | | | | |
| LOCAL DISEASES. | | | | | | | | | |
| Catarrh and bronchitis | | 18 | | 5 | | 15 | | 5 | |
| Pneumonia | | 1 | 1 | | | | | | |
| Pleurisy | | 4 | | 2 | | 1 | | | |
| Diarrhœa and dysentery | | 47 | | 14 | | 17 | | 9 | |
| Hernia | | 2 | | 1 | | | | | |
| Gonorrhœa | | 8 | | 1 | | 2 | | 4 | |
| Other local diseases | | 115 | 2 | 39 | | 30 | | 17 | |
| Alcoholism | | 3 | | 2 | | | | 2 | |
| Total disease | | 365 | 3 | 98 | | 111 | | 57 | |
| VIOLENT DISEASES AND DEATHS. | | | | | | | | | |
| Gunshot wounds | | 2 | | | | | | | |
| Other accidents and injuries | | 56 | 1 | 15 | | 14 | | 11 | |
| Total violence | | 58 | 1 | 15 | | 14 | | 11 | |

# JACKSON, MISSISSIPPI.

REPORT OF ACTING ASSISTANT SURGEON THEODORE ARTAUD, UNITED STATES ARMY.

Jackson, the capital of the State of Mississippi, is situated on Pearl River, on the line of the Jackson, New Orleans and Great Northern Railroad, about 183 miles north by east of New Orleans. Latitude, 32° 18′ north; longitude, 13° 7′ west. The altitude above the level of the Gulf is about 175 feet.

The military post of Jackson occupies an elevated spot of about 15 acres on the west and adjoining the corporate limits of the city. It was established in the spring of 1867, and the necessary buildings, which are all of wood, were erected in the course of the summer.

The soldiers' quarters are for three companies, and consist of two buildings, the one 300 feet, the other 150 feet in length. They are 25 feet in width, 12 feet high to the eaves, and 18 feet to the ridge, and are raised from 2 to 3 feet from the ground upon posts. In the center of the large building are two kitchens and two mess-rooms, each being 25 by 20 feet. The remainder of the building serves as dormitories for two companies. These are provided with single iron bunks, large wood-stoves, and ridge ventilation, in addition to eight windows to each dormitory. The building is whitewashed outside and inside, and kept neat and clean. The smaller building is similar, except that an office and store-room are partitioned off at one end, and that the kitchen and mess-room occupy a detached building, extending back from the center of the main barrack. The average air-space per man is 761 feet.

There are six sets of officers' quarters. They are small separate cottages, raised on brick piers. Each set consists of two rooms in addition to kitchens and separate store-rooms or servants' rooms, except that of the commanding officer, which includes three rooms. The rooms vary from 18 by 18 feet to 16 by 10 feet, and are 10 feet in height.

A post bakery was built in October, 1873.

The guard-house is a log building, 24 by 18 by 18 feet, divided into two rooms for prisoners and one for the guard. These are lighted by five small windows, and warmed by three stoves in winter. The ventilation is imperfect; the average occupancy, seven.

The hospital consists of a main building, 100 by 20 feet, and 18 feet in height to the ridge, with an extension back from the center 40 by 14 feet. The ward, 72 by 20 feet, occupies the center of the main building. This ward contains fourteen beds, although the space is sufficient for twenty. Sixteen feet at the northern end of the building is partitioned off and subdivided into a dispensary and steward's room, which are of equal dimensions. A space of 12 feet at the other end, formerly separated as a smaller ward, is now used for a bath-room. The rear building is divided into store-room, dining-room, and kitchen. A veranda runs along the entire front and rear of the main building and the south side of the projecting portion.

The sinks, four in number, conveniently located, are buildings 7 by 12 feet, over pits 7 feet deep, which are frequently disinfected with carbolic acid and lime. The contents are removed at intervals to a pit at a distance from the camp and further disinfected.

The soil being a light, sandy, porous loam, does not retain water to stagnate upon the surface, and three surface-drains are found sufficient to carry off all surplus moisture. The camp is frequently and thoroughly policed by fatigue parties and by prisoners from the guard-house and by convicts from the State penitentiary.

The water-supply is obtained from cisterns and hauled about a mile in tanks from the Pearl River.

*Meteorological report, Jackson, Miss., 1873–'74.*

| Month. | 1870–'71. Temperature. Mean. | Max. | Min. | Rain-fall in inches. | 1871–'72. Temperature. Mean. | Max. | Min. | Rain-fall in inches. | 1872–'73. Temperature. Mean. | Max. | Min. | Rain-fall in inches. | 1873–'74. Temperature. Mean. | Max. | Min. | Rain-fall in inches. |
|---|---|---|---|---|---|---|---|---|---|---|---|---|---|---|---|---|
| July | | | | | | | | | | | | | 81.75 | 94* | 64* | 6.52 |
| August | | | | | | | | | | | | | 81.61 | 101* | 61* | 7.02 |
| September | | | | | | | | | | | | | 77.47 | 101* | 41* | 2.12 |
| October | | | | | | | | | | | | | 62.27 | 99* | 18* | 2.02 |
| November | | | | | | | | | | | | | 55.58 | 86* | 15* | 4.02 |
| December | | | | | | | | | | | | | 51.34 | 81* | 10* | 1.74 |
| January | | | | | | | | | | | | | 51.24 | 73* | 20* | 4.64 |
| February | | | | | | | | | | | | | 54.87 | 80* | 20* | 2.50 |
| March | | | | | | | | | | | | | 62.56 | 88* | 32* | 10.08 |
| April | | | | | | | | | | | | | 62.03 | 84* | 29* | 23.80 |
| May | | | | | | | | | 73.62 | 88* | 55* | 4.20 | 76.59 | 100* | 41* | 1.14 |
| June | | | | | | | | | 79.78 | 90* | 66* | 5.02 | 83.49 | 101* | 60* | 2.68 |
| For the year | | | | | | | | | | | | | 66.73 | 101 | 10 | 68.28 |

* These observations are made with self-registering thermometers. The mean is from the standard thermometer.

*Consolidated sick-report, Jackson, Miss., 1870–'74.*

| Year | 1870–'71. Cases. | Deaths. | 1871–'72. Cases. | Deaths. | 1872–'73. Cases. | Deaths. | 1873–'74. Cases. | Deaths. |
|---|---|---|---|---|---|---|---|---|
| Mean strength { Officers | 7 | | 7 | | 6 | | 6 | |
| { Enlisted men | 133 | | 105 | | 98 | | 106 | |
| **Diseases.** | | | | | | | | |
| GENERAL DISEASES, A. | | | | | | | | |
| Small-pox and varioloid | | | | | 3 | 2 | | |
| Typho-malarial fever | 3 | | | | | | | |
| Remittent fever | 12 | | 5 | | 2 | | 6 | |
| Intermittent fever | 150 | 1 | 93 | 1 | 80 | 1 | 268 | 1 |
| Yellow fever | | | 25 | 18 | | | | |
| Diphtheria | | | | | 1 | | | |
| Other diseases of this group | 6 | | 2 | | | | 3 | |
| GENERAL DISEASES, B. | | | | | | | | |
| Rheumatism | 7 | | 9 | | 11 | | 26 | |
| Syphilis | 17 | | 11 | | 14 | | 12 | |
| Consumption | 2 | 1 | | | | | | |
| Other diseases of this group | | | | | | | 1 | |
| LOCAL DISEASES. | | | | | | | | |
| Catarrh and bronchitis | 9 | | 7 | | 9 | | 5 | |
| Pneumonia | | | 1 | | | | 1 | |
| Pleurisy | | | 1 | | 1 | | | |
| Diarrhœa and dysentery | 22 | | 26 | | 41 | | 46 | |
| Hernia | | | | | 1 | | | |
| Gonorrhœa | 4 | | 4 | | 8 | | 6 | |
| Other local diseases | 33 | 1 | 36 | 1 | 56 | 1 | 61 | 1 |
| Alcoholism | 1 | | 3 | | 15 | | 18 | |
| Total diseases | 266 | 3 | 223 | 20 | 242 | 4 | 453 | 2 |
| VIOLENT DISEASES AND DEATHS. | | | | | | | | |
| Gunshot wounds | 3 | | 6 | | 1 | | | |
| Other accidents and injuries | 36 | | 33 | | 22 | 1 | 59 | |
| Total violence | 39 | | 39 | | 23 | 1 | 59 | |

# JACKSON BARRACKS, LOUISIANA.

INFORMATION FURNISHED BY SURGEON B. A. CLEMENTS AND ASSISTANT SURGEON V. B. HUBBARD, UNITED STATES ARMY.

The post of Jackson Barracks is situated on the left bank of the Mississippi River, three miles below the center of the city of New Orleans, La., in latitude 29° 57′ north, longitude 12° 57′ west; altitude, 10 feet. The land was purchased in 1833, and the buildings erected in 1834–'35, the purpose probably being the defense of the people of New Orleans and vicinity in the event of a servile insurrection.

The buildings are well constructed of brick and granite. The quarters for enlisted men consist of four separate buildings, two stories high, each 53 by 32 feet, and surrounded with a spacious veranda. They are heated by open fire-places, and lighted and ventilated by large windows. The dormitories are all on the second floor. Each contains 20,187 cubic feet of air-space, with an average occupancy of about 45 men, giving 440 cubic feet of air-space per man. The doors and windows are large, and during a great part of the year the majority of the men sleep on the veranda. The dormitories are fitted up with iron bedsteads and bed-sacks, the straw of which is changed once a month.

The post is designed to accommodate four companies of infantry, and its arrangement, including that of the hospital, is shown by Figure 27.

A, headquarters; B, chaplain's quarters; C C, officers' quarters; D, quartermasters' quarters; E, surgeon's quarters; F, assistant surgeon's quarters; H H H H, barracks; I, prison; K, commissary store-house; L, barrack bakery; M, engine-house; N N N, hospital; O, tower; P, dining-room; R, kitchens; S, hospital bakery; T, ordnance-sergeant and hospital steward's quarters; V V, privies; W, laundry.

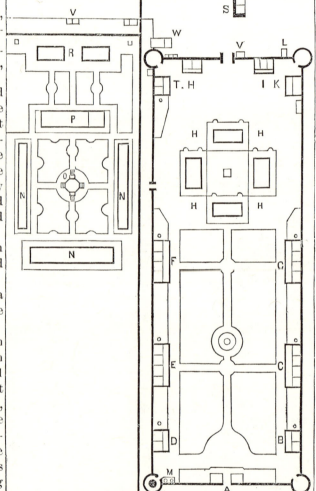

There are no wash or bath rooms, and the men wash near the cisterns. There are two large sinks, built of brick, about 8 feet deep, sloping on all sides toward the bottom, and lined with cement; they are cleaned through a trap opening from the level of the ground into the sink. They are disinfected twice daily; are provided with two urinals each, and are good and convenient.

The kitchens and mess-rooms are all on the first floor of the buildings, well adapted and furnished with the usual furniture.

Quarters for married soldiers are in a building similar to those occupied by the troops, 45 by 21 feet, and two stories high.

The officers' quarters are contained in seven two-story buildings, two of which measure 42 by 21 feet, and five 82 by 21 feet, divided into rooms about 18 feet square. They are very substantially built, though now somewhat out of repair. There are forty-eight rooms in all, of which one-half are on the first floor, and one half on the second, the former being used for kitchens and dining-rooms, and the latter for living apartments.

Figure 27.—Scale, 195 feet to 1 inch.

The building designed for quarters of commanding officer fronts the river, and has four rooms on the second floor and four on the lower. The buildings for other officers' quarters are on the long sides of the post, opposite, and similar to each other. The two nearest the commanding officer's quarters contain each two rooms up-stairs and two down, with a small yard adjacent. There are two more buildings on each side of the post, each containing four rooms on the upper and lower floors, with small yards at each end.

As the main wall of the post forms one of the sides of the rooms in the lower stories of the officers' quarters, and appears to have been made with a view to defense alone, there are no windows except at the front in these lower rooms; hence they are deficient in ventilation, and generally dark. River-water is supplied to the rooms, both up and down stairs, through pipes leading from the large tank in the tower at the southwest angle of the post. There is one cistern to each building. Water closets are situated in the yards; they are brick sinks, cleaned through a trap in the floor. The want of natural drainage of course prevents the use of water in them.

The quartermaster and commissary store-house is a two-story building, 42 by 32 feet, constructed of granite and brick. A similar building, 32 by 14 feet, is used as an engine-house, and another, 42 by 21 feet, is occupied as quarters by the band. In addition, at each of the four angles of the main wall surrounding the post, there is a circular brick tower, 29 feet in diameter, and used as store-houses, &c.

The guard-house is a building 65 by 21 feet, and similar in construction to those described. Only the lower story of the building is used for guard purposes, and the cells consist of three of the following dimensions, viz: One, $20\frac{3}{4}$ feet long, 17 feet wide, and $11\frac{2}{3}$ feet high; two, $9\frac{2}{3}$ feet long, $8\frac{3}{4}$ feet wide, and $11\frac{2}{3}$ feet high. The ventilation of all is defective, and of the large cell very bad, there being no openings at all on one side of it, and on another only a grating above the door.

There is no provision for warming the building in winter. The three cells afford an aggregate air-space of 5,817 cubic feet, and at times as many as 56 men have been crowded into them at once, leaving but 103 cubic feet of air-space per man. The bad effects of this overcrowding are greatly aggravated in the event of sickness, even of a slight character, appearing among the prisoners. Recovery is almost impossible without removal from confinement. There are two large and well-constructed sinks for the use of the men. They are disinfected daily and kept in good order.

The hospital buildings and grounds are immediately adjacent to the post proper, and occupy about the same space. The buildings were erected in 1849, and are constructed of wood, two stories high, and arranged in the shape of a square, open at the angles. (See figure.) In front and nearest the river is an ornamental garden handsomely and thickly shaded with magnolia, cedar, pine, and other trees. The buildings are in number and dimensions as follows, viz: Three, 168 by 31 feet; one, 112 by 31 feet; two, 50 by 25 feet. The first three were intended for wards, the second for mess-rooms, quarters for nurses, &c., and the last mentioned for kitchens and quarters. Only one of the largest buildings is now occupied as a hospital. It is surrounded by a spacious veranda. There are two wards on the second floor, containing fourteen beds each, with a superficial area of 158 feet, and a cubic air-space of 1,554 feet to each bed. Sufficient ventilation is afforded by windows extending from near the ceiling to within 3 feet of the floor. The patients wash in basins at a sink on the veranda; but there is also an excellent bath-room recently constructed on the same floor and adjoining the wards. The hospital sink is at a distance of 75 yards; but earth-closets and close-stools are in use for patients unable to leave the building. In the center of the square formed by the four principal buildings is an octagonal structure, 27 feet in diameter, intended and used for a dispensary and office. An apartment in one of the detached buildings is used for the double purpose of kitchen and mess-room. The dead-house is a temporary hut, 13 by 8 by 10 feet in size, provided with table and buckets. Extensive repairs have been made during the present year on the building occupied as a hospital; the others are old and mostly so dilapidated that the demolition of a part of them has been recommended.

There is a post library kept in one of the hospital wards. It is made up of the *débris* of former general hospitals in the department, and numbers about 500 volumes, but few of which are standard works.

There is a large iron reservoir, containing about 40,000 gallons, in the tower at the southwest angle of the post, into which the water is pumped from the river by a steam-engine, and forced through pipes to all the post and hospital buildings; there are numerous fire-plugs throughout the grounds, and recently a better arrangement and larger amount of hose than formerly. There is one cistern of about 8,000 gallons capacity to each building of the officers' quarters, and two of 8,000 gallons each to each set of company quarters. There are also six cisterns, of 12,000 gallons capacity each, in the court of the hospital-buildings, and three others, capacity 8,000 gallons each,

18 M P

at the sutler's store, bakery, and ordnance-sergeant's quarters. The supply of water from the reservoir is only limited by the capacity of the steam-engine, and there is always an abundant supply of cistern water.

The general surface of the whole vicinity is but 10 feet above the level of the sea. The almost inappreciable natural drainage is from the river to the swamps in the rear, and is almost wholly inefficient. The grounds of the post proper, and the immediately adjacent hospital-grounds, are elevated artificially about 30 inches at the highest parts. Large brick-lined drains extend through the whole area of the post and hospital grounds, and are very skillfully constructed and adapted to the artificial elevation of the surface. There are no sewers. The drains discharge in the rear of the post, toward the swamps, and are entirely efficient in draining the post proper. Slops, offal, and excreta are dumped into the Mississippi River.

There are no arrangements for bathing, either in summer or winter. Good swimmers bathe after night in the river, in summer, but it is attended with danger.

Notwithstanding the extent of the reservation and the fertility of the soil, no vegetable gardens are cultivated at the post.

*Consolidated sick-report, Jackson Barracks, New Orleans, La., 1870–'74.*

| Year | | 1870–'71. | | 1871–'72. | | 1872–'73.* | | 1873–'74. | |
|---|---|---|---|---|---|---|---|---|---|
| Mean strength | { Officers | 12 | | 13 | | 18 | | 11 | |
| | { Enlisted men | 206 | | 233 | | 328 | | 208 | |
| Diseases. | | Cases. | Deaths. | Cases. | Deaths. | Cases. | Deaths. | Cases. | Deaths. |
| GENERAL DISEASES, A. | | | | | | | | | |
| Small-pox and varioloid | | | | | | | | 1 | 1 |
| Typhoid fever | | | | | | 1 | | 1 | |
| Remittent fever | | 3 | 1 | 3 | | 2 | | 5 | |
| Intermittent fever | | 96 | | 133 | | 176 | | 189 | |
| Yellow fever | | 8 | 3 | 1 | | | | | |
| Cholera | | | | 1 | | | | | |
| Other diseases of this group | | 7 | | 1 | | 13 | | 2 | |
| GENERAL DISEASES, B. | | | | | | | | | |
| Rheumatism | | 20 | | 18 | | 11 | | 9 | |
| Syphilis | | 23 | | 24 | | 29 | | 22 | |
| Consumption | | 2 | 2 | | | 2 | | 2 | |
| Other diseases of this group | | 1 | | 5 | | 1 | | 1 | |
| LOCAL DISEASES. | | | | | | | | | |
| Catarrh and bronchitis | | 21 | | 30 | | 117 | | 52 | |
| Pneumonia | | | | | 1 | 1 | 1 | | |
| Pleurisy | | 1 | | 2 | | 1 | | | |
| Diarrhœa and dysentery | | 107 | | 99 | | 129 | 2 | 83 | |
| Hernia | | | | | | 2 | | 1 | |
| Gonorrhœa | | 14 | | 25 | | 12 | | 5 | |
| Other local diseases | | 138 | 2 | 102 | 1 | 68 | 1 | 49 | |
| Alcoholism | | 15 | | 8 | 1 | 65 | | 37 | |
| Unclassified | | | | 2 | | | | | |
| Total disease | | 456 | 8 | 454 | 2 | 630 | 4 | 459 | 1 |
| VIOLENT DISEASES AND DEATHS. | | | | | | | | | |
| Gunshot wounds | | 1 | 2 | | | | | | |
| Other accidents and injuries | | 53 | | 65 | | 67 | | 58 | 1 |
| Suicide | | | 1 | | | | | | |
| Total violence | | 54 | 3 | 65 | | 67 | | 58 | 1 |

* Nine months only.

# POST OF FORTS JACKSON AND SAINT PHILIP, LOUISIANA.

### REPORT OF ASSISTANT SURGEON P. F. HARVEY, UNITED STATES ARMY.

Fort Jackson, the more important of the two forts constituting this post, is situated on the right bank of the Mississippi River, 32 nautical miles by river from the Gulf of Mexico, about 22 miles above the light-house at the head of the passes, and 65 miles in a southeast direction below New Orleans. The flag-staff of the fort is located in latitude 29° 21′ 30″.68 north, and longitude 12° 23′ 21″.46 west. The altitude of the post above the sea is but a few feet.

The quarantine station, for the protection of the State, is distant five miles up the river.

The reservation was made February 9, 1842, and comprises sections 5, 6, 7, 8, and 9, of township 20, range 30 east, of the southeastern district of Louisiana. It is composed entirely of swamp-lands, and during seasons of high water is almost completely inundated. That portion containing the fort, quarters, and other buildings, is leveed on all sides, but notwithstanding the protection thus afforded, there are times when the water rises so high as to become a source of great inconvenience in going about the garrison.

The soil is alluvial, and is covered during the greater part of the year with rank tropical vegetation. In the levee inclosure this growth is mowed from time to time and burned.

The soil is fertile, but to render it secure for tillage the greatest possible care is required in the erection and supervision of levees, in which the slightest leak readily becomes a crevasse.

Rain and river waters are used exclusively. The supply of the former is obtained from wooden reservoirs, built over ground adjoining the officers' quarters, barracks, and hospital. Of these there are seven capable of containing about 5,000 gallons each.

The fort is located on the bank of the river. The parade inside the fort and the surface of the river have generally a common level. The fort is a bastioned work surrounded by a wet ditch, with a second wet ditch exterior to the covered-way.

The quarters, barracks, and hospitals, at both Forts Jackson and Saint Philip, are built on brick piers between two and three feet high. The barracks consist of one frame building, lathed and plastered inside. The building is divided in the center by a hall, 24 by 11 feet, into two equal compartments, each measuring 70 by 24 feet, with a general height of 13½ feet. A covered gallery, 11 feet wide, surrounds the building.

The buildings for officers' quarters are four in number, a one-story frame building, 82 by 16 feet, containing four rooms and a kitchen, and three cottages, 45 by 18 feet, with ceilings 14 feet high.

The guard-house is situated in the fort. It comprises three rooms, viz: the guard-room, 13½ by 14½ feet; the prison, 17 by 20 feet; and the dungeon, 14½ by 7 feet, all having an average height of 8 feet; warmed, when occupied, by means of fire-places, and ventilated by one embrasure, 3 by 2 feet, and three doors.

The hospital, situated on the bank of the river, is 135 by 25 feet, constructed of boards placed vertically and battened; the ward, 65 by 24 feet, occupying the center. At one end are two lavatories, kitchen, dining-room, and pantry; the dispensary, steward's room, and store-room occupy the other.

The post was vacated July 7, 1871.

For a more detailed description see Circular No. 4, of 1870, page 168.

---

# FORT JEFFERSON, FLORIDA.

REPORTS OF ASSISTANT SURGEON S. A. STORROW, UNITED STATES ARMY, AND ACTING ASSISTANT SURGEON W. E. DAY, UNITED STATES ARMY.

Fort Jefferson is situated on Garden Key, one of the Tortugas group of islets, being the most southwestern part of the so-called Florida reefs. Latitude, 24° 37′ 47″ north; longitude, 5° 47′ west; about five hundred miles southeast of Fort Barrancas and seventy-five miles west-northwest from Key West. The light-house on Garden Key was built in 1825, and the building of the fort was commenced in 1846.

The key contains seven acres, five of which are within the walls of the fort, the remainder being a narrow spit of sand and coral.

The average height above the sea is 3½ feet, but an excavation over 2½ feet in depth develops the primitive coral and the salt-water of the Gulf. The soil consists of pulverized coral and sand.

The fort is a double-casemated, hexagonal structure of brick. The quarters for enlisted men are in a three-story brick building, 350 by 45 feet, which is not finished. The kitchens are in brick buildings in rear of the barracks, and there is a good bakery in one of the bastion casemates.

The married soldiers' quarters are in casemates, which are not well adapted for the purpose, being constantly damp from percolation from the parapet.

The officers' quarters are in a brick building, 272 by 42 feet, and three stories in height. It contains seventy-two rooms, averaging 15 by 18 feet, and 14 feet in height. The quarters are well finished and conveniently arranged. All buildings at the post are heated when necessary by open fire-places.

There is no bath-room at the post, either for officers or men. The temperature of the sea rarely falls below 70° F., hence it is almost always available for bathing purposes.

The casemates on each side of the sally-port have been used as a guard-house.

Five rooms in the barracks were used as a hospital during the last years of the occupancy of the post. Three of the rooms are large, having each a cubic capacity of 12,000 feet, and the remaining two are small rooms at the end of the halls, used as store-rooms. The large room on the first floor was used as office and dispensary; that on the second floor as a ward for twelve beds; while the room on the third floor was occupied by the hospital steward, when not required by the sick.

The water supply is from three sources: first, a steam condensing apparatus; second, cisterns within the fort which receive the drainage from the various buildings; and third, cisterns outside the fort. The condensed water is sweet and pure. The water in the cisterns under the casemates, which receive the drainage from the terre-plein, is so contaminated with lime salts as to be nearly unfit for use.

The main sewer follows the internal circumference of the fort, forming the same outline, having exits at the alternate bastions by lateral sewers which open into the moat without, below low-water mark. The depression of the exits below the main sewer is not sufficient to secure a ready transit of débris. The vaults of the privies are of little less depth than the sewer. The opening between is trapped, but this does not prevent the return of offensive gases into the water-closets.

It will be seen at once how imperfect must be the sewerage where the entrance and exit are so nearly on a level. To obviate this difficulty the sewers are flushed from the privies by a stream of water thrown through hose by steam power. This partially remedies the evil, but at all times a sheet of paper saturated with a solution of acetate of lead will blacken if suspended above the privy-seat.

There are no gardens at the post except a small one in the center, which is kept up more as a curiosity than for any practical benefit.

Few or no fresh vegetables are to be had at the post, and for those exorbitant prices are charged.

Interments are made on Bird Key, three-fourths of a mile from the post. This place is unfit for the purpose, in consequence of the encroachment of the ocean upon the shifting coral sands of which it is composed.

The prevalent diseases are malarial fevers, usually mild, and catarrhal affections.

The post is occasionally visited by yellow fever in epidemic form.

The garrison was removed to Barrancas, Fla., January 11, 1874, and the post is now in charge of an ordnance-sergeant.

*Meteorological report, Fort Jefferson, Fla., 1870–'74.*

| Month. | 1870–'71. | | | | 1871–'72. | | | | 1872–'73. | | | | 1873–'74. | | | |
|---|---|---|---|---|---|---|---|---|---|---|---|---|---|---|---|---|
| | Temperature. | | | Rain-fall in inches. | Temperature. | | | Rain-fall in inches. | Temperature. | | | Rain-fall in inches. | Temperature. | | | Rain-fall in inches. |
| | Mean. | Max. | Min. | | Mean. | Max. | Min. | | Mean. | Max. | Min. | | Mean. | Max. | Min. | |
| July | 84.68 | 94* | 74* | 3.84 | 86.27 | 94⁴ | 80 | 1.66 | 84.98 | 93* | 70* | 4.64 | 82.69 | 91* | 71* | 5.74 |
| August | 85.63 | 95* | 76* | 1.78 | 87.06 | 9s* | 76 | 4.66 | 84.80 | 92* | 76* | 1.80 | 82.79 | 94* | 72⁴ | 3.34 |
| September | 84.75 | 95* | 72* | 6.04 | 84.88 | 100* | 71 | 3.92 | 83.73 | 91* | 76* | 4.08 | 82.84 | 93* | 72* | 2.90 |
| October | 80.28 | 90* | 72 | 4.02 | 81.15 | 89* | 65* | 3.64 | 79.04 | 87* | 69⁴ | 3.32 | 77.67 | 88* | 69* | 5.64 |
| November | 74.20 | 85* | 63 | 2.40 | 77.25 | 89* | 63⁰ | 0.90 | 74.61 | 88* | 57* | 2.12 | 72.33 | 87* | 56* | 2.16 |
| December | 69.69 | 85* | 48 | 0.74 | 71.95 | 85* | 52* | 1.58 | 70.92 | 80* | 54 | 0.78 | | | | |
| January | 68.56 | 82* | 58 | 0.16 | 68.60 | 85* | 48* | 2.18 | 68.22 | 81 | 57 | 3.62 | | | | |
| February | 71.03 | 82* | 57 | 1.16 | 69.65 | 84* | 55* | 5.12 | 70.67 | 81 | 60 | 0.08 | | | | |
| March | 74.03 | 85* | 65 | 1.20 | 72.58 | 88* | 50* | 0.72 | 69.77 | 83 | 55 | 0.04 | | | | |
| April | 74.41 | 90* | 62 | 0.22 | 80.42 | 91* | 66* | 0.88 | 75.95 | 90* | 58* | 2.04 | | | | |
| May | 80.07 | 92* | 70 | 3.24 | 82.16 | 95* | 59* | 0.76 | 80.97 | 92* | 71* | 0.18 | | | | |
| June | 85.41 | 95* | 76 | 3.10 | 84.87 | 92* | 72* | 2.32 | 83.23 | 93* | 75⁴ | 0.40 | | | | |
| For the year | 77.73 | 95* | 48 | 27.90 | 78.90 | 100* | 48* | 28.34 | 77.22 | 93* | 54 | 23.10 | | | | |

\* These observations are made with self-registering thermometers. The mean is from the standard thermometer.

*Consolidated sick-report, Fort Jefferson, Fla., 1870–'74.*

| Year | | 1870–'71. | | 1871–'72. | | 1872–'73. | | 1873–'74.* | |
|---|---|---|---|---|---|---|---|---|---|
| Mean strength { Officers | | 10 | | 9 | | 5 | | 3 | |
| { Enlisted men | | 101 | | 121 | | 69 | | 47 | |
| Diseases. | | Cases. | Deaths. | Cases. | Deaths. | Cases. | Deaths. | Cases. | Deaths. |
| GENERAL DISEASES, A. | | | | | | | | | |
| Typhoid fever | | | | | | 1 | 1 | | |
| Remittent fever | | 10 | | | | | | | |
| Intermittent fever | | 10 | | 20 | | 7 | | 3 | |
| Yellow fever | | | | | | | | 25 | 13 |
| Other diseases of this group | | 13 | | 17 | | 5 | | | |
| GENERAL DISEASES, B. | | | | | | | | | |
| Rheumatism | | 19 | | 15 | | 2 | | | |
| Syphilis | | 9 | | 8 | | | | | |
| Consumption | | 4 | | 1 | | 1 | | | |
| Other diseases of this group | | 5 | | 10 | | | | 1 | |
| LOCAL DISEASES. | | | | | | | | | |
| Catarrh and bronchitis | | 31 | | 15 | | 10 | | 5 | |
| Pleurisy | | | | 2 | | | | | |
| Diarrhœa and dysentery | | 24 | | 70 | 1 | 38 | | 5 | |
| Hernia | | 2 | | 1 | | | | | |
| Gonorrhœa | | 6 | | | | | | | |
| Other local diseases | | 83 | | 86 | | 80 | | 34 | |
| Alcoholism | | | | | | | | 2 | |
| Unclassified | | 1 | | | | | | | |
| Total disease | | 217 | | 245 | 1 | 144 | 1 | 75 | 13 |
| VIOLENT DISEASES AND DEATHS. | | | | | | | | | |
| Accidents and injuries | | 34 | | 61 | | 56 | | 11 | |
| Total violence | | 34 | | 61 | | 56 | | 11 | |

\* Six months only; last report December, 1873.

---

# FORT JOHNSTON, NORTH CAROLINA.

REPORTS OF ASSISTANT SURGEON D. WEISEL AND OF ACTING ASSISTANT SURGEON S. S. BOYER,
UNITED STATES ARMY.

Fort Johnston is on the west bank of Cape Fear River, four miles from its mouth; latitude, 34° north; longitude, 1′ 2″ west; elevation above the sea, 20 feet.

It was erected by the British between 1744 and 1750, being named in honor of Gabriel Johnston, governor of the Province of North Carolina, and jurisdiction over it was ceded to the United States by an act of the general assembly, dated July 17, 1794.

In 1798 it was ordered by the commissioners of the town of Smithville that lot No. 67 be leased for the use of the troops of the United States for the purpose of erecting a hospital thereon for the term of fourteen years, the rent to be one ear of Indian corn annually.

The reservation is irregular in shape, measuring on the east side 452 feet; on the west, 474 feet; on the north, 339 feet; on the south, 490 feet. The surface is level, the soil poor. Fish are abundant. There is no fort on the reservation.

The barrack is a one-story frame building, with a veranda on the southeast side, 100 by 25 by 14 feet, divided into three rooms, i. e., two section-rooms and central office. Each section-room is 39 feet 6 inches by 23 feet 2 inches by 12 feet, warmed by stoves and ventilated by windows and by central shafts from the ceiling to the roof. Each man has about 550 cubic feet of air-space. The bedsteads are of iron, and single. No wash or bath room is connected with the barrack. A latrine is built on the river at low-water mark, the ebbing and flowing of the tide preventing the excreta from accumulating. At high tide the water comes within two feet of the seats.

The kitchen and mess-room are in a one-story frame building, 46 by 22 feet, the former being a room 21 by 12 feet, the latter taking up the remaining space, 33 by 21 feet. One large cooking-stove is used in the preparation of food.

The laundresses' quarters is a one-story frame building, recently enlarged, allowing two rooms to each laundress.

The officers' quarters are in a brick building of two stories, with wings of one story, containing 12 rooms in all. It is old, damp, in bad condition, and inconveniently arranged, furnishing only two sets of quarters, and is not fit for residence. (For dimensions of rooms see Circular No. 4.)

The office of the commanding officer is a brick building, 22 by 20 feet, with one room. One of the store-houses is located alongside the Government wharf; it is 94 by 29 feet, and divided into four rooms, two of which are occupied by the quartermaster and commissary as an office. Of the other two rooms, one is for commissary's and the other for quartermaster's stores. The second store-house is situated about the central part of the reservation. It is a brick building, one story high, and is the old "block-house" erected in the earliest history of the post.

The guard-house is 22 by 18 by 10 feet, with a porch facing the river. The guard-room is 12 by 18 feet, and two rooms open into it; one is the lockup, 12 by 10 feet; the other the cell, 10 by 6 feet. The rooms are heated by stoves, and ventilated through the windows.

The hospital is located on the northeast side of the reservation. It is a frame building 52 by 28 by 26 feet. The central part is two stories high, and contains a ward on the upper floor 16 by 26 by 9½ feet. In the rear of the ward, at the head of the stairs, are two rooms, one on each side; the one to the right upon entering the ward is the store-room, 12 by 10 feet; the other is the bath-room, 12 by 6 feet. On the first floor are four rooms and a hall, the latter being 26 by 12 feet, with stairs leading to the second story. To the left of the hall are two rooms. At the northwest end of the hall is a space 6 by 4 feet, inclosed by a counter; this is the dispensary. Shelves and drawers are constructed along the walls on three sides. Underneath the stairs is a closet. There are two rooms northwest of the hall; the first is the dining-room, 14 by 12 feet; the second the kitchen, 12 by 12 feet. The ward has a capacity of twelve beds; air-space per man, 748 cubic feet. Bathing and washing are done in the bath-room, which is provided with a bath-tub and wash-stand. There are no water-closets in the hospital; a latrine is situated on the river-bank, 30 yards distant.

The dead-house is a frame building, 14 by 8 by 9 feet, located on the northwest side of the reservation.

The post bakery is a frame building, 9 by 8 feet, with an oven 7 by 6 feet, capable of baking 140 rations at once. There is no laundry, chapel, or school-house upon the reservation.

The water-supply upon the reservation is from a well and cisterns. The former is 20 feet in depth, and located 15 rods from the barracks. One of the latter is located in the rear of the officers' quarters, and has a capacity for 5,000 gallons, although it seldom contains that quantity at one time. The other is at the hospital. In both, the water is raised by a pump and distributed by hand.

Should the quantity become insufficient, it could be obtained from wells in the vicinity. Its quality is slightly brackish. From the porosity of the soil, the natural drainage is good.

A bath-house, 20 by 18 feet, is erected upon the river-beach, at low-water mark. The boards on each side are half an inch apart, thus allowing the water to enter. There is a partition running nearly the whole breadth of one side above water, which separates the building into two parts; the first is divided into four small dressing-rooms, the second contains the water. The men bathe daily in summer.

The means of communication with Wilmington, distant 30 miles, is by water, but is irregular. The mail is semi-weekly. The post is surrounded by the town of Smithville, essentially a pilot-town of about 800 inhabitants. It is a pleasant and healthy place, but isolated.

*Meteorological report, Fort Johnston, N. C., 1870–'74.*

| Month. | 1870–'71. | | | | 1871–'72. | | | | 1872–'73. | | | | 1873–'74. | | | |
|---|---|---|---|---|---|---|---|---|---|---|---|---|---|---|---|---|
| | Temperature. | | | Rain-fall in inches. | Temperature. | | | Rain-fall in inches. | Temperature. | | | Rain-fall in inches. | Temperature. | | | Rain-fall in inches. |
| | Mean. | Max. | Min. | | Mean. | Max. | Min. | | Mean. | Max. | Min. | | Mean. | Max. | Min. | |
| July | | | | | 81.38 | 92 | 66 | 1.53 | 83.33 | 95* | 67* | 5.50 | 81.80 | 94* | 66* | 6.50 |
| August | | | | | 81.09 | 91 | 71 | 6.93 | 81.69 | 99* | 57* | 6.20 | 81.61 | 94* | 63* | 8.71 |
| September | | | | | 72.50 | 91 | 50 | 4.06 | 76.68 | 89* | 53* | 5.90 | 78.07 | 95* | 57* | 12.73 |
| October | | | | | 68.34 | 86* | 50* | 4.17 | 63.54 | 82* | 32* | 3.50 | 65.28 | 90* | 28* | 2.25 |
| November | | | | | 55.69 | 79* | 22* | 3.20 | 52.57 | 76* | 9* | 4.60 | 55.36 | 84* | 24* | 1.71 |
| December | | | | | 45.63 | 68* | 13* | 3.60 | 41.64 | 65* | 9* | 3.60 | 51.02 | 73* | 12* | 3.75 |
| January | 48.81 | 72 | 25 | 1.00 | 42.66 | 60* | 20* | 3.11 | 45.55 | 68* | 15* | 6.20 | 51.12 | 76* | 18* | 6.56 |
| February | | | | | 45.24 | 68* | 24* | 3.00 | 48.96 | 64* | 25* | 4.24 | 49.89 | 65* | 28* | 6.11 |
| March | 61.48 | 80 | 40 | 6.80 | 47.63 | 68* | 24* | 5.70 | 50.26 | 69* | 14* | 1.80 | 58.08 | 80* | 27* | 4.29 |
| April | 66.27 | 76 | 50 | 3.00 | 62.88 | 77* | 38* | 0.90 | 62.11 | 81* | 33* | 3.10 | 63.90 | 77* | 35* | 1.84 |
| May | 71.77 | 86 | 52 | 5.37 | 73.01 | 85* | 54* | 2.66 | 71.58 | 87* | 50* | 12.35 | 72.02 | 92 | 45* | 4.21 |
| June | 80.70 | 89 | 66 | 3.72 | 78.87 | 90* | 59* | 2.50 | 78.34 | 92* | 55* | 2.80 | 81.63 | 95 | 65* | 4.09 |
| For the year | | | | | 62.91 | 92 | 13* | 41.36 | 63.02 | 99* | 9* | 59.79 | 65.81 | 95* | 12* | 62.75 |

* These observations are made with self-registering thermometers. The mean is from the standard thermometer.

*Consolidated sick-report, Fort Johnston, N. C., 1870–'74.*

| Year | 1870–'71. | | 1871–'72. | | 1872–'73. | | 1873–'74. | |
|---|---|---|---|---|---|---|---|---|
| Mean strength { Officers | 3 | | 3 | | 3 | | 4 | |
| { Enlisted men | 70 | | 40 | | 36 | | 52 | |
| Diseases. | Cases. | Deaths. | Cases. | Deaths. | Cases. | Deaths. | Cases. | Deaths. |
| GENERAL DISEASES, A. | | | | | | | | |
| Typho-malarial fever | | | | | | | 2 | |
| Remittent fever | | | | | 3 | | 8 | |
| Intermittent fever | 41 | | 27 | | 11 | | 14 | |
| GENERAL DISEASES, B. | | | | | | | | |
| Rheumatism | 8 | | 5 | | 3 | | 2 | |
| Syphilis | 3 | | | | 2 | | 5 | |
| Consumption | 1 | | | | | | | |
| LOCAL DISEASES. | | | | | | | | |
| Catarrh and bronchitis | 10 | | 3 | | | | 1 | |
| Diarrhœa and dysentery | 10 | | 8 | | 6 | | 4 | |
| Hernia | 1 | | | | | | | |
| Gonorrhœa | 2 | | 1 | | | | | |
| Other local diseases | 58 | | 25 | | 11 | | 10 | |
| Alcoholism | 7 | | 4 | | | | 3 | |
| Total disease | 141 | | 73 | | 36 | | 49 | |
| VIOLENT DISEASES AND DEATHS. | | | | | | | | |
| Accidents and injuries | 14 | | 26 | | 11 | 1 | 9 | |
| Total violence | 14 | | 26 | | 11 | 1 | 9 | |

## KEY WEST BARRACKS, FLORIDA.

### REPORT OF ASSISTANT SURGEON HARVEY E. BROWN, UNITED STATES ARMY.

Key West, a corruption of the Spanish name "Cayo Hueso," or Bone Island, is one of the chain of coral islands which extends from Cape Florida to the Tortugas, and constitutes the Florida reef. It is situated in latitude 24° 30′ north; longitude, 3° 37′ west from Washington. It is about seven miles long and one broad, and the highest point is not more than 10 feet above the level of the sea. The geological formation is a coralline base, with a superimposed stratum of limestone several feet in thickness, formed by the disintegration of the coral. This limestone at the surface, and especially where it is exposed to the air, is hard and dense, but two or three feet below the surface it becomes almost as soft as clay. The soil is thin, composed of disintegrated limestone, coral, sand, marine shells, and decaying vegetable matter, from which grows a thick chaparral or brush, which covers all the uninhabited portions of the Key. Where this brush is cleared away, and the soil is sufficiently thick, nearly all the tropical fruits and vegetables can be produced with the utmost facility, it being the paucity of the soil, rather than its poverty, that prevents the general cultivation of the whole island.

The Key is reputed to have been in former times a favorite resort of the buccaneers. About 1820 a settlement was formed consisting chiefly of fishermen, wreckers, and sponge-gatherers from the Bahamas, and a few emigrants from New York.

The city of Key West is situated on the north side of the island, fronting a safe and capacious harbor, and contains about eight thousand inhabitants, of whom white Americans form a comparatively small proportion, the remainder being Bahama negroes, Cuban refugees, and white natives of the Bahamas and their descendants, classified here under the general title of "Conchs." The Cubans number now several thousand, and have all arrived within a few years. They are chiefly employed in the manufacture of cigars, which has, during the past five years, become a very important and lucrative industry. The white inhabitants are chiefly engaged in wrecking, (a business formerly very profitable, but now of slight importance,) and in sponge-gathering.

At the entrance to the harbor and on the west of the town is Fort Taylor, an extensive casemated work, built of brick. It is at present unoccupied, except by the ordnance-sergeant in charge.

On the outskirts of the town to the east are the United States Barracks. The land upon which they are situated was purchased in 1833, (having then been occupied for about two years,) the sum paid being $2,958, and the tract conveyed embracing $14\frac{79}{100}$ acres. This being found insufficient, in 1837 a further purchase of eight acres was made with all the buildings and improvements thereon, for which there was paid the sum of $6,000. This latter purchase embraces the land upon which the post hospital is now built.

Prior to 1844 the barracks consisted of temporary structures, but in that year the present buildings were erected by Major E. B. Ogden, quartermaster, United States Army, and have long been regarded as among the best of their kind in the country.

The officers' quarters consist of five one-story frame buildings, each 34 feet deep by 24 broad, with attic and basement. Each house is surrounded on all sides by a piazza 12 feet broad. The basement is divided into a kitchen 17 feet 6 inches deep by 21 feet 4 inches broad and 8 feet height of ceiling, and two small rooms, one for a servants' bed-room and the other for a pantry. The first floor consists of a parlor 22 feet 6 inches broad by 18 feet 6 inches deep, and of a dining-room 22 feet 6 inches by 14 feet, the height of the ceiling being 11 feet. In the attic are two large bed-rooms, one 25 feet by 23 feet, and the other 26 feet 6 inches by 23 feet, the height of the ceiling varying somewhat with the slope of the roof, but being 9 feet at its highest point. These two rooms are separated by a hall in which is a large closet, and in each of the bed-rooms are smaller closets. The stairway from the first floor to the attic is on the piazza outside of the house. The windows (or rather doors, as they all extend to the floor) in the first story are twelve in number, and so arranged as to give the greatest possible amount of ventilation. In every respect these quarters are models of their kind, well built, cool and comfortable, and admirably adapted for a single family, but not capable of being divided so that two officers can occupy one house with any degree of privacy. To each set of officers' quarters is attached a large cistern, the water from which is brought to the house by pipes.

The men's barracks consist of two frame buildings, one story with basement, each 90 feet long by 34 broad. The squad-room is 70 feet long by 32 feet 6 inches broad and 12 feet high, the remainder of the space being occupied by the company offices and first sergeant's quarters, which is 18 feet by 32 feet 6 inches and 12 feet high. The basement is occupied by the company mess-rooms, kitchens and store-rooms. The buildings, like the officers' quarters, are entirely surrounded by a wide piazza. They are well lighted and are properly constructed for ventilation; nevertheless the amount of air-space per man can hardly be deemed sufficient for a tropical climate, being but about 500 cubic feet per man for a company of fifty men. A further objection to these barracks consists in the location of the kitchens so that the heat, &c., therefrom will rise into the squad-rooms. In all southern stations the kitchens should be located in a separate building in the rear and sufficiently apart from the barrack.

Between the two barracks is the guard-house, a stone building 34 by 24 feet, divided into a guard-room and prison-room. It is sufficiently well-adapted for the purpose, but, like all our garrison-prisons, does not afford sufficient air-space per man. The cells are simply unfit to confine any human being in. I have never known them to be used.

The storehouses for the commissary and quartermaster are large and roomy, and amply sufficient for the purpose. So is the stable, which is situated on the south side of the reservation.

The laundresses' quarters consist of a long frame building on the southwest of the reservation, divided into five sets of quarters, each 18 by 14 by 8.6 feet. They are in good repair. Other buildings at the post are the adjutant's and quartermaster's offices, carriage-house, and carpenter and blacksmith shops. An addition to the barracks of the greatest value, in a sanitary point of view, is a large and roomy bath-house built over the water north of the parade-ground, where the men have unlimited facilities for salt-water bathing.

The present hospital building is situated on the west side of the reservation, and was erected in 1861. The building is of similar construction to the officers' quarters, one main story with attic and basement and surrounded by a wide piazza, its total dimensions being 90 by 34 feet, (or, including the piazza, 114 by 58 feet.) The main floor is divided into two wards, dispensary, and wash-room. The height of the ceiling is 11 feet 6 inches. One ward is 31 by 32, and the other 38 by 32 feet, giving over 1,200 cubic feet of air without crowding the ward. The surgeon's office is 18 feet 6 inches by 17 feet, and the dispensary 13 by 15 feet. The attic is unfinished and is occupied for storage. Good store-rooms might be built in this part of the hospital at a small expense, and would be a desirable addition. In the basement are the hospital steward's quarters, consisting of one large room, 30 by 20, and 8 feet 6 inches to the ceiling, and two smaller rooms, each 15 by 15 feet, the hospital kitchen, 30 by 19 feet, dining-room, 30 by 13, and attendants' room, 30 by 15.6, all of these rooms being 8 feet 6 inches to the ceiling. At the northeast corner, under the piazza, a wash-house has recently been built, 13.6 by 11 by 9.6 feet. The hospital is excellently well ventilated, and, with the repairs that have recently been put upon it, may be said to be in very good condition. Better storage room is, however, very desirable, as all kinds of medical supplies deteriorate very rapidly in this climate.

The water supply of the post is entirely from cisterns, and is ample and of the best quality. The total capacity is as follows:

Gallons.

Hospital, 2 cisterns, 18,161 gallons each .................................................. 36,322
Officers' quarters, 5 cisterns, 10,400 gallons each ....................................... 52,000
Barracks, 4 cisterns, 29,082 gallons each ................................................. 116,328
At stables and laundresses' quarters, 3 cisterns, 13,127 gallons each ................... 39,381

244,031

There is, in addition, a condenser at Fort Taylor which can supply upward of 5,000 gallons per day, but no occasion has recently arisen for its use.

The post is unquestionably a very healthy one. Yellow fever prevails in certain years as an epidemic, invariably a foreign importation from Havana, the result of a vicious quarantine system, and propagated on arrival by filth, in which the town probably exceeds any other in the country, except, perhaps, Sabine, Texas. Apart from this, there may be said to be no prevailing diseases. Even the ordinary intestinal disorders, so common at southern stations, have been entirely absent at this post this summer. A fruitful source of disease is, however, the intemperate habits of many of the men. The city of Key West affords unlimited opportunities for indulgence in bad whisky, and a large percentage of the sick owe their disability to over-indulgence. The only case of venereal disease I have seen since my arrival was in a recruit who brought the disease with him from New York.

It is rather a singular fact that functional and organic diseases of the heart are extremely common among the men. The cause of this I have not been able to ascertain as yet, but I am now examining the question, and trust to be able to give a satisfactory explanation of it in the future. I have seen four cases of angina pectoris within two or three months, and of simple functional disorder, (palpitation,) certainly as many as fifteen cases.

The market is an expensive and very poor one, although under arrangements which are now being made it is likely to be much improved in the future. Beef is furnished the troops at 20 cents per pound. It is brought on ice from Galveston, and is of fine quality, but the steamers arriving but once a week renders it impossible to have a constant supply. Subsistence stores are furnished from New Orleans, and are, ordinarily, of good quality; it would be better on the score of economy, quality of stores, and time of transportation, that they should be shipped from New York. Medical stores are procured on half-yearly requisitions from the medical purveyor in New York, and are always of the best quality and arrive in good condition.

The means of access to and departure from the island consist in a weekly line of steamers from New York to Galveston, which touch here on Wednesdays from Galveston, and on Thursdays or Fridays from New York; in a semi-monthly line from Baltimore for New Orleans, touching both ways, but very irregular in their trips; and in a weekly line from New Orleans, via Cedar Keys, for Havana, which are supposed to arrive from New Orleans on Mondays and return on Thursdays, but which are also very irregular. Letters from Washington and points north should always be forwarded " via New York steamer." The time from Washington is six or seven days; from headquarters of the department from seven to ten days.

*Meteorological report, Key West, Fla., 1870–'74.*

| Month. | 1870–'71. | | | | 1871–'72. | | | | 1872–'73. | | | | 1873–'74. | | | |
|---|---|---|---|---|---|---|---|---|---|---|---|---|---|---|---|---|
| | Temperature. | | | Rain-fall in inches. | Temperature. | | | Rain-fall in inches. | Temperature. | | | Rain-fall in inches. | Temperature. | | | Rain-fall in inches. |
| | Mean. | Max. | Min. | | Mean. | Max. | Min. | | Mean. | Max. | Min. | | Mean. | Max. | Min. | |
| | ° | ° | ° | | ° | ° | ° | | ° | ° | ° | | ° | ° | ° | |
| July................ | 87.73 | 96 | 81 | 7.42 | 85.30 | 94 | 78 | 9.42 | 83.78 | 93 | 78 | 7.10 | 85.05 | 94 | 77 | 4.55 |
| August.............. | 87.84 | 98 | 80 | 1.30 | 86.36 | 94 | 81 | 3.26 | 84.80 | 94 | 77 | 3.06 | 84.29* | 97* | 74* | 2.89 |
| September............ | 85.78 | 98 | 77 | 9.22 | 84.54 | 93 | 77 | 9.48 | 84.47 | 93 | 80 | 8.66 | 82.40* | 94* | 74* | 7.10 |
| October ............. | 80.99 | 93 | 72 | 8.22 | 81.72 | 92 | 76 | 5.50 | 79.05 | 90 | 72 | 6.70 | 74.59* | 85* | 65* | 1.70 |
| November............ | 73.68 | 84 | 58 | 3.32 | 77.23 | 88 | 66 | 4.78 | 74.25 | 89 | 57 | 4.90 | 72.09* | 84* | 52* | 0.60 |
| December ............ | 69.86 | 84 | 48 | 5.24 | 72.34 | 84 | 57 | 4.40 | 71.20 | 85 | 56 | 0.00 | 71.04* | 82* | 51* | 2.00 |
| January.............. | 69.83 | 83 | 57 | 0.96 | 69.13 | 82 | 53 | 2.80 | 66.99 | 87 | 55 | 11.90 | 69.32* | 84* | 52* | 1.50 |
| February............ | 73.84 | 86 | 62 | ........ | 69.49 | 82 | 59 | 10.00 | 74.46 | 88 | 60 | 0.00 | 73.89* | 86* | 50* | 1.50 |
| March............... | 76.73 | 88 | 67 | 0.00 | 73.69 | 89 | 60 | 1.70 | 72.80 | 90 | 57 | 0.00 | 75.72* | 89* | 54* | 0.00 |
| April............... | 79.11 | 91 | 66 | 0.00 | 80.63 | 89 | 75 | 0.00 | 78.60 | 90 | 65 | 1.80 | 75.06* | 90* | 50* | 0.80 |
| May................ | 80.91 | 91 | 69 | 5.74 | 81.89 | 92 | 74 | 0.70 | 83.76 | 95 | 75 | 1.00 | 80.00* | 94* | 60* | 3.50 |
| June ................ | 85.78 | 92 | 76 | 2.40 | 84.45 | 94 | 74 | ......... | 84.91 | 97 | 63 | 0.00 | 84.13* | 97* | 72* | 5.50 |
| For the year .... | 79.34 | 98 | 48 | ........ | 78.89 | 94 | 53 | ........ | 78.50 | 97 | 55 | 45.12 | 75.63 | 97* | 50* | 32.04 |

*These observations are made with self-registering thermometers. The mean is from the standard thermometer.

*Consolidated sick-report, Key West, Fla., 1870–'74.*

| Year | 1870–'71. | | 1871–'72. | | 1872–'73. | | 1873–'74.* | |
|---|---|---|---|---|---|---|---|---|
| **Mean strength** { Officers / Enlisted men | 7 / 115 | | 4 / 90 | | 6 / 96 | | 4 / 71 | |
| Diseases. | Cases. | Deaths. | Cases. | Deaths. | Cases. | Deaths. | Cases. | Deaths. |
| GENERAL DISEASES, A. | | | | | | | | |
| Small-pox and varioloid | | | 1 | | | | | |
| Remittent fever | | | 1 | 1 | | | 2 | |
| Intermittent fever | 60 | | 29 | | 29 | | 5 | |
| Yellow fever | | | 1 | 1 | | | | |
| Other diseases of this group | | | | | 1 | | 4 | 1 |
| GENERAL DISEASES, B. | | | | | | | | |
| Rheumatism | 6 | | 8 | | 17 | | 4 | |
| Syphilis | 2 | | | | 5 | | | |
| Consumption | 1 | | 2 | 1 | 1 | | | |
| Other diseases of this group | | | | | | 1 | | |
| LOCAL DISEASES. | | | | | | | | |
| Catarrh and bronchitis | 27 | | 26 | | 33 | | 15 | |
| Pneumonia | | | | | | | 2 | 1 |
| Diarrhœa and dysentery | 45 | | 34 | | 37 | | 52 | |
| Hernia | | | 2 | | 1 | | | |
| Gonorrhœa | | | | | 1 | | 3 | |
| Other local diseases | 151 | | 75 | | 80 | | 63 | 2 |
| Alcoholism | 6 | | 11 | | 11 | | 20 | |
| Unclassified | | | | | 1 | | | |
| Total disease | 298 | | 190 | 3 | 217 | 1 | 170 | 4 |
| VIOLENT DISEASES AND DEATHS. | | | | | | | | |
| Gunshot wounds | | | 1 | | 1 | | | |
| Other accidents and injuries | 9 | | 4 | | 22 | | 25 | |
| Total violence | 9 | | 5 | | 23 | | 25 | |

* September, 1873, no report.

# LANCASTER, KENTUCKY.

### REPORT OF ACTING ASSISTANT SURGEON SAMUEL L. S. SMITH, UNITED STATES ARMY.

Lancaster, the county-seat of Garrard County, Kentucky, is pleasantly situated in a rich agricultural region, 113 miles distant from Louisville, by the Louisville and Nashville Railroad. The town is one of the oldest in the State, and was originally settled by emigrants from Lancaster, Pa.

The military post, established in 1871, occupies a parallelogram of about ten acres on the eastern edge of the town. The buildings found upon the grounds when first occupied were one brick residence and one log house, each one story in height. Other structures have been added to these as necessity required. The present company barracks consist of the brick house just mentioned, 48 by 16 feet, divided into three nearly equal rooms, the ceiling of which has a uniform height of 10 feet. One room is used as an office and orderly room, and the others as quarters for the men. In the rear of, and communicating with, this house is a rough frame structure, 40 by 20 feet, used as the main dormitory. It is furnished with single bedsteads of wood and iron combined. The air-space is about 320 cubic feet per bed, but, as some of the men occupy tents in summer, and others have families, the air-space is practically somewhat greater.

The kitchen, mess-room, and provision store-room are located in a convenient one-story wooden building. The post lavatories and privies are in the rear of the kitchen and placed under proper shelter.

The guard-house, in the rear of the barracks, consists of a one-story log house, about 16 feet square, divided into two rooms, one for the guard and the other for the prisoners. It is lighted by a window in each gable, and warmed by a coal-stove.

The post library, kept in a hospital-tent properly floored and framed, comprises from 800 to 1,000 volumes of well selected English and American works. The Louisville, Cincinnati, and other daily and weekly papers are taken and placed on file, and every opportunity afforded the men for mental improvement.

The laundresses' quarters are about 100 yards in rear of the barracks, in a rough frame building divided into five rooms.

There are no officers' quarters at the post, and private quarters are rented for that purpose in the town.

The post hospital is located opposite the garrison grounds in a one-story rented frame building, containing four rooms and a good dry cellar. The principal room occupied as a ward is 17 by 15 by 8½ feet. The ward opens upon a veranda at the side of the house and has space for six beds, which is more than necessary—the average occupancy being three.

The hospital kitchen and mess-room are in a detached rough frame building. The hospital inclosure contains about two acres, one-half of which is kept as a lawn for the benefit of convalescents, and the remainder cultivated as a hospital and company garden.

The surface of the ground slopes from the barracks in all directions to such an extent as to render artificial drainage unnecessary. A covered sewer, however, has been laid from the kitchen to carry off the waste-water.

The water-supply of the post is derived from a fine adjacent spring, and from a well on the garrison grounds, well protected from contamination and surface-drainage. There is no cistern on the hospital grounds, and all the water used is brought from the spring by the prisoners and kept in barrels. Buckets are placed on the veranda for use.

In sinking wells a chalybeate water is usually obtained after passing the first limestone, so strongly astringent as to be unpalatable and useless for culinary purposes. The springs that flow from the base of the black slate of the knob formation are generally chalybeate or magnesian in character; and a number of these, in the vicinity of Crab Orchard, fourteen miles distant, have long been recognized as possessing medicinal properties.

The water of the principal "Epsom Springs" in this locality, from which the "Crab Orchard Salts" of the United States Dispensatory are manufactured, was analyzed by Dr. Robert Peter, of Lexington, and found to contain, in 1,000 grains of this water, evaporated to dryness at 212°:

| | |
|---|---|
| Carbonate of lime, grains | 0.506 } Held in solution by |
| Carbonate of magnesia, grains | .375 } carbonic acid. |
| Carbonate of iron | a trace. |
| Sulphate of magnesia, grains | 2.989 |
| Sulphate of lime, grains | 1.566 |
| Sulphate of potash, grains | .298 |
| Sulphate of soda, grains | .398 |
| Chloride of sodium, grains | 1.000 |
| Silica, grains | .021 |
| Bromine | a trace. |
| | 7.153 |

Although the sulphate of magnesia is the chief saline ingredient of these springs, the presence of the other saline constituents with the carbonate of iron, modifies greatly the well-known action of this salt, and adapts the waters to a greater variety of medicinal purposes than could be attained by a solution of sulphate of magnesia alone.

In the manufacture of "Crab Orchard Salts" the water is evaporated in iron kettles to a certain density, and allowed to stand for some time in wooden vessels. The clear liquid is then drawn off from the mixed deposit of carbonates of lime and magnesia, and oxide of iron, thrown down by boiling, and again evaporated to full dryness. The salts obtained by this method consist of a moist, granular powder, with a slight tinge of brownish, like the whitest Havana sugar.

The analysis of Dr. Peter revealed the following composition:

| | |
|---|---|
| Sulphate of magnesia | 63.19 |
| Sulphate of soda | 4.20 |
| Sulphate of potash | 1.80 |

Sulphate of lime ........................................................................ 2.54
Chloride of sodium ...................................................................... 4.77
Carbonate of lime, magnesia, iron, and silica ........................................... .89
Bromine .......................................................................... a trace.
Water of crystallization and loss ..................................................... 22.61

100.00

The "Crab Orchard Salts" were much employed by the physicians of this section before they became an officinal article. They are said to be less drastic and more tonic than unmixed Epsom salts.

*Consolidated sick-report, Lancaster, Ky., 1870–'74.*

| Year | 1870–'71.* | | 1871–'72. | | 1872–'73. | | 1873–'74. | |
|---|---|---|---|---|---|---|---|---|
| Mean strength { Officers | 2 | | 3 | | 2 | | 3 | |
| { Enlisted men | 22 | | 52 | | 49 | | 49 | |
| Diseases. | Cases. | Deaths. | Cases. | Deaths. | Cases. | Deaths. | Cases. | Deaths. |
| GENERAL DISEASES, A. | | | | | | | | |
| Typhoid fever | | | | | | | 1 | |
| Typho-malarial fever | | | | | | | 3 | |
| Remittent fever | | | 3 | | 5 | | 10 | |
| Intermittent fever | 2 | | 6 | | 11 | | 8 | |
| Cholera | | | | | | | 4 | 3 |
| Other diseases of this group | | | 3 | | 5 | | 2 | |
| GENERAL DISEASES, B. | | | | | | | | |
| Rheumatism | 7 | | 7 | | 6 | | 3 | |
| Syphilis | 2 | | 3 | | 5 | | 6 | |
| Consumption | | | | | | | | |
| Other diseases of this group | | | | | | | 1 | |
| LOCAL DISEASES. | | | | | | | | |
| Catarrh and bronchitis | 1 | | 21 | | 11 | | 9 | |
| Pneumonia | 1 | | 3 | | | | | |
| Pleurisy | | | | | 1 | | | |
| Diarrhœa and dysentery | 12 | | 21 | | 20 | | 35 | |
| Hernia | 1 | | 1 | | | | | |
| Gonorrhœa | 16 | | 20 | | 5 | | 2 | |
| Other local diseases | 16 | | 55 | | 39 | | 26 | |
| Alcoholism | 1 | | 1 | | 1 | | 4 | |
| Total disease | 59 | | 144 | | 109 | | 114 | 3 |
| VIOLENT DISEASES AND DEATHS. | | | | | | | | |
| Gunshot wounds | 1 | | | | | | | |
| Other accidents and injuries | 13 | | 19 | | 14 | | 17 | |
| Homicide | | | | | | | | 1 |
| Total violence | 14 | | 19 | | 14 | | 17 | 1 |

* Four months only.

# LEBANON, KENTUCKY.

## REPORT OF ASSISTANT SURGEON ELY M'CLELLAN, UNITED STATES ARMY.

Lebanon, the county-seat of Marion County, Kentucky, is located on the Knoxville branch of the Louisville and Nashville Railroad, 67 miles southeast from Louisville.

The present military post of Lebanon was organized September 21, 1868. It occupies 7 acres of high and well-drained ground, on the northern outskirts of the town. The ground is rented. The buildings were erected by the United States, and are arranged to form three sides of an open square. The officers' quarters are in a wooden building, 60 by 30 feet, subdivided into 8 equal rooms. Quarters for two officers are also rented in the immediate vicinity of the post.

The barrack is a one-story wooden building on the pavilion plan, 81 feet long, 29 feet wide,

9½ feet to the eaves, and 16½ to the ridge. The interior of the building is not ceiled, the walls having but a single thickness of boards. Ventilation is effected by six doors, thirteen windows, and four brick flues in the ridge. The present occupancy is 44 enlisted men. Iron bedsteads are used, and the air-space per man is 800 feet. In the rear of the barrack, and connected with it by a small porch, is a building containing the kitchen and mess-room, also a small building containing the lavatory and bath-room. Between the last-named building and the barrack is a well five feet in diameter and 43 feet deep, from which water is obtained for all domestic purposes. The water is free from other impurities than that derived from the limestone through which it passes. No sep-arate quarters have been provided for the married soldiers, but small rooms in various parts of the buildings have been arranged for the authorized laundresses.

Adjoining the barracks on the north is a house 20 by 22 feet, and 12 feet high, which is used as a hospital ward. This room is plastered, and has four doors and four windows. An inclosed shed 29 feet long, 12 feet wide, and 7 feet high is divided into three equal rooms for kitchen, store-room, and dispensary. There is also at the post a hospital-tent, and a full supply of hospital furniture.

The guard-house is a wooden building 24 by 16 feet, lighted and ventilated by two windows and one door.

The privies at the post are wooden buildings erected over deep pits, which, during the summer months, are constantly disinfected with lime, copperas, and fresh earth.

In addition to the well above mentioned, water for ordinary purposes is collected in tanks from the roofs of the buildings.

The post garden, cultivated exclusively for the use of the enlisted men, comprises about 2¾ acres, and yields a plentiful return of the usual culinary vegetables.

*Consolidated sick-report, Lebanon, Ky., 1870–'74.*

| Year | 1870–'71. | | 1871–'72. | | 1872–'73. | | 1873–'74. | |
|---|---|---|---|---|---|---|---|---|
| Mean strength { Officers / Enlisted men | 3 / 52 | | 4 / 51 | | 4 / 61 | | 4 / 58 | |
| Diseases. | Cases. | Deaths. | Cases. | Deaths. | Cases. | Deaths. | Cases. | Deaths. |
| GENERAL DISEASES, A. | | | | | | | | |
| Remittent fever | 12 | | 8 | | 6 | | | |
| Intermittent fever | 20 | | 9 | | 26 | | 23 | |
| Cholera | | | | | | | 1 | 1 |
| Other diseases of this group | 1 | | 6 | | 2 | | | |
| GENERAL DISEASES, B. | | | | | | | | |
| Rheumatism | 2 | | 8 | | 6 | | 2 | |
| Syphilis | 3 | | 7 | | 4 | | 2 | |
| Consumption | | | | | | | 3 | |
| Other diseases of this group | | | | | | | 1 | |
| LOCAL DISEASES. | | | | | | | | |
| Catarrh and bronchitis | 1 | | 4 | | 29 | | 46 | |
| Pneumonia | 1 | | | | 2 | | 3 | |
| Pleurisy | 1 | | | | | | | |
| Diarrhœa and dysentery | 25 | | 15 | | 17 | | 52 | |
| Hernia | 1 | | | | | | | |
| Gonorrhœa | 1 | | 1 | | 5 | | 10 | |
| Other local diseases | 26 | | 33 | | 38 | | 35 | |
| Alcoholism | 3 | | 15 | | 12 | | 15 | |
| Total disease | 97 | | 106 | | 147 | | 193 | 1 |
| VIOLENT DISEASES AND DEATHS. | | | | | | | | |
| Gunshot wounds | 1 | | 3 | 1 | | | | |
| Other accidents and injuries | 14 | | 10 | | 25 | | 22 | |
| Total violence | 15 | | 13 | 1 | 25 | | 22 | |

# LITTLE ROCK, ARKANSAS.

INFORMATION FURNISHED BY ACTING ASSISTANT SURGEON W. A. CANTRELL, UNITED STATES ARMY.

The post of Little Rock, embraced within the limits of the city of Little Rock, is situated on the Arkansas River, about 300 miles from its mouth, in latitude 34° 43′ north; longitude 15° 7′ west.

This point had been a regular place for crossing the Arkansas River by the Indians from time immemorial; for, although the river was nowhere fordable, yet the hills set in on both sides in such a manner as to direct the great Indian trail north and south over the present site of the city. The place takes its name from a prominent rock, which projects upon the water's edge, and was called Little Rock in contradistinction from a larger rocky promontory about three miles higher up on the opposite side.

The steep, rocky bank, which originally rose sheer from the water's edge, gradually increases in height, in ascending the stream, from 20 to about 60 feet, and extending southward and westward within the city limits, the land attains a still higher elevation, being at its highest point about 150 feet above the level of the river, the ascent being everywhere gradual. The surface is a slight deposit of vegetable mold, superimposed upon strata of sandstone excellent for building purposes, very hard, and of light gray and brown colors, and upon slate which approaches the surface in the northwestern part of the city, and is there exposed in thick layers upon the bank of the river.

The reservation, comprising 36 acres of ground, is situated in the southeastern part of the city, and was purchased in 1836. Two years later the building of the post commenced. Five large brick buildings, consisting of an armory, commanding officer's quarters, a barrack for one company, ordnance store-rooms and workshop, and quartermaster's and commissary store-room, were erected. Also a magazine, brick stables, and out-houses.

The post was continuously occupied as a military station until February 18, 1861, when it was evacuated, and the governor of Arkansas, with his militia, took charge of and held the post until it was retaken by the United States forces under command of Major-General Steele, on the 10th of September, 1863.

A general hospital was established shortly after the recovery of the post, and maintained until December, 1866.

The building originally erected for an armory is at present occupied as quarters for the enlisted men. It is a two-story brick building, 87 by 40½ feet, with a double veranda in front, but none in the rear. It contains 10 rooms, each 20½ by 18 feet, and 6 rooms, each $8\frac{1}{6}$ by $6\frac{1}{2}$, exclusive of kitchen and mess-room, which are in the basement. The smaller rooms are used only for storing knapsacks and personal property of the men. The large rooms are used as dormitories, affording the present garrison of 74 men an air-space of 1,230 cubic feet per man. Sufficient ventilation is obtained from doors and windows. The men sleep upon single iron bedsteads and mattresses filled with straw. The sinks are placed 60 feet in rear of the quarters. Refuse matter is transported in carts about half a mile to a ravine, which is washed out by the rains.

Married soldiers are quartered in frame buildings located 373 feet in rear of the men's quarters. Their quarters are commodious and comfortable, giving two large rooms to each family.

The present quarters for officers are two brick buildings two stories in height, having basement kitchens and double verandas in front and single verandas in the rear.

The guard-house is built of brick, and ceiled at the level of the eaves with boards; ventilated and lighted by two grated windows and one iron grated door. The building contains a guard-room, 23¼ by 26½ feet, and 10⅓ feet high, and five cells, each 10½ by 4⅓ feet, and 10⅓ feet high. The cells are ventilated by means of apertures in the doors.

The hospital is a frame building, 160 by 30 feet, situated in the southeast corner of the reservation. It was formerly a ward of the general hospital, and was removed in sections to its present location. It is larger than is now necessary, affording abundant room for dispensary, office, clothes-room, store-room, dining-room, bath-room, kitchen, steward's quarters, and two large well-ventilated and lighted wards holding twenty-five beds. The area per bed is 85 feet and the cubic air-space 1,000 feet. But one ward is in use as such. It is provided with excellent ridge ventilation and is warmed by wood-stoves and lighted by windows and candles. A detached frame building, 16 by 13 feet, at the distance of 40 yards, is provided as a post-mortem room. The bath-room contains two bath-tubs and other necessary furniture. A large privy was built during the last year about 35 yards in rear of the hospital, and is kept in good order. Two earth-closets are also in use.

The post is supplied with excellent water from five wells, sunk from 30 to 60 feet beneath the surface. The water obtained is cool, clear, and soft, being entirely free from all impurities. The wells, together with a large cistern, abundantly supply the demands of the post. The ground upon which the post is situated being rolling, the natural drainage is excellent.

*Consolidated sick-report, Little Rock, Ark., 1870–'74.*

| Year | | 1870–'71. | | 1871–'72. | | 1872–'73. | | 1873–'74. | |
|---|---|---|---|---|---|---|---|---|---|
| Mean strength { Officers | | 5 | | 3 | | 14 | | 4 | |
| { Enlisted men | | 68 | | 56 | | 209 | | 85 | |
| Diseases. | | Cases. | Deaths. | Cases. | Deaths. | Cases. | Deaths. | Cases. | Deaths. |
| GENERAL DISEASES, A. | | | | | | | | | |
| Cerebro-spinal fever | | | | | | 1 | | | 1 |
| Typhoid fever | | | | | | 4 | | | |
| Typho-malarial fever | | 2 | | | | 2 | | | |
| Remittent fever | | 10 | | 2 | | 8 | | 88 | |
| Intermittent fever | | 68 | | 115 | | 143 | | 73 | |
| Other diseases of this group | | 8 | | 1 | | 73 | | 2 | |
| GENERAL DISEASES, B. | | | | | | | | | |
| Rheumatism | | 3 | | 7 | | 26 | | 11 | |
| Syphilis | | 10 | | 1 | | 21 | | 25 | |
| Consumption | | | 1 | | | 1 | | 1 | |
| Other diseases of this group | | | | | | | | 2 | |
| LOCAL DISEASES. | | | | | | | | | |
| Catarrh and bronchitis | | 2 | | 12 | | 56 | | 27 | |
| Pneumonia | | | | 1 | | 5 | | | |
| Pleurisy | | | | 1 | | 4 | | | |
| Diarrhœa and dysentery | | 6 | | 20 | | 91 | 1 | 36 | |
| Hernia | | | | | | 3 | | 1 | |
| Gonorrhœa | | 10 | | 6 | | 5 | | | |
| Other local diseases | | 25 | | 44 | | 159 | | 62 | 1 |
| Alcoholism | | 3 | | 6 | | 16 | | 13 | |
| Total disease | | 147 | 1 | 216 | | 618 | 1 | 341 | 2 |
| VIOLENT DISEASES AND DEATHS. | | | | | | | | | |
| Gunshot wounds | | 1 | | | | 3 | | | |
| Other accidents and injuries | | 20 | | 22 | | 57 | | 36 | |
| Suicide | | | | | | | | | |
| Total violence | | 21 | | 22 | | 60 | | 36 | |

# FORT LIVINGSTON, LOUISIANA.

Construction commenced in 1833. On Grand Terre Island, at the entrance of Barataria Bay, ninety-five miles from New Orleans, in latitude 29° 15′ north, longitude 12° 52′ west. Not occupied.

---

# FORT MACOMB, LOUISIANA.

Erected in 1825–'27, and named Fort Wood; changed to Fort Macomb, June 23, 1851. The fort stands on the right bank of Chef Menteur Pass, twenty-five miles from New Orleans, in latitude 30° 5′ north, longitude 12° 48′ west, approximately. In charge of an ordnance-sergeant.

# FORT MACON, NORTH CAROLINA

REPORTS OF ASSISTANT SURGEON E. COUES, AND OF ACTING ASSISTANT SURGEONS H. C. YARROW
AND S. T. WEIRICK, UNITED STATES ARMY.

Fort Macon is situated in latitude 34° 4′ north, longitude 23′ east.  It occupies the eastern
extremity of Borden or Bogue Island, commanding Beaufort Harbor, one of the southern outlets of
Pamlico Sound.  The town of Beaufort lies about two miles off, a little east of north, across the
harbor.  Morehead City, at the same distance westwardly, is the terminus of the Atlantic and
North Carolina Railroad.  Fort Johnston, some eighty miles distant, is the nearest military post.

The island is a mere sand-bar, lying nearly due east and west, separated from the mainland by
a narrow, shallow sound, (Bogue Sound.)  It is twenty-six miles long, with an average width of
less than a mile.  The sea-front is a gently undulating beach, flanked by extensive sand-hills, which
slope gradually to a low, flat marsh on the sound side, a narrow strip of comparatively fertile soil
intervening.  The sand-hills are constantly shifting, and the marsh is mostly overflowed at high
tide.  Part of the island is wooded, but the eastern extremity is treeless for several miles.  The
neighboring island of Shackleford has the same general character ; the adjoining mainland is low,
and consists chiefly of sandy tracts, pine barrens, and swamps.  Beaufort Harbor is shallow, and
obstructed by numerous extensive shoals ; the channel, navigable for vessels of ordinary tonnage,
is narrow and tortuous ; it sweeps around the point of the island close to the fort.  Vessels reach
the wharf at the railroad terminus, but only those of lightest draught go to Beaufort.  The bottom,
as well as the coast-line, is subject to constant change, and hydrographic surveys can be relied upon,
in detail, for only comparatively short periods.  There are no rocks whatever in the vicinity, except
those that have been brought hither.  The beach consists of pure sand mixed with shelly detritus.

The present fort has been in imminent danger from the encroachment of the sea, the water
having reached to the base of the glacis.  It is preserved by a system of stone jetties, by means of
which the beach was carried some 200 yards or more away from the fort.  Although they have thus
far answered their design, the fort must still be regarded as in an exposed and precarious condition.
The channel, as already stated, sweeps rapidly close inshore around the point of the island, with
constant erosive action.  The trend of the land lays it open to the prevailing and most violent
winds.  The open sea beats directly upon the beach, and the sand-hills are always shifting.  As
long as the fort is not defended by extensive and permanent masonry, care should be taken to disturb the surface as little as possible, since every formed or forming sand-hill is something of a natural protection.  The more grass and weeds are allowed to grow about the fort the better, as they
help to bind down the sand.

The reservation comprises about one mile of the end of the island.  The soil is poor, and most
of the land is uncultivated.  For the botany of the vicinity see Circular 4, page 84.

The waters give employment and support to a large part of the population, and furnish important additions to the Army ration.  A dozen or more of small or medium-sized fish may always be
taken at the wharf, and fishing for these is the chief amusement of the troops.  Of larger fish the
" sheephead," two species of drum, and the sea-trout, are abundant in season and easily secured.
Blue-fish are abundant late in summer, and trolling for them furnishes the most agreeable and
healthful exercise that is had here.  The most important fishing, however, in a commercial point of
view, is that of the mullet, (*Mugil*,) vast shoals of which make their appearance late in the fall.
They are only taken in the seine, and the annual catch for Carteret County is estimated at $70,000.

The humidity of the atmosphere is usually great, and the dew-point correspondingly high.  At most seasons articles of dress, books, the solid extracts, &c., rapidly gather mold, and instruments must be constantly cleaned. The prevailing winds are between south and west; these usually blow with great violence during most of February, March, and April, and are subject to sudden shift- ings. One effect of the shifting to the northward, in summer at least, is the wafting of the malaria from the swamps of the mainland, for the salt marsh itself is not, I am satisfied, appreciably miasmatic.

The fort stands on the eastern extremity of the reservation, at from 250 to 400 yards from the (present) water-mark, but very high tides flood the level shingle nearly to the foot of the glacis. The glacis has a long and gradual slope on the sea-front, but is short and abrupt on the sound side. The bottom of the ditch is just about at high-water mark. During unusually high tides it is flooded a foot or more in depth by water that enters from the marsh through a culvert into a drain running under the glacis. The parade-wall, of brick, incloses an irregularly pentagonal area of about half an acre. The parade is about 3 feet above the level of the ditch; its longest diagonal is 183 feet, the shortest 100 feet.

There are no barracks at the post; with the exception of a few married soldiers the troops are quartered in the casemates, a part of which have been furnished with iron-grated doors and win- dows to further fit them for prison-cells, for which they are in other respects well adapted; all are of solid masonry throughout, plastered and ceiled overhead, and with board flooring laid over the brick-work. They are nearly of the usual tunnel-shape, with low perpendicular walls and arched ceilings; they measure 38 by 18 feet in superficial area, by 15 feet to the ridge; they are warmed by an open fire-place, lighted in the rear by embrasures and port-holes, and in front by a door and window of ordinary dimensions, opening directly into the parade; ventilation is further provided for by two chimney-like openings in the ridge. There are twenty-four casemates of this descrip- tion, six of which are used as men's quarters, five as officers' quarters, two respectively as prison- cells, company mess-rooms, company offices, and store-rooms for quartermaster and commissary property, one respectively as adjutant's office, ordnance store-room, guard-house, bakery, and kitchen. The triangular spaces left between contiguous casemates at three of the five angles of the fort are partly used as magazines and partly as cook-rooms, a brick wall separating them into two compartments. With the usual garrison of two companies the men are overcrowded; the dimensions of the casemates afford only 10,260 cubic feet, without taking into consideration the arch of the ceiling, by which, with the bunks, boxes of clothing, &c., the capacity is further diminished materially. With 20 men in each casemate—there never have been fewer, and some- times more—the air-space per man is only about 500 cubic feet. It may be said that the case- mates will only accommodate 10 or 12 men, with due regard to hygiene, and, even when not crowded, cannot be considered as eligible quarters. In spite of the several openings above mentioned, the ventilation is defective. When the doors and windows are closed it is insufficient, as is readily per- ceived on entering a casemate at midnight; when open, there is generally a strong draught of air directly through from one end to the other. Most of the casemates are, moreover, extremely damp.

Suitable barracks remain an especial desideratum, and in case of an epidemic it would proba- bly be necessary to evacuate the fort.

The men sleep in iron bunks. There are no bath or wash-rooms—the men wash under a shed in the ditch at the postern gate. The kitchens are cramped in space, but otherwise eligible. The two mess-rooms answer every purpose, and are supplied with proper fixtures. There are no water- closets. A large and well-constructed sink is located on the edge of the marsh, within high-water mark, so that the excreta are constantly carried away by the tide.

This is a prison fort, the number of convicts being about twenty.

But few changes or improvements have been made at the post, and it is in rather a dilapidated condition.

The married soldiers' quarters are in very bad condition, with the exception of two houses recently erected for the ordnance and commissary sergeants.

There are four small wooden cottages for officers' quarters, insufficient for the wants of the post, without conveniences, and in bad repair.

The hospital, built since last report, is a two-story building of yellow pine, built in accordance with plan No. 2, Circular No. 3, plate 3, Surgeon-General's Office, 1871. It is in fair condition, and with a few changes, which have been authorized, may be considered as satisfactory.

Drinking-water is obtained from two wells, situated at the end of the glacis; it is daily distributed in barrels by the prisoners. Within the fort are four cisterns that collect the water from the inner parapet. This water is only used for washing. There is no distribution of water from the cisterns.

The porosity of the soil and the slope of the glacis render the natural drainage unusually effective. The level parade-ground within is drained by a system of five sewers, opening by six culverts, one for each side of the pentagon, and one in the middle. The several drains center here, whence a single sewer conducts under the sally-port to the ditch, and the water flows thence through a tunnel under the outer parapet and glacis into the marsh. The drains are constructed of wood and masonry; they have scarcely pitch enough inside of the fort, but are otherwise well adapted; nothing offensive is allowed to be poured into them; all slops and garbage are twice daily removed by the prisoners, in barrels, and thrown far out upon the beach, where they are partly devoured by birds and crabs, and partly washed away by the tide; the most wholesome regulations in this regard have always been enforced.

The sea affords constant bathing facilities in summer. There is no special provision for bathing in winter.

There are no post, hospital, or officers' gardens. There is daily (except Sunday) communication by rail with large cities north, and a weekly line of steamships from New Berne (28 miles distant) to New York. The daily mail is quite regular. Letters require between two and three days to reach Washington and New York.

There are now no aborigines in the vicinity, but tribes formerly living here have left their traces in at least one "Kjoekkenmoedding," (that on Harker's Island,) in which pieces of pottery and various implements may be found.

In spite of some obvious violations of hygienic principles that have been noted above, the general sanitary condition of the post is good; the locality is, perhaps, unusually healthy for one on the southern coast; the sudden changes of temperature are the chief drawbacks; these, joined to the humidity of the atmosphere, operate unfavorably in pulmonary complaints. Phthisis makes rapid progress when fairly established, while common colds and coughs are apt to prove tedious and troublesome, even when they do not have more serious terminations. Pneumonia requires close attention. It is difficult to specify any as the prevailing diseases; there have been no epidemics for some years at the fort itself; its isolation appears to confer comparative immunity, and would be an efficient furtherance of quarantine and other sanitary measures. An importation of yellow fever from New Berne to Beaufort a few years since did not spread, and subsided with comparatively small mortality; the residents assert that it is not known to have originated there. A moderate amount of malarial fever occurs in summer; it is of a mild form, and the type tends toward suppression of the chill, and corresponding lengthening of the febrile state; it is most probable that what little miasma is experienced is wafted by northerly winds from inland swamps; the marsh itself appears non-malarious. Nearly all the bowel diseases, of which there is a moderate amount, have proven of a transient character, yielding readily; though occasionally cases of dysentery, dependent upon or associated with malarial conditions, have been found intractable,

*Consolidated sick-report, Fort Macon, N. C., 1870–'74.*

| Year | 1870–'71. | | 1871–'72. | | 1872–'73. | | 1873–'74. | |
|---|---|---|---|---|---|---|---|---|
| Mean strength { Officers / Enlisted men | 6 / 82 | | 5 / 91 | | 5 / 101 | | 6 / 99 | |
| Diseases. | Cases. | Deaths. | Cases. | Deaths. | Cases. | Deaths. | Cases. | Deaths. |
| **GENERAL DISEASES, A.** | | | | | | | | |
| Typhoid fever | | | 1 | | 1 | | | |
| Remittent fever | 5 | | 1 | | | | 2 | |
| Intermittent fever | 1 | | 33 | | 16 | | 7 | |
| Other diseases of this group | 4 | | | | 1 | | 3 | |
| **GENERAL DISEASES, B.** | | | | | | | | |
| Rheumatism | 12 | | 22 | | 10 | | 9 | |
| Syphilis | 4 | | 15 | | 3 | | 1 | |
| Other diseases of this group | | | | | 1 | | | |
| **LOCAL DISEASES.** | | | | | | | | |
| Catarrh and bronchitis | 9 | | 78 | | 29 | | 22 | |
| Pleurisy | | | | | 1 | | | |
| Diarrhœa and dysentery | 36 | | 76 | | 41 | | 24 | 1 |
| Gonorrhœa | 4 | | 14 | | 9 | | 2 | |
| Other local diseases | 54 | | 80 | | 105 | 1 | 60 | |
| Alcoholism | 1 | | 2 | | 4 | | 9 | |
| Total disease | 130 | | 322 | | 221 | 1 | 139 | 1 |
| **VIOLENT DISEASES AND DEATHS.** | | | | | | | | |
| Gunshot wounds | 2 | | | | | | 1 | |
| Drowning | | | | 1 | | | | |
| Other accidents and injuries | 28 | | 45 | | 25 | | 17 | |
| Total violence | 30 | | 45 | 1 | 25 | | 18 | |

*Consolidated sick-report, (prisoners,) Fort Macon, N. C., 1870–'74.*

| Year | 1870–'71. | | 1871–'72. | | 1872–'73. | | 1873–'74. | |
|---|---|---|---|---|---|---|---|---|
| Mean strength ...... Enlisted men | 11 | | 14 | | 49 | | 15 | |
| Diseases. | Cases. | Deaths. | Cases. | Deaths. | Cases. | Deaths. | Cases. | Deaths. |
| **GENERAL DISEASES, A.** | | | | | | | | |
| Remittent fever | | | | | 1 | | | |
| Intermittent fever | 3 | | 6 | | 7 | | 9 | |
| Other diseases of this group | | | 2 | | | | | |
| **GENERAL DISEASES, B.** | | | | | | | | |
| Rheumatism | 8 | | 9 | | 23 | | 4 | |
| Syphilis | | | 3 | | 1 | | 2 | |
| Consumption | | | 1 | | | | | |
| Other diseases of this group | | | 1 | | 5 | | | |
| **LOCAL DISEASES.** | | | | | | | | |
| Catarrh and bronchitis | 1 | | 15 | | 22 | | 2 | |
| Diarrhœa and dysentery | 19 | | 17 | | 103 | | 6 | |
| Hernia | | | 1 | | 1 | | | |
| Other local diseases | 12 | | 24 | | 110 | | 19 | |
| Alcoholism | | | | | | | 2 | |
| Total disease | 43 | | 79 | | 273 | | 44 | |
| **VIOLENT DISEASES AND DEATHS.** | | | | | | | | |
| Accidents and injuries | 6 | | 10 | | 37 | 1 | 5 | |
| Total violence | 6 | | 10 | | 37 | 1 | 5 | |

# FORT MARION, FLORIDA.

Originally established by the Spaniards in 1756, and called the " Castle of St. Mark;" name changed to Fort Marion January 7, 1825. At St. Augustine, Fla.; latitude, 29° 48′ north; longitude, 4° 32′ west. The works are in charge of an ordnance-sergeant.

# FORT McREA, FLORIDA.

Construction commenced in 1833. On Foster's Bank, opposite Fort Pickens, at the entrance to Pensacola Bay. It is now unoccupied.

---

# MOBILE, ALABAMA.

## REPORT OF ASSISTANT SURGEON J. K. CORSON, UNITED STATES ARMY.

The post of Mobile is located on the west bank of the Mobile River, at its entrance into the bay, and within the limits of the city of the same name, in latitude 30° 42′ north, and longitude 11° 1′ west, and at a distance of about one mile from the river.

The mean annual temperature of the locality is 67° F.; the temperature at the post, however, is influenced by the heat-absorbing character and color of the soil, which is a loose, dark sand, with little organic matter; and experiments with a thermometer placed on the surface of this soil within the post have shown a difference equal to 31° over that indicated by the instrument in its usual position.

The present city of Mobile has a population of over 50,000 inhabitants, nearly one-half of whom are colored.

The post consists of fourteen detached wooden buildings, the windows and doors facing north and south, except in the hospital, where the greater number of the windows are on the eastern and western sides. The inclosure is on a level plain, 30 feet only above the river-level; on this plain numerous slight depressions afford stations for stagnant water in a direction northward, until, at that end of the town, they settle down into a continuous marsh or swamp, which stretches for some 36 to 40 miles along either bank of the river into the interior of the State.

The men's quarters consist of two wooden buildings, each 85 by 50 feet, two stories high, with a veranda 10 feet wide on the southern side. They are well ventilated by numerous windows on the north and south sides, and by ridge ventilators and shafts from the apex of the roof, and gave, when occupied by the band and two companies, an air-space of 779 cubic feet per man. They were furnished with the new pattern iron bedstead.

A kitchen, 23 by 11 feet, and a mess-room communicating therewith, 20 by 23 feet, completed each set of quarters. Two long, low, one-storied, wooden buildings are divided into six rooms in each building, or twelve rooms of 14½ by 15 feet, for the married soldiers of the post. These quarters are unhealthy, dilapidated, and unfit for their purpose. The store-house of the quartermaster and commissary is 42 by 40 feet, two stories high, with a small gallery in front, and a cellar, size of the buildings, underneath. It is too small for the purposes required, and much of the quartermaster's property had to be stored elsewhere. The bakery is 17½ by 14 feet, with a good oven. The officers' quarters consist of three detached two-story wooden buildings, with verandas in front and behind, and contain in each building four small sets of quarters of two rooms, each room being 15 feet square; each set of quarters has a small kitchen, and servant's room behind, and sink and well in the yard.

The hospital is a detached two-story wooden building, 80 by 60 feet, commodious and well constructed. Its site is not good, being placed almost on top of the main drain of the post. Into this sewer run the deposits of some one hundred and fifty persons daily, and however well and perfectly disinfected, it appears to be certainly the worst spot in the inclosure for a hospital.

Exteriorly, a gallery, 10 feet wide, runs round both stories of the building, adding greatly to the comfort of patients and occupants in a southern climate. The building is raised 4 feet from the ground.

On the upper floor are two wards, 40 by 25 feet, by 15 feet high, ceiled and plastered, with ventilators in ceiling. The windows also have ventilating panes at top. The hospital-sink is outside, 12 yards off, fitted with zinc-lined movable boxes, daily taken away, cleaned out, and disinfected, as are all the sinks at the post.

On the lower floor are the dispensary, 24 by 14½ feet; medicine and liquor room, 9 by 12 feet; the steward's room, 15 by 12 feet; two store-rooms, 15 by 12 feet, and 13 by 9 feet, respectively, the latter two designed for matron's quarters, and a post-mortem or dead room, but not so used. On the eastern side of the lower floor, and separated by a hall, 10 feet wide, are the principal store-room, 24 by 9 feet; the mess-room, 24 by 14½ feet; kitchen, 14½ by 15 feet; with a pantry, 9 by 9 feet, and a bath-room, 9 by 8½ feet. All these rooms on the lower floor are 9 feet high.

Water in abundance is supplied by artesian wells, eight in number, and by cisterns attached to each of the larger occupied buildings in the post. The well-water is of slightly acid reaction, containing the salts of the protoxide of iron, and yields a white precipitate when tested with nitrate of silver or liquor calcis. It is without odor, colorless, but exhibits an oily pellicle or scum floating on its surface when exposed for any length of time in a shallow vessel. These qualities, however, do not forbid its use.

The drainage of the post is effected by ditches, 5 feet deep, running east and west along the outside of the fence, and conveying their contents, very imperfectly, into the Mobile River.

The soil being dry and pervious to water, the want of sufficient elevation is the only cause of the defective sewerage which exists outside of the post and throughout the city, many of the streets of which are flooded during the heavy rains. Slops, offal, and excreta of the post, instead of being left to drain away, or filter into these ditches, have been carefully carried away daily to a distance and burned, buried, or destroyed.

Mobile is subject to periodical visitations of yellow fever, though its inhabitants maintain that it has always been imported. By a table published in 1871, the following information is given as to the years of epidemic, and the number of deaths:

| Years. | 1839. | 1843. | 1847. | 1853. | 1854. | 1855. | 1858. | 1867. | 1870. |
|---|---|---|---|---|---|---|---|---|---|
| Number of deaths*............ | 657 | 311 | 75 | 886 | 36 | 39 | 319 | 92 | 180 |

* In a population ranging from 20,000 up to 50,000 in year 1870.

These statistics, however, are not believed to be quite accurate.

In September, 1873, this scourge again appeared, having been imported direct from Shreveport, La., but through the unceasing exertions and watchfulness of the medical authorities of the town, its vastly improved sanitary condition and hygiene, and the unusual diminution of temperature from the middle of August, the disease happily did not attain to an epidemic, and the deaths were only 19. The troops were, however, as on former occasions, immediately removed to Mount Vernon Barracks, Alabama, where it is said yellow fever never existed, and where, the arsenal having been abandoned as such, the troops find comfortable and healthy quarters.

*Meteorological report, Mobile, Ala., 1872–'74.*

| Month. | 1870–'71. | | | | 1871–'72. | | | | 1872–'73. | | | | 1873–'74. | | | |
|---|---|---|---|---|---|---|---|---|---|---|---|---|---|---|---|---|
| | Temperature. | | | Rain-fall in inches. | Temperature. | | | Rain-fall in inches. | Temperature. | | | Rain-fall in inches. | Temperature. | | | Rain-fall in inches. |
| | Mean. | Max. | Min. | | Mean. | Max. | Min. | | Mean. | Max. | Min. | | Mean. | Max. | Min. | |
| July........ | | | | | | | | | 81.72 | 96* | 71* | 13.37 | 82.51 | 98* | 69* | 8.75 |
| August......... | | | | | | | | | 82.42 | 96* | 70* | 1.69 | 80.59 | 94* | 70* | 10.35 |
| September......... | | | | | | | | | 77.03 | 94* | 62* | 2.11 | 76.43 | 91* | 61* | 8.07 |
| October........ | | | | | | | | | 66.10 | 85* | 42* | 2.77 | | | | |
| November......... | | | | | | | | | 54.54 | 75* | 27* | 5.65 | | | | |
| December......... | | | | | | | | | | | | | | | | |
| January......... | | | | | | | | | 46.66 | 69* | 19* | 4.16 | | | | |
| February......... | | | | | | | | | 56.57 | 75* | 35* | 3.15 | | | | |
| March ......... | | | | | | | | | 57.28 | 77* | 31* | 3.86 | | | | |
| April......... | | | | | | | | | 65.99 | 85* | 44* | 0.88 | | | | |
| May......... | | | | | 76.37 | 96* | 51* | 3.69 | 74.68 | 92* | 55* | 11.47 | | | | |
| June......... | | | | | 81.72 | 95* | 68* | 6.33 | 79.82 | 95* | 68* | 9.87 | | | | |
| For the year....... | | | | | | | | | | 96* | | | | | | |

* These observations are made with self-registering thermometers. The mean is from the standard thermometer.

*Consolidated sick-report, Mobile, Ala., 1870–'74.*

| Year | | 1870–'71. | | 1871–'72. | | 1872–'73. | | 1873–'74. * | |
|---|---|---|---|---|---|---|---|---|---|
| Mean strength | Officers | 6 | | 7 | | 9 | | 8 | |
| | Enlisted men | 96 | | 108 | | 124 | | 109 | |
| Diseases. | | Cases. | Deaths. | Cases. | Deaths. | Cases. | Deaths. | Cases. | Deaths. |
| GENERAL DISEASES, A. | | | | | | | | | |
| Remittent fever | | 3 | 1 | 4 | | 19 | | 2 | |
| Intermittent fever | | 57 | | 46 | | 38 | | 11 | |
| Yellow fever | | 5 | 1 | | | | | | |
| Other diseases of this group | | 3 | | 3 | | 8 | | | |
| GENERAL DISEASES, B. | | | | | | | | | |
| Rheumatism | | 1 | | 5 | | 4 | | 3 | |
| Syphilis | | 10 | | 18 | | 17 | | 5 | |
| Consumption | | 4 | | 1 | | | | | |
| Other diseases of this group | | 4 | | 1 | | | | | |
| LOCAL DISEASES. | | | | | | | | | |
| Catarrh and bronchitis | | 12 | | 6 | | 6 | | | |
| Pleurisy | | 2 | | | | 1 | | | |
| Diarrhœa and dysentery | | 37 | | 33 | | 18 | | 8 | |
| Hernia | | | | 3 | | | | | |
| Gonorrhœa | | 9 | | 2 | | 3 | | | |
| Other local diseases | | 50 | 1 | 49 | | 51 | 2 | 15 | |
| Alcoholism | | 5 | | 13 | | 11 | | 2 | |
| Total disease | | 202 | 3 | 184 | | 176 | 2 | 46 | |
| VIOLENT DISEASES AND DEATHS. | | | | | | | | | |
| Gunshot wounds | | | | 1 | | 1 | | | |
| Other accidents and injuries | | 22 | | 29 | | 20 | | 2 | |
| Suicide | | | | | | | 1 | | |
| Total violence | | 22 | | 30 | | 21 | 1 | 2 | |

* Consolidated with Mount Vernon Barracks, September, 1873.  Two months only.

# FORT MORGAN, ALABAMA.

Fort Morgan was commenced in 1819, and first garrisoned March 7, 1834.  It is located on Mobile Point, at the entrance of Mobile Bay, in latitude 30° 14′ north; longitude 10° 57′ west.  It is now in charge of an ordnance-sergeant.

# FORT MOULTRIE, SOUTH CAROLINA.

A fort was established during the revolutionary period on Sullivan's Island, in the main entrance to Charleston Harbor, between 5 and 6 miles from the city, in latitude 32° 45′ 30″ north; longitude 2° 48′ 14″ west; and named Fort Moultrie.  The works are now in charge of an ordnance-sergeant.

# MOUNT VERNON BARRACKS, ALABAMA.

REPORTS OF ASSISTANT SURGEON J. K. CORSON, AND ACTING ASSISTANT SURGEON R. M. REYNOLDS,
UNITED STATES ARMY.

This post, formerly an arsenal, is in latitude 31° 6′ north; longitude 11° 5′ west; 28 miles, by rail, north of Mobile, and three miles from the west bank of the Mobile River; altitude above high water in the river, 155 feet.

A post was first established in this vicinity in 1799, and was called Fort Stoddart.  In 1804 this was the most prominent post in Alabama, having been made a port of entry and seat of a court of admiralty. In the following year Congress constituted the "Bigbee" settlements a revenue district, which created great dissatisfaction among the settlers on the river, as causing double taxation—their exports and imports paying duty to the Federal Government at Fort Stoddart, and again to the Spanish government at Mobile. From this and other causes the "Bigbee" settlers formed several plans to capture Mobile, without the concurrence of the Federal Government. The last attempt, led by a settler named Kemper, failed, and most of the party were captured by the Spaniards. About November, 1811, General Wilkinson sent Colonel Cushing with troops to protect Mobile from the designs of the settlers. They built a cantonment at Mount Vernon, consisting of log huts chinked with clay. The post was a general rendezvous for the Federal army during the Creek campaign, and was occupied by General Jackson while preparing for offensive operations against Pensacola and the defense of Mobile.

By an act of Congress approved May 24, 1828, the building of an arsenal at this point was authorized, and the reservation was approved by the President March 10, 1830.

July 1, 1873, under orders from the Secretary of War, the post was turned over for occupation by troops, and by General Orders No. 78, War Department, Adjutant-General's Office, dated Washington, July 25, 1873, the designation of the post was changed to that of Mount Vernon Barracks, Alabama.

About 35 acres of the reservation are inclosed by a well-built brick wall, 16 feet high, in the shape of a horseshoe, with an inverted crescent completing the inclosure. The buildings are arranged with this wall to form, with their connecting fences, an inner circle and crescent, corresponding to the outer wall.

The quarters for enlisted men are in a three-story brick building, 120 feet 6 inches by 40 feet 6 inches, height of stories 10 feet. The dormitories are furnished with single iron bedsteads, and give about 1,000 cubic feet space per man. The lower floor is brick-paved, and divided into kitchens and mess-hall. There is no wash-house or lavatory, and no proper privies.

Three buildings are used as officers' quarters; two of brick, two stories high, with piazza above and below on the north and east sides. Each contains two rooms 20 by 17 feet, two 20 by 15 feet, two 15 by 15 feet, bath-room and hall, with an adjoining building one and a half stories high, 30 by 14 feet, for kitchen, &c. Water is supplied by a hydraulic ram.

The third building is of brick, two-stories high, 56 by 42 feet, and was formerly the ordnance barrack. It has piazzas in front and half the depth of the sides, and four rooms on each floor. The kitchen for this building is with the post bakery in a one-story brick building, 45 by 23 feet, in rear of the quarters.

The storehouses and offices are in four brick buildings, each 30 by 50 feet and one story high.

The guard-house is of brick, 40 by 34 feet, the guard-room being 21 by 16 feet, by 12 feet high. The prisoners' room 16 by 10 feet.

Facing the guard-house, on the south side of the main entrance, is a building of the same size and shape intended for a hospital, and used as a dispensary, steward's room, and store-room. The patients were removed from this on account of dampness and unfitness, and are in a one-story frame cottage about 30 yards distant, giving two wards, each 25 by 20 feet, which contain 8 beds. A new hospital should be constructed at this post.

At the back of the adjutant's office is a deep ravine, in the lowest part of which a hydraulic ram was placed in 1855. From the ram, which is still used although nearly worn out, iron pipes run to a central reservoir in the middle of the parade, and thence to the various buildings, the waste-pipes going to the gardens of the post. Most of these pipes have been cut off on account of failing power. The water is from never-failing springs of good quality, estimated supply 3 gallons per minute. The reservoir contains 1,500 gallons, is three-eighths of a mile from and 125 feet above the ram, and high enough to furnish water to the second stories of the quarters.

There is a bath-house within the inclosure, now out of repair, supplied by springs. There are four large cisterns, but only one in order.

The natural and artificial drainage is good, but sinks are needed for the men's and laundresses' quarters. There is no inclosed cemetery. The post is a healthy one; the principal diseases are malarial in character.

Communication is maintained with Mobile by the river, and by the Mobile and Alabama Grand Trunk Railroad. Mount Vernon station on the latter is about half a mile distant from the barracks. There is but one train daily each way. There are two regular boats a week each way on the river, which is three miles from the post. In going up they are tolerably regular, leaving Mobile generally Tuesday and Saturday evenings. No regular time can be depended on for their return, as their destination up the river is not always the same. During the cotton season the number of boats on the river is considerably increased.

*Consolidated sick-report, Mount Vernon Barracks, Ala., 1870–'74.*

| Year | 1870-'71 Cases | Deaths | 1871-'72 Cases | Deaths | 1872-'73 Cases | Deaths | 1873-'74.* Cases | Deaths |
|---|---|---|---|---|---|---|---|---|
| Mean strength { Officers | 2 | | 2 | | 2 | | 7 | |
| { Enlisted men | 13 | | 8 | | 8 | | 92 | |
| **Diseases.** | | | | | | | | |
| GENERAL DISEASES, A. | | | | | | | | |
| Remittent fever | | | | | | | 1 | |
| Intermittent fever | 9 | | 6 | | 4 | | 49 | |
| Other diseases of this group | | | | | | | 2 | |
| GENERAL DISEASES, B. | | | | | | | | |
| Rheumatism | 1 | | | | | | 8 | |
| Syphilis | | | | | | | 5 | |
| Other diseases of this group | | | | | | 1 | | |
| LOCAL DISEASES. | | | | | | | | |
| Catarrh and bronchitis | 2 | | 1 | | 4 | | 27 | |
| Pneumonia | | | | | | | 1 | |
| Pleurisy | | | | | | | 1 | |
| Diarrhœa and dysentery | 7 | | 3 | | 1 | | 18 | |
| Other local diseases | 6 | | | | 6 | | 51 | 1 |
| Alcoholism | 2 | | 1 | | 1 | | 18 | |
| Total disease | 27 | | 11 | | 17 | | 181 | 1 |
| VIOLENT DISEASES AND DEATHS. | | | | | | | | |
| Accidents and injuries | | | 1 | | | | 33 | |
| Total violence | | | 1 | | | | 33 | |

* Consolidated with Mobile, Ala., in September, 1873.

# NASHVILLE, TENNESSEE.

## REPORT OF ASSISTANT SURGEON W. D. WOLVERTON, UNITED STATES ARMY.

The post of Ash Barracks is located near the northern limits of the city of Nashville; latitude, 36° 10' north; longitude, 10° west, and about 450 feet above low-water mark at Mobile. It is on high ground on the west bank of the Cumberland River, which is about one mile distant. The post was established in 1866, and constructed mainly from material obtained from the demolition of Cumberland Barracks. The surrounding country is undulating, the soil a clay loam mixed with fine gravel, from three to six feet deep, resting on stratified fossiliferous limestone.

About 9 acres are occupied by the post, being leased for a term of years by the Government. The water-supply is from the city water-works, and by an engine and reservoirs is distributed to every building.

With the exception of the hospital the buildings were originally made with flat roofs. In 1870 these were raised in the center and shingled, leaving the old roofs to serve as ceilings. The buildings are all of boards, with battened joints.

The barracks are five two-story buildings 128 by 23 feet, first stories 8, and second stories 10½ feet high. The dormitories are in the second story, are furnished with single iron bedsteads, and allow from 600 to 750 cubic feet per man. The lower floors are divided into kitchens, mess-rooms, lavatories, store-rooms, &c.

The married soldiers' quarters are three frame buildings, one 12 by 46 feet, containing two sets, one 12 by 24 feet, and one 20 by 30 feet.

The officers' quarters are seven frame buildings; one 40 by 42 feet, surrounded by a veranda and containing five rooms, used as quarters by the commanding officer; two, each 43 by 38 feet, one of which is surrounded by a veranda, the other but on three sides; said buildings each contain two sets of quarters, of three rooms each; the next building is two stories high, with a veranda on three sides and a double one in front, each story divided into six rooms, or four sets of quarters of three rooms each; the next is 33 by 37 feet, has a veranda on all sides, contains but one set of quarters of four rooms; the next building is two stories high, 32 by 78 feet, containing eight rooms to each story or eight sets of quarters of two rooms each, has a veranda in rear, and a double one in front; four rooms on the first floor are used as headquarters of post; the last of these buildings is 50 by 41 feet, containing nine rooms, or three sets of quarters of three rooms each, having a veranda on three sides. Kitchens are placed either at the sides or in rear of the building.

The guard-house is a frame building one-story high, with a veranda in front; it is 20 by 62 feet, and contains eight rooms, viz: a guard-room, prison-room, four cells, a room for the officer of the guard, and a store-room. Ventilation is effected by doors and windows, and heating by a wood-stove in the guard-room. The prison-room contains 3,312 cubic feet air-space, and each of the four cells has a capacity of 108 cubic feet.

The present post hospital was erected in the autumn of 1867. It is constructed chiefly of old lumber obtained by tearing down Cumberland Barracks. The outside is covered with rough boards set vertically. The joints are battened, and the whole washed with lime and yellow ochre. The walls of the wards, lavatories, water-closets, and intervening halls are ceiled with pieces of old flooring, and painted. The kitchen is lined with rough boards and whitewashed, and the other parts of the building are covered with machine-planed boards, battened and painted as on the outside. The central building, two stories in height, 35 by 30 feet, contains on the first floor, on the right of the main entrance, the office; on the left, the dispensary. In the rear of the latter, and separated from it by a hall 6 feet wide, is a room for attendants. Each of the three is 14 feet square. The remainder of the rear of the building is occupied by the dining-room, 14 by 19 feet. In the rear of the attendants' and dining rooms is an extension of one story, 13 by 23 feet, for a kitchen and small mess-room. The second floor of the center building is divided into an isolation ward, 12 by 14 feet, steward's room, matron's room, spare room, and two small store-rooms.

On each side of the center building is a wing 24 by 37 feet divided into a ward, 24 by 33 feet, a closet, and lavatory or bath-room. Each ward is ventilated by five windows and a ventilating shaft, and warmed by a large coal-stove. The number of beds in each is twelve. The entire hospital building, except the rear of the central portion, is surrounded by a veranda 8 feet in width. The hospital grounds are limited, extending only 20 feet beyond each end of the building and the rear of the kitchen. Along the rear fence are placed the dead-house, coal and wood shed, privy, and wash-house. The latter is 16 by 18 feet, and furnished with stationary boiler and tubs. The drainage is conveyed underground to the main sewer, which discharges into a covered cesspool 250 feet from the hospital.

The post library contains some 596 volumes, consisting of novels, histories, and biographies. The post bakery is a wooden building, 20 by 40 feet, one story high.

The quartermaster's and commissary buildings are frame buildings, each one story high; that of the quartermaster is 40 by 220 feet, and contains nine rooms, which are used for offices and storage purposes; the commissary building is 20 by 60 feet, and divided into four rooms; the building next to the commissary storehouse is a blacksmith-shop, 20 by 34 feet. A workshop, 25 by 100 feet, stands on the same line with the blacksmith-shop, and contains three rooms.

The stables are two in number, one of which is 50 by 156 feet, and the other 35 by 268 feet. Some 40 feet from the quartermaster's building stands a frame building, 32 by 40 feet, which is used as an engine-house, and contains a stationary steam-engine, used for sawing wood and forcing water into water-tanks, which are placed on an elevated platform near the engine-house. There are two of them, each having a capacity of 10,000 gallons of water.

The sinks are three in number; the one intended for the enlisted men stands 40 feet in rear of the center building, on the southwest side; it is 12 by 50 feet, contains thirteen seats and two urinals, and is so arranged that the refuse can be forced out of the vault with a pump and conveyed away from the post on carts. The other two sinks are for the use of the married soldiers and their families. The hospital sink is 6 by 14 feet, built over a vault from 15 to 20 feet in depth, and stands in the back yard of the hospital. The sinks for the use of the officers and their families are small and inconvenient, standing in rear of the quarters, and so close to the buildings as to render them obnoxious as well as unhealthy to the inmates.

The natural and artificial drainage is good. The site of the post is on elevated ground, declining on three sides; the whole is drained by a system of under-drains leading into cesspools remote from the post. There is no post garden.

The general sanitary condition of the post could scarcely be better, considering the location and general character of the surrounding country.

*Consolidated sick-report, Nashville, Tenn., (white troops,) 1870–'74.*

| Year. | | 1870–'71. | | 1871–'72. | | 1872–'73. | | 1873–'74. | |
|---|---|---|---|---|---|---|---|---|---|
| Mean strength { Officers | | 9 | | 9 | | 10 | | 9 | |
| { Enlisted men | | 181 | | 169 | | 164 | | 134 | |
| Diseases. | | Cases. | Deaths. | Cases. | Deaths. | Cases. | Deaths. | Cases. | Deaths. |
| GENERAL DISEASES, A. | | | | | | | | | |
| Typhoid fever | | 1 | ...... | 1 | ...... | 8 | ...... | 1 | ...... |
| Typho-malarial fever | | 1 | ...... | ...... | ...... | 4 | 3 | ...... | ...... |
| Remittent fever | | 8 | ...... | 4 | ...... | 13 | ...... | 4 | ...... |
| Intermittent fever | | 274 | ...... | 69 | ...... | 46 | ...... | 25 | ...... |
| Cholera | | ...... | ...... | ...... | ...... | 1 | ...... | ...... | ...... |
| Other diseases of this group | | 21 | ...... | 21 | ...... | 3 | ...... | 3 | ...... |
| GENERAL DISEASES, B. | | | | | | | | | |
| Rheumatism | | 17 | ...... | 13 | ...... | 10 | ...... | 21 | ...... |
| Syphilis | | 56 | 1 | 30 | ...... | 43 | 1 | 17 | 1 |
| Consumption | | 6 | ...... | 2 | ...... | 2 | ...... | ...... | ...... |
| Other diseases of this group | | 1 | ...... | 5 | ...... | ...... | ...... | ...... | ...... |
| LOCAL DISEASES. | | | | | | | | | |
| Catarrh and bronchitis | | 41 | ...... | 44 | ...... | 30 | ...... | 12 | ...... |
| Pneumonia | | 5 | 1 | 3 | ...... | 3 | 1 | 1 | ...... |
| Pleurisy | | 3 | ...... | 3 | ...... | 1 | ...... | 1 | ...... |
| Diarrhœa and dysentery | | 57 | ...... | 59 | 1 | 33 | ...... | 24 | 1 |
| Hernia | | 1 | ...... | ...... | ...... | ...... | ...... | ...... | ...... |
| Gonorrhœa | | 23 | ...... | 10 | ...... | 2 | ...... | 5 | ...... |
| Other local diseases | | 114 | ...... | 90 | 2 | 52 | 1 | 31 | ...... |
| Alcoholism | | 12 | ...... | 6 | ...... | 4 | ...... | 1 | ...... |
| Unclassified | | ...... | ...... | ...... | ...... | 1 | ...... | ...... | ...... |
| Total disease | | 641 | 2 | 360 | 3 | 256 | 6 | 146 | 2 |
| VIOLENT DISEASES AND DEATHS. | | | | | | | | | |
| Gunshot wounds | | ...... | ...... | 1 | ...... | 2 | 1 | ...... | ...... |
| Other accidents and injuries | | 64 | ...... | 59 | ...... | 65 | 1 | 29 | ...... |
| Total violence | | 64 | ...... | 60 | ...... | 67 | 2 | 29 | ...... |

# NEWBERRY, SOUTH CAROLINA.

### REPORT BY ASSISTANT SURGEON W. H. KING, UNITED STATES ARMY.

The town of Newberry is situated in the center of the district of the same name, latitude 34° 14′ north; longitude 3° 38′ west, forty-seven miles due west from Columbia, on the Columbia and Greenville Railroad. Four buildings are occupied by the troops, necessary offices, &c., at this station. One wooden building, 2½ stories high, containing eight square rooms, two attic bed-rooms, and three basement rooms, is used as a barrack. This house is in the suburbs of Newberry, surrounded by fine old trees, and has an inclosure about it of some four acres, containing a good well of water. Small frame buildings, formerly used as negro-quarters, afford ample room for kitchen, laundresses' quarters, &c. This building-site has been admirably selected on elevated ground, the front of the main edifice facing north. Barracks for a single company, so commodious and in every way so suitable as these, could hardly be erected.

Two small frame cottages, in close proximity to the building above described, are also rented by the United States Government, one as quarters for officers, the other containing the dispensary and necessary rooms for storage of hospital stores, &c., as well as offices for commanding officer, quartermaster, commissary, and adjutant of the post. One other small frame building is used as quarters for officers.

*Consolidated sick report, Newberry, S. C., 1871–'74.*

| Year | | 1871–'72. | | 1872–'73. | | 1873–'74. | |
|---|---|---|---|---|---|---|---|
| Mean strength ................................................ { Officers ............ | | 3 | | 4 | | 3 | |
| { Enlisted men ....... | | 45 | | 59 | | 47 | |
| | | Cases. | Deaths. | Cases. | Deaths. | Cases. | Deaths. |
| Diseases. | | | | | | | |
| GENERAL DISEASES, A. | | | | | | | |
| Cerebro-spinal fever ..................... | | | | | | 1 | |
| Remittent fever ....................................... | | 3 | | 2 | | 12 | |
| Intermittent fever ..................................... | | 48 | | 48 | | 15 | |
| Other diseases of this group ....................... | | 1 | | 4 | | 3 | |
| GENERAL DISEASES, B. | | | | | | | |
| Rheumatism ......................................... | | 1 | | 2 | | 1 | |
| Syphilis ............................................ | | 1 | | 3 | | 4 | |
| Consumption ........................................ | | 1 | | 3 | 1 | | |
| Other diseases of this group ....................... | | | | 1 | | | |
| LOCAL DISEASES. | | | | | | | |
| Catarrh and bronchitis ............................. | | 5 | | 4 | | 11 | |
| Pneumonia .......................................... | | | | 1 | | | |
| Pleurisy ............................................ | | | | 1 | | | |
| Diarrhœa and dysentery ............................ | | 29 | | 10 | | 18 | |
| Gonorrhœa .......................................... | | 1 | | | | 3 | |
| Other local disease ................................. | | 14 | 1 | 19 | | 29 | |
| Alcoholism ......................................... | | 1 | | | | | |
| Total diseases ................................ | | 105 | 1 | 98 | 1 | 97 | |
| VIOLENT DISEASES AND DEATHS. | | | | | | | |
| Gunshot wounds ..................................... | | | | 1 | | | |
| Other accidents and injuries ....................... | | 14 | | 10 | | 5 | |
| Total violence ............................... | | 14 | | 11 | | 5 | |

# NEWPORT BARRACKS, KENTUCKY.

## REPORTS OF SURGEONS G. PERIN AND E. SWIFT, UNITED STATES ARMY.

Newport Barracks are on the left bank of the Ohio River, at the junction of the Licking, in the town of Newport, Kentucky ; latitude, 39° 5′ north; longitude, 7° 29′ 4′′ west; altitude, 588 feet. The reservation contains about six acres, and the mean elevation above low water in the Ohio River is about $55\frac{1}{2}$ feet. The post has been for several years occupied as a depot for recruits. The buildings are for the most part old, in bad repair, and insufficient for the number of men who have been stationed at the post.

The barracks are two three-story brick buildings, the lower floors used as kitchens and mess-rooms, the two upper floors as dormitories. The dimensions of two dormitories are $83\frac{1}{2}$ by 25 by 12 feet, and of the other two $58\frac{8}{12}$ by 28 by 12 feet. Two-story double iron bunks are used, with the customary bedding.

Wash-rooms have been added to three of the dormitories. There are no arrangements for water-closets connecting with the barracks, the only sink for enlisted men being the one over the sewer, at the southwest angle of the garrison. The barracks for the soldiers are satisfactory when not crowded to excess. The kitchens and mess-rooms are in the basements of the barracks ; the kitchens are supplied with excellent ranges, of capacity to cook for about 500 men.

Quarters for laundresses and married soldiers are in a three-story block at the southwest angle of the garrison. This block is built of brick, with porches on the north side ; access to the second and third floors is by means of stairways on the porches. The stories are divided in such manner as to give six rooms on each floor. The upper rooms are $13\frac{1}{2}$ by 15 by 12 feet, the basements $13\frac{1}{2}$ by 15 by 8 feet. Five families, who have two rooms each, reside in this building.

There are two sets of officers' quarters at the northeast angle of the garrison, fronting the Ohio River. These have a hall and nine rooms each. They are so arranged as to be assignable only to field-officers. They are built of brick, with a porch in front.

There are two sets of officers' quarters on the east side of the garrison, fronting the parade. These sets have four rooms and basements to each.

All the quarters are heated by open fires, and scantily supplied with water hauled in carts. They have cisterns, but these do not afford sufficient quantity. There are neither water-closets nor bath-rooms in the officers' quarters. Each set is supplied with a sink in the yard. These sinks have vaults, varying in depth from 6 to 15 feet.

The arsenal building is a two-story brick structure, 84½ by 36 feet, occupied as store-rooms and offices.

The guard-house, on the west side of the parade-ground, is a two-story brick building, the upper story being partly occupied by the prisoners, and the lower as a guard-room and place for storage of fuel. The capacity of the upper floor is 56 by 39 by 14 feet. One room, 12 by 15 feet, is taken from this floor for the officer of the guard, and the remainder is allotted to the prisoners. Of this space, one room, 19 by 30 by 14 feet, has been added recently. The guard-house is now ample and well adapted for the purpose. It is ventilated by windows on all sides, and warmed by stoves.

During the year 1874 a new hospital has been constructed at this post, the plan and dimensions of which are shown in Figures 28 and 29.

A, general dining-room, 15 by 19 feet; B, dining-room, 15 by 15 feet; C, kitchen, 15 by 15 feet; D, store-room, 15 by 13 feet; E, lunatic cell, 14 by 15 feet; F, dead-house; G, fuel; H, laundry ironing-room, 15 by 19 feet; I, open cellar; J, laundry (wash-room); K, tubs; L, heater; M, principal stairs; N, back or kitchen stairs; O, corridor; P, Q, ash-pit; R, S, foundations to earth-closet; T, lift, or elevator; U, closet; V, boiler; W, ice-chest; X, brick pier; Y, area; Z, areas, 2 feet below parade-ground.

A, office, 17 by 15 feet 4 inches; B, dispensary, 15½ by 15 feet 4 inches; C, spare room; D, library 15½ by 15 feet 4 inches; E, ward, 52 by 25 feet; F, ward, 39 by 25 feet; G, principal staircase; H, hall, 6 feet wide, (passage to ward F, 4 feet 8 inches wide, staircase hall, 8 feet wide;) I, earth-closet, 6½ by 9 feet; J, earth-closet, 10½ by 6½ feet; K, water-closet and bath-room, 5 by 9 feet 8 inches; L, elevator, 3 by 6 feet 4 inches; M, closet, 6½ by 4 feet; N, kitchen-stairs; O,

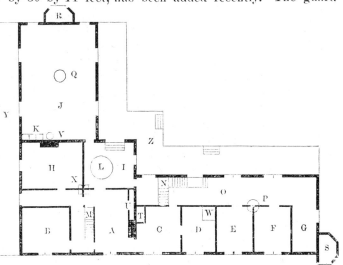

Figure 28.—Plan of basement.

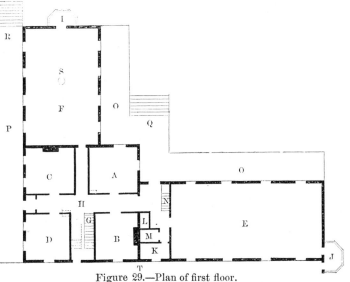

Figure 29.—Plan of first floor.

P, veranda 9½ feet wide; Q, steps; (veranda 5 feet above parade-ground;) R, steps to porch facing Ohio River; S, stove in ward; T, Licking River front.

The building is of brick, located on the northwest corner of the garrison and exposed greatly to the prevailing winds of winter, especially the administration portion, with its broad halls intersecting each other at right angles, through which a northwester will have a clear sweep. Pipes to convey hot and cold water to bath-rooms, and for gas, have been placed everywhere in the building requiring them.

The post bakery is in the basement of the block occupied as quarters for the families of soldiers.

The chapel is a frame structure, 45 by 28 by 13⅔ feet, between the officers' quarters and the hospital, on the east side of the parade. It is also occupied as a school-house.

The stable is at the northwest angle of the garrison, 49 by 28 feet, built of brick, and is one story and a half high.

There is no post library.

Water is supplied by means of pipes to all the buildings.

There is no organized system for extinguishing fire.

The drainage of the grounds is surface. As the Ohio River front of the garrison is several feet higher than the southern front, and the eastern side much higher than the west, these inequalities are made available in the arrangement of surface drains. An underground sewer, traversing the parade from east to west, and emptying into the Licking River, communicates with the vaults of the sinks on the east side of the garrison.

The sanitary condition of the post at present is satisfactory. The prevailing diseases are febrile intermittents, diarrhœa, and syphilis. It would not be correct, however, to ascribe the prevailing diseases to this locality, as the men received at this depot are usually affected by the diseases incident to the place where they have been living. They do not remain here long enough to exhibit the operation of local causes.

The men composing the permanent party are very healthy. Their duties being purely military, such as drill and guard, they are not exposed to the same causes of disease as soldiers belonging to regiments.

*Meteorological report, Newport Barracks, Ky., 1870–'74.*

| Month. | 1870–'71. | | | | 1871–'72. | | | | 1872–'73. | | | | 1873–'74. | | | |
|---|---|---|---|---|---|---|---|---|---|---|---|---|---|---|---|---|
| | Temperature. | | | Rain-fall in inches. | Temperature. | | | Rain-fall in inches. | Temperature. | | | Rain-fall in inches. | Temperature. | | | Rain-fall in inches. |
| | Mean. | Max. | Min. | | Mean. | Max. | Min. | | Mean. | Max. | Min. | | Mean. | Max. | Min. | |
| | ° | ° | ° | | ° | ° | ° | | ° | ° | ° | | ° | ° | ° | |
| July.................. | 79.00 | 93 | 64 | 1.74 | 75.59 | 96 | 58 | 3.61 | 77.62 | 92 | 67 | 5.10 | 77.28 | 93 | 65 | 2.56 |
| August................ | 73.61 | 93 | 60 | 1.93 | 76.05 | 94 | 63 | 5.33 | 77.51 | 96 | 60 | 2.00 | 76.31 | 93 | 65 | 3.46 |
| September............ | 72.27 | 89 | 58 | 0.11 | 64.65 | 85 | 38 | 1.15 | 68.33 | 92 | 43 | 2.27 | 68.33 | 88 | 47 | 1.84 |
| October.............. | 59.75 | 79 | 42 | 2.67 | 58.11 | 81 | 36 | 0.94 | 54.47 | 86 | 33 | 2.20 | 52.27 | 78 | 27 | 2.07 |
| November............ | 46.40 | 73 | 28 | 1.50 | 42.82 | 70 | 18 | 2.26 | 37.56 | 62 | 4 | 0.53 | 38.41 | 60 | 12 | 1.94 |
| December............ | 32.24 | 60 | −5 | 1.92 | 29.48 | 58 | 0 | 3.84 | 26.76 | 48 | −8 | 1.65 | 37.77 | 62 | 15 | 5.40 |
| January............. | 35.04 | 65 | 13 | 1.82 | 27.26 | 47 | 0 | 0.77 | 27.85 | 62 | −3 | 1.73 | 36.24 | 70 | 6 | 2.75 |
| February............ | 37.66 | 67 | 19 | 4.40 | 31.27 | 58 | 3 | 0.77 | 32.90 | 53 | 2 | 2.40 | 36.39 | 61 | 10 | 4.48 |
| March............... | 50.54 | 76 | 33 | 4.11 | 31.57 | 61 | 9 | 0.96 | 39.29 | 70 | 3 | 1.21 | 43.46 | 68 | 24 | 3.60 |
| April................ | 58.82 | 80 | 39 | 1.74 | 56.79 | 84 | 30 | 4.65 | 52.03 | 84 | 34 | 2.01 | 47.92 | 73 | 30 | 3.55 |
| May................. | 66.58 | 88 | 44 | 4.95 | 66.06 | 85 | 44 | 3.97 | 65.78 | 85 | 46 | 3.61 | 67.86 | 90 | 50 | 1.70 |
| June................ | 75.07 | 90 | 59 | 1.63 | 73.07 | 91 | 62 | 3.50 | 76.99 | 94 | 59 | 2.80 | 78.84 | 94 | 55 | 2.00 |
| For the year ........ | 57.25 | 93 | −5 | 28.52 | 52.73 | 96 | 0 | 31.75 | 53.09 | 96 | −8 | 27.51 | 55.09 | 94 | 6 | 35.35 |

*Consolidated sick-report, (white,) Newport Barracks, Ky., 1870–'74.*

| Year | | 1870–'71. | | 1871–'72. | | 1872–'73. | | 1873–'74. | |
|---|---|---|---|---|---|---|---|---|---|
| Mean strength { Officers | | 7 | | 7 | | 6 | | 7 | |
| { Enlisted men | | 328 | | 357 | | 347 | | 359 | |
| Diseases. | | Cases. | Deaths. | Cases. | Deaths. | Cases. | Deaths. | Cases. | Deaths. |
| GENERAL DISEASES, A. | | | | | | | | | |
| Small-pox and varioloid | | | | 7 | 1 | 9 | 4 | | |
| Typhoid fever | | 3 | | 5 | 1 | 6 | | 16 | 4 |
| Typho-malarial fever | | 2 | | | | | | | |
| Intermittent fever | | 239 | | 290 | | 261 | | 221 | |
| Other diseases of this group | | 33 | | 66 | | 65 | | 22 | |
| GENERAL DISEASES, B. | | | | | | | | | |
| Rheumatism | | 26 | | 14 | | 27 | | 24 | |
| Syphilis | | 43 | | 45 | | 63 | | 46 | |
| Consumption | | 3 | 1 | 4 | 3 | 6 | 3 | 8 | |
| Other diseases of this group | | 5 | | 2 | | 11 | 1 | 3 | |
| LOCAL DISEASES. | | | | | | | | | |
| Catarrh and bronchitis | | 95 | | 124 | | 198 | | 157 | |
| Pneumonia | | 6 | | 11 | | 7 | 1 | 13 | |
| Pleurisy | | 1 | | | | | | 1 | |
| Diarrhoea and dysentery | | 105 | 1 | 77 | | 117 | | 110 | 1 |
| Hernia | | 5 | | 1 | | 2 | | 1 | |
| Gonorrhoea | | 73 | | 61 | | 52 | | 49 | |
| Other local diseases | | 140 | 2 | 104 | | 144 | 1 | 119 | 2 |
| Alcoholism | | 23 | | 20 | | 13 | | 16 | |
| Total disease | | 802 | 4 | 831 | 5 | 981 | 10 | 797 | 7 |
| VIOLENT DISEASES AND DEATHS. | | | | | | | | | |
| Gunshot wounds | | 1 | | 1 | 1 | 1 | | | |
| Other accidents and injuries | | 53 | | 64 | | 56 | | 52 | |
| Homicide | | | | | | | | | 1 |
| Suicide | | | | | 2 | | | | |
| Total violence | | 54 | | 65 | 3 | 57 | | 52 | 1 |

*Consolidated sick-report, (colored,) Newport Barracks, Ky., 1870–'73.*

| Year | | 1870–'71.* | | 1871–'72.† | | 1872–'73.‡ | |
|---|---|---|---|---|---|---|---|
| Mean strength Enlisted men | | 19 | | 30 | | 13 | |
| Diseases. | | Cases. | Deaths. | Cases. | Deaths. | Cases. | Deaths. |
| GENERAL DISEASES, A. | | | | | | | |
| Small-pox and varioloid | | | | 1 | 1 | 1 | 1 |
| Typhoid fever | | | | | | 1 | |
| Intermittent fever | | 5 | | 19 | | 2 | |
| Other diseases of this group | | 5 | | 10 | | | |
| GENERAL DISEASES, B. | | | | | | | |
| Rheumatism | | | | | | 1 | |
| Syphilis | | 3 | | 3 | | 2 | |
| Other diseases of this group | | | | | | 1 | |
| LOCAL DISEASES. | | | | | | | |
| Catarrh and bronchitis | | 6 | | 18 | | 5 | |
| Pneumonia | | 1 | 1 | 9 | | | |
| Diarrhoea and dysentery | | 8 | | 5 | | 6 | |
| Gonorrhoea | | 10 | | 4 | | 2 | |
| Other local diseases | | 4 | | 5 | | 3 | |
| Total disease | | 42 | 1 | 74 | 1 | 24 | 1 |
| VIOLENT DISEASES AND DEATHS. | | | | | | | |
| Accidents and injuries | | 5 | | 3 | | | |
| Total violence | | 5 | | 3 | | | |

* Ten months only.    † Eight months only.    ‡ Six months only.

## FORT PICKENS, FLORIDA.

The construction of Fort Pickens was commenced 1828, on the western extremity of Santa Rosa Island, in latitude 30° 19' north; longitude, 10° 13' 54'' west. It was first garrisoned October 21, 1834. It is the principal defensive work at the entrance of the Bay of Pensacola. Owing to the great strength of the fort, and the gallant defense made by its garrison, it was enabled to resist all the efforts of the confederate forces during the late war, although Fort Barrancas, Fort McRae, and the navy-yard speedily fell into their hands, and their armaments were turned against Fort Pickens, in addition to numerous batteries of mortars and heavy guns employed for its reduction.

The fort, although little injured as a defensive work by the long siege, has not been garrisoned since the war, and is poorly adapted for the accommodation of troops in time of peace. The case-mates are damp, and in bad condition, and the ordnance-sergeant in charge has been allowed to build a small frame house outside the fort as a residence for his family.

The provision for water-supply is two brick cisterns inside the fort, having together a capacity of 150,000 gallons.

## FORT PIKE, LOUISIANA.

This fort was commenced in 1819, first occupied in 1821, and then called the Petite Coquille. The name was changed to Fort Pike November 8, 1827. It is located at the Rigolets, on the northern margin of the island of Petites Coquilles, thirty-five miles northeast of New Orleans, in latitude 30° 10' 50'' north; longitude, 12° 40' 15'' west.

The island is of rhomboid form, about three miles long, and at its greatest breadth two miles. It is bounded west by Lake Pontchartrain; north and northeast by the Rigolets; east, southeast, and south by Lake Catharine; and southwest by an unnamed bayou. The island is a large marsh, overflowed by spring tides, and the only dry ground is artificial, embracing the fort, barrack-ground, a narrow shell road three-quarters of a mile long, and at the end of it a raised shell bank, where stands the hospital.

The island seems to have been originally formed of a congeries of small shells, with an admixture of earthy deposit, based upon a substratum of argillaceous earth, rendered black or blue by the oxide of iron. The botany and zoology of the post are of little interest; no plants grow in the marsh but the marsh grass.

The fort, situated on the Rigolets, one mile from the entrance of the lake, is built on a foundation of cypress logs, sunk in the marsh, over which lies a layer of cemented shell. It is a triangular brick fortification, with a segment of a circle for base. It opens toward the Rigolets, from which it is separated by a breakwater. On the land side it is protected by an inner and outer moat.

The citadel of the fort is a building 70 feet long by 24 feet deep, two stories high; the lower story is casemated, and contains six divisions, used as kitchens; the upper story has been occupied as officers' quarters, containing six rooms, each 12 by 24 feet. The three bastions have small frame buildings, used as offices. On the east side of the outer moat are the quarters of the troops, a single-story frame building, 314 by 19 feet, and 11 feet high, running from east to west.

On the site known as the "Spanish Fort" is situated the post hospital. It is at a distance of three-quarters of a mile from the fort, and directly on the shore of Lake Pontchartrain. There have been, at different intervals, hospital-buildings at this place, but they were all destroyed by fire or blown down by gales. The present hospital was commenced in 1868, the plan of the same having been previously made by an officer of the quartermaster's department under the directions of the commanding officer. Neither capacious wards nor ventilation were provided for, the largest room of the house being 15 by 16 feet, the average 15 by 10 feet. Upon the suggestion of the medical officer two additional wings were erected, according to the directions laid down in the Surgeon General's Circular No. 4, 1867, retaining the original structure as an administration building.

The water-supply is by tanks for catching rain-water, which have seldom failed, and when they have the deficiency has been made good by using a condenser.

## CASTLE PINCKNEY, SOUTH CAROLINA.

This fortification was originally established during the revolutionary war, but the present works were begun in 1828. It is located on the southern point of Shute's Folly Island, at the mouth of Cooper River, Charleston Harbor, in latitude 32° 46′ 25″ north; longitude, 2° 51′ 25″ west. The works are now in charge of an ordnance-sergeant.

## FORT PULASKI, GEORGIA.

This post is on Cockspur Island, at the head of Tybee Roads, commanding both channels of the Savannah River; latitude, 32° 2′ north; longitude, 3° 51′ west.

For history and detailed description see Circular No. 4, page 148. The post was turned over to the Engineer Department for repair and alteration in October, 1873.

*Consolidated sick-report, Fort Pulaski, Ga., 1870–'74.*

| Year | | 1870–'71. | | 1871–'72. | | 1872–'73. | | 1873–'74.* | |
|---|---|---|---|---|---|---|---|---|---|
| Mean strength { Officers / Enlisted men | | 7 / 97 | | 8 / 93 | | 5 / 104 | | 6 / 102 | |
| Diseases. | | Cases. | Deaths. | Cases. | Deaths. | Cases. | Deaths. | Cases. | Deaths. |
| GENERAL DISEASES, A. | | | | | | | | | |
| Typhoid fever | | 2 | 1 | | | | | | |
| Remittent fever | | 4 | | 4 | | 15 | | 20 | |
| Intermittent fever | | 14 | | 11 | | 26 | | 7 | |
| Other diseases of this group | | 8 | | 4 | | 4 | | | |
| GENERAL DISEASES, B. | | | | | | | | | |
| Rheumatism | | 11 | | 14 | | 7 | | 5 | |
| Syphilis | | 1 | | 1 | | 3 | | | |
| Consumption | | 1 | | 1 | | 2 | | | |
| Other diseases of this group | | 4 | | 3 | | 2 | | 3 | |
| LOCAL DISEASES. | | | | | | | | | |
| Catarrh and bronchitis | | 7 | | 1 | | 12 | | 5 | |
| Pneumonia | | 6 | | 5 | | 3 | | 1 | |
| Pleurisy | | 6 | | 11 | | 6 | | | |
| Diarrhœa and dysentery | | 33 | | 42 | | 17 | 1 | 7 | |
| Hernia | | | | | | 2 | | 1 | |
| Gonorrhœa | | 2 | | 1 | | 1 | | | |
| Other local diseases | | 95 | | 42 | | 42 | | 14 | |
| Alcoholism | | 3 | | | | | | | |
| Total disease | | 197 | 1 | 140 | | 142 | 1 | 63 | |
| VIOLENT DISEASES AND DEATHS. | | | | | | | | | |
| Gunshot wounds | | | | | | | 1 | | |
| Drowning | | | | | 1 | | | | |
| Other accidents and injuries | | 20 | | 36 | | 25 | | 4 | |
| Total violence | | 20 | | 36 | 1 | 25 | 1 | 4 | |

*Four months only; post closed October 25, 1873.

22 M P

*Consolidated sick-report, Fort Pulaski, Ga., (prisoners,) 1870–'74.*

| Year | 1870–'71. | | 1871–'72. | | 1872–'73. | | 1873–'74.* | |
|---|---|---|---|---|---|---|---|---|
| Mean strength .....................Enlisted men...... | 56 | | 105 | | 50 | | 23 | |
| Diseases. | Cases. | Deaths. | Cases. | Deaths. | Cases. | Deaths. | Cases. | Deaths. |
| GENERAL DISEASES, A. | | | | | | | | |
| Typhoid fever............................................ | ...... | ...... | 1 | ...... | 1 | 1 | ...... | ...... |
| Remittent fever........................................... | 3 | ...... | 3 | ...... | 3 | ...... | 7 | ...... |
| Intermittent fever........................................ | 15 | ...... | 53 | ...... | 19 | ...... | 2 | ...... |
| Other diseases of this group ......................... | 3 | ...... | 3 | ...... | 1 | ...... | ...... | ...... |
| GENERAL DISEASES, B. | | | | | | | | |
| Rheumatism.............................................. | 13 | ...... | 40 | ...... | 10 | ...... | 2 | ...... |
| Syphilis ................................................... | 3 | ...... | 8 | ...... | ...... | ...... | 1 | ...... |
| Consumption ............................................ | 1 | ...... | 2 | ...... | ...... | ...... | ...... | ...... |
| Other diseases of this group ......................... | 3 | ...... | 1 | ...... | 1 | ...... | ...... | ...... |
| LOCAL DISEASES. | | | | | | | | |
| Catarrh and bronchitis .................................. | 2 | ...... | 11 | ...... | 5 | ...... | 1 | ...... |
| Pneumonia................................................ | 9 | ...... | 8 | ...... | 4 | ...... | ...... | ...... |
| Pleurisy.................................................... | ...... | ...... | 2 | ...... | ...... | ...... | ...... | ...... |
| Diarrhœa and dysentery................................ | 32 | 1 | 51 | ...... | 27 | 1 | ...... | ...... |
| Hernia..................................................... | 1 | ...... | 2 | ...... | 4 | ...... | ...... | ...... |
| Other local diseases..................................... | 85 | 1 | 58 | ...... | 20 | ...... | 7 | ...... |
| Total disease ........................... | 170 | 2 | 243 | ...... | 95 | 2 | 20 | ...... |
| VIOLENT DISEASES AND DEATHS. | | | | | | | | |
| Accidents and injuries................................... | 24 | ...... | 82 | ...... | 18 | ...... | 2 | ...... |
| Total violence ........................... | 24 | ...... | 82 | ...... | 18 | ...... | 2 | ...... |

*Four months only; post closed October 25, 1873.

---

# RALEIGH, NORTH CAROLINA.

### REPORTS OF ASSISTANT SURGEON F. LE BARON MONROE AND OF ACTING ASSISTANT SURGEON J. B. WHITE, UNITED STATES ARMY.

The post is situated one mile east of the center of the city of Raleigh ; latitude, 35° 47' north ; longitude, 1° 43'' west, and 317 feet above the sea level. The inclosure for the garrison measures 332 by 746 feet.

The barracks are three frame buildings, each 90 by 26 by 15 feet, originally erected for hospital wards. A fourth building of like size is used for married soldiers' quarters, mess-room, and kitchen, and two others for store-houses. One company has two-story wooden bunks, the others iron bed-steads.

There are six buildings available for officers' quarters, two of which were erected in 1871, and are in good condition.

The hospital is an old frame building recently repaired, and is sufficient for the wants of the post. The water-supply is from a well, and is of good quality. The drainage is good. The post is a healthy one, but malarial diseases have increased in the vicinity of late years.

*Meteorological report, Raleigh, N. C., 1870–'74.*

| Month. | 1870–'71. | | | | 1871–'72. | | | | 1872–'73. | | | | 1873–'74. | | | |
|---|---|---|---|---|---|---|---|---|---|---|---|---|---|---|---|---|
| | Temperature. | | | Rain-fall in inches. | Temperature. | | | Rain-fall in inches. | Temperature. | | | Rain-fall in inches. | Temperature. | | | Rain-fall in inches. |
| | Mean. | Max. | Min. | | Mean. | Max. | Min. | | Mean. | Max. | Min. | | Mean. | Max. | Min. | |
| | ° | ° | ° | | ° | ° | ° | | ° | ° | ° | | ° | ° | ° | |
| July ..... | | | | | | | | | | | | | 85.24 | 103 | 70 | 3.34 |
| August .... | | | | | | | | | | | | | 79.39 | 98 | 69 | 7.42 |
| September ... | | | | | | | | | | | | | 70.72 | 93 | 52 | 3.23 |
| October ..... | | | | | | | | | | | | | 57.43 | 77 | 31 | 3.23 |
| November .... | | | | | | | | | | | | | 47.04 | 68 | 27 | 5.40 |
| December ... | | | | | | | | | | | | | 44.77 | 72 | 16 | 0.75 |
| January ..... | | | | | | | | | | | | | 45.88 | 74 | 17 | 1.73 |
| February ... | | | | | | | | | | | | | 44.79 | 77 | 29 | 3.15 |
| March ..... | | | | | | | | | | | | | 52.15 | 77 | 29 | 1.33 |
| April ..... | | | | | | | | | | | | | 56.05 | 80 | 37 | 6.07 |
| May ..... | | | | | | | | | | | | | 68.48 | 91 | 44 | 5.75 |
| June ..... | | | | | | | | | 79.52 | 96 | 59 | 1.54 | 80.62 | 99 | 57 | 2.17 |
| For the year ..... | | | | | | | | | | | | | 61.04 | 103 | 16 | 43.56 |

*Consolidated sick-report, Raleigh, N. C., 1870–'74.*

| Year ..... | 1870–'71. | 1871–'72. | 1872–'73. | 1873–'74. |
|---|---|---|---|---|
| Mean strength ..... { Officers ..... | 7 | 7 | 8 | 10 |
| { Enlisted men ..... | 95 | 99 | 111 | 132 |

| Diseases. | 1870–'71. | | 1871–'72. | | 1872–'73. | | 1873–'74. | |
|---|---|---|---|---|---|---|---|---|
| | Cases. | Deaths. | Cases. | Deaths. | Cases. | Deaths. | Cases. | Deaths. |
| GENERAL DISEASES, A. | | | | | | | | |
| Typho-malarial fever ..... | | | 2 | | | | 1 | 2 |
| Remittent fever ..... | 2 | | 2 | | 11 | | 27 | 1 |
| Intermittent fever ..... | 28 | | 10 | | 14 | | 5 | |
| Other diseases of this group ..... | 9 | | 4 | | 2 | | 2 | |
| GENERAL DISEASES, B. | | | | | | | | |
| Rheumatism ..... | 10 | | 5 | | 17 | | 5 | |
| Syphilis ..... | 37 | | 9 | | 15 | | 13 | |
| Consumption ..... | | | | | | | 1 | |
| Other diseases of this group ..... | 2 | | 1 | | | | | |
| LOCAL DISEASES. | | | | | | | | |
| Catarrh and bronchitis ..... | 7 | | 15 | | 11 | | 16 | |
| Pneumonia ..... | | | | | 1 | 1 | | |
| Pleurisy ..... | | | | | | | 2 | |
| Diarrhœa and dysentery ..... | 71 | | 16 | | 21 | | 39 | |
| Hernia ..... | | | | | | | | |
| Gonorrhœa ..... | 11 | | 3 | | 12 | | 10 | |
| Other local diseases ..... | 61 | | 70 | | 59 | | 50 | 2 |
| Alcoholism ..... | 7 | | 5 | 1 | 12 | | 46 | 2 |
| Total disease ..... | 245 | | 142 | 1 | 175 | 1 | 217 | 7 |
| VIOLENT DISEASES AND DEATHS. | | | | | | | | |
| Gunshot wounds ..... | 1 | | | | | | | |
| Other accidents and injuries ..... | 38 | | 28 | | 27 | | 34 | |
| Total violence ..... | 39 | | 28 | | 27 | | 34 | |

# SAVANNAH, GEORGIA, (OGLETHORPE BARRACKS.)

## REPORT OF ASSISTANT SURGEON H. M. CRONKHITE, UNITED STATES ARMY.

The city of Savannah, Ga., stands upon the right or south bank of the Savannah River, about 18 miles from the sea, in latitude 32° 5' north; longitude, 4° 5' west. Its site is a sandy plateau elevated about 40 feet above low-water mark, surrounded on all sides, at the distance of a few miles, by low swampy grounds.

The present post of Oglethorpe Barracks was established about 1834, and occupies a square in the central part of the city, bounded on the north by Liberty street, on the east by Drayton street, on the south by Harris street, and on the west by Bull street. The square is surrounded by a brick wall 10 feet high, except where the buildings stand upon the line of the street. The buildings are placed around the four sides, facing inward upon an open space left as parade-ground.

There are five sets of quarters for officers; of these, two sets are upon Bull street, and three sets upon Liberty street. Each set upon Bull street has two stories, and is 55 feet long, 24 feet wide, and 21 feet in height. There is also a veranda 10 feet wide, resting upon circular brick pillars, extending along the front. These sets are separated in the lower story by the Bull-street sally-port, 10 feet wide; but in the upper story they are connected. Each has a middle hall with a circular stairway, and contains four rooms—two above and two below. These rooms are each 18 feet square. Besides, there is a basement for kitchen, servants' room, &c.; also a bath-room over the sally-port. The building is of brick, with a slate roof, and is in good condition.

The officers' quarters upon Liberty street are in the second story of a brick building, the first story of which is occupied as a store-house by the post quartermaster and post commissary. This building is 62 feet long and 32 feet wide, and also has a veranda, 10 feet wide, resting upon circular brick pillars extending along the front.

The sets of quarters in this building are separated by halls extending crosswise; each contains two rooms, 15 feet square and 12 feet high. There are two bath-rooms for these quarters under the veranda in front of the store-room. It has been recommended by the general commanding this department that the store-room be altered into kitchens and dining-rooms for these quarters.

The building for enlisted men's quarters is upon Drayton street. It is 130 feet long, 31 feet wide, and 40 feet high. In front of it also is a veranda similar to those above described. It has two stories and a basement. The lower story is separated in the center by a sally-port, 10 feet wide, and is divided into four sets of quarters, each containing two rooms, for married men and laundresses. These rooms are each 26 feet long, 15 feet wide, and 13 feet in height. In the upper story there are two rooms, each 57 feet long, 26 feet wide, and 14 feet high. They are occupied for company quarters. There is also a small room in the center, over the sally-port, used for the post library. The basement contains the company kitchens, mess-rooms, store-rooms, &c. This building is of brick, has a slate roof, and is in good condition.

The post hospital is a frame building, upon Harris street, 82 feet long, 40 feet wide, and 19 feet high. It stands upon a brick foundation, 11 feet in height. In front and at each end the framework projects 10 feet beyond the foundation. This projection is supported by square brick pillars. In rear the framework projects 7 feet. The projection here rests upon the brick wall which surrounds the post. In front there is a veranda 50 feet long and 10 feet wide; another on the east end, of the same width, 20 feet long; and another in the rear, upon Harris street, 50 feet long and 7 feet wide. The verandas were included in the general dimensions of the building as above given. There are two wards, each 27 feet long, 23 feet wide, and 19 feet high, ventilated by doors and windows. The ground-floor contains a dispensary and store-room, each 21 feet long, 14 feet wide, and 11 feet high; also a kitchen and mess-room, each 21 feet long, 12 feet wide, and 11 feet high. Above, on the east end, are two small rooms, each 10 feet square. On the west end are also two rooms, each 14 feet long and 10 feet wide. The hospital bath-room is in the upper part of a separate small building at the east end of the hospital. It is 7 feet long and 5 feet wide. An elevated covered way leads to it from the veranda on the east. It is in bad condition, and very unfit for its purpose. The hospital has a slate roof. Its framework is old and much decayed. Its drainage is poor and insufficient.

To the east of the hospital, on Harris street, is the guard-house. It is a frame building, in fair condition, 36 feet long, 30 feet wide, and 30 feet high. It has two stories. The upper story contains one large room, 35 feet long, 29 feet wide, and 12 feet high. This room is at present occupied by a company laundress. The lower story contains a guard-room, 35 feet long, 14 feet wide, and 15 feet high; a prisoners' room, 15 feet long, 10 feet wide, and 15 feet high; another room, for prisoners, 10 feet long, 7 feet wide, and 15 feet high; also 3 cells, each 8 feet long, 5 feet wide, and 15 feet high.

To the west of the hospital, on Harris street, is a brick building of two stories, 30 feet long, 20 feet wide, and 23 feet high. It contains four rooms, two above and two below, separated by a stairway in the center. Each room is 17 feet long, 12 feet wide, and 11 feet high. It was erected as quarters for the hospital steward and hospital matron. It is now occupied by the hospital steward and the commissary sergeant of the post. It has a tin roof. It is in good condition.

On Liberty street, to the west of the building for officers' quarters, is a two-story frame building for officers. It is 35 feet long and 27 feet wide, with a stairway in the center. It contains four rooms, each of which is 25 feet long and 15 feet wide. It has a tin roof and is in good condition.

The stable is 43 feet long, 22 feet wide, and 21 feet high. It is a brick building with a slate roof, and in good condition. The post bakery and carpenter-shop are in a building 30 feet long, 24 feet wide, and 11 feet high. The building is of brick, with a tin roof. Its condition is good.

The bath-house for the enlisted men is a frame building 30 feet long, 12 feet wide, and 16 feet high, with a tin roof. It is in good condition. It contains four rooms, each 7 feet long, 5 feet wide, and 16 feet high. Earth commodes are used by the enlisted men.

The post uses the water of the Savannah River, received from the aqueduct which supplies the city. All the buildings have water-pipes, but in some the drainage-pipes are inadequate and in bad repair. In general, the drainage of the post is bad. The health of the post is usually good. The prevailing diseases are of malarial origin.

*Meteorological report, Savannah, Ga., 1870–'74.*

| Month. | 1870–'71. Temperature. Mean. | Max. | Min. | Rain-fall in inches. | 1871–'72. Temperature. Mean. | Max. | Min. | Rain-fall in inches. | 1872–'73. Temperature. Mean. | Max. | Min. | Rain-fall in inches. | 1873–'74. Temperature. Mean. | Max. | Min. | Rain-fall in inches. |
|---|---|---|---|---|---|---|---|---|---|---|---|---|---|---|---|---|
| July | 86.96 | 98 | 76 | 4.18 | 84.86 | 99 | 68 | 1.80 | 83.88 | 99* | 72 | 4.24 | 81.62 | 96* | 70* | ...... |
| August | 84.71 | 98 | 74 | ...... | 82.41 | 98 | 74 | 12.90 | 80.79 | 93* | 69 | 12.30 | 80.64 | 93* | 70* | 4.55 |
| September | 77.25 | 88 | 68 | 0.28 | 73.22 | 88* | 49* | 3.78 | 76.99 | 90* | 68 | 2.09 | 76.87 | 97* | 64* | 1.94 |
| October | 68.13 | 88 | 50 | 3.28 | 68.97 | 83* | 50* | 2.95 | 65.08 | 85* | 44 | 3.95 | 64.40 | 83* | 36* | 0.35 |
| November | 53.90 | 80 | 35 | 0.00 | 60.05 | 81* | 40 | 1.29 | 54.64 | 75* | 28 | 2.20 | 55.17 | 76* | 27* | 3.82 |
| December | 39.22 | 73 | 15 | 13.26 | 49.61 | 75* | 27 | 0.55 | 47.21 | 74* | 28 | 1.05 | 52.77 | 80* | 26* | 2.62 |
| January | 49.36 | 68 | 35 | 0.00 | 46.74 | 74* | 26 | 3.81 | 49.09 | 71* | 18 | 3.03 | 52.37 | 75* | 27* | 0.60 |
| February | 56.84 | 75 | 38 | 1.50 | 49.72 | 73* | 32 | 1.60 | 55.09 | 74* | 33 | 0.60 | 54.64 | 79* | 36* | 7.00 |
| March | 64.56 | 80 | 44 | 2.65 | 54.43 | 79* | 37 | 3.94 | 54.58 | 77* | 27 | 3.10 | 63.49 | 85* | 37* | 0.90 |
| April | 68.66 | 86 | 50 | 2.65 | 67.48 | 89* | 52 | 2.26 | 66.29 | 87* | 41* | 4.20 | 68.64 | 83* | 47* | 1.45 |
| May | 74.14 | 89 | 53 | 0.65 | 76.25 | 92* | 61 | 2.75 | 74.13 | 88* | 55* | 2.10 | 75.04 | 95* | 59* | 3.85 |
| June | 82.21 | 96 | 70 | 3.25 | 80.00 | 96* | 72 | 7.99 | 80.20 | 94* | 60* | 3.75 | 83.61 | 97* | 68* | 7.05 |
| For the year | 67.19 | 98 | 15 | ...... | 66.14 | 99 - | 26 | 45.62 | 65.66 | 99* | 18 | 42.61 | 67.44 | 97* | 26* | ...... |

* These observations are made with self-registering thermometers. The mean is from the standard thermometer.

*Consolidated sick-report, Oglethorpe Barracks, Savannah, Ga., 1870–'74.*

| Year | | 1870–'71. | | 1871–'72. | | 1872–'73. | | 1873–'74. | |
|---|---|---|---|---|---|---|---|---|---|
| Mean strength { Officers<br>{ Enlisted men | | 4<br>56 | | 5<br>49 | | 3<br>54 | | 4<br>58 | |
| Diseases. | | Cases. | Deaths. | Cases. | Deaths. | Cases. | Deaths. | Cases. | Deaths. |
| GENERAL DISEASES, A. | | | | | | | | | |
| Typhoid fever | | 1 | ...... | 1 | ...... | 2 | 1 | ...... | ...... |
| Remittent fever | | ...... | ...... | 2 | ...... | 2 | ...... | 8 | ...... |
| Intermittent fever | | 13 | ...... | ...... | ...... | 6 | ...... | 6 | ...... |
| Other diseases of this group | | 3 | ...... | 3 | ...... | 3 | ...... | 1 | 1 |
| GENERAL DISEASES. B. | | | | | | | | | |
| Rheumatism | | 5 | ...... | ...... | ...... | 3 | ...... | 2 | ...... |
| Syphilis | | 2 | ...... | ...... | ...... | 3 | ...... | 8 | ...... |
| Consumption | | 1 | ...... | ...... | ...... | 1 | 1 | 1 | 1 |
| Other diseases of this group | | 1 | ...... | 1 | ...... | 1 | ...... | ...... | ...... |

*Consolidated sick-report, Oglethorpe Barracks, Savannah, Ga., 1870–'74—Continued.*

| Year | | 1870–'71. | | 1871–'72. | | 1872–'73. | | 1873–'74. | |
|---|---|---|---|---|---|---|---|---|---|
| Mean strength { Officers | | 4 | | 5 | | 3 | | 4 | |
| { Enlisted men | | 56 | | 49 | | 54 | | 58 | |
| Diseases. | | Cases. | Deaths. | Cases. | Deaths. | Cases. | Deaths. | Cases. | Deaths. |
| LOCAL DISEASES. | | | | | | | | | |
| Catarrh and bronchitis | | 5 | | | | | | | |
| Diarrhœa and dysentery | | 8 | | 2 | | 4 | | 10 | 1 |
| Hernia | | 1 | | | | | | | |
| Gonorrhœa | | 8 | | | | | | 4 | |
| Other local diseases | | 32 | | 6 | | 24 | | 27 | 1 |
| Alcoholism | | 5 | | | | | | | |
| Unclassified | | | | | | | | 1 | |
| Total disease | | 85 | | 15 | | 49 | 2 | 68 | 4 |
| VIOLENT DISEASES AND DEATHS. | | | | | | | | | |
| Accidents and injuries | | 4 | | 6 | | 11 | | 10 | |
| Total violence | | 4 | | 6 | | 11 | | 10 | |

# SAINT AUGUSTINE, FLORIDA.

### REPORTS OF ASSISTANT SURGEONS G. M'C. MILLER AND A. DELANY, UNITED STATES ARMY.

This post, or Saint Francis Barracks, is at the southeast edge of the town of Saint Augustine, near the Matanzas River; latitude, 29° 40′ north; longitude, 4° 32′.

The Matanzas River is really an arm of the sea, about twenty miles long, separated from the Atlantic Ocean by Anastasia Island, its northern end with the mouth of North River forming the Bay of Saint Augustine. The Atlantic Ocean is about two miles distant. The average elevation of the town above the sea-level is from 10 to 15 feet. On the west of the town is a small stream, the Saint Sebastian, flowing through salt marshes, and beyond these spread the pine forests. Jacksonville, the nearest place of importance, is distant 40 miles by land and 70 by water. Saint Augustine has about 1,800 inhabitants, about one-half of whom are of Spanish descent. In winter it receives several hundred health-seekers, chiefly consumptives. The picturesque, antique, Spanish aspect of the town, its plaza, cathedral, and ancient and castellated fort, its historical associations, and many other things, make this place a very attractive one. The summers are cool, the winters mild.

The post was occupied in July, 1871. The ground occupied is two rectangular strips, separated by Marine street.

The barrack is a frame building of two stories, 135 by 24 feet; the upper story divided into four dormitories, 33 by 23 feet, and 9 feet high, two being occupied by each company.

The lower story is divided into six rooms, giving a kitchen, mess-room, and office to each company. The rooms are plastered, and the dormitories are well lighted and ventilated.

The laundresses' quarters are in a building 126 by 30 feet, and one and a half stories high. The walls of the lower story are of coquina stone, (a shell conglomerate,) of the upper of wood, with shingle roof.

This building also contains the laundry, bakery, and guard-house.

Officers' quarters are in a building of two and a half stories, formerly a Franciscan monastery. The walls are of coquina stone, plastered inside and out; roof of wood. The building is H-shaped, the lateral rectangles 90 by 25 feet, the connecting one 70 by 42 feet, and contains 29 rooms. Four of these are used as offices. The rooms in the lateral wings (eight in each) are 22 by 20 feet, and 11 feet high. A covered porch, 8 feet wide, runs along the second story in front and rear.

The buildings occupied for a post hospital are of wood, raised on pillars 2½ feet above the ground.

The main building is 64 by 24 feet, containing an office and dispensary, each 13 by 10 feet, and a ward, 50 by 24 feet, 13 feet high to eaves, and 22 feet to ridge, with ridge ventilation. The kitchen is a separate building, 16 by 18 feet; another, 10 by 12 feet, is a store-room; and another, 31 by 14 feet, is the steward's quarters. All these buildings are unceiled and roughly constructed.

The water-supply is from four cisterns and three wells. One cistern holds 12,000 gallons; two, 4,000 each; and one, 3,300 gallons. The wells are shallow.

The natural drainage is not good, the surface being level.

The health of the command has been good. The merits of the climate and of the place as a health resort have probably been overrated. The atmosphere is damp and the climate is enervating.

*Consolidated sick-report, Saint Augustine, Fla., 1871–'74.*

| Year | | 1871–'72. | | 1872–'73. | | 1873–'74. | |
|---|---|---|---|---|---|---|---|
| Mean strength { Officers | | 3 | | 7 | | 5 | |
| { Enlisted men | | 40 | | 84 | | 100 | |
| Diseases. | | Cases. | Deaths. | Cases. | Deaths. | Cases. | Deaths. |
| GENERAL DISEASES, A. | | | | | | | |
| Typhoid fever | | | | 3 | | 2 | |
| Remittent fever | | 1 | | | | | |
| Intermittent fever | | 89 | | 8 | | 22 | |
| Other diseases of this group | | 1 | | 5 | | 3 | |
| GENERAL DISEASES, B. | | | | | | | |
| Rheumatism | | 13 | | 3 | | 7 | |
| Syphilis | | 17 | | 4 | | | |
| Consumption | | 4 | | | 1 | 1 | 1 |
| Other diseases of this group | | 2 | | 2 | | 1 | |
| LOCAL DISEASES. | | | | | | | |
| Catarrh and bronchitis | | 8 | | 7 | | 1 | |
| Pneumonia | | | | | | 4 | |
| Pleurisy | | | | | | 3 | |
| Diarrhœa and dysentery | | 13 | | 13 | | 25 | |
| Hernia | | | | 1 | | 1 | |
| Gonorrhœa | | 3 | | 6 | | | |
| Other local diseases | | 51 | | 39 | | 38 | |
| Alcoholism | | 4 | | 16 | | 8 | |
| Total disease | | 206 | | 107 | 1 | 116 | 1 |
| VIOLENT DISEASES AND DEATHS. | | | | | | | |
| Accidents and injuries | | 22 | | 22 | | 17 | |
| Total violence | | 22 | | 22 | | 17 | |

# SHIP ISLAND, MISSISSIPPI, (FORT MASSACHUSETTS.)

Ship Island is one of a line of low sand islands lying a few miles from the main-land and extending from Lake Borgne to Mobile Bay. This island is in latitude 30° 14′ north; longitude, 11° 50 west, and is six or seven miles in length from east to west. The west end consists of hummocks of fine, white sand interspersed with marshy spots. The east end widens out into a space of about one square mile, covered with pine trees, and inclosing several shallow lagoons. A large part of the island is overflowed during heavy gales from the south.

Early in 1861 the island was occupied by confederate troops, and considerable progress was made in the erection of a formidable work designated Fort Twiggs. The island was evacuated on the 18th of September in the same year, and was taken possession of two days later by a United States naval force under command of Capt. Melancthon Smith, of the steamer Massachusetts. It was thenceforward made a base of military operations in the Gulf. The present works were commenced in 1862, and are now in charge of an ordnance sergeant.

## FORT SUMTER, SOUTH CAROLINA.

Fort Sumter, commenced in 1828, stands upon a sand-bank near the center of Charleston Harbor, about five miles from the city; in latitude, 32° 45' north; longitude, 2° 49' 12'' west. Sullivan's Island, on which is Fort Moultrie, lies to the northeast on the other side of the main channel, Morris Island to the south, and James Island on the west. The foundations of the fort are of northern granite, and were laid with great difficulty, owing to the unstable character of the ground.

As is well known, it sustained the first attack of the war of 1861, from which it suffered severely. Since the close of the war what remained has been almost entirely demolished to make room for alterations and repairs. The works are now in the hands of the Engineer Department for that purpose.

## FORT TAYLOR, FLORIDA.

Fort Taylor, commenced in 1844, is situated on the southwest shore of Key West Island, near Whitehead's Point, and about one mile from the center of the city of Key West; in latitude 24° 33' north; longitude, 4° 45' west. The works have never been completed, nor formally turned over for the occupation of troops. The armament is in charge of an ordnance-sergeant, and the fort was garrisoned during the late war.

The quarters are for five companies, and in casemates. The officers' quarters are partly in casemates and partly in a brick structure over the casemates, on the land or gorge point. There is no provision, other than that afforded by the casemates, for hospital, guard-house, store-house, or bakery. The cistern capacity of the fort is immense, one large cistern under each casemate, but not surface drainage enough to supply them. The deficiency was supplied during the war by a condenser.

In connection with Fort Taylor are two structures, designated as the "Advanced Towers." Tower No. 1 is situated on the southern coast of the island about a mile and a half from Fort Taylor. Tower No. 2 is on the same coast, on the southeastern extremity of the island. Their construction was commenced in 1861, for the better defense of the south shore of the island, and is not yet completed.

## YORKVILLE, SOUTH CAROLINA.

### REPORTED BY ASSISTANT SURGEON A. C. GIRARD, UNITED STATES ARMY.

Yorkville, the county seat of York County, is situated in the northern part of the State, upon an elevated ridge forming a continuation of King's Mountain, and lying between the Catawba and Broad Rivers, about ten miles distant from each. The town is distant about eighty miles from Columbia, the State capital, and ten from the North Carolina line, in latitude 34° 55' north, longitude 4° 5' west, approximately. The ridge is of granite, overlaid with slates containing veins of auriferous quartz. The location is pleasant and healthy, a cool mountain breeze generally prevailing through the day in summer, and previous to the war of the rebellion the town was a frequent summer resort for the wealthier inhabitants of the low districts.

Troops were stationed at Yorkville in March, 1871, to assist the civil authorities in maintaining order and enforcing the authority of the courts. The garrison is still maintained, but, as the necessity is presumed to be temporary, no post-buildings have been erected. The troops are quartered in a large brick building, formerly a hotel, located on the main street, near the center of the town. It is capable of accommodating two companies without crowding. The lower story is occupied by the quartermaster and commissary of subsistence store-houses, 64 by 20½ feet on one side of the hall; on the other is the guard-room, 21 feet square, and prison-room, 19 by 21 feet. The second story has on one side of the hall a dormitory 64 by 20½ feet, and 12½ feet high, giving for the present occupation an area of 62½ feet and a cubic space of 787 feet per man. On the other side of the hall is a smaller dormitory, the adjutant's office, and company orderly room. The third story is at present occupied only by the barber, the tailor, and by camp and garrison equipage. The men sleep on single iron bunks. A large and commodious kitchen and dining-room, each 34 by 24½ feet, are contained in the first story of a rear wing. In the rear of this kitchen is a bakery, 16½ by 10 feet, dark and ill-suited to the purpose.

The officers live in rented houses and boarding-houses, and sometimes in a hotel in the vicinity.

The building used as a hospital, originally a dwelling-house, is a two-story wooden building, 44 by 24 feet, containing seven rooms, situated nearly opposite the barracks on the same street, and on the edge of a ravine which drains the northwest side of the town. The lower story is divided by a central hall, on one side of which are the office and dispensary, each 19 by 11 feet, and on the other the kitchen and mess-room combined, 38 by 11 feet. The four rooms of the second story, each 19 by 11 by 10 feet, are used, two as wards, one as store-room, and the other as steward's room. The wards have a capacity of three beds each, all of which are generally occupied. Arrangements have been made for placing one of the lower panels of each door upon hinges, and to lower the upper sashes of the windows for ventilation. The condition of the building is fair, and, considering the circumstances, it is well adapted to its purpose. The privy is about 30 yards below the hospital on the edge of the ravine, and is claensed by the rain-fall.

The water used at the hospital is obtained from a well in the court-house yard, 100 rods distant. Rain-water is also collected for cleansing purposes.

23 M P

# MILITARY DIVISION OF THE MISSOURI,

INCLUDING

## DEPARTMENTS OF TEXAS, OF THE MISSOURI, OF THE PLATTE, AND OF DAKOTA.

# DEPARTMENT OF TEXAS.

(Embracing the State of Texas, and Fort Sill, Indian Territory.)

POSTS.

| | | |
|---|---|---|
| Austin, Tex. | Duncan, Fort, Tex. | Richardson, Fort, Tex. |
| Bliss, Fort, Tex. | Griffin, Fort, Tex. | Ringgold Barracks, Tex. |
| Brown, Fort, Tex. | McIntosh, Fort, Tex. | San Antonio, Tex. |
| Clark, Fort, Tex. | McKavett, Fort, Tex. | Sill, Fort, Ind. T. |
| Concho, Fort, Tex. | Quitman, Fort, Tex. | Stockton, Fort, Tex. |
| Davis, Fort, Tex. | | |

NOTES ON THE DEPARTMENT OF TEXAS, BY SURGEON J. F. HAMMOND, UNITED STATES ARMY MEDICAL DIRECTOR.

The Military Department of Texas comprises the State of Texas and the Indian Territory. Texas is about 700 miles from north to south and 800 miles from east to west, forming an inclined plane of several plateaus, rising from the sea-level at the Gulf to a height of between three and four thousand feet at El Paso and the Llano Estacado. Large rolling prairies spread themselves over much of the State, and are covered with the ordinary prairie sedge, mesquite, buffalo, and gramma grasses. Portions are timbered in mots, or belts, of various dimensions and degrees of sparseness, in which the mesquite, cedar, dwarf post-oak, cotton-wood, pecan, and walnut are found; and in other parts are seen remains of mountains which, as they extend from the interior toward the seaboard, gradually sink into the plain, buried in their *débris*, from climatic action.

The mean temperature of the seasons, taken at nineteen posts in different parts of the State, during a series of years, is as follows:

Spring, 69°.12 F.; summer, 81°.76 F.; autumn, 68°.07 F.; winter, 52°.46 F.

The high temperature and prolonged warm season, the vicissitudes of the weather, the sudden and great falls of temperature, are very remarkable.

The following is the mean rain-fall during the same period, from fifteen of the same posts:

Spring, 6.93 inches; summer, 8.48 inches; autumn, 8 inches; winter, 4.67 inches.

The rain-fall is very irregular, uncertain, and partial. It is generally heaviest in May or June and in October. The large quantity of water that falls at times in two or three days, or in a few hours, the suddenness with which the streams rise and the height to which they attain, and the great extent and danger of and destruction by the floods, and the damage from hail-storms, are almost incredible. Between 28° and 33° N. and 22° W. there are numerous streams of water, but they are generally small and shallow, and many of them becoming nearly or quite dry in summer are not reliable for irrigation, and their margins are prolific of malaria. In consequence of which, and from protracted droughts and hail, vegetable-gardens are not to be relied on; and farming is precarious and unsatisfactory.

There are in the department fifteen military posts, one of which, Fort Sill, is in Indian Territory, and the other fourteen in Texas. They are extended along the line of the Rio Grande, from Brownsville to El Paso, and from Eagle Pass to Fort Sill, for protection from incursions of the

Indians on the one hand, and from Mexico on the other. They are garrisoned by three regiments of cavalry and four regiments of infantry. The sites generally have been selected with a view to dryness, a due water-supply, and to natural drainage. The barracks proper evince some knowledge of the rules of building, but little of the principles of hygiene which should be applied in the construction of every habitation. They may consist of separate buildings, and be arranged in lines, but no thought is given to the position of the building in relation to the direction of the sun's rays, nor to the prevailing winds, nor to the local sources of malaria, nor of atmospheric moisture; nor to the proper space between barracks, nor to the proper elevation of the ground-floor above the ground, and the ventilation beneath the floor; nor to the proper height of the ceiling, nor proper breadth of the barracks; nor to the cubic air-space and the superficial area per man; nor to the number of men which should be quartered in a barrack, aside from considerations of the prescribed allowance of air-space per man—the number quartered being almost invariably too great; nor to the proper ventilation—the outlets and the inlets; nor to the warming of the barracks, nor to the most suitable material of which to construct them, &c., &c. In short, they are mere approximations, more or less remote, to the best plan of promoting the health of men in barracks. When it is remembered that " it has been proven, over and over again, that nothing is so costly in all ways as disease, and nothing is so remunerative as the outlay which augments health," and that the loss to the Government by sickness in the Army amounts to about 481,800 days' work in one year, this should not be so, especially when it may be estimated that at least fifty per cent. of the sickness is probably due to the faulty habitations of the men, which might be avoided by little, if any, greater outlay of money than at present. The quarters, generally, for officers are comfortable and ample, when the garrison is not larger than was estimated for in planning the post.

Nine of the post-hospitals in the department are built on plans given in Circular No. 4, April 27, 1867, or Circular No. 3, November 23, 1870, or Circular No. 2, July 27, 1871, from the Surgeon-General of the Army, which plans embody all the principles of hygiene applicable, in habitations for the sick, to the present time. There is a regulation-hospital at each of the posts in the department where there is most sickness. The greatest obstacle that the post-surgeon has to contend with is the frequent and sudden changes of hospital nurses. They have barely learned their duties well when they are removed, and are generally replaced by men unaccustomed to the duties. It not only lessens materially the comfort of the sick, but renders uncertain the regularity, and consequently the success of the treatment prescribed, prolongs the duration of the illness and endangers the lives of the men, and may cause death in some instances.

The service in this department is essentially frontier-service, and includes garrison-duty, duty with scouting parties of from ten men or less, to three or four or more companies, for from two or three days to two or three months at a time, and escort duty. Officers coming here for a tour of service should provide themselves accordingly. There is little time or opportunity for the enjoyment of luxuries. There is no society for them outside of the garrison or of the Army, and it is the opportunity for them to avoid living beyond their means. A good supply of substantial clothing for hot and for cold weather, (the undress-uniform is generally worn in garrison,) among which may be included blankets, bed-linen, towels, and napkins, is important. Letter-paper, envelopes, and pens should be brought along; slat-cots, with legs to fold up, for bedsteads and lounges; and hair-mattresses and pillows are most suitable. Washstands and ottomans can be extemporized from boxes and barrels. Chairs, not glued together, or camp-stools, are the best, because less costly to transport. Bare floors in summer, and matting or oil-cloths in winter, are more healthy and more appropriate than carpets. But all articles necessary for housekeeping, including china and glass and cutlery, may be obtained by specie in the large towns in the State, and transported by contractors' trains at moderate rates to any of the military posts. Nothing of the kind is to be found for sale at the posts, unless by accident. If possible, they should bring servants.

Through the Commissary Department, any article of diet that is prepared for transportation, can now be obtained from New Orleans, or Saint Louis, or Chicago in any quantities, at the lowest rates, and delivered at the posts monthly, if desired.

Medical officers should bring with them their medicines for private practice.

## TABLE OF DISTANCES IN THE DEPARTMENT OF TEXAS.

| | Saint Louis | New Orleans | San Antonio | Austin | Fort Bliss | Fort Brown | Fort Clark | Fort Concho | Fort Davis | Fort Duncan | Fort Gibson | Fort Griffin | Fort McIntosh | Fort McKavett | Fort Quitman | Fort Richardson | Ringgold Barracks | Fort Sill | Fort Stockton |
|---|---|---|---|---|---|---|---|---|---|---|---|---|---|---|---|---|---|---|---|
| Saint Louis | Saint Louis. | | | | | | | | | | | | | | | | | | |
| New Orleans | 725 | New Orleans. | | | | | | | | | | | | | | | | | |
| San Antonio | 935 | 575 | San Antonio. | | | | | | | | | | | | | | | | |
| Austin | 977 | 517 | 77 | Austin. | | | | | | | | | | | | | | | |
| Fort Bliss | 1368 | 1273 | 701 | 778 | Fort Bliss. | | | | | | | | | | | | | | |
| Fort Brown | 1241 | 580 | 322 | 369 | 1023 | Fort Brown. | | | | | | | | | | | | | |
| Fort Clark | 1182 | 701 | 126 | 203 | 827 | 427 | Fort Clark. | | | | | | | | | | | | |
| Fort Concho | 896 | 804 | 229 | 306 | 472 | 551 | 355 | Fort Concho. | | | | | | | | | | | |
| Fort Davis | 1146 | 1055 | 479 | 556 | 223 | 758 | 827 | 250 | Fort Davis. | | | | | | | | | | |
| Fort Duncan | 1236 | 759 | 171 | 248 | 872 | 382 | 45 | 400 | 650 | Fort Duncan. | | | | | | | | | |
| Fort Gibson | 418 | 866 | 489 | 573 | 964 | 814 | 776 | 492 | 742 | 826 | Fort Gibson. | | | | | | | | |
| Fort Griffin | 756 | 781 | 369 | 322 | 612 | 696 | 309 | 140 | 390 | 540 | 353 | Fort Griffin. | | | | | | | |
| Fort McIntosh | 1172 | 725 | 165 | 242 | 866 | 257 | 170 | 394 | 644 | 125 | 875 | 534 | Fort McIntosh. | | | | | | |
| Fort McKavett | 951 | 750 | 175 | 252 | 527 | 497 | 301 | 55 | 303 | 353 | 658 | 195 | 340 | Fort McKavett. | | | | | |
| Fort Quitman | 1286 | 1194 | 619 | 696 | 82 | 941 | 745 | 390 | 140 | 797 | 925 | 530 | 784 | 445 | Fort Quitman. | | | | |
| Fort Richardson | 676 | 701 | 331 | 257 | 692 | 657 | 575 | 220 | 470 | 627 | 273 | 80 | 495 | 275 | 610 | Fort Richardson. | | | |
| Ringgold Barracks | 1225 | 700 | 306 | 383 | 777 | 117 | 290 | 535 | 785 | 265 | 934 | 717 | 141 | 481 | 773 | 637 | Ringgold Barracks. | | |
| Fort Sill | 720 | 943 | 674 | 597 | 988 | 859 | 800 | 516 | 766 | 850 | 307 | 376 | 615 | 571 | 906 | 296 | 844 | Fort Sill. | |
| Fort Stockton | 1066 | 974 | 399 | 476 | 302 | 721 | 525 | 170 | 80 | 577 | 663 | 310 | 564 | 225 | 220 | 410 | 705 | 675 | Fort Stockton. |

# AUSTIN, TEXAS.

### REPORTED BY ASSISTANT SURGEON J. V. D. MIDDLETON, UNITED STATES ARMY.

Austin, the capital of Texas and county-seat of Travis County, is situated on the left bank of the Colorado River, 400 miles from its mouth, and 213 miles from Galveston by railroad. Latitude, 30° 15′ north; longitude, 20° 44′ west.

The town is built on a succession of hills, between Waller and Shoal Creeks; the most elevated point, known as Capitol Hill, is 640 feet above the level of the sea, and 150 feet above the bank of the river. The houses are built chiefly of wood and stone, one story high, and, with the exception of those on Main and Pecan streets, are very much scattered.

The town is surrounded by hills, which are covered with grass, evergreen, chaparral, and live-oak, and from many prominent points the view is very picturesque. The valleys and plains are extremely fertile and highly cultivated. The soil consists of a black calcareous loam, admirably adapted for gardening purposes. The geological formation, in general, belongs to the lower chalk and upper oolite.

The country is abundantly supplied with water, very clear; but holding a large quantity of lime in solution, and thus rendered objectionable for drinking and washing. Nearly every house, however, has a cistern; and as there are several public ones in the town, there is no difficulty in obtaining a bountiful supply of good rain-water at all times.

The climate of this section of Texas is quite salubrious. Although the sun is extremely hot in summer, the temperature of the atmosphere is much modified by the southeasterly breeze that blows almost continuously during the twenty-four hours. A remarkable feature of this climate is the suddenness with which the north wind arises in the winter, constituting "the norther;" the temperature of the atmosphere is sometimes reduced from 80° to 30° in a few hours, and is very trying to both animal and vegetable life.

The military post is situated southeast of the city, about one mile distant from the capitol. The buildings are frame structures, most of which were erected in 1868 for Government workshops, and used as such until 1870, when the headquarters of the department were moved to San Antonio. They occupy about five acres, and are arranged in the form of a square. The officers' quarters and commissary building occupy the north side; the barracks for enlisted men, hospital, and storehouse are on the south; on the east the adjutant's office, reading-room, and married soldiers' quarters; and the surgeon's office, storehouse and stables occupy the west.

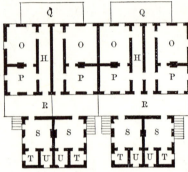

The officers' quarters consist of frame buildings divided into four sets, the arrangement of which is shown in Figure 30. H, main hall, 5 feet 6 inches wide; O, parlors, 13 feet 8 inches by 15 feet 10 inches; P, chambers, 13 feet 8 inches by 13 feet; Q, front porch, 8 feet wide; R, rear porch, 8 feet 2 inches wide; S, kitchens, 12 feet 10 inches by 13 feet 10 inches; T and U, store-rooms, pantry, &c. Each double house, (outside measurement,) 26 feet front, 29 feet 3 inches deep. Rear buildings, 25 feet 7 inches wide, 22 feet deep. Whole depth from front to rear, 59 feet 5 inches.

Figure 30.

### Meteorological report, Austin, Tex., 1870-'74.

| Month. | 1870-'71. | | | | 1871-'72. | | | | 1872-'73. | | | | 1873-'74. | | | |
| | Temperature. | | | Rain-fall in inches. | Temperature. | | | Rain-fall in inches. | Temperature. | | | Rain-fall in inches. | Temperature. | | | Rain-fall in inches. |
| | Mean. | Max. | Min. | | Mean. | Max. | Min. | | Mean. | Max. | Min. | | Mean. | Max. | Min. | |
|---|---|---|---|---|---|---|---|---|---|---|---|---|---|---|---|---|
| July | 82.65 | 97 | 71 | 3.05 | 87.05 | 105 | 71 | 0.00 | 85.72 | 104* | 71* | 2.08 | 82.55 | 104* | 67* | 4.64 |
| August | 81.98 | 96 | 72 | 4.33 | 86.23 | 105 | 71 | 2.02 | 86.06 | 106* | 67* | 1.10 | 81.76 | 105* | 65* | 1.08 |
| September | 79.66 | 95 | 63 | 2.25 | 75.84 | 97 | 57 | 3.64 | 80.32 | 104* | 57* | 0.00 | 76.99 | 102* | 54* | 10.05 |
| October | 68.12 | 86 | 46 | 12.44 | 68.57 | 89 | 47 | 8.06 | 67.48 | 96* | 37* | 1.68 | 62.97 | 98* | 30* | 2.10 |
| November | 60.04 | 90 | 32 | 3.46 | 55.37 | 83 | 31 | 5.64 | 51.56 | 91* | 18* | 2.60 | 58.97 | 89* | 26* | 2.46 |
| December | 45.53 | 75 | 10 | 0.98 | 43.74 | 84 | 21 | 0.38 | 42.07 | 79* | 10* | 6.88 | 53.25 | 80* | 20* | 0.20 |
| January | 47.76 | 78 | 20 | 1.18 | 40.64 | 75* | 12* | 2.00 | 45.27 | 79* | 9* | 3.45 | 51.14 | 80* | 22* | 0.50 |
| February | 52.81 | 80 | 27 | 1.80 | 51.74 | 83* | 21* | 0.68 | 55.36 | 85* | 23* | 0.10 | 53.28 | 80* | 25* | 1.34 |
| March | 62.57 | 90 | 39 | 2.06 | 52.96 | 81* | 27* | 4.64 | 63.05 | 93* | 30* | 3.67 | 62.30 | 87* | 30* | 5.26 |
| April | 68.34 | 92 | 35 | 1.15 | 72.04 | 90* | 32* | 3.67 | 66.17 | 102* | 28* | 1.84 | 63.07 | 89 | 36 | 1.26 |
| May | 72.69 | 91 | 58 | 4.72 | 74.35 | 98* | 46* | 3.03 | 74.12 | 100* | 44* | 4.50 | 75.65 | 99 | 57 | 1.04 |
| June | 81.61 | 104 | 67 | 0.37 | 82.74 | 102* | 66* | 8.32 | 80.38 | 101* | 62* | 7.76 | 81.71 | 100 | 70 | 2.08 |
| For the year | 75.31 | 104 | 10 | 40.79 | 65.94 | 105 | 12* | 42.08 | 66.46 | 106* | 9* | 35.66 | 66.97 | 105* | 20* | 32.01 |

\* These observations are made with self-registering thermometers. The mean is from the standard thermometer.

### Consolidated sick-report, (white,) Austin, Tex., 1870-'74.

| Year | 1870-'71. | | 1871-'72. | | 1872-'73. | | 1873-'74. | |
| Mean strength { Officers | 8 | | 2 | | 2 | | 3 | |
| { Enlisted men | 90 | | 50 | | 54 | | 67 | |
| Diseases. | Cases. | Deaths. | Cases. | Deaths. | Cases. | Deaths. | Cases. | Deaths. |
|---|---|---|---|---|---|---|---|---|
| GENERAL DISEASES, A. | | | | | | | | |
| Small-pox and varioloid | | | | | 1 | | | |
| Cerebro-spinal fever | 1 | 1 | | | | | | |
| Remittent fever | 4 | | 4 | | 4 | | 1 | |
| Intermittent fever | 16 | | 9 | | 1 | | 38 | |
| Dengue | | | | | | | 31 | |
| Other diseases of this group | 1 | | | | 1 | 1 | 1 | |

*Consolidated sick-report, (white,) Austin, Tex., 1870-'74—Continued.*

| Year | 1870-'71. | | 1871-'72. | | 1872-'73. | | 1873-'74. | |
|---|---|---|---|---|---|---|---|---|
| Mean strength { Officers / Enlisted men | 8 / 90 | | 2 / 50 | | 2 / 54 | | 3 / 67 | |
| Diseases. | Cases. | Deaths. | Cases. | Deaths. | Cases. | Deaths. | Cases. | Deaths. |
| GENERAL DISEASES, B. | | | | | | | | |
| Rheumatism | 4 | | 3 | | 9 | | 8 | |
| Syphilis | 4 | | 5 | | 1 | | 6 | |
| Consumption | 2 | 1 | | | | | | |
| Other diseases of this group | | | | | 1 | | | |
| LOCAL DISEASES. | | | | | | | | |
| Catarrh and bronchitis | 6 | | 1 | 1 | 5 | | 2 | |
| Pneumonia | | | 1 | | | | 1 | |
| Pleurisy | | | | | 2 | | | |
| Diarrhœa and dysentery | 29 | | 11 | | 10 | | 28 | |
| Hernia | 1 | | | | | | | |
| Gonorrhœa | 5 | | 5 | | 4 | | 4 | |
| Other local diseases | 45 | 1 | 23 | 1 | 22 | | 43 | 1 |
| Alcoholism | 14 | | 2 | | 5 | | 10 | |
| Total disease | 132 | 3 | 64 | 2 | 66 | 1 | 173 | 1 |
| VIOLENT DISEASES AND DEATHS. | | | | | | | | |
| Drowning | | | | | | | | 1 |
| Other accidents and injuries | 37 | | 18 | | 12 | | 8 | |
| Total violence | 37 | | 18 | | 12 | | 8 | 1 |

*Consolidated sick-report, (colored,) Austin, Tex., 1870-'74.*

| Year | 1870-'71.* | | 1871-'72.* | | 1872-'73.† | |
|---|---|---|---|---|---|---|
| Mean strength ... Enlisted men | 3 | | 22 | | 5 | |
| Diseases. | Cases. | Deaths. | Cases. | Deaths. | Cases. | Deaths. |
| GENERAL DISEASES, A. | | | | | | |
| Small-pox and varioloid | | | | | 4 | |
| Typhoid fever | | | 1 | | | |
| Remittent fever | | | | | 1 | |
| Intermittent fever | 2 | | | | | |
| GENERAL DISEASES, B. | | | | | | |
| Syphilis | | | 1 | | | |
| Consumption | | | | | 1 | 1 |
| LOCAL DISEASES. | | | | | | |
| Catarrh and bronchitis | 2 | | 1 | | 2 | |
| Pneumonia | | | 2 | | 2 | 1 |
| Pleurisy | | | | | | |
| Gonorrhœa | 1 | | | | | |
| Total disease | 5 | | 5 | | 10 | 2 |
| VIOLENT DISEASES AND DEATHS. | | | | | | |
| Gunshot wounds | 3 | | | | | |
| Total violence | 3 | | | | | |

* Four months only.    † Six months only.

# FORT BLISS, TEXAS.

REPORTED BY ACTING ASSISTANT SURGEON E. H. BOWMAN, UNITED STATES ARMY.

Fort Bliss is located on Concordia Ranch, 3 miles northeast from the town of El Paso, Tex., in latitude, 31° 46′ 5″ north; longitude, 29° 28′ west; at an altitude of 3,600 feet above the waters of the Gulf, and 10 feet above the high-water of the Rio Grande. It is much exposed to malaria

24 M P

from the bottom-lands of that river.   The depression of the ancient river-bed is close to the post on the west.   It is usually kept full of water for purposes of irrigation, but when the supply fails through drought, the river-bed and adjacent grounds crack to a great depth, and much malaria is developed.

The post is located on a bed of sand and gravel, destitute of loam.   North of the post is an expanse of small sand-knolls which, at the distance of 2½ miles, pass into the sand and gravel hills which form the southern terminus of the mesa, or great plain between the El Paso and the Huaco Mountains.

The river-bottom, when sufficiently irrigated, produces two crops annually, but the uplands are almost destitute of vegetation.   Advancing from the river, a band of drift is encountered, from 2 to 3 miles in width, composed of sand, gravel, and bowlders, without any appearance of fertile soil. It bears only scattering tufts of stunted chaparral and cactus, with an occasional dwarf mesquite.

The Mesa is a vast elevated plain, which at its southern border is, if possible, more barren than the drift, but farther north the influence of the mountains, causing a greater precipitation of moisture, has developed more fertility, and a short grass is produced, which, carefully gathered by hand, constitutes the principal supply of hay for the post.

There are no springs or ponds in the vicinity, except the pond made by the old river-bed, which is a muddy nuisance.   The water found a few feet below the surface is so brackish and alka- line as to be unfit for use.   Water is, in consequence, brought from the Rio Grande in a water- wagon, a distance of three-fourths of a mile.   There are no facilities for bathing, and very insuffi- cient means for subduing fire.   Although there is ground belonging to the post which, with irriga- tion, would be suitable for a garden, none is cultivated.

The ground occupied by the post is about 10 acres in extent, and is rented by the Govern- ment.   The buildings consist of three large adobe structures and several small ones, some of which are outside the limits of the ground held by the Government.   The buildings are all one story high, with earthen roofs and floors.

Two of the main buildings are situated in line on the north of the parade-ground, with a street between them of 60 feet width.   Each has a front of about 125 feet; one has eleven, the other twelve rooms.   Each has a court in the center; they are occupied as quarters by the quartermas- ter and commissary, as adjutant's office, as store-rooms of quartermaster's and commissary's stores, quarters for the troops, kitchens, guard-house, &c.   The rooms are large, the ceiling 14 to 16 feet high, with a sufficient number of doors and windows for light and ventilation.   On the north side of the west building, and adjoining by an adobe wall, 10 feet high, are the post bakery, carpenter- shop, and blacksmith-shop, the three, with the side walls, inclosing a second court, which is used for storing lumber, charcoal, &c.   On the north side of the east building, and adjoining, is the corral, inclosed by an adobe wall, 10 feet high.   On the south side of the parade-ground and near the southwest corner, is the other large building, containing eighteen rooms.   The quarters of the commanding officer and post-surgeon are in this building.   The quarters for troops have a capacity for two hundred men, with an air-space of 500 cubic feet per man.   They are warmed by fire- places, and well ventilated by doors, windows, and roof ventilation.   The quarters for laundresses are two small buildings outside, one of adobe, two rooms; the other built in what is called the "jacal" style.

The hospital was originally built as a dwelling-house, and is not on the Government reserva- tion, but is sufficiently near for convenience.   The building is in good condition.   Its greatest length is from east to west, 72 feet.   There is an extension of two rooms on the north side.   The east end of the main building is occupied by a store-room, 17 by 15 feet.   Next to this is the steward's room, 11 by 15 feet; then the dispensary, 23 by 15 feet; and lastly, the dining-room, 12 by 15 feet.   Directly in rear of the dining-room is the kitchen, of the same dimensions.   East of the kitchen, and in rear of the dispensary, is the ward, of the same dimensions as the latter. The ward contains six beds, allowing to each 800 cubic feet of air.   There is no bath-house, wash- room, or dead-house.   The privy is in the rear, and consists of a vault with wooden superstructure.

*Meteorological report, Fort Bliss, Tex., 1870–'74.*

| Month. | 1870–'71. | | | | 1871–'72. | | | | 1872–'73. | | | | 1873–'74, | | | |
|---|---|---|---|---|---|---|---|---|---|---|---|---|---|---|---|---|
| | Temperature. | | | Rain-fall in inches. | Temperature. | | | Rain-fall in inches. | Temperature. | | | Rain-fall in inches. | Temperature. | | | Rain-fall in inches. |
| | Mean. | Max. | Min. | | Mean. | Max. | Min. | | Mean. | Max. | Min. | | Mean. | Max. | Min. | |
| July | 78.28 | 105* | 65 | 1.43 | 82.64 | 107* | 66 | 1.20 | 80.16 | 107* | 65 | 2.72 | 84.93 | 109* | 58* | 0.56 |
| August | 76.96 | 101* | 60 | 4.01 | 71.57 | 107* | 56 | 0.82 | 80.61 | 101* | 66 | 0.04 | 80.31 | 103* | 61* | 0.98 |
| September | 73.88 | 100* | 74 | 0.00 | 70.71 | 98* | 53 | 2.64 | 74.39 | 97* | 51 | 0.58 | 78.33 | 103* | 51* | 0.50 |
| October | 63.44 | 94* | 40 | 0.05 | 61.54 | 90* | 38 | 0.01 | 62.02 | 93* | 31 | 0.32 | 66.54 | 99* | 34* | 0.00 |
| November | 54.14 | 85* | 26 | 0.00 | 50.33 | 76* | 20 | 0.00 | 47.85 | 77* | 11 | 0.06 | 53.21 | 82* | 25* | 1.02 |
| December | 44.38 | 77* | 13 | 0.60 | 47.13 | 74* | 15 | 0.28 | 44.59 | 74* | 21 | 1.08 | 45.49 | 70* | 15* | 0.00 |
| January | 44.97 | 76* | 12 | 0.59 | 39.30 | 72* | 11 | 0.10 | 42.52 | 71* | −19 | 0.64 | 48.66 | 75* | 14* | 0.37 |
| February | 51.56 | 78* | 29 | 0.00 | 50.26 | 81* | 12 | 0.00 | 50.56 | 76* | 25 | 0.00 | 47.57 | 73* | 18* | 0.34 |
| March | 57.16 | 84* | 20 | 0.20 | 55.03 | 85* | 18 | 0.00 | 60.75 | 89* | 35 | 0.30 | 57.15 | 85* | 27* | 0.06 |
| April | 63.62 | 95* | 28 | 0.00 | 62.98 | 98* | 32 | 0.00 | 63.05 | 88* | 28 | 0.36 | 59.32 | 95* | 28* | 0.52 |
| May | 73.59 | 101* | 52 | 0.33 | 73.37 | 107* | 42 | 0.05 | 74.09 | 95* | 50 | 0.04 | 75.94 | 103* | 41* | 0.00 |
| June | 83.83 | 112* | 66 | 1.54 | 82.05 | 103* | 67 | 1.83 | 80.73 | 105* | 50* | 1.34 | 84.79 | 105* | 54* | 0.26 |
| For the year | 63.83 | 112* | 12 | 8.75 | 62.24 | 107* | 11 | 6.93 | 63.44 | 107* | −19 | 7.48 | 65.19 | 109* | 14* | 4.61 |

* These observations are made with self-registering thermometers. The mean is from the standard thermometer.

*Consolidated sick-report, Fort Bliss, Tex., (colored,) 1870–'74.*

| Year | 1870–'71. | | 1871–'72. | | 1872–'73. | | 1873–'74. | |
|---|---|---|---|---|---|---|---|---|
| Mean strength ... Enlisted men | 64 | | 86 | | 55 | | 58 | |
| Diseases. | Cases. | Deaths. | Cases. | Deaths. | Cases. | Deaths. | Cases. | Deaths. |
| **GENERAL DISEASES, A.** | | | | | | | | |
| Remittent fever | 28 | | 8 | | | | | |
| Intermittent fever | 22 | | 11 | | 8 | | 4 | |
| Other diseases of this group | 2 | | 4 | | | | 1 | |
| **GENERAL DISEASES, B.** | | | | | | | | |
| Rheumatism | 12 | | 11 | | 2 | | 1 | |
| Syphilis | 2 | | 3 | | 2 | | 3 | |
| Consumption | | | | 1 | 1 | 1 | | |
| **LOCAL DISEASES.** | | | | | | | | |
| Catarrh and bronchitis | 3 | | 1 | | 4 | | | |
| Pneumonia | 7 | 1 | 2 | 1 | | | 1 | 1 |
| Pleurisy | | | | | 1 | | 4 | |
| Diarrhœa and dysentery | 29 | | 15 | | 8 | | 6 | |
| Hernia | 2 | | | | | | | |
| Gonorrhœa | 3 | | 4 | | 7 | | 9 | |
| Other local diseases | 31 | 1 | 46 | | 12 | | 15 | |
| Alcoholism | | | | | 1 | | | |
| Total disease | 141 | 2 | 105 | 2 | 46 | 1 | 44 | 1 |
| **VIOLENT DISEASES AND DEATHS.** | | | | | | | | |
| Gunshot wounds | 1 | | 1 | | 1 | | 1 | |
| Other accidents and injuries | 11 | | 6 | | 13 | | 21 | |
| Total violence | 12 | | 7 | | 14 | | 22 | |

# FORT BROWN, TEXAS.

### REPORT OF ASSISTANT SURGEON WILLIAM J. WILSON, UNITED STATES ARMY.

The Government reservation upon which the post of Fort Brown is built is a tract of land containing in all 358½ acres, situated on the Rio Grande immediately adjacent to the city of Brownsville, Tex., in latitude 25° 53' 16" north, and longitude 20° 93' west, and with an elevation of about 50 feet above the level of the sea. On the opposite side of the river, and distant about one mile, is the Mexican city of Matamoras. The topography of the post and vicinity is shown in the plate opposite.

The reservation consists of low, flat prairie-land covered with chaparral, a small stunted growth of underbrush or small timber, mostly consisting of mesquite and wausatchie. This prairie-land consists mostly of an alluvial deposit, underlaid at a depth of about 6 feet with a quicksand some 4 to 6 feet in depth. It is very fertile during favorable seasons, producing two crops of corn or cotton annually. Cotton here, as in Mexico, is perennial, and sometimes reaches the height of 15 or 20 feet. Sugar-cane grows in great luxuriance. The castor-bean seems a native of the soil, and can be produced with very little trouble, and in great abundance. These are the principal crops raised in this vicinity.

There is a considerable variety and abundance of game—the bob-white or quail, plover, and several varieties of wild duck; the teal, the black duck, the gray or spoonbill, a few mallard, and still fewer canvas back, visit this neighborhood, and are easily obtained on the ponds or lagoons about here. Wild geese and brant are plentiful, and deer can be obtained at a distance of from 6 to 12 miles from Brownsville. The fish that are obtained here are brought from Brazos Santiago, a distance of some 28 miles; they consist of bass, mullet, flounders, oysters, and redfish. The June-fish, weighing sometimes some 300 to 500 pounds, is also caught and obtained from there. In the Rio Grande and in the lagoon inside the reservation, the silver bass and the mud catfish, buffalo, and perch, weighing from 5 to 6 pounds, are caught. Of wild animals there are few, the principal being the catamount, and the prairie-wolf or coyote. Of reptiles, there are the rattlesnake, moccasin-snake, the adder, the black snake or racer, and the chicken-snake.

Inside the reservation is the lagoon, evidently an old channel of the Rio Grande. It is of an elliptical form, about 150 yards in width, and in some places from 10 to 14 feet in depth. It incloses a small island, containing $25\frac{1}{2}$ acres, which was prior to 1846 heavily covered with timber, but this timber was at that time cut down by United States troops to prevent the Mexicans from stealing up to attack Fort Brown. The national cemetery, containing space for 2,000 graves, is there located. In the center of the island is a flag-staff, and circularly arranged around it are the graves of officers of the regular and volunteer army. Extending south from the flag-staff, and laid out in plats 75 by 15 feet, separated by walks, is the space reserved for the graves of enlisted men. Each plat is intended for 50 graves.

The post of Fort Brown has accommodation for one battery of artillery, one company of cavalry, and four companies of infantry. These different quarters are separated from each other by a very considerable distance. The four sets of infantry quarters are situated on the northern boundary of the reservation, merely separated by a wall from the city of Brownsville. The artillery quarters are almost at the extreme southern end, while the cavalry are stationed about midway between. In close proximity to each of these barracks are the officers' quarters.

The infantry officers' quarters consist of seven houses, situated along the northern border of the lagoon, opposite to and distant from the infantry barracks about 175 yards. The commanding officer's house is a one-and-a-half story frame building, 39 by 33 feet, elevated on brick piers about two feet above the ground. It contains on the ground-floor four rooms, each 16 by 16 by 12 feet, with a hall 6 feet wide. There are four attic rooms on the second story, each similar in size to those below, but only about 8 feet in height. A covered porch, 7 feet wide, is in front of the house. The porch at the rear of the house is 12 feet wide, and by means of a lattice-work at the sides is converted into a dining-room. In the rear of this is a kitchen, 16 by 12 feet. Extending backward for about 60 feet, and inclosed by a lattice-work, is a yard, and at the lower end of this is a small water-closet, 11 by 11 feet, situated over a brick vault about 8 feet in depth. Underneath the stairs leading to the second story is a small closet or pantry. The three houses for captains are almost similar in size to this, but each house contains two sets of quarters, i. e., two rooms, 15 by 16 feet, on the ground-floor, attics above, a small dining-room and kitchen, and yard in the rear.

The lieutenants' quarters are similar in plan, but the rooms are only 14 by 15 feet, on account of the staircase running up between the rooms. A brick walk, 4 feet wide, runs along the front of the officers' quarters, and up to each house. The intervening ground is nicely sodded with Bermuda grass, as is also the remainder of the ground between these quarters and the main barracks.

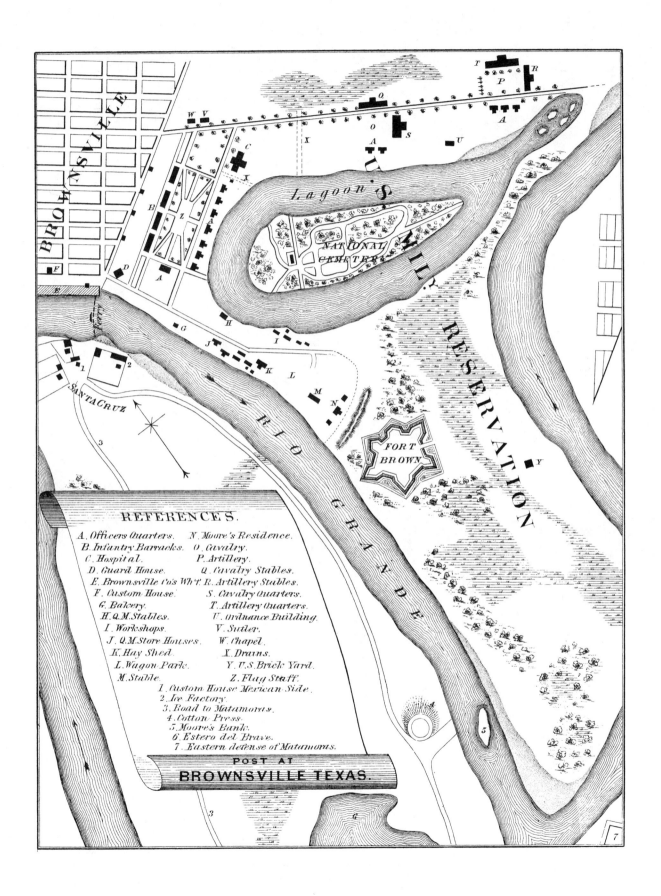

BROWNSVILLE

U.S. MLY. RESERVATION

*Lagoon*

NATIONAL CEMETERY

RIO GRANDE

SANTA CRUZ

FORT BROWN

## REFERENCES.

A. Officers Quarters.
B. Infantry Barracks.
C. Hospital.
D. Guard House.
E. Brownsville Co's Wh't
F. Custom House.
G. Bakery.
H. Q.M. Stables.
I. Workshops.
J. Q.M. Store Houses.
K. Hay Shed.
L. Wagon Park.
M. Stable.

N. Moore's Residence.
O. Cavalry.
P. Artillery.
Q. Cavalry Stables.
R. Artillery Stables.
S. Cavalry Quarters.
T. Artillery Quarters.
U. Ordnance Building.
V. Sutler.
W. Chapel.
X. Drains.
Y. U.S. Brick Yard.
Z. Flag Staff.

1. Custom House Mexican Side.
2. Ice Factory.
3. Road to Matamoras.
4. Cotton Press.
5. Moore's Bank.
6. Estero del Brave.
7. Eastern defense of Matamoras.

## POST AT BROWNSVILLE TEXAS.

7

The cavalry officers' quarters are situated adjacent to the cavalry barracks, and distant about 150 feet; they are built of brick, on the same plan as described for the infantry officers' quarters, and consist of two houses, each having a covered veranda, 7 feet wide, in front.

The artillery officers' quarters are situated almost on the extreme southern end of the reservation, and about half a mile distant from the infantry quarters and hospital. They consist of three brick buildings, built on exactly the same plan as the cavalry officers' quarters.

All the officers' quarters are much in need of repair.

The infantry barracks consist of four two-story frame buildings, each 34 by 163 feet, elevated on brick piers some 3 feet above the level of the ground, and with a covered porch, 7 feet wide, on either side on each story. The lower story, 9 feet high, is divided into an office, 11¼ by 55 feet; first sergeant's room, 11¼ by 22¾; reading-room, 11½ by 19¼; lavatory, 11¼ by 22; day-room, 11¼ by 55; mess-room, 23 by 49½; kitchen, 13½ by 29; cook's room, 9 by 10½; and commissary store-room, 9 by 18 feet. The upper story, 8½ feet in height, is reached by a staircase, is used as a dormitory for the men, and is fitted up with a sufficient number of single iron bedsteads, ranged down both sides of the room. The building is ventilated by twenty-eight windows in each story, and also by ridge ventilators through lattice-work in the ceiling of the dormitory. Situated as these quarters are, almost north and south, they are freely exposed to the prevailing winds, and thorough ventilation as a consequence ensues. In each of these dormitories there is an air-space per man, for an average strength of 50 men, of about 650 cubic feet.

The cavalry barrack is a one-story brick building, 26 by 200 feet, elevated some 3 feet above the surface of the ground, and surrounded by a covered veranda, 9 feet in width. This building is divided by an archway, 12 feet in width, into two large rooms, each 24 by 92 by 14 feet, used as day-rooms for the men, and also as dormitories. Each room of the barrack is sufficiently ventilated by doors at each end, and by 12 windows, six on each side, and also by ridge ventilator, through lattice-work in the ceiling. Projecting backward from the center of the building is a large mess-room, 40 by 40 feet, divided into two rooms by four open arches. There are two small store-rooms, one 14½ by 10 feet, the other 19 feet eight inches by 10 feet, at one end of the mess-room, in which commissary stores are kept. One of these was intended for a kitchen, but was inadequate for the purpose, and a small, temporary wooden building was erected in rear of all, in which the cooking is done, and answers the purpose. This barrack, for an average strength of 80 men, gives an air-space of 775 cubic feet per man.

The artillery barrack is a one-story building, 26 by 300 feet, elevated some 3 feet above the ground, and entirely surrounded by a covered veranda, 9 feet in width. By a covered archway, 12 feet wide, it is divided into two rooms, each 24 by 142 by 14 feet, which are used both as day-rooms and dormitories by the men. Projecting backward from the center of the building is the dining-saloon, 50 by 60 feet, at one end of which is a kitchen, 23 feet 9 inches by 14 feet 3 inches, store-room, 12 feet 9 inches by 14 feet 3 inches, and sergeant-major's room, 8 by 14 feet 3 inches. The dining-room proper is, by four open arches and a passage, 5 feet wide, divided into two rooms, 21 by 48 feet.

To all these barracks privies are provided, situated some little distance in the rear, and all built on the same general plan, being small, frame buildings, elevated some 3 feet above the ground, with a trough which slides underneath, and can be drawn out as often as necessary, emptied, washed out, and disinfected. The privies attached to the cavalry and artillery barracks are, like the quarters, built of brick.

Close to the gate of the principal entrance to the reservation is the guard-house—44 by 35 feet—constructed of hewn logs, with a veranda, 9 feet wide, all around. It is divided into a guard-room, 18 by 21 feet, one prison-room of the same dimensions, and another, 18 by 23 feet, and six cells, 4 by 8 feet. In the prison-rooms, which are without floors, raised platforms are erected, upon which the prisoners sleep. The guard-room and cells are floored. Holes are cut in the doors and ceilings for ventilation, and secured with iron bars. Those in the ceiling communicate with a small dome-shaped ventilator at the top, and also with lattice-work around the sides, beneath the eaves. The average number of prisoners confined is 32. The guard-room is warmed in winter by a wood-stove, but there are no means of warming any other part of the building. The building is highly objectionable, being an unsightly structure at the main entrance of the garrison, and entirely too small for the number of troops at the post.

The post-hospital is a handsome brick building, completed in 1869, in accordance with the plans of Circular No. 4, Surgeon-General's Office, for the year 1867. A covered veranda, 9 feet wide, surrounds the entire building. Extending laterally from the executive building, and separated from it by a covered archway, 10 feet 3 inches in width, are the wards, each of which is 24 by 66 by 14 feet, intended for twenty-four beds. These wards afford sufficient accommodation for the sick of the command, and seem admirably adapted for hospital purposes. A constant breeze (sometimes almost too strong) blows through each ward, thus securing perfectly free ventilation. Each ward is ventilated by thirteen windows and one door on the side, and a door on each end; there is also ventilation through the ridge by lattice-work in the ceilings. The windows are 11½ feet high by 5 feet wide, and are furnished with venetian blinds, opening down to the floor. In the winter months a large wood-stove is used in each ward, which gives sufficient heat. The fuel used is the "mesquite," the same as supplied to the post, an excellent fuel, making almost too hot a fire. The hospital is lighted by candles and lard-oil lamps in each ward.

The married soldiers and laundresses are quartered in twenty-four wooden shanties.

There are no gardens cultivated at the post.

The water-supply is raised from the Rio Grande by a steam-engine into eight large receiving-tanks. From these it is drawn into other tanks, in which the mud separates, and from which it is distributed by water-carts to all parts of the garrison. In addition to this supply, two large cisterns for rain-water were constructed in 1873, by which the post is now supplied with an abundance of pure drinking-water.

*Meteorological report, Fort Brown, Tex., 1870-'74.*

| Month. | 1870-'71. | | | | 1871-'72. | | | | 1872-'73. | | | | 1873-'74. | | | |
|---|---|---|---|---|---|---|---|---|---|---|---|---|---|---|---|---|
| | Temperature. | | | Rain-fall in inches. | Temperature. | | | Rain-fall in inches. | Temperature. | | | Rain-fall in inches. | Temperature. | | | Rain-fall in inches. |
| | Mean. | Max. | Min. | | Mean. | Max. | Min. | | Mean. | Max. | Min. | | Mean. | Max. | Min. | |
| | ° | ° | ° | | ° | ° | ° | | ° | ° | ° | | ° | ° | ° | |
| July | 84.39 | 94* | 70* | 0.75 | 84.15 | 94* | 71* | 0.40 | 84.10 | 93 | 76 | 1.92 | 83.37 | 94* | 63* | 1.10 |
| August | 83.81 | 94* | 70* | 0.10 | 83.76 | 97* | 72* | 1.40 | 82.58 | 96 | 72 | 4.19 | 82.09 | 95* | 67* | 1.98 |
| September | 81.26 | 95* | 64* | 2.53 | 78.95 | 91* | 51* | 2.80 | 79.39 | 92 | 66 | 4.56 | 80.56 | 91 | 66* | 15.35 |
| October | 74.61 | 90* | 49* | 1.00 | 71.73 | 88* | 57* | 8.50 | 72.16 | 89 | 51 | 0.61 | 71.33 | 88 | 51* | 2.81 |
| November | 67.99 | 91* | 33* | 0.70 | 67.64 | 84* | 42* | 1.77 | 62.02 | 84 | 37 | 1.60 | 65.30 | 82 | 41* | 1.71 |
| December | 56.24 | 89* | 23* | 0.30 | 58.92 | 86* | 32* | 0.05 | 59.48 | 81 | 29 | 1.98 | 63.12 | 80 | 37* | 2.10 |
| January | 59.01 | 77* | 29* | 0.90 | 54.72 | 79* | 30* | 0.05 | 55.39 | 82 | 20 | 0.00 | 59.72 | 85 | 30* | 0.86 |
| February | 65.52 | 81* | 38* | 0.00 | 62.41 | 83 | 34 | 0.00 | 67.81 | 88 | 45 | 0.15 | 64.32 | 84 | 41* | 1.48 |
| March | 69.06 | 93* | 43* | 0.30 | 68.42 | 84 | 39 | 1.64 | 69.90 | 86 | 47 | 0.47 | 72.41 | 86 | 55* | 1.90 |
| April | 74.09 | 99* | 45* | 0.10 | 76.24 | 91 | 56 | 0.82 | 71.12 | 91 | 49 | 0.59 | 68.27 | 86 | 44* | 0.30 |
| May | 77.21 | 94* | 57* | 3.40 | 80.02 | 93 | 62 | 0.27 | 79.42 | 98* | 60* | 0.96 | 74.37 | 87 | 48* | 1.34 |
| June | 82.29 | 102* | 63* | 0.78 | 82.55 | 93 | 71 | 1.78 | 82.08 | 95* | 66* | 0.43 | 80.74 | 91 | 69* | 1.50 |
| For the year | 72.96 | 102* | 23* | 10.86 | 72.46 | 97* | 30* | 19.48 | 72.12 | 98* | 20 | 20.46 | 72.13 | 95* | 30* | 32.43 |

* These observations are made with self-registering thermometers. The mean is from the standard thermometer.

*Consolidated sick-report, Fort Brown, Tex., (white troops,) 1870-'74.*

| Year | | | 1870-'71. | | 1871-'72. | | 1872-'73. | | 1873-'74. | |
|---|---|---|---|---|---|---|---|---|---|---|
| Mean strength | { Officers | | 15 | | 11 | | 16* | | 17† | |
| | { Enlisted men | | 306 | | 191 | | 108 | | 1‡ | |
| Diseases. | | | Cases. | Deaths. | Cases. | Deaths. | Cases. | Deaths. | Cases. | Deaths. |
| GENERAL DISEASES, A. | | | | | | | | | | |
| Remittent fever | | | 46 | ...... | 25 | ...... | 10 | ...... | 5 | ...... |
| Intermittent fever | | | 120 | ...... | 60 | ...... | 12 | ...... | 1 | ...... |
| Dengue | | | ...... | ...... | ...... | ...... | 102 | ...... | ...... | ...... |
| Other diseases of this group | | | 3 | ...... | 7 | ...... | 6 | ...... | 3 | ...... |

* Ten months only, officers.      † Eight months only, officers.      ‡ Four months only, enlisted men.

*Consolidated sick-report, Fort Brown, Tex.—Continued.*

| Year | 1870–'71. | | 1871–'72. | | 1872–'73. | | 1873–'74. | |
|---|---|---|---|---|---|---|---|---|
| Mean strength ........... { Officers ........... / Enlisted men ...... | 15 / 306 | | 11 / 191 | | 16 / 108 | | 17 / 1 | |
| Diseases. | Cases. | Deaths. | Cases. | Deaths. | Cases. | Deaths. | Cases. | Deaths. |
| GENERAL DISEASES, B. | | | | | | | | |
| Rheumatism ................... | 53 | ...... | 26 | ...... | 26 | ...... | ...... | ...... |
| Syphilis ................... | 74 | ...... | 25 | ...... | 25 | ...... | ...... | ...... |
| Consumption ................... | ...... | ...... | 3 | 1 | 1 | 2 | ...... | ...... |
| Other diseases of this group ......... | 1 | ...... | 1 | 1 | ...... | ...... | ...... | ...... |
| LOCAL DISEASES. | | | | | | | | |
| Catarrh and bronchitis ......... | 29 | ...... | 7 | ...... | 38 | ...... | 3 | ...... |
| Pneumonia ................... | 3 | 1 | 1 | ...... | ...... | ...... | ...... | ...... |
| Pleurisy ................... | ...... | ...... | ...... | ...... | 3 | ...... | ...... | ...... |
| Diarrhœa and dysentery ......... | 67 | 2 | 64 | ...... | 67 | ...... | 2 | ...... |
| Hernia ................... | 1 | ...... | 5 | ...... | 1 | ...... | ...... | ...... |
| Gonorrhœa ................... | 9 | ...... | 13 | ...... | 14 | ...... | ...... | ...... |
| Other local diseases ......... | 123 | 1 | 87 | ...... | 94 | ...... | 3 | ...... |
| Alcoholism ................... | 19 | ...... | 19 | 1 | 5 | ...... | ...... | ...... |
| Total disease ......... | 548 | 4 | 343 | 3 | 404 | 2 | 17 | ...... |
| VIOLENT DISEASES AND DEATHS. | | | | | | | | |
| Gunshot wounds ............... | 1 | ...... | 1 | ...... | 2 | ...... | ...... | ...... |
| Drowning ................... | ...... | ...... | ...... | 1 | ...... | ...... | ...... | ...... |
| Other accidents and injuries ......... | 44 | ...... | 55 | ...... | 45 | ...... | 1 | ...... |
| Total violence ......... | 45 | ...... | 56 | 1 | 47 | ...... | 1 | ...... |

*Consolidated sick-report, Fort Brown, Tex., (colored troops,) 1872–'74.*

| Year | 1872–'73.* | | 1873–'74. | |
|---|---|---|---|---|
| Mean strength ...................... Enlisted men ...... | 237 | | 266 | |
| Diseases. | Cases. | Deaths. | Cases. | Deaths. |
| GENERAL DISEASES, A. | | | | |
| Small-pox and varioloid ......... | 1 | ...... | 1 | ...... |
| Remittent fever ................... | 19 | ...... | 24 | ...... |
| Intermittent fever ............... | 9 | ...... | 28 | ...... |
| Dengue ................... | 29 | ...... | ...... | ...... |
| Other diseases of this group ......... | 12 | ...... | 46 | ...... |
| GENERAL DISEASES, B. | | | | |
| Rheumatism ................... | 65 | ...... | 93 | ...... |
| Syphilis ................... | 77 | ...... | 121 | ...... |
| Consumption ................... | ...... | 1 | ...... | 1 |
| LOCAL DISEASES. | | | | |
| Catarrh and bronchitis ......... | 94 | ...... | 130 | ...... |
| Pneumonia ................... | 1 | ...... | 1 | ...... |
| Pleurisy ................... | 2 | ...... | ...... | ...... |
| Diarrhœa and dysentery ......... | 73 | ...... | 132 | ...... |
| Hernia ................... | ...... | ...... | 5 | ...... |
| Gonorrhœa ................... | 99 | ...... | 72 | ...... |
| Other local diseases ......... | 145 | ...... | 211 | ...... |
| Unclassified ................... | ...... | ...... | ...... | ...... |
| Total disease .... | 626 | 1 | 864 | 1 |
| VIOLENT DISEASES AND DEATHS. | | | | |
| Gunshot wounds ............... | ...... | ...... | 3 | ...... |
| Other accidents and injuries ......... | 48 | ...... | 58 | ...... |
| Homicide ................... | ...... | ...... | ...... | 1 |
| Total violence ......... | 48 | ...... | 61 | 1 |

* Ten months only ; first report September, 1872.

# FORT CLARK, TEXAS.

REPORTS OF ACTING ASSISTANT SURGEON D. JACKSON AND ASSISTANT SURGEON P. MIDDLETON,
UNITED STATES ARMY.

Fort Clark, Tex., is situated in Kinney County, in latitude 29° 17′ north, longitude 23° 18′ west, at an approximate elevation of 1,000 feet above the level of the sea. It is 125 miles west of San Antonio, and about 45 miles north of Fort Duncan, at Eagle Pass, on the Rio Grande.

The site of the post is a rocky ridge of limestone, embraced in a curve of Las Moras Creek at its head, the post being about 400 yards south of the Las Moras Spring, from which the creek takes its rise. There is, west of the post, 30 miles distant on the El Paso and San Antonio road, a small settlement containing about a dozen families. There are but few settlers in the county; they are scattered along the Rio Grande and Nueces River. From the spring the Las Moras takes an easterly direction, curving south, then west, and keeping this general direction until it reaches the Rio Grande, distant about 18 miles. For about 8 miles the creek is skirted with a belt of heavily-timbered land, varying in width from a few yards to 70 or 80 rods.

This bottom-land is very fertile, and 500 acres are susceptible of irrigation; but a great part of this is liable to overflow during the summer freshets, greatly diminishing the value of the land in an agricultural point of view. Brackettsville, a small village, is situated between the reservation and the El Paso road.

This post was established in 1852, with a view of protecting the southwest frontier against depredations by Mexicans and Indians, as well as for the protection of the road. Since the re-occupation of the post in 1866, (it having been abandoned in 1861,) the Indians operating in this region have been the Lipan and Kickapoo tribes, whose homes are in Mexico.

There is no reservation. The ground occupied is leased by the Government.

The land lying from southeast to southwest of the post for the most part is low and gently undulating, and the flats well covered with mesquite, while that from northwest to northeast is high and rocky, with but little timber, except on the banks of streams. On the north the high-lands dividing this scope of country from the Nueces bound the view, while on the east and south-east is seen, some 20 miles distant, what is called the Turkey Creek range of mountains, ridges of from 100 to 200 feet in height. The Las Moras, Piedro Pinto, Elm Creek, and Turkey Creek ranges of mountains are all elevations of from 100 to 200 feet in height, and from one-half to one mile in circumference, all visible and within 20 miles of the post; they are all on this side of the Nueces "Divide," and are near the sources of the streams from which they receive their names. A range of mountains in Mexico is seen, in clear weather, west of this place; they are upward of 100 miles distant, and extend parallel to the Rio Grande and to a point opposite to the mouth of the San Félipe Creek.

Beds of bitumen are found on the Nueces, probably of little or no value. Grass is abundant, and the country is adapted to stock-raising only. Along some of the streams, such as the Rio Frio, Nueces, &c., are to be found, though not very plentifully, cypress, walnut, oak, elm, sycamore, mulberry, willow, and pecan. In the region of the Nueces and the mountain regions cedar grows abundantly. Prairie flats are usually covered with mesquite or post-oak. Large quantities of mulberry timber is to be found below the reservation along the Las Moras. The cactus is in great variety, and abundant throughout the barrens and higher regions.

The principal wild animals are the wolf, black bear, panther, wild cat, lynx, leopard, lion, gopher, red squirrel, raccoon, polecat, civet cat, red deer, and antelope. Buffalo rarely come down so far. Wild turkey, duck, grouse, plover, &c., are found, and all the streams have abundance of fish—trout, sunfish, bass, catfish, and buffalo.

All the rivers and creeks in this vicinity contain good water, originating from mountain springs; the most famous in this section, and, I believe, the largest in Texas, being the San Félipe Spring, 30 miles west of this. The Las Moras Spring, about 400 yards north of the post, is a sort of pond about one-eighth of an acre in area, from which issues the Las Moras Creek, a rather sluggish stream, having an average breadth for the first mile of about 20 yards; for the rest of its course its breadth is 6 yards; depth from 3 to 4 feet, with marshy banks.

The prevailing winds are east-southeast.

When the wind varies in force and direction, it is always the premonition of a "norther," which occurs about once every ten days during the winter season, i. e., from the beginning of November to the end of March. During these northers the wind usually blows with great violence from the northwest, north, or northeast, but most severely from the northwest, during which it is impossible to travel over the plains; in summer they are less frequent and not so violent.

The seasons are usually divided into "wet" and "dry," or summer and winter, the former commencing in April and ending in October, and consequently the dry or winter months being November, December, January, February, and March.

There is no fort proper. The post is built in a quadrangle, one of whose sides, the northeast, runs nearly parallel to the Las Moras Creek, from which it is distant from 75 to 100 yards, and on an elevated ridge of nearly bare limestone rock, 40 or 50 feet above the level of the creek.

The post has been much enlarged within the last four years, and now covers about 20 acres.

The barracks are ten one-story stone buildings, each 110 by 24 by 10 feet, shingled, floored, plastered, and with a porch in front 10 feet wide. They are warmed by fire-places, and fitted with iron bunks.

The kitchens and mess-rooms are about 30 feet in rear of the barracks; they are stockade buildings, each 46 by 18 feet, plastered but not floored. Six of these have been completed.

Nine new buildings are now completed for officers' quarters; they are built of stone, two stories high, with porch in front, and with back buildings.

The quarters for commanding officer has a central hall 10 feet wide, with four rooms, each 15 by 18 feet, on each floor. The remaining 8 buildings are each 55 by 34 feet, and divided into two sets of quarters, each having three rooms on each floor. They are well finished and in good condition.

The commissary storehouse is a new stone building one story high, 180 by 26 feet, floored and plastered, with a cellar 8 feet deep under its whole length.

The grain-house is of stone, 110 by 30 feet.

The guard-house is of stone, 80 by 26 feet, divided into three rooms, the center or guard-room 20 by 26 feet; the remaining two are each 30 by 26 feet; one is occupied by general prisoners, the other contains 6 cells.

The hospital is of stone, on the plan prescribed by Circular No. 2, Surgeon-General's Office, July, 1871, consisting of a central administration building and two wings, of which but one is finished. The wards are each 60 by 24 by 14 feet, and, except by the roof, do not connect with the main building. Each ward has eight windows, each 8 by 4 feet 10 inches, and ridge ventilation.

Earth-closets are used throughout the command.

All the water used at the post is taken from the head-waters of the Las Moras, which rises about 400 yards distant; it is transported by water-wagons, and received and stored in barrels.

It is understood that a system of water-works is to be furnished, which will certainly be a great improvement on the present plan.

The spring is gradually filling up, and the question of preserving the purity and quantity of the water-supply will soon become of much importance.

The post being on a limestone ledge, with not more than an inch or two of soil, and some 40 or 50 feet above the level of the creek, and embraced in a curve of the same, it is evident that the natural drainage itself is ample; offal, slops, and excreta are carted off some distance to leeward of the post, and dumped out on the prairie. There are no special arrangements for bathing; sheltered and secluded spots along the creek are usually selected, both in summer and winter, for this purpose.

The cemetery is located south of the post about 200 yards, near the creek.

The garden has been a failure. Fresh vegetables sell at almost fabulous prices, and, except onions, which are brought from Mexico, are very scarce.

*Meteorological report, Fort Clark, Tex., 1870–'73.*

| Month. | 1870–'71. | | | | 1871–'72. | | | | 1872–'73. | | | | 1873–'74. | | | |
|---|---|---|---|---|---|---|---|---|---|---|---|---|---|---|---|---|
| | Temperature. | | | Rain-fall in inches. | Temperature. | | | Rain-fall in inches. | Temperature. | | | Rain-fall in inches. | Temperature. | | | Rain-fall in inches. |
| | Mean. | Max. | Min. | | Mean. | Max. | Min. | | Mean. | Max. | Min. | | Mean. | Max. | Min. | |
| July | 82.88 | 97 | 71 | 1.92 | 90.52 | 109 | 75 | 0.00 | 83.26 | 99 | 68* | 3.70 | 81.37 | 101* | 68 | 1.70 |
| August | 81.45 | 96 | 71 | 10.10 | 89.29 | 113 | 73 | 2.46 | 83.78 | 100 | 69* | 0.52 | ...... | ...... | ...... | ...... |
| September | 79.79 | 98 | 65 | 2.22 | 81.09 | 103 | 61 | 3.69 | 79.93 | 100 | 60* | 1.76 | ...... | ...... | ...... | ...... |
| October | 68.30 | 88 | 43 | 4.58 | 69.31 | 94 | 46 | 3.26 | 70.18 | 98 | 43* | 0.25 | ...... | ...... | ...... | ...... |
| November | 62.46 | 88 | 37 | 1.86 | 59.01 | 85 | 30 | 0.32 | 52.68 | 86 | 10* | 1.64 | ...... | ...... | ...... | ...... |
| December | 47.92 | 76 | 12 | 0.30 | 52.46 | 82 | 23 | 0.00 | 46.67 | 78 | 22* | 4.32 | ...... | ...... | ...... | ...... |
| January | 52.89 | 78 | 25 | 1.21 | 48.32 | 76 | 24 | 0.03 | 45.63 | 74 | 1* | 0.32 | ...... | ...... | ...... | ...... |
| February | 59.42 | 84 | 33 | 0.23 | 54.57 | 84 | 22* | 0.45 | 55.33 | 82 | 29* | 0.24 | ...... | ...... | ...... | ...... |
| March | 66.11 | 90 | 34 | 0.07 | 60.68 | 90 | 31* | 0.06 | 64.14 | 89 | 30* | 1.56 | ...... | ...... | ...... | ...... |
| April | 71.54 | 96 | 42 | 0.12 | 72.87 | 99 | 45* | 0.56 | 68.60 | 97* | 30* | 0.44 | ...... | ...... | ...... | ...... |
| May | 79.90 | 102 | 56 | 2.07 | 76.74 | 98 | 51* | 1.12 | 78.53 | 106* | 56 | 3.74 | ...... | ...... | ...... | ...... |
| June | 86.67 | 107 | 73 | 0.13 | 83.13 | 100 | 63* | 3.90 | 80.51 | 99* | 59 | 7.68 | ...... | ...... | ...... | ...... |
| For the year | 69.94 | 107 | 12 | 24.81 | 69.83 | 113 | 22* | 15.85 | 67.43 | 106* | 1* | 26.17 | ...... | ...... | ...... | ...... |

* These observations are made with self-registering thermometers. The mean is from the standard thermometer.

*Consolidated sick-report, Fort Clark, Texas, (white,) 1870–'74.*

| Year | | 1870–'71. | | 1871–'72. | | 1872–'73.* | | 1873–'74.† | |
|---|---|---|---|---|---|---|---|---|---|
| Mean strength { Officers { Enlisted men | | 13 ...... | | 14 ...... | | 19 299 | | 23 628 | |
| Diseases. | | Cases. | Deaths. | Cases. | Deaths. | Cases. | Deaths. | Cases. | Deaths. |
| GENERAL DISEASES, A. | | | | | | | | | |
| Small-pox | | ...... | ...... | ...... | ...... | 1 | ...... | 1 | ...... |
| Typhoid fever | | ...... | ...... | ...... | ...... | 2 | 1 | 1 | 1 |
| Remittent fever | | ...... | ...... | ...... | ...... | ...... | ...... | 2 | 1 |
| Intermittent fever | | 1 | ...... | 3 | ...... | 34 | ...... | 126 | ...... |
| Yellow fever | | ...... | ...... | ...... | ...... | ...... | ...... | 1 | ...... |
| Other diseases of this group | | ...... | ...... | 1 | ...... | 6 | ...... | 6 | 1 |
| GENERAL DISEASES, B. | | | | | | | | | |
| Rheumatism | | ...... | ...... | ...... | ...... | 7 | ...... | 45 | ...... |
| Syphilis | | ...... | ...... | ...... | ...... | 3 | ...... | 5 | ...... |
| Consumption | | ...... | ...... | ...... | ...... | 3 | ...... | 3 | ...... |
| Other diseases of this group | | ...... | ...... | ...... | ...... | 4 | ...... | 4 | ...... |
| LOCAL DISEASES. | | | | | | | | | |
| Catarrh and bronchitis | | 1 | ...... | ...... | ...... | 1 | ...... | 27 | ...... |
| Pneumonia | | ...... | ...... | ...... | ...... | ...... | ...... | 1 | ...... |
| Pleurisy | | ...... | ...... | ...... | ...... | 1 | ...... | 5 | ...... |
| Diarrhœa and dysentery | | ...... | ...... | 2 | ...... | 41 | 1 | 162 | 1 |
| Hernia | | ...... | ...... | ...... | ...... | 2 | ...... | 4 | ...... |
| Gonorrhœa | | ...... | ...... | ...... | ...... | 1 | ...... | 5 | ...... |
| Other local diseases | | 3 | 1 | 6 | ...... | 52 | 1 | 269 | 1 |
| Alcoholism | | ...... | ...... | ...... | ...... | 1 | ...... | 6 | ...... |
| Total disease | | 5 | 1 | 12 | ...... | 159 | 3 | 672 | 5 |
| VIOLENT DISEASES AND DEATHS. | | | | | | | | | |
| Gun-shot wounds | | ...... | ...... | ...... | ...... | 4 | 1 | 4 | ...... |
| Other accidents and injuries | | 1 | ...... | 1 | ...... | 36 | ...... | 165 | ...... |
| Homicide | | ...... | ...... | ...... | ...... | ...... | ...... | ...... | 3 |
| Total violence | | 1 | ...... | 1 | ...... | 40 | 1 | 169 | 3 |

* Eight months only. † Eleven months only.

*Consolidated sick-report, Fort Clark, Texas, (colored,) 1870–'74.*

| Year | 1870–'71. | | 1871–'72. | | 1872–'73. | | 1873–'74.* | |
|---|---|---|---|---|---|---|---|---|
| Mean strength, enlisted men | 274 | | 275 | | 179 | | 44 | |
| Diseases. | Cases. | Deaths. | Cases. | Deaths. | Cases. | Deaths. | Cases. | Deaths. |
| GENERAL DISEASES, A. | | | | | | | | |
| Typhoid fever | | | 2 | 1 | | | | |
| Remittent fever | | | 6 | | 7 | | | |
| Intermittent fever | 45 | | 37 | | 20 | | 4 | |
| Other diseases of this group | 9 | | 2 | | 20 | | | |
| GENERAL DISEASES, B. | | | | | | | | |
| Rheumatism | 16 | | 18 | | 2 | | | |
| Syphilis | 23 | | 16 | | 1 | | 3 | |
| Consumption | 1 | 1 | 7 | 2 | | | | |
| Other diseases of this group | | | 3 | | 2 | | | |
| LOCAL DISEASES. | | | | | | | | |
| Catarrh and bronchitis | 15 | | 11 | 1 | 8 | | | |
| Pneumonia | | | 3 | 1 | 2 | | | |
| Pleurisy | 2 | | 1 | | 3 | | | |
| Diarrhœa and dysentery | 69 | | 53 | 1 | 21 | 1 | 6 | |
| Hernia | | | 1 | | 1 | | | |
| Gonorrhoea | 6 | | | | | | 2 | |
| Other local diseases | 119 | 1 | 62 | 2 | 22 | | 6 | |
| Alcoholism | 2 | | | | | | | |
| Unclassified | 2 | | | | | | | |
| Total disease | 309 | 2 | 222 | 8 | 109 | 1 | 21 | |
| VIOLENT DISEASES AND DEATHS. | | | | | | | | |
| Gun-shot wounds | 8 | | 6 | 1 | 3 | | 1 | |
| Other accidents and injuries | 127 | | 71 | | 30 | | 4 | |
| Homicide | | 2 | | 1 | | | | |
| Suicide | | | | | | 2 | | |
| Total violence | 135 | 2 | 77 | 2 | 33 | 2 | 5 | |

\* Four months only.

# FORT CONCHO, TEXAS.

REPORTS OF ASSISTANT SURGEONS W. M. NOTSON AND W. F. BUCHANAN, UNITED STATES ARMY.

Fort Concho is situated at the junction of the North and Main Concho Rivers; latitude, 31° 30′ north; longitude, 23° 17′ west. The surrounding country is a flat, treeless prairie, not susceptible of cultivation except on the bottom-lands where irrigation can be effected. The arrangement of the post is shown by figure 31.

The officers' quarters are five cottage buildings of stone; four erected for captains' quarters, and one for major or lieutenant-colonel. The quarters are built with two rooms facing the parade, separated by a broad hall; in the rear of the west room is a kitchen. The rooms are commodious, about 15 feet square, well lighted, without closets or shutters. The larger quarters are built upon the same plan, with one additional room in the L, which is about 4 feet higher. All of the buildings have attics, and are heated by open fires. Each kitchen is provided with a pantry.

The commissary's and quartermaster's storehouses are built upon the same plan, and are of the same dimensions, about 100 feet in length, 30 in width, and about the same to the peak of the roof, each building forming one large room, with one little closet about 10 feet square walled off for office purposes. The flooring is of large irregular slabs of stone, cemented with ordinary mortar. The wood-work—rafters, beams, &c.—as in all the other buildings, is of pecan, a peculiarly intractable variety of our northern hickory, which by its twisting, curling, and shrinking hardly promises a permanence of the symmetry of the buildings in which it has been used.

The guard-house is a stone building, with hipped roof, 67 by 25 feet, containing a guard-room 19 feet 10 inches by 23 feet 10 inches, not ceiled. Prison-room, 23 feet by 21 feet 6 inches, ceiled; height, 11 feet; and 8 cells, each 7 feet 10 inches by 3 feet 10 inches, arched; 9 feet high, with slat-doors, opening into a passage 3 feet wide, and a grated opening, 9 by 12 inches, opposite.

The hospital is a stone building, on the plan given in Circular No. 4, Surgeon-General's Office, 1867, for 24 beds. The flooring has been completed, ventilating-boxes placed in the wards, and a good cistern constructed, which last has been of great use. The hospital is now in good condition·

There are 5 corrals, 4 cavalry, each 300 by 75, and 1 quartermaster's, 400 by 225 feet, with stone walls, around which are sheds.

AA, barracks; B, guard-house; CC, storehouses; DD, officers' quarters completed; E, officers quarters requiring only plaster and paint; FF, GG, officers' quarters to be erected or completed; H, hospital; K, LL, corrals; M, proposed chapel and school-house; N, proposed chaplain's quarters; O and P, proposed quarters for officers; R, adjutant's office; S, proposed granary; T, shops; V, proposed front wall to be four feet high; main entrance in center; WW, sinks.

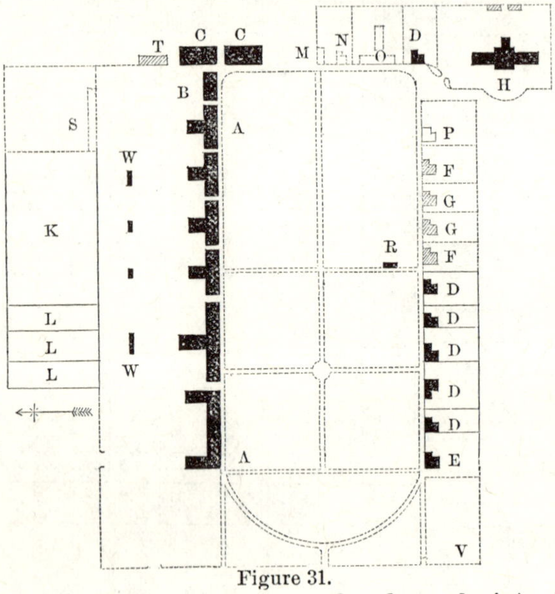

Figure 31.

The barracks are two stone buildings, 180 by 27 and 100 by 27 feet, 11 feet to eaves and 21 feet to ridge, with piazza, 9 feet wide, around each. These afford accommodation for two companies each. One of them has two L's in rear containing each a mess-room 20 by 54, a kitchen 20 by 15, and an orderly room 14 by 13 feet; the other has but a single L. Each dormitory contains 31,016 cubic feet air-space, is unceiled, with ridge and eaves ventilation—fitted with iron bedsteads, and for a full company gives 368 cubic feet air-space per man. There are four other barracks intended for one company each and similarly arranged.

The nearest supply depot is San Antonio, distant 225 miles. When the rainy season sets in, communication is almost entirely suspended.

The water-supply is hauled from the Concho River. Cisterns should be constructed for this post. Game is abundant in the vicinity. Buffalo exist in countless herds during the winter and spring, and deer and antelope at all seasons. The large gray wolf and the coyote are abundant, and the fox, the badger, and peccary can easily be found when desired. The prairie for miles in every direction being one vast "dog town," the prairie-dog holes interfere somewhat with the pursuit of the chase. Water-fowl of every kind, from the large white swan to the green-winged teal, abound upon the rivers. Wild turkey and quail, both the brown of Virginia and the blue or tufted quail of New Mexico, can be found anywhere upon the streams. Immense catfish, weighing even as much as 75 pounds, with eels of proportionate size, and a trout, called in this country a bass, with smaller fish, reward the angler for very little exertion. It may be some drawback that a country supplied so lavishly with game is equally generously furnished with venomous reptiles and insects. A prairie-dog town is the well-known habitat of the rattlesnake, as also the rocky borders of the streams. Tarantulas and lesser spiders lurk under every cactus shrub, and the centipede brings forth its interesting brood in every pile of chips or lumber about one's quarters. Small scorpions, from two to three inches in length, are found, though less frequently than either the centipede or tarantula. Indians, believed to be chiefly Comanches and Kiowas, commit frequent depredations in the vicinity.

*Meteorological report, Fort Concho, Tex., 1872–'74.*

| Month. | 1870–'71. | | | | 1871–'72. | | | | 1872–'73. | | | | 1873–'74. | | | |
|---|---|---|---|---|---|---|---|---|---|---|---|---|---|---|---|---|
| | Temperature. | | | Rain-fall in inches. | Temperature. | | | Rain-fall in inches. | Temperature. | | | Rain-fall in inches. | Temperature. | | | Rain-fall in inches. |
| | Mean. | Max. | Min. | | Mean. | Max. | Min. | | Mean. | Max. | Min. | | Mean. | Max. | Min. | |
| | | | | | | | | | ° | ° | ° | | ° | ° | ° | |
| July | | | | | | | | | | | | | 86.85* | 102* | 64* | 0.92 |
| August | | | | | | | | | 82.32 | 101 | 65 | 2.60 | 83.18* | 102* | 61* | 1.46 |
| September | | | | | | | | | 75.22 | 102 | 49 | 0.85 | 80.93* | 107* | 50* | 0.44 |
| October | | | | | | | | | 64.33 | 97 | 33 | 0.66 | 70.27* | 100* | 34* | 0.50 |
| November | | | | | | | | | 51.89 | 82 | 18 | 1.66 | 56.25* | 86* | 29* | 0.25 |
| December | | | | | | | | | 41.75 | 80 | 20 | 0.53 | 48.85* | 81* | 31* | 0.00 |
| January | | | | | | | | | 54.38 | 80 | 2 | 0.16 | 47.14* | 80* | 18* | 0.25 |
| February | | | | | | | | | 53.52 | 86 | 18 | 0.33 | 53.01* | 82* | 28* | 0.25 |
| March | | | | | | | | | 60.73 | 88 | 30 | 1.60 | 57.11* | 92* | 27* | 1.14 |
| April | | | | | | | | | 62.65 | 87 | 25 | 0.00 | 64.30* | 91* | 34* | 0.39 |
| May | | | | | | | | | 74.29 | 98 | 44 | 6.36 | 79.92* | 99* | 51* | 3.29 |
| June | | | | | | | | | 81.43* | 100* | 66* | 6.40 | 87.61* | 104* | 72* | 3.05 |
| For the year | | | | | | | | | | | | | 67.95* | 107* | 18* | 11.94 |

\* These observations are made with self-registering thermometers. The mean is from the standard thermometer.

*Consolidated sick-report, (white troops,) Fort Concho, Tex., 1870–'74.*

| Year | 1870–'71. | | 1871–'72. | | 1872–'73. | | 1873–'74. | |
|---|---|---|---|---|---|---|---|---|
| Mean strength { Officers | 17 | | 11 | | 19 | | 14 | |
| { Enlisted men | 437 | | 190 | | 242 | | 62 | |
| Diseases. | Cases. | Deaths. | Cases. | Deaths. | Cases. | Deaths. | Cases. | Deaths. |
| GENERAL DISEASES, A. | | | | | | | | |
| Typhoid fever | | | 2 | 1 | | 1 | 1 | |
| Typho-malarial fever | | | 1 | | | | 1 | 1 |
| Remittent fever | 21 | 1 | 3 | | 50 | | 2 | |
| Intermittent fever | 147 | 1 | 43 | | 50 | | 18 | |
| Other diseases of this group | 13 | | 6 | | 1 | | 2 | |
| GENERAL DISEASES, B. | | | | | | | | |
| Rheumatism | 52 | | 64 | | 12 | | 3 | |
| Syphilis | 14 | | 7 | | 7 | | | |
| Consumption | 2 | | 1 | | | | | |
| Other diseases of this group | 3 | | 4 | | 15 | | 3 | |
| LOCAL DISEASES. | | | | | | | | |
| Catarrh and bronchitis | 59 | | 78 | | 30 | | 3 | |
| Pneumonia | 8 | | 1 | | 2 | 1 | | |
| Pleurisy | 4 | | 3 | | 3 | | | |
| Diarrhœa and dysentery | 253 | 5 | 119 | | 64 | | 20 | |
| Hernia | 2 | | 2 | | 5 | | | |
| Gonorrhœa | 5 | | 2 | | 8 | | | |
| Other local diseases | 259 | | 130 | | 99 | | 32 | |
| Alcoholism | 17 | | 10 | | 4 | | 5 | |
| Total disease | 859 | 7 | 476 | 1 | 300 | 2 | 90 | 1 |
| VIOLENT DISEASES AND DEATHS. | | | | | | | | |
| Gunshot wounds | 7 | 1 | 7 | 1 | 2 | 1 | 1 | 1 |
| Other accidents and injuries | 153 | 3 | 118 | | 102 | | 26 | |
| Homicide | | 2 | | | | | | |
| Suicide | | | | | | 1 | | |
| Total violence | 160 | 6 | 125 | 1 | 104 | 2 | 27 | 1 |

*Consolidated sick-report, (colored troops,) Fort Concho, Tex., 1870–'74.*

| Year | 1870–'71.* | | 1871–'72. | | 1872–'73.† | | 1873–'74. | |
|---|---|---|---|---|---|---|---|---|
| Mean strength..........................................Enlisted men...... | 25 | | 27 | | 62 | | 165 | |
| Diseases. | Cases. | Deaths. | Cases. | Deaths. | Cases. | Deaths. | Cases. | Deaths. |
| GENERAL DISEASES, A. | | | | | | | | |
| Remittent fever............. | 1 | ...... | 1 | ...... | 1 | ...... | 8 | 1 |
| Intermittent fever............. | ...... | ...... | 15 | ...... | 6 | ...... | 26 | ...... |
| Other diseases of this group............. | ...... | ...... | 3 | ...... | 1 | ...... | 20 | ...... |
| GENERAL DISEASES, B. | | | | | | | | |
| Rheumatism............. | 1 | ...... | 9 | ...... | 1 | ...... | 11 | ...... |
| Syphilis............. | 3 | ...... | ...... | ...... | 2 | ...... | 1 | ...... |
| Consumption............. | ...... | ...... | 1 | 1 | ...... | ...... | ...... | ...... |
| Other diseases of this group............. | ...... | ...... | ...... | ...... | 1 | ...... | 4 | ...... |
| LOCAL DISEASES. | | | | | | | | |
| Catarrh and bronchitis............. | 1 | ...... | 16 | ...... | ...... | ...... | 20 | ...... |
| Pneumonia............. | ...... | ...... | 1 | ...... | ...... | 1 | 2 | 1 |
| Pleurisy............. | ...... | ...... | 2 | ...... | ...... | ...... | 7 | ...... |
| Diarrhœa and dysentery............. | ...... | ...... | 25 | ...... | 13 | ...... | 88 | ...... |
| Hernia............. | ...... | ...... | ...... | ...... | 1 | ...... | 2 | ...... |
| Gonorrhœa............. | ...... | ...... | ...... | ...... | ...... | ...... | 4 | ...... |
| Other local diseases............. | ...... | ...... | 24 | 1 | 11 | ...... | 97 | 1 |
| Alcoholism............. | ...... | ...... | ...... | ...... | ...... | ...... | 1 | ...... |
| Unclassified............. | ...... | ...... | ...... | ...... | ...... | ...... | 1 | ...... |
| Total disease............. | 6 | ...... | 97 | 2 | 37 | 1 | 292 | 3 |
| VIOLENT DISEASES AND DEATHS. | | | | | | | | |
| Gunshot wounds............. | 1 | ...... | 7 | ...... | 2 | ...... | 11 | ...... |
| Other accidents and injuries............. | 1 | ...... | 9 | ...... | 4 | ...... | 74 | ...... |
| Homicide............. | ...... | ...... | ...... | ...... | ...... | ...... | ...... | 1 |
| Total violence............. | 2 | ...... | 16 | ...... | 6 | ...... | 85 | 1 |

* Three months only.          † Seven months only.

---

# FORT DAVIS, TEXAS.

### REPORT OF ASSISTANT SURGEON D. WEISEL, UNITED STATES ARMY.

Fort Davis is located near Limpia Creek, Presidio County, Tex., in latitude 30° 36' 23'' north, longitude 26° 33' 45'' west, 479 miles northwest of San Antonio, and 220 miles southeast of El Paso. The altitude above the sea is 4,700 feet.

The post was established in 1854, for the purpose of keeping in check the predatory bands of the Apaches and Comanches, who could easily be interrupted from this point at the various crossings of the Rio Grande, to and from Mexico. The location was selected on account of its healthy and delightful climate, its defensibility, and its communication, by a fine natural road, with San Antonio and El Paso.

The post is at the mouth of a cañon about three-fourths of a mile long, about 400 yards wide at its mouth, and gradually narrowing to its termination in a recess in the mountain. The mountains on either side are formed of metamorphic rocks, are about 250 feet high, very rough and precipitous, and covered with grass and small oak trees. The surrounding country is wild and barren, with no trees excepting a few live-oaks in the cañon in rear of the post, and a few cotton-woods on the Limpia.

The officers' quarters are located in a line running north and south across the mouth of the cañon. These are nineteen in number, one story, a covered porch in front and rear along the entire building, a separate house for each officer, and distant from each other 24 feet, the commanding officer's in the center, each third building a captain's set, and on either side a lieutenant's set; each of these consists of a main building, 48 by 21 feet, containing two rooms, each 15 by 18 feet and 14 feet high, with a hall between, 12 by 18 feet; in addition, the commanding officer's has a wing, 41 by 21 feet, containing two rooms, each 15 by 15 feet; in all four rooms. The captain's set have each a wing, 21 by 18 feet, containing one room, 15 by 15 feet. To three sets, additional rooms of adobe have been added at the cost of the occupants. Four sets are built of native limestone from a quarry in the vicinity; the rest are of adobe. All have shingle roofs, and are warmed by open fire-places. East of, and in a line parallel with, the officers' quarters, with a parade of 500 feet in width intervening, are located the barracks, two separate buildings, distant from each other 30 feet, built of adobe, plastered inside and out and ceiled, a wide covered porch extending entirely around. Each barrack is 186 feet long and 27 feet wide, and contains two dormitories, separated by a passage-way, 27 by 12 feet, which leads to a building, 86 by 27 feet, containing the mess-room, 50 by 24 feet, the kitchen, 20 by 24 feet, and store-room, 10 by 24 feet. Each dormitory is 24 by 82 feet and 12 feet high, containing 23,760 cubic feet of air-space. They are warmed by open fire-places, and ventilated by large windows, four in the opposite sides of each room, and by a large ventilator in the ceiling, 20 by 4 feet. The men sleep upon iron bedsteads, having wooden slats. Five large and commodious sinks are placed 200 feet in rear of the quarters, and are kept well disinfected.

On the north side of the parade, midway between the barracks and officers' quarters, are the executive offices, three rooms, each 15 by 18 feet. On the south side of the parade, and opposite the executive offices, is the guard-house, built of limestone, 54 by 22 feet, and containing the guard-room, 13 by 15 feet and 11 feet high, three cells, each 4½ by 9 feet, and the prisoners' room, 15 by 16 feet. The cells are between the prisoners' room and the guard-room, and a passage, 6 feet wide, by the cells, communicates with these two rooms. It is warmed by an open fire-place, and ventilated by holes, 12 by 3 inches, in the upper part of the walls, and a large ventilator in the ceiling. In the rear of the barracks, at a distance of about 700 feet, are the quartermaster's and company stables and corrals. The former occupies a space 367 by 300 feet, inclosed by walls built of adobe, 10 feet high. Along two of these walls are the stables, well roofed, but otherwise open, the climate being such that additional shelter for the stock is not required. Separated from this, 70 feet, are the company stables, inclosing a space 350 by 450 feet, constructed like those just described, with stalls on all sides, capable of accommodating 400 horses.

The quartermaster's and commissary store-houses are located respectively north and south of the corrals, 100 feet distant. They are each 110 feet long by 27 feet wide, constructed of adobe and not ceiled.

The post-bakery is situated south of the commissary's store-house, and consists of one room, 40 by 16 feet, and one oven, with a capacity of 600 loaves.

Work was commenced on a new hospital in October, 1874. It is to be of adobe, with stone corners and tinned roof, on a stone foundation; the plan being that given for a provisionary hospital in Circular No. 3, Surgeon-General's Office, 1870.

The hospital now in use is a temporary adobe building, 50 by 19 feet, and contains one ward, 35 by 17 feet, with a capacity of fourteen beds, and the dispensary, 13 by 15 feet. It is plastered inside and whitewashed, well lighted and ventilated by numerous small holes in the lower and upper part of the walls. There is an L addition containing the dining-room, 8 by 10 feet, and the kitchen, 12 by 16 feet.

The post is supplied with water distributed by means of a water-wagon from the Limpia Creek, a small stream running through Limpia cañon and the northern part of the reservation. It is always clear, pure, and cool, not very hard, containing carbonate of lime and a small amount of organic matter, during the season of heavy rains, which is probably washed from the mountain at the foot of which it runs. Observation and experience show that it does not affect those using it in any manner, and no means of purification have been resorted to. There is also a large spring within the limits of the post, the water from which is harder than that from the Limpia. This water, it appears, was once, for some reasons unknown, condemned as unfit for potable purposes. It does not contain either organic or alkaline matter sufficient to render it unhealthy; and if it did, the cause was probably neglect during the long time the post was unoccupied. For extinguishing fire, a sufficient number of barrels and buckets are kept constantly filled with water, and placed at proper and convenient places.

The general conformation of the ground, gradually sloping from the post, is such that but little artificial drainage is necessary. Slops and refuse are collected in barrels, and emptied some distance from the post.

The married soldiers and laundresses occupy small adobe buildings scattered about the post.

On the south side of the parade is the guard-house, built of limestone, 66 by 22 feet, containing the guard-room, 13 by 15 feet and 11 feet high, three cells, each 4½ by 9 feet, and two prison-rooms. A passage, 6 feet wide, separates the cells from the guard-room. The guard-room is warmed by a stove, and ventilated by two windows and one door; the cells are ventilated by holes, 12 by 3 inches, in the upper part of the walls and openings in each door. One prison-room is ventilated by a large roof-ventilator and holes in the walls; the other by the door and holes in the walls above and below.

*Meteorological report, Fort Davis, Tex., 1870–'74.*

| Month. | 1870–'71. Temperature. | | | 1870–'71. Rain-fall in inches. | 1871–'72. Temperature. | | | 1871–'72. Rain-fall in inches. | 1872–'73. Temperature. | | | 1872–'73. Rain-fall in inches. | 1873–'74. Temperature. | | | 1873–'74. Rain-fall in inches. |
|---|---|---|---|---|---|---|---|---|---|---|---|---|---|---|---|---|
| | Mean. | Max. | Min. | | Mean. | Max. | Min. | | Mean. | Max. | Min. | | Mean. | Max. | Min. | |
| | ° | ° | ° | | ° | ° | ° | | ° | ° | ° | | ° | ° | ° | |
| July | 73.54 | 93 | 60 | ......... | ..... | ..... | ..... | ......... | 73.47 | 95* | 56* | 4.35 | ..... | ..... | ..... | ......... |
| August | 70.73 | 89 | 49 | 6.33 | ..... | ..... | ..... | ......... | 74.39 | 98* | 53* | 2.80 | 72.95 | 98* | 45* | 3.12 |
| September | 69.28 | 93* | 52 | 5.12 | ..... | ..... | ..... | ......... | 72.68 | 96* | 43* | 0.20 | 71.46 | 94 | 30* | 0.45 |
| October | 61.10 | 85* | 38 | 0.00 | ..... | ..... | ..... | ......... | 60.12 | 89* | 31* | 1.00 | 63.19 | 87 | 26* | 1.80 |
| November | 55.14 | 85* | 24 | 0.00 | ..... | ..... | ..... | ......... | 47.29 | 78* | 10* | 0.24 | ..... | ..... | ..... | ......... |
| December | 45.34 | 76* | 15 | ......... | ..... | ..... | ..... | ......... | 48.06 | 79* | 18* | 1.86 | 47.31 | 70 | 10* | 0.00 |
| January | 43.49 | 81* | 14 | ......... | ..... | ..... | ..... | ......... | 45.33 | 74 | —15* | 1.12 | ..... | ..... | ..... | ......... |
| February | 50.40 | 83* | 23 | 0.00 | ..... | ..... | ..... | ......... | 53.77 | 76 | 21* | 0.00 | ..... | ..... | ..... | ......... |
| March | 52.11 | 87* | 22 | ......... | ..... | ..... | ..... | ......... | 58.45 | 87* | 28* | 0.22 | ..... | ..... | ..... | ......... |
| April | 65.14 | 92* | 40 | 0.00 | ..... | ..... | ..... | ......... | 61.81 | 89* | — 2* | 0.00 | ..... | ..... | ..... | ......... |
| May | 75.35 | 94* | 45 | ......... | ..... | ..... | ..... | ......... | 72.82 | 96* | 38* | 0.76 | ..... | ..... | ..... | ......... |
| June | 76.63 | 106* | 59 | ......... | 76.94 | 98* | 54* | 1.71 | 73.87 | 107* | 45* | 6.82 | ..... | ..... | ..... | ......... |
| For the year | 61.52 | 106* | 14 | ......... | ..... | ..... | ..... | ......... | 61.84 | 107* | —15* | 19.37 | ..... | ..... | ..... | ......... |

*These observations are made with self-registering thermometers. The mean is from the standard thermometer.

*Consolidated sick-report, (white,) Fort Davis, Tex., 1870–'74.*

| Year | 1870–'71. | | 1871–'72. | | 1872–'73. | | 1873–'74. | |
|---|---|---|---|---|---|---|---|---|
| Mean strength { Officers | 13 | | 10 | | 13 | | 12 | |
| { Enlisted men | ..... | | ..... | | ..... | | 1* | |
| Diseases. | Cases. | Deaths. | Cases. | Deaths. | Cases. | Deaths. | Cases. | Deaths. |
| GENERAL DISEASES, A. | | | | | | | | |
| Remittent fever | 3 | ...... | 3 | ...... | 2 | ...... | ...... | ...... |
| Intermittent fever | 1 | ...... | ...... | ...... | ...... | ...... | ...... | ...... |
| Other diseases of this group | ...... | ...... | ...... | ...... | 3 | ...... | ...... | ...... |
| GENERAL DISEASES, B. | | | | | | | | |
| Rheumatism | ...... | ...... | ...... | ...... | ...... | ...... | 3 | ...... |
| LOCAL DISEASES. | | | | | | | | |
| Catarrh and bronchitis | 4 | ...... | 1 | ...... | 2 | ...... | 3 | ...... |
| Pleurisy | 1 | ...... | ...... | ...... | ...... | ...... | ...... | ...... |
| Diarrhœa and dysentery | 3 | ...... | 5 | ...... | 1 | ...... | ...... | ...... |
| Other local diseases | 5 | ...... | 4 | ...... | 5 | ...... | 4 | ...... |
| Alcoholism | ...... | ...... | ...... | ...... | 1 | ...... | ...... | ...... |
| Total disease | 17 | ...... | 13 | ...... | 14 | ...... | 10 | ...... |
| VIOLENT DISEASES AND DEATHS. | | | | | | | | |
| Accidents and injuries | 2 | ...... | ...... | ...... | 1 | ...... | ...... | ...... |
| Total violence | 2 | ...... | ...... | ...... | 1 | ...... | ...... | ...... |

* Two months only.

*Consolidated sick-report, (colored,) Fort Davis, Tex., 1870–'74.*

| Year | 1870–'71. | | 1871–'72. | | 1872–'73. | | 1873–'74. | |
|---|---|---|---|---|---|---|---|---|
| Mean strength..............Enlisted men...... | 316 | | 145 | | 216 | | 204 | |
| Diseases. | Cases. | Deaths. | Cases. | Deaths. | Cases. | Deaths. | Cases. | Deaths. |
| GENERAL DISEASES, A. | | | | | | | | |
| Remittent fever | 6 | | 3 | | 11 | | 2 | |
| Intermittent fever | 2 | | 4 | | 6 | | 9 | |
| Other diseases of this group | | | 5 | | 24 | | 19 | |
| GENERAL DISEASES, B. | | | | | | | | |
| Rheumatism | 9 | | 7 | | 24 | | 38 | |
| Syphilis | 7 | | 9 | | 2 | | | |
| Consumption | 1 | | | 1 | | 2 | 1 | |
| Other diseases of this group | 2 | | 2 | | 3 | | 5 | |
| LOCAL DISEASES. | | | | | | | | |
| Catarrh and bronchitis | 12 | | 24 | | 45 | | 33 | |
| Pneumonia | 1 | 1 | 2 | | | | | |
| Pleurisy | | | | | 20 | | 11 | |
| Diarrhœa and dysentery | 9 | | 13 | | 71 | 5 | 53 | |
| Hernia | 1 | | | | 2 | | | |
| Gonorrhœa | | | 4 | | 4 | | 9 | |
| Other local diseases | 25 | | 15 | | 44 | | 114 | |
| Total disease | 75 | 1 | 88 | 1 | 256 | 7 | 294 | |
| VIOLENT DISEASES AND DEATHS. | | | | | | | | |
| Gun-shot wounds | 3 | | 6 | 1 | 5 | | 3 | |
| Other accidents and injuries | 21 | | 22 | | 62 | 1 | 44 | |
| Homicides | | 2 | | | | | | |
| Total violence | 24 | 2 | 28 | 1 | 67 | 1 | 47 | |

# FORT DUNCAN, TEXAS.

### REPORT BY ASSISTANT SURGEON W. R. STEINMETZ, UNITED STATES ARMY.

Fort Duncan, Tex., is situated in Maverick County, on the east bank of the Rio Grande River, about 650 miles from its mouth; latitude, 28° 50' north; longitude, 23° 30' west. The location is on a tract of land of about 5,000 acres, for which the Government pays $130 per month. The lease expires January 1, 1876. About a mile east of the post is a range of hills, with spurs projecting toward the river. This post was first occupied in 1849 by Companies A and F, First Infantry, under command of Captain Scott, First Infantry, brevet major United States Army. Coming from Austin, Tex., the command first encamped at Paquache, on the river, thirty miles below this post. After exploration the companies marched here, and, arriving on March 26, 1849, pitched their tents where now stand the barracks of Companies D, Twenty-fourth, and A, Twenty-fifth Infantry. During the year 1850 preparations were made to build a permanent post. The first buildings erected were the commissary store-house and hospital, then the commanding officer's quarters, which is now the last house on the western end of the officers' line. The next in order were two barracks, one on the northeast and the other on the southwest of the parade-ground. On a line with the one on the northeast was built the bake-house; the latter is still in use, while the first-mentioned barrack has been destroyed. Other buildings were subsequently erected, but in what order is not known.

In 1851 the post was made the headquarters of the First Infantry, Colonel Morris commanding. In 1861 the post was abandoned, and in 1868 it was again occupied by the United States, when the buildings were found much injured, the doors, windows, and all portable property having been carried off or destroyed.

The soil consists mainly of fine sand or sandy loam. The consequence is that the appearance of the surface is constantly changing.

During the dry seasons these alterations are produced by the often-prevailing high winds, which raise portions of the loose soil in the form of thick clouds of dust; during the rainy season they are still more apparent and sudden, by means of currents of water, which take up large

26 M P

portions of earth and deposit them in the bottom-lands near the Rio Grande, or carry them along into the stream. From this cause quite a number of large and deep ravines, or arroyos, have been produced in the immediate vicinity, some of which, if allowed to extend much farther, bid fair to endanger the foundations of some of the buildings of the post.

The surface of the mountainous ridge running east from the post is thickly covered with sand and lime stones, while a peculiar kind of soft and exceedingly porous sandstone is found in the bed of the river and on its right or Mexican bank.

Both the hard and soft stones are admirably adapted for building-purposes, but especially is this the case with the latter variety, from the fact that it is light and can be cut into any required shape.

Within a few miles of the post, outcrops, and even extensive layers, of bituminous coal exist, which, however, appears to be of inferior quality, being strongly impregnated with iron-ore and sulphur. Here, as throughout the entire State, flourishes the everlasting thorny mesquite tree; also the cottonwood, pecan, wild plum, and mulberry, while only occasionally the traveler has an opportunity to find shelter beneath the foliage of the live-oak. Several species of the cactus in immense quantities grow in and around the post.

The country is abundantly supplied with game. Herds of deer and antelopes can be found within a comparatively short distance from the post; the rabbit, the coyote, as also the large gray wolf, are met with almost anywhere on the prairie, while the mountainous regions are inhabited by the black bear, Mexican lion, leopard, panther, wild-cat, &c. Deserving a prominent place here among the mammalia is the bat, which on account of its excessive numbers at this post becomes a great nuisance.

The feathered tribe is represented by the Mexican eagle, hawk, buzzard, crow, crane, chaparral cock, wild-turkey, goose and duck, quail, plover, scissor-tail, mocking-bird, redbird, blackbird, thrush, and swallow; the latter are in large numbers, and in the spring and summer frequently become a source of annoyance by building their nests under the roof of the porches of the officers' quarters and hospital. Rattlesnakes, king-snakes, and rattlesnake-pilots abound among the rocks, long grasses, and weeds, while the tarantula can be seen early every morning to crawl from its hole in search of its prey; and almost every building is the abode of small scorpions and enormous centi pedes.

The river contains only a small variety of fish, among which are the cat, buffalo, perch, gar, and sun-fish; these are, however, in great abundance.

After heavy rains, during the months of May and June, a peculiar red bug is seen crawling over the parade-ground; it is about the size of a pea, has eight legs, and is of a beautiful scarlet color.

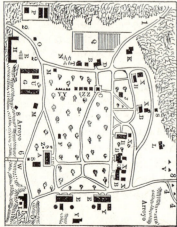

Figure 32.

Figure 32 shows arrangement of the post: A, hospital; B, officers' quarters; C, adjutant's office; D, quartermaster's department and acting commissary of subsistence; E, barracks; F, library; G, cavalry stables; H, quartermaster's corral; I, post-trader; J, magazine; K, blacksmith-shop; L, ordnance-sergeant's quarters; M, guard-house; N, artillery; O, scales; P, hay-yard; Q, wood-yard; R, wagon-stand; S, sinks; T, bakery; U, forage; V, laundresses' quarters; W, bridge over arroyo; X, officers' kitchens; Y, barrack kitchens; Z, thermometer house; YY, band quarters; ZZ, non-commissioned staff quarters; 1, road to Laredo; 2, road to Fort Clark and San Antonio; 3, road to Seminole Indian village; 4, road to Rio Grande; 5, road to Rio Grande; 6, road to Eagle Pass.

The barracks are two in number; one is built of stone, the other of adobes, each is 130 by 36 feet; occupied by four companies, giving only the following air-space per man: cavalry barracks, 463 cubic feet; infantry barracks, 542 cubic feet; they are warmed by fire-places and stoves, lighted by windows, and ventilated at the eaves. The non-commissioned staff and band of the Twenty-fourth Infantry, the headquarters of said regiment being temporarily at the post, occupy a line of tents on the northeast of the camp, parallel with the barracks.

There are two new stone kitchens, 48 by 18 feet, in rear of the barracks, each containing two apartments of unequal size, the larger of which is used as a mess-room; they have board floors and shingle roofs; a third kitchen is in process of erection. One of the cavalry companies uses as kitchen and mess-room a small stone building, with a shed attached, located in rear of the barracks. The laundresses occupy three lines of tents, which are framed and floored, and pitched in rear of the officers' quarters.

The officers' quarters are one-story houses, with shingle roofs, situated on two different lines, which form the south boundary of the parade-ground; these lines run respectively N. N. E. to S. S. W., and E. N. E. to W. S. W.; intersecting each other some four hundred feet east of the post, where they form an acute angle. Commencing on the east, the first building is of stone, 50 by 24 feet; contains three rooms; has a veranda on its north and east sides, and a stone kitchen detached.

The second set of quarters, located on the same line, and some two hundred and twenty feet from the first, is the residence of the commanding officer, consisting of two adobe buildings, containing four rooms, with a stone kitchen attached; the main house has a portico, 12 feet wide, on two sides. These quarters are of recent construction, the adobe buildings having been erected in 1871, while the stone kitchen was built about a year and a half ago. The next in order is situated on the second line, and is known as the "long house;" it faces east; is 80 by 18 feet; contains three rooms, and has a veranda on its north and east sides, and a stone kitchen in rear. The two remaining buildings are located on the same line with the one last described, but face north; both are of stone; the one nearest to and some 150 feet distant from the "long house," is 50 by 30 feet; it contains two rooms, besides a small addition on each end, built of adobes, and has a stone kitchen in rear. Seventy-five feet from it stands the last building, which finishes the officers line to the west; it is 64 by 23½ feet, and contains three comfortable rooms; it has a small addition, built of adobes, on its east end, and two stone kitchens in rear.

The two last-described buildings have verandas only on their north sides; with two exceptions the houses are raised from one to four feet from the ground.

The sinks are pits, except the one of the guard-house, which consists of a movable wooden box; this box is removed every morning, washed out and replaced, when its bottom is covered with dry earth.

The store-house is a large stone building, two stories high, 30 by 51 feet; the lower story which is altogether used for commissary and subsistence stores, has an addition, 23 by 18 feet, on its east side, and two entrances, one from the west and the other from the south; good ventilation, with a constant current of fresh air, is kept up by means of large grated openings in the walls. A large staircase in front gives access to the second story, which is divided into two rooms of unequal size; the larger affords storage for quartermaster's supplies, and camp and garrison equipage, while the smaller is used as an office by the post quartermaster and commissary. Between, and on a line with, the cavalry stables stands a small stone house, 48 by 27 feet, only one story high, which is used for storing corn and oats. The guard-house is a substantial stone building, 48 by 27 feet, with a stone floor and shingle roof. It is divided into three apartments, the center of which is used by the guard, while the two other rooms are the cells; the middle room has a fire-place; the two cells are not provided with any means of warming. Ventilation is effected by means of grated windows. Average occupancy during the last year was 12.

The magazine is a small stone building, 26 by 20 feet, situated between the first line of officers' quarters and the main road, about sixty feet from the latter. The only entrance, on its north side, is supplied with a double door; the outer door is made of good solid boards, while the inner consists of strong lattice-work. The object of this is, to give full access of the outer dry air to the interior, by leaving the outer door open, whenever the state of the atmosphere permits.

On a line with the bakery, and between it and the commissary store-house, is a new stone building, which was erected only a few months ago, as quarters of the commissary sergeant; its dimensions are 16½ by 24 feet. Quite remote from the rest of the houses, some three hundred and ninety feet in rear of the second line of officers' quarters, stands an old stone building, 20 by 30 feet, covered with a thatched roof; this has been assigned to the ordnance-sergeant as quarters.

Directly opposite the commissary store-house, and some sixty yards west of it, is located the adjutant's office. It is a small stone house, 18 feet 4 inches square, covered with a shingle roof, lighted by two windows, and warmed by a fire-place.

The post hospital stands on an elevated point northwest of the parade-ground, and consists of two substantial stone buildings, which apparently were intended to accommodate twelve patients; they are one story high, and covered by shingle roofs. The larger of the two buildings runs nearly due east and west, facing south; is 83 feet long by 29 feet wide; has a boarded ceiling, and is divided by two plastered walls into three apartments. The room in the east end of the house is 25 by 20 feet, and is subdivided by a boarded partition into two smaller rooms of unequal size, the dimensions of which are, respectively, 20 by 16 feet and 20 by 9 feet. The larger of the two is the dispensary and office, while the smaller is used as store-room. The apartment in the west end is of the same dimensions, and is also subdivided by a plastered partition in exactly the same manner as the former; the larger of its divisions is used as isolation or surgical ward, as circumstances may demand, while the smaller is used as additional store-room. Between these two rooms, in the center of the building, is the main ward, being 40 by 25 feet, by 12½ feet high, with a capacity of 12,500 cubic feet of air; its means of light and ventilation are four windows and a door on each side, several openings in the ceiling, and at each end of the room an open fire-place, which, however, on some days, smoke fearfully. Its air-space is barely sufficient for twelve beds, being only 1,042 cubic feet per man.

The whole building is surrounded by a portico, 14 feet wide, which within the last year has been repaired so far as the floor is concerned, while the roof over it is still in a bad condition, leaking very much, and should be re-shingled. The second building, located 21 feet from the former, and at a right angle with it, runs nearly north and south; it is 60 feet long by 20 feet wide, and contains three rooms; the first, on the north, is the kitchen; it is furnished with a cupboard, table, refrigerator, and chairs. The next is the mess-room; it has no fixtures, but is furnished with a table and chairs; this room and the kitchen are of equal dimensions, each being 18 feet 8 inches by 18 feet. The third and last is the steward's room, which is a new addition to the two rooms last described, and was erected, by joining it to the outer wall of the mess-room, as late as last spring, (1873.) The dimensions of this room are as follows: east side, 20 feet; west side, 19 feet 1 inch; north end, 20 feet; south end, 20 feet 10 inches; its southeast corner is seventeen inches nearer to the main building than the southwest corner. The consequence of these differences between the lengths of the opposite sides and ends of the room is, that it has three obtuse and one acute angles, which gives it an awkward shape.

The dispensary is supplied with the necessary shelving for the medicine-bottles, with a counter and a closet for storing instruments, liquor, and hospital-clothing; one of the store-rooms is provided with a closet for crockery, &c., while the other has only some rough shelving.

The thermometer-box stands on an open space, about one hundred feet east of the main building; it consists of a wooden box, 2 feet square by 2 feet high, nailed to a solid post 4½ feet from the ground; its sides are perforated by numerous augur-holes, while its bottom consists of lattice-work; it is also covered by what is called a hipped roof. The rain-gauge stands in an excavation made in the top of the same post, to which the box is nailed, at a height of 8½ feet from the ground.

The hospital sink is a stone building, 10 by 7½ feet, with a pit, situated in rear of the buildings; there are no bath or wash rooms, dead-house, lavatories, or urinals. The drainage of the hospital-grounds, as also of the entire camp, is natural and sufficient. There is no sewerage.

The means of extinguishing fire are fire and water buckets and four water-barrels, kept filled with water, and placed at convenient positions around the hospital. The bakery is a stone building, 23 by 35 feet, situated on the eastern boundary of the post; the oven is of sufficient capacity to bake three hundred loaves.

The stables, situated at the northeast corner of the post, are three in number, two for cavalry horses and one for the quartermaster's animals; the latter was totally demolished on the 23d of May, 1873, by a tornado which passed over this section of the country, and its re-erection has not yet been completed. One of the cavalry stables was also injured at the same time, but has since been repaired and is in use again.

The post library consists of about one hundred and seventy volumes of miscellaneous books, which are kept in two hospital tents situated on the parade-ground a short distance southeast of the hospital, and used as library and reading-room; the latter is open to the garrison from guard-mount until tattoo. Several daily and weekly papers are received. There are also two literary societies at the post, composed of members of the two cavalry companies.

The main water-supply is the Rio Grande River, from which water is hauled in a tank and distributed around the camp. The water is quite sweet and good in winter, but during the summer months becomes very muddy. It can be easily made clear by means of alum, sliced almonds, or other kernels containing hydrocyanic acid, which rapidly precipitate the impurities to the bottom of the barrels; there are also four cisterns, three in rear of the company barracks, and one on the officers' line. Owing to the comparatively great amount of rain which fell during the past year, (1873,) these cisterns have been well supplied with water.

The refuse matter is carted off some distance from the post, and deposited in a ravine, or along the Rio Grande, and all combustible matter burned.

There are no regular arrangements in regard to bathing, except for the prisoners, who are required to bathe in the river every Sunday morning when the weather permits.

Owing to the necessity of constant irrigation, it is very difficult to have a post garden; several attempts were made at different times to raise some vegetables in the bottom-land in rear of the barracks, without avail; the garrison is, however, well supplied with fresh vegetables and fruit brought from Mexico, and sold at reasonable prices.

Two mails per week are received from San Antonio, Tex., the nearest city of any size; from there nearly all supplies are received. It requires from two to three days for a mail to reach department headquarters, and from ten to twelve days to reach Washington, D. C.

The population of Eagle Pass, the adjoining town, amounts to about 1,500 inhabitants, consisting of Americans, Germans, and principally of Mexicans. Their chief occupation is mercantile business and stock-raising. The late epidemic of small-pox in the winter of 1872 and 1873 decimated the population of both Eagle Pass and the Mexican town which lies on the right bank of the river directly opposite the post, and called Piedras Negras, (Black Rock,) to such an extent that even the Mexicans were thereby frightened, who believe that variola is a disease which every one ought to have once in his life. Both towns were built since the establishment of the post of Fort Duncan.

Some three miles south of Piedras Negras is a small Mexican town, called Villa de Fuentes. It is situated on a beautiful little creek, about one and a half miles from the right bank of the Rio Grande. This creek furnishes the place all the year round with an ample supply of excellent fresh and sweet water, and the inhabitants make ready use of it for the purpose of irrigating their gardens. They are thereby enabled to raise quite a variety of vegetables, as cabbage, carrots, lettuce, turnips, sweet-potatoes, beets, corn, onions, and others which they bring to the camp and sell at reasonable prices. The general sanitary condition of the post, so far as climate and locality are concerned, is very good. In summer, bowel affections; in autumn, malarial fevers in one form or another; and during the winter months pulmonary complaints, come more especially to the notice of the medical officer. They are, however, rarely of a severe type, and as a general thing readily yield to proper medication. This climate has been found to be very favorable for the treatment of wounds and incipient phthisis, while it does not seem well adapted for far-advanced cases of pulmonary consumption. During the winter of 1872–'73, small-pox in a serious epidemic form raged in this vicinity; some few cases appeared also in the garrison, but by the prompt adoption of the necessary precautions, the epidemic was prevented from spreading among the troops.

*Meteorological report, Fort Duncan, Tex., 1873-'74.*

| Year. | 1870-'71. | | | | 1871-'72. | | | | 1872-'73. | | | | 1873-'74. | | | |
|---|---|---|---|---|---|---|---|---|---|---|---|---|---|---|---|---|
| | Temperature. | | | Rain-fall in inches. | Temperature. | | | Rain-fall in inches. | Temperature. | | | Rain-fall in inches. | Temperature. | | | Rain-fall in inches. |
| | Mean. | Max. | Min. | | Mean. | Max. | Min. | | Mean. | Max. | Min. | | Mean. | Max. | Min. | |
| | ° | ° | ° | | ° | ° | ° | | ° | ° | ° | | ° | ° | ° | |
| July | | | | | | | | | | | | | 84, 73 | 105 | 70 | 2. 84 |
| August | | | | | | | | | | | | | 84. 43 | 100 | 71 | 4. 05 |
| September | | | | | | | | | | | | | 79. 16 | 97 | 60 | 4. 10 |
| October | | | | | | | | | | | | | 70. 91 | 94 | 44 | 0. 44 |
| November | | | | | | | | | | | | | 57. 55 | 92 | 33 | 1. 40 |
| December | | | | | | | | | | | | | 54. 31 | 82 | 30 | 1. 00 |
| January | | | | | | | | | | | | | 51. 53 | 82 | 23 | 0. 30 |
| February | | | | | | | | | | | | | 60. 01 | 83 | 36 | 0. 20 |
| March | | | | | | | | | | | | | 67. 33 | 96 | 43 | 4. 00 |
| April | | | | | | | | | | | | | 69. 31 | 94 | 51 | 0. 00 |
| May | | | | | | | | | | | | | 79. 39 | 101 | 62 | 1. 50 |
| June | | | | | | | | | 81. 39 | 106 | 68 | 6. 61 | 84. 59 | 100 | 72 | 0. 68 |
| For the year | | | | | | | | | | | | | 70. 27 | 105 | 23 | 20. 51 |

*Consolidated sick report, (white,) Fort Duncan, Tex., 1871-'74.*

| Year | | 1870-'71. | | 1871-'72. | | 1872-'73.* | | 1873-'74. | |
|---|---|---|---|---|---|---|---|---|---|
| Mean strength { Officers | | 12† | | 12† | | 8 | | 8 | |
| { Enlisted men | | | | | | 52 | | 60 | |
| Diseases. | | Cases. | Deaths. | Cases. | Deaths. | Cases. | Deaths. | Cases. | Deaths. |
| GENERAL DISEASES, A. | | | | | | | | | |
| Remittent fever | | | | | | | | 4 | |
| Intermittent fever | | | | | | 5 | | 11 | |
| Other diseases of this group | | | | | | | | 4 | |
| GENERAL DISEASES, B. | | | | | | | | | |
| Rheumatism | | | | | | 1 | | 8 | |
| Syphilis | | | | | | 3 | | 6 | |
| Other diseases of this group | | | | | | 1 | | 2 | |
| LOCAL DISEASES. | | | | | | | | | |
| Catarrh and bronchitis | | | | | | 2 | | 14 | |
| Pneumonia | | | | | | 2 | | 1 | |
| Pleurisy | | | | | | | | 1 | |
| Diarrhœa and dysentery | | | | | | 5 | | 22 | 1 |
| Hernia | | | | | | 1 | | 2 | |
| Gonorrhœa | | | | | | 1 | | 2 | |
| Other local diseases | | | | 3 | | 12 | 1 | 36 | |
| Alcoholism | | | | | | | | 2 | |
| Total disease | | | | 3 | | 33 | 1 | 115 | 1 |
| VIOLENT DISEASES AND DEATHS. | | | | | | | | | |
| Gunshot wounds | | | | 1 | | 1 | | 2 | |
| Other accidents and injuries | | | | | | 5 | | 31 | 1 |
| Total violence | | | | 1 | | 6 | | 33 | 1 |

　　* Three months only.　　　　　　　　　† Officers of colored troops only.

*Consolidated sick report, (colored,) Fort Duncan, Tex., 1870-'74.*

| Year | | 1870-'71. | | 1871-'72. | | 1872-'73. | | 1873-'74. | |
|---|---|---|---|---|---|---|---|---|---|
| Mean strength Enlisted men | | 199 | | 206 | | 154 | | 113 | |
| Diseases. | | Cases. | Deaths. | Cases. | Deaths. | Cases. | Deaths. | Cases. | Deaths. |
| GENERAL DISEASES, A. | | | | | | | | | |
| Small-pox and varioloid | | | | | | 8 | 2 | | |
| Typho-malarial fever | | | | 3 | | | | | |
| Remittent fever | | 12 | | 39 | | 10 | | 4 | |
| Intermittent fever | | 17 | | 25 | | 29 | | 11 | |
| Other diseases of this group | | 1 | | 12 | | 58 | | 5 | |

*Consolidated sick-report, (colored,) Fort Duncan, Tex., 1870–'74—Continued.*

| Year | 1870–'71. | | 1871–'72. | | 1872–'73. | | 1873–'74. | |
|---|---|---|---|---|---|---|---|---|
| Mean strength ...............Enlisted men...... | 199 | | 206 | | 154 | | 113 | |
| Diseases. | Cases. | Deaths. | Cases. | Deaths. | Cases. | Deaths. | Cases. | Deaths. |
| GENERAL DISEASES, B. | | | | | | | | |
| Rheumatism | 19 | ...... | 14 | ...... | 17 | ...... | 26 | ...... |
| Syphilis | 18 | ...... | 17 | ...... | 8 | ...... | 5 | ...... |
| Consumption | | | | 1 | | | | |
| Other diseases of this group | 1 | ...... | 2 | ...... | 4 | ...... | | |
| LOCAL DISEASES. | | | | | | | | |
| Catarrh and bronchitis | 12 | ...... | 33 | ...... | 31 | ...... | 25 | ...... |
| Pneumonia | 4 | ...... | 5 | 1 | 8 | 1 | 4 | 1 |
| Pleurisy | 7 | ...... | 3 | ...... | | | | |
| Diarrhœa and dysentery | 53 | ...... | 75 | ...... | 49 | ...... | 18 | ...... |
| Hernia | | | | | | | 1 | |
| Gonorrhœa | 30 | ...... | 8 | ...... | 3 | ...... | 4 | ...... |
| Other local diseases | 89 | ...... | 92 | 1 | 96 | 1 | 59 | ...... |
| Alcoholism | ...... | ...... | 1 | ...... | 1 | ...... | 2 | ...... |
| Unclassified | ...... | ...... | 1 | ...... | | | | |
| Total disease | 263 | ...... | 330 | 3 | 322 | 4 | 164 | 1 |
| VIOLENT DISEASES AND DEATHS. | | | | | | | | |
| Gunshot wounds | 2 | 1 | 2 | ...... | 1 | ...... | | |
| Drowning | | | | | | | | 1 |
| Other accidents and injuries | 19 | ...... | 51 | ...... | 62 | ...... | 54 | ...... |
| Homicide | | | | | | 1 | | |
| Total violence | 21 | 1 | 53 | ...... | 63 | 1 | 54 | 1 |

# FORT GRIFFIN, TEXAS.

INFORMATION FURNISHED BY ASSISTANT SURGEONS HENRY M'ELDERRY AND WILLIAM E. STEINMETZ, UNITED STATES ARMY.

Fort Griffin is situated in latitude 32° 51' north, longitude 21° 57' west, about half a mile from the west bank of the Clear Fork of the Brazos River, and fifteen miles from the main stream. The ground rises from the bank of the Clear Fork in a succession of terraces, some of which, in a distance of four miles, attain a considerable height. The fort is located upon the first prominent line of terraces, on a plateau of about a mile square and 100 feet above the water of the fork.

The vegetable kingdom is poorly represented in the vicinity of the post. Of trees, there are found the post and live oak, the ash, mesquite, pecan, and cottonwood. There are also several species of the cactus.

The wild animals found in this vicinity are the cougar, or Texas wild cat, the gray and white wolf, coyote, black wolf, gray and red fox, skunk, raccoon, black bear, opossum, gray and fox squirrel, prairie dog, mule rabbit, American buffalo, antelope, deer, and peccary or Mexican hog.

The birds are the eagle, (bald and Mexican,) wild turkey, goose, duck, buzzard, owl, scissor-tail, Arkansas fly-catcher, common robbin, bluebird, mocking-bird, red-winged blackbird, common crow, quail, white crane, sandhill crane, plover, and snipe.

Rattlesnakes, (common and prairie,) copperheads, and meadow snakes, the horned toad, striped and green lizards, snapping and common box turtle, centipedes, and tarantulas are found.

The fish are the bass, cat, gar, perch, and buffalo.

The post was established July 31, 1867. Quarters were extemporized from such materials as the country afforded, and have never been replaced by permanent or suitable buildings, although the garrison consists at present of five companies. A log house, consisting of two rooms with a hall between, was hauled from a deserted ranch for the quarters of the commanding officer, and a similar building was brought in for the hospital. Small temporary houses were built for the men. A line of officers' quarters was put up, consisting of a room and a kitchen each. These buildings have suffered the natural deterioration incident to an occupancy of seven years, and now afford insufficient protection to the inmates. The enlisted men occupy the small houses above mentioned, except one company quartered in a picket-house. All these quarters are full of cracks, admitting dust, rain, and snow. They are furnished with substantial iron bunks of excellent pattern, are warmed by open fire-places, and have an average air-space of 264 feet per man.

The married soldiers are quartered in small frame huts, picket-houses, wall and common tents, or a combination of the four.

About 35 yards from the southwest end of each row of company quarters are the kitchens and mess-rooms—rough frame buildings, of the following dimensions: kitchen, 20 by 20 feet; mess-room, 20 by 60 feet.

The sinks for the companies are three in number, situated about 150 yards distant from the quarters, and are supplied with movable boxes, perforated in the bottom to allow the fluid portion to drain away; the solid portion retained in the boxes is removed by the prisoners every morning after reveille. The boxes, after being washed and disinfected, are replaced.

The guard-house is an old frame building, 14 by 32 feet, and poorly adapted to its purpose. It is divided into two apartments, one for the guard, the other for prisoners; it is ventilated at the ridge, and by means of one grated window on its front side. The prison-room is heated by a stove, the guard-room by an open fire-place. A small house, 9 by 14 feet, 12 feet from the guard-house, is used by the non-commissioned officers of the guard. The average occupancy during last year, when there were five companies at the post, was seventeen.

The post hospital stands on one of the prominent bluffs forming the plateau of the fort. It consists of four distinct buildings; the first is a dilapidated log building, which, shortly after the establishment of the post, was hauled in from an old, deserted ranch. It contains the steward's room, dispensary, and a store-room. This building is covered with a dirt roof, is very much dilapidated, leans considerably to one side, and leaks badly. In its present condition, the old store-room is unsuited for any purpose except storing such articles as will not be damaged by the rain and dirt which is continually falling off the walls and roof. The second building is a frame one, joined to the first at a right angle; is 12 by 34 feet, and is divided into apartments of unequal size, the larger of which, the one adjoining the dispensary, with which it is connected by a door, is 14 by 24 feet, and is used for the mess-room. The smaller, being 10 by 14 feet, is used as a kitchen. The third building stands on the opposite (northwest) side of and 6 feet from the log building, at right angles with it. It is an old frame house, formerly used as the adjutant's office, and is divided into two rooms; the smaller, at the southeast end, is the office of the surgeon in charge; the other, the store-room, is provided with shelves for the medicines, and a closet, in which are kept the poisons and most expensive drugs. On a line with, and 10 feet from the log building, stands the pavilion ward, erected of lumber, raised 18 inches above the ground, on stone supports; it is 44 by 20 by 12 feet, has four windows on each side, and a door at each end; at the northeast end two small rooms are partitioned off, one the wardmaster's, and the other the wash and bath room. The ward proper is 20 by 33 feet, is heated by two sheet-iron stoves, and ventilated by two shafts, through which pass the stove-pipes. This building is plastered, but not ceiled; it has a shingle roof. The capacity of the ward is 7,920 cubic feet of air-space; it contains twelve beds, giving an air-space of 660 cubic feet to each man. In order to secure an upward current of air, several small holes are made in the floor under the stove. The crevices between the boards of the floor, at the ends of the building, and between the shingles of the roof, furnish a sufficient amount of ventilation. The privy for the hospital is placed 60 feet from the ward, and is provided with two sets of movable boxes lined with zinc, placed one within the other. The smaller boxes are perforated in the bottom; through these orifices the fluid excretum passes into the bottom box, leaving the solid portion in the top. These boxes are emptied every morning immediately after reveille, by the prisoners, thoroughly cleaned and disinfected.

The dead-house is a small frame building, 14 by 14 feet, situated on the side of the hill, about 300 yards from the ward; it has a large window on each side, and is ventilated at the eaves; it is furnished with a good post-mortem table. This building and the ward are the best buildings belonging to the hospital. An attempt was made to dig a cellar, but had to be abandoned, as the ground was too rocky. An application for the erection of a new hospital at this post has been disapproved for the reason that it is probable that the post will soon be removed.

The principal water-supply is from Collins's Creek, a small stream emptying into Clear Fork; it is hauled to the post in a wagon built for that purpose. During the winter the water can be used for almost any purpose, but during the summer it has a bad taste, and is unfit for drinking. During the hot weather a cart is sent to the spring on the bank of the Clear Fork, which furnishes a supply of water sufficient for drinking purposes. Behind each set of quarters are several water-barrels which are filled every morning. There is no cistern or reservoir at the post. The only means of extinguishing fire are the water-barrels and the water-wagon, which is kept over night filled with water. For immediate use in the hospital a dozen fire-buckets are kept constantly filled with water. Owing to the circumstance that the plateau on which the fort stands has an inclination on all sides, the natural drainage is sufficient to relieve the ground of all surplus water. There are no artificial drains.

The offal, slops, and excreta of the post, as also all the refuse matter of the stables, are carted away every day by the prisoners, and taken to the flat to the west, and about half a mile from the camp.

There are no arrangements or regulations in regard to bathing. During the summer the men bathe in Collins's Creek and Clear Fork.

There are no gardens at the post, owing to the great difficulty in raising vegetables in this locality, during the dry season, it being necessary to keep up constant irrigation.

The only means of communication with any town are Government trains.

*Meteorological report, Fort Griffin, Tex., 1870–'74.*

| Month. | 1870–'71. | | | | 1871–'72. | | | | 1872–'73. | | | | 1873–'74. | | | |
|---|---|---|---|---|---|---|---|---|---|---|---|---|---|---|---|---|
| | Temperature. | | | Rain-fall in inches. | Temperature. | | | Rain-fall in inches. | Temperature. | | | Rain-fall in inches. | Temperature. | | | Rain-fall in inches. |
| | Mean. | Max. | Min. | | Mean. | Max. | Min. | | Mean. | Max. | Min. | | Mean. | Max. | Min. | |
| | ° | ° | ° | | ° | ° | ° | | ° | ′ ° | ° | | ° | ° | ° | |
| July | 82.89 | 98 | 62 | 7.50 | 89.71 | 105 | 64* | 0.36 | 83.35 | 102* | 61* | 3.87 | 85.45 | 106* | 48* | 0.63 |
| August | 81.74 | 99 | 52* | 4.40 | 87.21 | 108 | 55* | 0.45 | 84.01 | 103* | 59* | 0.74 | 83.87 | 104* | 50* | 0.44 |
| September | 76.27 | 98 | 50* | 5.05 | 76.56 | 98 | 44* | 0.15 | 77.98 | 101* | 46* | 1.81 | 77.23 | 100* | 38* | 1.64 |
| October | 65.82 | 90 | 40* | 3.75 | 64.52 | 96 | 29* | 5.05 | 63.77 | 93* | 30* | 0.58 | 65.07 | 96* | 16* | 0.28 |
| November | 58.03 | 88 | 22* | 0.90 | 51.96 | 86 | 9* | 1.00 | 46.53 | 83* | 11* | 0.80 | 54.58 | 86* | 11* | 0.56 |
| December | 37.10 | 76 | − 7* | 3.35 | 43.07 | 82 | 7* | 0.00 | 37.08 | 78* | − 1* | 1.32 | 45.62 | 76* | 9* | 0.91 |
| January | 41.90 | 76 | 10* | 0.65 | 37.64 | 66 | 5* | 2.21 | 38.81 | 76* | − 4* | 0.26 | 42.85 | 80* | 15 | 1.30 |
| February | 50.01 | 86 | 20* | 1.30 | 47.19 | 80 | 12* | 1.00 | 46.30 | 79* | 10* | 0.79 | 45.51 | 76* | 20 | 1.82 |
| March | 58.57 | 92 | 30* | 1.43 | 53.35 | 90* | 24* | 0.20 | 57.36 | 92* | 14* | 0.08 | 56.09 | 85* | 30 | 0.90 |
| April | 64.90 | 100 | 38* | 0.55 | 64.88 | 93* | 31* | 2.60 | 62.92 | 97* | 27* | 0.63 | 58.17 | 90* | 32 | 1.09 |
| May | 68.99 | 98 | 42* | 5.50 | 73.90 | 96* | 39* | 3.30 | 72.71 | 98* | 39* | 2.57 | 75.04 | 99* | 51 | 2.46 |
| June | 81.28 | 105 | 57* | 0.00 | 81.79 | 102* | 57* | 2.15 | 80.13 | 104* | 55* | 3.24 | 81.64 | 100* | 60 | 1.80 |
| For the year | 63.96 | 105 | − 7* | 34.38 | 64.31 | 108 | 5* | 18.47 | 62.57 | 104* | − 4* | 16.69 | 64.26 | 106* | 9* | 13.83 |

* These observations are made with self-registering thermometers. The mean is from the standard thermometer.

*Consolidated sick-report, (white,) Fort Griffin, Tex., 1870–'74.*

| Year | | 1870–'71. | | 1871–'72. | | 1872–'73. | | 1873–'74. | |
|---|---|---|---|---|---|---|---|---|---|
| Mean strength { Officers | | 17 | | 15 | | 11 | | 11 | |
| { Enlisted men | | 330 | | 211 | | 205 | | 125 | |
| Diseases. | | Cases. | Deaths. | Cases. | Deaths. | Cases. | Deaths. | Cases. | Deaths. |
| GENERAL DISEASES, A. | | | | | | | | | |
| Cerebro-spinal fever | | 1 | | | | 1 | | | |
| Typhoid fever | | 1 | 1 | | | | | | |
| Remittent fever | | 15 | | 3 | | 7 | | 2 | |
| Intermittent fever | | 115 | | 55 | | 40 | | 21 | |
| Cholera | | | | | | | | | 1 |
| Other diseases of this group | | 24 | | | | 5 | | 4 | |

27 M P

*Consolidated sick-report, (white,) Fort Griffin, Tex., 1870–'74—Continued.*

| Year | 1870–'71. | | 1871–'72. | | 1872–'73. | | 1873–'74. | |
|---|---|---|---|---|---|---|---|---|
| Mean strength { Officers / Enlisted men } | 17 / 330 | | 15 / 211 | | 11 / 205 | | 11 / 125 | |
| Diseases. | Cases. | Deaths. | Cases. | Deaths. | Cases. | Deaths. | Cases. | Deaths. |
| GENERAL DISEASES, B. | | | | | | | | |
| Rheumatism | 29 | | 25 | | 26 | | 12 | |
| Syphilis | 20 | | 1 | | 4 | | 1 | |
| Consumption | | | 3 | 1 | 1 | | | |
| Other diseases of this group | | | 25 | | 1 | | | |
| LOCAL DISEASES. | | | | | | | | |
| Catarrh and bronchitis | 31 | | 32 | | 35 | | 22 | |
| Pneumonia | 1 | | 18 | | 8 | | 1 | 1 |
| Pleurisy | 5 | | 5 | | 5 | | | |
| Diarrhœa and dysentery | 183 | 2 | 90 | 2 | 82 | 1 | 57 | |
| Hernia | 1 | | 1 | | 1 | | | |
| Gonorrhœa | 8 | | 1 | | 7 | | | |
| Other local diseases | 190 | 2 | 176 | | 136 | 3 | 64 | |
| Alcoholism | 5 | | 2 | | 6 | | | |
| Unclassified | | | 2 | 1 | 1 | 1 | 11 | |
| Total disease | 628 | 5 | 439 | 5 | 365 | 5 | 195 | 2 |
| VIOLENT DISEASES AND DEATHS. | | | | | | | | |
| Gunshot wounds | 6 | | 5 | | 1 | 2 | 3 | |
| Drowning | | 1 | | | | | | |
| Other accidents and injuries | 146 | 2 | 70 | | 58 | 1 | 15 | |
| Homicide | | 1 | | 1 | | 3 | | |
| Total violence | 152 | 4 | 75 | 1 | 59 | 6 | 18 | |

*Consolidated sick-report, (colored,) Fort Griffin, Tex., 1870–'71.*

| Year | 1871–'72.* | | 1872–'73.† | | 1873–'74. | |
|---|---|---|---|---|---|---|
| Mean strength .... Enlisted men | 66 | | 22 | | 120 | |
| Diseases. | Cases. | Deaths. | Cases. | Deaths. | Cases. | Deaths. |
| GENERAL DISEASES, A. | | | | | | |
| Cerebro-spinal fever | | 1 | | | | |
| Typhoid fever | | | | 1 | | |
| Remittent fever | | | | | 2 | |
| Intermittent fever | 8 | | 2 | | 31 | |
| Other diseases of this group | 2 | | | | 35 | |
| GENERAL DISEASES, B. | | | | | | |
| Rheumatism | 5 | | 4 | | 10 | |
| Syphilis | 2 | | | | 6 | |
| Consumption | 1 | | | | 1 | |
| Other diseases of this group | 2 | | 1 | | | |
| LOCAL DISEASES. | | | | | | |
| Catarrh and bronchitis | 15 | | 5 | | 21 | |
| Pleurisy | 1 | | | | | |
| Diarrhœa and dysentery | 26 | | 7 | 1 | 41 | |
| Gonorrhœa | 7 | | 1 | | | |
| Other local diseases | 25 | | 16 | | 43 | |
| Alcoholism | | | | | 2 | |
| Total disease | 94 | 1 | 36 | 2 | 192 | |
| VIOLENT DISEASES AND DEATHS. | | | | | | |
| Gunshot wounds | 1 | | | | 6 | |
| Drowning | | | | | | 2 |
| Other accidents and injuries | 16 | | 3 | | 16 | 1 |
| Homicide | | | | 1 | | 1 |
| Total violence | 17 | | 3 | 1 | 22 | 3 |

\* 7 months only          10 months only.

# FORT McINTOSH, TEXAS.

REPORTED BY ACTING ASSISTANT SURGEON J. P. ARTHUR, UNITED STATES ARMY.

Fort McIntosh is located on the left bank of the Rio Grande, in latitude 27° 45′ north; longitude 22° 47′ west; 165 miles from San Antonio, and 242 miles from Austin, the nearest railroad station. It is three-fourths of a mile northwest of the old Spanish town of Laredo, in Texas. The post occupies a tract of 600 acres, partially surrounded by a bend of the river, and elevated 380 feet above the waters of the Gulf of Mexico.

The fort proper is a star-shaped earth-work, occupying an area of one acre upon a bluff some 50 feet above the waters of the Rio Grande. The post now occupied is distant about half a mile from the fort, being lower down the river, and about 400 yards from the bank. It is completely surrounded by chaparral or thickets of mesquite.

The elevated plain upon which the post and the town of Laredo stand, extends back about two miles from the river, where it is bounded by a range of low hills. In these hills granite and sandstone of good quality for building are obtained. A fair quality of lime is burned about ten miles above the post, and bituminous coal in small quantities is found in the banks of the river a few miles from the post. The soil is of a loose, sandy character, with a depth of from 15 to 30 feet, resting upon a basis of cretaceous limestone. In low places, receiving the washings of the hills, it is fertile, and produces corn, sweet-potatoes, melons, and garden vegetables in abundance.

In 1868 orders were received at the post for the construction of new buildings sufficient for two companies; but for some reason work was suspended after the completion of the hospital, guard-house, bakery, and quartermaster's store-house. The present garrison consists of one company, which is quartered in the store-house. This is built of sandstone and covered with shingles; is 60 by 25 feet, and 13 feet high, and is provided with ridge ventilation and attached kitchen and mess-room built of adobes. The men sleep in the single room of this building, on bunks of the new pattern of wood and iron combined. The air-space per bed is 406 feet. The heating is by stoves. Refuse is carried in a cart to the arroyos or small streams beyond the limits of the post.

The married soldiers and laundresses occupy tents, and the officers are quartered in spare rooms of the hospital building.

The hospital is substantially built of sandstone with shingle roof, 136 by 40 feet, one story high and 15 feet from floor to ceiling. There is a veranda the entire length front and rear. Halls extend through the building, dividing it into three sections, the first of which contains five rooms varying in size from 10 by 15 feet to 15 feet square; the second, four rooms 15 feet square, and the third is the ward, 40 by 25 feet. The dispensary and steward's room are at the end of the ward, and are each 11 by 8½ feet. The ward contains 12 beds, giving 1,250 cubic feet of air-space to each. The kitchen is a detached building of stone 20 by 15 feet. It stands in the rear of the hospital, and the intervening space is covered with an awning of canvas. Near the kitchen is a small detached bath-room. Eight of the smaller rooms in the hospital-building have open fire-places, and all have sufficient windows to insure ventilation. The ward is heated by stoves and furnished with ridge ventilation. The dry-earth closet is in use in the ward, as also a bath-tub placed behind a screen. The hospital sink is located 30 yards to the rear. The building, fixtures, and furniture are in good condition.

The guard-house is also of sandstone with shingle roof. It is 42 by 16½ feet, one story high, and contains a room for the guard, 16½ by 15 feet; a prison-room of the same dimensions, and four cells, 6 by 3 feet. The guard-room is warmed by an open fire-place. A fair degree of ventilation is obtained for both guard and prisoners by means of windows.

The post is supplied with water hauled from the Rio Grande. In summer and early autumn, owing to the heavy rains, the water is very muddy and has to stand several hours before it is at all fit to drink. A little alum stirred about in a barrel of this muddy water will precipitate the suspended matter and render it in a few minutes as clear as spring-water. A piece of the prickly-pear has the same effect.

There are no stage-coaches or other public means of conveyance. Heavy freight is carried in ox-carts, and officers and soldiers are furnished transportation on horseback or in Government wagons.

*Meteorological report, Fort McIntosh, Tex., 1870–'74.*

| Month. | 1870–'71. Temperature. Mean. | Max. | Min. | Rain-fall in inches. | 1871–'72. Temperature. Mean. | Max. | Min. | Rain-fall in inches. | 1872–'73. Temperature. Mean. | Max. | Min. | Rain-fall in inches. | 1873–'74. Temperature. Mean. | Max. | Min. | Rain-fall in inches. |
|---|---|---|---|---|---|---|---|---|---|---|---|---|---|---|---|---|
| July | 85.79 | 99 | 77 | ? | 91.96 | 108 | 75 | 0.00 | 89.19 | 101* | 76* | 0.00 | 86.91 | 100 | 75 | 1.25 |
| August | 83.75 | 94 | 77 | 2.76 | 88.91 | 109 | 76 | 3.20 | 87.38 | 101* | 74* | 2.22 | 87.13 | 98 | 79 | 2.81 |
| September | 84.61 | 94 | 70 | 1.24 | 83.55 | 96 | 58 | 4.50 | 85.35 | 99* | 67* | 0.34 | 82.91 | 96 | 69 | 3.54 |
| October | 76.61 | 86 | 55 | 0.00 | 72.74 | 85 | 47 | 0.00 | 76.32 | 98* | 49* | 0.40 | 73.44 | 91 | 53 | 0.71 |
| November | 67.24 | 87 | 32 | 0.00 | 58.30 | 86 | 35 | 0.00 | 62.26 | 96 | 30 | 1.37 | 67.39 | 79 | 52 | 0.42 |
| December | 49.06 | 81 | 19 | 0.00 | 53.36 | 74 | 33 | 0.00 | 56.62 | 93 | 31 | 3.75 | 65.44 | 82 | 50 | 1.42 |
| January | 50.63 | 79 | 27 | 0.00 | 46.38 | 70 | 26 | 0.00 | 58.49 | 85 | 22 | 0.03 | 60.91 | 79 | 42 | 0.08 |
| February | 61.32 | 80 | 39 | 0.00 | 53.42 | 87 | 30 | 1.65 | 68.53 | 100 | 43 | 0.10 | 66.31 | 86 | 52 | 0.21 |
| March | 67.17 | 90 | 46 | 0.00 | 67.12 | 91 | 37 | 0.56 | 72.93 | 98 | 47 | 0.64 | 73.02 | 89 | 57 | 0.81 |
| April | 73.84 | 105 | 37 | 0.00 | 79.77 | 108* | 55* | 1.30 | 79.77 | 100 | 54 | 1.25 | 73.87 | 93 | 55 | 0.08 |
| May | 82.83 | 110 | 57 | 1.40 | 84.47 | 105* | 56* | 1.78 | 82.89 | 109 | 65 | 0.25 | 80.59 | 94 | 62 | 1.50 |
| June | 89.17 | 106 | 75 | 0.80 | 86.25 | 101* | 70* | 5.00 | 86.31 | 99 | 75 | 6.32 | 89.28 | 99 | 76 | 4.16 |
| For the year | 72.67 | 110 | 19 | ...... | 72.18 | 109 | .26 | 17.99 | 75.50 | 109 | 22 | 16.67 | 75.60 | 100 | 42 | 16.99 |

\* These observations are made with self-registering thermometers. The mean is from the standard thermometer.

*Consolidated sick-report, (white,) Fort McIntosh, Tex., 1870–'74.*

| Year | 1870–'71. Cases. | Deaths. | 1871–'72.* Cases. | Deaths. | 1872–'73.† Cases. | Deaths. | 1873–'74. Cases. | Deaths. |
|---|---|---|---|---|---|---|---|---|
| Mean strength { Officers | 6 | | 3 | | 4 | | 2‡ | |
| { Enlisted men | 124 | | 40 | | 36 | | ...... | |
| **Diseases.** | | | | | | | | |
| GENERAL DISEASES, A. | | | | | | | | |
| Typhoid fever | ...... | ...... | 2 | 1 | 1 | ...... | ...... | ...... |
| Typho-malarial fever | ...... | ...... | ...... | 1 | ...... | ...... | ...... | ...... |
| Remittent fever | 1 | ...... | 1 | ...... | ...... | ...... | ...... | ...... |
| Intermittent fever | 17 | ...... | 4 | ...... | 1 | ...... | 1 | ...... |
| Other diseases of this group | 2 | ...... | 1 | ...... | 1 | ...... | ...... | ...... |
| GENERAL DISEASES, B. | | | | | | | | |
| Rheumatism | 17 | ...... | 3 | ...... | 1 | ...... | ...... | ...... |
| Syphilis | 11 | ...... | 4 | ...... | ...... | ...... | ...... | ...... |
| Consumption | 2 | ...... | ...... | ...... | ...... | ...... | ...... | ...... |
| Other diseases of this group | 1 | ...... | ...... | ...... | ...... | ...... | 1 | ...... |
| LOCAL DISEASES. | | | | | | | | |
| Catarrh and bronchitis | 3 | ...... | 2 | ...... | ...... | ...... | ...... | ...... |
| Pleurisy | ...... | ...... | 1 | ...... | ...... | ...... | ...... | ...... |
| Diarrhœa and dysentery | 66 | ...... | 20 | 1 | 4 | ...... | ...... | ...... |
| Gonorrhœa | 2 | ...... | 1 | ...... | ...... | ...... | ...... | ...... |
| Other local diseases | 93 | 1 | 18 | ...... | 3 | ...... | 2 | ...... |
| Alcoholism | 2 | ...... | 4 | ...... | ...... | ...... | ...... | ...... |
| Unclassified | 1 | ...... | ...... | ...... | ...... | ...... | ...... | ...... |
| Total disease | 218 | 1 | 61 | 3 | 11 | ...... | 4 | ...... |
| VIOLENT DISEASES AND DEATHS. | | | | | | | | |
| Gunshot wounds | 1 | ...... | ...... | ...... | ...... | ...... | 1 | ...... |
| Other accidents and injuries | 65 | ...... | 20 | ...... | ...... | ...... | ...... | ...... |
| Total violence | 66 | ...... | 20 | ...... | ...... | ...... | 1 | ...... |

\* 11 months only.     † 4 months only.     ‡ Officers of colored troops only.

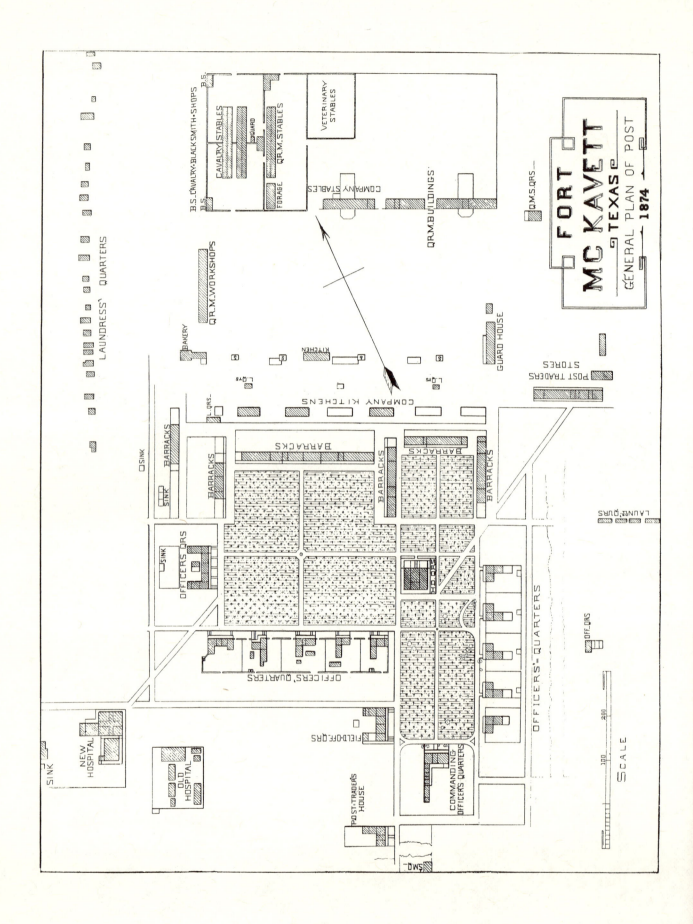

LAUNDRESS' QUARTERS

B.S. CAVALRY·BLACKSMITH·SHOPS
B.S.
B.S.
CAVALRY STABLES
GUARD
QR.M.STABLES
FORAGE
VETERINARY STABLES
COMPANY STABLES
QRM.BUILDINGS

QR.M.WORKSHOPS
BAKERY
KITCHEN
L.Qrs
L.Qrs
L.Qrs
COMPANY KITCHENS
L.QRS.
GUARD HOUSE
POST TRADERS STORES
Q.M.S.QRS.

SINK
SINK
BARRACKS
BARRACKS
BARRACKS
BARRACKS
SINK
BARRACKS
BARRACKS
BARRACKS
OFFICERS QRS
H.D.QRS.
LAUNR.QURS

SINK
NEW HOSPITAL
OLD HOSPITAL
OFFICERS' QUARTERS
FIELD·O·OF.QRS
POST·TRADERS HOUSE
COMMANDING OFFICERS QUARTERS
OFFICERS' QUARTERS
OFF.QRS
SMQ

SCALE
100    200

# FORT
# MC KAVETT
### TEXAS
GENERAL PLAN OF POST
1874

*Consolidated sick-report, (colored troops,) Fort McIntosh, Tex., 1871–'74.*

| Year | | 1871–'72.* | | 1872–'73. | | 1873–'74. | |
|---|---|---|---|---|---|---|---|
| Mean strength ........................................................Enlisted men...... | | 47 | | 94 | | 59 | |
| Diseases. | | Cases. | Deaths. | Cases. | Deaths. | Cases. | Deaths. |
| GENERAL DISEASES, A. | | | | | | | |
| Small-pox and varioloid.................................................... | | 2 | ...... | 3 | ...... | ...... | ...... |
| Typhoid fever............................................................ | | 1 | ...... | ...... | ...... | ...... | ...... |
| Typho-malarial fever..................................................... | | ...... | ...... | 1 | ...... | ...... | ...... |
| Intermittent fever....................................................... | | 2 | ...... | 9 | ...... | 2 | ...... |
| Other diseases of this group.............................................. | | 1 | ...... | 3 | ...... | ...... | ...... |
| GENERAL DISEASES, B. | | | | | | | |
| Rheumatism.............................................................. | | 2 | ...... | 16 | ...... | 7 | ...... |
| Consumption............................................................. | | ...... | ...... | ...... | 1 | 1 | 1 |
| LOCAL DISEASES. | | | | | | | |
| Catarrh and bronchitis.................................................... | | 2 | ...... | 13 | ...... | 7 | ...... |
| Pneumonia............................................................... | | 2 | ...... | ...... | ...... | ...... | ...... |
| Pleurisy................................................................. | | ...... | ...... | ...... | ...... | 1 | ...... |
| Diarrhœa and dysentery.................................................. | | 11 | ...... | 73 | ...... | 20 | ...... |
| Gonorrhœa............................................................... | | ...... | ...... | 3 | ...... | ...... | ...... |
| Other local diseases...................................................... | | 18 | ...... | 92 | ...... | 20 | ...... |
| Total disease............................................................. | | 41 | ...... | 213 | 1 | 58 | 1 |
| VIOLENT DISEASES AND DEATHS. | | | | | | | |
| Gunshot wounds........................................................... | | ...... | ...... | 3 | 1 | ...... | ...... |
| Drowning................................................................. | | ...... | ...... | ...... | ...... | ...... | 1 |
| Other accidents and injuries............................................... | | 4 | ...... | 48 | ...... | 14 | ...... |
| Total violence............................................................ | | 4 | ...... | 51 | 1 | 14 | 1 |

* First report March, 1872, for 4 months.

---

# FORT McKAVETT, TEXAS.

### REPORTS OF ACTING ASSISTANT SURGEON R. SHARPE AND ASSISTANT SURGEON S. M. HORTON UNITED STATES ARMY.

Fort McKavett is situated on a bluff on the right or south bank of the San Saba, about two miles from its source; latitude, 30° 50′ north; longitude, 23° 17′ west; altitude, 2,000 feet. It is one hundred and eighty miles nearly west from Austin, the nearest railroad station, and about the same distance northwest from San Antonio. Fredericksburgh is one hundred miles from the post. The nearest post is Fort Concho, distant fifty-three miles. The surrounding country is hilly, covered with dwarf-oak. The post was established in 1852, abandoned in 1860, and re-occupied in 1868. The general arrangement is shown in the plate opposite. The barracks consist of one building, 324 by 20 feet; one, 101 by 23 feet; one, 157 by 20 feet; one, 80 by 20 feet; all of stone; one frame building, 140 by 20 feet, and one picket-building, 156 by 22 feet. All of these buildings are of one story, 10 feet high to the eaves. A space of from 5 to 8 inches is left open at the eaves the whole length of the building, which ordinarily affords sufficient ventilation. The dormitories are fitted with single iron-bedsteads, and allow about 485 cubic feet air-space per man.

Each bed has a wooden chest, so made that the top projects over the head of the bunk, with a shelf over it. These chests have been found to be very convenient.

There are no lavatories or bath-rooms. The men wash out of doors; and during nine months in the year can bathe in the lake.

The kitchens and mess-rooms are separate buildings, about 22 by 15 feet, and insufficient in number.

The married soldiers' quarters are picket-huts and wall-tents, inconvenient, shabby, and in bad condition.

The commanding-officer's quarters consist of a stone building, 51 by 35 feet, two stories high, with an L, 38 by 16 feet. The main building has lower and upper halls, and a lower veranda front and rear; the latter one extending along the L partly inclosed with lattice-work. These quarters are elegant in every respect. They contain two large rooms on each floor; also a dining-room, pantry, kitchen, and servants' room on the first floor, and a cellar cut in solid rock beneath the main portion. The quarters of the field-officers are in a one-story stone building, with two Ls. It contains four rooms and a pantry for each field-officer. The main portion of this double set is 77 by 18 feet, with a veranda in front running the whole length. Each of the two Ls is 45 by 18 feet. There are four captains' quarters, all of stone; each is 36 by 15 feet, one story, comprising two rooms, and an L, 15 by 16 feet, containing one room; a veranda extends the whole length in front. One of these quarters has a kitchen, 15 by 12 feet; the others have no kitchens. The plan of these quarters, had they all of them kitchens, would be excellent, but they are built of uneven and mis-shaped stones, of the most varied sizes, all put up in the utmost confusion as to making any joints; the walls not pointed and the mortar inferior and subject to washing out by rains. Two out of three fires in each smoke so badly when the winds blow, which they do nearly daily in the latter part of fall, the entire winter, and early spring, that the occupants are well-nigh blindfolded whenever fires are made in them. These fire-places are all small. The quartermaster received stoves during the year sufficient to give one to each of these quarters. In rear of the line of captains' quarters is a frame building, 40 by 20 feet, one story high, containing three rooms, which comprise one set of quarters for a married lieutenant. One stone building, 98 by 15 feet, one story, with an L at each end running back, with a veranda in front the whole length, contains eight rooms for four lieutenants, two of whom are married officers. These quarters have good fire-places. Other officers' quarters are one stone building, 61 by 15 feet, one story high, with an L at each end running back; one of these is 21 by 13 feet, the other is 15 by 19 feet. This building contains five rooms, and in it live one married and one single lieutenant. In front it has a shed-roof; in rear is a frame kitchen with two small rooms in it. A one-story building, 53 by 14 feet, with an L in rear, 23 by 15 feet, shed-roof in front, and containing four rooms with large fire-places, affords quarters for a captain and one lieutenant; a tent is used for kitchen purposes. One building, of stone, one story high, 48 by 15 feet, with an L, 31 by 15 feet, has four rooms for the post surgeon and one lieutenant, both married. In rear is a frame building with two rooms as kitchens; a shed-roof is in front. A one-story stone building, 36 by 15 feet, with L, 31 by 15 feet, has four rooms for one captain. Another similar building, 46 by 16 feet, L 27 by 13 feet, with shed-roof in front, contains five rooms for one married and one single lieutenant. All the officers' quarters on the south side of the parade-ground are one story high, and have low floors, and ceilings of canvas.

The officers' quarters are, with the exception of the commanding officer's quarters, restricted to the literal requirements of the Regulations, with no conveniences whatever that are found at many military posts in the way of attics or basements. But three of the lieutenants' quarters have any outbuildings, such as wood-sheds or shelters of any kind. With but few exceptions there are no closets and but few shelves, which would take the place of wardrobes, cupboards, &c.

The headquarters-building at the post is a stone structure, 56 by 42 feet, by 10 feet high to the eaves from the floor, which is raised a little over 2 feet from the ground, situated on the eastern side of the main parade-ground. A veranda extends along the front and sides. This building contains six rooms, of nearly equal size, viz, the commanding officer's office, adjutant's office, sergeant major's and clerk's office, the post school-room, the court-martial room, and the post library, the latter used at night for school for the enlisted men.

The commissary store-house is built of stone, one story, 120 by 22 feet, and 10 feet from the floor, which is raised 4 feet from the ground, to the eaves; contains a large store-room and a small room for an office at one end. The L, 60 by 30 feet, contains at the farther end a counter for issuing and a small room with shelving. It is an excellent building for the purpose. The quartermaster's store-house is also of stone, one story, 140 by 23 feet, and 10 feet from the floor, which is raised 4 feet from the ground, to the eaves. It contains in the middle a small room for an office. The rest of the building is store-room. In addition there is one 90 by 20 feet, and 8½ feet high to the eaves, for stores, paints, tools, &c. The carpenter, wheelwright, saddler, and blacksmith shops are comprised in a stone building, 98 by 20 feet, and one story high. This building is on the west side of the post. A store-house for forage, 18 by 22 feet, is situated at the end of the guard-house.

During the last two years a small stone building, 21 by 18 feet, by 10 feet high to the eaves directly in rear of the commanding officer's quarters, was built. It was intended to be used as a guard-house for pickets on that side of the post, and was designed to have a turret on top as a lookout for Indians. It is occupied by the sergeant major Tenth Infantry.

The post guard-house referred to in Circular No. 4, December 5, 1870, is now too small to accommodate the number of prisoners at the post, and give them proper air-space per man. It is a stone structure, 60 by 22 feet, outside measurement, by 10 feet high to the eaves; contains a prison-room, 28 by 16 feet, one room for the guard, and six cells. The two rooms are floored, with raised platforms on both sides of each, on which the guard and the prisoners sleep. It is warmed by fire-places, except in the room containing the cells, which has no means of heating. Ventilation is good when the general prison-room is not overcrowded. Daylight is admitted by small windows with gratings, and is sufficient. The average occupancy by prisoners is 30, giving only 194 cubic feet of air to each prisoner. The commanding officer is as helpless as the post surgeon is to remedy this evil, so far. There has been no lumber or other material at the post whereby the guard-house could be extended. Lumber and other materials for many necessary purposes were urgently asked for more than a year ago, but without success.

The new hospital is of stone throughout. It is a modification of the administration building, and one ward of a twenty-four-bed hospital of the plan approved by the Surgeon General United States Army, in Circular No. 3, dated Washington, D. C., November 23, 1870. The modification of this plan is the following, viz: The administration building is but one story high. To compensate for the want of a second story a store-room, 15 by 18 feet, and a dead-house, 14 by 14 feet, both in one building, 10 feet high to the eaves, of stone, have been erected in the rear of the hospital ward. The northern half of the hall, running north and south, of the administration building, has been closed in and shelved, to be utilized as a store-room for liquors, instruments, &c.; a large wooden cupboard is to be placed in the nurse's room for linen; a sink, a stone building, with two compartments, 8 by 6 feet each, has been made on the earth-closet principle in rear of the southern end of the ward, in line with the store-room and dead-house; a bath-room, 7 by 9 feet, is to be made on the rear veranda of the ward at its south end and adjoining the earth-closet attached to the ward; it is to accommodate two bath-tubs. An isolation ward could not be had, but it was not seen how it could be helped with the limited appropriation given for the construction of the hospital. The reasons for the above modification of the original plan, approved by the Surgeon General, were the following, viz, want of appropriation sufficient to make any more extensive or elaborate outside store-room and dead-house, and an isolation ward, and a large bath-room, of stone, and the apparent insecurity and instability of the foundation-walls of the administration building, already made more than a year before the resumption of work on this hospital, to sustain as much as the weight of two stories high of stone wall upon them. For eighteen months the rains had washed out much of the mortar, in fact, injured the most of it contained in the foundation walls throughout. The amount of money already expended on the work of the hospital, so far, being so great, as stated above, and the limited appropriation given with which to complete the whole structure, being insufficient to do anything but make a modification of the hospital within the limits already specified, in the way of contraction in size of buildings and economy in expenditure of money, the modification thus reported was made.

The dimensions of the rest of the new hospital are the same as laid down in the plan approved by the Surgeon-General United States Army, in Circular No. 3, November 23, 1870, except that the verandas are but 8½ feet wide, and the administration building is separated from the ward by an open porch or veranda, 10 feet wide. All the floors of the hospital are raised 2½ feet from the ground with ample ventilation beneath. The ward is 50 by 24 feet, by 12 feet high from the floor to the ceiling. This hospital altogether is a good building and an ornament to the post. It is believed that it will be very well adapted to this climate and prove to be commodious, convenient, and comfortable in every way. Ridge ventilation is used for the ward, the ridge being 25 feet long with a box opening in the center of the ceiling, and lattice-work in the ceiling extending both ways from this opening. Between the ceiling and the ridge, half-way up the shaft, regular dampers have been made to open and shut by pulleys and cords extending down the interior side of the ward; from this opening, with a collar in it, a sheet-iron tube runs to the top of the ridge above which an artificial wooden chimney extends 4 feet, and is lined by block tin; there are 3 inches of space all around between this tube and the stove-pipe from the stove which heats the ward; a wooden shaft surrounds this tube.

The bakery is of stone, a new building recently erected, 41 by 24 feet by 8 feet high, containing an oven-room with two ovens, each 15 by 8 feet, and the bread-room, 20 feet square. The ovens, floor and sides, are made of small, flat, sawn bricks or blocks of soap-stone, and the arches, 2 feet high, are of fire-brick; capacity, seven hundred and fifty rations of bread each. It is not believed that there is anywhere in the Department of Texas a better oven than the one described.

The stables of the two companies stationed at the post consist of, for each company, two rows of stalls, each row 160 feet long by 10½ feet wide; the rows of stalls separated by a high stone wall, and each double row covered by one continuous roof. The stable-yards are surrounded by a high stone wall, forming an excellent corral. In each of two corners of the yard is a small stone building for a blacksmith-shop—one for each company; in the yard is also a similar building for a small guard-house. The quartermaster's stables are in a stable-yard adjoining that of the cavalry companies, which yard is also surrounded by a high stone wall. These stables consist of two long rows of stalls, the rows separated by a high, close picket-fence or wall, and each row with the partition between them being 124 by 11 feet; both rows have continuous roofs; in the inclosure is a one story frame forage-house, 60 by 20 feet; in the cavalry-stable yard are two stone forage-houses, each 28 by 13 feet, and one story high.

The water from the spring, used for drinking and washing purposes, is very hard water, containing much salts of lime, among others, a vast amount of the carbonate of lime, producing thick incrustations on the inside of all boilers and kettles in which it has been for a short time boiled. Even a tin-cupful once boiled deposits a slight crust of the white carbonate, besides throwing down a loose, whitish sediment of saltish taste. Nitrate of silver causes instantly deep whitish cloudiness on adding it to this water before boiling. This water is most refreshing and healthy all of the time for drinking purposes.

There are no drains at the post. An immediate descent from the post in every direction but one makes good natural drainage. All sewage is removed daily in barrels to the ravine, 600 yards below the post, where the rains wash it down and flood it into the San Saba River. The sinks of the barracks are 65 yards in rear of the same; they are disinfected daily, and the troughs emptied daily from 500 to 800 yards away in the ravine. Dry earth is chiefly used as a disinfectant, and with good results.

The post gardens, comprising in all at the post 30 acres, yielded, during the preceding years, a good supply of water-melons, cantaloupes, tomatoes, squashes, and pumpkins. Sweet potatoes are also raised, but attempts to cultivate Irish potatoes have proved perfect failures. One of the gardens referred to is cultivated by the musicians of the band, and is set apart for the use of the band, the post hospital, the commanding officer, and the commissioned staff at the post. There is no officers' mess at the post, or room available for such a purpose. This is a very serious want felt by many, and at times by nearly all, of the officers. If it were possible to get good servants this want would not be so serious, but female servants are most difficult to get from either Austin, San Antonio, or Fredericksburgh, as it is deemed disreputable for them to come to a garrison filled with soldiers. The command is well supplied with the best of food at all times. Fresh beef is issued daily, and is very good. Good coffee, rice, hominy, sugar, pease, beans are issued to the troops. Fifty barrels of Irish potatoes were during the year brought from Dennison, Tex., and sold by the commissary for 2½ cents per pound; very recently they were retailed by hucksters at $9 per bushel. Sweet potatoes are purchased for $1.50 per bushel. Water-cress grows abundantly all the year round at the springs and on the banks of the San Saba River, and is used extensively by both the officers and enlisted men. Fresh butter, 50 cents per pound; chickens, 50 cents each, and milk at 10 cents per quart, are purchased throughout the year. Fresh eggs are difficult to obtain, but can be purchased in Fredericksburgh for 30 cents per dozen.

The cost of furniture in Austin and San Antonio, added to the cost of transportation to the post, makes all such articles excessively dear in price. The great difficulty of getting any lumber to the post but by paying fabulous prices for it, so as to get furniture made here, debars a few officers from being able to have articles of furniture sufficient to give them the feeling of bare respectability in the appearance of their dwellings.

There are one ambulance, a Dougherty wagon, and a spring-wagon, with top for ambulance purposes, all in good condition, all new; eight ambulance-mules in good condition; five horse-litters, ten hand-litters, and two Tompkins wheeled litters in hospital.

The post is reached by tri-weekly stages from Austin and San Antonio; the El Paso coaches changing for the McKavett stage, a smaller vehicle, 16 miles below the post, at Mr. Coglin's stage-ranch.

The elevated location of the post, the dryness of the atmosphere, the delightful breezes of morning and evening, throughout the latter part of the spring, the entire summer and fall, the middle portions of the days during a great part of this time being excessively warm, and the sunlight excessively bright, which, with the dry winds blowing incessantly, tries the eyes to the utmost when out of doors; the pure, fresh drinking-water from a most excellent spring, bubbling up at the foot or base of the bluff, just west of the post, through limestone rock of indefinite thickness, and in consideration of the very favorable reports of former years as to the small amount of sickness occurring in this vicinity: these have all combined to give this post and locality the name of being exceedingly healthy. The cause of the excessive amount of disease existing at the post during the past year is believed to be malarial poisoning. The depressing and debilitating influence of this poison renders men, it seems, beyond doubt, much more susceptible to the slighter causes operating at all times to diarrhœa and dysentery. The post is in close proximity to the low, moist, bottom-land, just north and northwest of the post, and bordering the San Saba River, which runs close by, and bordering also the two lakes in the immediate vicinity of the post, the larger one formed by an artificial dam in the course of this river; the other between the river and the post, formed by the large dam retaining the water from the springs. The post is located on the high bluff above these lakes and this bottom-land. These lakes are used for irrigating, by cross-channels or acequias running in every direction, about 20 acres of post and company gardens in this bottom. The sluggish back waters from these lakes, with the most prolific, dense, and rank vegetation bordering them and existing in them in the numerous shallow places, produce the most favorable conditions imaginable for the generation of malarial poisoning. Dense, low fogs rest on the bluff and banks below the post in the early mornings of summer and fall until after sunrise each day. By far the great majority of cases of diarrhœa and dysentery require the administration of quinine before convalescence. The dams of the lakes could be easily torn down, but the letting out of the water in them would only lay bare, exposed to the air, the foulest marshy beds at the bottoms of the lakes, serving only to intensify the miasm, besides ruining the gardens. The constant labor of three times as many men as the command now consists of could not keep in check the luxuriant vegetation of summer that borders and exists in the shallow portions of these lakes and covers this extensive low bottom-land. In May, 1873, it rained on 15 days of the month. Nearly everything planted in the lower portions of the company gardens was washed away. The surface of the bottom-lands mentioned above was soaked with water the entire month.

In relation to the causes of typhoid fever that existed in the months of June, September, and October, 1873, the following facts are submitted, viz, the air-space per man in the barracks of Company M, Ninth Cavalry, was 432 cubic feet. That company was absent from the post from June 15 to August 5, 1873, and it was during the absence of that company that one of their men, left behind at the post, and who had been sleeping in the company kitchen, contracted this disease. It was one of the two most virulent cases of typhoid fever that occurred at the post. Before the departure of the company and after their return, there were no other cases. The air-space per man in the barracks of Company F, Ninth Cavalry, during the year was 443 cubic feet. No case at all was received from that company. The other most virulent and quickly fatal case came from the barracks of Company C, Tenth Infantry, where the man slept prior to his contracting typhoid fever. The average air-space per man in that barrack was 512 cubic feet, which was from 20 to 40 cubic feet per man more than the men in the other barracks not named above enjoyed. The post guard-house, with an average cubic air-space per man of only 194 cubic feet during the summer and fall, furnished no cases at all of typhoid fever. One of the men, who had a relapse from which he died, was exceedingly depressed on account of the desertion of his brother from the post; another, from the same company, contracted the disease after having slept in his company-kitchen; another had been sleeping in the bread-room of the post-bakery before coming on sick-report with the disease; another one had been working and sleeping in his company garden prior to his contracting the disease. In June, upon recommendation of the medical officer, the floors in nearly all of the barracks were taken up, the surface of the ground beneath thoroughly scraped off, the rubbish and filth cleaned away, after which carbolic acid was freely sprinkled upon the ground. That did not prevent subsequent cases from arising in the least. The water-barrels at the post were cleaned out every third day; the water-wagon was thoroughly cleaned out and kept clean. As to sleep, the men retired at taps from 8 to 9 o'clock p. m. during the warm season but reveille was sounded, as stated, from 3 to 5 o'clock a. m. throughout the summer and early fall. The electrical conditions of the atmosphere could not be ascertained. Headaches were very frequent, nearly daily. Enlisted men, not on sick-report, applied for medicines at the hospital for relief of this affection. Officers and their families complained frequently of this. In addition to the depressing influences of malarial poisoning, some agency in the general atmosphere may be supposed to exist, owing to locality, no doubt. A very intelligent officer, after an absence of seven weeks from the post, on his return from Fort Griffin noticed a close atmosphere and an indefinable, unhealthy odor, upon approaching the low valley in this immediate vicinity, on his road to the post, so appreciably different from the atmosphere in the country above and farther out.

*Meteorological report, Fort McKavett, Tex., 1872–'74.*

| Months. | 1870–'71. Temperature. Mean. | Max. | Min. | Rain-fall in inches. | 1871–'72. Temperature. Mean. | Max. | Min. | Rain-fall in inches. | 1872–'73. Temperature. Mean. | Max. | Min. | Rain-fall in inches. | 1873–'74. Temperature. Mean. | Max. | Min. | Rain-fall in inches. |
|---|---|---|---|---|---|---|---|---|---|---|---|---|---|---|---|---|
| July | | | | | | | | | | | | | 84.39 | 105 | 50* | 3.93 |
| August | | | | | | | | | 84.84 | 102 | 73 | 0.42 | 81.78 | 100 | 66* | 2.74 |
| September | | | | | | | | | 82.12 | 100 | 55 | 0.60 | 77.01 | 98 | 49* | 5.03 |
| October | | | | | | | | | 65.28 | 91 | 36 | 1.09 | 64.67 | 90 | 31* | 0.64 |
| November | | | | | | | | | 49.03 | 80 | 20 | 2.70 | 54.83 | 85 | 19* | 0.52 |
| December | | | | | | | | | 43.66 | 78 | 11 | 1.96 | 50.78 | 75 | 19* | 0.28 |
| January | | | | | | | | | 44.37 | 78 | 6 | 0.08 | 47.21 | 77 | 14* | 1.82 |
| February | | | | | | | | | 53.41 | 82 | 23 | 0.40 | 49.53 | 80 | 17* | 0.28 |
| March | | | | | | | | | 61.07 | 89 | 29 | 2.16 | 60.83 | 85 | 27* | 2.00 |
| April | | | | | | | | | 65.34 | 100 | 34 | 0.18 | 61.13 | 88 | 27* | 0.68 |
| May | | | | | | | | | 74.77 | 100 | 49 | 6.30 | 74.66 | 92 | 42* | 3.50 |
| June | | | | | | | | | 79.47 | 102* | 55* | 3.22 | 79.92 | 96 | 62* | 1.11 |
| For the year | | | | | | | | | | | | | 65.56 | 105 | 14* | 22.53 |

* These observations are made with self-registering thermometers. The mean is from the standard thermometer.

*Consolidated sick-report, (white,) Fort McKavett, Tex., 1870–'74.*

| Year | 1870–'71.* Cases. | Deaths. | 1871–'72.† Cases. | Deaths. | 1872–'73.‡ Cases. | Deaths. | 1873–'74. Cases. | Deaths. |
|---|---|---|---|---|---|---|---|---|
| Mean strength { Officers | 15 | | 15 | | 16 | | 16 | |
| Enlisted men | 15 | | 1 | | 158 | | 308 | |
| **GENERAL DISEASES, A.** | | | | | | | | |
| Typhoid fever | | | | | 2 | | 4 | 3 |
| Typho-malarial fever | 2 | | | | | | 2 | |
| Remittent fever | 4 | | | | 4 | | 11 | |
| Intermittent fever | 1 | | 2 | | 23 | | 130 | |
| Other diseases of this group | | | | | 13 | | 53 | |
| **GENERAL DISEASES, B.** | | | | | | | | |
| Rheumatism | | | 2 | | 17 | | 36 | |
| Syphilis | | | | | 3 | | 3 | |
| Consumption | | | | | | 1 | | |
| Other diseases of this group | | | | | 1 | | 9 | |

*One month only.        † Two months only.        ‡ Ten months only.

*Consolidated sick-report, (white,) Fort McKavett, Tex., 1870–'74—Continued.*

| | 1870–'71. | | 1871–'72. | | 1872–'73. | | 1873–'74. | |
|---|---|---|---|---|---|---|---|---|
| Year | Cases. | Deaths. | Cases. | Deaths. | Cases. | Deaths. | Cases. | Deaths. |
| Mean strength { Officers | 15 | | 15 | | 16 | | 16 | |
| { Enlisted men | 15 | | 1 | | 158 | | 308 | |
| **LOCAL DISEASES.** | | | | | | | | |
| Catarrh and bronchitis | | | | | 32 | | 59 | |
| Pneumonia | | | | | 4 | | 2 | |
| Pleurisy | | | | | 65 | 2 | 121 | 1 |
| Diarrhœa and dysentery | | | 1 | | | | | |
| Hernia | | | | | 1 | | 3 | |
| Gonorrhœa | | | 4 | | 61 | | 175 | 2 |
| Other local diseases | | | | | 20 | | 28 | |
| Alcoholism | | | | | | | | |
| Total disease | 7 | | 9 | | 246 | 3 | 636 | 6 |
| **VIOLENT DISEASES AND DEATHS.** | | | | | | | | |
| Gunshot wounds | | | | | 4 | | 2 | |
| Other accidents and injuries | | | 2 | | 23 | | 91 | 1 |
| Homicide | | | | | | | | |
| Total violence | | | 2 | | 27 | | 93 | 1 |

*Consolidated sick-report, (colored,) Fort McKavett, Tex., 1870–'74.*

| | 1870–'71. | | 1871–'72. | | 1872–'73. | | 1873–'74.* | |
|---|---|---|---|---|---|---|---|---|
| Year | Cases. | Deaths. | Cases. | Deaths. | Cases. | Deaths. | Cases. | Deaths. |
| Mean strength ...... Enlisted men | 298 | | 381 | | 114 | | 90 | |
| **GENERAL DISEASES, A.** | | | | | | | | |
| Typhoid fever | 1 | 1 | 1 | | 1 | 1 | | |
| Typho-malarial fever | 1 | | 1 | | | | | |
| Remittent fever | 11 | | 2 | | | | 1 | |
| Intermittent fever | 42 | | 21 | | 15 | | 12 | |
| Other diseases of this group | 26 | | 2 | | 7 | | 11 | |
| **GENERAL DISEASES, B.** | | | | | | | | |
| Rheumatism | 30 | | 4 | | 11 | | 9 | |
| Syphilis | 26 | | 19 | | 8 | | 4 | |
| Consumption | 3 | 1 | | 2 | | | 2 | 1 |
| Other diseases of this group | 1 | | 1 | | 2 | | | |
| **LOCAL DISEASES.** | | | | | | | | |
| Catarrh and bronchitis | 19 | | 6 | | 21 | | 9 | 1 |
| Pneumonia | 1 | 1 | 1 | | | | | |
| Pleurisy | 10 | | 1 | | | | | |
| Diarrhœa and dysentery | 72 | | 27 | | 34 | 2 | 21 | |
| Hernia | 1 | | | | | | 1 | |
| Gonorrhœa | 7 | | 6 | | | | 1 | |
| Other local diseases | 82 | 1 | 47 | 5 | 29 | | 45 | |
| Unclassified | 1 | | | | | | | |
| Total disease | 334 | 4 | 139 | 7 | 128 | 3 | 116 | 2 |
| **VIOLENT DISEASES AND DEATHS.** | | | | | | | | |
| Gunshot wounds | 11 | 1 | 7 | 1 | 8 | | 3 | |
| Other accidents and injuries | 46 | | 61 | | 37 | | 7 | |
| Total violence | 57 | 1 | 68 | 1 | 45 | | 10 | |

* Seven months only.

# FORT QUITMAN, TEXAS.

INFORMATION FURNISHED BY ACTING ASSISTANT SURGEONS JOHN J. CULVER AND D. HERSHEY, UNITED STATES ARMY.

Fort Quitman is situated in latitude 31° 10′ north; longitude, 28° 37′ west, 418 miles due west from Austin, or 696 miles by the usual routes of travel. The camp is 400 yards from the Rio Grande, from which the water-supply is taken.

The country in every direction is a rolling-sand prairie, covered with stunted mesquite bushes and wild cactus, which often attains a great height. Beyond the prairie, and at one point within ten miles of the post, are steep, rocky mountains, destitute of all vegetation. Several attempts have been made to cultivate a post-garden, but all have failed on account of the heat, drought, and sterility of the soil.

All the buildings at the post are constructed of adobes with earth roofs. There are two barracks, each 74 by 36 by 10 feet, which have been made comfortable by recent repairs. They are warmed by open fire-places, and sufficiently ventilated by doors and windows. The air-space for the present garrison is 500 cubic feet per man.

There are at the post six sets of officers' quarters, consisting of four or five rooms each, which have been made quite comfortable within the last three years, in part, however, by the individual exertions of the occupants.

The married soldiers and laundresses occupy an old set of officers' quarters.

The hospital is 72 by 26 by 12 feet, and divided into a dispensary, office, ward, store-room, and kitchen. The arrangement is inconvenient, and the general style and finish of the most inferior character. No part of the building is either floored or ceiled. The capacity of the ward is 8 beds, giving 55 square feet and 550 cubic feet to each bed. The building is warmed by open fire-places. Two bath-tubs are kept for the use of the hospital. The sink is about 25 yards from the hospital, and is kept disinfected with lime and dry earth.

The guard-house is divided by a hall into two rooms of 3,168 cubic feet of space each, one for the guard and the other for the prisoners. There are in addition four cells. The warming is by open fire-places; the ventilation, by doors and windows, and the average occupancy, 2⅔.

Milk, and sometimes butter, eggs, and chickens, can be procured in the immediate vicinity of the post. Fresh vegetables, grapes, peaches, pears, melons, &c., can usually be obtained during the summer months, but they are hauled over a dusty road 50 or 75 miles from the Mexican towns of San Ignatius, Guadalupe, San Elizario, and El Paso. Milk costs 50 cents per gallon; butter from 70 cents to $1 per pound; eggs, 50 cents per dozen; chickens, $1 per pair; and fresh vegetables range from 8 to 10 cents per pound.

The inhabitants of the surrounding country are Mexicans and Pueblo and Apache Indians.

*Meteorological report, Fort Quitman, Texas.*

| Month. | 1870-'71. | | | | 1871-'72. | | | | 1872-'73. | | | | 1873-'74. | | | |
|---|---|---|---|---|---|---|---|---|---|---|---|---|---|---|---|---|
| | Temperature. | | | Rain-fall in inches. | Temperature. | | | Rain-fall in inches. | Temperature. | | | Rain-fall in inches. | Temperature. | | | Rain-fall in inches. |
| | Mean. | Max. | Min. | | Mean. | Max. | Min. | | Mean. | Max. | Min. | | Mean. | Max. | Min. | |
| July | 81.91 | 100 | 70 | 3.84 | | | | | | | | | 85.61 | 109 | 63 | 0.50 |
| August | 80.25 | 98 | 67 | 5.31 | | | | | | | | | 80.90 | 103 | 69 | 2.42 |
| September | 76.70 | 98 | 54 | 5.90 | | | | | | | | | 79.23 | 102 | 58 | 0.06 |
| October | 64.44 | 90 | 32 | 1.20 | | | | | | | | | 66.09 | 59 | 32 | 0.34 |
| November | 54.07 | 90 | 22 | 0.00 | | | | | | | | | 52.36 | 83 | '26 | 1.18 |
| December | 41.65 | 73 | 13 | 0.70 | | | | | | | | | 43.93 | 79 | 10 | 0.00 |
| January | 42.72 | 75 | 11 | 0.16 | | | | | | | | | 47.29 | 78 | 24 | 0.30 |
| February | 48.28 | 82 | 18 | 0.00 | | | | | | | | | | | | |
| March | | | | | | | | | | | | | | | | |
| April | 63.95 | 99 | 33 | 0.00 | | | | | | | | | | | | |
| May | 76.24 | 101 | 57 | 0.26 | | | | | | | | | | | | |
| June | | | | | | | | | 80.53 | 109 | 58 | 4.59 | | | | |
| For the year | | | | | | | | | | | | | | | | |

*Consolidated sick-report, (white,) Fort Quitman, Tex., 1870–'74.*

| Year | 1870–'71. | | 1871–'72. | | 1872–'73. | | 1873–'74. | |
|---|---|---|---|---|---|---|---|---|
| Mean strength..........Officers...... | 7 | | 4 | | 3 | | 2 | |
| Diseases. | Cases. | Deaths. | Cases. | Deaths. | Cases. | Deaths. | Cases. | Deaths. |
| GENERAL DISEASES, A. | | | | | | | | |
| Typhoid fever | 1 | | | | | | | |
| Intermittent fever | | | | | 1 | | | |
| LOCAL DISEASES. | | | | | | | | |
| Diarrhœa and dysentery | | | 2 | 1 | | | | |
| Other local diseases | | | 1 | | 2 | | 1 | |
| Total disease | 1 | | 3 | 1 | 3 | | 1 | |

*Consolidated sick-report, (colored,) Fort Quitman, Tex., 1870–'74.*

| Year | 1870–'71. | | 1871–'72. | | 1872–'73. | | 1873–'74. | |
|---|---|---|---|---|---|---|---|---|
| Mean strength..........Enlisted men...... | 184 | | 81 | | 72 | | 53 | |
| Diseases. | Cases. | Deaths. | Cases. | Deaths. | Cases. | Deaths. | Cases. | Deaths. |
| GENERAL DISEASES, A. | | | | | | | | |
| Remittent fever | 3 | | 1 | | 1 | | | |
| Intermittent fever | 20 | | 4 | | 9 | | 3 | |
| Other diseases of this group | 10 | | 3 | | 5 | | 2 | |
| GENERAL DISEASES, B. | | | | | | | | |
| Rheumatism | 11 | | 4 | | 1 | | 1 | |
| Syphilis | 4 | | 1 | | | | 1 | |
| Consumption | | | 1 | | 1 | | | |
| Other diseases of this group | 8 | | 1 | | | | 1 | |
| LOCAL DISEASES. | | | | | | | | |
| Catarrh and bronchitis | 22 | | 2 | | 5 | | 2 | |
| Pneumonia | 4 | | 5 | 2 | 2 | | | |
| Pleurisy | 4 | | 2 | | 1 | | | |
| Diarrhœa and dysentery | 63 | 1 | 17 | 2 | 21 | 1 | 4 | |
| Hernia | 1 | | | | | | | |
| Gonorrhœa | 5 | | 1 | | | | 3 | |
| Other local diseases | 79 | | 13 | | 23 | | 20 | 1 |
| Unclassified | | 1 | | | | | | |
| Total disease | 234 | 2 | 55 | 4 | 69 | 1 | 37 | 1 |
| VIOLENT DISEASES AND DEATHS. | | | | | | | | |
| Gunshot wounds | 4 | 2 | 1 | | 1 | | | |
| Other accidents and injuries | 42 | 1 | 15 | | 8 | | 7 | 1 |
| Homicide | | | | | | | | 2 |
| Total violence | 46 | 3 | 16 | | 9 | | 7 | 3 |

# FORT RICHARDSON, TEXAS.

REPORTS OF ASSISTANT SURGEONS J. H. PÁTZKI AND W. H. FORWOOD, UNITED STATES ARMY.

The post of Fort Richardson is located in Jack County, Texas, in latitude 33° 15′ north, and longitude 21° 15′ west, upon the south bank of Lost Creek, a tributary of the Trinity River, southwest from and about seven miles above the point at which it empties its waters into the west fork of that stream. The nearest range of hills is that known as Flat-Top Mountain, about twenty miles in a west-northwesterly direction, one of the low ranges of hills that divide the headwaters of the Brazos from those of the Trinity. These hills appear to be detached spurs of the Wichita Mountains, through which the Red River passes at about sixty miles northeast of the post, and which seem to form part of a mountain system from which diverge the lesser tributaries of the Brazos, the Trinity, and the Red Rivers. The village of Jacksborough, the county-seat of Jack County, is in the immediate vicinity of the post, being situated on the north bank of Lost Creek, and about one-half mile distant. The nearest settlements are Weatherford, the county-seat of Parker County, distant forty-two and a half miles in a southeasterly direction, on the direct mail-route to Waco and Austin; Decatur, in Wise County, distant forty miles east-southeast, on the road leading toward Jefferson and towns in Eastern Texas; and Montague, in Montague County, distant about forty miles in a northeasterly direction, and on the line of the overland mail-route from Fort Concho, in Texas, to Fort Smith, in Arkansas.

The nearest post is Fort Griffin, distant about seventy-five miles. Dallas, on the Texas Central, and Sherman, on the Missouri, Kansas and Texas Railroad, each distant about one hundred miles, are the nearest railroad-stations, and are connected with this point by tri-weekly stage. The projected route of the Texas Pacific road is within a few miles of the post.

The reservation on which the post is built is one mile square, located on a high rolling prairie, bounded on the northern side, for nearly its entire length, by Lost Creek, which runs in an easterly direction at that point,

The whole region appears to be underlaid with a stratum of rock, which is covered but thinly by soil, or crops out at the surface, except in the "bottoms" or small valleys watered by streams, which sometimes admit of cultivation. The adjacent country for many miles around the post is of the same general formation. Notwithstanding the thinness and barrenness of the soil, the grazing in the immediate vicinity is excellent, the grass being principally mesquite, a variety superior to ordinary prairie-grass. At Fort Belknap, thirty-two miles west of the post, on the east bank of the Brazos, bituminous coal of a quality resembling that of Western Pennsylvania, is found, and some small veins which crop out near the surface have been opened. Indications of considerable deposits of copper-ore have been seen within about seventy-five miles, in a northwesterly direction, some specimens of which, on being assayed, have proved very rich, and contain silver in considerable quantity.

The varieties of timber in the neighborhood are oak, pecan, and mesquite, but generally of a small and stunted growth, and unfit for building purposes, except the construction of picket or stockade-houses; the timber used in the building of the post having been procured on the Big Sandy, in Wise County, about thirty-eight miles due east from the post.

The mustang-grape and chickasaw-plum abound, and the pecan-nut, which grows upon the tree of that name, may be gathered in great quantities. The wild onion, a wholesome and palatable addition to the soup-ration, is found in small quantities on the prairies, and along the banks of the water-courses. Buffalo are found during the winter months within thirty or forty miles to the northwest of the post, but in the warm season are rarely seen south of Red River. Antelope and deer are numerous, and bear and panther occasionally met with. Of smaller animals, raccoons and rabbits are very plentiful. Of the latter the hare, or, as it is popularly known in this State, the mule-ear variety, is the most numerous. Wild turkeys exist along all the water-courses in incredible numbers, and prairie-chickens and wild ducks are seen at times. Fish cannot be obtained (except some small varieties in Lost Creek) nearer than the Brazos River, the nearest point of which is about thirty miles distant. In that stream they are very abundant, but of little variety, catfish, drum, buffalo, and gaspers (the latter nearly resembling the catfish) being about the only kinds found which are fit for food. Turtle abound in all the streams. Tarantulas, centipedes, and scorpions infest this whole region, and chameleons and horned-toads may be frequently met with. The copperhead, moccasin, puff-adder, and rattlesnake are found, the latter very frequently, but generally of small size. Besides these, there are several unimportant varieties of harmless serpents found in great numbers, such as the black-snake, chicken-snake, and common house-snake.

The heat of the summer months, reflected from the rocky soil, bare of shade trees, would be insupportable if it were not tempered by constant breezes from the southwest or southeast, and close, sultry nights are unknown even during the hottest weather. These winds contain but little moisture, owing to the character of the surface over which they sweep before reaching here. The rain-fall during this season is but scanty, yet sometimes so heavy as to render the labors of the farmer fruitless. The uncertainty of the climate in this respect, together with the thinness of the soil covering the rocky substratum, form the most serious obstacles to successful agriculture in this portion of Texas. From the beginning of November until the end of March "northers" are frequent and although usually of short duration, yet they sometimes prevail for days, the cold being intense during their continuance. Snow-storms occur but rarely, generally but one or two during the season, and the quantity of snow which falls is so slight that it soon disappears. Spring may be said to fairly commence early in April, and no degree of cold is experienced before the end of October. Horses and other domestic animals inured to the climate are exposed to the weather during the entire winter with impunity, the low temperature incident to the "northers" above referred to being about all the really cold weather experienced.

For the general plan and arrangement of the post, see Plate IV, Circular No. 4, page 186.

The barracks are nine buildings, constructed of pickets, cut 11 feet long, and set 2 feet in the ground, chinked with mud, and with shingle roofs. They are unceiled and unlined; in height, 9 feet to eaves, and 15 feet to ridge. Three of these buildings are 85 by 20 feet; four, 85 by 20 feet, with wing, 73 by 27 feet; one, 100 by 20 feet; and one, 114 by 27 feet. In rear of each is a building for kitchen and mess-hall, 50 by 18 feet, except for the last, which is of stone, 60 by 16 feet. Fifteen feet at one end of each set of quarters is partitioned off for office and company store-room. The dormitories are fitted with iron bedsteads, and give an average of about 500 cubic feet per man. Ventilation cannot be regulated, and draughts of cold and damp air come in through the crevices.

The floors are full of cracks and holes, through which refuse falls on the ground below.

The company sinks are two stockade-buildings, 22 by 60 feet, placed 300 feet in rear of the barracks. They have boxes; are provided with dry-earth, and cleaned every night, and are in excellent condition.

The quarters for married soldiers and laundresses have been removed to a suitable place on Lost Creek, and consist of about a dozen picket houses, known as "Sudsville."

The officers' quarters are ten buildings, five frame and five of pickets. The frame buildings are one and a half story cottages, ceiled and plastered, with porches in front and rear. The attics have never been finished and are not habitable. Four of these contain each four rooms; one 18 by 18, one 18 by 15, and two 15 by 15 feet. Four of the picket-buildings are 47 by 16, one 73 by 18 feet. These last are unceiled, with rough floors, and without porches. All of these quarters are heated by open fire-places, and ample light and ventilation are secured by windows.

Privies are erected 75 feet in rear of the quarters, having movable troughs, (similar to those in use at the barracks,) which, in accordance with existing regulations at the post, should be emptied and cleaned at an early hour each day.

The adjutant's office is a stockade-building of 47 by 16 feet, divided into three rooms, used as offices by the commanding officer, adjutant, and clerical force employed at post headquarters. The quartermaster's office is a stockade-building of 77 by 16 feet, and is divided into four rooms, two of them furnishing quarters for the post-quartermaster, one used as an office, and the remaining one as quarters for the veterinary surgeon and post quartermaster-sergeant. Both of these buildings are of the same height and description as the stockade-houses for officers, and are suitable for the purpose to which they are applied.

The quartermaster store-house and commissary building are built of sandstone, each 86 by 29 feet, and of a 19-foot story, with a space between them of 20 feet, which was originally designed to be arched and to form an entrance to the fort, it being the central point of its eastern side. This space has been, however, filled by a frame structure built flush with the two store-houses, making them parts of a continuous building. The lower part is used by the commissary officer as a store-room, and the upper floor as his office and a sleeping-room for his subordinates. An upper story or loft in both of the store-houses has been added by laying a floor on the joists, thus securing a space where light stores may be kept.

In addition to this, a stockade building, 90 by 18 by 9 feet, with canvas roof, was erected in 1870, adjoining the north end of the original stone structure, also a similar building, 120 by 27 feet. In 1872, a commissary store-house was built, 103 by 27 by 10 feet, with shingle roof.

The guard-house is built of stone and pickets, is too small, dark, damp, not ventilated, and is unfit for its purpose.

The hospital is built of sandstone, consisting of main building of two stories, 33 by 35 feet, and two wings, 44 by 24 feet, with kitchen, 12 by 20 feet, in rear of the main building. A veranda 12 feet wide surrounds the whole building. The plan of construction is that furnished from the Office of the Surgeon-General, (Circular No. 4, April 27, 1867,) except in a few particulars. Each ward is 33 by 24 feet; contains 12 beds; giving an air-space of 990 cubic feet to each patient, the ceiling being 15 feet high. The arrangement for warming the wards is very bad, for the reason that the pipe does not go out through the ventilator as it should; a long horizontal pipe is now suspended with wires obliquely across the room. Other parts of the building are warmed from fire-places. The bath-rooms, 11 by 9 feet, are furnished with bath-tubs and basins; there are no sink-pipes to carry off the water, and it has to be removed in buckets. Each ward is provided with an earth-closet or commode, which works satisfactorily; two sinks are located 100 feet in rear of the building. The roof of the hospital is very defective, owing to the inferiority of the shingles with which it is covered. There is no laundry, nor laundresses' quarters. The stockade building, 16 by 16 feet, formerly used as laundry, is without a roof, and is now only used for storing old boxes, &c., and for a dead-house.

The post bakery, 26 by 26 feet by 12 feet high to the eaves, is built of stone; has a good oven, with a capacity for 400 rations.

There are 4 stables, each 200 by 35 feet, and one 200 by 30 feet. The post library contains about 600 volumes.

The water-supply is obtained from Lost Creek, and from the several springs situated near its banks, all of which are near the post. The supply of water from this source is good and ample, although containing a slight excess of lime. No cisterns or reservoirs are constructed, although the large area of roofing on the hospital, store-houses, barracks, &c., would serve to collect large quantities of rain-water during the wet season. The post water-wagon (a tank of about 500 gallons capacity) is kept running constantly, by which the officers, troops, hospital, bakery, offices, and laundresses are supplied, and each cavalry company, having a cart of their own, can procure additional supplies for their own use when required. The water thus supplied is depended upon by the enlisted men mainly for cooking purposes, by some also for drinking, and by the officers exclusively for cleansing purposes. There are no means at hand for extinguishing fire except by pails filled with water kept standing in the passages and rooms of the various buildings, with the addition of a few Babcock fire-extinguishers, most of which are believed to be out of order. The natural drainage of the camp is so good that it has not been deemed necessary to improve it by artificial means. The creek cuts its course through the rocks and runs between steep banks shaded with fine trees, the narrow seam of which forms a pleasant relief from the monotonous prairie. It is at most places narrow and shallow, but expands at others into pond-like basins with beautifully clear water. To the great depth of some of these expansions the creek is supposed to owe its name, and they contain an ample supply of good water for the post during the dry season when the creek ceases to run. The heavy rains of the wet season swell the creek not unfrequently to the top of its banks. In 1871 and 1872, the banks of the creek were cut down and roads made by which the water-supply can now be obtained from a point above the drainage into the creek. Slops and refuse around the quarters are collected in barrels, and removed to a distance from the post, there to be buried; that from the stables and sinks is gathered to the same place with equal punctuality; the sink-boxes being drawn out at night and cleaned with a suitable instrument.

As it appears to be intended to continue Fort Richardson as a permanent post for a large garrison, it would be a most important improvement if earth-closets or similar contrivances could be arranged, to be cleaned under contract.

A large water-hole in Lost Creek, below the fort, is used by the troops for bathing purposes, and has never yet failed to have a sufficient depth of water. Except this place, however, no facilities for bathing, either natural or artificial, exist.

The cemetery, located nearly in the center of the reservation and about 400 yards east from the fort, is surrounded by a neat wall, 150 by 150 feet, with gate-ways.

The post garden, containing about two acres, is located on the bank of the creek in the north-western corner of the fort. It is cultivated by the labor of two enlisted men detailed for the purpose, the necessary seeds and implements being purchased from the commissary officer at the expense of the post fund. Sweet potatoes, Lima beans, beets, tomatoes, and lettuce have been produced in limited quantities, but, as before remarked, the irregularity and uncertainty of this climate present almost insurmountable obstacles to the successful prosecution of "truck-gardening" in average seasons.

Milk during the summer season averages about 10 cents per quart, and butter from 25 to 40 cents per pound, while during the winter the former article brings 25 cents per quart, and the latter from 50 to 60 cents per pound. These high prices, in a country where cattle are so abundant, are occasioned by the owners not feeding their stock, but allowing them to depend solely on the herbage they can pick up. Eggs and chickens are proportionately high, the former ranging from 30 to 75 cents per dozen, and the latter from 40 to 75 cents apiece, during the year. Fresh vegetables can seldom be obtained, and command enormous prices for the reasons given above.

The furniture of the barracks has been made by the troops of the garrison, and answers the purpose sufficiently well. That of the officers' quarters (with the exception of a few tables and wardrobes and the shelving in the five frame houses) has been obtained by them from a distance. Owing to the scarcity of lumber, and the small force of mechanics, the officers and men derive but little benefit from the provisions of General Order No. 31, Headquarters of the Army, Adjutant General's Office, Washington, March 21, 1870. The nearest point at which a general assortment of furniture can be procured is Weatherford, in Parker County, and as a matter of course it commands the high prices occasioned by scarcity of material, long and costly transportation, and want of competition.

The routes leading to the post are liable to frequent interruption, owing to the suddenness and rapidity with which the rivers and creeks become converted from almost dry ravines into impassable torrents, in which condition they remain for days after a heavy fall of rain. Bridges are rare, and but little labor being expended on roads in this region, their condition after a continued storm is such as to render teaming difficult.

Daily mails are received from the North and East by way of Dallas and the El Paso stage-line. The passenger-coach runs daily to Weatherford, (40 miles,) and on Tuesday, Thursday, and Saturday to this post, and the mail is brought on the alternate days by dog-cart.

The great majority of the inhabitants in the vicinity of the post are engaged in the cattle business, but little attention being paid to agriculture. The character of the population is such as is peculiar to a frontier country, but less marked by lawlessness than in some other parts of Texas.

Prior to the late war, the population of Jack County was about four-fold what it now is, the settlements having been deserted during the war, owing to the increased danger from Indians, at a time when the fighting-material was engaged elsewhere. The boldness of these predatory Indians is increasing from year to year, the scouting parties sent in pursuit of them failing to overtake or meet them, except in rare instances. It would appear that these bands are principally Kiowa Indians, who draw supplies from the United States Government at the reservations north of the Texas frontier, as the instances in which they have boasted of their exploits, after returning from a plundering and murdering expedition in this region, are numerous and well authenticated. The "Southern Comanches," whose hunting-grounds cover all of the unsettled territory of the State west of the Brazos, are also constantly committing depredations, but it is believed they rarely extend their operations so far east as this post. The settlers in the tiers of frontier counties being widely scattered, bands of savages, frequently numbering hundreds, cross into the State during the first of the moon, divide into small parties, and plunder the country (often fifty miles farther from this post) during the full of the moon, and in the wane pass out of the country and meet at some point far out of reach of pursuit, with large numbers of horses and scalps as the result of their raid. Each month, while the grass lasts, depredations are committed, the settlers living in constant dread Indian raids in 1871, 1872, and 1873 were very numerous. The fact is, that Indians, supposed to have been quietly located on their reservation around the agency at Fort Sill, have

29 M P

been galloping all over the northwestern counties of Texas, howling and shooting around the settlers' cabins, and carrying off hundreds of horses and a few children and scalps every summer. The Comanches, Kiowas, and Apaches raid in company, but as the former constitute about three-fourths of the whole they are the most frequently represented; and as their language is the one always used by the interpreters, and never that of the Kiowas or Apachés, it is very easy to see by what shrewd trick the latter have often been made to father the sins of the former. A train of twelve six-mule teams was captured near here in 1871, and the wagon-master and six of the teamsters killed. Six persons were killed by Indians in the immediate vicinity of this post during the past summer. But the main object of these raids is not to kill or destroy, but to get horses; and to do this, they come stealthily in small parties, and penetrate far in among the thrifty settlements.

The population of Jack County is now about 800. A better class of settlers are seeking location here, and if the danger from Indians could be removed, the surrounding country would speedily fill up with an industrious farming and grazing people.

*Meteorological report, Fort Richardson, Tex., 1872–'74.*

| Month. | 1870–'71. Temperature. Mean. | Max. | Min. | Rain-fall in inches. | 1871–'72. Temperature. Mean. | Max. | Min. | Rain-fall in inches. | 1872–'73. Temperature. Mean. | Max. | Min. | Rain-fall in inches. | 1873–'74. Temperature. Mean. | Max. | Min. | Rain-fall in inches. |
|---|---|---|---|---|---|---|---|---|---|---|---|---|---|---|---|---|
| | ° | ° | ° | | ° | ° | ° | | ° | ° | ° | | ° | ° | ° | |
| July | | | | | | | | | 85. 78 | 98 | 73 | 4. 32 | 83. 45 | 101* | 55* | 0. 64 |
| August | | | | | | | | | 85. 21 | 102* | 61* | 0. 38 | 82. 39 | 105* | 61* | 1. 96 |
| September | | | | | | | | | 78. 15 | 100* | 51* | 2. 08 | 76. 72 | 98* | 52* | 2. 38 |
| October | | | | | | | | | 64. 34 | 93* | 34* | 0. 91 | 61. 86 | 94* | 30* | 0. 18 |
| November | | | | | | | | | 42. 16 | 67* | 8* | 1. 30 | 55. 27 | 80* | 21* | 1. 94 |
| December | | | | | | | | | 36. 29 | 71* | 2* | 1. 02 | 46. 28 | 74 | 22* | 1. 54 |
| January | | | | | | | | | 39. 00 | 73* | −10* | 0. 16 | 44. 60 | 78* | 14* | 1. 34 |
| February | | | | | | | | | 45. 93 | 71* | 10* | 0. 84 | 46. 23 | 76 | 20* | 2. 14 |
| March | | | | | | | | | 58. 65 | 84* | 26* | 0. 96 | 56. 31 | 83* | 33* | 1. 04 |
| April | | | | | | | | | 67. 02 | 94* | 34* | 2. 00 | 56. 67 | 83* | 31* | 2. 80 |
| May | | | | | | | | | 72. 32 | 97* | 51* | 9. 88 | 73. 18 | 96 | 40* | 1. 30 |
| June | | | | | | | | | 78. 01 | 96* | 45* | 4. 12 | 79. 96 | 97 | 56* | 1. 65 |
| For the year | | | | | | | | | 62. 73 | 102* | −10* | 27. 97 | 63. 58 | 105* | 14* | 18. 91 |

*These observations are made with self-registering thermometers. The mean is from the standard thermometer.

*Consolidated sick-report, (white,) Fort Richardson, Tex., 1870–'74.*

| Year | | 1870–'71. | | 1871–'72. | | 1872–'73. | | 1873–'74. | |
|---|---|---|---|---|---|---|---|---|---|
| Mean strength | { Officers | 20 | | 23 | | 15 | | 17 | |
| | { Enlisted men | 368 | | 397 | | 281 | | 169 | |
| Diseases. | | Cases. | Deaths. | Cases. | Deaths. | Cases. | Deaths. | Cases. | Deaths. |
| GENERAL DISEASES, A. | | | | | | | | | |
| Cerebro-spinal fever | | | 1 | | | | | | |
| Typhoid fever | | 4 | | | 1 | 3 | | 1 | |
| Typho-malarial fever | | | | | | 2 | | | |
| Remittent fever | | 7 | 1 | 18 | 3 | 29 | | 1 | |
| Intermittent fever | | 309 | | 91 | 1 | 117 | | 46 | |
| Other diseases of this group | | 4 | | 3 | | 8 | | 1 | |
| GENERAL DISEASES, B. | | | | | | | | | |
| Rheumatism | | 10 | | 30 | | 13 | | 4 | |
| Syphilis | | 17 | | 12 | | 9 | | 6 | |
| Consumption | | 6 | 1 | 1 | | 2 | 1 | 1 | |
| Other diseases of this group | | 2 | | 28 | | 15 | | 1 | |

*Consolidated sick-report, (white,) Fort Richardson, Tex., 1871–'74—Continued.*

| Year | 1870–'71. | | 1871–'72. | | 1872–'73. | | 1873–'74. | |
|---|---|---|---|---|---|---|---|---|
| Mean strength { Officers / Enlisted men | 20 / 368 | | 23 / 397 | | 15 / 281 | | 17 / 169 | |
| Diseases. | Cases. | Deaths. | Cases. | Deaths. | Cases. | Deaths. | Cases. | Deaths. |
| LOCAL DISEASES. | | | | | | | | |
| Catarrh and bronchitis | 30 | ...... | 27 | ...... | 8 | ...... | 15 | ...... |
| Pneumonia | 3 | ...... | 2 | ...... | 23 | ...... | 1 | ...... |
| Pleurisy | 1 | ...... | 1 | ...... | 1 | 1 | 1 | ...... |
| Diarrhœa and dysentery | 81 | ...... | 101 | 3 | 57 | ...... | 34 | ...... |
| Hernia | 2 | ...... | 3 | ...... | | ...... | 1 | ...... |
| Gonorrhœa | 2 | ...... | 17 | ...... | 5 | ...... | 2 | ...... |
| Other local diseases | 142 | ...... | 106 | 2 | 102 | 2 | 96 | ...... |
| Alcoholism | 14 | 1 | 12 | 2 | 5 | 2 | 10 | ...... |
| Unclassified | ...... | 1 | 5 | | | | | |
| Total disease | 634 | 5 | 457 | 12 | 399 | 6 | 221 | ...... |
| VIOLENT DISEASES AND DEATHS. | | | | | | | | |
| Gunshot wounds | 12 | 3 | 7 | 2 | 9 | ...... | 1 | ...... |
| Drowning | ...... | 2 | ...... | | ...... | | ...... | ...... |
| Other accidents and injuries | 69 | 1 | 112 | ...... | 80 | ...... | 50 | ...... |
| Homicide | ...... | ...... | ...... | | ...... | 1 | ...... | ...... |
| Suicide | ...... | ...... | ...... | | ...... | | ...... | 1 |
| Total violence | 81 | 6 | 119 | 2 | 89 | 1 | 51 | 1 |

*Consolidated sick-report, (colored,) Fort Richardson, Tex., 1872–'74.*

| Year | 1872–'73.* | | 1873–'74. | |
|---|---|---|---|---|
| Mean strength .......Enlisted men | 146 | | 154 | |
| Diseases. | Cases. | Deaths. | Cases. | Deaths. |
| GENERAL DISEASES, A. | | | | |
| Typhoid fever | 1 | ...... | ...... | ...... |
| Remittent fever | | ...... | 1 | ...... |
| Intermittent fever | 1 | ...... | 16 | ...... |
| Other diseases of this group | | ...... | 43 | ...... |
| GENERAL DISEASES, B. | | | | |
| Rheumatism | | | 7 | ...... |
| Syphilis | | | 3 | ...... |
| Consumption | | ...... | 1 | ...... |
| Other diseases of this group | | ...... | 1 | ...... |
| LOCAL DISEASES. | | | | |
| Catarrh and bronchitis | | | 12 | ...... |
| Pneumonia | 1 | ...... | 3 | 2 |
| Pleurisy | | | 1 | |
| Diarrhœa and dysentery | 3 | ...... | 30 | ...... |
| Hernia | | | 1 | |
| Gonorrhœa | | ...... | 5 | ...... |
| Other local diseases | 4 | 1 | 93 | ...... |
| Total disease | 10 | 1 | 217 | 2 |
| VIOLENT DISEASES AND DEATHS. | | | | |
| Gunshot wounds | 1 | ...... | 2 | ...... |
| Other accidents and injuries | 15 | ...... | 79 | ...... |
| Total violence | 16 | ...... | 81 | ...... |

\* Five months only.

# RINGGOLD BARRACKS, TEXAS.

### REPORT OF ASSISTANT SURGEON P. F. HARVEY, UNITED STATES ARMY.

Ringgold Barracks, Tex., is situated on the left bank of the Rio Grande, in latitude 26° 23′ north, longitude 21° 50′ west, and half a mile southeast of Rio Grande City, a post village, port of entry, and capital of Starr County. With reference to adjacent military posts and towns the post is located 5 miles north of Camargo, Mexico, 110 miles north of Fort Brown, Tex., 120 miles southeast of Fort McIntosh, Tex., and 280 miles south of San Antonio, Tex. Its height above the level of the sea has been estimated by barometer at 521 feet, an estimate probably somewhat in excess of its true altitude.

The history of the post comprehends but little of general interest and may be summed up in the statement that it was first established October 26, 1848, at Davis Landing, by Companies C and G, First United States Infantry, commanded by Capt. J. H. La Motte, and called "Camp Ringgold." By General Order No. 8, Headquarters of the Army, of July 16, 1849, its designation was changed to "Ringgold Barracks." Troops were withdrawn therefrom March 3, 1859, and it was re-occupied December 29, 1859. Troops were again withdrawn March 7, 1861, and the post re-occupied June, 1865. Established at the time of hostility with Mexico, the site was evidently selected by reason of its proximity to Camargo as a suitable point for the surveillance of our neighbor's territory in that vicinity, and from its situation at the head of steam navigation as a convenient point for the distribution of supplies.

*Geology.*—The general aspect of the adjoining country is that of a plain, intersected by arroyos, covered with chaparral, and broken along the river by a range of abrupt hills. As we recede to the interior this character gives place to the prairie covered with luxuriant grass. Superficially the formation belongs to the tertiary period, although the hills present denudations which are referable to the preceding system. A short distance from the post, and in the vicinity of Las Cuevas, strata of cretaceous sandstone, 10 or 15 feet thick, are exposed, assisting at the latter place in the formation of the caves from which it takes its name. Some miles west from the post, the bluffs bordering the river are composed of yellowish sandstone, containing ferruginous nodules, and beds of enormous fossil oyster-shells, some of them 18 inches in length, are found in the same vicinity. Sprinkled copiously over the hills are deposits of sand, gravel, and pebbles. Composed of a diversity of material and smoothed and rounded by the process of attrition, they give evidence of having been transported here from remote sections by the operations of water. Among them may be found specimens of dendritic and fortification agate, septaria, jasper, bloodstone, and other siliceous minerals; breccia and calcareous conglomerates are occasionally met with.

The river-bed, aside from its shifting deposits of mud and sand, is composed of an argillaceous sandstone, in which concretions of impure carbonate of lime constitute a prominent ingredient. When the bed is exposed by low water, it is seen to be fissured in some places, giving to it a somewhat tessellated appearance. At such times curious veins of chalcedony, about one-half inch thick, and evidently produced by the infiltration of water holding siliceous matter in solution, are exposed and can be seen traversing the sandstone from the bank to the river. Petrefactions of wood are frequent, owing to the circumstances just mentioned. The interior portion of the hills consists mainly of carbonate of lime. Mica exists sparingly in some localities in the neighborhood. Thin incrustations or stains of a white color are noticeable on pebbles, glass, or other hard substances, exposed for any length of time to the washings from the hills, and are caused by the evaporation of water holding lime in solution, and lime is disseminated through the soil by the same process. Common salt is found by analysis in the soil, and in certain neighboring localities exists in abundance. About fifty miles east, in Hidalgo County, and some miles back from the river, there are several lagoons, the waters of which are strongly impregnated and the shores thickly incrusted with salt of merchantable quality. This is carted away by the Mexicans in large quantities, and forms an article of considerable traffic among them.

The soil of this region, as may be inferred, is generally arid and unfavorable to cultivation, but some part of it, along the river-bottoms, is rich friable loam, mixed indeed with sand, but not to such an extent as to prevent the culture of the most exhausting products. The most serious barriers to agriculture are the prolonged periods of drought and the excessive solar heat experienced during the seasons of planting and growth. At the cost of considerable labor and by some ingenuity, corn, pease, melons, squashes, &c., may be raised, but they do not arrive at the same excellence either as to size or taste as the same in more northern regions. It seems impossible to grow potatoes of an edible quality, and difficult to produce them of any kind in this soil. They, as indeed almost every vegetable used at this post, are supplied by the Subsistence Department. About the only exception to the above are the onions and beans, (frejoles,) which are abundant and excellent. During the winter months the markets are supplied with delicious oranges from Mexico. The material wealth of the country at large will receive but slight, if any, contribution from this section until nature or man does more for it in the way of increasing its fruitfulness. Railroads and artesian-wells would inaugurate a new and better condition of affairs undoubtedly, but they are expensive experiments. Holding out such meager inducements to the farmer or artisan, this vicinity has drawn principally from our country the non-producer, the adventurer, who chafes under the restraints of civilization, and others of that ilk, and until the more attractive parts of our continent are occupied, the prospect of a progressive class of immigration settling in these parts is extremely small.

A stranger is struck by the dwarfed appearance and paucity of vegetation, and the singularly uninteresting and uninviting appearance in general of the face of nature; but, notwithstanding, the flora of the country possesses several trees and plants highly interesting from their economic value.

A general survey shows the vegetation to be liliputian, meager, and armed freely with thorns, and consisting chiefly of mesquite and cactus.

The other plants, like the latter, present to the air the smallest surface compatible with their bulk, which adapts them to the seasons of heat and drought. In some of the alluvial bottoms bordering the river the mesquite, palo-blanco, roisache, and some other trees flourish well, and attain a considerable size, but elsewhere, and far more generally, the trees are small, and contain a scanty foliage. Grass is rarely or never seen during the dry season, the ground presenting a barren and parched appearance. The Mexicans feed their cattle upon the *opuntia*, or prickly-pear cactus, which is first subjected to fire for the removal of its thorns. This constitutes their exclusive food in some cases. The *opuntia* grows more abundantly in this neighborhood than any other variety of cactus. The cattle eat it as they roam through the chaparral, notwithstanding the needle-like spines with which it bristles. Their tongues are filled with the points, and our tables deprived of that commodity. Freed from its thorns, warmed and split open, the *opuntia* is used by the Mexicans as a cataplasm, and from my limited experience in its use, I judge that it fairly answers the purpose. It combines a slightly irritant with its emollient action, and for this reason is objectionable in some cases. The *petayah*, a species of small columnar cactus, which grows in tufts containing about a dozen stalks, usually about the roots of the mesquite or other trees, bears an edible berry, which is served on the table with milk, or wine and sugar, and possesses some of the characteristics of the strawberry.

A species of *Echinocactus*, the Turk's-head, grows sparsely in this vicinity. In Mexico, it is cut in slices, boiled in sugar, and sold as *dulce*. As it grows, it is armed with formidable spines of iron-like hardness, and so firmly fixed in its substance, and of such strength, as to readily pierce a horse's hoof, or the sole of an ordinary shoe.

Guaiacum wood, or *lignum-vitæ*, is furnished by a small tree of the genus.

The common growth of the country is the mesquite, (*Algarobia glandulosa*, Torry,) allied to the gum-producing acaciæ in its botanical affinities and habits, and first described by Dr. Edward James, about fifty years ago. The plants belonging to this genus are trees or shrubs, generally the latter, thorny, and bearing a thin, feathery-looking foliage. The fruit is a long, curved, somewhat compressed loment, containing a sweet pulp, in which the seeds are lodged. The matrix containing the seed is very nutritious, and is much used by the Mexicans for feeding cattle. A kind of beer is said to be manufactured from the pods by the Mexicans and Indians, both on the American and Mexican side, as also sugar, and a meal used for making cakes. A gum exudes where the bark is wounded, and concretes on exposure; it resembles gum-arabic in its physical characteristics, as it does also in its ultimate composition. Dissolved in water, it serves excellently as mucilage, and possesses demulcent properties of a high order. The mesquite is probably analogous to the algarobra bean, consumed in South Spain by horses, and used in England as a substitute for oil-cake; supposed also to have been the food of Saint John in the wilderness, and to have furnished the seed used originally as the carat-weight by jewelers. The sap-wood is light in color, while the duramen is hard, and of a reddish-brown color. The mesquite furnishes almost exclusively the wood used for fuel at the post and in the vicinity. One porch, the lower story of the hospital administration building, and the porches and lower stories of two of the barracks are floored with hexagonal blocks of the same wood, which makes a comely, vermin-proof, and almost indestructible pavement.

The American aloe, or maguey, (*Agave Americana*,) aptly styled by Prescott the "Miracle of Nature," grows sparsely in this vicinity, but not in sufficient quantity to be used in the fabrication of any of the commodities obtained from it in Mexico, although it would readily admit of cultivation. When cut the root and leaves yield a saccharine juice, which, by evaporation, is converted into sirup and even sugar, and by fermentation affords a vinous liquor. The flower-stalk is said to attain the height of 40 feet at the time of inflorescence, which, contrary to former belief, takes place in favorable localities once in about fifteen years. From this flower-stem the beverage called *pulque*, *octli*, or *agave wine* is obtained, and from the latter the ardent spirit called *mescal* is distilled. According to Assistant Surgeon (now Surgeon) G. Perin, United States Army, the fresh-expressed juice of the plant is an excellent antiscorbutic, much better than lime-juice. He gave it to the extent of about half a pint per day. Assistant Surgeon Moses found its use objectionable on account of its cathartic effects. Happily there has existed no necessity for its use for the purpose in question during my stay at this post, the improved dietary of the Army rendering the occurrence of scurvy highly improbable. A substitute for soap is obtained by evaporating the juice of the leaves to the consistence of a soft extract, which forms a lather with water. The fibers of the old leaves furnish a substitute for pins and needles; the cellular structure is woven into cloth, and is also used for thatching huts; and the root is cooked and used as food.

A species of Yucca, the Spanish bayonet, is met with here and there in this vicinity. The panicle of white flowers rising from its crown of lanceolate leaves is showy, and serves as a ready-made bouquet. The root, taken as far under ground as possible, is used as a substitute for soap.

A small shrub, called by the Mexicans *vrago*, grows abundantly in this vicinity, and possesses considerable interest from its domestic applications. From the end of a freshly-cut section, a sap exudes, possessing astringent properties, probably due to the presence of tannic acid and capable of making an indelible mark on linen. Handkerchiefs marked by the writer over a year ago still retain their marks with perfect distinctness. The linen at first shows no mark, but in the process of washing, the iron contained in the water unites with the tannin, producing the characteristic reaction. The plant is also used to cleanse the teeth and to harden the gums, and takes from that circumstance the name of Mexican tooth-brush.

The ebony tree is indigenous, but is neither large in size nor abundant in growth.

The peccary or Texas hog, Mexican leopard, wild-cat, armadillo, rabbit, squirrel, deer, beaver, raccoon, and coyote are the most common wild animals of the vicinity. The gar and cat-fish are the only fish found in the river at this point.

The birds are varied, and some of them very beautiful.

The snakes of the vicinity embrace several innocuous and two or three venomous species. The latter are prominently represented by the common rattlesnake, and the prairie rattlesnake, *Crotalophorus tergeminus*, Holbr. The former are a source of dread to the new-comer and the timid, and not without reason, as many have been killed within the purlieus of the post, and not unfrequently after nightfall they make their way into the quarters. One, recently killed in a neighboring *jacal*, measured at least six feet in length, and possessed upward of thirty rattles.

The centipede, (*Scolopendra*, several species,) tarantula, so called, but properly, I think, the crab-spider, (*mygale cancerides*,) scorpion, galley-worm, (*Julus*,) and numberless spiders find a favorite habitat and flourish without restraint in this locality, both numerically and in magnitude. Of ants the most formidable is the scarlet mutilla. The female, although destitute of wings, is armed with a powerful sting. The weapon is as long as the abdomen, and the writer testifies from personal experience to the poisonous wound it is capable of inflicting. The animal is a sand-borer. Other ants (*Formicidæ*) abound, the red, black, brown, &c., burrowing the ground and stripping trees of their foliage.

The river is the main source of supply of water for all purposes, and furnishes at best a very inferior article. During its low stage it is clear but saturated with salts of lime and other minerals, which impart to it a harsh, disagreeable taste; and during its high stage the amount of earthy and organic detritus borne along by its rapid current renders it turbid and offensive to taste and smell. It requires filtering to make it potable, and frequently must be allowed to settle some time before it is even fit for washing purposes. There are three cisterns at the post, but the water they contain is generally foul and unfit for any purpose but washing, owing to the infrequency of rain and high temperature. A thorough cleansing before the rainy season sets in, and afterward charcoal in bags suspended in the water, would remedy this.

There are no means of subduing fire at the hospital, and a cistern is very much needed for this and other reasons. There are no springs, wells, or ponds in the vicinity.

The climate in the aggregate is subtropical, but torrid heats prevail during the summer months. During the hotter periods of the year the mercury indicates a temperature of over 100° in the shade for weeks at a time occasionally. At such times hot, dry winds, comparable to the simooms of Arabia, blow from the parched plateaus of Mexico, wilting vegetation and compelling the closure of doors and windows to exclude the dust and heat. The prevailing winds for all seasons are from the southeast. Sudden storms of wind from the north, with or without rain, attended with rapid lowering of temperature, called wet or dry northers, are frequent in winter. The atmosphere is generally dry; beef used by the Mexicans is prepared and preserved by drying in the open air, desiccation taking place rapidly and thoroughly. The rain-fall is trivial, entirely inadequate for agricultural purposes. The rain-fall for the past season, however, was unusually great. Snow is unknown.

*Diarrhœa and dysentery* may be regarded as the prevailing diseases. They are generally of a mild grade and greatest frequency during the summer months, and are, no doubt, caused by errors in diet, drinking large quantities of water, and exposure to draughts of air while heated. The use of a diet largely composed of azotized matter, for which the negro manifests a predilection, during the heated term, also engenders bowel diseases.

*Rheumatism and neuralgia* prevail to a considerable extent. The effects of malaria have not been sufficiently marked to ascribe to it an undoubted genetic connection with these diseases, but from the curative action of quinine in some cases it is probable that it has been an element in their causation. But exposure to variation of temperature and the sudden arrest of cutaneous transpiration, acting on a system relaxed and enervated by the excessive summer-heat, is to my mind the most probable etiology. Many cases of well-marked hemicrania, *migraine* or nervous sick-headache, have been observed in this locality, induced, no doubt, by the solar glare and debilitating heats of summer, and yielding to antispasmodics and nerve tonics. The cooler seasons are exempt from this affection.

*Diseases of the lungs and air-passages* were of infrequent occurrence and mild grade.

*Catarrhal affections* were most prevalent during the winter months, and were due to climatic influences, sudden changes of temperature, and a neglect to guard against them by the proper precautions. It is not a rarity to observe a fall of 40° Fahrenheit in the course of twelve hours at this post, and greater variations occur occasionally.

*Malarial fevers* were rare among the troops, their immunity being largely due, no doubt, to the well-known idiosyncracies of the negro race, as diseases of this class were much more frequent when white troops formed the garrison. It would seem, however, that there is but little evolution of malaria in this vicinity, as the climate is dry, the vegetation scant, and the soil sandy and deficient in organic constituents.

The limits of the post are kept well policed and in good sanitary condition, but back of the cavalry stables, in the immediate vicinity of the post, the ground is covered with great quantities of refuse from stables and post, which, if left to be acted upon by the high temperature, will decay and furnish abundant food for disease. Recommendations have been made for its removal.

The post is divisible into two distinct portions, that which is left standing of the old post consisting of frame buildings, viz, a two-story barrack, now used as quartermaster's and commissary storehouse, and four one-story buildings, used as officers' quarters and divided into seven sets. They stand near the river, and are old, cheerless, and dilapidated. On this part of the reservation are also the post-trader's store, the workshops, quartermaster's corral, hay-yard, wood-pile, and officers' stables.

The new post, standing farther back from the river, is built of brick. Its construction was commenced in 1869, and it is still unfinished, the appropriation having been exhausted some time ago, and an appropriation of additional funds for its completion having been refused. It is composed of the following buildings: Four company-barracks; five buildings for officers' quarters, divided into nine sets; hospital, (incomplete;) bakery; guard-house, and adjutant's office. For plan of the post, see Plate opposite.

The barracks are each two stories high, 135 feet long by 40 feet wide, the latter inclusive of a porch in front and rear 9 feet wide, supported by Moorish arches. Each building contains, on the first floor, a reading-room, a wash-room, a dining-room, a squad-drill room, a store-room, a company office, and a room for the first sergeant. The second story is occupied as a dormitory. Iron bunks are used, and each soldier has a separate bed, provided with two blankets and one single bedsack filled with hay. All the rooms and the dormitory are amply provided with the necessary fixtures and furniture. Each barrack was intended for one company, but the increase of the command has made it necessary to quarter four of the smaller companies in two of the buildings, which has resulted in no special inconvenience, as they are sufficiently spacious to accommodate one hundred men each. Two sets are used by the infantry and two by the cavalry. Those of the infantry are built facing the line of officers' quarters. At right angles to these, and running back, are the two cavalry barracks, one at either extremity, forming three sides of an oblong square, the line of laundresses' tents completing the square, as shown in the diagram. The parade-ground lies between the officers' and infantry quarters, and is flanked on one side by the hospital and on the other by the adjutant's office, guard-house, and bakery. The kitchens in rear of the company barracks are two small pent-roof structures, detached from the main building and furnished with ranges and shelves. The cavalry quarters have their kitchens in the lower stories, adjoining the dining-room, an objectionable arrangement in this hot climate, for obvious reasons.

The officers' quarters are each 54 feet long and one and one-half stories high. Excepting the commanding officer's quarters, each building has two halls, each 7 feet wide, running through the center from front to rear. A partition separating the halls divides the building into halves, each half forming a set of quarters and containing four rooms, two on the lower and two on the upper floor, each 18 feet square. The commanding officer's house is 40 feet wide, 50 feet long, and has a hall 10 feet wide running through the center. It contains six rooms, each 18 by 18 feet, and one 18 by 36 feet. Each set of quarters is provided with dining-room, kitchen, and out-houses, communicating with the first floor by means of a covered and latticed way.

The bakery is 43 by 34 feet, has a porch in front 12 feet wide, and contains a sleeping-room, store-room, bake-room, and two ovens.

The guard-house is of the same dimensions as the bakery. It contains a guard-room, 20 by 16 feet, and a prison-room of the same size. There are, also, three cells between the two rooms, each 4 by 8 feet. The average occupancy is 20, giving about 250 cubic feet of air-space to each prisoner. The ventilation of the prison-room is effected by means of four small barred windows near the ceiling. It is entirely inadequate for the number of occupants.

The adjutant's office is an oblong building, recently built, and contains three rooms, each 18 by 18 feet.

The library is in a small brick building, situated in the old post, formerly used as a magazine. The library contains about 500 volumes, and receives most of the leading periodicals of the day.

The quartermaster's and commissary store-room is in the old company barracks, already spoken of, situated on the river bank. It is old, rickety, and infested with vermin. Aside from its insecurity, it is unfit for public stores, particularly commissary articles, on account of the damage and destruction wrought by insects. It is poor economy to delay the construction of a suitable store-house any longer.

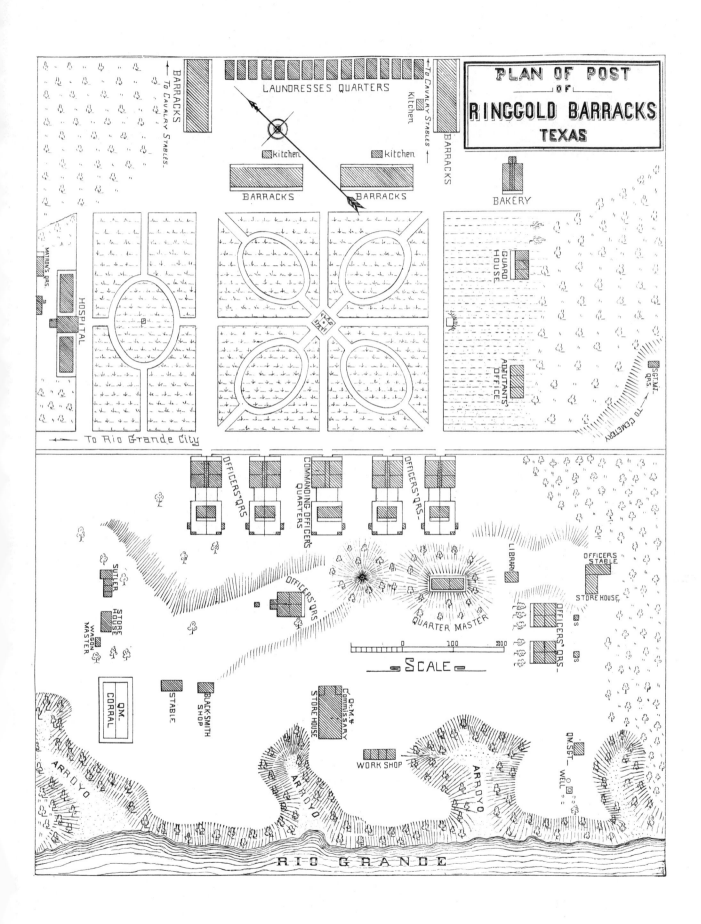

PLAN OF POST
OF
RINGGOLD BARRACKS
TEXAS

BARRACKS
To Cavalry Stables.

LAUNDRESSES QUARTERS

To Cavalry Stables →

Kitchen

BARRACKS

kitchen

kitchen

BARRACKS

BARRACKS

BAKERY

MATRON'S QRS.

HOSPITAL

FLAG STAFF

GUARD HOUSE

ADJUTANTS' OFFICE

SGT. MJ. QRS.

TO CEMETERY

← To Rio Grande City

OFFICERS' QRS

COMMANDING OFFICERS QUARTERS

OFFICERS' QRS.

OFFICERS' QRS.

SUTLER

STORE HOUSE

WAGON MASTER

OFFICERS' QRS

LIBRARY

OFFICERS STABLE

STORE HOUSE

OFFICERS' QRS.

QUARTER MASTER

0      100      200

SCALE

QM. CORRAL

STABLE

BLACK SMITH SHOP

STORE HOUSE

Q. M. & Commissary

WORK SHOP

QM.SGT.

WELL

ARROYO

ARROYO

ARROYO

RIO GRANDE

The stables, of which there are four, are temporary makeshifts, built of upright beams, supporting a brush roof.

The company sinks are pits dug at the rear of company quarters, and inclosed by an adobe wall. They are poor affairs, but the best that can be made with the material on hand.

The ration is ample in quantity and fair in quality. Special efforts should be made by the Subsistence Department to furnish remote stations, such as this, with a full assortment of supplies, as very little for the table can be obtained from any other source. Milk, eggs, and chickens can be bought at reasonable prices. Milk, 50 cents a gallon; eggs, 25 to 50 cents a dozen; chickens, 25 cents each.

There is no garden at the post. Efforts were made last spring to cultivate one, and a good-sized piece of ground was fenced in and worked, but without success.

The hospital was first occupied November 25, 1870. It is a brick structure, built in accordance with the approved plan from the Surgeon-General's Office. It is 190 feet long, and is surrounded by a porch 12 feet wide, supported by Moorish arches 15 feet high. It consists of a central administration building, 37½ by 36 feet, two stories high, flanked on each side by a ward, each 20 by 40 feet. The central building has on the first floor an office, dispensary, and store-room, each 14 by 14 feet, and a dining-room, 20 by 14 feet. Back of these is the kitchen, 12 by 14 feet. It contains a pantry. The second story has corresponding rooms, used as store-rooms, steward's room, and prison. The furniture and fixtures are ample throughout the building. Each ward contains 12 beds. Adjoining each ward is a store-room for men's clothing, and a wash-room, each 12 by 14 feet. Both wards are occupied, although only one is finished; the unfinished one requiring a ceiling and paving for the porch.

The laundresses are quartered in tents pitched on frame supports at the rear of the company barracks. The structures, variously patched with boards, barrel-staves, gunny-bags, &c., and occupying a conspicuous position, detract from the comely appearance of the garrison. They are open to the additional and weightier objection of being too poorly ventilated and lighted, and too cramped for healthful or comfortable occupation by human beings. The remedy is obvious, but not likely to be applied, from the difficulty of obtaining funds.

There is steam-communication by river between this post and Brownsville; thence by rail to Point Isabel, and from there by ocean-steamer to New Orleans. Steamers from New Orleans arrive semi-monthly. Mail from the north is received once per week; from Laredo, once; and from Brownsville, twice weekly. Seven to ten days are required for a letter to go to department headquarters, and two weeks or longer to go to Washington.

The inhabitants in this vicinity are mostly natives of Mexico, engaged in stock-raising, herding, small traffic, such as peddling, &c. Indian blood flows in their veins, as denoted by their swarthy complexion, high cheek-bones, and non-progressiveness.

*Meteorological report, Ringgold Barracks, Tex., 1870–'74.*

| Months. | 1870–'71. | | | | 1871–'72. | | | | 1872–'73. | | | | 1873–'74. | | | |
|---|---|---|---|---|---|---|---|---|---|---|---|---|---|---|---|---|
| | Temperature. | | | Rain-fall in inches. | Temperature. | | | Rain-fall in inches. | Temperature. | | | Rain-fall in inches. | Temperature. | | | Rain-fall in inches. |
| | Mean. | Max. | Min. | | Mean. | Max. | Min. | | Mean. | Max. | Min. | | Mean. | Max. | Min. | |
| July | 88.13 | 106 | 76 | 0.61 | 87.16 | 101 | 79 | 0.00 | 88.69 | 103* | 72* | 1.66 | 86.71 | 104* | 69* | 1.72 |
| August | 86.90 | 105 | 75 | 2.48 | 89.54 | 105 | 81 | 0.70 | 86.64 | 103* | 73* | 4.38 | 86.69 | 103* | 70* | 0.88 |
| September | 86.53 | 105 | 70 | 2.92 | 84.76 | 99 | 69 | 1.14 | 84.91 | 100* | 72* | 0.94 | 82.34 | 99 | 60* | 7.26 |
| October | 76.17 | 94 | 44 | 0.00 | 74.07 | 90 | 54 | 3.42 | 75.17 | 95* | 40* | 1.22 | 73.51 | 93 | 40* | 0.85 |
| November | 67.22 | 95 | 34 | 0.52 | 68.05 | 92 | 42 | 0.22 | 61.24 | 89* | 22* | 3.10 | 65.14 | 86 | 32* | 1.58 |
| December | 54.20 | 79 | 27 | 0.86 | 59.52 | 85 | 31 | 0.00 | 58.02 | 83* | 29* | 1.16 | 58.04 | 86 | 24* | 0.26 |
| January | 59.32 | 81 | 32 | 0.86 | 55.67* | 84* | 29* | 0.36 | 54.92 | 79* | 20* | 0.00 | 61.79 | 87 | 31* | 0.16 |
| February | 68.11 | 92 | 42 | 0.00 | 64.79 | 95* | 32* | 0.00 | 68.36 | 94* | 40* | 0.16 | 64.45 | 92 | 32* | 0.28 |
| March | 72.73 | 92 | 42 | 0.05 | 70.87 | 95* | 45* | 0.76 | 72.84 | 97* | 41* | 0.28 | 74.16 | 99* | 52* | 2.64 |
| April | 78.85 | 102 | 46 | 0.00 | 81.07 | 102* | 60* | 0.66 | 73.40 | 97 | 30* | 2.56 | 72.64 | 101 | 47* | 0.00 |
| May | 82.42 | 109 | 68 | 1.28 | 85.37 | 105* | 55* | 0.00 | 83.28 | 106 | 56* | 2.42 | 79.94 | 101 | 49* | 1.44 |
| June | 86.01 | 104 | 72 | 1.81 | 86.44 | 103* | 70* | 0.52 | 86.19 | 105* | 65* | 1.66 | 83.39 | 99 | 70* | 3.22 |
| For the year | 75.55 | 109 | 27 | 11.39 | 75.61 | 105* | 29* | 7.78 | 74.47 | 106 | 20* | 19.54 | 74.07 | 104* | 24* | 20.29 |

* These observations are made with self-registering thermometers. The mean is from the standard thermometer.

30 M P

*Consolidated sick-report, (white,) Ringgold Barracks, Tex., 1870–'74.*

| Year | 1870–'71. | | 1871–'72. | | 1872–'73.* | | 1873–'74.† | |
|---|---|---|---|---|---|---|---|---|
| Mean strength { Officers / Enlisted men } | 12 / 250 | | 8 / 133 | | 10 / 64 | | 15 / 1 | |
| Diseases. | Cases. | Deaths. | Cases. | Deaths. | Cases. | Deaths. | Cases. | Deaths. |
| GENERAL DISEASES, A. | | | | | | | | |
| Typhoid fever | 3 | 1 | | | | | | |
| Typho-malarial fever | | | 1 | | | 1 | | |
| Remittent fever | 133 | 3 | 11 | | | | 3 | |
| Intermittent fever | 21 | 1 | 42 | | 13 | | 2 | |
| Other diseases of this group | 4 | | 3 | | | | | |
| GENERAL DISEASES, B. | | | | | | | | |
| Rheumatism | 10 | | 11 | | 4 | | | |
| Syphilis | 7 | | 9 | | 3 | | | |
| Consumption | 2 | | 5 | | | | | |
| Other diseases of this group | 1 | | 7 | | | | 1 | |
| LOCAL DISEASES. | | | | | | | | |
| Catarrh and bronchitis | 5 | | 5 | | | | | |
| Pleurisy | 4 | | 9 | | | | 1 | |
| Diarrhœa and dysentery | 43 | | 73 | | 24 | | 2 | |
| Hernia | | | 6 | | 3 | | | |
| Gonorrhœa | 7 | | 3 | | | | | |
| Other local diseases | 104 | 4 | 74 | | 15 | | 11 | |
| Alcoholism | 10 | | 11 | | 4 | | 1 | |
| Total disease | 354 | 9 | 270 | | 66 | 1 | 21 | |
| VIOLENT DISEASES AND DEATHS. | | | | | | | | |
| Gun-shot wounds | 1 | | | | | | | |
| Drowning | | 1 | | 1 | | | | |
| Other accidents and injuries | 35 | | 44 | 1 | 9 | | 1 | |
| Homicide | | 1 | | | | | | |
| Total violence | 36 | 2 | 44 | 2 | 9 | | 1 | |

\* Six months only.  † Two months only.

*Consolidated sick-report, (colored,) Ringgold Barracks, Tex., 1871–'74.*

| Year | 1871–'72.* | | 1872–'73. | | 1873–'74. | |
|---|---|---|---|---|---|---|
| Mean strength — Enlisted men | 47 | | 182 | | 332 | |
| Diseases. | Cases. | Deaths. | Cases. | Deaths. | Cases. | Deaths. |
| GENERAL DISEASES, A. | | | | | | |
| Small-pox and varioloid | | | | | 1 | 1 |
| Typho-malarial fever | | | 2 | 1 | | |
| Remittent fever | 1 | | 3 | | 10 | |
| Intermittent fever | 1 | | 14 | | 29 | |
| Other diseases of this group | | | 4 | | 29 | |
| GENERAL DISEASES, B. | | | | | | |
| Rheumatism | | | 13 | | 56 | |
| Syphilis | | | 5 | | 27 | |
| Other diseases of this group | | | 2 | | 7 | |
| LOCAL DISEASES. | | | | | | |
| Catarrh and bronchitis | 1 | | 8 | | 28 | |
| Pneumonia | | | | 1 | | |
| Pleurisy | | | 12 | | 6 | |
| Diarrhœa and dysentery | 4 | | 42 | | 75 | 1 |
| Gonorrhœa | | | 2 | | 28 | |
| Other local diseases | 1 | | 69 | | 181 | |
| Total disease | 9 | | 176 | 2 | 477 | 2 |
| VIOLENT DISEASES AND DEATHS. | | | | | | |
| Gun-shot wounds | | | 2 | | 5 | |
| Drowning | | | | | | 1 |
| Other accidents and injuries | 1 | | 18 | | 88 | |
| Total violence | 1 | | 20 | | 93 | 1 |

\* Two months only ; first report, May, 1872.

# SAN ANTONIO, TEXAS.

The town of San Antonio is situated in Bexar County, Texas, in latitude 29° 30′ north, longitude 21° 25′ west. It is the headquarters of the Military Department of Texas, and was also a military station up to August, 1873, when the troops were withdrawn. The post was within the corporate limits of the town. The buildings occupied were the Alamo, a strong inclosure, dating from 1744, and a number of private houses rented from citizens. For the history and topography of the place, see Circular No. 4, Surgeon-General's Office, December 5, 1870.

*Meteorological report, San Antonio, Tex., 1870–'73.*

| Month. | 1870–'71. | | | | 1871–'72. | | | | 1872–'73. | | | | 1873–'74. | | | |
|---|---|---|---|---|---|---|---|---|---|---|---|---|---|---|---|---|
| | Mean. | Max. | Min. | Rain-fall in inches. | Mean. | Max. | Min. | Rain-fall in inches. | Mean. | Max. | Min. | Rain-fall in inches. | Mean. | Max. | Min. | Rain-fall in inches. |
| July | 83.76 | 102* | 68* | 3.72 | 88.80 | 108* | 62* | 0.00 | 84.96 | 101* | 72 | 1.84 | 83.78 | 100* | 60* | 2.10 |
| August | 82.54 | 99* | 60* | 6.48 | 88.37 | 109* | 75 | 0.95 | 84.86 | 105* | 72 | 1.62 | | | | |
| September | 80.68 | 101* | 54* | 1.95 | 79.54 | 100* | 58 | 5.81 | 84.32 | 102* | 63 | 0.05 | | | | |
| October | 69.71 | 90* | 36* | 2.80 | 68.57 | 89* | 46 | 6.65 | 70.29 | 96* | 46 | 1.69 | | | | |
| November | 61.46 | 89* | 29* | 3.58 | 58.39 | 83* | 32 | 1.92 | 55.52 | 90* | 27 | 2.19 | | | | |
| December | 47.82 | 77* | 14* | 0.60 | 51.02 | 83* | 25 | 0.00 | 48.75 | 82* | 21 | 2.10 | | | | |
| January | 53.25 | 76* | 23* | 1.38 | 47.17 | 75* | 21 | 0.40 | 48.95 | 75* | 17 | 1.14 | | | | |
| February | 58.74 | 85* | 28* | 0.60 | 55.54 | 84* | 28 | 1.56 | 58.51 | 84 | 36 | 0.47 | | | | |
| March | 63.14 | 90* | 35* | 1.10 | 59.96 | 87* | 31 | 1.14 | 68.08 | 99 | 35 | 1.95 | | | | |
| April | 69.72 | 94* | 32* | 0.76 | 73.01 | 98* | 52 | 0.70 | 68.16 | 95 | 31* | 0.52 | | | | |
| May | 76.85 | 98* | 47* | 3.44 | 77.87 | 98* | 55 | 4.58 | 77.76 | 107 | 46* | 3.71 | | | | |
| June | 83.88 | 108* | 63* | 0.18 | 82.55 | 99* | 68 | 8.30 | 80.24 | 98 | 63* | 6.99 | | | | |
| For the year | 69.28 | 108* | 14* | 26.59 | 69.23 | 109* | 21 | 32.01 | 69.20 | 107 | 17 | 24.27 | | | | |

* These observations are made with self-registering thermometers. The mean is from the standard thermometer.

*Consolidated sick-report, (white,) San Antonio, Tex., 1870–'74.*

| Year | 1870–'71. | | 1871–'72. | | 1872–'73. | | 1873–'74. | |
|---|---|---|---|---|---|---|---|---|
| Mean strength { Officers / Enlisted men | 18 / 147 | | 19 / 127 | | 18 / 55 | | 8* / 26† | |
| Diseases. | Cases. | Deaths. | Cases. | Deaths. | Cases. | Deaths. | Cases. | Deaths. |
| GENERAL DISEASES, A. | | | | | | | | |
| Typhoid fever | | | 2 | 1 | 1 | 1 | | |
| Remittent fever | 2 | | 15 | | | | | |
| Intermittent fever | 27 | | 14 | | 5 | | 1 | |
| Other diseases of this group | 4 | | 3 | | 2 | | | |
| GENERAL DISEASES, B. | | | | | | | | |
| Rheumatism | 7 | | 9 | | 4 | | | |
| Syphilis | 16 | | 20 | | 3 | | | |
| Consumption | 3 | 1 | | | 1 | | | |
| LOCAL DISEASES. | | | | | | | | |
| Catarrh and bronchitis | 22 | | 8 | | 1 | | | |
| Pneumonia | | | 1 | | | | | |
| Pleurisy | | | 1 | | | | | |
| Diarrhœa and dysentery | 34 | | 60 | | 15 | | 2 | |
| Hernia | | | | | 1 | | | |
| Gonorrhœa | 17 | | 13 | | | | | |
| Other local diseases | 63 | | 47 | 2 | 23 | | 1 | |
| Alcoholism | 8 | | 5 | | 2 | | | |
| Total disease | 203 | 1 | 198 | 3 | 58 | 1 | 4 | |
| VIOLENT DISEASES AND DEATHS. | | | | | | | | |
| Gunshot wounds | 1 | | 1 | | | | | |
| Drowning | | 2 | | 1 | | 1 | | |
| Other accidents and injuries | 30 | | 35 | | 9 | | | |
| Suicide | | 2 | | | | | | |
| Total violence | 31 | 4 | 36 | 1 | 9 | 1 | | |

* Nine months only.          † Three months only.

*Consolidated sick-report, (colored,) San Antonio, Tex., 1870-'74.*

| Year | 1870-'71.* | | 1871-'72.† | | 1872-'73. | | 1873-'74.‡ | |
|---|---|---|---|---|---|---|---|---|
| Mean strength ...... Enlisted men | 16 | | 68 | | 56 | | 36 | |
| Diseases. | Cases. | Deaths. | Cases. | Deaths. | Cases. | Deaths. | Cases. | Deaths. |
| GENERAL DISEASES, A. | | | | | | | | |
| Small-pox and varioloid | | | 1 | | | | | |
| Typhoid fever | | | 1 | 1 | | | | |
| Remittent fever | | | 3 | | 2 | | 1 | |
| Intermittent fever | | | 4 | | 7 | | 8 | |
| Other diseases of this group | | | 7 | | 3 | | | |
| GENERAL DISEASES, B. | | | | | | | | |
| Rheumatism | | | 4 | | 2 | | | |
| Syphilis | | | 5 | | 7 | | 2 | |
| Consumption | | | 1 | | 3 | | 1 | |
| Other diseases of this group | | | 1 | 1 | 1 | | | |
| LOCAL DISEASES. | | | | | | | | |
| Catarrh and bronchitis | | | 2 | | 3 | | 11 | |
| Pneumonia | | | | | 1 | 1 | | |
| Diarrhœa and dysentery | 3 | 2 | 2 | | 5 | | 13 | |
| Gonorrhœa | | | 1 | | 2 | | 5 | |
| Other local diseases | 3 | | 6 | | 20 | 1 | 5 | |
| Alcoholism | | | 1 | | | | | |
| Total disease | 6 | 2 | 39 | 2 | 56 | 2 | 46 | |
| VIOLENT DISEASES AND DEATHS. | | | | | | | | |
| Gunshot wounds | | | 1 | | | | | |
| Other accidents and injuries | 1 | | 4 | | 10 | | 4 | |
| Total violence | 1 | | 5 | | 10 | | 4 | |

* Six months only.     † Seven months only.     ‡ Ten months only.

# FORT SILL, INDIAN TERRITORY.

REPORTED BY ASSISTANT SURGEONS H. S. KILBOURNE AND J. MORRIS BROWN, UNITED STATES ARMY.

Fort Sill is situated on the Comanche, Kiowa, and Apache reservation, Indian Territory, in latitude 34° 40', longitude 21° 22' west. The elevation above the sea is 1,700 feet. Fort Richardson is distant 110 miles south, Fort Griffin 150 miles southwest, and Camp Supply 190 miles northwest. The Washita River is 30 miles north, and Red River 45 miles south. Fort Sill was located by General Grierson in June, 1868, under the name of " Camp Wichita ;" the name was changed to Fort Sill July 2, 1869. It was selected by Major-General Sheridan as a base of operations against the Cheyennes and Kiowas in his winter campaign of 1868-'69, and from that date has been the military center of the reservation of the Comanches, Kiowas, and affiliated bands of the Wichitas, Keechies, Wacoes, and Caddoes. The reservation is in the form of a quadrangle, 9 miles in length by 4 miles wide. Within its boundaries are included the confluence of the Cache and Medicine Bluff Creeks, with the rich timber and bottom lands skirting those streams, the hills called Medicine Bluffs, the Indian commissary building, lime-kilns, quarries, &c.

The Wichita range of mountains extends from the northwest corner of the reservation westward about 50 miles. The intervening country, as far as the Red River, is traversed by a net-work of streams which rise in these mountains. The general prairie surface is loam and marl, with various admixtures of sand and gravel. The subsoil is a reddish clay, mixed with sand. The bed-rock is a light-gray limestone, generally far below the surface, but cropping out occasionally in the hills and at points along Cache Creek. It makes a good quality of lime and a fine building-material.

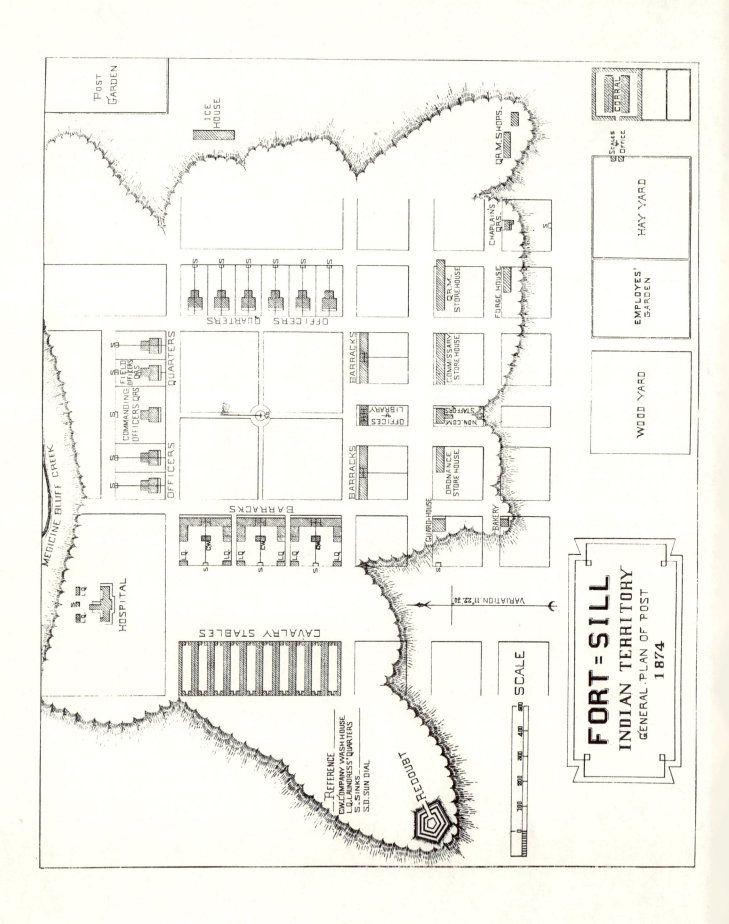

FORT-SILL
INDIAN TERRITORY
GENERAL PLAN OF POST
1874

Quarries within a mile of the post furnish the rock in any desirable quantities. The soil of the creek-bottoms is very fertile.

The largest and finest forest-trees are the oaks, cotton-wood, and pecans, found in the bottoms. The two former are sufficiently numerous to furnish lumber for building-purposes. There are three varieties of the oak, also hackberry, ash, black walnut, elm, and mesquite; among the small trees and shrubs are dogberry and willow. Among the fruits are the wild plum, wild grape, and black-berry; strawberries are found in small quantities. The edible plants are what is known as the prairie pea, the artichoke, and the fruit of one sort of cactus, of which latter there are several varieties. The taraxacum and chenopodium, the latter in large quantities, are seen about the post. There are also a large variety of flowering plants.

The following is a list of wild animals found on the reservation and vicinity: Buffalo, bear, elk; antelope, white-tailed deer, panther, gray wolf, wild rabbit, coyote or prairie-wolf, wild cat, otter, squirrel, coon, and a few others of small size.

Among the birds are the wild turkey, wild goose, wild duck, (four varieties;) prairie-hen or grouse, snipe, quail, meadow-lark, blackbird, and swallow. Cache and Medicine Bluff Creeks furnish the following kinds of fish in small quantities: Catfish, white-fish, sunfish, eels, and garfish; the latter stream has also a few trout in the mountains. Thirteen sorts of game have been killed, besides fish, in one week, among the headwaters of West Cache Creek, where all the above varieties are plentiful in their season.

Fort Sill is situated at the junction of Cache and Medicine Bluff Creeks, in the center of the post reservation. The latter is an area of one square mile in the center of the United States military reservation. The ground occupied by the buildings is a plateau of irregular outline, sloping in all directions, and about one-fourth of a mile square in extent. Its elevation above the low water of the adjacent streams is about 50 feet. The outline of the post and arrangement of the buildings are shown by the plate opposite.

All the buildings of the post are constructed of the gray limestone mentioned above, and when fully completed, will furnish accommodation for ten companies. Of five buildings designed for barracks only four are complete. Each building is double and one story in height. The dimensions are 200 by 27 feet, with a height of 12 feet to the eaves. Each division is intended for one company, and is divided into a barrack-room 84 feet in length and an orderly-room 27 by 12 feet. The barrack-room has an air-space of about 388.57 cubic feet per man for a company of 100 men; but, as the companies at the post actually average only 60 men, the present air-space is about 647.61 cubic feet per man. The orderly-room is subdivided into two rooms, respectively, 12 by 15 feet and 12 feet square. The dormitories and orderly-rooms are well ventilated by the doors and windows, and two of the barrack-buildings have ridge ventilation in addition. Three barracks, situated on the west side of the parade, have covered porches in front 10 feet wide, and extensions backward at each end. Each of these is divided into a kitchen 27 by 17 by 9 feet, and mess-room 37 by 27 by 9 feet. The mess-rooms and kitchens are well lighted by windows, but have no special arrangements for ventilation. In the yard in rear of each barrack is a small building intended for laundresses' quarters and wash-rooms. The former, of which there are two to each company, are 15 by 13 by 9 feet, and the latter 17 by 8 by 9 feet. The two barracks on south side of the parade, not yet entirely completed, have only temporary kitchens, and one end of the barrack-room is used for mess-room. In rear of the barracks are separate privies for each company, constructed on the principle of the earth-closet. The dormitories are insufficiently warmed by two wood-stoves in each. The men sleep on single iron bunks.

The buildings for officers' quarters are twelve, of which nine contain each two sets of quarters entirely separated from each other, making, in all, twenty-one sets of quarters. In twelve sets of quarters there are two rooms, each 15 by 15 feet; a hall, 8 by 30 feet; a covered porch, 12 feet square, used as a dining-room; and a kitchen, 10 by 12 feet, with attic over kitchen and covered porch used as servants' room. Six sets of quarters differ from the above in having large attic-rooms in the front part of the house. One set of quarters, those of the chaplain, consists of two rooms and a kitchen. One building has four rooms, each 15 by 18½ feet; hall, 10 by 30 feet; covered porch, used as a dining-room, 12 by 19 feet; kitchen, 12 feet square; two large attic-rooms in front part of the building, and three attic-rooms over kitchen, and covered porch. The quarters of the commanding officer are in a building a story and a half high. It contains on the ground-floor four rooms, each 18½ by 18 feet; hall, 10 by 36 feet; covered porch, used as a dining-room, 12 by 19 feet, and a kitchen, 12 feet square. On the second floor, the hall and rooms are of the same size. The officers' quarters are all well lighted, but have no other ventilation than that afforded by the doors and windows; all have covered porches in front, 10 feet wide; and all except two have fire-places in the front rooms.

The guard-house is a large one-story stone building, with basement. The basement is divided into five cells, of which four are 7 by 16 by 12 feet, and one, 12 by 16 by 12 feet, and a general prison-room, 16 by 26 by 12 feet. The main floor is divided into four rooms, of which two are 16 by 12 by 12 feet, and the others, 16 by 26 by 12 feet. There is no means of heating the basement; the rooms on the main floor are heated by stoves. The ventilation throughout is by windows.

The hospital is built on the plan of Circular No. 2, Surgeon-General's Office, 1871, with a capacity of twenty-four beds. It was commenced in October, 1871, and is not yet entirely finished, although parts of it have been occupied for more than a year.

An ice-house, 150 by 30 by 15 feet, is in process of construction. There is no school-house or laundry yet. A room has been temporarily partitioned off from the unfinished barrack for a chapel.

About 40 acres have been in cultivation during the last three years, and a sufficient supply of early vegetables has been raised. Owing to the drought, gardens are generally abandoned about the 1st of August. Canned vegetables and fruits are furnished by the Subsistence Department, but the supply of fresh vegetables for winter-use is insufficient. The nearest settlement from which they can be obtained is about seventy-five miles distant.

There is no special provision for a lavatory in the barracks or hospital; the hospital bath-room is unfinished, and there are no facilities at the post for enabling the men to bathe, if they were so disposed. The water-supply is principally brought in wagons from the Cache Creek. There is one cistern at the hospital, with a capacity of about 480 barrels.

*Meteorological report, Fort Sill, Indian Territory, 1870–'74.*

| Month. | 1870–'71. | | | | 1871–'72. | | | | 1872–'73. | | | | 1873–'74. | | | |
|---|---|---|---|---|---|---|---|---|---|---|---|---|---|---|---|---|
| | Temperature. | | | Rain-fall in inches. | Temperature. | | | Rain-fall in inches. | Temperature. | | | Rain-fall in inches. | Temperature. | | | Rain-fall in inches. |
| | Mean. | Max. | Min. | | Mean. | Max. | Min. | | Mean. | Max. | Min. | | Mean. | Max. | Min. | |
| July .............. | 82.14 | 105 | 64 | 4.55 | 86.04 | 109 | 71 | 0.19 | 83.43 | 105* | 64* | 6.14 | 83.27 | 106* | 50* | 2.90 |
| August .............. | 78.64 | 106 | 62 | 3.03 | 85.38 | 109 | 64 | 0.54 | 84.03 | 105* | 61* | 2.51 | 81.59 | 104* | 59* | 3.90 |
| September .......... | 74.99 | 98 | 55 | 7.24 | 75.23 | 103 | 49 | 0.30 | 76.63 | 102* | 46* | 3.03 | 72.37 | 97* | 46* | 3.80 |
| October .............. | 56.17 | 84 | 40 | 5.56 | 62.62 | 93 | 36 | 1.73 | 66.12 | 94* | 35* | 1.16 | 60.25 | 96* | 21* | 3.25 |
| November ........... | 46.97 | 62 | 39 | 0.14 | 46.35 | 74 | 10 | 0.84 | 42.77 | 82* | 8* | 0.19 | 51.19 | 84* | 19* | 1.30 |
| December........... | 37.20 | 72 | −11 | 2.70 | 39.09 | 75* | 8* | 0.00 | 32.55 | 66* | − 3* | 1.60 | 41.43 | 72* | 16* | 3.08 |
| January............... | 39.25 | 74 | 10 | 0.00 | 35.96 | 64* | 4* | 1.08 | 33.74 | 70* | −20* | 1.05 | 39.28 | 77* | 11* | 0.80 |
| February ............ | 45.86 | 77 | 15 | 1.63 | 45.32 | 80* | 11* | 0.18 | 41.08 | 74* | 5* | 1.15 | 41.12 | 75* | 7* | 2.90 |
| March .............. | 53.48 | 88 | 30 | 4.52 | 53.03 | 82* | 26* | 0.03 | 54.90 | 90* | 20* | 1.60 | 52.27 | 81* | 24* | 0.96 |
| April ................ | 63.85 | 95 | 35 | 0.77 | 64.72 | 90* | 30* | 3.41 | 60.20 | 97* | 27* | 0.80 | 53.72 | 87* | 29* | 3.79 |
| May ................ | 69.39 | 88 | 46 | 5.59 | 72.68 | 97* | 43* | 4.44 | 70.84 | 98* | 41* | 7.12 | 72.09 | 97* | 39* | 3.70 |
| June ................ | 82.91 | 101 | 68 | 3.62 | 81.75 | 103* | 56* | 1.37 | 78.53 | 96* | 60* | 3.85 | 79.20 | 96* | 54* | 3.14 |
| For the year .... | 60.90 | 106 | −11 | 39.35 | 62.35 | 109 | 4* | 14.11 | 60.40 | 105* | −20* | 30.20 | 60.65 | 106* | 7* | 33.52 |

* These observations are made with self-registering thermometers. The mean is from the standard thermometer.

*Consolidated sick-report, (white,) Fort Sill, Indian Territory, 1870–'74.*

| Year | 1870–'71.* | | 1871–'72.† | | 1872–'73.‡ | | 1873–'74. | |
|---|---|---|---|---|---|---|---|---|
| Mean strength { Officers ........... / { Enlisted men ...... | 19 / 161 | | 23 / 4 | | 19 / 67 | | 16 / 47 | |
| Diseases. | Cases. | Deaths. | Cases. | Deaths. | Cases. | Deaths. | Cases. | Deaths. |
| GENERAL DISEASES, A. | | | | | | | | |
| Typho-malarial fever ........... | | | 1 | 1 | | | | |
| Remittent fever ........... | | | | | 1 | | | |
| Intermittent fever ........... | 139 | 1 | 12 | | 23 | | 29 | |
| Other diseases of this group........... | | | | | 4 | | 3 | |
| GENERAL DISEASES, B. | | | | | | | | |
| Rheumatism ........... | 3 | | 5 | | 8 | | 6 | |
| Syphilis ........... | | | | | 1 | | 2 | |
| Consumption ........... | | | 2 | | | | | |
| Other diseases of this group........... | | | | | | | 1 | |
| LOCAL DISEASES. | | | | | | | | |
| Catarrh and bronchitis ........... | 10 | | 13 | | 11 | | 15 | |
| Pneumonia........... | 1 | 1 | | | | | | |
| Pleurisy ........... | | | 2 | | | | | |
| Diarrhœa and dysentery ........... | 29 | | | | 8 | | 13 | |
| Hernia ........... | | | | | | | 2 | |
| Other local diseases ........... | 9 | | 6 | | 9 | | 29 | |
| Total disease........... | 191 | 2 | 41 | 1 | 65 | | 101 | |
| VIOLENT DISEASES AND DEATHS. | | | | | | | | |
| Gunshot wounds ........... | 1 | 1 | 1 | | | | 1 | |
| Other accidents and injuries ........... | 3 | | 1 | | 4 | | 8 | |
| Total violence........... | 4 | 1 | 2 | | 4 | | 9 | |

* Six months only.          † Three months only.          ‡ Five months only.

*Consolidated sick-report, (colored,) Fort Sill, Indian Territory, 1870–'74.*

| Year | 1870–'71. | | 1871–'72. | | 1872–'73. | | 1873–'74. | |
|---|---|---|---|---|---|---|---|---|
| Mean strength ...... Enlisted men ...... | 494 | | 506 | | 341 | | 316 | |
| Diseases. | Cases. | Deaths. | Cases. | Deaths. | Cases. | Deaths. | Cases. | Deaths. |
| GENERAL DISEASES, A. | | | | | | | | |
| Typhoid fever ........... | 1 | 1 | | | | | | |
| Typho-malarial fever........... | 1 | | 1 | 3 | 1 | | 1 | |
| Remittent fever ........... | 293 | | 11 | | | | | |
| Intermittent fever ........... | | | 247 | | 113 | | 82 | |
| Other diseases of this group........... | 5 | | 14 | | 53 | 1 | 25 | |
| GENERAL DISEASES, B. | | | | | | | | |
| Rheumatism ........... | 11 | | 49 | | 53 | 1 | 57 | |
| Syphilis........... | 16 | | 5 | | 14 | 2 | 9 | |
| Consumption ........... | | 2 | 6 | 1 | | | | 1 |
| Other diseases of this group........... | 8 | | 11 | | 5 | | 7 | |
| LOCAL DISEASES. | | | | | | | | |
| Catarrh and bronchitis ........... | 54 | | 229 | | 152 | | 101 | |
| Pneumonia........... | 3 | 3 | 2 | | | | 3 | |
| Pleurisy........... | 1 | | 5 | | 2 | | 3 | |
| Diarrhœa and dysentery ........... | 114 | 1 | 141 | | 78 | | 59 | |
| Hernia ........... | | | 2 | | 2 | | 6 | |
| Gonorrhœa ........... | 1 | | 1 | | 8 | | 1 | |
| Other local diseases........... | 46 | 2 | 202 | 1 | 189 | | 162 | 2 |
| Total disease ........... | 548 | 9 | 926 | 5 | 670 | 4 | 516 | 3 |
| VIOLENT DISEASES AND DEATHS. | | | | | | | | |
| Gunshot wounds ........... | 8 | 3 | 21 | | 6 | 1 | 6 | 1 |
| Drowning ........... | | 2 | | | | | | |
| Other accidents and injuries........... | 63 | | 125 | | 118 | | 83 | |
| Homicide ........... | | 1 | | | | | | 1 |
| Total violence ........... | 71 | 6 | 146 | | 124 | 1 | 89 | 2 |

# FORT STOCKTON, TEXAS.

REPORTS OF ASSISTANT SURGEON P. J. A. CLEARY AND ACTING ASSISTANT SURGEON E. ALEXANDER, UNITED STATES ARMY.

Fort Stockton, Tex., is situated on Comanche Creek, on the line of the great Comanche trail, latitude, 30° 50′ north; longitude, 25° 35′ west, with an elevation of 4,950 feet above sea-level. It is on a line of travel across a vast dry and barren prairie, far removed from any city or town, and is thirty-five miles southwest from the nearest river, the Pecos, and fifty miles north of the nearest mountains, a continuation of the Guadalupe chain, which runs in a southeast direction to the Rio Grande. The nearest post is Fort Davis, seventy-four miles southwest. Fort Concho is one hundred and seventy miles east-northeast, Fort Clark lies two hundred and sixty-six miles southeast, and Fort Quitman two hundred and two miles west-southwest. The nearest town is Presidio del Norte, in Mexico, one hundred and forty-seven miles southwest. The nearest American town of any importance is Fredericksburgh, three hundred and seventy miles west, with a population of about 7,000. San Antonio is three hundred and ninety-two miles southeast. The place was first occupied as a military post in December, 1858. In May, 1861, it was abandoned. Was re-occupied by United States troops in July, 1867.

The reason for establishing a military post here was to guard the mail-route from San Antonio to El Paso. It is also a valuable link in the chain of forts which protect emigrants, merchandise, &c., going to or coming from California and Chihuahua, against the attacks and depredations of hostile Indians. Before the post was established, and also prior to its re-occupation by the Ninth Cavalry, the Comanche Indians lived here, and, being far from any settlement, held almost undisputed possession of the road, rendering it exceedingly dangerous to all who attempted to travel on it, and issuing in bands to the settlements, drove off stock, and found here a safe retreat and plenty of water. But at present, though they yet roam about in thieving bands, the road is comparatively safe, as they very rarely attack the mail or a passing train.

There is no Government reservation, the post being located on land belonging to a citizen. The land gradually rises from the creek, so that the center of the post is about fifty feet above it. The land on the opposite bank of the creek is much lower and almost perfectly level, so that when there is a heavy rain the creek overflows it to a distance of half a mile from its bank. For the most part the land in the neighborhood is flat, though in some places it is gently sloping for miles, terminating abruptly in extensive valleys. Elevations, called "table-lands," surround the post, varying from seven to twenty miles distant. They are from 100 to 500 feet high, with an area varying from three to twenty miles. Their surface is flat, and covered with coarse grass and several species of cactus. Their sides are abrupt and rocky. But few mineral products have as yet been found in the vicinity. Gypsum has been found in several places in and near the post, about 3 feet below the surface, but not in such quantities as to warrant an outlay in procuring it. The soil for the most part is sandy and strongly alkaline, containing chloride of sodium, sulphate of potash, &c., and cannot be farmed except by irrigation, but when cultivated in the vicinity of the creek and of a large spring, where it can be thoroughly irrigated, it produces corn, melons, and garden vegetables generally. Wheat and oats have not been successfully cultivated yet, though the effort this year promises to be a success; neither have potatoes nor cabbage.

There are no indigenous trees at or in the vicinity of the post, except one cotton-tree in the post garden. Mesquite-bush covers the entire surface. There is a water-cress which abounds in the creek, and which is an excellent antidote for scorbutus, as is also a species of cactus called the "Turk's head."

In winter, there is an abundance of ducks, and sometimes of wild geese, on the creek, while the marsh is frequented by cranes, herons, and a large number of water-hens.  In the spring, immense flocks of curlew visit the creek and remain about six weeks, and recently a species of partridge, called the Mexican, or California partridge, has made its appearance in the vicinity, and is increasing so rapidly that it will soon be an attraction for the sportsman.

There are but two kinds of fish found in the creek, the perch and catfish; but fishing is carried on to such an extent by the soldiers and Mexicans that they rarely attain over a pound in weight Turtle are plenty, and are often caught, weighing from twelve to fifteen pounds.

The only water at this post is from the creek, which rises about half a mile south of the post and runs nearly due north for about four miles, when it sinks into the ground, forming a kind of marsh or swamp.  In the first half mile of its course it is fed by six fine, clear springs, has an average width of about 40 feet, and a depth of 5 feet.  About eight miles west from the post are what are called the "Leon Holes," three large springs, having an average diameter of 30 feet and a depth of 20 feet.  From them issues a stream which irrigates a large tract of land cultivated chiefly by Mexicans.  Eighteen miles east from the post, on the mail-route to Fort Concho, is the Escondido Spring.  It is about 10 feet square; its stream runs a short distance and forms a miniature lake about 50 by 8 feet; its water is strongly impregnated with sulphur, but is cool and pleasant.  About twelve miles northeast from the post, on the "Horsehead"-crossing road to Concho, is a large spring, called the "Antelope."  There is a salt-lake about thirty-five miles to the northeast, near the Pecos River, whence excellent rock-salt can be obtained.  The supply is almost inexhaustible.  Frequently large quantities of it are taken to Mexico by trains returning from San Antonio.

The barracks consist of three adobe buildings with stone foundations.  Each building is 80 by 24 feet, and two of them have wings for kitchen and mess-room, each wing being 40 by 24 feet. They are roofed with thatch, except the wings, which are partly roofed with canvas and partly with thatch.  The barracks have a capacity of 700 cubic feet air-space per man.  Each building is warmed by one large fire-place, the fuel being "mesquite-root," and is lighted and ventilated by eight large windows and two doors.  Each building is intended to accommodate a full company, but seldom contains over fifty men.  The men sleep on straw-ticks and wooden bunks.  Each company has good kitchens and separate mess-rooms.

Quarters for married soldiers and laundresses are adobe buildings of two rooms, 12 by 14 feet each, and well adapted.

The officers' quarters comprise seven buildings, built of adobe, with stone foundations and shingle roofs, and a porch front and rear, boarded floors, plastered and whitewashed inside, and well finished; they are each one story high.  The dimensions of the rooms are 18 by 15 by 14 feet, and are heated by a fire-place in each room, and supplied with water every morning by a water-wagon, from which barrels are filled.  There are neither water-closets nor bath-rooms.

The guard-house is built of rock, with shingled roof, and is located on the south side of the parade-ground, in view of the officers' quarters.  It is 56 by 16 feet, and is divided into two rooms, one for the guard, and the other for the prisoners.  That for the guard is ventilated by means of one door, one window, and a fire-place.  The cell where the prisoners are confined is ventilated by two openings in the wall, each 18 by 14 inches; it is not lighted except by these apertures, and is not heated except by the exhaled air of its occupants.  Its means of ventilation are such that its capacity ought to be two, though it is generally occupied by twelve prisoners.

The hospital was completed in 1871, built of adobe with stone foundation, shingled roof, and porch.  For arrangement of rooms see figure 33.

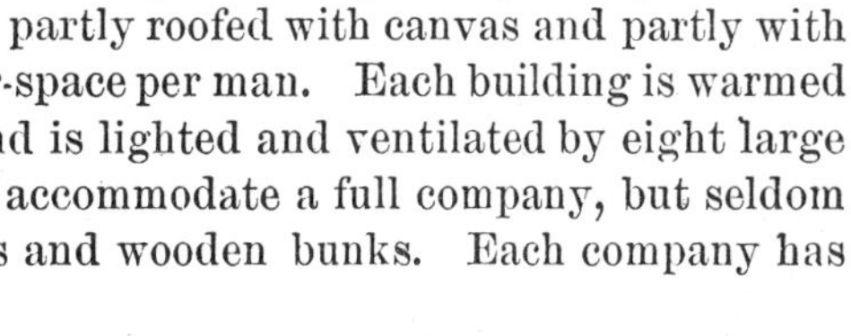

A, ward, 40 by 20 feet; A, ward, 20 by 20 feet; D, office, 10 by 20 feet; E, steward's room, 10 by 10 feet; F, dining-room, 10 by 20 feet; O, dispensary, 10 by 10 feet; P, shingled porch, 101 by 10 feet.

Figure 33.  (40 feet to 1 inch.)

A detached building, 14 by 42 feet, in rear of the hospital, divided into three rooms, serves for kitchen and attendant's room.  The large ward contains eight beds, allowing 1,440 cubic feet air-space to each. The smaller ward is used as a store-room.  There are no means of ventilation; fire-places are used. The water-closet is 35 yards in rear of the hospital, and constructed to introduce the dry-earth

31 P M

system. There is no bath-room or lavatory, no post-mortem room or dead-house. An excellent spring is located about 30 paces from the building, and the creek is distant only 40 paces, toward which drainage and sewerage are effected by the natural slope of the ground.

The post bakery is of adobe, 22 by 18 feet, with shingled roof.

A school-room has been erected for enlisted men and children.

The stables are situated 100 yards in the rear of the men's quarters, between them and the creek; it was intended to complete three large buildings for the purpose, but two of them have not been finished and will not be; the remaining one is an excellent building for the purpose. It is 250 by 30 feet, has stone foundation and adobe walls, with shingled roof. There are 100 apertures, each 18 by 10 inches, for the purpose of ventilation, in addition to two large doors at the ends and one large door on each side.

There is no post library.

The post is supplied with water from the creek and from the springs which flow into it, but there are no cisterns or reservoirs. The water is hauled every morning in a large wagon, and distributed into barrels kept for the purpose. The quantity of water is abundant; it is decidedly alkaline, but is not unhealthy; one likes it very well a short time after using it, though at first it is rather unpleasant to the taste. It has not been analyzed, but it contains chloride of sodium and probably nitrate of soda and sulphur, with salts of lime and magnesia. The only means of extinguishing fire are the barrels of water kept outside the quarters of the officers and men for drinking purposes.

The drainage of the post is effected by the gradual slope of the ground toward the creek. It ·has a fall of about 50 feet in 1,000 yards, so that no water whatever remains on the surface at the post. The only artificial drainage consists of a ditch on the west side, in rear of the officers' quarters, and emptying into a ravine, which carries its water to the creek. This ditch prevents the rains from running over the parade-ground, or into the officers' quarters, barracks, and stables. The excreta of the men accumulate in neighboring ravines, which are thoroughly washed by heavy rains. The offal or rubbish of the post is carried off on carts by police parties, and conveyed to a distance beyond the post.

There are no special arrangements for bathing, but the men, and all who desire, bathe in the creek, parts of which are well adapted for the purpose.

The cemetery is located one mile north from the post.

There is a post garden which has an area of 20 acres, and is cultivated by men detailed for the purpose. It is located about four miles north from the post, and is rendered productive by an excellent system of irrigation, the water being obtained from the creek. It furnishes abundance for the entire command. The value of the garden is almost inestimable, from the fact that vegetables cannot be obtained from the citizens in the vicinity except in small quantity, small variety, and at enormous prices. The amount of articles of food procurable from the post commissary is abundant, and, for the most part, they are of good quality. Although the supply of milk is abundant, it is high, chiefly, I presume, because it is sold only by two persons at the post. It is 20 cents per quart; butter is $1 per pound; eggs, 75 cents to $1 per dozen; chickens, from $1 to $1.50 each.

The only means of communication with the nearest large city is by the stage-coach, which is generally regular, though liable to interruption from Indians and floods; last year during the summer it was frequently interrupted by floods for two weeks at a time. The mail arrives and departs twice weekly.

It requires seven days for a letter to reach department headquarters at Austin, Tex., and fifteen days to reach Washington, although letters have been received here from Washington in twelve days; but so short a time is the exception.

The inhabitants of the vicinity are chiefly Mexicans, a cross between the Spaniard and Indian, which seems to have deteriorated both races; their occupation is farming and laboring work, such as making adobes at the post.

The general sanitary condition of the post is and has been excellent. In the winter and spring, in consequence of the "northers," catarrh is the prevalent affection; during the summer and autumn there are many cases of mild diarrhœa, and a few of intermittent fever. The only apparent cause of the diarrhœa is indiscretion in eating fresh vegetables, especially watermelons and cucumbers. The cases, however, are mild, and yield readily to treatment. The beneficial effects of the atmosphere and climate of this place on pulmonary affections, and particularly on phthisis pulmonalis, cannot be too highly extolled. The atmosphere is warm, dry, and pure. Many people come to the State to have their "consumption" cured, but generally arrive when the disease is too far advanced, and, moreover, do not come far enough west.

*Meteorological report, Fort Stockton, Tex., 1870–'74.*

| Month. | 1870–'71. | | | | 1871–'72. | | | | 1872–'73. | | | | 1873–'74. | | | |
|---|---|---|---|---|---|---|---|---|---|---|---|---|---|---|---|---|
| | Temperature. | | | Rain-fall in inches. | Temperature. | | | Rain-fall in inches. | Temperature. | | | Rain-fall in inches. | Temperature. | | | Rain-fall in inches. |
| | Mean. | Max. | Min. | | Mean. | Max. | Min. | | Mean. | Max. | Min. | | Mean. | Max. | Min. | |
| July | 81.81 | 98 | 68 | 1.90 | 84.77 | 104 | 71 | 1.06 | 80.51 | 105* | 64* | 4.68 | 82.05 | 111* | 49* | 0.22 |
| August | 78.87 | 98 | 68 | 8.96 | 84.14 | 100 | 72 | 0.42 | 79.16 | 102* | 58* | 0.30 | 81.84 | 108* | 60* | 1.04 |
| September | 75.71 | 95 | 61 | 3.68 | 76.01 | 96 | 61 | 1.51 | 75.01 | 100* | 44* | 0.22 | 77.58 | 109* | 53* | 0.00 |
| October | 66.49 | 92 | 46 | 0.60 | 64.01 | 91 | 34 | 0.18 | 62.55 | 90* | 24* | 0.68 | 66.37 | 102* | 34* | 1.32 |
| November | 57.16 | 88 | 27 | 0.28 | 53.86 | 86 | 20 | 0.23 | 48.50 | 84* | 14* | 1.56 | 53.96 | 86* | 25* | 3.14 |
| December | 45.16 | 88 | 6 | 1.22 | 49.47 | 84 | 10 | 0.08 | 44.02 | 78* | 13* | 0.16 | 49.32 | 84* | 15* | 0.74 |
| January | 47.32 | 84 | 13 | 0.08 | 39.18 | 74 | 4 | 0.19 | 42.63 | 79* | —3* | 0.16 | 50.57 | 88* | 21* | 0.00 |
| February | 50.79 | 88 | 20 | 0.00 | 52.04 | 82 | 16 | 0.12 | 50.05 | 87* | 21* | 0.00 | 51.95 | 84* | 20* | 0.00 |
| March | 54.99 | 98 | 28 | 0.10 | 58.99 | 93 | 32 | 0.08 | 58.83 | 95* | 24* | 0.00 | 59.86 | 88* | 34* | 0.83 |
| April | 64.61 | 99 | 34 | 0.00 | 67.85 | 105* | 32* | 0.00 | 62.18 | 99* | 22* | 0.00 | 59.63 | 96* | 27* | 0.25 |
| May | 71.09 | 97 | 48 | 0.98 | 77.83 | 111* | 43* | 0.40 | 73.36 | 102* | 40* | 0.92 | 74.02 | 97* | 32* | 0.05 |
| June | 80.49 | 100 | 68 | 0.52 | 81.97 | 108* | 56* | 1.70 | 80.38 | 112* | 54* | 4.40 | 81.74 | 108* | 54* | 3.11 |
| For the year | 64.54 | 100 | 6 | 18.32 | 65.84 | 111* | 4 | 5.97 | 63.77 | 112* | —3* | 14.98 | 65.74 | 111* | 15* | 10.70 |

* These observations are made with self-registering thermometers. The mean is from the standard thermometer.

*Consolidated sick-report, (white,) Fort Stockton, Tex., 1873–'74.*

| Year | | 1873–'74.* |
|---|---|---|
| Mean strength | { Officers | 8 |
| | { Enlisted men | 49 |

| Diseases. | Cases. | Deaths. |
|---|---|---|
| GENERAL DISEASES, A. | | |
| Intermittent fever | 5 | |
| GENERAL DISEASES, B. | | |
| Syphilis | 3 | |
| LOCAL DISEASES. | | |
| Catarrh and bronchitis | 1 | |
| Pleurisy | 1 | |
| Diarrhœa and dysentery | 10 | |
| Other local diseases | 8 | |
| Alcoholism | 5 | |
| Total disease | 33 | |
| VIOLENT DISEASES AND DEATHS. | | |
| Accidents and injuries | 3 | |
| Total violence | 3 | |

* Enlisted men 10 months only.

*Consolidated sick-report, (colored,) Fort Stockton, Tex., 1870–'74.*

| Year | 1870–'71. | | 1871–'72. | | 1872–'73. | | 1873–'74. | |
|---|---|---|---|---|---|---|---|---|
| Mean strength ..........Enlisted men...... | 201 | | 226 | | 177 | | 146 | |
| **Diseases.** | Cases. | Deaths. | Cases. | Deaths. | Cases. | Deaths. | Cases. | Deaths. |
| GENERAL DISEASES, A. | | | | | | | | |
| Typhoid fever.......... | | | 1 | 1 | | | 1 | 1 |
| Remittent fever....... | 3 | | | | | | 4 | |
| Intermittent fever.... | 32 | | 3 | | 2 | | 6 | |
| Other diseases of this group.... | 6 | | 1 | | 4 | 1 | 1 | |
| GENERAL DISEASES, B. | | | | | | | | |
| Rheumatism........ | 38 | | 6 | | 1 | | 9 | |
| Syphilis ......... | 7 | | 4 | | 3 | | 12 | |
| Consumption ......... | | | | | 1 | 1 | 4 | |
| Other diseases of this group..... | 3 | | 4 | | 1 | | 1 | |
| LOCAL DISEASES. | | | | | | | | |
| Catarrh and bronchitis.... | 28 | | 16 | | 11 | | 4 | |
| Pneumonia..... | | | | | 1 | | | |
| Pleurisy...... | | | | | | | 3 | |
| Diarrhœa and dysentery .... | 53 | | 63 | 2 | 11 | | 9 | |
| Hernia ..... | 1 | | 2 | | | | | |
| Gonorrhœa ..... | 1 | | 1 | | 3 | | 25 | |
| Other local diseases ..... | 80 | 1 | 73 | 1 | 28 | 1 | 24 | 1 |
| Total disease ..... | 252 | 1 | 174 | 4 | 66 | 4 | 103 | 2 |
| VIOLENT DISEASES AND DEATHS. | | | | | | | | |
| Gunshot wounds.... | 6 | | | 2 | 2 | | 3 | |
| Other accidents and injuries.... | 39 | 1 | 30 | | 15 | | 20 | |
| Homicide...... | | | | 2 | | | | |
| Total violence..... | 45 | 1 | 30 | 4 | 17 | | 23 | |

# DEPARTMENT OF THE MISSOURI.

---

(Embracing the States of Missouri, Kansas, and Illinois, and the Territories of Colorado and New Mexico, and Fort Gibson and Camp Supply, Indian Territory.)

### POSTS.

| | | |
|---|---|---|
| Bayard, Fort, N. Mex. | Larned, Fort, Kans. | Selden, Fort, N. Mex. |
| Craig, Fort, N. Mex. | Leavenworth, Fort, Kans. | Stanton, Fort, N. Mex. |
| Cummings, Fort, N. Mex. | Lyon, Fort, Colo. T. | Supply, Camp, Ind. T. |
| Dodge, Fort, Kans. | McRae, Fort, N. Mex. | Tulerosa, Fort, N. Mex. |
| Garland, Fort, Colo. T. | Riley, Fort, Kans. | Union, Fort, N. Mex. |
| Gibson, Fort, Ind. T. | Rock Island Arsenal, Ills. | Wallace, Fort, Kans. |
| Harker, Fort, Kans. | Saint Louis Arsenal and Barracks, Mo. | Wingate, Fort, N. Mex. |
| Hays, Fort, Kans. | Santa Fé, N. Mex. | |

### TABLE OF DISTANCES IN THE DEPARTMENT OF THE MISSOURI.

| | Chicago | Saint Louis | Fort Leavenworth | Fort Bayard | Fort Craig | Fort Dodge | Fort Garland | Fort Hays | Fort Larned | Fort Lyon | Fort McRae | Fort Riley | Rock Island Arsenal | Santa Fé | Fort Selden | Fort Stanton | Saint Louis Arsenal | Camp Supply | Fort Tulerosa | Fort Union | Fort Wallace | Fort Wingate |
|---|---|---|---|---|---|---|---|---|---|---|---|---|---|---|---|---|---|---|---|---|---|---|
| Chicago | Chicago. | | | | | | | | | | | | | | | | | | | | | |
| Saint Louis | 281 | Saint Louis. | | | | | | | | | | | | | | | | | | | | |
| Fort Leavenworth | 492 | 311 | Fort Leavenworth. | | | | | | | | | | | | | | | | | | | |
| Fort Bayard | 1633 | 1437 | 1285 | Fort Bayard. | | | | | | | | | | | | | | | | | | |
| Fort Craig | 1455 | 1259 | 1059 | 226 | Fort Craig. | | | | | | | | | | | | | | | | | |
| Fort Dodge | 845 | 652 | 370 | 798 | 620 | Fort Dodge. | | | | | | | | | | | | | | | | |
| Fort Garland | 1189 | 979 | 728 | 578 | 352 | 351 | Fort Garland. | | | | | | | | | | | | | | | |
| Fort Hays | 774 | 572 | 286 | 896 | 718 | 80 | 442 | Fort Hays. | | | | | | | | | | | | | | |
| Fort Larned | 786 | 598 | 314 | 861 | 683 | 65 | 483 | 46 | Fort Larned. | | | | | | | | | | | | | |
| Fort Lyon | 1027 | 817 | 535 | 642 | 449 | 185 | 193 | 249 | 295 | Fort Lyon. | | | | | | | | | | | | |
| Fort McRae | 1487 | 1291 | 1091 | 156 | 32 | 652 | 384 | 750 | 715 | 516 | Fort McRae. | | | | | | | | | | | |
| Fort Riley | 620 | 410 | 134 | 1050 | 872 | 311 | 569 | 153 | 252 | 407 | 904 | Fort Riley. | | | | | | | | | | |
| Rock Island Arsenal | 182 | 243 | 311 | 1529 | 1347 | 671 | 1014 | 598 | 598 | 851 | 1379 | 444 | Rock Island Arsenal. | | | | | | | | | |
| Santa Fé | 1295 | 1099 | 870 | 415 | 189 | 721 | 163 | 623 | 562 | 340 | 221 | 712 | 1169 | Santa Fé. | | | | | | | | |
| Fort Selden | 1540 | 1344 | 1159 | 126 | 100 | 705 | 452 | 803 | 768 | 681 | 58 | 957 | 1432 | 289 | Fort Selden. | | | | | | | |
| Fort Stanton | 1402 | 1206 | 927 | 512 | 286 | 567 | 402 | 665 | 630 | 411 | 318 | 819 | 1276 | 239 | 386 | Fort Stanton. | | | | | | |
| Saint Louis Arsenal | 293 | 12 | 323 | 1449 | 1271 | 664 | 991 | 584 | 610 | 829 | 1303 | 422 | 255 | 1111 | 1356 | 1218 | Saint Louis Arsenal. | | | | | |
| Camp Supply | 931 | 736 | 461 | 758 | 612 | 91 | 437 | 171 | 152 | 271 | 644 | 397 | 757 | 496 | 665 | 522 | 748 | Camp Supply. | | | | |
| Fort Tulerosa | 1517 | 1321 | 1042 | 285 | 107 | 682 | 406 | 780 | 745 | 526 | 139 | 934 | 1405 | 236 | 192 | 335 | 1333 | 674 | Fort Tulerosa. | | | |
| Fort Union | 1195 | 999 | 762 | 521 | 295 | 597 | 304 | 465 | 563 | 234 | 327 | 612 | 1069 | 106 | 395 | 345 | 1011 | 446 | 322 | Fort Union. | | |
| Fort Wallace | 905 | 695 | 420 | 765 | 587 | 216 | 308 | 134 | 180 | 115 | 619 | 285 | 731 | 507 | 798 | 534 | 707 | 302 | 649 | 327 | Fort Wallace. | |
| Fort Wingate | 1465 | 1269 | 1078 | 481 | 227 | 931 | 371 | 728 | 693 | 548 | 259 | 882 | 1352 | 208 | 355 | 305 | 1281 | 604 | 164 | 270 | 597 | Fort Wingate. |

# FORT BAYARD, NEW MEXICO.

## REPORT OF ASSISTANT SURGEON WILLIAM J. WILSON, UNITED STATES ARMY.

Fort Bayard is situated in almost the extreme southwestern corner of New Mexico, latitude 30° 40′ north, longitude 31° 25′ west, at an altitude of 6,022 feet. It is distant about eighty miles from Janos, the nearest settlement on the Mexican frontier, and about the same distance from Apache Pass, on the Arizona border. The Government reservation contains almost sixteen square miles.

The post was first established in 1866, its site being selected by Col. N. H. Davis, Inspector-General United States Army. At present it is a four-company post, two of cavalry and two of infantry being stationed here.

That portion of the reservation upon which the post is built is a valley almost surrounded by hills of granite, in which gold and silver are found. About a mile south of the post is the Mexican village of Central City, consisting of a number of adobe shanties, inhabited by gamblers, saloon-keepers, and prostitutes, all of whom prey upon the soldiers and support themselves mainly therefrom. About ten miles west is Silver City, the county seat of the county, and a flourishing mining town, having an American population of about 500, and about an equal number of Mexicans. It was first laid out in 1871, and now has four quartz-mills and three furnaces in operation. Silver exists in large quantities in the mountains around the town, and the mines are being rapidly developed. The village of Pinos Altos, now almost fallen into ruin, is also about ten miles distant from the post. There are several rich gold mines in its neighborhood, but owing to a scarcity of water they are at present very little worked.

Another little mining village has, within the past two years, sprung up at Lone Mountain, four miles south, and owes its existence to the presence of silver. Its inhabitants, about 200 in number, are nearly all miners. Gold, silver, copper, iron, and lead are found in great abundance, but no coal.

The country around is badly suited for agriculture, as the climate is so dry that vegetables can only be raised by irrigation, and the springs or streams available for this purpose are far distant from each other. It is much better suited for stock-raising, as the grass is good and highly nutritious for animals, and there is an immense range for cattle around the immediate vicinity of the water.

The principal wild animals found are the black and cinnamon bear, the wolf, coyote, fox, deer, and antelope. The wild turkey, wild duck, quail, lark, robin, and mocking-bird are also observed.

On the north, northwest, and east, the post is surrounded by high mountains, open on the south and southeast. Pine, cedar, and oak are found in large quantities on the surrounding hills. The climate is delightful, but there is very little rain except during the rainy season, which lasts from about the end of June till the middle of September, when more or less rain falls nearly every day, sometimes in torrents. The winds are generally from the west, northwest, and south, and seldom severe. Changes in temperature are very gradual. On account of the altitude of the post and the dryness of the atmosphere, the heat of summer is never oppressive, while the nights are always deliciously cool. The winter season is very mild, one or two slight falls of snow occurring generally in February, and lasting but one or two days.

In bronchitis, either acute or chronic, this climate is unfavorable either for cure or relief. The air is too rarified and too stimulating, and acts almost as an irritant to the bronchial mucous membrane. I have also observed in even slight cases of catarrh attended with cough, that they are very intractable. I have seen several cases of phthisis, and have one at the present time under my charge, but I have not seen any beneficial results produced by this climate. They have all gone on from bad to worse, and finally died. I believe that it is only in the very early stages of tubercular disease that this, or any other climate, can exert a beneficial influence.

I have a theory of my own with regard to the disease, and which I believe I have seen exemplified by several cases; and that is, that there are, so to speak, two classes of cases, one of which is characterized or accompanied by a dry, hacking cough, but with little expectoration, and a tendency to hæmoptysis. In the other, there is copious secretion from the bronchial mucous membrane. This latter class would be benefited by a mild, dry climate not subject to sudden changes, and of a lower altitude than this, say, 2,000, or 3,000, or 4,000 feet. The former class would lead a life of torture here, and this climate, or one similar to it, would only add to the mischief already done. They would be benefited by a mild, moist climate, in close proximity to the sea. Phthisis is almost unknown among the Mexican population here, notwithstanding their filthy habits—probably on account of their living nearly all the time out of doors, and being natives of the soil and accustomed to this climate. I know that horses brought here from the States and cattle introduced here go down in condition for the first year until they are acclimated, and I believe that the human race require also a certain time for acclimation.

The post is on the side of a small hill, sloping to the east, near the center of the reservation. The buildings are in course of construction, and will be of adobe, with shingled roofs; the post, when completed, will form a parallelogram, 650 by 400 feet.

The barracks, accommodating three companies, are adobe buildings, each one story high, consisting of a hall, 23 by 12 feet, in the center, with a squad-room, 23 by 30 feet, on either side. There is a room, 23 by 12 feet, for the first sergeant at the end of each of the squad-rooms. They are warmed by stoves, well ventilated, and allow to each man about 584 cubic feet air-space. Single iron bedsteads are used in these quarters. One company is quartered in a log building, with shingle roof, almost as old as the post, and much out of repair; but it is contemplated to erect a new set of quarters instead, to be similar to those above described. Temporary sinks are in rear of each barrack. Large kitchens, store-rooms, and dining-rooms are in one-story adobe buildings in rear of each company quarters. Laundresses occupy old log-shanties, which are much out of repair.

Seven new sets of officers' quarters are in course of completion, one as commanding-officer's quarters, the others intended each for two officers. They are of adobe, with shingle roof, and consist each of a hall, bedroom, dining-room, with pantry attached and cellar underneath, and a kitchen. There will also be an attic-story when completed. An inclosed yard, with walls of stone or adobe, will also be attached to each house, with wood-shed, water-closet, bath-room, chicken-coop, and servants' room. A covered porch will also extend in front of each building. The rooms are 16 by 16 feet, by 14 feet high. Some of the old log huts, previously used as quarters, are still occupied by officers.

The storehouses are two adobe buildings, 120 by 26 feet, by 10 feet high, of sufficient capacity and in good repair. Under the commissary storehouse is a cellar, 50 by 20 feet, by 8 feet high. The intervening space between these storehouses is occupied by the sally-port, on each side of which was the guard-house, until a new building was erected for that purpose. Above this guard-house and sally-port, and forming the second story of the building, are the adjutants' offices and a small store-room for tools, &c.

The guard-house, built of stone, is probably the finest building for that purpose in the Territory. It contains a guard-room, prison-room, and cells, a large court-yard, and two large water-closets, urinals, &c. A stone wall, 12 feet high, surrounds the court-yard. The guard-house is well ventilated and kept in excellent order and cleanliness. The building is now used as a kind of military prison; its average occupancy is thirty-five. A magazine has been recently erected; it is a circular building, of stone and adobe, two stories, with a door opening only into the upper story and covered with a tin roof painted. It has a rough coat of plaster on the outside.

The hospital, erected in 1869, is of adobe, with shingle roof, and consists of an executive building, one and a half stories high, and one wing or ward, one story high, intended for twelve beds. The executive building, 42 by 42 feet, is divided into the office, 14 by 14½ feet; dispensary, 14 by 14½ feet; store-room, 12 by 18 feet, and dining-room, 22 by 18 feet, with a kitchen and pantry, 23 by 16 feet, attached in rear. The ward is 47½ by 25½ feet. The ceiling in all the rooms is

14 feet high. A bath and wash room, and a nurse-room, each 9 by 9 feet, are cut off from one end of the ward, though the partitions do not reach the ceiling. Air-space in the ward, 1,062 cubic feet per bed. Ventilation is ample, by six windows and two doors, and by the ventilating shaft which runs from below the floor to the roof. The ward is warmed by a stove, the offices by fire-places. One large double privy is situated at some distance from the hospital. It is a frame building, with a large vault; into this dry earth is thrown. The building can be moved when necessary. An earth-closet with a close stool are in the bath-room, which also contains a bath-tub, &c. Although recommendations have been made for another wing or ward to the hospital building, the present size is deemed quite sufficient as far as the wants of the sick are concerned. There is, however, no steward's room, nor dead-house, nor is there sufficient store-room. A porch in front of the building has also been applied for. The post bakery is built of stone and sufficient in size. The corrals are surrounded by adobe walls, with stalls covered with brush.

The post library contains 177 well-selected volumes. One of the cavalry companies has by far the largest and best company library I have as yet seen in the Army.

Until the summer of 1872, the water-supply, though sufficient, was of a very bad quality, Coming from a spring, it passed through a swamp where cows, horses, and pigs used to wallow, and there was every reason to believe that even fecal matter was washed into it during the rainy season. As a consequence, bowel complaints were very numerous, and even some deaths from that cause occurred during the summer of 1871. Since then the spring has been enlarged and lined with a wooden casing, from which wooden pipes are laid a distance of 450 yards to a tank, where the water passes through a filter of charcoal and sand, and from thence is delivered by a water-wagon to the barracks, quarters, and other buildings of the post. The water is now excellent, and there is hardly a trace of diarrhœa, which ceased almost immediately on the completion of these water-works. There are no facilities for bathing. The cemetery is 300 yards northwest of the post. Each company cultivates a garden, and large quantities of vegetables are raised; potatoes do not succeed well. Once or twice each year wagons are sent by the post commissary to Santa Fé, where potatoes of a very fine quality can be procured, and which are principally raised in Colorado. These cost about 3 cents per pound. Very fine and large onions are also brought here, principally from the neighborhood of El Paso, and cost about 6 cents per pound. Grapes are received from Las Cruces or Messilla, on the Rio Grande, and cost 25 cents per pound. Apples come from Chihuahua in small quantities, and cost about 3 cents to 5 cents each. The post commissary supply is large and contains nearly every article of subsistence stores needed for family use. A tri-weekly mail is received, once by coach and twice on horseback. The nearest railroad point is Granada, or Pueblo, Colo., distant about 700 miles. The mails are very insecure, and it is rare that any article of value reaches its destination to or from this point. About fourteen days are required for letters to go through to Washington, about ten days to department headquarters, and five days to district headquarters at Santa Fé. Communication is had by ambulance or by private conveyance, and by stage-coach which runs from Silver City to Santa Fé once a week each way. The stage leaves Silver City and this post every Sunday morning, arriving in Santa Fé on Thursday evenings, (distant about 400 miles.) On its return trip it leaves Santa Fé on Monday mornings and arrives here on Fridays, generally about noon. The fare to this place is $89. From Santa Fé to the railroad at Pueblo, about 300 miles, the fare is $60. Expressage from the States costs about $1 per pound.

The Indians, up till the year 1873, were pretty bad, even in the immediate neighborhood of the post; but at present, owing to treaties that have been made with them, confining them to their reservations, and the frequent scouts sent out from this post, there is little damage done by them The roads around here are traveled without fear of danger, as the country is being pretty rapidly settled up, owing to the large discoveries of silver and other metals. A great number of Americans, and those, too, of a good class, are locating in this part of New Mexico, and the Indians and Indian troubles are bound to disappear before them. The surveyed route for the Texas Pacific Railroad passes about 30 miles south of Fort Bayard. This will be the nearest point.

*Meteorological report, Fort Bayard, N. Mex., 1870–'74.*

| Month. | 1870–'71. Temperature. Mean. | Max. | Min. | Rain-fall in inches. | 1871–'72. Temperature. Mean. | Max. | Min. | Rain-fall in inches. | 1872–'73. Temperature. Mean. | Max. | Min. | Rain-fall in inches. | 1873–'74. Temperature. Mean. | Max. | Min. | Rain-fall in inches. |
|---|---|---|---|---|---|---|---|---|---|---|---|---|---|---|---|---|
| July | 69.46 | 86 | 59 | 2.96 | 74.17 | 96 | 60 | 0.09 | 72.49 | 91* | 50* | 2.85 | 77.21 | 96* | 30* | ?.02 |
| August | 69.52 | 87 | 57 | 3.57 | 71.85 | 97 | 62 | 0.19 | 69.54 | 87* | 50* | 3.37 | 69.19 | 87* | 50* | 11.73 |
| September | 63.89 | 88 | 42 | 0.73 | 68.21 | 86 | 57 | 2.27 | 65.11 | 82* | 40* | 1.25 | 67.25 | 85* | 41* | 1.30 |
| October | 54.86 | 80 | 30 | 0.01 | 55.01 | 81 | 32 | 0.75 | 56.76 | 81* | 12* | 0.15 | 57.37 | 86* | 29* | 0.00 |
| November | 45.57 | 70 | 24 | 0.00 | 44.21 | 64 | 25 | 1.30 | 42.05 | 70 | 3* | 0.04 | 47.33 | 70* | 20* | 0.70 |
| December | 33.82 | 65 | 10 | (?) | 41.26 | 62 | 25 | 0.25 | 41.67 | 68 | 21* | 2.08 | 38.34 | 63* | 11* | 0.74 |
| January | 35.96 | 62 | 8 | 0.64 | 31.12 | 58 | 13 | 0.85 | 39.39 | 64 | −8* | 0.48 | 41.27 | 64* | 9* | 1.79 |
| February | 37.03 | 64 | 18 | 0.05 | 39.85 | 70* | 18* | 0.72 | 39.18 | 60 | −1* | 1.91 | 36.62 | 58* | 2* | 5.68 |
| March | 46.51 | 70 | 21 | (?) | 42.22 | 70* | 15* | 0.27 | 50.23 | 75 | 20* | 0.87 | 43.57 | 66* | 12* | 1.72 |
| April | 52.60 | 76 | 32 | 0.10 | 49.43 | 80* | 15* | 0.66 | 53.09 | 77* | 9* | 0.04 | 48.17 | 77* | 14* | 2.32 |
| May | 64.19 | 86 | 45 | 0.00 | 64.54 | 92* | 35* | 0.11 | 61.43 | 78* | 30* | 0.29 | 62.49 | 89* | 29* | 0.90 |
| June | 75.32 | 100 | 56 | 0.05 | 72.72 | 92* | 45* | 1.26 | 73.05 | 98* | 35* | 1.10 | 74.07 | 92* | 40* | 0.30 |
| For the year | 54.06 | 100 | 8 | | 54.97 | 97 | 13 | 8.72 | 55.33 | 98* | −8* | 14.43 | 55.24 | 96* | 2* | 30.20 |

* These observations are made with self-registering thermometers. The mean is from the standard thermometer.

*Consolidated sick-report, Fort Bayard, N. Mex., 1870–'74.*

| Year | | 1870–'71. | | 1871–'72. | | 1872–'73. | | 1873–'74. | |
|---|---|---|---|---|---|---|---|---|---|
| Mean strength { Officers | | 6 | | 10 | | 8 | | 10 | |
| { Enlisted men | | 189 | | 190 | | 197 | | 220 | |
| Diseases. | | Cases. | Deaths. | Cases. | Deaths. | Cases. | Deaths. | Cases. | Deaths. |
| GENERAL DISEASES, A. | | | | | | | | | |
| Typhoid fever | | 1 | 1 | | 1 | | | | |
| Remittent fever | | 4 | | 22 | | 1 | | | |
| Intermittent fever | | 9 | | 28 | | 60 | | 32 | |
| Other diseases of this group | | 7 | | 3 | | 4 | | 7 | |
| GENERAL DISEASES, B. | | | | | | | | | |
| Rheumatism | | 8 | | 6 | | 3 | | 5 | |
| Syphilis | | 11 | | 2 | | 5 | | 8 | |
| Consumption | | | | | | 2 | 1 | | |
| Other diseases of this group | | 2 | | 1 | | | | | |
| LOCAL DISEASES. | | | | | | | | | |
| Catarrh and bronchitis | | 1 | | 11 | | 42 | | 12 | |
| Pneumonia | | 2 | | 1 | | 3 | 1 | 1 | |
| Pleurisy | | | | | | 1 | 1 | 1 | |
| Diarrhœa and dysentery | | 70 | | 42 | 2 | 106 | | 52 | |
| Gonorrhœa | | 11 | | 9 | | 6 | | 2 | |
| Other local diseases | | 44 | 1 | 39 | 1 | 49 | | 28 | |
| Alcoholism | | 4 | | 7 | | 3 | | 7 | |
| Total disease | | 174 | 2 | 171 | 4 | 285 | 3 | 155 | |
| VIOLENT DISEASES AND DEATHS. | | | | | | | | | |
| Gunshot wounds | | 2 | 1 | 1 | | 1 | | 3 | |
| Other accidents and injuries | | 36 | | 44 | 1 | 49 | 1 | 38 | 1 |
| Homicide | | | 1 | | | | | | |
| Suicide | | | | | | | 1 | | 1 |
| Total violence | | 38 | 2 | 45 | 2 | 50 | 1 | 41 | 2 |

# FORT CRAIG, NEW MEXICO.

INFORMATION FURNISHED BY LIEUT. COL. C. SUTHERLAND, ASSISTANT MEDICAL PURVEYOR, AND BY ACTING ASSISTANT SURGEONS W. R. BREWER, H. G. TIEDEMANN, AND J. F. BOUGHTER, UNITED STATES ARMY.

Fort Craig is situated in the county of Socorro, N. Mex., on the right or west bank of the Rio Grande del Norte; latitude, 33° 38′ north; longitude, 30° west; altitude, 4,314 feet above the sea. It is about ten miles above a well-known landmark in that vicinity, known as Fra Christobal,

32 M P

the commencement of the Jornada del Muerto. This Jornada is about eighty miles in length on the eastern side of the river, and mostly dry during the year. The nearest military post is Fort McRae, thirty-two miles to the south. Paraja, eight miles south, on the east side of the river, and San Marcial, three miles north, on the west bank, are the only neighboring towns.

The post was established on the abandonment of Fort Conrad, distant nine miles north, April 1, 1854, the buildings having been in process of erection some months previous. The object of Fort Craig was to afford protection against the inroads of the numerous bands of Apaches that roamed at large throughout the lower portion of New Mexico, from the Pecos to the Gila Rivers. The fort served also the purpose of protecting a road running to the lower portion of the Territory on the west side; this road, not much traveled ten years ago, is now principally used.

The reservation embraces an area of a little over thirty-eight square miles; the fort overlooks the river from the edge of a plain which extends for miles to the base of the western range of mountains. To the south, southwest, west, and north of the fort, the mountains are mainly basaltic, and partially covered with timber and scrub bushes. There is a large "mesa" nearly opposite and northeast of the fort, rising very abruptly from the river-bank, which is of volcanic origin, and whose summit is crowned with an extinct crater.

The soil of the bottom-lands is fertile, producing excellent vegetables and cereals, while that of the uplands affords only pasturage for stock.

Of wild animals, the grizzly, brown, and black bears, panther, wild-cat, weasel, large and small wolves, are the most important. Black and white tailed deer, as well as antelope, are abundant in the mountain regions. Swans, pelicans, wild geese, brant, and almost every species of duck abound on the river, as well as sand-hill cranes, blue herons, bitterns, and several species of snipe. At some distance from the post, and principally in the mountains, are found turkey, quail, blackbird, meadow-lark, robins, doves, sparrows, bluebird, cardinal bird, snow-bird, and many others. The river abounds in catfish, buffalo, and white fish. Beavers and muskrats are found in great numbers within a mile of the post.

The climate is variable; in summer the heat is very great; in winter there is a slight frost, and some little snow. This season is disturbed by the great storms of dust which blow, from the west principally, over this post, as well as over all the lower posts of New Mexico, thereby marring what would otherwise be a very delightful climate at that time of the year. The dust at times is stifling. The prevailing winds in summer are southwest; during winter, from the north. The fort is placed nearly equidistant from the northern and southern boundaries of the reservation, and is 72 feet above the Rio Grande.

The buildings are, with few exceptions, constructed of adobe, and are arranged around a rectangular area, 1,050 by 600 feet. For the general arrangement of the post, see Figure 34.

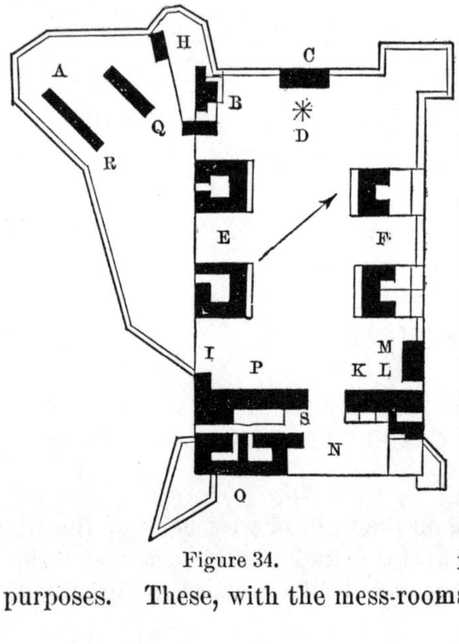

Figure 34.

A, casemates; B, commanding officer's quarters; C, guard-house; D, initial point; E, soldiers' quarters; F, officers' quarters; H, P, Q, R, store-houses; I, trader's store; K, married soldiers' quarters; L, hospital; M, unfinished hospital; N, corral; O, stables; S, shops.

The post was designed for two companies. The barracks are two in number, built of adobe, in the form of a hollow square, each inclosing a plazita. Each barrack contains two dormitories, 51 by 20 by 12⅔ feet, with a wide hall extending from the front of the building to the inclosed court in the rear. The buildings are badly designed; the ventilation is defective, and they cannot be heated. The dormitories have each two windows in front and one in the outer end; at the adjoining ends a door opens from each into the hall. Air-space per man, 786 cubic feet; single iron bedsteads are used. Movable sinks have been built 200 yards distant. The kitchens are comfortable and well floored rooms, furnished with stoves and open fire-places for cooking purposes. These, with the mess-rooms, non-commissioned officers' quarters, laundresses' quarters, and wood and coal rooms, are located to the rear of the dormitories, and complete the square inclosing the court.

The officers' quarters are three one-story buildings, built of adobe, plastered within and without; the flooring of all is composed of impure gypsum; the roofs are flat and of the same material. A portico, supported by wooden columns, extends the entire length of the western front of two, and eastern front of one of them. The arrangement of the rooms is shown by figure 35.

A, veranda; B, hall, 12 by 20 feet; C, D, rooms, each 20 feet square; E, F, rooms, each 14 by 18 feet; G, servant's room, 10 by 14 feet; H, dining-room, 14 by 26 feet; I, kitchen, 14 by 16 feet; J, store-room, 10 by 13 feet; K, yard, 15 by 21 feet; L and M, out-houses.

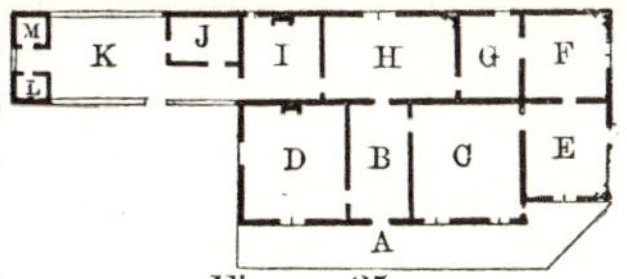

Figure 35.

All the rooms are 12½ feet high. These quarters are heated by open fire places, and well lighted by windows. There are no bath-rooms.

The guard-house is located in the center of one side of the post; the sally-port passes through it. On one side of the sally-port is the guard-room, 20 by 17 feet, and in rear of this the prison-room. This room has no floor, and the dust being very annoying, the ground is sprinkled frequently, producing constant dampness. On this damp ground the prisoner must sleep. On the south side, near the ceiling, are two openings, each 10 by 18 inches, and on the north side two, each 3 by 6 inches, with one barred window, 18 by 25 inches. The room is heated by a wood-stove. The average daily occupancy during 1873 was 7.46, the maximum 20.

In one corner of the guard-room is a trap-door opening upon a stairway which leads down to the cells where prisoners are kept in solitary confinement. The cells are six in number, three on each side of the passage-way. Each cell is 5 feet 7 inches long, 2 feet 10 inches wide, and 4 feet 10 inches high, giving a cubic space of 76 feet. Eight auger-holes and the chinks around the doors are the only means of admitting air and light into the cells. The whole amount of air and light admitted into the dungeons passes through two openings not to exceed in area 4 square feet. These cells are seldom occupied, but are considered as available for use.

The hospital buildings are as described in Circular No. 4, page 246. The new hospital ward has never been finished. But four beds are placed in each of the old wards, giving an allowance of 1,300 cubic feet to each.

Water is obtained from the Rio Grande, about one mile distant, and distributed by a water-wagon. The natural drainage is good. The whole post is dilapidated and in bad condition, no repairs or changes having been made for several years.

There are no systematic arrangements for bathing, either in summer or winter; the men avail themselves of the river during the hot months, at their own discretion. In the cold months, the wash-tubs of the laundresses are used for that purpose by the men.

Attempts have been made to cultivate gardens, but with little success. With the exception of the very small quantity of vegetables raised, none have been used by the troops. It has been recommended that potatoes be provided for winter use; but the chief commissary of the district reports that his department will not countenance such purchase.

The furniture of the barracks, though meager, is quite sufficient for the wants of the men. There are no benches or chairs; the men rolling up their bedding each morning to the head of the bunk, employing the foot of it as a seat.

A daily mail is received. A letter to Washington is from ten to twelve days in transit. Supplies for the post are transported by wagon from Granada, Colo.

The nearest railroad stations are Pueblo and Las Animas.

*Meteorological report, Fort Craig, N. Mex., 1870–'74.*

| Month. | 1870–'71. Mean. | Max. | Min. | Rain-fall in inches. | 1871–'72. Mean. | Max. | Min. | Rain-fall in inches. | 1872–'73. Mean. | Max. | Min. | Rain-fall in inches. | 1873–'74. Mean. | Max. | Min. | Rain-fall in inches. |
|---|---|---|---|---|---|---|---|---|---|---|---|---|---|---|---|---|
| July | 78.16 | 98 | 59 | 2.45 | 77.30 | 99 | 54* | 1.13 | | | | | 85.05 | 104* | 57* | 0.10 |
| August | 74.53 | 96 | 59 | 3.61 | | | | | | | | | 75.26 | 96* | 56* | 1.80 |
| September | 69.14 | 91 | 42 | 1.00 | 71.03 | 93 | 52 | 2.33 | | | | | 73.17 | 94* | 46* | 1.35 |
| October | 58.36 | 85 | 34 | 1.05 | 56.35 | 87* | 30* | 0.69 | 57.43 | 80 | 30* | 0.52 | 60.34 | 89* | 25* | 0.07 |
| November | 48.01 | 72 | 20 | 0.04 | 46.73 | 72* | 27* | 0.00 | 40.12 | 70 | 10 | 0.02 | 50.20 | 73* | 23* | 0.39 |
| December | 30.79 | 63 | −2 | 0.36 | 36.27 | 68 | 12 | 0.00 | 41.16 | 66 | 23 | 0.60 | 39.33 | 74* | 8* | 0.04 |
| January | 35.59 | 60 | 16 | 0.23 | 28.64 | 69* | 5* | (?) | 37.23 | 66 | 5 | 0.02 | 42.15 | 74* | −3* | 0.73 |
| February | 43.83 | 76 | 20 | (?) | 37.61 | 71 | 17 | 0.70 | 41.67 | 70 | 24 | 0.16 | 41.84 | 66* | 10* | 1.14 |
| March | | | | | 34.20 | 76* | 28* | 0.00 | 51.08 | 84 | 24 | 0.40 | 52.07 | 81* | 26* | 0.99 |
| April | | | | | 56.85 | 87 | 29 | 0.07 | 52.23 | 84 | 28 | 0.18 | 55.28 | 91* | 20* | 0.74 |
| May | | | | | 72.01 | 103* | 41* | 0.11 | 65.75 | 93 | 44 | 0.13 | 70.81 | 102* | 36* | 0.32 |
| June | | | | | 76.34 | 102* | 52* | 1.15 | 78.71 | 102 | 64 | 1.21 | 82.39 | 110* | 51* | 0.52 |
| For the year | | | | | | | | | | | | | 60.66 | 110* | −3* | 8.19 |

* These observations are made with self-registering thermometers. The mean is from the standard thermometer.

*Consolidated sick-report, Fort Craig, N. Mex., 1870–'74.*

| Year | | 1870–'71. Cases. | Deaths. | 1871–'72. Cases. | Deaths. | 1872–'73. Cases. | Deaths. | 1873–'74. Cases. | Deaths. |
|---|---|---|---|---|---|---|---|---|---|
| Mean strength | { Officers | 6 | | 5 | | 4 | | 3 | |
| | { Enlisted men | 139 | | 72 | | 75 | | 46 | |
| **Diseases.** | | | | | | | | | |
| GENERAL DISEASES, A. | | | | | | | | | |
| Typhoid fever | | 1 | | 1 | | 2 | | | |
| Typho-malarial fever | | 1 | | | | | | | |
| Remittent fever | | | | | | | | 1 | |
| Intermittent fever | | 12 | | 7 | | 8 | | 5 | |
| Other diseases of this group | | 4 | | 2 | | 4 | | 3 | |
| GENERAL DISEASES, B. | | | | | | | | | |
| Rheumatism | | 7 | | 10 | | 11 | | 3 | |
| Syphilis | | 19 | | 11 | | 14 | | 2 | |
| Other diseases of this group | | 4 | | | | | | | |
| LOCAL DISEASES. | | | | | | | | | |
| Catarrh and bronchitis | | 7 | | 13 | | 2 | | 4 | |
| Pneumonia | | | | | | | | 1 | |
| Pleurisy | | 3 | | | | | | 2 | |
| Diarrhœa and dysentery | | 17 | | 12 | 1 | 13 | | 4 | |
| Hernia | | | | | | 1 | | | |
| Gonorrhœa | | 7 | | 2 | | 5 | | 3 | |
| Other local diseases | | 27 | 1 | 20 | | 25 | 1 | 19 | |
| Alcoholism | | 8 | | 16 | | 22 | | 5 | |
| Total disease | | 117 | 1 | 94 | 1 | 107 | 1 | 52 | |
| VIOLENT DISEASES AND DEATHS. | | | | | | | | | |
| Gunshot wounds | | 2 | | | | 1 | | 1 | |
| Other accidents and injuries | | 21 | | 21 | | 28 | | 15 | |
| Homicide | | | 1 | | 1 | | | | 1 |
| Suicide | | | | | | 1 | | | |
| Total violence | | 23 | 1 | 21 | 1 | 29 | | 16 | 1 |

## FORT CUMMINGS, NEW MEXICO.

Fort Cummings is situated on the northeast side of Cook's Mountain, near the mouth of Cook's Cañon, in Grant County, N. Mex.; latitude, 32° 20′ north; longitude, 30° 45′ west; altitude, 4,750 feet. It is fifty-three miles west of the Rio Grande, and twenty miles east of the Rio Mimbres, the nearest water after leaving the post.

The general arrangement of this post is shown in Figure 36.

A, store-rooms; B, company and adjutant's offices; C, quartermaster's office; D, corral; E, shops; F, sally-port; G, prison; H, sheds; I, guard-house; J, officers' quarters; K, commanding officer's quarters; L, hospital; M, unfinished room; N, company quarters; P, sinks.

The post was abandoned in August, 1873. For full description see Circular No. 4, page 238.

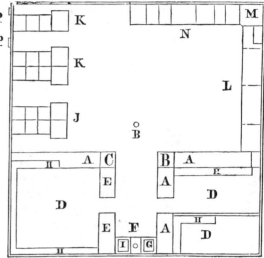

Figure 36—Scale 125 feet to 1 inch.

*Meteorological report, Fort Cummings, N. Mex., 1870–'74.*

| Month. | 1870–'71. | | | | 1871–'72. | | | | 1872–'73. | | | | 1873–'74. | | | |
|---|---|---|---|---|---|---|---|---|---|---|---|---|---|---|---|---|
| | Temperature. | | | Rain-fall in inches. | Temperature. | | | Rain-fall in inches. | Temperature. | | | Rain-fall in inches. | Temperature. | | | Rain-fall in inches. |
| | Mean. | Max. | Min. | | Mean. | Max. | Min. | | Mean. | Max. | Min. | | Mean. | Max. | Min. | |
| | ° | ° | ° | | ° | ° | ° | | ° | ° | ° | | ° | ° | ° | |
| July | 79.85 | 100 | 64 | 6.50 | 82.52 | 99 | 69 | 2.84 | 75.25 | 95* | 58* | 3.58 | 80.57 | 102* | 56* | 1.27 |
| August | 78.01 | 100 | 65 | 8.99 | 69.69 | 101 | 70 | 1.83 | 75.83 | 95* | 54* | 3.58 | ........ | ...... | ...... | ...... |
| September | 76.58 | 102 | 60 | 0.44 | 76.56 | 97 | 63 | 2.88 | 71.40 | 89* | 47* | 0.31 | ........ | ...... | ...... | ...... |
| October | 67.69 | 95 | 40 | 0.12 | 68.92 | 106 | 42 | 0.72 | 59.21 | 87* | 23* | 0.13 | ........ | ...... | ...... | ...... |
| November | 59.33 | 82 | 36 | 0.00 | 58.56 | 90 | 30 | 0.14 | 46.52 | 72* | 3* | 0.00 | ........ | ...... | ...... | ...... |
| December | 44.53 | 78 | 20 | 2.00 | 58.04 | 94 | 37 | 0.10 | 45.81 | 71* | 24* | 4.95 | ........ | ...... | ...... | ...... |
| January | 47.78 | 73 | 20 | 0.68 | 51.13 | 95 | 28 | 0.22 | 42.73 | 67* | − 5* | 2.00 | ........ | ...... | ...... | ...... |
| February | 53.57 | 77 | 32 | 0.15 | 56.12 | 83* | 21* | 0.00 | 45.91 | 66* | 13* | 0.62 | ........ | ...... | ...... | ...... |
| March | 53.60 | 82 | 33 | 0.05 | 58.13 | 100* | 23* | 0.00 | 56.20 | 81* | 24* | 0.32 | ........ | ...... | ...... | ...... |
| April | 59.80 | 83 | 39 | 0.00 | 62.43 | 88* | 33* | 0.20 | 57.98 | 82* | 10* | 0.15 | ........ | ...... | ...... | ...... |
| May | 72.70 | 94 | 56 | 0.00 | 73.81 | 102* | 44* | 0.11 | 67.31 | 85* | 36* | 0.05 | ........ | ...... | ...... | ...... |
| June | 83.68 | 107 | 65 | 1.40 | 82.93 | 99* | 56* | 0.44 | 77.14 | 106* | 45* | 1.27 | ........ | ...... | ...... | ...... |
| For the year | 64.76 | 107 | 20 | 20.33 | 66.57 | 106 | 21* | 9.48 | 60.11 | 106* | − 5* | 16.96 | ........ | ...... | ...... | ...... |

* These observations are made with self-registering thermometers. The mean is from the standard thermometer.

## FORT DODGE, KANSAS.

### REPORT BY ASSISTANT SURGEON W. S. TREMAINE, UNITED STATES ARMY.

Fort Dodge is situated on the north bank of Arkansas River, on the old Santa Fé trail; latitude, 37° 43′ 15″ north; longitude, 23° west. It is at the foot of a range of limestone bluffs, about

75 feet high, on a strip of bottom-land, consisting of blackish clay mixed with sand, and formed by washings from the bluffs.  The width of this strip is about 800 feet.

The position is weak in a military point of view, being commanded by the bluffs, and liable to surprise on account of the numerous ravines in the rear.  In a sanitary point of view the location is bad, the low land being difficult to drain, and flanked by a creek and low marshy ground.  Malarial diseases are frequent during the autumn months.  A much better location, but a few hundred yards distant, would be on an elevated plateau, with good natural drainage and commanding an extensive view of the surrounding country.  The meadow-lands on the right and left of the post and on the opposite bank of the river, here about 500 yards wide, furnish excellent grazing.  The upland in the vicinity is covered with buffalo-grass.  No timber is found within fifteen miles.  Buffalo, antelope, deer, and rabbits abound, and wild ducks in large numbers frequent the river and adjacent ponds.

The average monthly temperature for 1873 was 52° Fah.; maximum, 105°; and minimum, 21° below zero.

For history of the post see Circular No. 4, Surgeon-General's Office, 1870.

The barracks are three buildings, two of stone, one of adobe, weather-boarded, each 130 by 30 feet, by 9 feet high in the clear, with an L, 50 by 30 feet, containing dining-room and kitchen.  The dormitory, 118 feet long, contains forty-four iron single bunks, allowing 613 cubic feet per man.  This applies to the infantry companies, their average strength being about forty-five.  In the cavalry the average occupancy is seventy, giving a cubic air-space per man of 394 feet.  Ventilation is effected by opposite windows and doors; heating by wood-stoves.  In the rear is a well, and attached to the kitchen is a wooden shed, with trough for washing.  The latrines are about 30 yards distant.  Laundresses and married soldiers live in dug-outs and sod buildings along the river-bank.

Officers' quarters are contained in six one-story buildings, located on the north and west sides of the parade.  The first, a cottage building, frame, with an L, is 55 by 40 feet, and divided into two dwellings, consisting of a hall and two rooms, 19 by 18 feet by 10 feet high; two attic-rooms; a kitchen, 8 by 15 feet; and dining-room, 10 by 15 feet, in L; with servants' room over them in the attic of the L.  Each room is warmed by a fire-place, and lighted by two windows.  A veranda is in front.  These are captains' quarters.  An adobe cottage, of one story, weather-boarded, and divided into two dwellings, containing each two rooms, 17 by 17 feet, by 9 feet high, a small kitchen and dining-room in L, are also occupied as captains' quarters.

The commanding-officer's house, a stone building, one and a half stories high, and arranged for a field-officer, consists of a central hall with two rooms on each side, 18 by 18 feet by 10 feet high, a kitchen and pantry in the L, and four attic rooms.  In rear of this building is a frame building, weather-boarded, with coach-house and four stalls.

Three sets of double frame-buildings for lieutenants have been completed, and are on the west side of the parade.  Each is 45 by 22 feet, with an L, 25 by 32 feet, divided into two dwellings, containing a hall and two rooms, 15 by 15 feet; two small attic rooms; kitchen, 14½ by 11 feet; and dining-room, 14½ by 11 feet by 9 feet high, in the L.

Verandas are on the front of each of these buildings.  All the officers' quarters have good-sized yards, inclosed by a board fence.  There is also a small quadrangular inclosure in front of each set of officers' quarters, made with a lattice-work of laths.  Inside of these inclosures osage-orange has been planted, which will in time make hedges.

The store-houses, two in number, located on the west side of the parade, are built of sand-stone, 130 by 30 feet each, and separated by a wooden shed, 110 by 27 feet, which is used as a forage-house.  At the north end of each building two rooms are partitioned off as offices.

The guard-house is a temporary wooden shed, 28 by 18 feet, divided into two prison-rooms, one 13 by 17 feet, the other 16 by 13 feet; each room is 7 feet high, lighted and ventilated by two windows, unglazed, and warmed by a stove in each room.  Average daily occupancy for the past two months, $17\frac{15}{16}$.  This guard-house is a disgraceful place to confine prisoners, and the attention of the proper authorities has been repeatedly called to its condition.  About 10 feet distant from the above building is another shed, 27 by 15 feet by 7 feet high, occupied by the guard, lighted by two small windows, and warmed by a stove.

The hospital, located at the northwest-corner of the parade, is built of stone, one story high, and finished and occupied in February, 1868. The arrangement of the hospital is bad, as will be seen by reference to Figure 37.

A, ward, 26 by 43 feet; B, wash-room, 6¾ by 7 feet; D, dispensary, 15½ by 16½ feet; K, kitchen, 10 by 18 feet; M, dining-room, 10½ by 17 feet; N, bed-room, 10 by 15½ feet; O, office, 15½ by 16½ feet; S, store-room, 10 by 15½ feet.

The ward is a passage-way between the dispensary and steward's room on the one hand, and the kitchen, dining, and attendants' rooms on the other, thus separating the administration. The building is heated by stoves, and lighted by candles and lard-oil lamps. The ward, containing 12 beds, is plastered and hard-finished, lighted and ventilated by nine windows on opposite sides; no other means of securing ventilation is provided, and the top sash of the windows is not made to lower; the air-space per bed, however, is ample, being 1,040 cubic feet. The wash-room adjoining contains a bath-tub and basins. Situated 75 feet to the west is a frame building, 76 by 24⅓ feet, which is occupied by patients. During the year 1873 this build-ing was fitted up and divided as follows: a ward, 27 feet 5 inches by 23 feet 7 inches, by 10 feet high, ceiled and floored with hard-pine, with bath-room and water-closet attached; steward's room, 13½ feet by 13 feet 1 inch; matron's room, 13 feet 1 inch by 10 feet 2 inches, by 10 feet high; store-room, 21½ feet by 9 feet 10 inches; and post-mortem room, 23 feet 7 inches by 22 feet 5 inches. A veranda surrounds the building on the south and west. The hospital-grounds are inclosed by a fence 7 feet high.

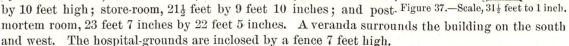

Figure 37.—Scale, 31½ feet to 1 inch.

The post bakery, built of stone, contains two ovens, capable of baking 500 rations of bread per diem.

The cavalry corral, 464 feet east of the cavalry quarters, is an inclosure 200 feet long, by 150 feet wide, surrounded by a sod wall, 8 feet high, with a shed-roof on three sides, and capacity for one troop of cavalry horses. In 1873, this corral being out of repair, shed-stables were built adjoin-ing it, of the following dimensions: Each 68 by 120 feet, with forage-house and harness-rooms, and affording shelter to the horses of one company of cavalry and eighty mules.

The post library is kept at the adjutant's office, and comprises 225 volumes, principally the works of celebrated novelists of the day.

The water-supply is obtained for drinking-purposes from wells, and for washing and extin-guishing fires from the Arkansas River; for the latter purpose, buckets and axes are kept in the barracks and store-houses. The supply from the wells is plentiful, and of excellent quality.

The drainage of the post is effected by a drain from each of the company quarters, discharging into a larger drain which empties into the river. Slops and refuse are carted into the river below the post, and carried off by the current. During the summer months the men bathe in the river, but in winter there are no facilities.

Radishes, string-beans, and lettuce have been raised in the hospital garden. It is believed that if a systematic and determined effort mas made to cultivate a post garden it would be success-ful, as the soil is rich and fertile near the river. The difficulties to be overcome are the natural dryness of climate and the attacks of insects and grasshoppers. Watering the plants with a diluted solution of coal-oil has proved most successful in meeting the latter difficulty.

The furniture of officers' quarters consists principally of plain bedsteads, tables, and chairs, made at the post. The cost of transportation from Saint Louis or Leavenworth makes it difficult to obtain other furniture except at a very great expense.

Since the completion of the Atchison, Salina and Santa Fé Railroad, January 1, 1873, the route of supply for this post is from Fort Leavenworth, distant 368 miles, via Kansas Pacific Railroad, to Topeka, thence by Atchison, Salina and Santa Fé Railroad to Dodge City, (a village 5 miles west.) The above railroad strikes the Arkansas Valley at Hutchinson, 134 miles east of Fort Dodge, and continues up the valley to Granada, Colo., 130 miles west; a daily train runs each way. The telegraph line sends a loop in, and there is an office of the Western Union Telegraph Company at the post. The nearest point on the railroad is distant $1\frac{7}{10}$ miles; the station is at Dodge City. The completion of the railroad to this post has given it the importance formerly attached to Fort Hays. It is now the point from which the Cheyenne, Arapahoe, Kiowa, and Comanche Indians are watched.

The garrison is therefore increased, during the summer months, by three or four companies of cavalry, which are kept continually scouting the country south of the river; an additional company of infantry also furnishes a guard to each station west on the line of railroad. The garrison consisted in July, 1874, of five companies of cavalry and four of infantry; one company of cavalry and two of infantry were quartered in the barracks, the other companies in tents.

While this could hardly be said to be a malarious country, yet the greater number of cases is seen to be from diarrhœa, dysentery, or intermittents. In the winter months diseases of the respiratory organs abound. Cholera was brought to the post July 9, 1867, by a detachment of colored troops, *en route* to New Mexico. The first case appeared among the troops July 21st, and the disease continued until the 31st day of that month, when it disappeared as suddenly as it commenced. This is the only epidemic that has been at the post. Since 1870, the health of the garrison has been good; there have been no epidemics. Mild malarial diseases, diarrhœa, and, in the winter months, catarrh of a mild type are prevalent. During the construction of the railroad and adjoining village of Dodge City, many cases of typho-malarial fevers occurred among the workmen, most of which were treated in hospital. The cool and cold bath was found to be an effectual mode of treatment. Owing to the dryness of the climate and the elevation, (about 2,600 feet above sea-level,) Fort Dodge may be considered a favorable climate for the early stages of pulmonary consumption, and in fact for most of the diseases incident to the "strumous diathesis." Many such cases have been benefited by residence here.

*Consolidated sick-report, (colored,) Fort Dodge, Kans., 1870–'72.*

| | 1870–'71. | | 1871–'72.* | |
|---|---|---|---|---|
| Year | | | | |
| Mean strength ......................................Enlisted men...... | 78 | | 1 | |
| Diseases. | Cases. | Deaths. | Cases. | Deaths. |
| GENERAL DISEASES, A. | | | | |
| Intermittent fever | 9 | | | |
| Other diseases of this group | 1 | | | |
| GENERAL DISEASES, B. | | | | |
| Rheumatism | 19 | | | |
| Syphilis | 1 | | | |
| Consumption | 1 | | 1 | |
| Other diseases of this group | 1 | | | |
| LOCAL DISEASES. | | | | |
| Catarrh and bronchitis | 9 | | | |
| Diarrhœa and dysentery | 33 | | | |
| Other local diseases | 48 | 1 | | |
| Alcoholism | 1 | | | |
| Total disease | 123 | 1 | 1 | |
| VIOLENT DISEASES AND DEATHS. | | | | |
| Gunshot wounds | 1 | | | |
| Other accidents and injuries | 50 | | | |
| Total violence | 51 | | | |

\* One month only.

*Consolidated sick-report, (white,) Fort Dodge, Kans., 1870-'74.*

| Year | 1870-'71. | | 1871-'72. | | 1872-'73. | | 1873-'74. | |
|---|---|---|---|---|---|---|---|---|
| Mean strength { Officers.......... { Enlisted men...... | 10 162 | | 9 168 | | 11 195 | | 16 286 | |
| Diseases. | Cases. | Deaths. | Cases. | Deaths. | Cases. | Deaths. | Cases. | Deaths. |
| GENERAL DISEASES, A. | | | | | | | | |
| Typhoid fever ...... | 2 | 1 | 3 | 1 | 1 | 1 | ...... | ...... |
| Typho-malarial fever...... | 2 | | ...... | | ...... | | ...... | |
| Remittent fever ...... | 2 | | ...... | | ...... | | ...... | |
| Intermittent fever...... | 42 | | 84 | | 106 | | 83 | |
| Other diseases of this group ...... | 13 | 1 | 5 | | 21 | | 29 | |
| GENERAL DISEASES, B. | | | | | | | | |
| Rheumatism ...... | 19 | ...... | 25 | ...... | 28 | ...... | 23 | ...... |
| Syphilis ...... | 8 | ...... | 13 | ...... | 3 | ...... | 5 | ...... |
| Consumption ...... | 1 | 1 | ...... | | 2 | 1 | 1 | ...... |
| Other diseases of this group ...... | ...... | | 3 | | ...... | | 4 | |
| LOCAL DISEASES. | | | | | | | | |
| Catarrh and bronchitis...... | 45 | ...... | 59 | ...... | 46 | ...... | 77 | ...... |
| Pneumonia ...... | 1 | ...... | 3 | 2 | 1 | ...... | ...... | |
| Pleurisy...... | 2 | | ...... | | ...... | | ...... | |
| Diarrhœa and dysentery...... | 50 | ...... | 100 | ...... | 41 | ...... | 105 | ...... |
| Hernia ...... | 1 | | ...... | | ...... | | ...... | |
| Gonorrhœa ...... | ...... | | 7 | ...... | 6 | ...... | 5 | ...... |
| Other local diseases ...... | 148 | ...... | 119 | ...... | 108 | ...... | 169 | ...... |
| Alcoholism...... | 12 | ...... | 3 | ...... | 3 | ...... | 17 | ...... |
| Unclassified...... | ...... | | ...... | | 1 | | ...... | |
| Total disease ...... | 348 | 3 | 424 | 3 | 367 | 2 | 518 | ...... |
| VIOLENT DISEASES AND DEATHS. | | | | | | | | |
| Gunshot wounds ...... | ...... | | 2 | ...... | 4 | ...... | 6 | ...... |
| Other accidents and injuries...... | 64 | ...... | 84 | ...... | 75 | ...... | 80 | ...... |
| Homicide ...... | ...... | | ...... | | ...... | 1 | ...... | |
| Suicide...... | ...... | 1 | ...... | | ...... | | ...... | 1 |
| Total violence ...... | 64 | 1 | 86 | ...... | 79 | 1 | 86 | 1 |

# FORT GARLAND, COLORADO TERRITORY.

## REPORT OF ASSISTANT SURGEON P. MOFFATT, UNITED STATES ARMY.

Fort Garland is located in Southern Colorado. Latitude, 37° 23′ north; longitude, 27° 20′ west; altitude, 7,805 feet above the sea. The reservation, comprising a little less than four square miles, lies between Sangre de Cristo and Ute Creeks, in the northeast portion of San Luis Park.

The San Luis is the southern of the Colorado parks; through it, entering at the northwest and flowing south, runs the Rio Grande del Norte, while from its mountain boundaries numerous streams either empty their waters into the great river or sink and become lost upon its plains. Throughout the park isolated volcanic buttes are found, resembling islands upon the surface of the sea. The mountains surrounding this valley are rugged, and attain to such a height that on almost every side snow is to be seen the year round. A conspicuous group to the north and west of the post, in the range of the Sierra Blanca, and designated locally as "*Old Baldy*," reach an elevation of 14,206 feet above the sea. This group is a prominent landmark from all surrounding sides, resembling in general contour the Spanish peaks 100 miles to the east.

The perennial snows of Old Baldy sustain some half a dozen elevated lakes in the recesses between its summit and base; and these again are the feeders of Ute Creek, from which the water-supply of Fort Garland is derived.

Upon Ute Creek is the site of old Fort Massachusetts, erected in 1850. From its unfavorable location in the cañon it was abandoned, and Fort Garland erected in its stead, in 1857. That locality was selected for the reason that it was in close proximity to the point where an important Indian trail passed over the mountain ridge which divides the valley of the Arkansas from that of the Rio Grande.

33 M P

The fort effectually commands the pass (which, however, is no longer traveled by the Indians,) as well as other points at which wagon-roads have been constructed over the divide.

The character of the country in this vicinity, as over all the mountainous regions of Colorado Territory, is not such as to admit of cultivation, except in mere spots on the margins of the streams.

Cattle-men state that a weed grows among the grass—particularly in damp ground—which is poisonous to horned cattle and horses, and destroys many of them. From the manner in which they describe its effects upon animals, it must be of the nature of a narcotic; and they state that cattle after having eaten it may linger for many months, or for a year or two, but invariably die at last from its effects. The animal does not lose in flesh apparently, but totters on its limbs and becomes crazy. While in this condition a cow will lose her calf, and never find it again; and will not recognize it if presented to her. The eyesight becomes affected, so that the animal has no knowledge of distances, but will make an effort to step or jump over a stream or an obstacle while at a distance off, but will plunge into it or walk up against it upon arriving at it.*

The wild animals of the vicinity are the black, cinnamon, and grizzly bears, elk, deer, antelope, panther, wild cat, gray wolf, coyote, prairie-dog, and mountain-sheep.

In the fall and early spring all varieties of wild ducks, geese, swan, and crane, are to be found upon the meadows of the Rio Grande, with an occasional snipe and Virginia rail.

The streams abound in trout, beaver, otter, and mink, with a few muskrats.

The climate is dry, and favorable to most diseases of the respiratory and digestive organs, but unfavorable to rheumatism.

The spring seasons are very short, and hard frosts are liable to occur early in the summer—in one year as early as the month of July.

The post consists of a parallelogram, inclosing a parade, with quarters for officers and men, arranged on its several sides.

The barracks are two buildings, one story high, built of adobe, with mud roofs; each is 119 feet 6 inches by 33 feet 3 inches, and is 15 feet 4 inches to the center of the roof, which slopes toward the parade. The interior is plastered with mud, and whitewashed with lime; contains the company office and store-room, 20 feet 8 inches by 33 feet 3 inches; two squad-rooms, 37 feet 6 inches by 33 feet 3 inches, and the kitchen, 24 feet 6 inches by 33 feet 3 inches. The latter is also used as a mess-room. Each barrack is intended to accommodate one company. The squad-rooms are warmed by stoves and open fire-places, and lighted by four large windows, two at either end of the room, by which ventilation is also procured.

The air-space per man, for a company of 50 men, is about 1,100. cubic feet. The dormitories are furnished with single iron bedsteads of the usual pattern. As there are no wash or bath rooms, ablutions are made in the squad-room or in the open air.

The sinks are wooden buildings placed over an *acequia*, through which a large volume of water constantly flows, carrying *débris* into Ute Creek, below the post.

A spacious kitchen and mess-room for each barrack is furnished with a large cooking-stove and open fire-place, and fully meets all demands. Quarters for the band are in a building west of the general barracks and parade-ground. This building is very imperfectly constructed, being divided into a number of poorly lighted and ventilated compartments, some of which are without floors.

Married soldiers are quartered in a building of much the same character, situated to the east and north of the general inclosure, at a distance of about 100 paces.

The officers' quarters extend along the north side of the parade, are seven in number, and built of adobe.

The rooms are ceiled with pine boards and covered with earth, after the old Mexican custom. They are well lighted and ventilated; have large, open fire-places and boarded flooring. On the south side of the parade are two long buildings used as offices and store-rooms. In one of these is the guard-house, which is badly arranged, being cramped as to space, and ill ventilated. The cells in its rear are ventilated only by a small opening in the roof—no arrangements for floor ventilation existing.

---

* This plant is understood to be the *Oxytropis Lamberti*.

The guard-room is warmed by means of a large stove, and the prison-room by an open fire-place; there are no means provided for heating the cells, and in the winter the occupants suffer from extreme cold.

The hospital-building is situated north of the post, and to the left and rear of the officers' quarters. This building was put up in 1866, and the adobes used were not properly dried before the walls were built. The meteorological register shows the season in which the work was performed to have been unusually wet and stormy. The beams used were too small and set too far apart to bear properly the weight of the roof. When the walls commenced to settle, which was soon after the completion of the building, and when the post was garrisoned by New Mexican volunteers, no care seems to have been taken properly to repair the damage. In the wards, kitchen, and dining-room, the majority of the beams are broken, requiring supports to be placed under them; and in the largest ward no less than five of these supports are required. The rear wall of the plazita, which is 20 feet in height and 2 feet in thickness, requires supports to be placed against it from the outside. Of the two wards, each containing six beds, the larger has a superficial area of 97.22 feet, and an air-space of 1,069.44 feet to each bed; the smaller has an area of 84.22 feet, and an air-space of 926.85 feet. The dispensary is well arranged and adapted to the purpose. There is no bath-room in the hospital; a small room is used as a lavatory. A small wooden building, standing over a deep pit, is the hospital water-closet; its drainage is good, and it is constantly disinfected by lime.

The post-bakery is a room 21 feet 8 inches by 29 feet 5 inches, containing two ovens built of adobe, having a capacity of one hundred rations at a baking.

The stables are situated 126 feet due east from the post, and consist of three long corrals built of adobe, each $229\frac{1}{2}$ by $44\frac{1}{2}$ feet. These corrals contain long sheds, which are used as stables for public animals, and inclosed stables for officers' horses. The space between the sheds is raised and the floors of the sheds slope from within out. In the rear of each shed is a wooden drain sunk to the level of the ground, and empties upon a gravel-bank east of the corral.

The water-supply is excellent in quantity, being obtained from the Ute Creek by an *acequia*; it flows around the parade, at each corner of which is a well. The water is pure and cold, flowing from the rocky sides of the Sierra Blanca over a rocky, sandy bed directly into the post.

There are no means of extinguishing a fire at the post beyond buckets and ladders and two of "Babcock's fire-extinguishers." The drainage of the post is naturally perfect, being built upon a large gravel-bed, which has little or no covering, and through which water is reached only at a great depth.

There is no artificial sewerage at the post.

On the Sangre de Cristo Creek very fine bathing and swimming arrangements have been established. For winter-bathing no arrangements have been made.

The post-garden consists of about six acres of ground, one-half of which is devoted to enlisted men, the balance to officers and the hospital. It is cultivated by a detail from the garrison; and all garden-produce that requires but a short season can be raised here. The crop of the past season comprised radishes, potatoes, turnips, carrots, tomatoes, beets, and squash. Only a moderate success was achieved, and in the case of some articles the effort was a failure.

Government wagons and ambulances or private conveyances are almost the only means of communication with Butte Valley Station, in the Huerfano, whence daily stages run to Pueblo to the north, and Santa Fé to the south. A "buck-board," semi-weekly, carrying the mail, is the only public conveyance between San Luis Park and the Arkansas Valley. From the post to Butte Valley Station, where stage can be taken, is forty-five miles; and thence to Pueblo, the present terminus of the Denver and Rio Grande Railway, narrow-gauge, is forty-two miles. It is expected that this railway will be pushed forward by another year in the direction of Santa Fé, so as to be within forty or fifty miles of this point. Travel over the road between this place and Butte Valley Station, on the stage-road, is at times impracticable, or attended with great hardship, on account of the piercing cold and deep snow in going over the divide by the Sangre de Cristo Pass or any of the other passes. As Pueblo is in regular communication, via Denver City, with the general railway system of the country, the difficulties and delays of traveling, or in regard to mail matter, do not extend beyond that point; but, in consequence of failures in the connections, mail-matter which ought to reach this place from New York or Washington in seven days, and sometimes does so, may require two weeks.

The population of San Luis Park is estimated at about 7,500 souls, including the number in and about the post of Fort Garland. The character of the people of Colorado, excluding the Mexicans, is, I am persuaded, superior on an average to that of the people in most of the western Territories. There is an amount of thrift and enterprise about them which promises well for the development of the country; and a laudable public spirit is exhibited by the people at large, in the support of schools, churches, and kindred institutions.

The sanitary condition of Fort Garland is favorable, and has been so during the past year. No epidemic has prevailed, and no tendency to any one disease has been manifested, except it be a liability to sub-acute and chronic rheumatism. Venereal diseases, formerly very prevalent among the command at Fort Garland, are now rarely met with, and then mostly imported.

In the last few years this region has acquired quite a degree of notoriety as a sanitarium for persons suffering from various forms of chronic disease—more particularly in cases involving pulmonary affections. Great numbers of invalids come to this Territory yearly from the Atlantic States, and many from foreign countries, in search of health. This region promises fair to become to health-seekers the Italy and Switzerland of the American Continent, and the Rocky Mountains to vie with the Alps and Appenines as a resort for those in search of a new lease of life.

In considering the sanitary effects of a sojourn or permanent residence in this country—including not this point only, but all the elevated portions of the Southwest—two distinct points are to be taken cognizance of; one is the change in occupation, manner of life, and social relations to which the individual is introduced, and which he is led to adopt upon arriving in this country; the other has reference to climatic and other conditions peculiar to the locality, to which he is subjected.

In the case of the tourist traveling for pleasure or for health, the drudgery of business has been suspended, and recreation is made the object of life for the time; or the indolent and luxurious life of the city has been exchanged for the novelties, exercise, and less sumptuous fare of " the mountains." In the case of those who have settled permanently in the country, they too have adopted occupations and habits of life materially different from what they were accustomed to before coming here. It is quite a usual thing in these mountainous regions to find people living a pastoral life, or prospecting for ledges, amidst the rudest surroundings, and in the most primitive style, who had been reared in affluence and fashion in some of the larger cities of the East or of Europe. The number of the population who prepare their victuals over the camp-fires, or in the rudest cabins, and who work, eat, and sleep in the open air, is by no means inconsiderable. Closely-built buildings, heated with stoves, are the exception, out of the larger towns. Most of the habitations are so constructed as to admit of free ventilation, and are warmed by the primitive back-log upon the hearth, or the little fire-place in one corner of the room, where the wood is burned on end, after the Mexican manner. It is my opinion that no small degree of the undoubted benefits of residence n these mountainous regions, is, in certain forms of disease, attributable to these causes. From what I have observed, it is by those who place themselves under such circumstances, more frequently than by those who endeavor to approximate as closely as possible to the personal surroundings of older communities, that improvement in health is enjoyed. As a general thing the more thoroughly the person can approximate his occupation and manner of life to the state of existence known as " roughing it," the better the result.

The principal distinguishing feature of Fort Garland and vicinity, in a sanitary point of view, is its great altitude. Little perceptible effect is observed upon the respiration of persons in good health as a general thing, but some individuals do complain of a want of breath on slight exertion. The respiration is somewhat increased in frequency, and the action of the chest deeper than at ordinary altitudes. This is rendered necessary from the fact that a greater volume of air is required to furnish a given quantity of oxygen to the economy in this place, where the barometer indicates a pressure of only about 22.50 inches, than at ordinary levels. To this increased mechanical action or play of the lungs, and distention of the parenchymatous-tissue, may be attributed part of the beneficial effects of high altitudes in certain diseases of these organs. The effect of this place upon the circulation is quite as marked as upon the respiration. The pulse of fifteen persons, all in good health, was carefully noted. In every case the person was in a state of quiet at the time of the examination, the subjects being either seated or in the recumbent posture. Three of the number were females. The average per minute of the fifteen was, in round numbers, ninety, lacking only the slightest fraction. In examining the pulse for diagnostic purposes, I had, prior to these observations, and almost unconsciously, dropped into the habit of allowing an increase of ten to fifteen in frequency over the usual rate per minute without attaching any significance there to. A very noticeable feature in connection with the pulse is its rapid rise in frequency upon exertion. The pulses of four persons in perfect health were noted while at rest, and again after a brisk walk on level ground of a hundred yards, with an increase in frequency, respectively, of 28, 42, 35, and 23 per minute. This rapid action of the heart and excitability upon exertion is in accordance with the increased rapidity of the respiration, but it constitutes a very serious objection to this place as a residence for those laboring under cardiac disease, or any affection in which it forms a complication. I have not seen cases of this nature here, but from what I have observed in other localities of considerable altitude, I am satisfied of the truth of this remark Altitude seems to have an effect upon those suffering from heart-disease something similar to. the exertion of ascending a stair or walking up hill. In any case in which this condition exists as a complication, whatever may be the benefit otherwise, I am satisfied the embarrassment caused to the heart will be a serious offset, if not an insuperable obstacle, to any real improvement.

I believe Fort Garland will be found unfavorable as a residence for those suffering from dilatation of the heart, fatty degeneration, and valvular lesions, and, in short, from any of the forms of cardiac disease.

Vesicular emphysema, and that form of chronic bronchitis associated with disease of the heart, I believe unsuited to a residence here, or in any locality possessing this altitude. The other forms of chronic bronchitis, chronic pneumonia, and phthisis are the diseases, par excellence, for which I believe this region peculiarly well fitted.

A case is under my observation at present at this post of a man who left the Atlantic coast a little over one year ago, and came to Colorado for his health. Before leaving the East he had suffered three alarming hemorrhages from the lungs, and his case was considered grave in the extreme. Since coming to this region he has much improved, and has had no repetition of the hemorrhage. A permanent residence in this country will, in all probability, confer length of years upon a life which was considered doomed before he left his home in the East. Another case has come under my observation in contrast with this, where a man came to this region in the third stage of pulmonary tuberculosis ten months ago. He was not improved by coming here; but, on the contrary, the increased labor imposed upon the portion of lung still remaining caused a constant uncomfortable feeling of want of breath. At an unexpected moment, after he had been in this country some months, violent pulmonary hemorrhage occurred, and the man died within ten minutes.

*Meteorological report, Fort Garland, Colo., 1870–'74.*

| Month. | 1870–'71. Temperature. | | | 1870–'71. Rain-fall in inches. | 1871–'72. Temperature. | | | 1871–'72. Rain-fall in inches. | 1872–'73. Temperature. | | | 1872–'73. Rain-fall in inches. | 1873–'74. Temperature. | | | 1873–'74. Rain-fall in inches. |
|---|---|---|---|---|---|---|---|---|---|---|---|---|---|---|---|---|
| | Mean. | Max. | Min. | | Mean. | Max. | Min. | | Mean. | Max. | Min. | | Mean. | Max. | Min. | |
| | ° | ° | ° | | ° | ° | ° | | ° | ° | ° | | ° | ° | ° | |
| July | 67.50 | 90 | 47 | 7.30 | 68.06 | 97 | 50 | 1.00 | 62.80 | 82 | 45 | 10.30 | 66.24 | 87 | 35* | 0.80 |
| August | 66.29 | 90 | 52 | 7.50 | 63.89 | 87 | 43 | 1.25 | 61.61 | 90 | 41 | 5.68 | 63.82 | 82 | 39* | 0.48 |
| September | 60.14 | 80 | 35 | 0.90 | 58.23 | 83 | 40 | 2.90 | 50.46 | 70 | 26 | 0.83 | 59.18 | 78 | 25* | 0.18 |
| October | 48.99 | 80 | 27 | 1.30 | 41.19 | 70 | 19 | 1.40 | 38.15 | 60 | 3 | 0.10 | 43.61 | 74 | 9* | 0.50 |
| November | 41.36 | 72 | 20 | 0.15 | 28.31 | 58 | 0 | 7.10 | 20.95 | 50* | -35?* | 0.00 | 32.78 | 60 | 5* | 0.01 |
| December | 15.68 | 70 | -26 | 3.35 | 29.19 | 54 | 0 | 1.75 | 18.79* | 50* | -20* | 0.00 | 19.88 | 52 | -15* | 0.20 |
| January | 19.93 | 59 | -15 | 1.20 | 18.37 | 52 | -14 | 2.25 | 13.17 | 40* | -40* | 0.00 | 19.40 | 48 | -23* | 0.50 |
| February | 23.96 | 50 | -12 | 1.45 | 26.62 | 58 | - 9 | 2.75 | 15.23 | 40* | -10* | 2.25 | 15.29 | 38 | -23* | 2.80 |
| March | 35.15 | 58 | 11 | 2.80 | 32.86 | 59 | 4 | 3.65 | 29.45 | 55* | 5* | 0.00 | 31.35 | 58 | 0* | 0.50 |
| April | 41.68 | 67 | 17 | 2.45 | 40.93 | 69 | 16 | 2.78 | 30.08* | 60* | 0* | 1.75 | 34.27 | 67 | 8* | 0.15 |
| May | 53.81 | 93 | 36 | 1.45 | 52.74 | 83 | 30 | 6.25 | 45.54 | 70* | 14* | 0.00 | 51.12 | 76 | 25* | 0.08 |
| June | 66.89 | 92 | 50 | 0.25 | 60.45 | 81 | 45 | 7.75 | 60.80 | 86 | 35* | 1.58 | 63.77 | 84 | 30* | 0.20 |
| For the year | 45.11 | 93 | -26 | 30.10 | 43.40 | 52 | -14 | 40.83 | 37.25 | 86 | -40* | 22.49 | 41.73 | 87 | -23* | 6.40 |

* These observations are made with self-registering thermometers. The mean is from the standard thermometer.

NOTE.—The observations at Fort Garland are not reliable. Mean temperatures from 1872 to 1873 are especially doubtful, as also the rain-fall for 1873–'74, provided the record of the rain-fall for the three previous years be approximately correct.

*Consolidated sick-report, Fort Garland, Colo., 1870–'74.*

| Year | | 1870–'71. | | 1871–'72. | | 1872–'73. | | 1873–'74. | |
|---|---|---|---|---|---|---|---|---|---|
| Mean strength........ { Officers ........... | | 5 | | 5 | | 5 | | 5 | |
| { Enlisted men ....... | | 108 | | 71 | | 87 | | 104 | |
| | | | | | | | | | |
| Diseases. | | Cases. | Deaths. | Cases. | Deaths. | Cases. | Deaths. | Cases. | Deaths. |
| GENERAL DISEASES, A. | | | | | | | | | |
| Typhoid fever.... | | 3 | | | | | | | |
| Typho-malarial fever... | | | | 1 | | | | | |
| Remittent fever.... | | 14 | | 13 | | | | 1 | |
| Intermittent fever :... | | 11 | | | | | | 4 | |
| Diphtheria... | | | | | | 1 | | | |
| Other diseases of this group... | | 42 | | 8 | | 7 | | 39 | |
| GENERAL DISEASES, B. | | | | | | | | | |
| Rheumatism ... | | 35 | | 23 | | 25 | | 22 | |
| Syphilis ... | | 24 | | 12 | | 8 | | 6 | |
| Consumption ... | | 1 | | | | 1 | | 2 | |
| Other diseases of this group... | | 6 | | | | 3 | | 1 | |
| LOCAL DISEASES. | | | | | | | | | |
| Catarrh and bronchitis... | | 122 | | 34 | | 94 | | 41 | |
| Pneumonia... | | 2 | | | | | | 1 | |
| Pleurisy... | | | | | | | | 2 | |
| Diarrhœa and dysentery ... | | 82 | | 33 | | 41 | | 34 | |
| Hernia ... | | 1 | | | | | | | |
| Gonorrhœa ... | | 5 | | 5 | | 3 | | 2 | |
| Other local diseases ... | | 130 | 1 | 63 | | 75 | | 60 | |
| Alcoholism... | | 33 | | 45 | | 22 | | 24 | |
| Total disease... | | 511 | 1 | 237 | | 280 | | 239 | |
| VIOLENT DISEASES AND DEATHS. | | | | | | | | | |
| Gunshot wounds ... | | 3 | | 2 | | 1 | | | |
| Other accidents and injuries ... | | 72 | | 41 | 1 | 36 | | 57 | |
| Homicide... | | | | | | | | | 2 |
| Total violence... | | 75 | | 43 | 1 | 37 | | 57 | 2 |

# FORT GIBSON, CHEROKEE NATION, INDIAN TERRITORY.

### REPORTS OF ASSISTANT SURGEON ALFRED DELANY, AND OF ACTING ASSISTANT SURGEON H. S. KILBOURN, UNITED STATES ARMY.

Fort Gibson is located on the east bank of the Neosho or Grand River, 3 miles northeast of its confluence with the Arkansas; latitude, 35° 48' 10'' north; longitude, 18° west, and 600 feet above the level of the sea. The reservation is an irregular rectangle, 6 miles long from north to south, containing an area of eight square miles and four hundred and twenty-one acres. (See plate opposite.) The reservation lines include the national cemetery, which is situated near the southeast corner. The general configuration of the surface of the reserve is very irregular. It is well watered and timbered.

Tahlequah, the territorial seat of government, is 17 miles distant, in a northeasterly direction. The nearest military post is Fort Smith, Arkansas, 65 miles distant, in a southeasterly direction, on the dividing line between Arkansas and the Territory. The site is the western terminus of a high rolling prairie, which extends in an easterly direction from the fort to the Menard Mountain, distant about 3 miles. On the north side of the fort the prairie descends rapidly to a narrow strip of bottom, which has a river margin of 1½ miles. On the south side it generally slopes to a plain, which is fifty feet below the fort, and distant about 400 yards. This plain extends back from the river more than 300 yards, where it is terminated by a ridge of land, the commencement of the prairie. To the south and west this plain is continuous with an extensive river-bottom, which extends to the Arkansas River, 3 miles, and along this river, in a southeasterly direction, more than 4 miles to the Bayou Menard; it has an average breadth of 3 miles, and contains several lakes. The southern half of this plain is covered with forest trees and a very dense undergrowth.

On the west side of Grand River lies another extensive bottom, irregularly triangular in form,

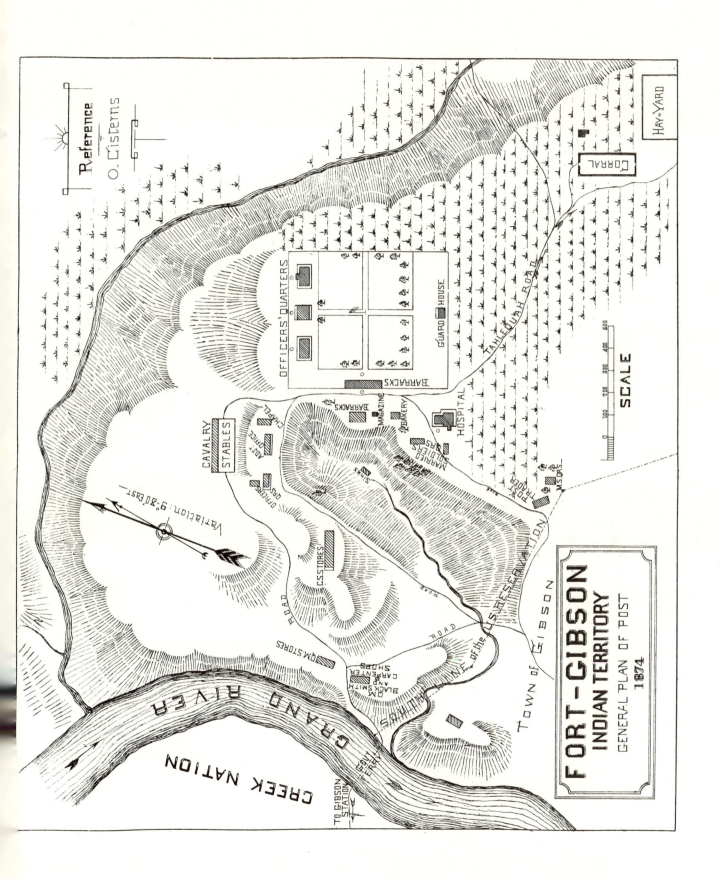

which is limited by the Arkansas River on the southwest, the Grand River on the east, and the Verdigris River on the west; it has an average breadth of 2 miles, and is heavily timbered. The soil is sandy, underlaid by limestone, and varies in depth from a few inches to several feet. There is scarcely an acre of land, except upon the ranges of high hills, that is not arable and susceptible of cultivation; the soil will produce abundantly all kinds of cereals, vegetables, fruits, cotton, and tobacco. The principal crops now raised are corn, wheat, potatoes, and oats; fruits, (apples, pears, and peaches,) of the finest quality, are very plentiful. Timber is scarce, growing only in the bottoms, along the rivers and bayous, and on the mountains, but there very densely. It consists chiefly of oak, walnut, hickory, pecan, and cotton-wood. Wild prairie grass grows rank and heavy, and is cut for hay in large quantities. None of the cultivated varieties, or clover, have been sown. The country is well watered, and abounds in springs; near the post, however, water is only found at great depths, and is strongly impregnated with lime. There are innumerable salt springs of the purest quality on the Illinois, Grand, and Canadian Rivers, some of which are extensively worked.

The fort is more than 100 feet above ordinary low-water mark in the Grand River.

The barrack is built of dark yellow sandstone, of two stories, with mess-rooms and kitchens below, and squad-rooms and orderly-rooms above. Though calculated to afford quarters for two companies, this building is at present occupied by only one company, giving in the dormitories, which are ceiled, about 900 cubic feet per man. The old commissary warehouse is now occupied as quarters by one company. This structure is of stone, one story, a basement and a loft; first floor is occupied as squad-room, basement as mess-room and kitchen. Air space in squad-room per man, about 500 cubic feet. There is no special arrangement for ventilation in either of these buildings. The new pattern iron bunks (single) are used in the dormitories; gun-racks have been removed, and the arms are kept in one of the office rooms in each barrack. A new barrack sink consists of a stone vault surmounted by a wooden out-building, and is located 75 yards in rear of the quarters.

Married soldiers' quarters within the limits of the garrison are tents and log out-buildings.

There are five sets of quarters for officers. The commanding officer's quarters are built of dark sandstone, one story and a half high, with an English basement. This house contains thirteen rooms, including the attic and basement. Those of the first floor and basement are built on opposite sides of a hall, 10 feet wide, extending through the building. All the rooms are large, well lighted, and, excepting those of the attic, have open fire-places. The other sets of quarters are built in pairs. They are frame, with stone foundations. Two of them have basements; the remaining two have, in lieu thereof, a small cellar each. There are six rooms in each house, including the kitchen. These quarters are substantially built houses, having high, airy rooms, open fire-places, and large doors and windows.

Each single set of quarters is now occupied by two officers. The post surgeon occupies a room in the hospital for lack of suitable quarters.

The store-house of the chief quartermaster and commissary of the district is a handsome stone building, 150 feet by 42 feet, and one story high; about 50 yards south of the officers' quarters is a narrow stone building, 50 feet long, used as offices by the district and post commanders.

The commissary store-house stands 50 feet south of the barracks and parallel to them. It is a substantial stone structure, 30 feet by 36 feet, two stories high, and has a cellar. This building is dry, freely ventilated, and is admirably adapted to the purpose for which it is used.

In addition to the buildings described may be mentioned the saw-mill, the blacksmith-shop, and the officers' mess-hall. An ice-house has been erected which will hold sufficient ice to supply the demands of the garrison throughout the summer season.

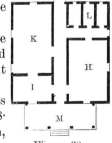

The guard-house is a square wooden building, with no special arrangements for ventilation, and ill adapted for the purpose, being too small. See Figure 38. Outside measurement, 35 feet 6 inches by 35 feet 6 inches. H, guard-room, 14 feet 3 inches by 21 feet 6 inches; I, officer of the guard's room, 8 feet 4 inches by 14 feet 3 inches; K, prisoners' room, 25 feet 2 inches by 14 feet 3 inches; L, cells, 8 feet deep—

Figure 38.

three in the space of 14 feet 3 inches; M, veranda, 24 feet long by 8 feet wide. It is now unoccupied, and the rooms in the office-building are used as guard-room. These are warmed and ventilated by fire-places. Average occupancy, 4.

During the year 1871, a new hospital was erected. It is of pine lumber, and consists of an administration building and one ward, arranged as a wing, on the north side of the former, and is built on the plan proposed in Circular No. 4, dated April 27, 1867, Surgeon-General's Office, for a post hospital of twelve beds. A veranda surrounds the entire building, excepting the back building, or kitchen, and the central window on each side of the ward has been converted into a door with a sash above it. The ward is ventilated entirely by the ridge, as provided in the plan for summer ventilation. No shaft or jacket has been provided for winter ventilation. A cistern, of sufficient capacity to supply water for all purposes, is sunk in the angle formed by the wing and back building. A privy with a stone vault has been built. In the dimensions of the hospital, and arrangement of the rooms, &c., the plan was strictly followed, but in the matter of fixtures it is yet incomplete. No sinks and drains to the kitchen and wash-rooms were made; but the building, generally speaking, is well adapted to its purpose.

The stable is located on the northwest side of the officers' quarters, and to the leeward of them, as well as the men's quarters; it is built in the form of a square, and consists simply of sheds divided into stalls. Refuse from the stable is carted to the distance of over a mile from the post.

Two cisterns, one in front and the other in the rear of the barracks, each having a capacity of 8,000 gallons, are chiefly depended upon for the supply of water, though many prefer, for drinking, the water of the Grand River, which, when confined to its sandy and rocky bed, is beautifully clear, very agreeable to the taste, and remarkably free from organic matter. For cooking purposes however, the cistern-water is usually employed.

There is no system of sewerage at the post. The configuration of the surface on which the fort is located, being a gradual declination to all sides, secures good drainage. All refuse at the post is collected and carted away daily.

The cemetery is situated about a mile and a half from the garrison. The post-garden consists of about ten acres of land, from which the garrison and hospital are amply supplied with all kinds of vegetables, especially potatoes.

The nearest quartermaster and subsistence depots are at Fort Leavenworth, Kansas, two hundred and ninety-seven miles distant. The route of supply is by the Arkansas River, which is open about six months in the year, and the best method of transporting supplies is by steamboat. Communication between the post and the nearest town is by boat, when there is sufficient water in the Arkansas River.

Fort Gibson has been called the "charnel-house of the frontier," and it may reasonably be supposed that when the fort was located on the plain to the south the ratio of sick was greater than at present; for, while citizens and others who live in the village on the site of the old fort, and those who live in the bottoms bounded by the Arkansas and Verdigris Rivers, suffer almost constantly from malarial fevers or in some other manner manifest symptoms of malarial poisoning, the troops suffer much less, and are usually able to attribute an attack to special exposure. The quartermaster's employés, who occupy quarters built on the slope to the south of the fort and about 35 feet above the village plain, suffer less than the villagers, but vastly more than the troops.

The Grand River is subject to an annual rise, which usually takes place in June or July. The bottoms are then subject to an overflow. When the water subsides the soil is left saturated with moisture, and the reeking, slimy surface, rich in decomposing vegetable matter, sends forth that poison which is supposed to be the cause of malarial fevers.

*Meteorological report, Fort Gibson, C. N., Ind. Ter., 1872–'74.*

| Month. | 1870–'71. | | | | 1871–'72. | | | | 1872–'73. | | | | 1873–'74. | | | |
|---|---|---|---|---|---|---|---|---|---|---|---|---|---|---|---|---|
| | Temperature. | | | Rain-fall in inches. | Temperature. | | | Rain-fall in inches. | Temperature. | | | Rain-fall in inches. | Temperature. | | | Rain-fall in inches. |
| | Mean. | Max. | Min. | | Mean. | Max. | Min. | | Mean. | Max. | Min. | | Mean. | Max. | Min. | |
| | ° | ° | ° | | ° | ° | ° | | ° | ° | ° | | ° | ° | ° | |
| July.......... | | | | | | | | | | | | | 82.91 | 100* | 54* | 2.13 |
| August......... | | | | | | | | | | | | | 83.45 | 104* | 56* | 1.53 |
| September...... | | | | | | | | | | | | | 71.37 | 96* | 44* | 7.71 |
| October........ | | | | | | | | | | | | | 57.08 | 88* | 18* | 2.80 |
| November....... | | | | | | | | | | | | | 51.12 | 80* | 21* | 2.02 |
| December....... | | | | | | | | | | | | | 40.48 | 70* | 16* | 3.42 |
| January........ | | | | | | | | | | | | | 39.77 | 74* | 11* | 3.43 |
| February....... | | | | | | | | | | | | | 41.86 | 69* | 19* | 3.34 |
| March......... | | | | | | | | | | | | | 52.05 | 78* | 29* | 2.75 |
| April......... | | | | | | | | | 57.49 | 86* | 23* | 5.18 | 54.66 | 79* | 31* | 5.55 |
| May........... | | | | | | | | | 68.74 | 80* | 32* | 5.10 | 71.72 | 94* | 40* | 2.32 |
| June.......... | | | | | | | | | 78.32 | 101* | 56* | 2.96 | 81.22 | 94* | 56* | 3.11 |
| For the year ...... | | | | | | | | | | | | | 60.64 | 104* | 11* | 40.16 |

* These observations are made with self-registering thermometers. The mean is from the standard thermometer.

*Consolidated sick-report, (white,) Fort Gibson, C. N., Ind. Ter., 1870–'74*

| Year ..... | 1870–'71. | | 1871–'72.* | | 1872–'73.† | | 1873–'74. | |
|---|---|---|---|---|---|---|---|---|
| Mean strength ..... { Officers ............... | 10 | | 7 | | 10 | | 6 | |
| { Enlisted men ...... ....... | 143 | | 110 | | 116 | | 120 | |
| Diseases. | Cases. | Deaths. | Cases. | Deaths. | Cases. | Deaths. | Cases. | Deaths. |
| GENERAL DISEASES, A. | | | | | | | | |
| Typhoid fever......... | 1 | | | | | | 4 | |
| Remittent fever......... | 2 | | | | | | | |
| Intermittent fever......... | 196 | | 63 | | 40 | | 137 | |
| Other diseases of this group......... | 2 | | 2 | 1 | 1 | | 8 | |
| GENERAL DISEASES, B. | | | | | | | | |
| Rheumatism ......... | 7 | | 3 | | 1 | | 10 | |
| Syphilis ......... | 2 | | 1 | | 1 | | 14 | |
| Other diseases of this group......... | 2 | | | | | | 10 | |
| LOCAL DISEASES. | | | | | | | | |
| Catarrh and bronchitis......... | 38 | | 6 | | 8 | | 29 | |
| Pneumonia......... | 1 | | | | | | | |
| Diarrhœa and dysentery......... | 70 | | 42 | 1 | 8 | | 36 | |
| Hernia......... | 3 | | | | | | | |
| Gonorrhœa......... | 6 | | 3 | | | | 11 | |
| Other local diseases ......... | 85 | | 31 | | 15 | | 60 | 1 |
| Alcoholism ......... | 9 | 1 | 1 | 1 | | | 7 | |
| Total disease ......... | 424 | 1 | 152 | 3 | 74 | | 326 | 1 |
| VIOLENT DISEASES AND DEATHS. | | | | | | | | |
| Gunshot wounds ......... | 3 | | | | | | 2 | 2 |
| Drowning ......... | | | | | | | | 5 |
| Other accidents and injuries......... | 103 | | 23 | | 2 | 1 | 45 | |
| Total violence......... | 106 | | 23 | | 2 | 1 | 47 | 7 |

* Five months only.        † Three months only.

34 M P

*Consolidated sick-report, (colored,) Fort Gibson, C. N., Ind. Ter., 1872–'73.*

| Year | 1872–'73.* |
|---|---|
| Mean strength..............................................................Enlisted men...... | 149 |

| Diseases. | Cases. | Deaths. |
|---|---|---|
| GENERAL DISEASES, A. | | |
| Remittent fever .................................................................. | 18 | ...... |
| Intermittent fever .............................................................. | 93 | ...... |
| Other diseases of this group ................................................ | 2 | ...... |
| GENERAL DISEASES, B. | | |
| Rheumatism ...................................................................... | 16 | ...... |
| Syphilis ........................................................................... | 27 | ...... |
| Consumption ..................................................................... | 1 | ...... |
| Other diseases of this group ................................................ | 5 | ...... |
| LOCAL DISEASES. | | |
| Catarrh and bronchitis ....................................................... | 14 | ...... |
| Pleurisy ........................................................................... | 1 | ...... |
| Diarrhœa and dysentery....................................................... | 17 | ...... |
| Gonorrhœa ......................................................................... | 10 | ...... |
| Other local diseases............................................................ | 62 | 1 |
| Alcoholism ........................................................................ | 1 | ...... |
| Unclassified ...................................................................... | 1 | ...... |
| Total disease ............................................................. | 268 | 1 |
| VIOLENT DISEASES AND DEATHS. | | |
| Gunshot wounds.................................................................. | 5 | ...... |
| Other accidents and injuries.................................................. | 27 | ...... |
| Total violence ............................................................ | 32 | ...... |

* Eleven months only.

# FORT HARKER, KANSAS.

Fort Harker is situated on the Kansas Pacific Railroad; latitude, 38° 45′ north; longitude, west; altitude, 1,856 feet.

For history and description of post, see report of Surgeon B. E. Fryer, United States Army, in Circular No. 4, pp. 290–298.

The post was abandoned in April, 1872.

*Meteorological report, Fort Harker, Kans., 1870–'72.*

| Month. | 1870–'71. | | | | 1871–'72. | | | | 1872–'73. | | | | 1873–'74. | | | |
|---|---|---|---|---|---|---|---|---|---|---|---|---|---|---|---|---|
| | Temperature. | | | Rain-fall in inches. | Temperature. | | | Rain-fall in inches. | Temperature. | | | Rain-fall in inches. | Temperature. | | | Rain-fall in inches. |
| | Mean. | Max. | Min. | | Mean. | Max. | Min. | | Mean. | Max. | Min. | | Mean. | Max. | Min. | |
| | ° | ° | ° | | ° | ° | ° | | ° | ° | ° | | ° | ° | ° | |
| July.................... | | | | | 78.79 | 106* | 55* | 4.81 | | | | | | | | |
| August................. | 72.47 | 106 | 48 | (?) | 76.17 | 105* | 44* | 0.80 | | | | | | | | |
| September ............ | 65.21 | 95 | 42 | 7.46 | 66.51 | 97* | 35* | 1.05 | | | | | | | | |
| October............... | 52.73 | 85 | 35 | 6.25 | 55.23 | 94* | 26* | 0.05 | | | | | | | | |
| November............. | 38.76 | 79* | 15* | 0.00 | 32.60 | 75* | 6* | 1.50 | | | | | | | | |
| December............. | 21.05 | 76* | –13* | 6.25 | 23.67 | 52* | –5* | 0.20 | | | | | | | | |
| January............... | 27.08 | 76* | –10* | 2.43 | 25.22 | 52* | –10* | 0.00 | | | | | | | | |
| February ............. | 39.35 | 85* | –10* | 5.25 | 33.14 | 67* | –4* | 0.39 | | | | | | | | |
| March................. | 45.91 | 89* | 11* | 2.08 | 38.74 | 73* | –15* | 0.00 | | | | | | | | |
| April................. | 55.43 | 95* | 25* | 0.97 | 55.32 | 91* | 28* | 1.11 | | | | | | | | |
| May................... | 64.23 | 87* | 36* | 0.78 | | | | | | | | | | | | |
| June.................. | 77.55 | 101* | 52* | 3.27 | | | | | | | | | | | | |
| For the year....... | | | | | | | | | | | | | | | | |

* These observations are made with self-registering thermometers. The mean is from the standard thermometer.

# FORT HAYS, KANSAS.

REPORTS OF SURGEON A. F. MECHEM AND ASSISTANT SURGEON J. H. JANEWAY, UNITED STATES ARMY.

Fort Hays, in the central part of the State of Kansas—latitude, 38° 59' north; longitude, 22° west; 1,893 feet above the level of the sea—is located on a slightly elevated piece of ground a quarter of a mile from Big Creek, a branch of the Smoky Hill Fork of the Kansas River; ten miles north of the Smoky Hill Fork, and fifteen miles south of the Saline River, another branch of the Kansas.

The nearest mountains are from two hundred to two hundred and fifty miles distant, in a westerly direction. The nearest post, Fort Larned, is forty-one miles southeast; Fort Dodge, about eighty miles south, and Fort Wallace, one hundred and twenty-seven miles west.

Hays City, about three-quarters of a mile from the post, is the nearest station of the Kansas Pacific Railroad.

Old Fort Hays, on Big Creek, fifteen miles east of this post, was established in the autumn of 1866 to protect the employés of the Kansas Pacific Railroad Company from the attacks of Indians, and at first was named Fort Fletcher, in honor of ex-Governor Fletcher, of Missouri; but afterward, in the winter of 1866–'67, the name was changed to Fort Hays, in honor of Major-General Isaac G. Hays, who was killed at the battle of the Wilderness. During the summer of 1867, it became necessary to abandon the site first chosen on account of a destructive overflow of Big Creek at that point. The present site of Fort Hays was selected by Brevet Major-General Gibbs, United States Army, major Seventh United States Cavalry, June 22, 1867, by authority of Major-General Hancock, commanding the Department of the Missouri.

The reservation is irregularly triangular, extreme length six miles, extreme breadth three and a half miles, and contains about 7,500 acres. This tract of land and country in the immediate vicinity are situated in a shallow basin surrounded by a low limestone ridge, the distance from the post to the ridge varying from two to five miles. The surface of the reservation is gently undulating, and is traversed by numerous gullies running from the ridge to the creek, which convey the surface-drainage of the reservation and the ground about the post.

The geological formation includes a series of groups constituting the secondary mountain formation of the cretaceous system. This formation occurs at greater or less depths on the reservation, but crops out throughout the whole extent of the ridge which surrounds the post.

Overlying the cretaceous strata from above downward, we have dark, sandy loam, fine siliceous loam of a buff color, yellow clay, and hard marly clay. Selenite, breccia, and conglomerates are found thinly scattered over the ground in the vicinity of the post. The soil is tolerably fertile in the bottoms, but unproductive, not so much for want of rain as on account of the dry scorching winds which sweep the plains during the summer season.

The trees grow almost exclusively along the banks of the streams, as there are but few other localities which are protected from the annual fires which sweep the plains. A few elms have been found in the ravines and cedars on the cliffs. The elm surpasses all other trees, both in beauty and number, on the bank of the creek near the post.

The wild animals found near the post are three varieties of the common bat, the American wild-cat, gray wolf, coyote, long-tailed weasel, common mink, American badger, raccoons, skunk, American otter, American beaver, striped gopher, prairie dog, wood-rats, yellow-haired porcupine, common American hare, prairie hare, jackass rabbit, American elk, antelope, two varieties of the genus cervus, and the American buffalo.

The birds are the turkey-buzzard, duck-hawks, pigeon-hawk, sparrow-hawk, great horned owl, screech-owl, burrowing-owl, sapsucker, black woodcock, red-headed woodpecker, red-shafted flicker, whippoorwill, nighthawk, belted kingfisher, bee-martin, robin, cliff-swallow, mocking-bird, red-bird, cowbird, red-winged blackbird, western lark, crow blackbird, crow, blue jay, Carolina dove, wild turkey, dusky grouse, prairie-chicken, sand-hill crane, killdeer, wild-goose, long-billed curlew, blue-winged teal, mallard.

The fish found in Big Creek, near the post, belong principally to the *Cyprinidæ* or carp family ; the common shiner, (*Leuciscus americanus;*) brook minnows, (*Leuciscus atronacus;*) chub suckers, (*Catostomi.*)   Besides these are the catfish or common horned-pout.   The crustaceans are repre- sented by the crawfish, and the mollusks by the *Unio* or fresh-water clam, both found in the creek. There are but few streams in this region.   Big Creek, the only one within ten miles, is a clear running stream, from 10 to 20 feet wide, with gravelly bottom and good fall.   Four wells, from 30 to 50 feet deep, were dug at different points about the post in July and August, 1867, and walled with lime- stone.   No springs have been found in the vicinity, and the nearest ponds, about two miles distant, are near the creek, containing water only for a short time after heavy rains.

The prevailing winds for the greater part of the year are from the south; in the fall and winter northerly winds prevail.   The winds are dry and scorching in the summer and early fall, cold and piercing in the winter and early spring.   The barracks, for four companies, consist of four frame buildings erected in the winter of 1867–'68, by citizen carpenters in the employ of the quarter- master.   These buildings are temporarily constructed of pine lumber, with single-cased wooden walls, boards nailed on vertically, and the joints battened.   They are not ceiled or plastered.   Each barrack is 118 feet long by 24 feet wide, 10 feet high from floor to eaves, and 6 feet from eaves to ridge.

The plan of one of these barracks is shown in Figure 39.

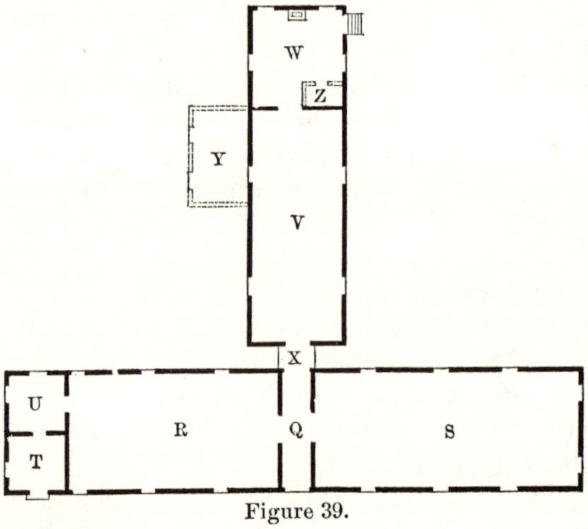

Figure 39.

Q, entry; R, squad-room, 42 by 24 feet; S, squad- room, 55 by 24 feet; T, first sergeant's room, 13 by 13 feet; U, store-room, 13 by 11 feet; V, mess-room, 60 by 20 feet; W, kitchen, 20 by 21 feet; X, covered way; Y, proposed wash-house; Z, proposed pantry.

The dormitories are fitted with single iron bunks, and allow about 600 cubic feet to each.

The sinks are in rear of, and lower than, the barracks, about 50 yards distant, and consist of pits covered with small frame buildings.   These sinks are moved occasionally, and the excreta in the pits thickly covered with dry earth.   In rear of each bar- rack is a frame building, 66 by 20 feet, containing the mess-room, 46 by 20 feet, and kitchen, 20 by 20 feet; height from floor to eaves, 10 feet, from eaves to ridge of roof, 6 feet.

The plan of the commanding officer's quarters is shown in Figure 40.

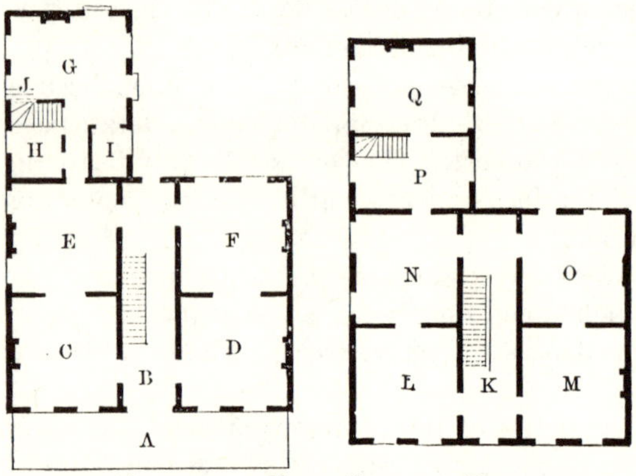

A. First story.—A, porch, 8 by 38 feet; B, hall, 8 by 31 feet; C, parlor, 15 by 15 feet; D, bedroom, 15 by 15 feet; E, dining-room, 15 by 15 feet; F, bed- room, 15 by 15 feet; G, kitchen, 17 by 13 feet; H, pantry; I, stores; J, back stairs.

B. Second story.—K, hall and staircase; L, bedroom, 15 by 15 feet; M, bedroom, 15 by 15 feet N, bedroom, 15 by 15 feet; O, bedroom, 15 by 15 feet; P, lumber-room, 17 by 10 feet; Q, servants' room, 17 by 13 feet.

A.              Figure 40.              B.

The married soldiers' quarters consist of four frame buildings of the same character as the barracks, each building containing four sets of quarters of two rooms each, the rooms being 12 feet square.   Some of the quarters have temporary sheds in the rear, which are used as kitchens.   There are nine buildings at this post used as officers' quarters.   They are tolerably well constructed of unseasoned pine lumber, which, having shrunk since the erection of the buildings, allows the rain and snow to drive in, particularly when accompanied by high winds.   All the officers' quarters are plainly finished, weather-boarded frame buildings, painted on the outside.   The interior walls and ceilings were at first hard-finished, but have since been lime-washed.   Seven of the buildings are one story and a half high, with porches in front, the remaining two being one story high without porches.

The plan of one of the other sets of officers' quarters is shown in Figure 41.

S, porch, 8 by 39 feet; T, hall, 7 by 15 feet; U, parlor, 15 by 15 feet; V, chamber, 15 by 15 feet; W, dining-room, 13 by 15 feet; X, kitchen, 15 by 16 feet; Y, pantry; Z, kitchen closet.

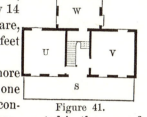

Figure 41.

The one-story buildings have each four rooms on the first floor; in one, two rooms are 14 by 9 feet; the dining-room, 16 by 14 feet; kitchen, 14 by 14 feet—height to ceiling 10 feet. In the other two rooms, one 15 feet square, and one 8 by 11 feet—height to ceiling 8 feet; two other rooms, 13 by 11 feet—height to ceiling, 7½ feet; kitchen, 15 by 10 feet.

The quarters are conveniently arranged for one family, or two or more officers without families; but when it becomes necessary for more than one family to live in a single set of quarters, it has been found exceedingly inconvenient. To obviate this in some measure temporary shed-rooms have been erected in the rear of front rooms of some of the quarters.

In the story and a half buildings, and chaplain's quarters, the front rooms are heated by means of wood fires in fire-places, the other rooms by means of wood-burning stoves. They are ventilated by means of the fire-places, and the wind passing through openings about the windows and doors.

The water for officers' use is brought from the creek in a water-wagon and emptied into barrels placed near the quarters. There are no bath-rooms.

The quartermaster's store-houses consist of three one-story frame buildings, each 96 by 24 feet, built parallel to each other, at an interval of 10 feet, all joined the whole length by narrow roofs, with less pitch than the main roofs. The quartermaster's offices, &c., are in a one-story frame building, 96 by 24 feet.

The commissary office and store-house are in a one-story frame building, 150 by 34 feet. These buildings are in rear of the company barracks, outside of the parade ground and diagonally in front of the officers' quarters, on sloping ground, lower than the officers' quarters or soldiers' barracks.

The guard-house is built of stone. The plan is shown in Figure 42.

A, room for officer of the guard, 10 by 20 feet; B, guard-room, 20 by 38 feet; C, prison-room, 20 by 35 feet; D, cells, 5 by 7 feet.

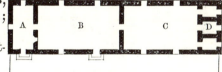

Figure 42.

The heating and ventilation of this building are not satisfactory.

The post hospital is a frame building, one story, built of pine lumber, with jointed weather-boarding, constructed in Saint Louis, Mo., shipped to this post, and erected in November, 1867; since which time, however, many additions and alterations in the original building have been made rendering it more suitable for the purpose for which it was intended. The arrangement of the hospital is shown in Figure 43.

E, vestibule, 12 by 8 feet; F, south ward, 24 by 40 feet; G, north ward, 24 by 40 feet; H, office, 9 by 12 feet; I, dispensary, 9 by 12 feet; J, attendant's room, 9 by 13 feet; K, store-room, 9 by 10 feet; L, knapsack-room, 9 by 8 feet; M, hall and passage, 5 feet wide, (passage, 7 feet 6 inches;) N, cook's room, 9 by 11 feet; O, dining-room, 12 by 24 feet; P, kitchen, 12 by 14 feet; Q, attendants' room, 12 by 12 feet; R, smoking and wash-room, 12 by 12 feet; S, store-room, 12 by 20 feet; T and

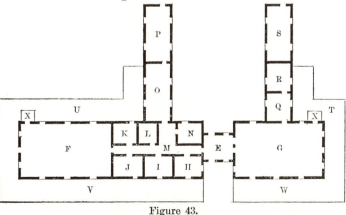

Figure 43.

U, rear veranda, 8 feet wide; W and V, front veranda, 8 feet wide; X X, earth-closets, 5 by 6 feet.

Early in the winter of 1872, a frame building, 104 by 24 feet, was removed to this place from Fort Harker. It is divided into a chapel, 40 by 20 feet, and a reading-room and hall, 64 by 24 feet.

The quartermaster's stables are located about 75 yards northeast of the nearest barrack. There are four frame buildings, each 175 by 28 feet, roughly weather-boarded, shingle-roofed, with ridge ventilation; or it may be considered as one frame-building, 175 by 112 feet, with a "double M" shingle roof, partitioned so as to form four parallel stables, the aisles between the stables having a gradual slope the whole length of the building, so that the stables are dry and well drained under all circumstances.

The cavalry-stables are about 100 yards west of the nearest barrack, on a gentle slope, lower than the post dwellings, and consist of a main building, 110 by 24 feet, with wings at the ends, each 86 by 24 feet. This building has stockade walls, plastered outside and inside, shingle-roofed, with louvre ventilation.

The most of the water used at the post is brought from the creek in a water-wagon. Besides this source of supply there are four wells, one near the quartermaster's corral, one near the barracks, one in the hospital yard, and another in rear of the officers' quarters. The supply of water is practically unlimited, as there is water in all the wells, and there is brought from the creek to the post between 1,500 and 2,000 gallons daily. The water from the creek ordinarily deposits very little organic sediment. After heavy rains the oxidizable organic matter is much increased, but not to such a degree as to produce any injurious effects. The water is impregnated to a limited extent with lime and magnesia, in combination with carbonic and sulphuric acids.

The natural drainage is excellent, the post being so located on a slight elevation that the drainage in every direction is from the site of the post.

All manure and refuse are carted to a point one mile west of the post, deposited in a ravine, and from time to time burned.

There are no arrangements for bathing in winter.

The cemetery is badly located between two ravines, which carry the drainage into the creek above the place where the water is procured for the post. Area of cemetery, 133,464 square feet, or a little more than three acres.

*Meteorological report, Fort Hays, Kans., 1870–'74.*

| Month. | 1870–'71. | | | | 1871–'72. | | | | 1872–'73. | | | | 1873–'74. | | | |
|---|---|---|---|---|---|---|---|---|---|---|---|---|---|---|---|---|
| | Temperature. | | | Rain-fall in inches. | Temperature. | | | Rain-fall in inches. | Temperature. | | | Rain-fall in inches. | Temperature. | | | Rain-fall in inches. |
| | Mean. | Max. | Min. | | Mean. | Max. | Min. | | Mean. | Max. | Min. | | Mean. | Max. | Min. | |
| July | 82.08 | 100 | 59 | 2.25 | 81.43 | 106 | 60 | 2.40 | 76.73 | 99 | 59 | 4.42 | 78.59 | 103 | 57 | 1.38 |
| August | 73.99 | 104 | 46 | 0.50 | 73.01 | 100 | 50 | 2.30 | 76.09 | 103 | 54 | 1.92 | 78.67 | 101 | 59 | 4.08 |
| September | 66.85 | 89 | 47 | 5.40 | 65.84 | 92 | 48 | 9.00 | 65.35 | 102 | 33 | 2.50 | 64.69 | 96 | 30 | 0.86 |
| October | 50.52 | 74 | 38 | 2.50 | 51.97 | 70 | 33 | 1.80 | 55.79 | 97 | 10 | 0.00 | 51.71 | 87 | 12 | 0.60 |
| November | 46.39 | 72 | 19 | 0.00 | 29.47 | 74 | — 2 | 1.63 | 34.15 | 74 | — 7 | 0.04 | 43.97 | 79 | 2 | 0.42 |
| December | 28.89 | 66 | —10 | 1.70 | 21.26 | 42 | — 5 | 5.00 | 20.22 | 63 | —15* | 0.34 | 24.67 | 45 | 1 | 2.18 |
| January | 37.19 | 64 | 18 | 0.10 | 21.92 | 42 | —13 | (?) | 23.65 | 60 | —15* | 0.38 | 29.69 | 62 | 5 | 1.32 |
| February | 36.55 | 62 | 5 | 5.80 | 31.57 | 68 | — 1 | (?) | 29.86 | 68 | —15* | 0.62 | 24.27 | 54 | —12 | 1.80 |
| March | 45.48 | 80 | 21 | 0.25 | 36.69 | 75 | 15 | (?) | 46.06 | 82 | 4 | 0.40 | 38.64 | 69 | 20 | 7.26 |
| April | 52.23 | 89 | 30 | 4.60 | 52.93 | 84 | 29 | 0.96 | 45.52 | 92 | 23 | 1.40 | 48.40 | 91 | 23 | 2.34 |
| May | 62.55 | 89 | 40 | 2.75 | 64.61 | 90 | 30 | 3.92 | 61.31 | 88 | 34 | 7.88 | 67.49 | 91 | 45 | 3.68 |
| June | 75.94 | 104 | 55 | 0.67 | 75.39 | 106 | 53 | 0.80 | 77.84 | 102 | 49 | 2.44 | 76.71 | 104 | 54 | 2.18 |
| For the year | 54.83 | 104 | —10 | 26.52 | 50.51 | 106 | —13 | ........ | 51.04 | 103 | —15 | 22.34 | 60.62 | 104 | —12 | 28.10 |

* These observations do not represent the actual minimum temperature, the thermometer being graduated to only 15°.

*Consolidated sick-report, Fort Hays, Kans., 1870–'74.*

| Year | 1870–'71. | | 1871–'72. | | 1872–'73. | | 1873–'74. | |
|---|---|---|---|---|---|---|---|---|
| Mean strength { Officers | 15 | | 15 | | 12 | | 10 | |
| { Enlisted men | 225 | | 176 | | 186 | | 227 | |
| **Diseases.** | Cases. | Deaths. | Cases. | Deaths. | Cases. | Deaths. | Cases. | Deaths. |
| GENERAL DISEASES, A. | | | | | | | | |
| Cerebro-spinal fever | | | | | 1 | | | |
| Typhoid fever | 2 | 1 | | | | 1 | | |
| Remittent fever | | | 1 | | | | 1 | |
| Intermittent fever | 26 | | 120 | | 29 | | 77 | |
| Other diseases of this group | 8 | | 23 | | 1 | | 5 | |
| GENERAL DISEASES, B. | | | | | | | | |
| Rheumatism | 7 | | 13 | | 20 | | 42 | |
| Syphilis | 5 | | 3 | | 6 | | 4 | |
| Consumption | | 1 | 3 | 2 | 4 | | 2 | |
| Other diseases of this group | 3 | | 1 | | | | | |
| LOCAL DISEASES. | | | | | | | | |
| Catarrh and bronchitis | 19 | | 29 | | 91 | | 226 | |
| Pneumonia | | | 6 | 1 | | | 2 | 1 |
| Pleurisy | 1 | | 3 | | 1 | 1 | | |
| Diarrhœa and dysentery | 28 | 1 | 36 | 1 | 68 | | 127 | |
| Hernia | | | 1 | | 4 | | 2 | |
| Gonorrhœa | 3 | | 5 | | 5 | | 5 | |
| Other local diseases | 66 | 2 | 110 | | 117 | | 255 | |
| Alcoholism | 3 | | 19 | | 25 | | 19 | |
| Unclassified | | | 1 | | | | | |
| Total disease | 171 | 5 | 374 | 4 | 372 | 2 | 767 | 1 |
| VIOLENT DISEASES AND DEATHS. | | | | | | | | |
| Gunshot wounds | 2 | | 4 | | 5 | 1 | 4 | |
| Other accidents and injuries | 77 | | 99 | 1 | 101 | 1 | 165 | |
| Homicide | | 1 | | | | 1 | | |
| Suicide | | | | | 1 | | | |
| Total violence | 79 | 1 | 103 | 2 | 106 | 3 | 169 | |

# FORT LARNED, KANSAS.

INFORMATION FURNISHED BY ASSISTANT SURGEONS W. H. FORWOOD, A. A. WOODHULL, AND S. G. COWDREY, UNITED STATES ARMY.

Fort Larned is situated on the right bank of Pawnee Fork, about seven miles from its confluence with the Arkansas; latitude, 38° 10′ north; longitude, 22° west; altitude above the sea, 1,932 feet. The post was established in September, 1859, for the protection of the Santa Fé trail, and was at first known as Camp Alert. Adobe buildings were constructed in 1860, and the post received its present name as a compliment to Colonel B. F. Larned, then Paymaster-General. The reservation, as declared by General Order No. 22, Headquarters Department of the Missouri, dated November 25, 1867, contains sixteen square miles. The Atchison, Topeka, and Santa Fé Railroad was completed to this point in August, 1872; since which time trains have been run regularly.

The town of Larned is on the east bank of Pawnee Creek, at its mouth; contains a depot, express, telegraph, and newspaper offices; is growing rapidly, and will probably be the county-seat.

The post is bounded on the north and west by the creek; on the south a flat prairie extends six miles to the Arkansas River. The bottom-land is covered with good grass, from which hay is obtained for the post. The post was rebuilt in 1867, the buildings being of sandstone and arranged around a square; the quarters for enlisted men being on the north. There are two buildings, each containing two sets of company-quarters. Three of the four squad-rooms are 40 feet square by 10 feet high. Between the ceilings of these rooms and the roof there is a free space, containing (in each building) about 30,000 cubic feet, and communicating with the external air by a series of openings under the eaves on the south side; said openings having in each building the aggregate area of 30 square feet. Each squad-room communicates with this loft by three rectangular openings in the middle line of the ceiling, having an aggregate area of 2,652 square inches.

The buildings for officers' quarters are three in number, built of sandstone, one story high, shingled roof, with a broad portico in front. One of these buildings is for the commanding-officer; it contains a hall, four rooms, each 14 by 16 feet, a kitchen, 19 by 16 feet, and a servants' room over the kitchen, which is the only up-stairs room at the post. Each of the other buildings is 84 by 33 feet, and contains four sets of quarters. They are traversed by two halls, 7 feet wide, each hall being common to two sets of quarters, so that each building is supposed to accommodate two captains and four lieutenants. The captains' quarters are in the ends, and consist of two rooms, each 16 feet wide by 14½ feet deep, and 12 feet high, and a kitchen, 19 by 10 feet, from which opens a servants' room. The two rooms communicate by folding-doors, and the kitchen opens into the back or bed room. Under the kitchen is a cellar, which has been deepened and floored, and been thus transformed into a kitchen, leaving the kitchen proper for use as a dining-room.

The hospital occupies the northeast half of the northeast barrack, and consists of two wards, each 39½ feet long and 32¼ and 27 feet wide. Dispensary, 23 by 17⅔ feet. Mess-room, 22 feet 10 inches by 16 feet 6 inches. Kitchen, 19 feet 6 inches by 16 feet. Store-room, 16 feet by 12 feet 3 inches. Attendants' room, 26 feet by 10 feet 6 inches; and a good cellar under the store-room. There is a portico in front 10½ feet wide.

The old hospital is now used as ordnance sergeant's quarters; the cellar is the magazine.

Wash-houses have been built for each set of company quarters. A new corral and small building for civilian employés were constructed in 1872. The quartermaster's and commissary store-houses are stone buildings, in good condition. The water-supply is mainly from the creek. There are several wells, from 15 to 40 feet deep, but the water in most of them is sulphurous, and unfit for use. The drainage of the post is superficial, and not good.

There are much better locations for a post about four miles down the creek, near the point at which stone was quarried for the buildings.

*Meteorological report, Fort Larned, Kans., 1870–'74.*

| Month. | 1870–'71. | | | | 1871–'72. | | | | 1872–'73. | | | | 1873–'74. | | | |
|---|---|---|---|---|---|---|---|---|---|---|---|---|---|---|---|---|
| | Temperature. | | | Rain-fall in inches. | Temperature. | | | Rain-fall in inches. | Temperature. | | | Rain-fall in inches. | Temperature. | | | Rain-fall in inches. |
| | Mean. | Max. | Min. | | Mean. | Max. | Min. | | Mean. | Max. | Min. | | Mean. | Max. | Min. | |
| July | 83.38 | 103 | 61 | 2.22 | 80.85 | 115 | 64 | 1.28 | 78.28 | 99 | 61 | 2.64 | 77.94 | 100 | 60 | 1.57 |
| August | 72.90 | 105 | 47 | 3.64 | 78.16 | 103 | 55 | 0.74 | 78.73 | 103* | 60 | 0.59 | 79.34 | 100 | 60 | 1.70 |
| September | 65.41 | 96 | 45 | 4.54 | 66.91 | 96 | 45 | 3.32 | 66.82 | 102* | 34 | 0.56 | 64.79 | 98 | 35 | 2.45 |
| October | 53.95 | 77 | 37 | 5.44 | 54.40 | 92 | 28 | 0.60 | 55.51 | 98* | 24 | 0.00 | 51.64 | 86 | 11 | 0.20 |
| November | 46.08 | 76 | 19 | 0.00 | 33.42 | 74 | 1 | 2.90 | 33.02 | 78 | 1 | 0.05 | 41.52 | 82 | 4 | 0.00 |
| December | 25.45 | 71 | −13 | 0.40 | 24.56 | 57 | − 1 | 0.18 | 20.39 | 65 | −15 | 0.31 | 27.48 | 57 | 0 | 0.19 |
| January | 28.58 | 65 | 1 | 0.45 | 25.82 | 52 | −12 | 0.00 | 23.14 | 65 | −17 | 1.05 | 27.71 | 61 | 2 | 0.27 |
| February | 33.44 | 73 | − 2 | 0.44 | 33.93 | 70 | 3 | 0.39 | 31.51 | 62 | − 6 | 0.05 | 24.50 | 50 | − 9 | 2.47 |
| March | 45.67 | 67 | 18 | 0.24 | 40.25 | 80 | 19 | 0.00 | 45.09 | 85 | 6 | 0.10 | 39.37 | 69 | 21 | 0.53 |
| April | 56.15 | 96 | 27 | 2.40 | 53.55 | 86 | 28 | 0.68 | 48.51 | 90 | 11 | 3.05 | 48.21 | 88 | 25 | 2.60 |
| May | 64.28 | 88 | 41 | 0.66 | 66.14 | 94 | 45 | 2.54 | 62.14 | 86 | 36 | 4.07 | 67.41 | 92 | 40 | 3.45 |
| June | 79.07 | 103 | 61 | 0.44 | 76.18 | 105* | 60 | 0.21 | 73.75 | 98 | 59 | 2.41 | 76.51 | 103 | 49 | 1.15 |
| For the year | 54.53 | 105 | −13 | 20.87 | 52.85 | 115 | −12 | 12.84 | 51.40 | 103* | −17 | 14.88 | 52.20 | 103 | − 9 | 16.58 |

* These observations are made with self-registering thermometers. The mean is from the standard thermometer.

*Consolidated sick-report, Fort Larned, Kans., 1870-'74.*

| Diseases. | 1870-'71. Cases. | Deaths. | 1871-'72. Cases. | Deaths. | 1872-'73. Cases. | Deaths. | 1873-'74. Cases. | Deaths. |
|---|---|---|---|---|---|---|---|---|
| Year | 1870-'71. | | 1871-'72. | | 1872-'73. | | 1873-'74. | |
| Mean strength { Officers | 5 | | 7 | | 6 | | 6 | |
| Enlisted men | 116 | | 104 | | 110 | | 120 | |
| **GENERAL DISEASES, A.** | | | | | | | | |
| Remittent fever | 13 | 1 | 1 | 1 | | | | |
| Intermittent fever | 30 | | 96 | | 19 | | 32 | |
| Other diseases of this group | 4 | | 4 | | 12 | | 2 | |
| **GENERAL DISEASES, B.** | | | | | | | | |
| Rheumatism | 4 | | 23 | | 10 | | 8 | |
| Syphilis | 4 | | 3 | | 3 | | 2 | |
| Consumption | 1 | | | | | 2 | | |
| Other diseases of this group | 1 | | 1 | | | | | |
| **LOCAL DISEASES.** | | | | | | | | |
| Catarrh and bronchitis | 10 | | 65 | | 14 | | 38 | |
| Pneumonia | | | 5 | 1 | | | 3 | |
| Pleurisy | | | 1 | | | | | |
| Diarrhœa and dysentery | 37 | 1 | 35 | | 26 | | 31 | |
| Hernia | | | | | | | 1 | |
| Gonorrhœa | 1 | | 1 | | 7 | | 4 | |
| Other local diseases | 40 | | 68 | 1 | 81 | | 63 | |
| Alcoholism | 1 | | 5 | | 29 | | 25 | |
| Total disease | 146 | 2 | 308 | 3 | 201 | 2 | 209 | |
| **VIOLENT DISEASES AND DEATHS.** | | | | | | | | |
| Gunshot wounds | 3 | 1 | 2 | 1 | 2 | | 2 | |
| Other accidents and injuries | 27 | 1 | 51 | | 49 | | 38 | |
| Total violence | 30 | 2 | 53 | 1 | 51 | | 40 | |

# FORT LEAVENWORTH, KANSAS.

INFORMATION FURNISHED BY SURGEON T. A. McPARLIN AND ASSISTANT SURGEON W. E. WATERS, UNITED STATES ARMY.

Fort Leavenworth is situated on the right bank of the Missouri River; latitude, 39° 20' north; longitude, 17° 30' west.

The following order was the first step toward establishing the post:

ADJUTANT-GENERAL'S OFFICE,
*Washington, March 7, 1827.*

*Ordered,* Colonel Leavenworth, of the Third Infantry, with four companies of his regiment, will ascend the Missouri, and when he reaches a point on the left bank near the mouth of the Little Platte River, and within a range of twenty miles above or below its confluence, he will select such a position as, in his judgment, is best calculated for the site of a permanent cantonment. The spot being chosen, he will construct, with the troops at his command, comfortable though temporary quarters, sufficient for the accommodation of four companies. This movement will be made as early as the convenience of the service will permit.

By order of Major-General Brown:

R. JONES, *Adjutant-General.*

On the 8th of May, 1827, Colonel Leavenworth reported that there was no proper site on the left or east bank of the river, but that there was one on the west bank, about twenty miles above the mouth of the Platte.

This recommendation was approved September 19, 1827, and by an order dated Adjutant-General's Office, November 8, 1827, the post was named Cantonment Leavenworth.

At first it was very unhealthy, a large part of the command being prostrated by malarial fevers, which in many cases were fatal.

35 M P

No steps were taken to secure a reservation until 1838, when President Van Buren declared as such a large tract of timber-land on the east side of the river opposite the fort. In 1830 a survey was made to define the boundary of the tract of land assigned to the Delaware Indians, which joined the post on the south, and in 1839 a second survey was made.

In the latter part of 1854, by direction of the Secretary of War, a survey was made to define the reservation, under the direction of Capt. F. E. Hunt, Fourth Artillery, and on this survey the reservation was declared by the President, October 10, 1854. The reservation on the east side of the river had its northern boundary changed in 1840, and a large part of it was relinquished in 1841, when that part of the State of Missouri was surveyed. It now comprises a somewhat square tract, bounded on the north and west by the river, containing 936 acres. The reservation on the west side contains 5,904½ acres, of which 138½ belong to the arsenal. The Secretary of the Interior, November 7, 1861, decided that a large part of the land lying between the post and the northern boundary of the reserve was land ceded to the United States by the Delaware Indians in the treaty of May 6, 1854.

Attorney-General Williams decided (April 19, 1872) that the land in question never was a portion of the territory allotted to the Delawares, and that while the United States has never parted with its title to the land in this reservation, the jurisdiction over the same has passed to the State of Kansas in the act admitting that State into the Union, and it will be necessary to obtain a cession of jurisdiction from the State. In 1860, Captain Van Vliet, post quartermaster, leased to a mining company the privilege of mining coal under the reservation for a period of sixteen years, the company agreeing to furnish free of charge all the coal required by the Government at the post, and to pay a royalty of ¼ cent per bushel on all other coal mined there. This lease was declared invalid without the approval of Congress. July 20, 1868, Congress authorized the sale of 20 acres of land in the southeast corner of the reservation to another company, and extended to it the same privileges, on the same conditions, for the same period. Although mining has been going on for several years, the Government has realized nothing beyond the amount received for the land, ($1,400,) as the company have avoided mining under the reservation.

The Missouri Pacific Railroad passes through the reserve on the bank of the river. The Kansas Central, a narrow-gauge road, crosses the reserve from east to west.

The Missouri Bridge Company were authorized by Congress to construct a railroad and wagon bridge on the reservation across the Missouri. This is an iron truss-bridge of three spans, used at present by the Chicago, Rock Island and Pacific Railroad.

The reservation and arrangement of the post are shown by the plate opposite, made from a tracing executed by Lieut. Ernest H. Ruffner, United States Engineers, from his own surveys.

The principal entrance to the post is from the south, through an ornamented wooden archway put up in 1871.

The parade, 517 by 514 feet, was graded in 1871, being cut down three feet on the west side, and filled about the same depth in the center, from which the magazine was removed.

The barracks for enlisted men consist of three two-story frame buildings, each 134 by 40 feet, with porticoes above and below on the eastern front; each building being intended for two companies, and each set of company quarters having barrack, orderly, and mess rooms, besides kitchen and store-room. Figure 44 shows the general arrangement of the building.

1, first floor; 2, second floor; A A, laundresses' quarters, 19 by 15 feet; B, bed-rooms, 9½ by 13 feet; C C, halls, 6 by 15 feet; D D, dining-rooms, 31½ by 39 feet; E E, kitchens, 18 by 20½ feet; F F, store-rooms, 10 by 18 feet; H H, sergeants' rooms, 13½ by 16¾ feet; I I, dormitories, 52 by 39 feet; K K, porches. Height of rooms—first floor, 10 feet; second floor, 11 feet.

The only means of ventilation in the dormitories are fire-places, windows, and doors.

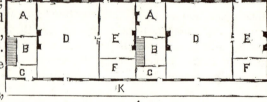

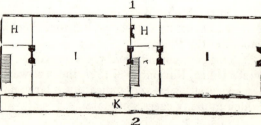

Figure 44.—Scale, 45 feet to 1 inch.

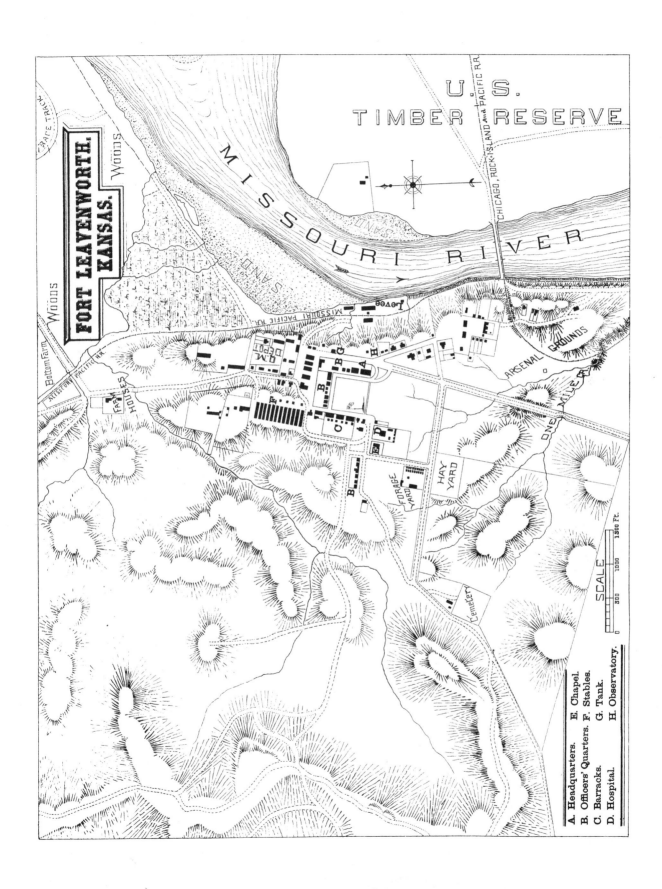

FORT LEAVENWORTH. KANSAS.

U. S.
TIMBER RESERVE

MISSOURI RIVER

A. Headquarters.      E. Chapel.
B. Officers' Quarters.  F. Stables.
C. Barracks.           G. Tank.
D. Hospital.           H. Observatory.

SCALE
0    500    1000    1500 Ft.

RACE TRACK

Woods

Woods

Bottom Farm      Woods

MISSOURI PACIFIC R.R.

FARM HOUSES

SAND

SAND

Levee

CHICAGO, ROCK-ISLAND and PACIFIC R.R.

ARSENAL GROUNDS

ONE MILE

R. M. DEPOT

HAY YARD

FORAGE YARD

Cemetery

On the north of the parade and facing it is a row of officers' quarters of various styles, erected at different periods, from 1828 to 1871. Commencing on the east, the first is a double Syracuse cottage, a two-story building with basement and attic, containing four sets of quarters.

Next come two one-story buildings, each containing two sets of quarters, each of which has two rooms, 18 by 19 feet, on the main floor, and others of the same size in the basement. The attics are divided into three small sleeping-rooms. Temporary summer-kitchens are attached to some of these. There are wide verandas in front and rear. These are supposed to be the first buildings erected in Cantonment Leavenworth, in 1828; they are log buildings, but have been neatly weather-boarded, and present a good appearance.

Two sets of field-officers' quarters consist of two-story frame houses, with hall in the middle, and two rooms on each side on both stories. There is a kitchen and pantry in the rear and a cellar under the back rooms, in which there is also a kitchen, and connected with a dumb-waiter. Bath-rooms are in the rear of the west first-story rooms. These quarters are heated by a wood-furnace in the basements and fire-places in all the rooms. The buildings are uniform in size and structure, with verandas in front, and were erected in 1871.

The post-commander usually occupies a large, double two-story brick building, containing four rooms on each floor, with halls in the middle. The kitchen, store-rooms, &c., are in the basement; the servants' rooms in the attic. Verandas are on both stories in front and rear. At the end of the row are two adjoining frame cottages, one story, each containing two sets of quarters similar to those previously described.

Facing west, and at right angles with these, are, first, two sets of field-officers' quarters in a long two-story and basement stone house, with wide windows in front. Next to these are two double Syracuse cottages, separated the usual distance, and like that previously noticed. They contain four sets of captains' and subalterns' quarters. On a continuation of this row is a large two-story brick building, partitioned off so as to constitute twelve sets of subalterns' quarters. A corresponding building constitutes the headquarters of the Department of the Missouri, where all the officers on the staff of the department commander have their offices, except the chief commissary, who has his in the store-house. In front of these quarters is a lawn, 22 feet wide, with a brick pavement between it and the carriage-way which passes around three sides of the parade. All the quarters here mentioned are supplied with water from cisterns in the rear of each set. There are no regularly constructed bath-rooms in any of these quarters, excepting those occupied by the post-commander and by the field-officers. All are furnished with stables, carriage-houses, fuel-houses, and sinks with covered ways thereto. This completes the description of the officers' quarters facing the parade, which has them on two sides, with the barracks on the third, and an open space to the south, in which stand four brass field-pieces for salutes, and the morning and evening guns. Between the parade and the arsenal there are two sets of officers' quarters, consisting of two one-story frame houses, without attics or basements. They are occupied by the officers of the personal staff of the department commander, who occupies the large frame building on the west side of the road to the arsenal, and east of the road to the city. The building has been remodeled and added to from time to time by the several officers who have commanded the department. A large yard surrounds the building on all sides, ornamented by a profusion of flowers and shade-trees.

It was the design of the present department commander to build a new garrison throughout, and the site selected for it is about 500 yards from the parade, in a southwesterly direction. The contemplated plan, however, has been carried out only so far as the erection of a row of officers' quarters, designated as the "West End." These consist of five buildings facing south, and similar in design and arrangements; quarters for captains and subalterns. They are two-story and basement buildings, each house containing four sets of quarters, with a common entrance for two. Each set contains two large rooms, and those on the lower floor, a small room in the rear. Kitchen and dining-room for each set in basement. The buildings are separated thirty feet, and have neat fence in front, inclosing flower-gardens. All are provided with back yards, fuel-houses, sinks, &c.

The post headquarters is a one-story brick building, L-shaped, containing office-rooms for the commanding officer, the adjutant, and the sergeant-major. A fourth large room in this building is arranged and fitted up as a court-martial room.

Fort Leavenworth, in addition to its organization as a military garrison, contains important depots, from which quartermasters' stores of all kinds and subsistence supplies are furnished the different posts of the department. There are large store-houses and shops pertaining to those depots. Of the former, the store-house of the depot commissary is a large two-story and basement stone building, situated next to the post commissary store-house. East of these are two large, massive, three-story stone buildings, store-houses for quartermasters' property, and north of the last described, is another two-story stone building, also for quartermasters' stores, and containing the offices of the depot quartermaster. In the vicinity of these are the various shops of the depot, carpenters, wheelwrights, blacksmiths, and saddlers. A number of frame buildings farther to the north are used as mess-rooms and quarters for employés.

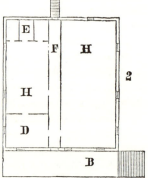

Contiguous to the post in a southeasterly direction is the United States arsenal, bearing the same name. The arsenal inclosure contains 138 acres. The first building was erected in 1859; there are now two store-houses, besides shops and offices, and two dwelling-houses, the officers' quarters. Recently, the arsenal has been transferred from the ordnance to the line of the latter for Army, and is now used as barracks for one company of infantry. The buildings of the quartermaster's depot have been fitted to receive military prisoners, and the quartermaster's department also now occupies a portion of the arsenal.

The guard-house is a massive structure of stone, 50 by 45 feet, and two stories high. The security of prisoners, even at the expense of their health, seems to have been the only consideration that governed its design and construction. No attention whatever seems to have been given to its ventilation; and the defect in this particular is now seriously felt, as it is made the military prison of the department, and often overcrowded.

Figure 45.

The arrangement of the guard-house is shown in Figure 45. 1, ground-floor; A and H, general prison-rooms, each $46\frac{2}{3}$ by 20 feet by $8\frac{5}{6}$ feet high; B, porch, 45 by 12 feet. 2, second story; B, porch, reached by outside stairs; D, provost-marshal's office, 16 by 12 feet; E, cells, 9 by 5 feet; F, hall, 50 by $4\frac{5}{6}$ feet; H, prison-room, $46\frac{2}{3}$ by 20 feet by $11\frac{7}{12}$ feet; H, prison-room, 34 by 21 feet by $11\frac{7}{12}$ feet.

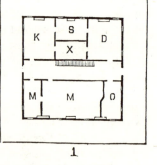

The cells are ventilated only by small auger-holes in the doors windows are the only means of ventilating the other rooms in the building. All the rooms are heated by stoves burning wood. In consequence of the large number of prisoners, the guard is now quartered in hospital-tents in the hospital inclosure west of the guard-house. The yard in the rear is inclosed by a high wooden fence, and in it are the sinks used by the guard and prisoners.

The hospital, situated east of the guard-house, and standing back from the road, surrounded by a lawn, in which grow locust and ot r trees, is one of the oldest buildings at the post, and, originally defective in plan, remains as at first constructed. The building is of brick, 50 by 50 feet, and two stories and an attic high. Verandas, 12 feet wide, are on all sides for both stories.

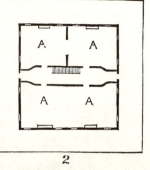

Figure 46 shows the plan of the building. 1, first floor; 2, second floor. A, wards, 50 by 20 feet, and $24\frac{1}{2}$ by 20 feet, respectively; D dispensary, 17 by 20 feet; M M, mess-rooms, 20 by 12, and 25 by 27 feet, respectively; K, kitchen, 16 by 20 feet; O, office, $15\frac{1}{2}$ by 10 feet; S, store-room; X, pantry.

Figure 46.

The front ward of the two smaller is used as a prison-ward, the windows and doors being secured by iron-grating. The ceilings are 14 feet high, allowing, in the large ward, which contains twelve beds, 1,167 cubic feet air-space per bed. The smaller wards contain six beds each, giving the same amount of air-space as to those in the large ward. A bath and wash-room has been constructed on the veranda in the rear, at the end of the hall; and at this point also a stairway descends to the first story. Earth-closets are used by patients in the hospital. Sinks are in the yard, and are well arranged. Water is supplied from a tank in the attic, which is filled from the cistern by a force-pump. Facilities for hot and cold water have been added. Babcock's fire-extinguishers are at hand. The attic story contains nurse-room, 20 by 13 feet; isolation ward, 23 by 20 feet, and a tank-room in rear; store-room, 23 by 20 feet; and steward's room, 20 by 13 feet. It is finished inside, and has dormer-windows.

The post-bakery is a frame building erected for the purpose in 1866, and is well adapted. Directly opposite the hospital is a frame one-story building, where a school is taught by Sisters of Charity, who come daily from Leavenworth for the purpose. It is attended by children of soldiers and employés. The school for officers' children is held in a one-story brick building, formerly the officers' mess, taught by a lady residing in the city. This is attended only by the smaller children, while an ambulance conveys to the city in the morning and back in the afternoon such children as desire to attend school there. One-half of the L-shaped building, in which is the school of officers' children, is fitted up as a chapel, with the arrangements necessary for the Episcopal service. There is also a Roman Catholic chapel, built by voluntary contributions.

East of the garrison, and on the edge of the hill overlooking the river, is a water-tank that holds 21,000 gallons, and covered by a brick building. This is not only to furnish water in case of fire, but from it the cisterns are replenished in the absence of rain. The water is pumped into the tank from the river by a steam-pump. There is a steam fire-engine at the post to extinguish fires, and a large number of Babcock fire-extinguishers are distributed throughout the garrison.

The drainage of the post is very good; natural declivities conduct the water off in all directions from the garrison, and no sewerage has been required. The sinks throughout the garrison consist of vaults dug in the rear of all the habitable buildings, which, when they become too foul, are filled up and new ones dug. Disinfectants are used regularly in all of these, particularly in the summer months, to keep up a constant acid reaction. All refuse at the post is carted about a mile from the garrison and thrown into the Missouri River.

The national cemetery, surrounded by a stone wall, and containing about 1,490 graves, is distant three-quarters of a mile southwest of the post.

In addition to the hospital-garden, there are gardens for all the companies, a post-garden, and one cultivated by the depot quartermaster for department headquarters.

*Meteorological report, Fort Leavenworth, Kans., 1870–'74.*

| Month. | 1870–'71. | | | | 1871–'72. | | | | 1872–'73. | | | | 1873–'74. | | | |
|---|---|---|---|---|---|---|---|---|---|---|---|---|---|---|---|---|
| | Temperature. | | | Rain-fall in inches. | Temperature. | | | Rain-fall in inches. | Temperature. | | | Rain-fall in inches. | Temperature. | | | Rain-fall in inches. |
| | Mean. | Max. | Min. | | Mean. | Max. | Min. | | Mean. | Max. | Min. | | Mean. | Max. | Min. | |
| | ° | ° | ° | | ° | ° | ° | | ° | ° | ° | | ° | ° | ° | |
| July | 80.33 | 99 | 65 | 6.30 | 79.85 | 99 | 65 | 5.64 | 77.62 | 93 | 50* | 10.06 | 76.28 | 98 | 54 | 3.12 |
| August | 73.65 | 98 | 55 | 7.50 | 73.77 | 98 | 55 | 1.00 | 75.89 | 96 | 48 | 6.83 | 77.29 | 104* | 51* | 1.40 |
| September | 67.88 | 95 | 43 | 4.68 | 63.49 | 94* | 37* | 1.85 | 64.22 | 95 | 32 | 4.02 | 62.49 | 95* | 34* | 2.53 |
| October | 57.57 | 80 | 34 | 8.65 | 57.25 | 93* | 20* | 4.00 | 51.55 | 90 | 26 | 0.10 | 47.64 | 82* | 17* | 0.91 |
| November | 45.09 | 74 | 17 | 0.70 | 35.98 | 78* | − 4* | 5.79 | 32.41 | 64 | 2 | 0.00 | 37.29 | 78* | 10* | 0.87 |
| December | 28.62 | 63 | −10 | 2.75 | 24.18 | 63* | − 5* | 4.60 | 29.64 | 58 | −16* | 2.85 | 30.58 | 71* | 6* | 6.51 |
| January | 30.45 | 68 | − 6 | (?) | 22.31 | 55* | −10* | 2.00 | 15.54 | 45 | −26 | 1.32 | 26.83 | 58* | − 2* | 1.44 |
| February | 38.15 | 78 | − 7 | 5.80 | 28.54 | 60* | −14* | 5.40 | 27.01 | 59 | − 8 | 1.35 | 27.13 | 48* | 0* | 1.07 |
| March | 47.76 | 73 | 20 | 5.06 | 35.51 | 74* | 9* | 4.10 | 40.75 | 75 | 4 | 1.80 | 38.35 | 69* | 15* | 1.50 |
| April | 55.60 | 86 | 27 | 3.79 | 52.96 | 84 | 13* | 4.50 | 47.36 | 88 | 29 | 4.30 | 47.12 | 82* | 19* | 1.40 |
| May | 68.74 | 91 | 50 | 2.53 | 64.99 | 87 | 21* | 8.15 | 61.75 | 86 | 45 | 5.03 | 67.55 | 93* | 41* | 1.00 |
| June | 75.78 | 94 | 56 | 5.44 | 75.59 | 97* | 49* | 3.64 | 74.49 | 96 | 57 | 3.02 | 75.36 | 93* | 48* | 3.55 |
| For the year | 55.80 | 99 | −10 | ........ | 51.19 | 99 | 14* | 50.67 | 49.38 | 96 | −26 | 40.68 | 51.16 | 104* | − 2* | 25.30 |

*These observations are made with self-registering thermometers. The mean is from the standard thermometer.

*Consolidated sick-report, Fort Leavenworth, Kans., 1870–'74.*

| Year | | 1870-'71. | | 1871-'72. | | 1872-'73. | | 1873-'74. | |
|---|---|---|---|---|---|---|---|---|---|
| Mean strength { Officers | | 20 | | 19 | | 27 | | 31 | |
| { Enlisted men | | 434 | | 302 | | 373 | | 383 | |
| **Diseases.** | | Cases. | Deaths. | Cases. | Deaths. | Cases. | Deaths. | Cases. | Deaths. |
| GENERAL DISEASES, A. | | | | | | | | | |
| Small-pox and varioloid | | | | 2 | | 4 | 1 | | |
| Typhoid fever | | 16 | 2 | | | 4 | 1 | | |
| Typho-malarial fever | | | | | | 1 | 1 | 1 | 1 |
| Remittent fever | | 34 | | 45 | | 43 | | 2 | |
| Intermittent fever | | 121 | | 59 | | 265 | | 147 | |
| Other diseases of this group | | 16 | | 21 | | 50 | | 83 | |
| GENERAL DISEASES, B. | | | | | | | | | |
| Rheumatism | | 20 | | 24 | | 53 | | 23 | |
| Syphilis | | 17 | | 27 | | 57 | | 33 | |
| Consumption | | | | 5 | 1 | 1 | | | |
| Other diseases of this group | | 1 | | 2 | | | | | |
| LOCAL DISEASES. | | | | | | | | | |
| Catarrh and bronchitis | | 49 | | 87 | | 126 | | 85 | |
| Pneumonia | | 2 | | 4 | 1 | 2 | | 11 | 1 |
| Pleurisy | | | | 4 | | | | | |
| Diarrhœa and dysentery | | 128 | 2 | 98 | | 174 | | 135 | |
| Hernia | | 1 | | | | 2 | | 1 | |
| Gonorrhœa | | 18 | | 14 | | 46 | | 15 | |
| Other local diseases | | 132 | | 93 | 2 | 187 | 1 | 239 | |
| Alcoholism | | 5 | | 15 | | 19 | | 35 | 1 |
| Unclassified | | | | | | 1 | | | |
| Total disease | | 560 | 4 | 500 | 4 | 1,031 | 3 | 810 | 5 |
| VIOLENT DISEASES AND DEATHS. | | | | | | | | | |
| Gunshot wounds | | 2 | 2 | 2 | | | | 1 | |
| Drowning | | | 1 | | | | | | |
| Other accidents and injuries | | 133 | | 75 | | 174 | 1 | 207 | 1 |
| Homicide | | | 3 | | | | | | 1 |
| Suicide | | | | | | | 1 | | |
| Total violence | | 135 | 6 | 77 | 1 | 174 | 1 | 208 | 2 |

(In October, 1870, there were 10 colored recruits at the above post, among whom was one case of quotidian intermittent fever.)

# FORT LYON, COLORADO.

### REPORT OF ASSISTANT SURGEON J. C. G. HAPPERSETT, UNITED STATES ARMY.

Fort Lyon is situated on the north bank of the Arkansas River, in latitude 38° 5′ 36″ north, longitude 26° 30′′ west, and is 3,800 feet above the sea-level. The reservation, as declared by the President September 1, 1868, contains nine square miles and 115 acres.

The town of West Las Animas, the present terminus of the Arkansas Valley Railroad, is five miles distant. This road connects with the Kansas Pacific Railroad at Kit Carson, 55 miles north. The town of Granada, at the terminus of the Atchison, Topeka and Santa Fé Railroad, is 55 miles east. The nearest spurs of the Rocky Mountains are about 100 miles west.

The geological formation is sandstone of the Lower Cretaceous period. Eight miles distant lime-stones of a later period, very rich in fossils, are found. Coal of poor quality has been discovered on Rule Creek, ten miles from the post.

Over 1,000 acres are under cultivation within ten miles of the post. The land is irrigated by a small canal, leading from Purgatory River, a small stream emptying into the Arkansas, two and a half miles west of the post. Large crops of cereals, vegetables, and melons are raised. Wild plums, currants, and gooseberries grow on the Purgatory River bottoms, and wild grapes are found in great abundance on both streams.

The following animals have been killed or seen within forty miles of the post, viz: buffalo, prong-horned antelope, elk, black-tailed deer, white-tailed deer, American panther, wild cat, white, gray, and dusky wolves, coyotes, cinnamon-bear, fox, weasel, mink, otter, skunk, badger, raccoon, gopher, prairie-dog, beaver, kangaroo-rat, Norway rat, porcupine, muskrat, mule-rabbit, sage-hare, wild horse.

Birds seen are the golden eagle, pigeon, sparrow and fish hawks, prairie-falcon, great horned

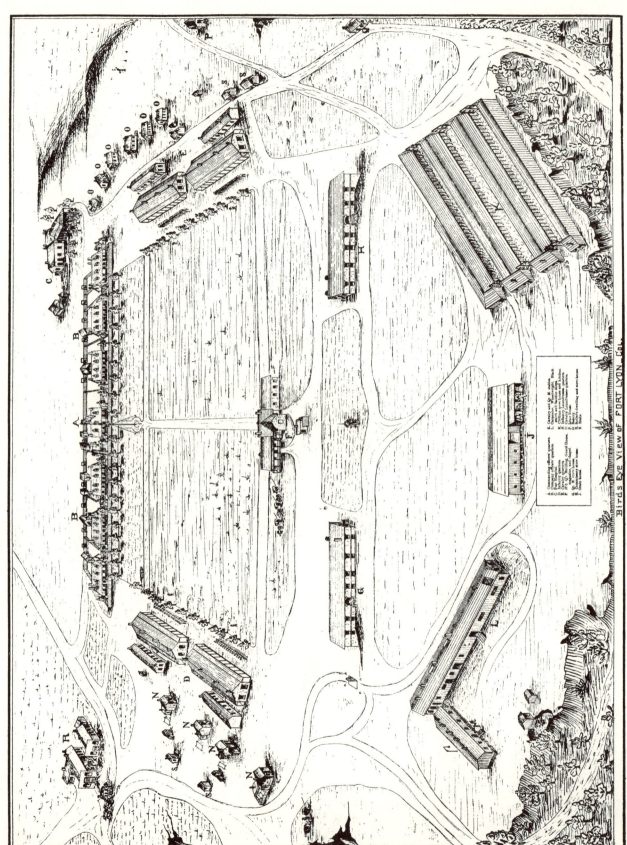

Birds Eye View of FORT LYON, Col.

A. Commanding officer's quarters.
B. Company officers quarters.
C. Infantry quarters.
D. Post Hospital.
E. Cavalry quarters.
E. R. Q. M. building, Guard House, magazine, and chapel.
G. Infantry store house.
H. Commissary store house.
J. Guest house.

E. Cavalry and Q. M. stables.
L. Carpenter, wheelwright, black smith and saddler shops.
M. Civilian store house and kitchen.
N. Infantry Laundresses quarters.
O. Cavalry Laundresses quarters.
P. Ice house.
Q. Lime house.
R. Sutlers dwelling and store house.
S. Stable.

owl, burrowing owl, woodpecker, kingfisher, robin, blue-bird, mocking-bird, skylark, sparrow, red-winged blackbird, meadow-lark, raven, magpie, turtle-dove, wild turkey, prairie-chicken, (rare, but increasing,) sandhill-crane, white heron, blue heron, killdeer, plover, wild goose, and ducks of various kinds.

The climate is mild; the nights mostly pleasant. A difference of 50° F. between the morning and 2 p. m. has been observed, though very seldom. Snows are seldom more than three inches in depth, and rapidly disappear.

The fort is located on a sandstone bluff, the highest point of which is 36 feet above the river. There is a stratum of sand and gravel, more or less impregnated with alkali, overlying the sandstone. A low bottom, from 100 to 200 yards wide, separates the bluff from the river. This is overflowed when the river is unusually high, which is very objectionable, but no place within the limits designated for the post could be found so free from disadvantages as this site. The bluff is 2,000 feet wide and 1,500 feet long, with a face of sandstone 10 feet high. There is a gradual slope from the center to the edge of the bluff, in all directions, making the surface drainage excellent.

This site was first occupied on the 9th day of June, 1867; the old site, twenty miles distant, being abandoned because of its unhealthy location and the increasing scarcity of wood.

The general arrangement of the post is shown in the "bird's eye view" given in the Plate opposite.

There are four sets of barracks for troops—two built of sandstone on the west side of the parade, and two of adobe on the east side. These buildings are 100 by 34 by 12 feet; one story high, covered with good shingle roofs, and divided into company offices, store-room, and dormitory. The inside walls are hard-finished. There are two ventilators in each dormitory, 18 inches square, twelve windows, two doors, (double,) opening outside. They are neatly furnished with single bedsteads, lockers, gun-racks, benches and tables, and supposed to accommodate fifty men each, which would allow 625 cubic feet air-space per man. The ventilation is insufficient. In rear of each set of barracks, and connected by a board walk, is a stone building 60 by 18 by 10 feet, having a good shingle roof, and divided into mess-room, wash-room, and company kitchen, with a good cellar under the latter. These buildings are all neatly plastered, well lighted, and supplied with furniture appropriate to the uses of each.

The sinks are vaults, over which are frame buildings, and are removed as often as required.

The quarters for married soldiers and laundresses are old frame shanties and stone buildings, used as the temporary quarters for officers during the time the post was in construction. Estimates have been approved and plans adopted for the erection of suitable quarters for laundresses.

The officers' quarters form the north side of the parade, and consist of seven adobe houses, that of the commanding officer being in the center, and making in all thirteen sets of quarters. They are all one and one-half stories high, and have good shingle roofs. The commanding officer's quarters has four rooms, 18 by 18 by 10 feet, and hall 7 feet wide, and kitchen 16 by 17 feet, on the first floor: The upper story contains four rooms, 14 by 18 feet. There are four sets of captains' quarters, containing two rooms and kitchen on the first floor, with hall running the entire length, and two rooms on the upper floor.

There are eight sets of lieutenants' quarters, having three rooms on the first floor, with hall running half through, and two rooms and hall on the second story. These quarters have no addition for a kitchen, and are a few feet smaller than the captains' quarters. They are all nearly finished; have fire-places in the rooms on the lower floor, and are very comfortable dwellings, though all need repair.

Each set of quarters has a neat porch in front, with a small yard inclosed by a handsome picket paling. In rear of each is a commodious yard, surrounded by a good board fence, and in most of the yards there is a stable and out-house for poultry. Shade trees have been planted in all the yards, and in front of the barracks. None of the buildings have bath-rooms.

Opposite the line of officers' quarters, and forming the south side of the parade, is the building originally erected for the post hospital, nearly in accordance with the plan adopted in 1867, and now used as headquarters of the post, containing office of commanding officer and adjutant, chapel, guard-house, reading-room, arsenal, and magazine. The building is of sandstone and much in need of repair.

The quartermaster and commissary buildings are similar in dimensions and appearance, built of sandstone in the most substantial manner, and are 100 by 42 feet, basement 9 feet high, and main floor 12 feet high.

Near to the edge of the bluff is a large and very fine forage-house, of frame.

The workshops are nearly new, and are also frame buildings, with frame mess-hall adjoining at right angles, for use of mechanics. Near the shops are small buildings for lime and charcoal.

There are two ice-houses near the bluff, on the eastern side of the post, the capacity of which is ample.

The post bakery is built of sandstone, 24 by 46 by 10 feet, and divided by a stone partition, which separates the ovens from the mixing-rooms. The ovens are of fire-brick, and much in need of repair; the capacity is 480 ration-loaves per day.

The quartermaster and cavalry stables are similar in appearance and construction, and are capable of comfortably sheltering two troops of cavalry horses and 150 public animals of the quartermaster's department. These stables are open, but have good roofs. There are, in these, two large tanks with water for the use of the animals. The offal is removed daily.

The post library numbers about 110 volumes, well selected. The reading-room is in the same building as the post headquarters, (formerly the hospital.)

One of the old buildings, formerly used as quarters for officers, has been fitted up as a theater and concert-room.

The post hospital was completed and occupied in October, 1871, and consists of an executive building (one story and attic) and two wings, built at right angles to the main building, one used as a ward and the other for mess-room, kitchen, and attendants' room.

The following description is condensed from the special report of Assistant Surgeon Woodhull, United States Army:

"The building is of rough-hewn sandstone, situated at the northerly angle of the post and outside the rectangle described by the other buildings. It faces the northeast, and is distant from the flag-staff 245 yards, and 190 yards from the nearest company quarters.

"The main building consists of four rooms, each about 13 feet square, used as an office, dispensary, stewards' room, and store-room respectively. Above is a plastered attic, 34 by 20 feet, and 6½ feet high, used for storage. On the southeasterly side a wing, furnishing a ward 47 by 24½ by 13 feet, (inside,) extends flush with the main building. The cubic capacity of this ward is 14,970 feet, and contains twelve beds, giving each a superficial space of 96 feet, and a cubic air-space of about 1,250. The front of the main building and the entire ward are surrounded by a covered veranda, 8 feet wide. On this veranda, at the extremity of the ward, are built two rooms, each 11 by 5½ feet, for earth-closet and bath-room. Each of these has a ventilating-shaft, and one contains a caldron for heating water.

"From the rear of the main building, at right angles to the ward, extends another wing, containing mess-room, 19 feet 4 inches by 13 feet 10 inches; kitchen, 19 feet 4 inches by 12 feet 8 inches; and laundry, 19 feet 4 inches by 10 feet 7 inches. The latter is used as room for attendants. Under the kitchen is an excellent cellar and wine-closet for storing liquors. The building is well lighted, the ward containing eight windows, and three of the doors being half glazed, with transoms above. The ventilation is by two boxed shafts, each 8 feet long, 2 feet wide, surmounted by a ridge ventilator. There are also two boxed openings, one near each end of the ward, connecting with the chimney in the center of the roof. Two boxes, one on each side, extend from the outside and open under the stove. The attic of the main building, used as a store-room, is reached by a movable step-ladder from the main store-room. There is also a hatchway above the intersection of the hall, through which bulky and heavy articles are raised by block and tackle. The double ventilating fire-place furnished for the hospital was abandoned, and the ward is now heated by large wood-stoves with sheet-iron drums. The fire-places in the other rooms smoke badly, and wherever possible small wood-stoves have been substituted.

"The original plan contemplated another ward, similar to that already described, and application was made to have it constructed, but this, as well as the estimate for repairs, was disapproved.

"The roof leaks badly, and, as a result, the plastering is in many places dropping off."

The entire water-supply is from the Arkansas River, from which it is hauled in large water-tanks and distributed about the post. These tanks are filled by a force-pump, under cover.

The water of the Arkansas River is always muddy, and, from April until August, during the usual season of high water, contains much mineral and organic matter. This objection is increased by the offal from both dwellings and stables in the town of Las Animas being dumped into the river about one-fourth of a mile above the point of supply for the post.

The average rain-fall (11 inches) would not justify the building of cisterns. One well was sunk, but the water was so strongly alkaline as to be unfit for use.

An acequia, or small canal, was completed in the summer of 1873, from a point on the Arkansas River, nearly six miles west of the post. This canal enters the post at the northwest angle, and furnishes branches, 1st, to the line of officers' quarters, (running just inside the front paling;) 2d, around the entire parade-ground, passing out at the southeasterly angle and running in front of the stables. The main acequia passes down the north side of the parade, parallel with the line of officers' quarters, passing out at the northeast angle, and continuing in the same line of direction in front of the hospital, and opening on the marsh on the east of the post. Just before it terminates, ditches intersect it, so as to furnish water for the company garden.

From faulty construction at the head of this ditch, it has frequently been without water, and the result has been a very decided increase in the sickness from malarial complications. It is proposed to remedy this defect the coming spring, and also to continue the canal through the marsh to the river, which will not only convey the surplus water of the acequia, but also drain a large tract of the marsh.

Shade-trees have been planted about the post, along the course of this canal.

Two companies planted gardens, which were watered from the acequia, and, considering the lateness of the season, were very successful. The experiment has proved, beyond doubt, the great advantage to be derived in the supply of vegetables, melons, &c., which grow in perfection.

The cemetery is about one mile west of the post, is 150 feet square, and inclosed by a very poor board fence. The graves have very neat head and foot boards.

The drainage of the post is entirely superficial, but excellent, and the offal removed in covered carts to the river daily.

This section of the country was formerly in possession of the Cheyennes and Arapahoes, but since the fight at Sand Creek, in 1864, no open hostility has occurred. They make frequent visits, but are mostly peaceable.

The country along the water-courses (the only place available) is now entirely settled, principally by Americans; and the soil yields abundant crops wherever irrigation can be secured.

Mails are received daily via the Arkansas Valley Railroad, two days and a half to Leavenworth, and five to Washington.

The prevailing diseases at this post are catarrhal and mild malarial fevers and rheumatism. Bowel affections prevail in summer, owing probably to the increased organic matter in the drinking-water.

*Meteorological report, Fort Lyon, Colo., 1870–'74.*

| Month. | 1870–'71. | | | | 1871–'72. | | | | 1872–'73. | | | | 1873–'74. | | | |
|---|---|---|---|---|---|---|---|---|---|---|---|---|---|---|---|---|
| | Temperature. | | | Rain-fall in inches. | Temperature. | | | Rain-fall in inches. | Temperature. | | | Rain-fall in inches. | Temperature. | | | Rain-fall in inches. |
| | Mean. | Max. | Min. | | Mean. | Max. | Min. | | Mean. | Max. | Min. | | Mean. | Max. | Min. | |
| July | 78.38 | 107* | 50* | 1.46 | 81.40 | 107* | 53* | 1.02 | 74.48 | 99* | 41* | 6.30 | 76.79 | 101* | 51* | 2.84 |
| August | 72.39 | 101* | 40* | 2.78 | 77.17 | 101* | 42* | 1.02 | 74.34 | 98* | 53* | 3.05 | 77.69 | 99* | 51* | 0.23 |
| September | 63.59 | 99* | 38* | 4.72 | 67.61 | 97* | 35* | 1.60 | 65.56 | 95* | 29* | 0.62 | 65.48 | 95* | 29* | 1.56 |
| October | 49.83 | 89* | 29* | 1.30 | 51.78 | 90* | 18* | 0.04 | 53.00 | 91* | 14* | 0.04 | 50.81 | 91* | 13* | 0.04 |
| November | 44.28 | 75* | 12* | 0.00 | 31.27 | 71* | – 3* | 0.51 | 32.36 | 74* | – 3* | 0.10 | 40.24 | 76* | 8* | 0.00 |
| December | 21.68 | 65* | –23* | 0.28 | 28.41 | 62* | – 1* | 0.04 | 24.81 | 65* | – 6* | 0.09 | 28.57 | 69* | – 3* | 0.07 |
| January | 32.32 | 72* | 4* | 0.07 | 24.43 | 67* | –15* | 0.03 | 26.60 | 66* | –22* | 0.04 | 27.76 | 69* | –14* | 0.18 |
| February | 35.62 | 72* | 3* | 0.06 | 35.21 | 75* | –12* | 0.60 | 31.23 | 66* | 2* | 0.04 | 26.97 | 68* | –22* | 0.86 |
| March | 43.44 | 79* | 12* | 0.38 | 39.78 | 75* | 11* | 0.14 | 45.36 | 81* | 11* | 0.02 | 40.05 | 71* | 10* | 0.68 |
| April | 53.28 | 87* | 18* | 0.96 | 52.65 | 85* | 26* | 1.82 | 46.72 | 86* | 12* | 0.30 | 43.89 | 89* | 11* | 2.02 |
| May | 65.29 | 91* | 31* | 1.34 | 62.42 | 96* | 23* | 2.24 | 58.89 | 91* | 22* | 4.82 | 63.71 | 95* | 28* | 5.42 |
| June | 79.04 | 104* | 49* | 0.63 | 72.48 | 100* | 49* | 1.94 | 73.44 | 102* | 51* | 1.62 | 75.03 | 103* | 46* | 0.11 |
| For the year | 53.26 | 107* | –23* | 13.98 | 52.05 | 107* | –15* | 11.00 | 50.56 | 102* | –22* | 17.04 | 51.42 | 103* | –22* | 14.01 |

* These observations are made with self-registering thermometers. The mean is from the standard thermometer.

*Consolidated sick-report, Fort Lyon, Colo., 1870–'74.*

| Year | | 1870–'71. | | 1871–'72. | | 1872–'73. | | 1873–'74. | |
|---|---|---|---|---|---|---|---|---|---|
| Mean strength { Officers | | 9 | | 10 | | 8 | | 10 | |
| { Enlisted men | | 168 | | 119 | | 148 | | 204 | |
| Diseases. | | Cases. | Deaths. | Cases. | Deaths. | Cases. | Deaths. | Cases. | Deaths. |
| GENERAL DISEASES, A. | | | | | | | | | |
| Small-pox and varioloid | | | | 2 | 1 | | | | |
| Typhoid fever | | 1 | | | | | | | |
| Remittent fever | | 2 | | 3 | | 1 | | | |
| Intermittent fever | | 42 | | 13 | | 39 | | 51 | |
| Other diseases of this group | | 13 | | 11 | | 36 | | 7 | |
| GENERAL DISEASES, B. | | | | | | | | | |
| Rheumatism | | 15 | | 6 | | 10 | | 17 | |
| Syphilis | | 1 | | 3 | | | | 6 | |
| Consumption | | 1 | | | | | | | |
| Other diseases of this group | | 1 | | | | 2 | | | |
| LOCAL DISEASES. | | | | | | | | | |
| Catarrh and bronchitis | | 37 | | 15 | | 7 | | 112 | |
| Pleurisy | | 2 | | | | | | | |
| Diarrhœa and dysentery | | 44 | | 32 | | 11 | | 69 | |
| Hernia | | | | | | | | 1 | |
| Gonorrhœa | | 1 | | 1 | | 1 | | 8 | |
| Other local diseases | | 59 | 1 | 35 | 1 | 44 | | 55 | |
| Alcoholism | | 5 | | 7 | | 2 | | 26 | |
| Total disease | | 224 | 1 | 128 | 2 | 153 | | 352 | |
| VIOLENT DISEASES AND DEATHS. | | | | | | | | | |
| Gunshot wounds | | 1 | | 1 | | | | 3 | |
| Other accidents and injuries | | 42 | 1 | 38 | | 40 | | 78 | |
| Homicide | | | | | 1 | | 1 | | 1 |
| Total violence | | 43 | 1 | 39 | 1 | 40 | 1 | 81 | 1 |

# FORT McRAE, NEW MEXICO.

INFORMATION FURNISHED BY ACTING ASSISTANT SURGEONS W. B. LYON AND R. H. M'KAY, UNITED STATES ARMY.

Fort McRae is situated near the southern border of Socorro County, New Mexico, 2½ miles east of the Rio Grande. Latitude, 33° 01' north; longitude, 30° 5' west; height above the sea, 4,500 feet.

It is in a wide cañon extending westward from the plain of the Jornada del Muerto to the Rio Grande, and is five miles from the head of the cañon. The Miembres range of mountains is 25 miles distant to the west, and 30 miles to the east are the San Andres Mountains. It is 32 miles south of Fort Craig, and 60 miles north of Fort Selden. The post was established in 1863, for the protection of the Jornada del Muerto from the depredations of the Miembres branch of the Apaches.

The crossing at the mouth of the cañon is the best on the river, and this was the principal pass through which the Indians drove their stolen stock. The fort also protects the Ojo del Muerto, (spring of the dead,) which, except at certain seasons, is the only water to be found near the Jornada, between Fort Selden and Paraja, a distance of 90 miles. The reservation is 2 miles square. The formation is quite recent, nearly the whole of the reservation having been simply washed out from the original level of the plain to the present broken slope to the river. The whole mesa is of recent water formation. A well sunk at Aleman, midway between Paraja and Fort Selden, passed through successive layers of soft sandstone, in which hard, flinty water-washed pebbles were imbedded.

Thirty feet from the surface well-preserved bones were found. At a depth of 100 feet a petrified walnut was discovered. Abundance of water was struck at a depth of 140 feet. Thin veins of coal crop out at several points near the river. A ten-foot layer of lava covers the mesa near the fort, extending to the mountain of Fra Christobal above, and the Sierra de Caballo below. The soil is covered with fine grama grass, but is not arable, as it cannot be irrigated. Cedar and ash grow in the neighboring ravines, groves of cottonwood on the river-bottoms, and there is a good supply of mesquite on the higher slopes. Many species of cacti abound. The principal wild animals are the antelope, deer, panther or Mexican lion, cinnamon bear, wolves, foxes, and beaver. The eagle, crane, wild turkey, ducks, and quail are found. The Rio Grande abounds with cat-fish. The climate is delightful, except in June and July, when the heat is excessive. Mean temperature 60° F., extremes 105° F. and 8° F. The rainy season sets in about the middle of July, and continues one or two months. Average amount of rain-fall about 9 inches. There is very little snow.

The buildings are all of adobe, and of but one story. The barracks, officers' quarters, and hospital buildings are plastered on the inside with lime; they have mud roofs, and jaspe or gypsum floors.

The commanding officer's quarters, barracks, guard-house, and hospital were built in 1866; the other buildings belonging to the post are new.

The barracks, for one company of soldiers, measures 120 by 27 feet, and is divided into two apartments, with a hall. The rooms are sufficiently warmed by one heating-stove in each, and lighted by three windows in the east and five in the west side; there are no means of ventilation except by the windows and doors, and the air-space per man is 260 cubic feet when the barracks are full. The bunks are iron and single. The hall leads back into the dining-room, immediately back of which are the kitchen and bakery.

Excellent quarters for officers have recently been completed, the outer walls of which are of adobe, and 27 inches in thickness. These quarters are lime-plastered, with jaspe floors and good cellar, and are heated by open fire-places. Each set contains four rooms and a hall; the rooms measure from 14 by 18 feet to 18 feet square. The commanding officer's quarters contain six rooms, each about 16 feet square.

The storehouse comprises two large rooms, 20 by 30 feet, with an office, 20 by 15 feet, between. This building is used by the commissary and quartermaster department, and is in excellent condition.

The guard-house is also of adobe, with jaspe floors; dimensions, 44 by 18 feet, and 10 feet high. The walls are mud-plastered and whitewashed. It comprises a guard-room, 14 by 14 feet, a prisoners' room, 14 by 18 feet, and a cell, 10 feet square; these rooms are 10 feet high, and are all warmed by open wood-fires. The ventilation of the guard-house is insufficient, consisting only of openings, 12 inches by 24 inches, in the north, south, and west walls, 7 feet and 8 inches from the floor. Prisoners sleep on the floor.

The hospital fronts on the parade-ground, facing east, is 95 by 25 feet, and, excepting the floors, is in fair condition. The ward is 30 by 14 feet, and contains five beds.

The water-supply of the post is by a water-wagon from the Ojo del Muerto, a spring near the post. The water is clear and slightly saline in taste. An analysis by Dr. J. F. Boughter gave the following result:

| | |
|---|---|
| Organic matter | 1.316 grains per gallon. |
| Salts of lime | 21.5 grains per gallon. |
| Salts of magnesia | 2.3 grains per gallon. |
| Salts of soda | 37 grains per gallon. |

When kept in barrels exposed to the air the water becomes very offensive, probably owing to the evolution of sulphureted hydrogen.

There is a weekly stage line to Santa Fé. The nearest post-office is Aleman, distant 17 miles. Mails are received twice a week. A letter should go to Fort Leavenworth in from 9 to 12 days. The inhabitants of the surrounding country are Mexican farmers, who are a very healthy class of people.

*Meteorological report, Fort McRae, N. Mex., 1870–'74.*

| Months. | 1870–'71. | | | | 1871–'72. | | | | 1872–'73. | | | | 1873–'74. | | | |
|---|---|---|---|---|---|---|---|---|---|---|---|---|---|---|---|---|
| | Temperature. | | | Rain-fall in inches. | Temperature. | | | Rain-fall in inches. | Temperature. | | | Rain-fall in inches. | Temperature. | | | Rain-fall in inches. |
| | Mean. | Max. | Min. | | Mean. | Max. | Min. | | Mean. | Max. | Min. | | Mean. | Max. | Min. | |
| | ° | ° | ° | | ° | ° | ° | | ° | ° | ° | | ° | ° | ° | |
| July | 80.91 | 100 | 65 | 4.11 | | | | | | | | | 87.35 | 116* | 55* | 0.05 |
| August | 76.66 | 100 | 63 | 3.67 | | | | | | | | | 78.58 | 107* | 59* | 2.50 |
| September | 72.34 | 98 | 49 | 0.95 | | | | | | | | | 75.22 | 103* | 44* | 1.38 |
| October | 60.17 | 87 | 35 | 0.95 | | | | | | | | | 62.31 | 90* | 20* | 0.08 |
| November | 45.34 | 70 | 22 | 0.00 | | | | | | | | | 49.57 | 78* | 22* | 0.30 |
| December | 34.56 | 59 | 4 | 0.54 | 39.50 | 63 | 17 | 0.10 | 43.11 | 68* | 13* | 1.10 | 38.57 | 69* | 11* | 0.00 |
| January | | | | | | | | | | | | | 42.89 | 72* | 3* | 0.01 |
| February | 41.39 | 70 | 15 | 0.00 | | | | | 45.75 | 71* | 16* | 0.12 | 36.49 | 68* | 9* | 0.09 |
| March | 52.73 | 80 | 17 | 0.00 | | | | | 57.42 | 88* | 14* | 0.40 | 54.58 | 81* | 19* | 0.60 |
| April | | | | | 64.12 | 91* | 32* | 0.00 | 60.32 | 95* | 22* | 0.20 | 55.60 | 89* | 25* | 2.20 |
| May | | | | | 77.75 | 109* | 45* | 0.45 | | | | | 71.07 | 98* | 37* | 0.15 |
| June | | | | | | | | | 79.24 | 120* | 46* | 0.39 | 79.47 | 104* | 50* | 0.10 |
| For the year | | | | | | | | | | | | | 60.97 | 116* | 3* | 7.46 |

* These observations are made with self-registering thermometers. The mean is from the standard thermometer.

*Consolidated sick-report, Fort McRae, N. Mex., 1870–'74.*

| Year | 1870–'71. | | 1871–'72. | | 1872–'73.* | | 1873–'74. | |
|---|---|---|---|---|---|---|---|---|
| Mean strength  { Officers | 3 | | 2 | | 1 | | 2 | |
| { Enlisted men | 61 | | 46 | | 45 | | 61 | |
| Diseases. | Cases. | Deaths. | Cases. | Deaths. | Cases. | Deaths. | Cases. | Deaths. |
| GENERAL DISEASES, A. | | | | | | | | |
| Remittent fever | | | | | 2 | | | |
| Intermittent fever | 7 | | 9 | | 8 | | 5 | |
| Other diseases of this group | 3 | | | | | | 4 | |
| GENERAL DISEASES, B. | | | | | | | | |
| Rheumatism | 2 | | 1 | | 1 | | 4 | |
| Syphilis | 3 | | 6 | | 3 | | 3 | |
| Other diseases of this group | | | | | 1 | | 1 | |
| LOCAL DISEASES. | | | | | | | | |
| Catarrh and bronchitis | 3 | | 5 | | 4 | | 7 | |
| Pneumonia | | | | | | | 3 | 1 |
| Pleurisy | 1 | | | | | | 2 | |
| Diarrhœa and dysentery | 4 | | 7 | | 6 | | 19 | |
| Gonorrhœa | 4 | | 6 | | 4 | | 4 | |
| Other local diseases | 31 | | 9 | | 10 | | 25 | |
| Alcoholism | 1 | | | | 2 | | 6 | |
| Total disease | 59 | | 43 | | 41 | | 83 | 1 |
| VIOLENT DISEASES AND DEATHS. | | | | | | | | |
| Drowning | | | | | | | 1 | 1 |
| Other accidents and injuries | 21 | 1 | 10 | | 9 | | 24 | |
| Total violence | 21 | 1 | 10 | | 9 | 1 | 24 | 1 |

* 10 months only.

## FORT RILEY, KANSAS.

Fort Riley is situated on a high plateau of prairie on the left bank of the Kansas River, immediately below the confluence of the Smoky Hill and Republican Forks. Latitude, 39° north; longitude, 19° 27′ west; elevation above the sea about 1,084 feet; above the bottom-land on the east between 50 and 60 feet. From 300 to 600 yards to the northwest is a ridge of secondary or rotten limestone bluffs, from 150 to 200 feet high, from which the post is separated by a small ravine, which serves as a drain. To the south and southwest the plateau slopes rapidly toward the Kansas River. On this slope runs the Kansas Pacific Railroad.

The valley of the Kansas at this point is nearly 3 miles wide, the distance from the river to the foot of the plateau on which the post is built being about 2,500 yards. The soil of the bottoms is a pale yellow loam, and very fertile.

The post was established in the spring of 1852, and was at first known as Camp Center, it being very nearly the geographical center of the United States, but was finally called by its present name after General B. C. Riley, United States Army.

The post is built around a parallelogram 553 by 606 feet. The barracks for enlisted men consist of six two-story buildings of hammered magnesian limestone, each intended for one company, and measuring 88 by 40 feet, with piazzas in front and rear for both stories. The first floor is subdivided into rooms for kitchen, dining-room, orderly-room, &c. The second floor consists of one room, 85 by 37 feet, and 11 feet 9 inches high, lighted and ventilated by six windows on each side, each 6 feet 6 inches by 3 feet 8 inches. At each end of the dormitory is a fire-place, which, however, is not used, stoves having been substituted. Each dormitory contains 37,740 cubic feet, which gives 686 cubic feet to each man on an average occupancy of 55. The latrines are from 100 to 300 feet distant, and have walled vaults about 20 feet in depth.

The guard-house is a two story stone building, 43 by 20 feet, arranged as shown in Figure 47.

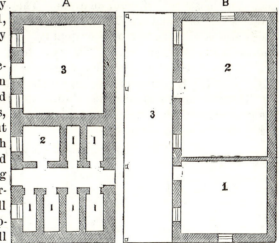

A, first floor; 1, cells, 3 by 7 feet; 2, cell, 7 by 7¼ feet; 3, prison, 16 by 7 feet. B, second floor; 1, guard-room, 14 by 17 feet; 2, guard-room, 16¾ by 25¼ feet; 3, porch, 10 feet wide.

A broad stairway leads to the porch in the second story, the porch being covered by an extension of the roof of the building. The commissary and quartermaster store-houses are two frame buildings, one story high, having basements or cellars about two-thirds their extent. The north end of each building is subdivided into several rooms designed for offices and sleeping apartments. The remaining portion constitutes one large room for storage purposes. The cellars are commodious, being well adapted for vegetables, &c. Each building is supplied with a hoist. The offices and other small rooms are plastered and whitened.

Figure 47.—Scale, 18 feet to 1 inch.

The ordnance building is a one-story stone building, 117 by 18 feet.

The magazine attached to the post is a brick structure, 16 feet square, and one story high, with a rock foundation.

The officers' quarters consist of six buildings of hammered stone, two stories in height, and measuring 60 by 40 feet, five being intended for two sets of quarters each, the sixth for the commanding officer. All of them have a piazza in front and rear for the lower story. The kitchens are separate buildings in the rear, each with a good cellar underneath. All the quarters are well finished.

This hospital is a stone building, which was modified and repaired in 1873, under the supervision of Surgeon B. J. D. Irwin, United States Army, and is now in good order and condition. Its plan, as modified, is shown in Figure 48. 1, first floor; 2, second floor.

A, ward, 60 by 22 feet, and $11\frac{1}{2}$ feet high; B, reading-room; C, lavatory and bath-room; D, dining-room; E, kitchen, $20\frac{1}{2}$ by $19\frac{1}{2}$ feet; F, dispensary, $17\frac{5}{6}$ by 20 feet; G, office, 18 by $21\frac{2}{3}$ feet; H, steward's room, $17\frac{2}{3}$ by 20 feet; I, store-room, $17\frac{2}{3}$ by $21\frac{2}{3}$ feet; K, earth-closet; L, covered porches, 10 feet wide; M, yard; N, bake-oven; height of rooms, 12 feet. Second-story rooms are each $17\frac{5}{6}$ by 20 feet, and 9 feet 10 inches high. The main ward contains fourteen beds; air-space, 1,131 cubic feet. It is ventilated on the ridge by a raised lattice-work.

There are five stables, built of stone, each 256 by 39 feet, running north and south, and parallel to each other. They are 62 feet apart, and contain over 100 stalls each.

Reading-rooms and libraries are attached to the post. They contain over 700 volumes.

The water-supply is from 19 cisterns, 5 wells, and from the river by means of water-wagons. The cisterns are about 30 feet deep by 12 feet in diameter, and have stone bottoms with cement walls. They receive the water from the various buildings, there being one to each barrack and to each double set of officers' quarters. They have no filters, but the water is of good quality. The wells have an average depth of 58 feet. The water is alkaline and of poor quality. The wells are in bad repair, and the water is seldom used. The water from the river, when the latter is high, is soft and of good quality, when it is allowed to settle; but when the river is low it contains many impurities, and is very disagreeable.

There is no system of artificial drainage, the elevation and slope of the grounds, and the numerous small ravines and gullies giving very good facilities for natural drainage.

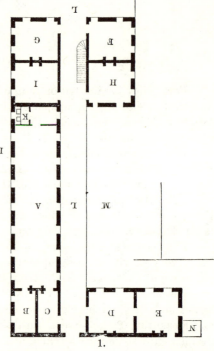

Figure 48.

*Meteorological report, Fort Riley, Kans., 1870–'74.*

| Month. | 1870–'71. | | | | 1871–'72. | | | | 1872–'73. | | | | 1873–'74. | | | |
|---|---|---|---|---|---|---|---|---|---|---|---|---|---|---|---|---|
| | Temperature. | | | Rain-fall in inches. | Temperature. | | | Rain-fall in inches. | Temperature. | | | Rain-fall in inches. | Temperature. | | | Rain-fall in inches. |
| | Mean. | Max. | Min. | | Mean. | Max. | Min. | | Mean. | Max. | Min. | | Mean. | Max. | Min. | |
| July | 83.11 | 104 | 62 | 1.74 | 79.76 | 100 | 63 | 7.38 | 79.18 | 101* | 54* | 7.19 | 78.46 | 97* | 50* | 2.71 |
| August | 73.28 | 102 | 48 | 5.24 | 76.49 | 99 | 56 | 4.11 | 78.28 | 99* | 49* | 4.83 | 80.55 | 103* | 49* | 0.90 |
| September | 67.21 | 90 | 51 | 5.84 | 66.82 | 91 | 42 | 0.79 | 65.53 | 99* | 38* | 6.74 | 65.61 | 97* | 31* | 1.91 |
| October | 55.33 | 80 | 28 | 5.17 | 56.55 | 91 | 28 | 0.93 | 55.57 | 90* | 25* | 2.53 | 50.79 | 84* | 9* | 0.66 |
| November | 43.00 | 72 | 16 | 0.07 | 34.30 | 75 | 2 | 4.71 | 33.08 | 71* | − 1* | 0.00 | 41.63 | 78* | 9* | 0.51 |
| December | 27.16 | 60 | −12 | 1.86 | 22.91 | 52 | − 7 | 0.32 | 18.86 | 59* | −16* | 0.64 | 26.80 | 67* | 4* | 2.04 |
| January | 27.62 | 61 | − 7 | 1.76 | 23.42 | 60* | −10* | 0.02 | 18.53 | 48* | −17* | 1.26 | 25.69 | 60* | − 4* | 0.44 |
| February | 34.43 | 71 | 0 | 2.06 | 31.09 | 67* | −11* | 0.69 | 29.26 | 63* | − 7* | 0.48 | 24.70 | 49* | 0* | 0.54 |
| March | 46.30 | 83 | 22 | 0.99 | 37.55 | 72* | 13* | 1.41 | 42.76 | 80* | 3* | 0.42 | 39.07 | 69* | 12* | 1.11 |
| April | 55.85 | 95 | 32 | 3.02 | 56.08 | 90* | 20* | 1.36 | 47.54 | 92* | 20* | 1.40 | 49.31 | 88* | 10* | 1.01 |
| May | 66.66 | 86 | 44 | 4.93 | 66.46 | 92* | 38* | 4.06 | 64.51 | 88* | 39* | 4.79 | 69.56 | 94* | 39* | 2.30 |
| June | 79.04 | 95 | 62 | 1.19 | 76.22 | 97* | 50* | 2.08 | 76.89 | 98* | 52* | 7.17 | 77.25 | 95* | 45* | 4.22 |
| For the year | 54.35 | 104 | −12 | 33.87 | 52.30 | 100 | −11* | 27.86 | 50.83 | 101* | −17* | 37.45 | 52.45 | 103* | − 4* | 18.35 |

* These observations are made with self-registering thermometers. The mean is from the standard thermometer.

*Consolidated sick-report, Fort Riley, Kans., 1870–'74.*

| Year | | 1870–'71. | | 1871–'72. | | 1872–'73. | | 1873–'74. | |
|---|---|---|---|---|---|---|---|---|---|
| Mean strength { Officers | | 15 | | 11 | | 9 | | 9 | |
| { Enlisted men | | 298 | | 203 | | 199 | | 137 | |
| Diseases. | | Cases. | Deaths. | Cases. | Deaths. | Cases. | Deaths. | Cases. | Deaths. |
| **GENERAL DISEASES, A.** | | | | | | | | | |
| Small-pox and varioloid | | | | | | 1 | | | |
| Typhoid fever | | 1 | | | | | | | |
| Remittent fever | | 1 | | | | 1 | | 1 | |
| Intermittent fever | | 115 | | 144 | | 42 | | 12 | |
| Other diseases of this group | | 28 | | 27 | | 86 | | 15 | |
| **GENERAL DISEASES, B.** | | | | | | | | | |
| Rheumatism | | 15 | | 16 | | 13 | | 19 | |
| Syphilis | | 2 | | 13 | | 4 | | 1 | |
| Consumption | | 1 | | | | 3 | | | |
| Other diseases of this group | | 10 | 1 | | | 1 | | 4 | |
| **LOCAL DISEASES.** | | | | | | | | | |
| Catarrh and bronchitis | | 45 | | 49 | | 49 | | 68 | |
| Pneumonia | | | | | | 3 | | 2 | |
| Pleurisy | | 1 | | 2 | | 1 | | | |
| Diarrhœa and dysentery | | 63 | | 59 | | 17 | | 65 | |
| Hernia | | 1 | | 1 | | | | | |
| Gonorrhœa | | 12 | | 16 | | 3 | | 5 | |
| Other local diseases | | 99 | | 96 | 1 | 82 | | 75 | |
| Alcoholism | | 10 | | 5 | | 7 | | 12 | |
| Unclassified | | 1 | | 1 | | | | | |
| Total disease | | 405 | 1 | 429 | 1 | 313 | | 279 | |
| **VIOLENT DISEASES AND DEATHS.** | | | | | | | | | |
| Gunshot wounds | | 5 | | 2 | 1 | 6 | | 2 | |
| Other accidents and injuries | | 174 | 3 | 141 | | 90 | | 52 | |
| Total violence | | 179 | 3 | 143 | 1 | 96 | | 54 | |

# ROCK ISLAND ARSENAL, ILLINOIS.

This post, an arsenal of construction, is situated on Rock Island, in the Mississippi River, latitude 41° 32′ north, longitude 13° 27′ west, and opposite Davenport, Iowa. It was first occupied and reserved during the war of 1812, and called Fort Armstrong. Being vacated by United States troops in 1836, the post was in charge of a civil agent until 1863, when it was occupied as a depot for rebel prisoners. Major Kingsbury, United States Army, at this time commenced the erection of a United States arsenal, and on the 7th of July, 1865, Maj. John A. Kress took command of the post, from which dates its occupancy as an established arsenal and armory.

In its early history Rock Island was the headquarters, the pleasure and fishing grounds of the Sac and Fox tribe of Indians. Here General Taylor at one time commanded. During the Black Hawk war, in 1832, General Scott made his headquarters at this place, where his command was decimated by cholera.

The island has a base of magnesian limestone, with superincumbent soil of great fertility.

The arsenal-building is a stone structure situated at the foot of the island.

The barrack is a two-story stone building with attic and basement, recently constructed at a cost of $95,000. It is supposed to be the most complete barrack-building in the United States. The building is 154 by 57 feet, and consists of a main part with two wings. A covered veranda extends the entire length on the east side. The basement contains the kitchen, with a large mess-room adjoining, store-rooms, the bakery, laundry, cellar-pantry, coal-room, and two furnaces. The second floor has four dormitories, each 20 by 36 feet; a bath-room, 12 by 20 feet; a library with reading-room, and an armory. Ventilation is effected by windows, transoms, and flues. The dormitories are warmed by hot-air furnaces in the basement. Single iron bunks are furnished; air-space per bed, 600 cubic feet. The sinks, fifteen in number, are supplied with iron pipes which extend to the river.

The married soldiers occupy the south wing of the barrack-building, which has been fitted up especially for them, with commodious and complete arrangements for laundry purposes in the basement.

The officers' quarters are four new stone buildings, and one temporary.frame.

The store-houses are also of stone, new, ample, and well adapted.

A building which is designed for the fire-engine, guard-house, post commissary and quartermaster's offices and store-house, was completed and occupied in July, 1874. It is of stone, two stories and attic. The guard-room is 23 by 30 feet, and has a bath-room and water-closet attached. There are five cells, two light and three dark; the former are, respectively, 6 by 8 feet, and 7½ by 8 feet; of the latter, one is 5 by 8 feet, the others 6 by 8 feet each. The cells are ventilated by registers, one at the top and one near the floor of each. Warming is by coal-stoves. A room for the officer of the day and officer of the guard is on the second floor.

The hospital is a temporary frame building, which will probably be replaced by a stone hospital. It is of two stories, built for hospital purposes in 1863, and is now in a very bad condition and almost untenantable. Its dimensions are 130 by 45 feet; a veranda 10 feet wide extends nearly around the building. The second floor is divided into twelve ward-rooms, six on either side, with a spacious hall extending through the center the entire length of the building. These rooms are 12 feet high, and have each two windows opening over the roof of the veranda. The windows afford ample ventilation. Each room contains two beds, allowing an air-space of 500 cubic feet. A bathroom adjoins the laundry. Two sinks are located 50 yards distant from the hospital; a large-sized commode is used for in-door patients.

The water-supply is abundant and good. A steam-engine pumps the water from the river into a reservoir of 1,000,000 gallons capacity. This reservoir is located on a height; water is distributed throughout the post by iron pipes. There is a steam fire-engine at the post.

*Meteorological report, Rock Island arsenal, Illinois, 1870–'74.*

| Month. | 1870–'71. | | | | 1871–'72. | | | | 1872–'73. | | | | 1873–'74. | | | |
|---|---|---|---|---|---|---|---|---|---|---|---|---|---|---|---|---|
| | Temperature. | | | Rain-fall in inches. | Temperature. | | | Rain-fall in inches. | Temperature. | | | Rain-fall in inches. | Temperature. | | | Rain-fall in inches. |
| | Mean. | Max. | Min. | | Mean. | Max. | Min. | | Mean. | Max. | Min. | | Mean. | Max. | Min. | |
| | ° | ° | ° | | ° | ° | ° | | ° | ° | ° | | ° | ° | ° | |
| July | 79.69 | 100 | 29 | 1 40 | 75.81 | 94 | 61* | 1.83 | 76.09 | 98* | 58* | 3.80 | 74.08 | 97* | 51* | 1.35 |
| August | 72.34 | 95 | 55 | 3.70 | 74.98 | 99 | 38* | 3.81 | 75.21 | 94* | 50* | 7.60 | 77.67 | 102* | 50* | 0.28 |
| September | 67.41 | 88 | 56 | 4.74 | 62.71 | 89* | 31* | 0.23 | 66.26 | 93* | 32* | 3.67 | 64.54 | 94* | 32* | 0.52 |
| October | 53.30 | 75 | 30 | 2.84 | 55.51 | 87* | 34* | 3.34 | 52.64 | 83* | 20* | 0.16 | 49.04 | 79* | 12* | 1.25 |
| November | 41.64 | 68 | 16 | 1.04 | 33.77 | 63* | — 2* | 2.29 | 30.35 | 57* | — 7* | 1.26 | 32.51 | 64* | 1* | 1.06 |
| December | 26.68 | 56 | — 8* | 0.66 | 20.11 | 44 | —10 | 5.68 | 14.93 | 48* | —26* | 0.29 | 27.08 | 62* | 5* | (?) |
| January | 25.28 | 64 | — 5 | 3.01 | 21.02 | 45 | —10* | 0.38 | 20.16 | 46* | —29* | 2.75 | 21.43 | 64* | —13* | 3.10 |
| February | 28.66 | 54 | —10 | 3.25 | 26.00 | 57 | — 9 | 0.22 | 20.16 | 46* | —21* | 0.30 | 24.34 | 47* | — 5* | 0.45 |
| March | 41.24 | 71 | 24 | 1.54 | 30.68 | 64* | 2* | 1.04 | 33.31 | 61* | —14* | 0.46 | 34.24 | 70* | 12* | 0.90 |
| April | 54.69 | 86 | 25* | 2.86 | 51.81 | 87* | 21* | 2.00 | 45.48 | 85* | 25* | 4.05 | 40.99 | 79* | 16* | 1.27 |
| May | 66.33 | 92 | 40 | 1.04 | 62.59 | 89* | 34* | 3.65 | 59.59 | 89* | 39* | 3.45 | 63.21 | 94* | 36* | 2.93 |
| June | 74.52 | 96 | 39* | 3.85 | 73.82 | 98* | 53* | 2.58 | 75.49 | 95* | 41* | 0.95 | 71.83 | 97* | 47* | 3.43 |
| For the year | 52.66 | 100 | — 8* | 29.93 | 49.07 | 99 | —10* | 27.05 | 47.11 | 98* | —29* | 28.74 | 48.41 | 102* | —13* | |

* These observations are made with self-registering thermometers. The mean is from the standard thermometer.

*Consolidated sick-report, Rock Island arsenal, Illinois, 1870–'74.*

| Year | | 1870–'71. | | 1871–'72. | | 1872–'73. | | 1873–'74. | |
|---|---|---|---|---|---|---|---|---|---|
| Mean strength { Officers | | 6 | | 5 | | 5 | | 4 | |
| { Enlisted men | | 75 | | 66 | | 73 | | 70 | |
| Diseases. | | Cases. | Deaths. | Cases. | Deaths. | Cases. | Deaths. | Cases. | Deaths. |
| GENERAL DISEASES, A. | | | | | | | | | |
| Cerebro-spinal fever | | | | | | 1 | | | |
| Remittent fever | | 24 | | 6 | | | | 1 | |
| Intermittent fever | | 13 | | 29 | | 118 | | 123 | |
| Other diseases of this group | | 11 | | 12 | | 8 | | 22 | |

*Consolidated sick-report, Rock Island arsenal, Illinois, 1870–'74—Continued.*

| Year | | 1870–'71. | | 1871–'72. | | 1872–'73. | | 1873–'74. | |
|---|---|---|---|---|---|---|---|---|---|
| Mean strength { Officers | | 6 | | 5 | | 5 | | 4 | |
| { Enlisted men | | 75 | | 66 | | 73 | | 70 | |
| Diseases. | | Cases. | Deaths. | Cases. | Deaths. | Cases. | Deaths. | Cases. | Deaths. |
| GENERAL DISEASES, B. | | | | | | | | | |
| Rheumatism | | 17 | ...... | 5 | ...... | 14 | ...... | 9 | ...... |
| Syphilis | | 6 | ...... | ...... | ...... | 1 | ...... | 5 | ...... |
| Other diseases of this group | | 5 | ...... | 1 | ...... | ...... | ...... | ...... | ...... |
| LOCAL DISEASES. | | | | | | | | | |
| Catarrh and bronchitis | | 48 | ...... | 33 | ...... | 40 | ...... | 65 | ...... |
| Pneumonia | | ...... | ...... | 2 | ...... | 3 | ...... | 2 | ...... |
| Pleurisy | | 9 | ...... | 4 | ...... | 1 | ...... | ...... | ...... |
| Diarrhœa and dysentery | | 49 | ...... | 21 | ...... | 16 | ...... | 63 | ...... |
| Gonorrhœa | | 3 | ...... | 1 | ...... | 4 | ...... | 5 | ...... |
| Other local diseases | | 125 | 1 | 88 | ...... | 22 | ...... | 56 | ...... |
| Alcoholism | | 8 | ...... | 1 | ...... | 2 | ...... | 1 | ...... |
| Unclassified | | ...... | ...... | 1 | ...... | ...... | ...... | ...... | ...... |
| Total disease | | 318 | 1 | 204 | ...... | 230 | ...... | 352 | ...... |
| VIOLENT DISEASES AND DEATHS. | | | | | | | | | |
| Accidents and injuries | | 44 | ...... | 24 | ...... | 18 | ...... | 15 | ...... |
| Total violence | | 44 | ...... | 24 | ...... | 18 | ...... | 15 | ...... |

# SAINT LOUIS BARRACKS, MISSOURI.

### REPORT OF SURGEON B. A. CLEMENTS, UNITED STATES ARMY.

The post of Saint Louis Barracks is situated on the right bank of the Mississippi River, in the southeastern part of the city of Saint Louis, Mo. It occupies an area of about 25 acres, fronting 950 feet on the river, and extending back about 1,100 feet toward Carondelet avenue, one of the main thoroughfares of the city, which is about 600 feet distant from the western limits of the reservation. Originally the reservation extended quite to Carondelet avenue, but a portion nearest to this street was, within a few years past, ceded to the city on the condition that it should be converted into a public park. The reservation was acquired by the United States in 1827 for an arsenal, and, soon after, the buildings were commenced. It continued to be used as an arsenal until January 16, 1871, when, in accordance with General Order No. 125, Adjutant-General's Office, Washington, December 15, 1870, it was occupied as a depot for the general mounted recruiting service, for which purpose it is still used.

The quarters for enlisted men are three buildings formerly used as ordnance store-houses. Two of these are each 70 by 40 feet, two stories high and well ventilated; the mess-rooms are immediately adjacent, and are of stone, 145 by 30 feet, with shingle roofs. The third building is of brick, three stories high, 107 by 69 feet, used as quarters for recruits. It is well ventilated, and the mess-room and kitchen occupy the ground-floor. There is a two-story brick building divided into two sets of quarters of four rooms each, for the non-commissioned staff, and four one-story cottages, detached, for other non-commissioned officers.

The laundresses' quarters consist of ten sets, in one long one story frame building, two rooms to each set, with a small yard in the rear of each. One one-story stone building, 66 by 40, with shingle roof, is used as quarters for the band.

The buildings for officers' quarters face toward the river, and from their front the ground slopes rapidly for some 60 yards to where an iron railing separates this space from the Iron Mountain Railroad and the river. This ground forms what might be called a lawn, and is shaded by a number of trees, principally locust, which are old and decaying. Three buildings and part of a fourth are used for quarters.

1. The commanding officer's quarters, 47 by 40 feet, two stories and basement, built of stone,

37 M P

and recently thoroughly repaired. There is a wing or back building, 100 by 19½ feet, containing kitchens, servants' rooms, water-closets, &c.

2. A stone building, 50 by 40 feet, two stories high, with a cellar, slate roof, and an iron veranda on three sides of both stories. There is to this building a wing, two stories high, of stone, with slate roof, for servants' rooms, kitchen, and water-closets, but the rooms are small.

3. Between the buildings just named is a large three-story stone building, formerly used as a storehouse, 120 by 40 feet in size, which was partly converted in 1872 into officers' quarters. There are some four sets of quarters in it, of two rooms each, but the arrangement is very poor, and there are no suitable kitchens and water-closets. The remainder of this building on the second floor is used as a post-library and reading-room.

4. A brick cottage, formerly the adjutant's office of the arsenal, converted into quarters for officers. The rooms are quite small. The size is 60 by 36 feet; the greater part of the length being cut up into small rooms for dining-room, servants, &c.

There is, also, a frame building, one story, intended for a chapel and a school-room, and used occasionally for dancing purposes.

The hospital consists of a brick building, two stories high, 42 by 30 feet in size, divided into four rooms on the first floor, and three on second. This is used for office, dispensary, kitchen, and mess-room, on the first floor, and store-room, steward's room, and prison ward, on the second. It is not well adapted for these uses, but is made to answer, without serious inconvenience, and is in a fair state of repair. Also of one frame building, one story high, 77 by 30 feet in size, divided equally into two wards. The capacity of the wards is 12 beds each, with a superficial area of 95 square feet per bed, and 1,140 cubic feet of air-space each. The wards have ridge ventilation, are well lighted and comfortable. There is but one bath-room for the two wards, and gas has, within a few weeks, been introduced.

The grounds of the hospital are 36 feet wide on each side, north and south, and 92 by 102 feet at the east end; the latter has been graded during the past year, and will be sown with grass-seed the coming spring. On the north side of the hospital-wards there is good turf, with a few trees. The hospital is situated on the south side of the post, and the locality is low and imperfectly drained.

The post is supplied amply with water from the city water-works, as well as with gas from the city.

The prevailing diseases are mainly intestinal affections in summer, malarious diseases in the fall, and inflammatory affections of the chest in the winter and spring.

*Consolidated sick-report, (white,) Saint Louis Barracks, Mo., 1870–'74.*

| Year | | 1870–'71. | | 1871–'72. | | 1872–'73. | | 1873–'74. | |
|---|---|---|---|---|---|---|---|---|---|
| Mean strength | Officers | 4 | | 6 | | 8 | | 7 | |
| | Enlisted men | 156 | | 328 | | 427 | | 273 | |
| Diseases. | | Cases. | Deaths. | Cases. | Deaths. | Cases. | Deaths. | Cases. | Deaths. |
| GENERAL DISEASES, A. | | | | | | | | | |
| Small-pox and varioloid | | | | 2 | | 23 | 3 | | |
| Typhoid fever | | 1 | | 1 | 2 | 6 | 2 | | |
| Remittent fever | | 20 | 1 | 4 | | 3 | | 8 | |
| Intermittent fever | | 91 | | 106 | | 134 | | 120 | |
| Cholera | | | | | | | | 1 | 1 |
| Diphtheria | | 2 | | | | 3 | | | |
| Other diseases of this group | | 34 | | 24 | | 46 | | 37 | |
| GENERAL DISEASES, B. | | | | | | | | | |
| Rheumatism | | 21 | | 22 | | 38 | | 18 | |
| Syphilis | | 9 | | 13 | | 23 | | 8 | |
| Consumption | | 4 | | 4 | 1 | 1 | | 1 | 1 |
| Other diseases of this group | | 1 | | 2 | | 8 | | 5 | |

*Consolidated sick-report, (white,) Saint Louis Barracks, Mo., 1870–'74—Continued.*

| | 1870–'71. | | 1871–'72. | | 1872–'73. | | 1873–'74. | |
|---|---|---|---|---|---|---|---|---|
| Year | | | | | | | | |
| Mean strength { Officers | 4 | | 6 | | 8 | | 7 | |
| { Enlisted men | 156 | | 328 | | 427 | | 273 | |
| Diseases. | Cases. | Deaths. | Cases. | Deaths. | Cases. | Deaths. | Cases. | Deaths. |
| LOCAL DISEASES. | | | | | | | | |
| Catarrh and bronchitis | 121 | ...... | 43 | ...... | 237 | ...... | 106 | ...... |
| Pneumonia | 1 | ...... | 3 | 2 | 9 | 2 | 4 | ...... |
| Pleurisy | 8 | ...... | ...... | ...... | 1 | 1 | ...... | ...... |
| Diarrhœa and dysentery | 130 | 1 | 45 | 1 | 101 | ...... | 173 | ...... |
| Hernia | 1 | ...... | ...... | ...... | 2 | ...... | 1 | ...... |
| Gonorrhœa | 29 | ...... | 11 | ...... | 22 | ...... | 15 | ...... |
| Other local diseases | 168 | ...... | 130 | 2 | 275 | ...... | 161 | 1 |
| Alcoholism | 14 | 1 | 17 | ...... | 23 | 1 | 16 | ...... |
| Unclassified | ...... | ...... | ...... | ...... | 4 | ...... | ...... | ...... |
| Total disease | 655 | 3 | 427 | 8 | 959 | 9 | 674 | 3 |
| VIOLENT DISEASES AND DEATHS. | | | | | | | | |
| Gunshot wounds | ...... | ...... | 3 | 1 | ...... | ...... | 1 | ...... |
| Other accidents and injuries | 67 | ...... | 107 | ...... | 150 | ...... | 105 | ...... |
| Total violence | 67 | ...... | 110 | 1 | 150 | ...... | 106 | ...... |

*Consolidated sick-report, (colored,) Saint Louis Barracks, Mo., 1871–'74.*

| | 1871–'72.* | | 1872–'73. | | 1873–'74. | |
|---|---|---|---|---|---|---|
| Year | | | | | | |
| Mean strength ..... Enlisted men | 43 | | 44 | | 37 | |
| Diseases. | Cases. | Deaths. | Cases. | Deaths. | Cases. | Deaths. |
| GENERAL DISEASES, A. | | | | | | |
| Small-pox and varioloid | 2 | ...... | 6 | 3 | 1 | ...... |
| Remittent fever | 1 | ...... | 2 | ...... | 1 | ...... |
| Intermittent fever | 8 | ...... | 11 | ...... | 2 | ...... |
| Diphtheria | ...... | ...... | ...... | ...... | 1 | ...... |
| Other diseases of this group | 3 | ...... | 8 | ...... | 11 | ...... |
| GENERAL DISEASES, B. | | | | | | |
| Rheumatism | 6 | ...... | 2 | ...... | 3 | ...... |
| Syphilis | 3 | ...... | 1 | ...... | 1 | ...... |
| Consumption | ...... | ...... | 1 | ...... | ...... | ...... |
| Other diseases of this group | ...... | ...... | 4 | ...... | ...... | ...... |
| LOCAL DISEASES. | | | | | | |
| Catarrh and bronchitis | 2 | ...... | 45 | ...... | 15 | ...... |
| Pneumonia | 1 | ...... | 2 | ...... | ...... | ...... |
| Diarrhœa and dysentery | 3 | ...... | 8 | ...... | 14 | ...... |
| Hernia | ...... | ...... | 2 | ...... | ...... | ...... |
| Gonorrhœa | 1 | ...... | 4 | ...... | 4 | ...... |
| Other local diseases | 16 | 1 | 21 | 1 | 21 | ...... |
| Alcoholism | ...... | ...... | 1 | ...... | ...... | ...... |
| Total disease | 46 | 1 | 118 | 4 | 74 | ...... |
| VIOLENT DISEASES AND DEATHS. | | | | | | |
| Gunshot wounds | ...... | ...... | ...... | ...... | 2 | ...... |
| Other accidents and injuries | 12 | ...... | 18 | ...... | 12 | ...... |
| Total violence | 12 | ...... | 18 | ...... | 14 | ...... |

* First report July, 1871.

## JEFFERSON BARRACKS, MISSOURI.

The post of Jefferson Barracks, Saint Louis County, Mo., is situated on the west bank of the Mississippi River, 475 feet above the level of the sea, in latitude 30° 28′ north, longitude 13° 14′ west. It is west of south of the city of Saint Louis, whose southern boundary, now formed by the river Des Peres, an insignificant stream, at times dry, is three miles distant. The Iron Mountain Railroad, passing along the river-bank directly through the post, commences at Saint Louis and terminates at Belmont, Mo., where a ferry across the river to Columbus, Ky., connects this road with railroads to Mobile and New Orleans. To the south and west, partially encircling the post, at a distance of about ten miles, runs the river Maramec, emptying into the Mississippi.

For history and description of the post see Circular No. 4, Surgeon-General's Office, December 5, 1870, page 275.

By General Orders No. 41, War Department, Adjutant-General's Office, Washington, April 25, 1871, the post, together with the lands appertaining thereto, were transferred to the Ordnance Department. The Saint Louis Arsenal was transferred to Jefferson Barracks, and the old arsenal site has been since known as Saint Louis Depot.

---

## SANTA FÉ, NEW MEXICO.

INFORMATION FURNISHED BY SURGEON C. T. ALEXANDER, UNITED STATES ARMY, AND ASSISTANT SURGEON D. L. HUNTINGTON, UNITED STATES ARMY.

The city of Santa Fé is pleasantly situated on an extensive plateau on the western slope of the Rocky Mountains, at an elevation of 6,850 feet above the level of the sea, and in latitude 35° 41′ north, longitude 28° 59′ west. To the north and east rise the foot-hills and peaks of the Rocky Mountain range; on the south the plateau is gradually lost in spurs of mountains shooting out of the main range, and on the west it terminates somewhat abruptly in the valley of the Rio Grande. The city is reached from the north by the stage road from the terminus of the Kansas Pacific Railroad, this terminus being about 400 miles distant. Fort Union, on this same road, lies to the east about 100 miles. To the south runs the main road to Albuquerque and Southern New Mexico, and less important roads leading to neighboring towns. The Rio Grande runs in a southwesterly direction from Santa Fé, about 18 or 20 miles distant at the nearest point. A small mountain-stream, a tributary of the Rio Grande, called the Rio de Santa Fé, nearly bisects the town.

The soil of Santa Fé and vicinity is dry, light and sandy, yet very fruitful. Irrigation is almost entirely relied upon, and extensive systems of acequias or canals surround the town, the water for this purpose being taken from the Santa Fé River, which has sufficient fall to afford facilities for the irrigation of the soil for miles around. Good crops of wheat, corn, beans, red pepper, and many of the vegetables are raised. Potatoes cannot be successfully cultivated in this vicinity. Until recently, but few fruits or berries have been raised, but late experiments in the culture of apples and the smaller fruits have been quite successful. The grape does not mature well; the frosts are too late and early.

The country for miles about Santa Fé is destitute of trees. The large growth is said to have been cut away, at an early date in the history of the place, for fuel and for better security against hostile Indians, and a subsequent growth of large trees has not appeared, though stunted cedars and pines are very common. This want of vegetation detracts much from the natural beauties of the town and vicinity. On the hills toward the mountains are found large pines and cedars. The piñon, a species of pine, furnishes the almost sole supply of fire-wood. It is brought for miles on the backs of donkeys and sold by the load, in the plaza, at from twenty-five cents to one dollar, according to the season of the year or severity of the winter. Coal is not brought to market.

The natural drainage of Santa Fé is excellent, and is materially assisted by the above-mentioned system of acequias. Still, little attention is paid to the subject, and many of the narrow streets and lanes of the city are excessively filthy.

The river-water is very extensively used for drinking purposes, and is excellent. Good water, but a little impregnated with lime, may be obtained by wells at a depth of from 10 to 40 feet.

The population of Santa Fé is about 6,000, of which the larger portion is Mexican and Indian, or an admixture of the two. The American element is rapidly increasing, and already has the chief influence in matters of trade and politics.

The place is irregularly built of adobe, and, when seen from the approaches to the town, has an exceedingly uninviting appearance. The houses are generally built on the Spanish plan, a quadrangle with an interior court-yard, the entrance being through a gateway, generally kept closed. The older portions of the town are built upon narrow lanes and passage-ways, rather than upon streets. The better portion is the more recent, and inhabited by the American residents. The plaza holds a conspicuous place as a business center, and about it and in its vicinity are the civil and military offices, Santa Fé being the headquarters of both the civil and military establishments.

The buildings formerly composing Fort Marcy, which was abandoned as a post in 1867, are still used in connection with the military headquarters, as quarters for guards, escorts, and detachments, and for store-houses; they are in fair repair and answer well the purpose indicated.

The quarters formerly allotted to officers and the barracks are occupied by the enlisted men of the band and detachment, also affording room for offices and store-rooms. These buildings are warmed by fire-places, and well lighted. In the band-quarters the air-space per man is 1,000 cubic feet, and in the detachment-quarters 936 cubic feet; in the former single bunks are used, while in the latter double bunks are furnished, and the bedding is both good and in sufficient quantity. Each detachment has its own mess-room; the kitchen is good, and the cooking is performed by men belonging to the detachment, and is inspected by the officer commanding.

The quarters of married soldiers and laundresses are those formerly occupied by officers, and the officers' quarters are the same as those occupied by the officers of the post, and are also used as offices for the non-commissioned staff. There are two sets of officers' quarters, built of adobe, one story high, plastered in and out, and have dirt roofs; there are three and four rooms to each set, with hall in the center. The rooms are 18 by 18 by 10 feet. The kitchens and servants' rooms are 14 by 14 by 10 feet. A porch extends the entire length in front of both sets.

The buildings are heated by fire-places, and lighted by windows, and ventilated by one door and one window to each room; they are supplied with water from a well in the yard; there is no water-closet or bath-room. The offices and store-houses are located on the east side of the parade-ground; they are built of adobe, with dirt roofs, and are in bad condition; one office, with two rooms, used as quartermaster and commissary offices. There are two commissary store-houses, each 114 by 18 by 10 feet, and two quartermaster's store-houses, one 105 by 24 by 10 feet, and the other 132 by 24 by 10 feet.

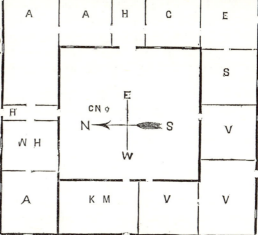

Figure 49.—Scale, 28 feet to 1 inch.

The guard-house is but little used; it is well ventilated, and is warmed by fire-places, and lighted by a large window; its average occupation is not one during the year.

The hospital is located upon grounds 201 by 120 feet, or 24,120 square feet in extent. The buildings are of adobe, and are of sufficient capacity to receive the usual per cent. of sick enlisted men, and well adapted for the purpose. They are built in the form of a square, measuring 77 feet on a side, and inclosing a court-yard, 47 feet square. The plan of the hospital is shown in Figure 49

A, ward, 15 by 32 feet; A, ward, 15 by 17 feet; A, ward, 14 feet 6 inches by 15 feet; C, surgery, 15 by 15 feet 6 inches; E, steward's room, 15 by 15 feet; H H, halls; K M, kitchen and mess-room, 14 by 25 feet; S, store-room, 15 by 15 feet; V, matron's quarters, 15 by 22 feet; V, matron's quarters, 15 by 15 feet; V, matron's quarters, 14 by 14 feet; W H, bath-room, 14 by 15 feet.

Nearly all of the rooms have windows and doors opening both to the outside of the building and to the court-yard within. The hospital is warmed by fire-places, which, in connection with the windows, are the only means of ventilation. The dispensary is large and convenient, and furnished with all the necessary fixtures. In the large wards, the air-space per bed is 798 feet; in the smaller wards, 840 feet.

The following extracts are from a letter by Surg. A. K. Smith, United States Army, relative to climatology and diseases at Santa Fé and vicinity:

"From an experience of fourteen months, and upon rational grounds, I cannot coincide in the popular belief that Santa Fé, and the contiguous localities of equal or superior altitude, are well adapted as a residence for persons suffering from pulmonary tuberculosis, heart disease, or any cause producing obstruction to free and ample respiration. The universal testimony is, so far as I can ascertain, that a stranger to the rarefied atmosphere, however sound his pulmonary and circulatory organs may be, is almost invariably affected by a great oppression in respiration upon his advent into this elevated country, accompanied naturally by an unwonted lassitude and indisposition for exertion. There have been, in the case of two or three of my acquaintances, ugly symptoms of a partial paralysis of the organs of locomotion and speech. A continued residence, however, is said to overcome these unpleasant effects in persons of sound and robust health, and from the number of Americans and Germans residing in the higher regions of New Mexico, who transact their business at no small expenditure of physical exertion, I believe this to be the case, and that in time an accommodation obtains between the lungs and the somewhat diminished quantity of oxygen.

"As regards the invalid whose breathing-apparatus is crippled by tubercular deposit, by chronic pneumonia, or whose blood, whatever may be the cause, requires full aeration, I deem it worse than useless for him to endeavor to regain health or even comfort in such localities. I regard my lungs (and my chest-measurement is 44 inches) as perfectly sound, and yet after reporting for duty in Santa Fé I could not, as a general rule, breathe comfortably, although at times, when a damp atmosphere prevailed, I could not notice any impediment to respiration. The past summer (1874) was exceptionally warm, and I was at intervals asthmatic to a terrible degree, crushed actually by a feeling of impending dissolution. The common advice to me was 'Wear it out; you will be all right next year.' No sooner, however, had I started East than my troubles, as I descended in altitude, lessened proportionately."

*Meteorological report, Santa Fé, N. Mex., 1870–'74.*

| Month. | 1870–'71. | | | | 1871–'72. | | | | 1872–'73. | | | | 1873–'74. | | | |
| | Temperature. | | | Rain-fall in inches. | Temperature. | | | Rain-fall in inches. | Temperature. | | | Rain-fall in inches. | Temperature. | | | Rain-fall in inches. |
| | Mean. | Max. | Min. | | Mean. | Max. | Min. | | Mean. | Max. | Min. | | Mean. | Max. | Min. | |
| | ° | ° | ° | | ° | ° | ° | | ° | ° | ° | | ° | ° | ° | |
| July .................. | 73.66 | 93 | 57 | 4.00 | 76.69 | 97 | 60 | 0.91 | 70.47 | 96 | 57 | 2.38 | 75.45 | 95 | 60 | 0.35 |
| August ............... | 71.31 | 91 | 57 | 3.32 | 74.48 | 97 | 60 | 2.89 | 68.87 | 88 | 59 | 2.30 | ........ | .... | .... | ........ |
| September ........... | 65.87 | 90 | 42 | 2.67 | 69.18 | 82 | 58 | 2.89 | 62.56 | 83 | 46 | 0.26 | ........ | .... | .... | ........ |
| October .............. | 52.09 | 82 | 32 | 1.14 | 56.60 | 73 | 38 | 0.77 | 54.21 | 82 | 22 | 0.10 | ........ | .... | .... | ........ |
| November............. | 44.18 | 65 | 26 | 0.17 | 44.57 | 60 | 25 | 1.46 | 29.59 | 60 | 3 | 0.00 | ........ | .... | .... | ........ |
| December ............ | 27.78 | 61 | − 3 | 0.61 | 39.65 | 58 | 17 | 1.01 | ........ | .... | .... | ........ | ........ | .... | .... | ........ |
| January .............. | 35.25 | 59 | 9 | 1.49 | 30.34 | 55 | 0 | 0.14 | 30.97 | 58 | − 8 | 0.97 | ........ | .... | .... | ........ |
| February............. | 35.34 | 55 | 12 | 0.20 | 33.99 | 62 | 15 | 0.08 | ........ | .... | .... | ........ | ........ | .... | .... | ........ |
| March................ | 43.56 | 65 | 18 | 0.51 | 42.05 | 70 | 18 | 0.18 | ........ | .... | .... | ........ | ........ | .... | .... | ........ |
| April ................ | 49.98 | 82 | 28 | 0.38 | 48.93 | 76 | 30 | 0.14 | ........ | .... | .... | ........ | ........ | .... | .... | ........ |
| May ................. | 64.08 | 85 | 45 | 0.85 | 61.58 | 92 | 39 | 0.35 | ........ | .... | .... | ........ | ........ | .... | .... | ........ |
| June ................. | 76.57 | 98 | 61 | 1.26 | 69.46 | 92 | 54 | 2.19 | 72.03 | 89 | 52 | 0.92 | ........ | .... | .... | ........ |
| For the year....... | 53.30 | 98 | − 3 | 16.60 | 53.96 | 97 | 0 | 13.01 | ........ | .... | .... | ........ | ........ | .... | .... | ........ |

*Consolidated sick-report, Santa Fé, N. Mex., 1870–'74.*

| Year | 1870-'71 | | 1871-'72 | | 1872-'73 | | 1873-'74 | |
|---|---|---|---|---|---|---|---|---|
| Mean strength { Officers | 10 | | 10 | | 9 | | 9 | |
| { Enlisted men | 49 | | 60 | | 48 | | 43 | |
| **Diseases.** | Cases. | Deaths. | Cases. | Deaths. | Cases. | Deaths. | Cases. | Deaths. |
| GENERAL DISEASES, A. | | | | | | | | |
| Intermittent fever | | | | | 4 | | | |
| Other diseases of this group | 1 | | 4 | | 6 | | 10 | |
| GENERAL DISEASES, B. | | | | | | | | |
| Rheumatism | | | 3 | | 3 | | 6 | |
| Syphilis | 4 | | 6 | | 7 | | 8 | |
| Consumption | | | | 1 | | | | |
| Other diseases of this group | | | | | 1 | | | |
| LOCAL DISEASES. | | | | | | | | |
| Catarrh and bronchitis | 6 | | 8 | | 9 | | 8 | |
| Pneumonia | | | 1 | | | | 1 | |
| Pleurisy | | | | | 3 | 1 | | |
| Diarrhœa and dysentery | 5 | | 11 | | 11 | | 4 | |
| Gonorrhœa | 6 | | 10 | | 5 | | | |
| Other local diseases | 13 | | 13 | | 16 | | 9 | |
| Alcoholism | | | 6 | | 7 | | 2 | 1 |
| Total disease | 35 | 1 | 62 | | 72 | 1 | 48 | 1 |
| VIOLENT DISEASES AND DEATHS. | | | | | | | | |
| Gunshot wounds | 1 | | 1 | | 1 | | | |
| Other accidents and injuries | 6 | | 10 | | 19 | | 8 | |
| Homicide | | | | | | 1 | | |
| Suicide | | | | | | 1 | | |
| Total violence | 7 | | 11 | | 20 | 2 | 8 | |

# FORT SELDEN, NEW MEXICO.

## REPORT OF ASSISTANT SURGEON CHARLES STYER, UNITED STATES ARMY.

Fort Selden is situated in a sandy basin one and a half miles from the Rio Grande, in Southern New Mexico; latitude, 32° 25′ north; longitude, 30° west; height above the sea, about 4,250 feet. At this point the river incloses an irregular crescent, upon which the fort is placed. Twenty-five miles east are the Organ Mountains, the Pechaco Mountains lying four miles to the west. The nearest posts are Fort McRae, 58 miles north; Fort Cummings, 55 miles west; and Fort Bliss, Tex., 67 miles south. The nearest towns are on the river to the southeast, being Leesburgh, 1½ miles distant; Dona Ana, 12 miles; Las Cruces, 18 miles; and Franklin, Tex., 65 miles. A good rope ferry across the Rio Grande is one and a half miles above the post.

The reservation is four miles square. The soil is sandy and sterile, resting on volcanic rocks. The ground rises gradually to the north for about four miles; on the south it slopes to the river-bottom. The cottonwood on the river, a coarse and scanty growth of grass on the reservation, with plenty of cacti and stunted mesquite comprise the botany of the vicinity. Deer, antelopes, and bears are found in the mountains. Wolves and skunks are annoyingly numerous about the post. At the river, beavers are plenty.

The post was established in May, 1865, for protection of settlers and of the post-road. It is not yet completed. The buildings are of adobe, plastered outside and in, and the plan of arrangement is shown in Plate No. 5 of Circular No. 4.

The dormitories measure 90 by 24 feet, and allow 950 cubic feet air-space per man. They are warmed by stoves. The bunks are one story.

The officers' quarters are all one-story buildings, with flat earth roofs. They are heated by fire-places.

The hospital is also one story, with dirt roof and floor, warmed by fire-places, and ventilated by these and by windows. It has two wards, each containing five beds, giving 1,440 cubic feet of air-space per man.

Sinks to all the buildings are ordinary latrines with deep vaults.

The water-supply is from the river, by a water-wagon. It is kept in barrels, there being no cisterns or reservoirs. The quantity supplied is ample, and the quality tolerably good. The natural drainage is good, and answers every purpose.

There is a mail six times a week, irregular. Time to department headquarters, from twelve to twenty days.

The sanitary condition of the post is good, and there are no prevailing diseases.

[Extract from a report on climate, by Assistant Surgeon Samuel S. Jessop, United States Army.]

"Lung troubles are comparatively rare at Fort Selden, as are all diseases of the respiratory organs, excepting catarrh, which I prefer to consider separately from bronchitis, as it mostly affects the mucous membranes of the nares, tonsils, and larynx, and, I think, seldom extends even to the trachea. It seems to be produced by the almost constant drifting of the irritating dust peculiar to this region, and few new-comers who are much exposed in the open air escape it. It gradually wears off, as they become acclimated. Women, from their in-door habits, are usually freer from it. The native New Mexicans are not at all affected by it. Many of them, however, suffer from a form of bronchitis, induced, it is thought, by their peculiar fashion of smoking the cigarita, i. e., by inhaling the smoke into their bronchial tubes, and exhaling it through their nostrils.

"The climate of this part of the valley of the Rio Grande will improve, and probably tend to the cure of, many patients afflicted with commencing phthisis, but only by a residence here, not a sojourn of a few months. I think I am within the mark in stating that it will take from eighteen months to two years to acclimate them. To those in advanced stages of consumption, no such benefit can accrue. Added to the annoyance of the dust-storms are the distance from home and the impossibility of obtaining many of the comforts, and especially the varieties in food, which the sick always crave. The prognosis is extremely serious if diarrhœa be a complication, and here I may observe that all cases of chronic diarrhœa appear to do badly at this post, and that, with my present convictions, I would not suffer, if it could be avoided, a patient laboring under this disease to remain at Fort Selden, or any point where the Rio Grande constituted the water-supply. The enervating nature of the climate has doubtless much to do with the ill success attending the treatment of such patients.

"As regards chronic bronchitis, I can only speak for New Mexico, and, for that disease, I con-sider the climate of this region as the best in the Territory."

*Meteorological report, Fort Selden, N. Mex., 1870–'74.*

| Month. | 1870–'71. | | | | 1871–'72. | | | | 1872–'73. | | | | 1873–'74. | | | |
|---|---|---|---|---|---|---|---|---|---|---|---|---|---|---|---|---|
| | Temperature. | | | Rain-fall in inches. | Temperature. | | | Rain-fall in inches. | Temperature. | | | Rain-fall in inches. | Temperature. | | | Rain-fall in inches. |
| | Mean. | Max. | Min. | | Mean. | Max. | Min. | | Mean. | Max. | Min. | | Mean. | Max. | Min. | |
| July | 79.52 | 93 | 68 | 5.20 | 83.81 | 104 | 73 | 2.30 | 80.85 | 104* | 49* | 1.19 | 82.96 | 103 | 64 | 0.20 |
| August | 76.52 | 90 | 64 | 4.00 | 82.30 | 105 | 71 | 1.05 | 78.73 | 102* | 52* | 0.85 | 77.58 | 97 | 65 | 2.24 |
| September | 70.65 | 88 | 48 | 0.70 | 74.24 | 94 | 56 | 2.75 | 71.67 | 94* | 39* | 1.10 | 75.86 | 99 | 52 | 0.30 |
| October | 59.76 | 87 | 36 | 0.65 | 60.48 | 91 | 35 | 0.00 | 59.57 | 93* | 18* | 0.25 | 63.35 | 94 | 30 | 0.11 |
| November | 48.17 | 75 | 24 | 0.00 | 46.39 | 71 | 21 | 0.00 | 44.16 | 76* | 4* | 0.00 | 50.73 | 79 | 25 | 0.26 |
| December | 35.91 | 68 | 9 | 0.25 | 44.07 | 68 | 12 | 0.00 | 45.55 | 74* | 12* | 2.70 | 42.24 | 69 | 17 | 0.04 |
| January | 38.75 | 66 | 9 | 0.00 | 37.26 | 62 | 9 | 0.15 | 41.13 | 72* | −12* | 0.03 | 45.92 | 71 | 18 | 0.59 |
| February | 44.64 | 72 | 14 | 0.00 | 47.64 | 80* | 15* | 0.00 | 46.73 | 74* | 11* | 0.00 | 44.60 | 70 | 16 | 0.55 |
| March | 54.03 | 82 | 20 | 0.00 | 53.74 | 83* | 15* | 0.00 | 58.39 | 86 | 29 | 0.00 | 53.33 | 81 | 28 | 0.26 |
| April | 60.89 | 88 | 37 | 0.00 | 62.00 | 93* | 27* | 0.00 | 58.68 | 88 | 27 | 0.01 | 56.11 | 90 | 30 | 0.62 |
| May | 72.74 | 100 | 55 | 0.22 | 74.44 | 106* | 33* | 0.00 | 76.04 | 92 | 37 | 0.02 | 72.00 | 98 | 48 | 0.01 |
| June | 85.43 | 105 | 66 | 0.60 | 81.71 | 104* | 52* | 0.09 | 78.86 | 105 | 56 | 0.28 | 83.80 | 103 | 66 | 0.18 |
| For the year | 60.58 | 105 | 9 | 11.62 | 62.34 | 106* | 9 | 6.34 | 61.69 | 105 | −12* | 6.43 | 62.37 | 103 | 16 | 5.36 |

* These observations are made with self-registering thermometers. The mean is from the standard thermometer.

*Consolidated sick-report, Fort Selden, N. Mex., 1870–'74.*

| Year | 1870–'71. | | 1871–'72. | | 1872–'73. | | 1873–'74. | |
|---|---|---|---|---|---|---|---|---|
| Mean strength { Officers / Enlisted men | 125 | | 4 / 100 | | 4 / 87 | | 5 / 103 | |
| Diseases. | Cases. | Deaths. | Cases. | Deaths. | Cases. | Deaths. | Cases. | Deaths. |
| GENERAL DISEASES, A. | | | | | | | | |
| Typhoid fever | 1 | | | | | | | |
| Typho-malarial fever | | | | | | | | |
| Remittent fever | 2 | | | | | 1 | | |
| Intermittent fever | 6 | | 8 | | 4 | | 14 | |
| Other diseases of this group | | | | | 2 | | 2 | |
| GENERAL DISEASES, B. | | | | | | | | |
| Rheumatism | 2 | | 3 | | 2 | | 6 | |
| Syphilis | 3 | | 4 | | 3 | | 5 | |
| Other diseases of this group | 1 | | | | | | 2 | |
| LOCAL DISEASES. | | | | | | | | |
| Catarrh and bronchitis | 9 | | 7 | | 10 | | 12 | |
| Pleurisy | | | | | 3 | | | |
| Diarrhœa and dysentery | 12 | | 23 | 2 | 8 | | 19 | 1 |
| Hernia | | | | | 1 | | 1 | |
| Gonorrhœa | 6 | | 8 | | 5 | | 8 | |
| Other local diseases | 25 | 1 | 20 | | 23 | | 56 | |
| Alcoholism | 1 | | 2 | | 2 | | 11 | |
| Total disease | 68 | 1 | 75 | 2 | 63 | 1 | 137 | 1 |
| VIOLENT DISEASES AND DEATHS. | | | | | | | | |
| Gunshot wounds | 2 | | | | 1 | | 2 | 1 |
| Other accidents and injuries | 25 | | 14 | | 18 | | 15 | |
| Suicide | | 1 | | | | | | |
| Total violence | 27 | 1 | 14 | | 19 | | 17 | 1 |

# FORT STANTON, NEW MEXICO.

REPORTS OF ASSISTANT SURGEON J. R. GIBSON AND ACTING ASSISTANT SURGEON A. T. FITCH, UNITED STATES ARMY.

Fort Stanton is situated on the Rio Bonitoa, mountain stream rising in the White Mountains; latitude, 33° 29′ 27″ north ; longitude, 28° 25′ 19″ west; altitude about 7,500 feet. Placita, a small Mexican village nine miles distant, is the only town in the vicinity.

This post was established in 1855 to control the Mescalero Apaches.

On the occupation of the Territory of New Mexico by the Texan troops, Fort Stanton was abandoned and fired by the United States troops in the year 1861, and, with the exception of the walls of the buildings and corrals, the post was destroyed. In the year 1862 a garrison of volunteer troops re-occupied the post, and by covering the walls with rafters and earth roofs made the quarters tenantable. In this condition the post was occupied until 1868, when repair and reconstruction were commenced.

The valley of the river at the site of the post is from one-half to three-quarters of a mile wide. Its banks ascend gradually until the plain of the valley is reached, which, at the site of the post, is about 75 feet above the bed of the stream.

The geological formation exhibits outcroppings of new red sandstone and magnesian limestone. Gold is found in limited quantity in the Jicarillo Mountains northwest, distant about 30 miles from the post. Pines, cedars, and cottonwoods abound. The game consists of bear, deer, antelope, wild turkeys, and quail. Trout are abundant in the stream.

The post was originally laid out in a rectangular form. In the middle of one side of the square, that next and parallel to the river, is situated the commanding officer's quarters. On the side facing this are two sets of company quarters, and one building in the center is designated for use as adjutant's office, guard-room, and cell. In each of the remaining sides of the square are three buildings, viz: One set of company quarters, a store-house, and one building designated as four sets of officers' quarters. All the buildings of the post are constructed of undressed stone, and originally shingled roofs. As before mentioned, these dilapidated walls were rudely and temporarily repaired on the re-occupation of the post, and, with earth roofs, (earth floors in the barracks,) constituted the quarters of the troops.

The post was ordered to be rebuilt in 1868, but the work was stopped in June, 1869, leaving most of the buildings unfinished.

The barracks are stone buildings, shingled, lathed, and plastered; well lighted and ventilated, and allow in the dormitories about 850 cubic feet per man.

The officers' quarters are in two stone buildings, each 90 by 35 feet, and divided into 8 rooms, with two halls. In rear of each of these buildings is another similarly divided, intended for use as kitchens and dining-rooms. There are no bath-rooms or water-closets. The commanding officer's quarters contain seven rooms.

The hospital buildings, described in Circular No. 4, are now used for laundresses' quarters.

The hospital is in one of the barrack buildings, which is unfinished. The squad room, 53 by 29 feet and 10 feet 9 inches high, is used as a ward. The room intended for the first sergeant is used as office and dispensary.

The wing, 75 feet in length, contains the steward's room, store-room, dining-room, and kitchen. There is no bath-room.

Water is brought to the post by an aqueduct which taps the river about three quarters of a mile above the post. The natural drainage of the post is good. The nearest supply-depot is Fort Union.

*Meteorological report, Fort Stanton, N. Mex., 1870–'72.*

| Month. | 1870–'71. | | | | 1871–'72. | | | | 1872–'73. | | | | 1873–'74. | | | |
|---|---|---|---|---|---|---|---|---|---|---|---|---|---|---|---|---|
| | Temperature. | | | Rain-fall in inches. | Temperature. | | | Rain-fall in inches. | Temperature. | | | Rain-fall in inches. | Temperature. | | | Rain-fall in inches. |
| | Mean. | Max. | Min. | | Mean. | Max. | Min. | | Mean. | Max. | Min. | | Mean. | Max. | Min. | |
| | ° | ° | ° | | ° | ° | ° | | ° | ° | ° | | ° | ° | ° | |
| July .................. | 68.63 | 89 | 56 | 4.45 | 74.12 | 91 | 50 | 5.50 | 69.52 | 90 | 52 | 4.78 | ...... | ...... | ...... | ...... |
| August ............... | 65.90 | 84 | 54 | 4.70 | 68.68 | 85 | 50 | 1.13 | 67.84 | 84 | 54 | 3.19 | ...... | ...... | ...... | ...... |
| September ........... | 61.49 | 81 | 45 | 0.94 | 63.21 | 87 | 45 | 2.10 | 60.95 | 80 | 46 | 3.27 | ...... | ...... | ...... | ...... |
| October .............. | 51.80 | 76 | 36 | 2.84 | 53.11 | 74 | 35 | 2.54 | 49.23 | 69 | 33 | 3.02? | ...... | ...... | ...... | ...... |
| November ............ | 46.15 | 69 | 21 | 0.00 | 45.62 | 64 | 20 | (?) | ...... | ...... | ...... | ...... | ...... | ...... | ...... | ...... |
| December ............ | 37.18 | 65 | 5 | 0.36 | 43.05 | 64 | 17 | 0.00 | ...... | ...... | ...... | ...... | ...... | ...... | ...... | ...... |
| January .............. | 37.93 | 64 | 6 | 1.68 | 35.16 | 65 | 10 | 0.66 | ...... | ...... | ...... | ...... | ...... | ...... | ...... | ...... |
| February ............. | 41.89 | 63 | 24 | 0.07 | 43.54 | 68 | 6 | 0.63 | ...... | ...... | ...... | ...... | ...... | ...... | ...... | ...... |
| March ................ | 47.00 | 68 | 16 | 4.28 | 44.45 | 68 | 11 | 0.37 | ...... | ...... | ...... | ...... | ...... | ...... | ...... | ...... |
| April ................. | 52.58 | 76 | 35 | 0.00 | 54.19 | 73 | 28 | 0.66 | ...... | ...... | ...... | ...... | ...... | ...... | ...... | ...... |
| May .................. | 62.05 | 84 | 42 | 0.65 | 64.97 | 93 | 32 | 0.00 | ...... | ...... | ...... | ...... | ...... | ...... | ...... | ...... |
| June ................. | 72.29 | 95 | 55 | 0.14 | 72.10 | 90 | 58 | 2.29 | ...... | ...... | ...... | ...... | ...... | ...... | ...... | ...... |
| For the year .... | 53.74 | 95 | 5 | 20.11 | 55.18 | 93 | 6 | ...... | ...... | ...... | ...... | ...... | ...... | ...... | ...... | ...... |

*Consolidated sick-report, Fort Stanton, N. Mex., 1870–'74.*

| Year ...................................................................... | 1870–'71. | | 1871–'72.* | | 1872–'73. | | 1873–'74. | |
|---|---|---|---|---|---|---|---|---|
| Mean strength.................................... { Officers........... <br> { Enlisted men...... | 6 <br> 117 | | 4 <br> 96 | | 5 <br> 116 | | 4 <br> 119 | |
| Diseases. | Cases. | Deaths. | Cases. | Deaths. | Cases. | Deaths. | Cases. | Deaths. |
| GENERAL DISEASES, A. | | | | | | | | |
| Typhoid fever................................................................ | ...... | ...... | ...... | ...... | ...... | ...... | 1 | 1 |
| Remittent fever ............................................................. | ...... | ...... | ...... | ...... | 8 | ...... | 1 | ...... |
| Intermittent fever .......................................................... | 8 | ...... | 5 | ...... | 2 | ...... | 10 | ...... |
| Other diseases of this group.............................................. | 2 | ...... | 4 | ...... | 4 | ...... | 18 | ...... |

*Consolidated sick-report, Fort Stanton, N. Mex., 1870–'74—Continued.*

| Year | 1870–'71. | | 1871–'72.* | | 1872–'73. | | 1873–'74. | |
|---|---|---|---|---|---|---|---|---|
| Mean strength... { Officers.............. } Enlisted men........ | 6 117 | | 4 96 | | 5 116 | | 4 119 | |
| Diseases. | Cases. | Deaths. | Cases. | Deaths. | Cases. | Deaths. | Cases. | Deaths. |
| GENERAL DISEASES, B. | | | | | | | | |
| Rheumatism........ | 13 | ...... | 4 | ...... | 6 | ...... | 8 | ...... |
| Syphilis......... | 6 | ...... | 2 | ...... | 3 | ...... | 7 | ...... |
| Consumption...... | 1 | ...... | | | | | | |
| LOCAL DISEASES. | | | | | | | | |
| Catarrh and bronchitis...... | 17 | ...... | 6 | ...... | 2 | ...... | 8 | ...... |
| Pneumonia........ | | | | | 4 | ...... | 2 | ...... |
| Diarrhœa and dysentery....... | 38 | ...... | 10 | ...... | 1 | ...... | 26 | ...... |
| Hernia...... | | | | | 1 | ...... | | |
| Gonorrhœa....... | 3 | ...... | 4 | ...... | | | 5 | ...... |
| Other local diseases....... | 74 | ...... | 29 | ...... | 8 | 1 | 23 | ...... |
| Alcoholism........ | 1 | ...... | | | 3 | ...... | 2 | ...... |
| Total disease...... | 163 | ...... | 64 | ...... | 42 | 1 | 111 | 1 |
| VIOLENT DISEASES AND DEATHS. | | | | | | | | |
| Gunshot wounds..... | 1 | ...... | | | | | 2 | 1 |
| Arrow wounds...... | ...... | 2 | | | | | | |
| Other accidents and injuries...... | 22 | ...... | 22 | ...... | 9 | ...... | 31 | 1 |
| Total violence...... | 23 | 2 | 22 | ...... | 9 | ...... | 33 | 2 |

* 11 months only.

# CAMP SUPPLY, INDIAN TERRITORY.

REPORTS OF ASSISTANT SURGEONS J. A. FITZGERALD AND W. H. GARDNER, UNITED STATES ARMY.

Camp Supply is situated in the western part of Indian Territory, on a low sandy bottom between Beaver and Wolf Creeks, 1½ miles southwest of their junction, to form the north fork of the Canadian; latitude, 36° 30′ north; longitude, 22° 27′ west.

The post was established in November, 1868, as a base of supplies for troops operating against hostile Indians. During the winter of 1868–'69 the most of the officers were quartered in tents and the troops in pits from 4½ to 5 feet deep, walled with cottonwood logs rising above the surface about 3 feet, and covered with logs, straw, and earth. During the latter part of 1869 five sets of company-quarters were built of logs placed upright in stockade, each set being 90 by 18 feet and 9 feet high. Several sets of officers' quarters were constructed in like manner. They all had earth floors and roofs, and were damp and uncomfortable.

This region has been for many years the winter-range of the buffalo, and the favorite haunt of the Kiowas, Cheyennes, and Arapahoes, especially the two latter. Thirty-five miles to the north the road to Fort Hays crosses the Cimarron, or Red Fork of the Arkansas, a broad, shallow stream, with scarcely any timber, except at the mouths of its few tributaries. The bottom-lands are usually broad, sandy tracts, covered in spots with an alkaline efflorescence, principally chloride of sodium. The several streams in the vicinity are tributaries of the Arkansas, and, when taking an easterly course, are invariably skirted on their northern banks by ridges of sand-hills, frequently of formidable proportions, indicating the force and direction of the prevailing winds. The surrounding country is a high, rolling prairie, with occasional ranges of hills, broken by cañon-like ravines, in which is a scanty growth of red cedar. It abounds in game, the principal animals being the buffalo, deer, antelope, black and cinnamon bear, gray wolf, coyote, panther, wild-cat, beaver, otter, raccoon, opossum, badger, weasel, and skunk. There is an impression among the scouts, trappers, and herders that the bite of a skunk is sure to be followed by hydrophobia, and several well-authenticated cases are mentioned of this result.

Among the most common birds are the wild turkey, geese, ducks of all kinds, grouse, snipe, and plover. The fish are the buffalo, cat, and sun fish, and in the small streams the black bass.

The parade is about 800 feet square. There are five sets of company quarters, built in 1873, being stockade-buildings, with shingle roofs and flooring of matched pine. Each consists of a main building 94 by 22 feet, 9 feet high at eaves and 16 feet at ridge, with two wings at right angles from the ends, each 70 by 22 feet. The dormitory consists of the main building, with about 20 feet of each wing, giving about 500 cubic feet air-space per man. The mess-room, kitchen, and wash-room are in one wing, the first sergeant's room and store-room in the other. Each barrack has 16 or 18 windows and 2 or 4 ventilators at the ridge. In the rear of each set of company quarters is a stockade-building 75 by 18 feet, containing quarters for three married soldiers.

The quarters for officers are in ten buildings; five of these contain two sets of quarters each; the others a single set each. They are all one-story stockade-buildings, similar to the quarters for the men. They all have floors of matched pine and shingled roofs. The walls inside, and the ceilings, are covered with canvas, which is neatly whitewashed. The walls are 11 feet high; the partitions are mostly made with canvas, set to suit the taste or convenience of the occupants; consequently there is no uniformity in the size of the rooms; but as there is no scarcity of quarters, such as they are, each officer has at least the regulation allowance of rooms. What they lack in elegance and finish, they make up in numbers; and, on the whole, are good quarters. These buildings front the eastern side of the parade. The office of the commanding officer and adjutant is a small stockade-building of one room, situated on the western side of the parade, and is similar in construction to the quarters.

The quartermaster's and commissary's offices and store-houses are about 300 feet in the rear (east) of the officers' quarters. They are two stockade-buildings with shingled roofs and matched-pine floors, and two buildings constructed of logs set upright in the ground, 5 or 6 feet apart, on which canvas is nailed to form the walls. They are roofed with canvas, and are not floored.

The guard-house is a stockade building 45 by 18 feet, 8 feet high to the eaves, has a canvas roof and clay floor, is ventilated by three doors, three windows, and a ventilator in the peak of the roof, and is not a remarkably comfortable habitation either in summer or winter, and holds out but few inducements for men to become inmates of it. It is located about 200 feet west of the adjutant's office, on the crest of the hill.

The hospital is situated about 600 feet southwest from the adjutant's office. It was built in 1873 on the Surgeon-General's plan for a provisional hospital for twelve beds. It is in good condition, but entirely too small for a five-company post.

The post bakery is 80 feet west of the guard-house. It is a stockade-building similar to the quarters, contains all needful appliances, and is capable of baking 1,000 rations of bread per day.

The cavalry stables are about 500 feet to the east of the south end of the row of officers' quarters. The quartermaster's stables and corral are west of north from the quartermaster's store-houses, about 800 feet distant.

Each year since the post was established attempts have been made to cultivate gardens, but beyond a few dwarfed melons, they have come to actually nothing. This is due to the sandy, porous nature of the soil, drought, and grasshoppers.

All the water for drinking and cooking is obtained from Wolf Creek. It contains (in its stage of greatest purity) 46 grains of solid matter per gallon, composed of 16 grains chloride of sodium, 10 grains sulphate of lime, 5 grains carbonate of lime, with sulphates of magnesia and soda, and a trace of alumina and oxidizable organic matter. The water from Beaver Creek is much worse in every respect, having a well-marked alkaline taste, and containing 57 grains of solid matter per gallon. Several wells have been sunk at the post, but the water of none of them is as good as that of Wolf Creek.

The situation of the post combines all the grave sanitary objections that could be urged against any place as the site for a military post, nearly all the ground occupied being so low (only five feet above the level of the streams) that not only is proper drainage impossible, but the water running down the adjacent hillside frequently collects to a depth of over two feet, and can only be got rid of by its evaporation or absorption by the soil. Besides this, its low situation and close proximity to two streams, expose it to malarial poison in its most concentrated form. On every side but the north, it is overlooked by sand-hills, over which in the summer comes the dry, parching wind, loaded with sand and dust, while in the winter its exposed northern aspect allows it to receive the full fury of the piercing northers.

The nearest mail-station is Dodge City, Kans., on the Atchison, Topeka and Santa Fé Railroad, 88 miles distant, north.

*Meteorological report, Camp Supply, Ind. Ter., 1873-'74.*

| Year. | 1870-'71. | | | | 1871-'72. | | | | 1872-'73. | | | | 1873-'74. | | | |
|---|---|---|---|---|---|---|---|---|---|---|---|---|---|---|---|---|
| | Temperature. | | | Rain-fall in inches. | Temperature. | | | Rain-fall in inches. | Temperature. | | | Rain-fall in inches. | Temperature. | | | Rain-fall in inches. |
| | Mean. | Max. | Min. | | Mean. | Max. | Min. | | Mean. | Max. | Min. | | Mean. | Max. | Min. | |
| July | | | | | | | | | | | | | 82.87 | 105 | 63 | 1.71 |
| August | | | | | | | | | | | | | 83.04 | 107 | 66 | 0.59 |
| September | | | | | | | | | | | | | 69.49 | 103 | 38 | 4.23 |
| October | | | | | | | | | | | | | 55.94 | 88 | 21 | 0.00 |
| November | | | | | | | | | | | | | 47.47 | 81 | 10 | 0.50 |
| December | | | | | | | | | | | | | 32.60 | 57 | — 2 | 0.44 |
| January | | | | | | | | | | | | | 32.52 | 66 | — 1 | 0.68 |
| February | | | | | | | | | | | | | 33.55 | 63 | 5 | 3.06 |
| March | | | | | | | | | | | | | 44.45 | 73 | 20 | 0.88 |
| April | | | | | | | | | | | | | 50.01 | 80 | 25 | 5.00 |
| May | | | | | | | | | | | | | 68.60 | 95 | 40 | 1.90 |
| June | | | | | | | | | | | | | 77.56 | 102 | 56 | 0.40 |
| For the year | | | | | | | | | | | | | 56.51 | 107 | — 2 | 19.39 |

*Consolidated sick-report, (white,) Camp Supply, Ind. Ter., 1870-'74.*

| Year | 1870-'71. | | 1871-'72. | | 1872-'73. | | 1873-'74. | |
|---|---|---|---|---|---|---|---|---|
| Mean strength { Officers | 14 | | 13 | | 12 | | 14 | |
| { Enlisted men | 156 | | 174 | | 156 | | 285 | |
| Diseases. | Cases. | Deaths. | Cases. | Deaths. | Cases. | Deaths. | Cases. | Deaths. |
| GENERAL DISEASES, A. | | | | | | | | |
| Typhoid fever | | | 1 | 1 | | | | |
| Remittent fever | | | 2 | | | | 1 | |
| Intermittent fever | 98 | | 99 | | 33 | | 62 | |
| Other diseases of this group | 6 | | 7 | | 25 | 1 | 20 | |
| GENERAL DISEASES, B. | | | | | | | | |
| Rheumatism | 8 | | 17 | | 8 | | 5 | |
| Syphilis | 8 | | 8 | | 4 | | 4 | |
| Consumption | | | | | | | 2 | |
| Other diseases of this group | 4 | | | | 3 | | 1 | 1 |
| LOCAL DISEASES. | | | | | | | | |
| Catarrh and bronchitis | 21 | | 24 | | 33 | | 57 | |
| Pneumonia | | | | | 2 | | 3 | |
| Pleurisy | | | 1 | | | | 1 | |
| Diarrhœa and dysentery | 85 | | 86 | 1 | 42 | | 51 | |
| Hernia | | | | | 1 | | | |
| Gonorrhœa | 1 | | 3 | | 4 | | 1 | |
| Other local diseases | 65 | 1 | 83 | | 86 | 1 | 104 | 1 |
| Alcoholism | 1 | | | | 1 | | 3 | |
| Total disease | 297 | 1 | 331 | 2 | 242 | 2 | 315 | 2 |
| VIOLENT DISEASES AND DEATHS. | | | | | | | | |
| Gunshot wounds | 1 | | 6 | 2 | 1 | | 2 | |
| Other accidents and injuries | 49 | | 75 | | 74 | 1 | 128 | |
| Suicide | | | | | | | | 2 |
| Total violence | 50 | | 81 | 2 | 75 | 1 | 130 | 2 |

*Consolidated sick-report, (colored,) Camp Supply, Ind. Ter., 1870–'73.*

| Year | 1870–'71. | | 1871–'72. | | 1872–'73.* | |
|---|---|---|---|---|---|---|
| Mean strength ...... Enlisted men ...... | 287 | | 107 | | 95 | |
| Diseases. | Cases. | Deaths. | Cases. | Deaths. | Cases. | Deaths. |
| GENERAL DISEASES, A. | | | | | | |
| Cerebro-spinal fever | 1 | 1 | | | | |
| Remittent fever | 3 | | | | | |
| Intermittent fever | 53 | | 25 | | 16 | |
| Other diseases of this group | 15 | | 4 | | 16 | |
| GENERAL DISEASES, B. | | | | | | |
| Rheumatism | 21 | | 7 | | 14 | 1 |
| Syphilis | | | 4 | | 1 | |
| Consumption | 1 | | | | | |
| Other diseases of this group | 2 | | 1 | | | |
| LOCAL DISEASES. | | | | | | |
| Catarrh and bronchitis | 21 | | 21 | | 22 | |
| Pneumonia | 1 | | 1 | | 1 | |
| Diarrhœa and dysentery | 101 | | 55 | | 29 | |
| Hernia | 1 | | 1 | | | |
| Other local diseases | 83 | | 27 | | 29 | |
| Unclassified | 2 | | | | | |
| Total disease | 305 | 1 | 146 | | 128 | 1 |
| VIOLENT DISEASES AND DEATHS. | | | | | | |
| Gunshot wounds | 10 | | | | 3 | |
| Other accidents and injuries | 87 | | 60 | | 72 | |
| Homicide | | 2 | | | | |
| Total violence | 97 | 2 | 60 | | 75 | |

\* 11 months only; May, 1873, last report.

# FORT TULEROSA, NEW MEXICO.

### INFORMATION FURNISHED BY ACTING ASSISTANT SURGEON H. DUANE, UNITED STATES ARMY.

Fort Tulerosa is on the left bank of the Rio Tulerosa, two miles below its headwaters, in a cañon varying from 600 to 1,000 yards in width; latitude, 33° 54' north; longitude, 31° 27' west; altitude, about 7,400 feet. The post was established in the spring of 1872, in connection with a reservation for the Apaches. The surrounding country is mountainous.

The valley shows many ruins of pueblos, and other signs that it was once thickly settled. About one-half mile northwest of the post are caves with cemented partition walls, and the remains of houses on which the roofs are yet apparent. Broken pottery, beads, stone arrow-heads, &c., are found in the vicinity. The Indians, consisting of bands of Mogollon, Coyotero and Miembres Apaches, were brought to this point in May, 1872, the agency being established about one and a half miles below the post, on the right bank of the stream. The Indians are strong and healthy, with no traces of syphilis; the number fed and clothed at the agency varies from 180 to 800.

The buildings are merely temporary shelters, constructed of logs or slabs, with earth-roofs, with the exception of one barrack, grain-house, and hospital, which are balloon frames, with shingle-roofs. The officers' quarters are built of adobes. The post was abandoned November 26, 1874.

*Meteorological report, Fort Tulerosa, N. Mex., 1873–'74.*

| Month. | 1870–'71. Temperature. | | | Rain-fall in inches. | 1871–'72. Temperature. | | | Rain-fall in inches. | 1872–'73. Temperature. | | | Rain-fall in inches. | 1873–'74. Temperature. | | | Rain-fall in inches. |
|---|---|---|---|---|---|---|---|---|---|---|---|---|---|---|---|---|
| | Mean. | Max. | Min. | | Mean. | Max. | Min. | | Mean. | Max. | Min. | | Mean. | Max. | Min. | |
| July | | | | | | | | | | | | | 76. 09 | 100* | 42* | 1. 30 |
| August | | | | | | | | | | | | | 67. 69 | 86* | 42* | 10. 48 |
| September | | | | | | | | | | | | | 61. 87 | 85* | 34* | 1. 76 |
| October | | | | | | | | | | | | | 50. 81 | 85* | 10* | 0. 00 |
| November | | | | | | | | | | | | | 43. 18 | 73* | 14* | 0. 38 |
| December | | | | | | | | | | | | | 29. 28 | 68* | − 7* | 7. 08 |
| January | | | | | | | | | | | | | 35. 12 | 72* | − 4* | 2. 24 |
| February | | | | | | | | | | | | | 30. 42 | 56* | −10* | 4. 94 |
| March | | | | | | | | | | | | | 38. 68 | 68* | 14* | 1. 38 |
| April | | | | | | | | | | | | | 41. 67 | 74* | 12* | 1. 34 |
| May | | | | | | | | | | | | | 57. 24 | 84* | 22* | (?) |
| June | | | | | | | | | | 56. 78 | 79* | 18* | 0. 55 | 57. 24 | 84* | 22* | (?) |
| June | | | | | | | | | | 73. 15 | 105* | 33* | 0. 96 | 68. 83 | 91* | 34* | 0. 30 |
| For the year | | | | | | | | | | | | | 50. 07 | 100* | −10* | |

\* These observations are made with self-registering thermometers. The mean is from the standard thermometer.

*Consolidated sick-report, Fort Tulerosa, N. Mex., 1871–'74.*

| Year | | 1871–'72.* | | 1872–'73. | | 1873–'74. | |
|---|---|---|---|---|---|---|---|
| Mean strength { Officers | | 3 | | 4 | | 4 | |
| { Enlisted men | | 103 | | 71 | | 94 | |
| Diseases. | | Cases. | Deaths. | Cases. | Deaths. | Cases. | Deaths. |
| GENERAL DISEASES, A. | | | | | | | |
| Remittent fever | | | | | | 1 | |
| Intermittent fever | | | | 8 | | 23 | |
| Other diseases of this group | | | | 1 | | 4 | |
| GENERAL DISEASES, B. | | | | | | | |
| Rheumatism | | 1 | | 6 | | 6 | |
| Syphilis | | | | 6 | | 8 | |
| Consumption | | | | 1 | | 1 | |
| LOCAL DISEASES. | | | | | | | |
| Catarrh and bronchitis | | | | 4 | | 5 | |
| Pleurisy | | | | 1 | | 1 | 1 |
| Diarrhœa and dysentery | | 17 | | 17 | | 21 | |
| Gonorrhœa | | 1 | | 1 | | 2 | |
| Other local diseases | | 2 | | 26 | | 34 | 1 |
| Alcoholism | | | | 6 | | 2 | |
| Total disease | | 21 | | 77 | | 108 | |
| VIOLENT DISEASES AND DEATHS. | | | | | | | |
| Gunshot wounds | | | | 2 | | 3 | |
| Other accidents and injuries | | 2 | | 19 | | 20 | |
| Total violence | | 2 | | 21 | | 23 | |

* One month only.

# FORT UNION, NEW MEXICO.

### REPORT OF ASSISTANT SURGEON P. MOFFATT, UNITED STATES ARMY.

Fort Union is situated in latitude 35° 54′ 21″ north; longitude, 27° 54′ 15″ west; altitude, 6,700 feet.

Santa Fé is one hundred miles southwest. The nearest railroad station is Las Animas, near Fort Lyon.

The most important settlements in the vicinity are Mora, eighteen miles to the west, and Las Vegas, twenty-eight miles distant, on the Santa Fé road.

The post is in a beautiful valley about twenty-five miles long by five and a half wide, having on the north and east a wooded range of hills known as Turkey Mountains, and on the west a low and rocky range running into table-land.

The craters of several extinct volcanoes are in the vicinity, and, on sinking wells in the vicinity of the arsenal, a stratum of lava is found of varying depths.

The water-supply is obtained partly from wells, and in part from an excellent spring about a quarter of a mile distant. That from the wells is hard, from lime in solution.

Twenty miles distant the road to Santa Fé crosses a ridge which is the divide between the tributaries of the Mississippi and the Rio Grande. Five miles northwest of Las Vegas are a number of hot springs, noted for their efficacy in rheumatism and chronic syphilitic complaints. The temperature is 140° Fahrenheit.

Among the useful wild plants found in the vicinity is the common hop, (*Humulus lupulus.*) This grows abundantly along the mountain-streams, and the product is of the best quality.

The following statement relative to the climate and its effects upon health is by Assistant Surgeon W. H. Gardner, United States Army:

"Fort Union is situated in a narrow valley on the eastern slope of the Rocky Mountains, and is about 6,700 feet above the level of the sea. The soil around it is composed of fine sand, with a slight admixture of yellowish clay, and is underlaid by trap-rock and irregular beds of dark lava, which have apparently overflowed from a volcano, now extinct, about thirty miles to the northward of the post.

"Wind from some quarter is almost constant, and the soil being light and sandy, is blown about in clouds of blinding, suffocating dust, that irritates the air-passages, and is the prevalent cause of catarrhs, pharyngitis, and bronchitis.

"The diurnal variation in temperature is very great, the thermometer frequently showing, at 6 a. m., but 60°, and at 2 p. m. showing 97°; even in mid-summer nights one or more blankets are always comfortable to sleep under. Now, from the foregoing causes, viz, the high elevation, the constant winds, the suffocating dust-storms, and the great diurnal variation in temperature, I do not believe this post *can* be favorable for any kind of lung disease, and, though my medical experience here is limited, I believe it will point to the same conclusion.

"The question of increased altitude as a source of disease has been one of great interest to me personally, and as I suffered as much from it myself as any other case I have seen, I will give you the history of my own case.

"Shortly after arriving at the post I was attacked with a fullness of the head, ringing in the ears, mental hebetude and confusion of ideas, dizziness, and headache. Thinking these symptoms might be caused by constipation, dyspepsia, or torpidity of the liver, I took a mercurial purgative, and followed it up with a dose of Rochelle salt, which relieved the fullness of oppression for a day or two, but it at once returned, the dizziness and confusion of ideas increased, and a feeling of numbness and tingling commenced in the fingers of the left hand, and gradually spread until it involved the whole left side, even the muscles of the tongue being involved in the paralysis, so that I could not articulate. There was also oppression of breathing, throbbing of the carotids, and slight dilation of the pupils. The only medicine handy at the time of the first attack was a bottle of chloroform; and thinking the symptoms might be due to spasm of the cerebral or pulmonary veins, I poured a dram or two on my handkerchief and inhaled it, when the disagreeable symptoms promptly subsided. The next day, on my visit to Doctor Moffatt, of our corps, (who, you will recollect, was lying here disabled with a broken leg,) I told him of my troubles, and he thought they were due to malarial poisoning, and advised me to commence a course of quinia and arsenic, which I at once did, taking twelve grains of quinia and one-tenth of a grain of arsenic each day. But in the course of five or six days, while under the full influence of these medicines, I had another attack, in all respects similar to the first, coming on after a hearty dinner; which was relieved by a prompt emetic. Shortly after this second attack I was sent for to attend a case of midwifery at Mora, (a little town in the mountains, fifteen miles northwest of the post, and about four hundred feet higher in altitude,) and while there alone I had another attack more severe and prolonged than the other two, and upon this occasion I certainly thought there would be another vacancy in the Medical Corps to fill, for I took emetics, bromide of potassium, and chloroform ad nauseam, without the least effect. The symptoms went off before morning, but when I got back to the post I brought the Darwinian theory to bear on the case. *Ita:* If the environment of an animal be suddenly changed, and the animal does not change its habits to suit its environment, it will be speedily eliminated. The only radical change in environment I could detect here was decreased atmospheric pressure from increased altitude, and consequently deficient oxygenation of the blood. The indication, therefore, was either to supply the deficiency of oxygen to the blood, or to reduce the volume of blood to the decreased amount of oxygen. The latter alternative seemed the easiest and the most certain. I therefore decreased the amount of my nitrogenous food, and made up the quantity by laxative vegetables and fruits, and have been in good health ever since. I have seen two cases since, in every respect similar to mine, and they have promptly succumbed to the treatment indicated; that is, decreasing the amount of blood to the decreased amount of oxygen, by cathartics and decreased animal food.

"Gonorrhœal and syphilitic affections are probably the greatest scourge we have to deal with, and particularly as affecting white males, for, as far as my own observation extends, I have not been called upon to treat a single native, man or woman, for either of these affections, nor in my practice among them (and I am the only physician within a radius of fifty miles) have I observed any evidence of constitutional syphilis. Now I do not wish to give this negative evidence as testimony to a fact, but I do believe that the whole Mexican population are so much under the influence of syphilization that the disease, when it does occur, is as much modified as small-pox is when it occurs after vaccination. Another reason why I have not been called upon to treat these cases may be from the fact that they use two native plants which have a very high local reputation in these diseases."*

---

* Surgeon A. K. Smith states that these plants are a species of the *clematis.*

Fort Union was established in August, 1851, and was first located on the present site of Fort Union arsenal. The reservation, nearly square, contains 51½ square miles. There is also a timber reservation of 50 square miles.

Fort Union includes the post proper, the depot, and Fort Union arsenal.

The arsenal is thus described by Capt. W. R. Shoemaker, ordnance officer in charge : " Fort Union arsenal is one mile west of Fort Union, on a reservation belonging to the Ordnance Department, and is inclosed by a wall forming a square of 1,000 feet each side. The buildings are, one barrack 100 by 26 feet with porticoes in front and rear ; one set officers' quarters 54 by 75 feet; an office 45 by 18 ; one main store-house 216 feet long, three smaller store-houses, shops, &c. All are of adobe with stone foundations. The water-supply is from a good well, and two cisterns of 18,000 gallons each."

Fort Union depot is thus described by Capt. G. C. Smith, assistant quartermaster, United States Army :

" The depot is adjacent to and north of the post. The buildings are, six sets used as offices and quarters ; five store-houses, shops, and corrals. The quarters are well built of adobes, laid on stone foundations, with tops finished with brick and roofs of tin. These sets are each 79 by 57 feet; the other three, each 56 by 55 feet. The store-houses are each 200 by 40 feet, except the southern one, which is one-half the width of the others. In the plaza, fronting the northern sets of depot quarters, are two cisterns holding 2,400 gallons each, the supply of which comes from the roofs of the store-houses."

Fort Union is a four-company post, the arrangement of the main part of which is shown in Figure 50.

A, officers' quarters ; B B B B, squad-room ; C C, mess-rooms ; D, forage-rooms ; E, bakery ; F, quartermaster's store-room ; H, issuing-room ; I, quartermaster's stables ; L, cavalry stables ; M, cavalry corral ; N, quartermaster's corral.

All the buildings are of adobe, one story high, on stone foundations, and, with the exception of the hospital, are all roofed with tin.

On the northeast side of the parade-ground, and directly opposite the line of officers' quarters, are the quarters of the men. Each set occupies three sides of a rectangle—within which is a small court-yard or open space with a well in the center. The main buildings are each 73 by 27 feet. They are used as squad-rooms and dormitories, and at the present time have an average occupancy of 30 men each, giving an air-space of about 700 cubic feet per man. The wings on one side of each set are used as orderly and company store-rooms ; those on the opposite side, for kitchens and dining-rooms. These quarters are really comfortable dwellings, although deficient in facilities for ventilation.

In rear of the blocks occupied by the men's quarters, and separated from them by a wide street, are situated the quarters of

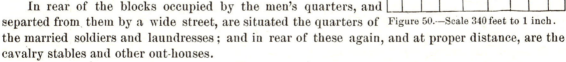

Figure 50.—Scale 340 feet to 1 inch.

the married soldiers and laundresses ; and in rear of these again, and at proper distance, are the cavalry stables and other out-houses.

On the southwest of the parade-ground are situated the quarters of officers, consisting of nine buildings in one row. Each building is divided by a single hall running from front to rear, on each side of which are three capacious rooms—except the middle building, (the commanding officers' quarters,) which has four—affording the regulation-allowance of quarters for an officer with the rank of captain. As in the case of most of the buildings here, the roofs were made too flat, so that they allow of leakage when violent rains occur, as they frequently do during the rainy season. In other respects the quarters are good ; they all have good yards and out-houses in the rear, and are upon the whole very comfortable residences.

The guard-house is situated in the line of the laundresses' quarters. The structure itself may

39 M P

be well suited for the purpose for which it was intended, but the location of it is inappropriate, as no extended view of the post can be had from its vicinity.

Sinks for the men and for the families of soldiers have been constructed at all available points, but the accommodations in this respect are not sufficient without the necessity of traveling to a greater distance than is likely to be done under all circumstances.

The post-hospital is situated outside of the garrison inclosure, and about 300 paces to the east of it. The hospital-building faces towards the southeast. It consists essentially of a central building 13½ feet wide, running back 130 feet, this being a hall 11½ feet wide inside. Attached to each side of this central hall are three wings, each 31 by 39 feet outside, the long axis parallel, and the short axis at right angles to, the hall. These wings are separated from each other by spaces 6½ feet wide. An adobe partition through the center of each wing, and at right angles to the hall, divides each of them into two rooms, 19 by 30 feet, by 12 feet 9 inches high; thus giving twelve rooms, each of the above dimensions. The two front wings are used as dispensary and store-rooms, the rear half of each posterior wing for kitchen and dining-room respectively. The two middle wings and the front rooms of the posterior wings are used as wards, making six wards, occupied by six beds each, giving 1,200 cubic feet of space to each occupant. In case of emergency, the capacity could readily be increased one-fourth by temporarily using some of the store-rooms as wards. The hospital differs from all other buildings at the post, in being roofed with shingles, and in having a roof with the usual pitch. Although not constructed upon the best plan, in a hygienic point of view, it is amply adequate to the requirements of a four-company post.

For the reason that this post is located on the thoroughfare to and from New Mexico, and that it is the base of supplies of the district, it occurs that there are at almost all times men in the hospital not belonging to the command at Fort Union, but who have been taken sick or hurt while *en route* to or from other points, and been detained at this post for treatment or discharge on surgeon's certificate of disability.

Fort Union is situated upon the stage-road between the railroad terminus, on the northeast, and the city of Santa Fé, on the southwest. A daily stage, conveying the mail, is received from each point. From this point mail communications can be had with Santa Fé in twenty hours; with department headquarters at Fort Leavenworth in four to six days, and with Washington in seven to nine days. A line of telegraph also passes this place *en route* from the railroad to Santa Fé along the stage-road, and having a station at this point.

Fort Union, as a frontier post, may be considered desirable, not so much from the natural surroundings as from the facilities, by stage, mail, and telegraph, of communication with the outside world.

One question I should like to add before closing: Are adobe quarters productive of rheumatism? I believe they are a fruitful source not only of rheumatism, but sciatica, and other forms of neuralgia.

*Meteorological reports, Fort Union, N. Mex., 1870–'74.*

| Month. | 1870–'71. | | | | 1871–'72. | | | | 1872–'73. | | | | 1873–'74. | | | |
|---|---|---|---|---|---|---|---|---|---|---|---|---|---|---|---|---|
| | Temperature. | | | Rain-fall in inches. | Temperature. | | | Rain-fall in inches. | Temperature. | | | Rain-fall in inches. | Temperature. | | | Rain-fall in inches. |
| | Mean. | Max. | Min. | | Mean. | Max. | Min. | | Mean. | Max. | Min. | | Mean. | Max. | Min. | |
| | ° | ° | ° | | ° | ° | ° | | ° | ° | ° | | ° | ° | ° | |
| July | 67.87 | 94* | 40* | 4.80 | 72.21 | 101 | 58 | 2.49 | 67.02 | 86* | 53 | 5.56 | 79.91 | 100* | 55 | 3.30 |
| August | 67.27 | 92* | 32?* | 1.75 | 68.67 | 93 | 50 | 5.31 | 67.34 | 87* | 53 | 4.94 | 66.89 | 88* | 57 | 7.38 |
| September | 62.34 | 90* | 28?* | 1.70 | 61.81 | 82 | 46 | 2.77 | 63.27 | 88* | 45 | ? | 63.19 | 86* | 42 | 0.84 |
| October | 51.75 | 80* | 17?* | 0.10 | 50.76 | 82* | 26 | 0.38 | 51.57 | 81* | 28 | 0.00 | 53.20 | 86* | 19 | 0.02 |
| November | 48.01 | 72* | 5* | 0.00 | 40.37 | 64* | 10 | 0.22 | 36.85 | 67* | 12 | 0.24 | 43.39 | 75* | 15 | 0.00 |
| December | 32.77 | 70* | 4* | 0.03 | 42.55 | 65* | 16 | 0.05 | 35.15 | 62* | 5 | 0.00 | 32.93 | 70* | 10 | 0.22 |
| January | 39.52 | 74* | 8* | 0.50 | 33.50 | 63* | −9 | 0.50 | 31.12 | 62* | −13 | ? | 36.16 | 63* | 1 | 0.54 |
| February | 37.15 | 65* | 5* | 0.00 | 38.99 | 64* | 12 | 0.54 | 34.32 | 58* | 19 | 0.30 | 29.91 | 55* | −7 | 1.26 |
| March | 42.41 | 70* | 5* | ? | 40.44 | 67* | 18 | 0.56 | 45.49 | 76* | 15 | 0.04 | 39.89 | 69* | 20 | 0.32 |
| April | 50.24 | 79* | 20* | 0.16 | 50.13 | 79* | 30 | 0.76 | 44.53 | 76* | 23 | 0.04 | 43.51 | 85* | 23 | 0.94 |
| May | 58.19 | 94* | 20?* | 0.20 | 59.78 | 94* | 35 | 3.46 | 57.29 | 81* | 33 | ? | 60.03 | 90* | 40 | 4.38 |
| June | 71.51 | 98* | 25?* | 1.02 | 67.65 | 90* | 50 | 4.05 | 66.67 | 95* | 45 | 3.38 | 70.57 | 100* | 51 | 1.10 |
| For the year | 52.42 | 98* | 4* | ........ | 52.23 | 101 | −9 | 21.09 | 50.05 | 95* | −13 | ........ | 51.63 | 100* | −7 | 20.30 |

* These observations are made with self-registering thermometers. The mean is from the standard thermometer.

*Consolidated sick-report, Fort Union, N. Mex., 1870-'74.*

| Year | | 1870-'71. | | 1871-'72. | | 1872-'73. | | 1873-'74. | |
|---|---|---|---|---|---|---|---|---|---|
| Mean strength { Officers<br>{ Enlisted men | | 12<br>310 | | 11<br>211 | | 9<br>155 | | 10<br>185 | |
| Diseases. | | Cases. | Deaths. | Cases. | Deaths. | Cases. | Deaths. | Cases. | Deaths. |
| GENERAL DISEASES, A. | | | | | | | | | |
| Small-pox and varioloid | | | | 2 | | | | | |
| Typhoid fever | | 9 | 4 | | | 3 | 1 | | |
| Remittent fever | | 27 | | | | 3 | | | |
| Intermittent fever | | 81 | | 24 | | 16 | | 21 | |
| Diphtheria | | | | | | 3 | | | |
| Other diseases of this group | | 42 | | 25 | | 14 | | 35 | |
| GENERAL DISEASES, B. | | | | | | | | | |
| Rheumatism | | 97 | | 24 | | 8 | | 26 | |
| Syphilis | | 59 | | 33 | | 16 | | 18 | |
| Consumption | | 3 | | 1 | | | | | |
| Other diseases of this group | | 8 | | 1 | | 4 | | 3 | |
| LOCAL DISEASES. | | | | | | | | | |
| Catarrh and bronchitis | | 133 | | 75 | | 14 | | 66 | |
| Pneumonia | | 4 | 1 | 1 | | 3 | | 1 | |
| Pleurisy | | 23 | | 9 | | 4 | | 5 | |
| Diarrhœa and dysentery | | 99 | 1 | 81 | | 33 | | 67 | |
| Hernia | | | | 5 | | | | 4 | |
| Gonorrhœa | | 31 | | 14 | | 3 | | 9 | |
| Other local diseases | | 250 | | 130 | 1 | 52 | | 117 | |
| Alcoholism | | 12 | | 16 | | 10 | | 7 | |
| Total disease | | 878 | 6 | 441 | 1 | 186 | 1 | 379 | |
| VIOLENT DISEASES AND DEATHS. | | | | | | | | | |
| Gunshot wounds | | 4 | | 2 | 1 | 7 | 1 | 5 | |
| Other accidents and injuries | | 92 | | 79 | 1 | 46 | | 55 | |
| Homicide | | | 1 | | 1 | | 1 | | 1 |
| Suicide | | | | | | | | | 1 |
| Total violence | | 96 | 1 | 81 | 3 | 53 | 1 | 60 | 2 |

# FORT WALLACE, KANSAS.

INFORMATION FURNISHED BY ACTING ASSISTANT SURGEONS M. M. SHEARER AND F. H. ATKINS, UNITED STATES ARMY.

Fort Wallace, situated on the line of the Kansas Pacific Railroad, two miles southeast of Wallace Station, is built upon a Government reservation fourteen miles square, lying upon the South Fork of the Smoky Hill River, in latitude 38° 55' north; longitude 23° 47' west; altitude, by barometer, above the sea, 3,320 feet.

At this point the river is a running stream, owing to the water received from a tributary that enters it about three miles to the west of the bluff upon which the post stands; beyond that, it sinks into its sandy bed, leaving occasional ponds, supplied by subterranean currents.

To the north, the plateau ascends gradually for several hundred yards, terminating in ravines that run to the river on the east of the garrison. On the east, south, and west the slope toward the stream is more abrupt.

The soil is good, but unproductive from want of water. No timber grows within sixty miles, and the surrounding country, a rolling prairie, is covered with buffalo grass.

In this vicinity the wild animals are the prong-horned antelope, black-tailed deer, elk, buffalo, wild horse, rabbit, and jack-rabbit, muskrat, beaver, otter, wolf, and weasel.

The reptiles consist of the rattlesnake, (very numerous,) the copperhead, (rare,) and black, milk, garter, and ring snakes, with the horned and common toad.

Birds: wild goose, canvas-back duck, mallard, teal, widgeon, spoonbill, pintail, black diver, black chin, (*Podiceps minor*,) crane, bittern, coot, plover, (three varieties, great, little yellow-legged, and golden—all numerous,) curlew, kingfisher, avocette, robin, finch, sparrow, wren, meadow-lark, crow, blackbird, red-winged blackbird, golden-winged blackbird, cow bunting, woodcock, brown thrush, bee martin or king bird, bobolink, woodpecker, yellow hammer, wild turkey, quail, and grouse.

Two of the barracks are constructed of a marl which can be easily worked with carpenters' tools. When fresh it is of a light pink color, but grows darker and hardens by exposure, owing to the presence of magnesium and iron. These buildings measure 118 by 25 feet, with a height of 11 feet 3 inches to the eaves, 17 feet 3 inches to the ridge, inside measurement, and have walls two feet thick. They are divided into dormitories, 100 feet in length, and into two small rooms, used by the first sergeants, and for store-rooms; thus affording a space of 490 cubic feet to each man of a company of infantry of minimum strength.

These barracks are ventilated by the ridge, and lighted by three windows upon the west, and two upon the east side, each window being arched, 7 feet 3 inches in height, and 3 feet in width. Additional light is admitted by glass in the upper part of all of the doors in the building.

The company quarters are warmed by stoves provided with drums, the pipe extending throughout the length of the rooms. Single iron bunks are used.

The remaining barracks, which are of wood, are somewhat wider than those just described, and constructed upon a similar plan. They are not provided with bath-rooms.

The kitchens and mess-rooms are close to the barracks, and are low wooden buildings, battened and shingled. One of them contains quarters for a married soldier, a shoemaker's shop, and a bath-room, warmed in winter, but unprovided with sufficient means for heating water. The mess-rooms are neatly painted, and kept scrupulously clean.

The frame buildings are shingled, and some of them lined with canvas.

A row of officers' quarters on the north fronts the guard-house and magazine on the south side of the parade-ground. The former, all one story high, (with the exception of that of the commanding officer, which has two stories,) are 40 feet by 20. A great improvement has been made in this row since the last report. At this time all the buildings are painted and sided, have verandas in front, and picket or latticed fences, either placed, or in process of construction. Two or three of the houses are adapted to the use of small families, having a wing for the kitchen and dining-room, and separate yards and out-houses. These quarters contain from four to nine rooms of good size, all of them plastered and painted. The ninth and last building in this row is used for offices of the commanding officer and adjutant, and the post library. The latter contains 206 volumes, (recently strongly rebound in the garrison,) and is in charge of the sergeant-major.

The store-houses, occupying the southwestern part of the camp, are durable stone buildings, 128 feet long, 24 feet wide, and 10 feet in height to the eaves. Both have ventilated cellars and skylights. The grain-house, which is of wood, will contain 15,000 bushels. All of these structures are in good condition.

A stone guard-house, 34 by 31 feet, with a veranda eight feet in width before it, fronts the parade on the south. It is divided into three rooms. The rear and largest room, 13 by 26 feet, and with a height of $8\frac{1}{6}$ feet, is intended for prisoners. Ventilation is by the peak, and the loosely-laid boards of the roof admit much air. The rooms in front are occupied by the guard, and there are besides two very small cells. This building is not large enough for the average number of its occupants, the usual number of prisoners for 1873 being nine, of whom five were discharged soldiers serving out long sentences. It also shares with the temporary hospital, next door to it, the serious inconvenience of having no sink, the prisoners having to be escorted three hundred yards to that of the nearest company.

As precautions against fire, several Babcock extinguishers are distributed through the garrison, ropes, hooks, and ladders are placed at convenient points, and buckets filled with water stand in most of the buildings. A supply of Johnson pumps is expected.

The post cemetery, half a mile distant upon the hill to the north, is a walled inclosure of about two acres, and has a cenotaph in the center commemorating the men slain by Indians in June, 1867. There are one hundred and forty-three graves, ninety-two of soldiers and fifty-one of citizens.

At present this post has no hospital building, that described in Circular No. 4, issued December 5, 1870, having been destroyed by fire March 12, 1872, during a heavy gale. The wing containing the kitchen and the steward's wooden cottage escaped. This wing has been recently refitted, glazed, plastered, &c., furnished with settees, platform, desk, railing, and turned into a chapel, (17 by 40 feet,) which was very much needed. It is well lighted and warmed. One of the sets of wooden company quarters has been occupied as a hospital since the destruction of the former one. It is a rough battened board house, forming a single ward, 100 feet long and 23 feet wide. The horizontal ceiling is 7½ feet high, and it is ventilated by traps and the ridge. Owing to the looseness of the boarding and the insecure state of the walls and the windows, the circulation of air is so great that in cold weather the two large box-stoves scarcely suffice to heat it comfortable, and when the wind is high are wholly inadequate to that purpose, so that much suffering would ensue if it contained many inmates in winter.

One end of the ward is partitioned off into a dispensary and store-room, but there is neither laundry, bath-room, sink, nor dead-house in connection with it, while the kitchen and dining-room are in an adjoining building of similar construction. The want of a dead-house has been the cause of considerable trouble, and the absence of a sink is a perpetual source of discomfort and detriment to patients. Further, this hospital is in the center of the camp, so that retirement and quiet are impossible. A small but complete building on the edge of the post, like the former one, is a necessity that should be at once supplied.

The configuration of the stream at this point has been somewhat altered by the construction of a dam some 6 or 8 feet high, and the formation of a pond, from which all the water and ice of the garrison are procured. There is a well, however, near the foot of the bluff, but as it does not descend below the bed of the stream and is fed entirely by surface drainage, the water is highly impregnated with minerals.

An attempt to sink an artesian well within the limits of the post has been made. After penetrating the alluvium and cretaceous drift the shale was reached at a depth of 36 feet, and after much labor penetrated 50 feet deeper, when the work was abandoned by the advice of a competent geological authority. The appearance of petroleum in the underlying stratum was observed.

All the water used here is hauled in wagons, and placed in barrels near the various buildings, and the ice, of which there is an abundant supply, is stored in houses estimated to contain from seven hundred to nine hundred tons.

As the fort is built on a gradual slope inclining toward the river, no artificial drainage is necessary, and the refuse matter from about the quarters, kitchens, stables, &c., is daily carted away.

The Smoky River flows within a short distance, and the men are compelled to bathe at least once a week in warm weather. Efforts to make a post garden have been unavailing.

Fort Leavenworth, Kans., four hundred and twenty miles distant, is the nearest quartermaster and commissary depot, and is connected by the Kansas Pacific Railroad with this post at all seasons of the year. Medical supplies come from Saint Louis, Mo., and are received in good condition. Four months' general supply is kept on hand. Between the fort and the nearest town the communication is by stage. A mail arrives every day from the East and West, with the exception of one for each direction. The time for a letter to pass between the post and department headquarters at Leavenworth is twenty-four hours.

Five ambulances, but two of which are in running order, afford the means of transporting the sick.

The inhabitants of the surrounding country are ranchmen and hunters, who gather much excellent hay in the river-bottoms, within ten or fifteen miles of the garrison; about nine hundred tons being harvested during 1873. In the fall they kill buffalo, and large shipments of hides and meat are made every year from Wallace Station, on the Kansas Pacific Railroad. During the winters of 1872 and 1873 nearly one hundred thousand hides were sent from this point. Traders and railroad employés make up the remainder of a population of about one hundred persons. There are no Indians within a hundred miles or more of the post.

Rheumatism in all of its forms is the prevailing disease here and in the adjoining country; and pneumonia, due to exposure and a poor diet, has been very prevalent among the citzens working upon the railroad. Colds, inflammation of the lungs, and pleural, hepatic, and intestinal disorders are of local origin. The prevailing diseases in the garrison generally arise from errors in diet and from cold and sudden changes of temperature.

Among the white troops cold has been the most prolific source of disease, giving rise to bronchial affections, pulmonary complaints, and inflammatory diarrhœa. It was observed that those colored troops coming from the South yielded most readily to the prevailing unhealthy influences, while those recruited in the North exhibited the same power of resistance to the effects of climate and exposure as the other portion of the garrison.

The climate is of great salubrity and extreme dryness. Snow falls rarely and in small quantity, seldom lying more than a day or two. High winds are common, and frequent gales of alarming force often blow for many hours. During the warm months the direction of winds is from the south and east, and this is reversed during cold weather. Malarial diseases do not originate here, all cases having their origin elsewhere. No scurvy, pneumonia, pleuritis, or phthisis had occurred during 1872 or 1873, and but six cases of dysentery were treated in that time. Influenza has also been very rare.

Doubtless, improved quarters, diet, and general surroundings have modified the extent and character of diseases both among citizens and soldiers.

*Meteorological report, Fort Wallace, Kans., 1872–'74.*

| Month. | 1870–'71. | | | | 1871–'72. | | | | 1872–'73. | | | | 1873–'74. | | | |
|---|---|---|---|---|---|---|---|---|---|---|---|---|---|---|---|---|
| | Temperature. | | | Rain-fall in inches. | Temperature. | | | Rain-fall in inches. | Temperature. | | | Rain-fall in inches. | Temperature. | | | Rain-fall in inches. |
| | Mean. | Max. | Min. | | Mean. | Max. | Min. | | Mean. | Max. | Min. | | Mean. | Max. | Min. | |
| | ° | ° | ° | | ° | ° | ° | | ° | ° | ° | | ° | ° | ° | |
| July........ | ...... | ...... | ...... | ...... | ...... | ...... | ...... | ...... | 73.94 | 81.33 | 61.66 | 5.45 | 80.33 | 106 | 59 | 1.58 |
| August...... | ...... | ...... | ...... | ...... | ...... | ...... | ...... | ...... | 78.67 | 85.00 | 65.33 | 1.31 | 80.65 | 103 | 54 | 1.26 |
| September.. | ...... | ...... | ...... | ...... | ...... | ...... | ...... | ...... | 67.69 | 83.00 | 53.66 | 0.25 | 66.50 | 96 | 30 | 0.21 |
| October.... | ...... | ...... | ...... | ...... | ...... | ...... | ...... | ...... | 58.63 | 75.33 | 43.00 | 0.05 | 55.95 | 93 | 24 | 0.30 |
| November... | ...... | ...... | ...... | ...... | ...... | ...... | ...... | ...... | 36.20 | 53.33 | 22.00 | (†) | 43.78 | 78 | 12 | 0.01 |
| December... | ...... | ...... | ...... | ...... | ...... | ...... | ...... | ...... | 26.47 | 46.66 | 2.33 | (;) | 30.48 | 76 | 4 | 0.07 |
| January.... | ...... | ...... | ...... | ...... | 27.65 | 42.66 | −3.33 | (*) | ...... | ...... | ...... | ...... | 28.97 | 69 | 1 | 0.09 |
| February... | ...... | ...... | ...... | ...... | 33.91 | 57.33 | 19.00 | 0.12 | ...... | ...... | ...... | ...... | 24.70 | 63 | −15 | 0.68 |
| March...... | ...... | ...... | ...... | ...... | 44.54 | 56.66 | 21.66 | 0.60 | ...... | ...... | ...... | ...... | 33.07 | 61 | 3 | 0.20 |
| April...... | ...... | ...... | ...... | ...... | 53.25 | 66.00 | 39.33 | 2.55 | ...... | ...... | ...... | ...... | 47.20 | 93 | 22 | 0.50 |
| May........ | ...... | ...... | ...... | ...... | 66.01 | 71.33 | 53.00 | 4.09 | ...... | ...... | ...... | ...... | 65.99 | 95 | 36 | 3.31 |
| June....... | ...... | ...... | ...... | ...... | 74.93 | 82.00 | 68.33 | 1.00 | 76.69 | 104.00 | 56.00 | 0.10 | 76.88 | 104 | 52 | 0.19 |
| For the year | ...... | ...... | ...... | ...... | ...... | ...... | ...... | ...... | ...... | ...... | ...... | ...... | 52.87 | 106 | −15 | 8.40 |

* Two days' snow.            † Three days' rain.            ; Six days' snow.

*Consolidated sick-report, Fort Wallace, Kans., 1870–'74.*

| Year | | 1870–'71. | | 1871–'72. | | 1872–'73. | | 1873–'74. | |
|---|---|---|---|---|---|---|---|---|---|
| Mean strength { Officers........... | | 8 | | 9 | | 5 | | 6 | |
| { Enlisted men...... | | 185 | | 164 | | 103 | | 118 | |
| Diseases. | | Cases. | Deaths. | Cases. | Deaths. | Cases. | Deaths. | Cases. | Deaths. |
| GENERAL DISEASES, A. | | | | | | | | | |
| Typhoid fever........ | | 3 | 1 | 4 | 1 | ...... | ...... | ...... | ...... |
| Remittent fever...... | | 26 | ...... | 5 | ...... | 9 | ...... | ...... | ...... |
| Intermittent fever... | | 54 | ...... | 33 | ...... | 26 | ...... | 7 | ...... |
| Other diseases of this group | | 8 | ...... | 7 | ...... | 12 | ...... | 6 | ...... |
| GENERAL DISEASES, B. | | | | | | | | | |
| Rheumatism.......... | | 35 | 1 | 25 | ...... | 16 | ...... | 10 | ...... |
| Syphilis............. | | 10 | ...... | 11 | ...... | 2 | ...... | ...... | ...... |
| Consumption......... | | 1 | ...... | ...... | ...... | ...... | ...... | 2 | ...... |
| Other diseases of this group | | ...... | ...... | 2 | ...... | ...... | ...... | ...... | ...... |
| LOCAL DISEASES. | | | | | | | | | |
| Catarrh and bronchitis | | 138 | ...... | 192 | ...... | 44 | ...... | 17 | ...... |
| Pneumonia........... | | ...... | ...... | ...... | ...... | ...... | ...... | 2 | 1 |
| Pleurisy............. | | ...... | ...... | ...... | ...... | 1 | ...... | 1 | ...... |
| Diarrhœa and dysentery | | 95 | ...... | 88 | ...... | 37 | ...... | 11 | ...... |
| Hernia............... | | 2 | ...... | ...... | ...... | ...... | ...... | ...... | ...... |
| Gonorrhœa........... | | 4 | ...... | 2 | ...... | 2 | ...... | 1 | ...... |
| Other local diseases. | | 128 | 2 | 108 | 1 | 65 | ...... | 39 | ...... |
| Alcoholism........... | | 3 | ...... | 2 | ...... | 2 | ...... | 6 | ...... |
| Total disease | | 507 | 4 | 480 | 2 | 216 | ...... | 102 | 1 |
| VIOLENT DISEASES AND DEATHS. | | | | | | | | | |
| Gunshot wounds...... | | 2 | ...... | 5 | ...... | ...... | ...... | 4 | ...... |
| Other accidents and injuries | | 94 | 2 | 123 | ...... | 62 | ...... | 34 | ...... |
| Homicide............. | | ...... | ...... | ...... | ...... | ...... | ...... | ...... | 1 |
| Suicide.............. | | ...... | 1 | ...... | ...... | ...... | ...... | ...... | ...... |
| Total violence | | 96 | 3 | 128 | ...... | 62 | ...... | 38 | 1 |

# FORT WINGATE, NEW MEXICO.

REPORTS OF ASSISTANT SURGEONS R. S. VICKERY AND J. V. DE HANNE, UNITED STATES ARMY.

Fort Wingate is situated in latitude 35° 20′ north; longitude, 31° 22′ west; altitude, 6,822 feet.

This post was formed about the beginning of August, 1838, by the arrival of troops with the Navajo tribe of Indians, who were moved by General Sherman from the reservation of Fort Sumner, New Mexico, where they had been for some years, back to this, their old country. At the same time old Fort Wingate, sixty miles southwest, was abandoned, and the troops moved to this point. The present fort is west-northwest of Albuquerque, on the Rio Grande, about one hundred and fifty miles from it by the road, and about forty-five miles southeast of old Fort Defiance. It is on the Pacific slope of the mountains, about twenty-three miles west of a slight elevation called the Dividing Ridge, and is situated on gently rising ground at the south side of a valley, about two miles in diameter, opening to the north. The valley is open and grassy, with some pine timber and scrubby oak scattered through it, and has well-wooded hills back of it. The mountains around are mostly red sandstone and clayey rock. The surface soil is clay and decayed sandstone mixed with gravel, the latter being in larger proportion near the head of the valley.

The wild animals found in this region are antelope, black-tailed deer, black bear, large gray wolf, coyote, wild cat, fox, (dark gray,) beaver. On the Nutria Creek, a tributary of the Zuñi River, about twenty miles to the south, are prairie-dogs, kangaroo-rats, pouch-rats, and field-mice, (white-footed.)

Birds: Wild turkey, wild duck, (teal,) large raven, blackbird, blue jay, (Canada,) wood blue-bird or rusty bluebird, woodpecker, (speckled,) woodpecker, (red-headed, large, slate-colored body with black spots,) woodpecker flicker, sparrow-hawk, (small,) hawk, (several varieties,) owls, (several species,) mourning-dove, fly-catcher, meadow-lark, magpie, snowbird, Rocky Mountain bluebird, and Rocky Mountain swallow.

There is very little game in the neighborhood of the post, it having been thinned out of late years by the Navajo Indians.

The climate is dry and equable; breezy and pleasant even in the hottest weather. There are no very high winds, except in March. Average difference between dry and wet bulb thermometer in summer, 10.59°; in winter, 4.43°. In March and April there are occasional high, dry winds from southwest and west, bringing much dust with them, and going down generally at sun-set. The nights are nearly always calm. The coldest winds in winter are from northwest and northeast, partly because the fort is not sheltered from these directions.

Spring begins about the middle of March. There are light snow-showers and frosts occasionally until the end of April, or early in May, making the season for planting late. Frosts sometimes set in in the latter part of September, keeping late corn from ripening fully.

The stream from the spring crosses the east angle of the plan. The buildings of the post are near the head of the valley.

The post was begun on a circular plan, which has been disapproved at district head-quarters, as giving too much space to defend, and as being too expensive. This plan is shown in Figure 51.

1, 2, 3, 4, 5, 6, officers' quarters; 7, store-house; 8, cavalry quarters; 9 infantry quarters; 10, guard-house; 11, 12, infantry quarters;

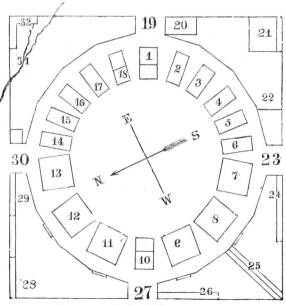

Figure 51.—Scale 300 feet to 1 inch.

13, store-house; 14, chaplain's quarters; 15, 16, 17, 18, officers' quarters; 19, 23, 27, 30, sally-ports; 20, 22, post trader; 21, hospital; 24, 26, cavalry quarters; 25, cavalry stables; 28, 29, infantry quarters; 31, stream; 32, wash-house.

The plan finally approved, and upon which the post has been constructed, is shown in Figure 52.

A, commanding-officers' quarters; B, C, D, E, finished officers' quarters; F, G, unfinished officers' quarters; H, hospital; I, adjutant's office; J, unfinished store-house; K, guard-house; L, M, barracks; N, corral, 200 by 125 feet, surrounded by mule-sheds, company-sinks, repair-shops, coal and corn rooms; P, unfinished corral, 240 by 75 feet; Q, quarters for employés; R, laundresses' quarters; S and T, cavalry stables, unfinished, 240 by 275 feet.

The barracks are two adobe buildings, with shingle roofs. The dormitories, of which there are two in each building, are 22 by 65½ feet by 13 feet high, floored and ceiled with boards, the walls plastered and white-washed. Each has two doors and seven windows, the latter 3 by 6½ feet. Double-tier bunks are used. There is no special provision for ventilation. The floors of the company barracks are raised about one foot from the ground in front, which, as the ground slopes back, raises the rear rooms from 4 to 6 feet. There is a small cellar under each company kitchen. The walls of the officers' quarters and company barracks are 18 inches thick, built of adobe, on stone foundation. The officers' quarters are all raised from 4 to 6 feet from the ground, giving space for a cellar under each. There are nine sets of officers' quarters,

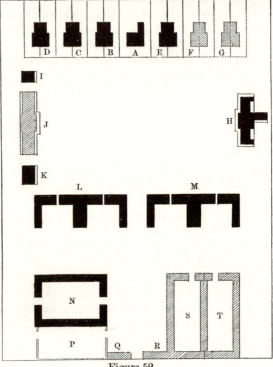

Figure 52.

each containing four rooms and a hall on the first floor, and two attic-rooms. The dimensions of the rooms are respectively, 18 by 16, 16 by 16 feet, 16 by 13 feet, 16 by 13½ feet, and are all 13 feet high. The walls and ceilings are plastered. The sets are in couples, separated by a partition. Each double-set has a porch and an inclosed space of about three-fifths of an acre.

There are four sets of adobe-cottages on stone-foundations, for married soldiers, each set containing two rooms 12 by 15 and 15 by 17 feet.

The hospital is a new building, on the plan for a hospital of twenty-four beds, given in Circular No. 2, Surgeon-General's Office, July 27, 1871. The walls are of adobes, on stone foundations, are 36 inches thick at the base, and 24 inches at the top. The ground-floor is from two to twelve feet above the surface, and the ventilation beneath is by grated openings in the foundation-wall.

The interior walls are of adobes, 18 inches thick. The building is plastered.

One of the great needs of this post is soft water. The supply for drinking and irrigation is from Bear Spring, a few yards distant, and is abundant, but the water is very hard. Cisterns are much needed. The natural drainage is good.

The nearest city is Santa Fé. A new road has been opened, almost due east, to the Rio Grande, crossing that river at San Félipe, about 28 miles north of Albuquerque. Distance to Santa Fé, via Albuquerque, 208 miles; to the same place, via San Félipe, 170 miles—a saving of 38 miles. The mails arrive once a week from Santa Fé, via the latter route. They are regular, though sometimes interrupted for a week or two in the spring by floods and snows. It requires about seven days for a letter to reach department headquarters, and from nine to ten days to Washington.

The inhabitants of the surrounding country are the Navajoes, numbering about 7,500, who are generally of good physique, and better-looking and more intelligent than most tribes of Indians. They were moved to this place from a former reservation, and about two months afterward the most of them were removed to old Fort Defiance, about 45 miles to the northwest. These Indians receive from Government, clothing, and a daily ration of half a pound of beef and half a pound of corn. They have small flocks of sheep and goats, and some ponies. They cultivated in 1869 4,000 or 5,000 acres of corn. Some of them work for the quartermaster and for private parties at this post. They are industrious and quick to learn, even some of the mechanical arts. The squaws make excellent woolen blankets, woven in a way peculiar to their tribe.

The nearest Pueblo village is Zuñi, about 40 miles south of the post. These Indians are an agricultural and a very peaceful people, living in fortified towns or pueblos.

*Meteorological report, Fort Wingate, N. Mex., 1870–'74.*

| Month. | 1870–'71. | | | | 1871–'72. | | | | 1872–'73. | | | | 1873–'74. | | | |
|---|---|---|---|---|---|---|---|---|---|---|---|---|---|---|---|---|
| | Temperature. | | | Rain-fall in inches. | Temperature. | | | Rain-fall in inches. | Temperature. | | | Rain-fall in inches. | Temperature. | | | Rain-fall in inches. |
| | Mean. | Max. | Min. | | Mean. | Max. | Min. | | Mean. | Max. | Min. | | Mean. | Max. | Min. | |
| | ° | ° | ° | | ° | ° | ° | | ° | ° | ° | | ° | ° | ° | |
| July | 72.33 | 99 | 55 | 3.88 | 71.78 | 97 | 55 | 2.37 | 72.27 | 97 | 52 | 1.10 | 77.82 | 90 | 65 | 0.26 |
| August | 69.78 | 102 | 50 | 3.23 | 69.19 | 86 | 57 | 1.20 | 69.56 | 97 | 58 | 3.15 | 70.77 | 82 | 61 | 2.65 |
| September | 63.86 | 97 | 30 | 0.73 | 63.95 | 80 | 48 | 2.80 | 63.17 | 84 | 41 | 0.50 | 66.62 | 80 | 53 | 3.60 |
| October | 51.00 | 95 | 25 | 1.50 | 47.21 | 73 | 21 | 1.20 | 51.15 | 84 | 18 | 2.75 | 53.13 | 77 | 23 | 0.50 |
| November | 39.36 | 62 | 21 | 0.15 | 36.17 | 59 | 10 | 1.33 | 36.33 | 68 | 8 | 0.00 | 44.05 | 59 | 26 | 0.55 |
| December | 26.41 | 62 | − 8 | 2.21 | 33.96 | 54 | 6 | 2.29 | 37.45 | 68 | 7 | 0.50 | 28.94 | 53 | 5 | 2.00 |
| January | 31.12 | 60 | 6 | 2.65 | 26.52 | 53 | −10 | 3.30 | 34.03 | 62 | − 5 | 0.75 | 32.08 | 48 | 2 | 1.85 |
| February | 33.16 | 56 | 15 | 5.05 | 35.86 | 65 | 8 | 1.59 | 32.62 | 58 | 3 | 11.25 | 29.67 | 45 | 3 | 0.44 |
| March | 41.14 | 65 | 14 | 0.58 | 42.50 | 69 | 20 | 0.63 | 47.95 | 57 | 18 | 0.00 | 37.62 | 59 | 5 | 0.55 |
| April | 50.75 | 76 | 26 | 1.80 | 44.85 | 73 | 22 | 1.99 | 49.21 | 74 | 18 | 0.15 | 39.19 | 73 | 24 | 0.07 |
| May | 58.16 | 86 | 33 | 0.31 | 57.68 | 90 | 35 | 3.00 | 60.23 | 77 | 43 | 0.20 | 62.64 | 78 | 32 | 0.30 |
| June | 73.04 | 96 | 52 | 0.00 | 67.06 | 91 | 50 | 2.25 | 71.59 | 88 | 49 | 3.15 | 74.27 | 90 | 62 | 0.03 |
| For the year | 50.84 | 102 | − 8 | 22.09 | 49.73 | 97 | −10 | 23.95 | 52.13 | 97 | − 5 | 23.30 | 51.40 | 90 | 2 | 12.80 |

*Consolidated sick-report, Fort Wingate, N. Mex., 1870–'74.*

| Year | | 1870–'71. | | 1871–'72. | | 1872–'73. | | 1873–'74. | |
|---|---|---|---|---|---|---|---|---|---|
| Mean strength | { Officers | 12 | | 9 | | 7 | | 7 | |
| | { Enlisted men | 276 | | 152 | | 152 | | 167 | |
| Diseases. | | Cases. | Deaths. | Cases. | Deaths. | Cases. | Deaths. | Cases. | Deaths. |
| GENERAL DISEASES, A. | | | | | | | | | |
| Typhoid fever | | 8 | | 1 | | 1 | | 2 | |
| Remittent fever | | 13 | | | | | | 1 | |
| Intermittent fever | | 15 | | 5 | | 5 | | 3 | |
| Other diseases of this group | | 25 | | 2 | | 11 | | 9 | |
| GENERAL DISEASES, B. | | | | | | | | | |
| Rheumatism | | 17 | | 18 | | 13 | | 15 | |
| Syphilis | | 38 | | 41 | | 33 | | 29 | |
| Consumption | | | | | | 1 | | | |
| Other diseases of this group | | 1 | | 2 | | 1 | | 3 | |
| LOCAL DISEASES. | | | | | | | | | |
| Catarrh and bronchitis | | 23 | | 8 | | 40 | | 46 | |
| Pneumonia | | 2 | 2 | | | 1 | | | |
| Pleurisy | | | | | | 1 | | 3 | |
| Diarrhœa and dysentery | | 46 | | 11 | | 12 | | 18 | 1 |
| Hernia | | | | | | | | 1 | |
| Gonorrhœa | | | | 4 | | 3 | | 5 | |
| Other local diseases | | 72 | | 51 | | 60 | | 76 | |
| Alcoholism | | 4 | | | | 4 | | 3 | |
| Total disease | | 264 | 2 | 143 | | 186 | | 214 | 1 |
| VIOLENT DISEASES AND DEATHS. | | | | | | | | | |
| Gunshot wounds | | 1 | | 3 | | 5 | 1 | 1 | |
| Other accidents and injuries | | 87 | 1 | 38 | | 28 | | 50 | |
| Total violence | | 88 | 1 | 41 | | 33 | 1 | 51 | |

40 M P

# DEPARTMENT OF THE PLATTE.

(Embracing the States of Iowa and Nebraska and the Territories of Utah and Wyoming.)

## POSTS.

Bridger, Fort, Wyo.
Brown, Camp, Wyo.
Cameron, Fort, Utah.
Cheyenne, Depot, Wyo.
Douglas, Camp, Utah.
Fetterman, Fort, Wyo.
Hartsuff, Camp, Wyo.

Laramie, Fort, Wyo.
McPherson, Fort, Nebr.
Medicine Bow, Wyo.
North Platte Station, Wyo.
Omaha Barracks, Nebr.
Robinson, Camp, Nebr.
Russell, D. A., Fort, Wyo.

Sanders, Fort, Wyo.
Sheridan, Camp, Nebr.
Sidney Barracks, Nebr.
Stambaugh, Camp, Wyo.
Steele, Fred, Fort, Wyo.

## TABLE OF DISTANCES IN THE DEPARTMENT OF THE PLATTE.

| | Saint Louis. | Omaha. | Fort Bridger. | Camp Brown. | Fort Cameron. | Fort D. A. Russell. | Camp Douglas. | Fort Fetterman. | Fort Fred Steele. | Fort Laramie. | Fort McPherson. | Omaha Barracks. | Camp Robinson. | Fort Sanders. | Sidney Barracks. | Camp Stambaugh. |
|---|---|---|---|---|---|---|---|---|---|---|---|---|---|---|---|---|
| Saint Louis | | | | | | | | | | | | | | | | |
| Omaha | 442 | | | | | | | | | | | | | | | |
| Fort Bridger | 1356 | 912 | | | | | | | | | | | | | | |
| Camp Brown | 1455 | 980 | 197 | | | | | | | | | | | | | |
| Fort Cameron | 1725 | 1288 | 386 | 573 | | | | | | | | | | | | |
| Fort D. A. Russell | 961 | 518 | 398 | 339 | 765 | | | | | | | | | | | |
| Camp Douglas | 1513 | 1068 | 178 | 352 | 225 | 544 | | | | | | | | | | |
| Fort Fetterman | 1130 | 688 | 560 | 654 | 934 | 172 | 712 | | | | | | | | | |
| Fort Fred Steele | 1056 | 697 | 220 | 306 | 594 | 183 | 365 | 351 | | | | | | | | |
| Fort Laramie | 1050 | 596 | 476 | 564 | 854 | 82 | 622 | 80 | 261 | | | | | | | |
| Fort McPherson | 728 | 283 | 641 | 729 | 1008 | 247 | 787 | 418 | 426 | 325 | | | | | | |
| Omaha Barracks | 447 | 5 | 917 | 985 | 1293 | 523 | 1073 | 693 | 702 | 601 | 288 | | | | | |
| Camp Robinson | 1146 | 704 | 589 | 685 | 950 | 187 | 743 | 176 | 367 | 96 | 434 | 709 | | | | |
| Fort Sanders | 1012 | 570 | 452 | 430 | 708 | 58 | 498 | 226 | 125 | 134 | 299 | 575 | 242 | | | |
| Sidney Barracks | 856 | 414 | 500 | 599 | 864 | 105 | 657 | 270 | 280 | 182 | 143 | 419 | 290 | 156 | | |
| Camp Stambaugh | 1401 | 948 | 165 | 32 | 519 | 454 | 320 | 622 | 274 | 532 | 697 | 753 | 631 | 398 | 545 | |

# FORT BRIDGER, WYOMING TERRITORY.

REPORT OF ASSISTANT SURGEON CHARLES SMART, UNITED STATES ARMY.

Fort Bridger is in Uintah County, Wyoming Territory, in a valley, or rather basin, through which the Black Fork of Green River runs. It is surrounded on all sides by table-lands, rising in a succession of benches. Latitude, 41° 18′ 12″ north; longitude 33° 29′ 38″ west; altitude 7,010 feet above the sea.

The Uintah Mountains, a spur of the Wasatch, with perpetual snow on the tallest peaks, are about fifty miles south. Carter Station, Union Pacific Railroad, is directly north, eleven miles distant. There are no towns of any importance nearer than Ogden, in Utah, one hundred and thirty-eight miles distant west, on the Union Pacific Railroad, and Salt Lake City, about the same distance south of west, by the old overland stage route.

In all the valleys and on the terrace-lands, extending over a wide range of country, are extensive alluvial deposits, indicating the existence of inland seas after the general upheaval of the great Rocky Mountain region. A characteristic feature of the country is the butte formations, where the earth's crust seems to have yielded to the subterranean pressure so gradually, or uniformly, as to allow an upheaval in regular form, constituting hills perfectly flat on the surface. On the sides of these buttes, or hills, as well as along the terraces of the table-lands, and where streams have washed their beds in the sides of bluffs, a remarkable uniformity in structure may be observed. Lowest of the strata thus exposed is a green sandstone, often of very considerable thickness, above it a shaly formation, then a drift deposit of pebbles and bowlders, and, above all, the alluvium on the surface. Coal of a bituminous character, similar to that found in many other parts of the Rocky Mountain region, has been discovered in several places within a few miles. It is used as fuel at the post, being procured from Rock Springs, about eighty miles distant eastward, on the railroad. Within three miles of the post is a large bed of siliceous limestone, with horizontal fractures, converting it into slabs of uniform thickness. It is easily obtained without blasting; and has been used of late in the erection of storehouses at the post, proving a good building-material. None of the precious or useful metals have been found in this region. There are but few indigenous trees. On the borders of the streams may be found a few aspen and small cottonwood trees, and a very thick growth of a herbaceous variety of willow. The soil is fertile and yields abundantly of all the cultivated vegetables whose growth is not prevented by the shortness of the season. Potatoes, turnips, and nearly all the summer table-vegetables have been successfully cultivated. Wheat, rye, barley, and oats have been raised, though the frequent failure of the crops rendered their cultivation, since the completion of the railroad, unprofitable. There are but few wild animals in the immediate vicinity. The sage-hen is very abundant. The wild goose, mallard, and green-winged teal ducks are found in limited numbers. The streams abound with trout, which are caught in great numbers during the summer and fall months. They weigh from six to twenty ounces each, and are marked with black spots.

The post was established in June, 1858. It is in the northwest corner of a reservation, which extends four miles north and south by one mile east and west. The reservation takes in all the grass-lands of the valley. Black Fork divides into five branches a short distance above the post, all uniting again within a mile below. One of the larger branches runs through the parade-ground from south to north, dividing it into two unequal parts. The buildings are but a few feet above the water-level, but the slope of the surface in and around the post is so regular that it is well drained.

The barrack-buildings are twelve in number—six on the north flank of the parade-ground, arranged in two rows, with a street running east and west between them, and six on the south flank, similarly arranged. Eleven of these are log-buildings, erected at the time the post was established; are each 76 feet long, those nearest the parade being 18 feet wide, the others 26 feet. On the parade-front are porches, extending the length of the buildings. The rear buildings are used partly as sleeping-rooms and in part as company mess-rooms, store-rooms, and kitchens. Six of these buildings were extensively repaired in 1873. The roofs were raised, so as to make the rooms 9 feet high; they were reshingled, newly floored, new window-frames and doors were put in, the old fireplaces were bricked up, and they now make very comfortable quarters for three companies, affording an average of 340 cubic feet of space per man in the dormitories. The ventilation is by the doors and windows and ventilating-shafts in the ceiling. Of the five other old log-buildings, three are occupied as laundresses' quarters, one as a carpenter and wheelwright shop, and one as a store-room. They have had very little repairing. The rooms are only 7 feet high.

In 1873 a new barrack-building was erected for the use of the band. It is a frame building, battened externally. The floor is raised 18 inches from the ground, the walls and ceiling are lathed and plastered; it is lighted freely by windows, ventilated by the doors and opposite windows, and affords ample space for the men who occupy it, the dormitory being $39\frac{1}{3}$ by $25\frac{2}{3}$ by 10 feet, giving to each of 13 men 770 cubic feet of space.

The quarters for the men are all furnished with single bedsteads of iron, with wooden slats, but, to permit the men to club their blankets during the protracted winter, they are arranged in pairs. The quarters are all heated by coal-stoves. The sinks are back of the rear rows of buildings; vaults are used, and as they fill up near the surface new ones are dug.

In 1873 a small one-story frame building was erected at the northwest angle of the parade-ground, for laundresses' quarters. The building is raised 18 inches from the ground, shingled, lathed and plastered, and is partitioned off into four sets, each consisting of two rooms, 12 by 10 by 10 feet, with door, window, and brick chimney in each room.

The officers' quarters consist of six log buildings, of uniform size, and like arrangement, placed about 40 feet apart, in a row, facing west, each containing four large rooms and a hall, and a frame building on the north flank, containing two sets of quarters, consisting of two large rooms and a kitchen each. These buildings were repaired in 1873. They were reshingled, floored, plastered and hard-finished, and in rear of each of the log buildings a frame attachment was put up, which differ in size and plan, but each contains a kitchen, servant's room, and closets. The open fireplaces were bricked up and coal-stoves furnished instead. The set occupied by the commanding officer, in addition to the kitchen, &c., in the rear, has a frame extension attached to each end— one used as a parlor, the other divided into bed-rooms.

A log building, with frame attachment, on the south flank, originally erected for officers' quarters, containing two large rooms and a kitchen, is now occupied as adjutant's office, regimental library, and printing-room.

Narrow ditches, extending from the stream above, run in front and through the yards in rear of the quarters, furnishing an abundant supply of pure water.

There are neither water-closets nor bath-rooms connected with the buildings. Detached privies are built in the yards.

The guard-house is a durable stone structure, lined with heavy timber, divided by a partition into a guard-room in front, 28 by 20 by 12 feet, and a prison-room in the rear, 24 by 20 by 10 feet. The guard-room has three large windows and a door in the outside walls, by which it is ventilated. The prison-room is ventilated only by four small barred windows near the eaves and by the door communicating with the guard-room. Two cells, of heavy timber, each $6\frac{1}{2}$ by 3 by 6 feet, are built against the partition. They afford only 117 cubic feet of space each, but the interstices between the timbers are so large, and the gratings of the doors so open, that the occupants are virtually occupants of the guard-room. The building is warmed by a large coal-stove in the guard-room.

The post-bakery is a log building, with two good brick ovens, faced with stone, having a capacity of 275 rations each daily.

The hospital consists of an L-shaped building 113 by 18 feet on the long side, running east and west, and an addition 62 by 20 feet, running north and south. The whole is built of logs. The extension to the south was built in 1869. The longer portion of the building is divided into a dispensary, two wards, attendants' room, bath-room, and lavatory, the wing into steward's room, store-room, dining-room, and kitchen. Extensive repairs were made in 1871. The roof of the largest ward was raised and renewed, the ceiling was arched and heightened to 10 feet in the center, or to an average of about 9 feet, a new floor was put down, and it was newly lathed and plastered. The capacity of the larger ward is ten beds, affording 680 cubic feet of space to each, and of the smaller ward is four beds, with 650 cubic feet to each. The wards are well ventilated by the doors and opposite windows and shaft in the roof, and are warmed by coal-stoves. During the year 1874 the wing of the building containing kitchen, dining-room, and store-room was shingled, ceiling raised to 9 feet, and, with the walls, lined with boards, as being more permanent than lath and plaster. These rooms were new-floored. The walls of the hospital were lime-chinked externally, and a new piazza was built on the east side of the wing, leading from the dispensary to the dining-room. Estimates have been made for other repairs and improvements to the hospital, consisting of setting up of walls of the main building, new ceiling, and shingling a portion of the same, &c.

A small ditch runs past the entire length of the hospital, furnishing water to it, and also to the officers' quarters beyond.

The water-supply is abundant and convenient, without labor in constructing cisterns, digging wells, or any artificial means of conducting it to the quarters other than a few surface-ditches along the regular slope, by which it is made to run convenient to all the barracks; and an abundant supply is thus obtained during the greater part of the year. In winter it must be carried in buckets from the stream that runs through the post. The stream furnishing the supply has its rise in the Uintah mountains, and is fed by never-failing mountain-springs, yielding water free from mineral impurities; and, running through a gravelly bed, it reaches the post almost as pure as at its source. The convenience of water in an unlimited quantity has prevented any serious accident from fire since the establishment of the post.

*Analysis of the water-supply from Black's Fork of Green River at Fort Bridger, Wyo.*

Clear, cool, pleasant to taste, and without odor.

3 litres evaporated for total solids gave .273 gram, of which .020 gram was dissipated by heat; the residue yielded .020 gram silica, .070 gram lime, .056 pyrophosphate of magnesia, and trace of iron and alumina.

2 litres yielded .030 gram "mixed alkali chlorides," which used 4.3 cubic centimeters deci-normal silver to precipitate the chlorine.

3 litres precipitated by barium chloride gave .015 gram of sulphate.

2 litres for chlorine used 1.4 cubic centimeters decinormal silver.

400 cubic centimeters treated with standard lime-water and acid (in presence of ammonium and calcium chlorides) gave .00045 gram of free carbonic acid, while the precipitate in the 400 cubic centimeters weighed .040 gram.

Total hardness, 5.8°; permanent hardness, 3.5°.

The following is deduced from the above:

|  | Gram per liter. | Grams per gallon. |
|---|---|---|
| Organic matter | .0066 | .462 |
| Lime | .0233 | 1.631 |
| Magnesia | .0067 | .469 |
| Potassium | .0024 | .168 |
| Sodium | .0040 | .280 |
| Silica | .0066 | .462 |
| Combined { Chlorine | .0025 | .165 |
| Combined { Sulphuric acid | .0017 | .119 |
| Combined { Carbonic acid | .0430 | 3.010 |
| Trace of iron, &c. | | |
| Total found | .0968 | 6.766 |
| Total by evaporation | .0910 | 6.370 |
| Free carbonic acid | .00113 | .079 |

or .575 cubic centimeter per litre.     or .167 cubic inch per gallon.

The natural drainage being good, no artificial drains or sewers have been made. The slops and offal from the kitchens are collected in barrels, and every morning hauled below the post and thrown into the stream.

There is an old cemetery in the valley half a mile northeast of the post, but it is no longer used.

A new one was started in 1868, on higher ground, about a mile and a quarter distant in a southerly direction. In both the graves of citizens who have died at or in the vicinity of the post largely predominate. There are but six graves of soldiers in the new cemetery.

The garden consists of an inclosure of about five acres, all of which, however, is not under cultivation. The products are divided proportionately among the companies, the hospital, and the officers, each paying at the end of the season a pro rata of the cost of seeds and garden-implements.

There is a daily mail from both east and west, and communications are received regularly and promptly, being only two days in reaching the post from Omaha.

The climate is temperate and salubrious the greater part of the year. The weather during the fall months is mild and delightful, excepting a few snow-storms of short duration. No severe weather occurs before the middle of December; after that time there are frequent storms and high winds. Cold weather continues late in the spring, and the grass does not begin to grow until May. Although the post is in a valley, with streams all around and through it, the atmosphere is comparatively dry, the reading of the wet and dry bulb thermometers varying from ten to fifteen degrees. The prevailing winds are from the west, and on an average blow from that quarter twenty-eight days in a month.

In investigating the amount and character of the sickness at this station, the records of the past eight years—1866–'73—have been examined. Although the post has been in existence since 1857, the records are complete only from the close of the war, when the volunteers were relieved by a regular garrison.

During these years 2,355 cases were entered on the registers, of which 6 died and 49 were discharged, an annual average of 1,932 cases per thousand of mean strength, with a mortality of 1 in 392 cases. This is a healthier record than the average of the army during the same period. The discharges, as a whole, have a greater bearing on the physique of the recruits received than on the diseases prevalent at the station; setting them aside, the other figures show to the advantage of Fort Bridger. If we express the sickness and mortality of the army, each as unity, Fort Bridger sick-roll will be represented by .81 and its mortality by .25.

Acute rheumatism, conjunctivitis, catarrh, quinsy, laryngitis, and phthisis, are specially the diseases of the station. These would seem, with the exception of the conjunctivitis, to be developed from climatic influences. The spread of the eye disease was the result of low ceilings, over-crowding, and deficient means for effecting personal cleanliness. It continued prominent on the records for three years, and disappeared with repairs and improvements, which furnished increased air-space, by heightening the ceiling of the barrack-rooms and abolishing double-tiered bunks. This point in the history of the post offers a good example of what sanitary science can accomplish. Non-professional men, in their superiority to such trifles, may smile at the doctor's insistance on air-space, ventilation, lavatories, and so on; but a disease completely expunged from the records by attention to these trifles proves the virtue there may be in them.

The intermittents are imported diseases. During my service at this station I have found no case which originated in the locality. On the contrary, the tendency in the imported cases is to longer intervals and ultimate recovery. Every monthly report which shows an unusual number of cases of this disease shows at the same time some change in the garrison. During succeeding months the number becomes smaller until a new company or a detachment of recruits brings a fresh influx of intermittent cases. In one notable instance, occurring in June, 1869, when the garrison was relieved by troops from Florida, forty intermittents were taken on sick-report in a strength of 199 men, or 200 per thousand for the month, while the average for the year is only 167. This, by the way, gives June a much higher figure as its ratio per thousand than it would have possessed without this accidental circumstance.

But, although the station seems free from intermittents, a remittent fever, susceptible to the action of quinine, is well recognized as being indigenous. It is known as a "mountain-fever." It has also been called a "modified typhoid"—typhoid without the enteric symptoms. The cases I have seen have rarely reached this typhoid condition. Soldiers, when indisposed, appear at surgeon's call for excuse from duty, when, if in civil life, they would not think of sending for medical advice. Most of the cases occurring in the garrison are thus seen at the first manifestations of the disease, and are returned to duty in three or four days after treatment by mercurial purges and twenty to thirty grains of quinine daily. If, however, the disease be permitted to run unchecked for a few days the patient falls into a condition undistinguishable from typhoid, and which cften proves fatal among miners, settlers, prospecting and surveying parties. During the past year I have treated three such cases, and in two of them the enteric symptoms were well marked. A fourth case occurred in the person of a soldier belonging to the post. He was on duty as post-gardener, and as such, being his own master, and requiring no excuse from duty, he permitted several days to pass without appearing at surgeon's call. In each of these cases, however, the disease began to yield as soon as the quinine affected the system—the amount required being proportionate to the delay in the commencement of its administration.

Pure typhoid fever occurred recently in a girl fifteen years old, living in the neighborhood. She is now convalescing. At first, her case was viewed as "mountain-fever," and quinine administered, but as it produced no beneficial effect, although strongly pushed, the diagnosis was altered to typhoid, doubtingly, until the eruption established its truth. One case of typhoid is on the records as occurring among the troops during the past eight years. Scurvy disappeared from the record with the opening of the Union Pacific Railroad, which brought the post into communication with Ogden and other depots of country produce.

Diarrhœa is an accidental disease, and owes its origin to causes within the control of the garrison. Two tides of this affection pass over the post annually; the one, beginning in August and ending with October, corresponds to the period of vegetable and fruit supply; the other, beginning in December and ending with the return of mild weather, is owing to a deteriorated condition of system in the men, produced by sleeping in unventilated barrack-rooms. In a report on the air of the dormitories of the post which I had the honor to furnish during the spring of the present year, this winter-diarrhœa was shown to be much more prevalent in the companies quartered in the better-finished and more air-tight buildings than in those occupying rooms which admitted of ventilation through the crevices of faulty construction. Ventilation, as recommended in that report, would do much to lessen sickness from this and allied diseases during future winters.

Acute and chronic bronchitis, pneumonia, and pleurisy are rare diseases at this station, only three of pleurisy and two of pneumonia having occurred during the eight years. This is a favorable showing; nor is it detracted from by the fact that four of the six deaths are set down to lung-affection. Two are reported as from congestion of the lung; but intemperance and exposure are added, materially qualifying the part which climate enacted in the deaths. The third was from abscess of the lung (latent) in a soldier prematurely old and broken down by long courses of dissipation. The fourth is from "acute phthisis," as a sequel to mountain-fever. Peritonitis is responsible for the fifth, (particulars not given,) and penetrating chest wound for the sixth.

Among the many citizens in the neighborhood, I have seen but one case of lung-inflammation, and it also comes under the category of intemperance and exposure.

In examining the diseases proper to the station, I have tabulated them in monthly ratios per thousand of mean strength, the better to show fluctuations during the progress of the year, and to compare such fluctuations with the climatic conditions.

*Table of monthly ratios per thousand of mean strength, average of eight years, 1866–'73.*

| Month. | Strength. | Remittent fever. | Catarrh. | Quinsy. | Laryngitis. | Acute bronchitis. | Chronic bronchitis. | Pleurisy. | Inflammation of lung. | Phthisis. | Acute rheumatism. | Chronic rheumatism. | Total climatic diseases. |
|---|---|---|---|---|---|---|---|---|---|---|---|---|---|
| January | 172 | 4.36 | 42.89 | 18.17 | 1.45 | 1.45 | .73 | ...... | ...... | .73 | 12.36 | .73 | 82.87 |
| February | 167 | .75 | 29.94 | 4.49 | .75 | ...... | ...... | .75 | ...... | .75 | 14.97 | 2.25 | 54.65 |
| March | 168 | 1.49 | 68.45 | 5.95 | .74 | 2.23 | .74 | ...... | ...... | 1.48 | 7.44 | ...... | 88.52 |
| April | 154 | 1.62 | 42.21 | 7.31 | .81 | ...... | ...... | ...... | .81 | .81 | 13.80 | 2.44 | 69.81 |
| May | 134 | 5.60 | 54.10 | 5.60 | ...... | ...... | ...... | .93 | ...... | 1.86 | 3.73 | 2.80 | 74.62 |
| June | 135 | 13.89 | 50.93 | 9.26 | ...... | ...... | ...... | ...... | ...... | 1.85 | 4.63 | 2.79 | 83.35 |
| July | 132 | 9.47 | 15.15 | 4.73 | ...... | .95 | .95 | ...... | ...... | .95 | 11.36 | 1.89 | 45.45 |
| August | 145 | 4.26 | 5.11 | .85 | ...... | ...... | ...... | ...... | ...... | ...... | 4.26 | 1.70 | 16.18 |
| September | 131 | ...... | 12.40 | .95 | ...... | ...... | ...... | ...... | .95 | ...... | 5.73 | .95 | 20.98 |
| October | 156 | ...... | 19.23 | 7.21 | .80 | 4.01 | ...... | ...... | .80 | 1.60 | 3.21 | 1.60 | 38.46 |
| November | 171 | 5.85 | 26.32 | 5.85 | ...... | 2.92 | ...... | ...... | ...... | .73 | 3.65 | 1.46 | 46.78 |
| December | 168 | .74 | 34.22 | 14.14 | .74 | 1.49 | ...... | ...... | ...... | ...... | 7.44 | ...... | 58.77 |
| Yearly | 153 | 48.03 | 400.95 | 84.51 | 5.29 | 13.05 | 2.42 | 2.48 | 1.76 | 10.76 | 92.58 | 18.61 | 680.44 |

In connection with the above, the following synopsis of the meteorology of the station is furnished. This table is an average from the records of the past fifteen years, with the exception of the figures indicating the air-pressure. The barometrical record was kept only for one year, 1869. Its monthly mean is singularly uniform.

I regret that the meteorological register does not furnish in this connection minute enough data with regard to the force of the wind. Three observations daily are given, the force of each being expressed by the figures 1, 2, 3, 4, &c., in accordance with instructions from Surgeon-General's Office. A force of 1 signifies a wind of less than five miles an hour; the average of 1 would therefore be about two and a half miles; while 2, signifying wind between five and ten miles an hour, would have an average meaning of seven and a half miles. The figure 2 in the register, sum of the forces of two observations, (1 + 1,) differs in value from the same figure 2 indicating force of one observation, and so for the higher numbers. The constant current, as given below, is the sum of the registered forces divided by the number of observations. It was found impossible to turn this with any degree of accuracy into miles per hour.

*Fort Bridger meteorological table, (average of fifteen years.)*

| | January. | February. | March. | April. | May. | June. | July. | August. | September. | October. | November. | December. | Annual. |
|---|---|---|---|---|---|---|---|---|---|---|---|---|---|
| Rain-fall, (inches) | .51 | .49 | .61 | .47 | 1.04 | .60 | .72 | .82 | .55 | .31 | .58 | .61 | .61 |
| Relative humidity | 70 | 40 | 51 | 63 | 64 | 55 | 52 | 53 | 57 | 63 | 60 | 48 | 56 |
| Barometer | 23.444 | .443 | .436 | .458 | .483 | .649 | .663 | .620 | .615 | .644 | .560 | .550 | 23.547 |
| Winds | 2.39 | 2.50 | 2.46 | 2.47 | 2.09 | 1.59 | 1.53 | 1.59 | 1.78 | 1.82 | 2.21 | 2.10 | 2.04 |
| Mean thermometer, (Fahrenheit) | 19°.08 | 21°.92 | 28°.51 | 37°.54 | 50°.08 | 59°.67 | 65°.95 | 64°.76 | 53°.75 | 41°.97 | 31°.01 | 20°.56 | 41°.23 |
| Average maximum, (Fahrenheit) | 46° | 46° | 55° | 68° | 76° | 84° | 87° | 86° | 80° | 75° | 62° | 46° | 68° |
| Average minimum, (Fahrenheit) | −17° | − 6° | − 2° | 13° | 26° | 33° | 43° | 39° | 26° | 12° | 1° | −11° | 13° |
| Average fluctuation | 63° | 52° | 57° | 55° | 50° | 51° | 44° | 47° | 54° | 63° | 61° | 57° | 55° |

From the above it is seen that catarrh, numerically considered, is pre-eminently the disease of the station—four out of every ten men being affected annually. It is difficult to appreciate why March should exceed the other months so remarkably in its production of this disease, unless it be attributed to the alternate freezing and thawing, caused by variations above and below the mean temperature of 28°.51 Fahrenheit. April, May, and June follow on the list; the gradual rise in temperature melts the snows of winter, necessitating precautions against damp feet from slush and mud, and furnishing more cases than the colder months. Another cause of the prominence of this disease during the months of rising temperature is the change which the warm mid-day hours call for in the soldier's clothing; the extra shirt is laid aside, and after sunset a slight chilliness ushers in the attack. July, August, September, and October have less of these cases; August notably so.

Pure cold seems to have much to do with the production of tonsillitis; December and January, the two coldest months, giving by far the largest numbers, although February, which takes rank next as to cold, gives fewer cases than the warmer months that follow, perhaps because the variation and humidity are relatively less. In this disease, also, June shows the effects of lessening the clothing. In August and September the disease is at its minimum.

I believe that these catarrhs and quinsies could be much reduced by a system of ventilation During four months of the year the temperature falls below zero at night. The great object of the men in quarters in such weather is to keep warm. The fires are well attended to, and every chink which admits fresh air, and can be reached, is carefully stopped up. With the thermometer so low, there is seldom any wind to promote change in the atmosphere of the room, and it soon becomes loaded with exhalations and depressingly warm, leading the men to sick-call from exposure at the reveille; properly-constructed ventilation, which would renew the air and prevent the rooms from becoming overheated, would relieve the sick-report of many a case which burdens it under existing arrangements.

Laryngitis appears in the colder months and early spring, and is unknown in the summer.

Rheumatic fever is scattered over the months without reference to season, wind, humidity, temperature, or its fluctuations; July, with its higher temperature and minimum of variation, having nearly as many cases as January with its lower temperature, and three times as many as October

41 M P

with its maximum of variation. The small number of chronic cases, which result from these acute attacks, is very noteworthy.

Summer is the season for the remittents, but they appear during all the other months except September and October.

I am not aware of any case of consumption which has originated in this neighborhood, but, although the country has been settled as now for some fifteen years, and several large families have been brought up, the population is too scanty to give this point by itself much weight. The prevailing impression among the citizens is, that the climate, though severe in the winter, is very beneficial to such cases of consumption as are able to stand it. Such ideas among the people are usually the reflection of professional opinion, and I state the above to indicate what has probably been that of my predecessors at the post.

Twelve entries of consumption appear on the registers; of these one died, as recorded above; eight were discharged, one returned to duty, and two are presumed to have been returned, although mutilation of a part of the records prevents certainty; at all events, they are not borne on the monthly reports as discharged or dead. Of the eight discharged one only is stated to have originated prior to entry into service; the other seven are reported as having been developed in the line of duty—that is, the men, whether affected with incipient phthisis or not before their arrival in this climate, were able to perform their duty while at the post, and broke down under the progress of the disease while exposed to the climatic influences of this station. To the twelve entries I have added in the table a thirteenth, appearing in May, 1871, as a discharge for "debility on account of catarrh." This gives 10.76 per thousand of mean strength of cases of consumption developed at Fort Bridger annually, to such extent as to cause withdrawal from duty for medical treatment, and 8.3 per thousand dead and discharged by reason of this disease, while only 3.5 per thousand required medical treatment in the Army as a whole.—(Records of 1866.)

These figures do not support the popular opinion with regard to Fort Bridger. Even allowing that three of the cases (2.43 per thousand) were so improved by the climate as ultimately to recover, the same climate is responsible for the attack which brought them to the hospital from the performance of duty, and it is also responsible for the death and discharge of the remaining ten, (8.33 per thousand,) while the temporary and permanent disablement from duty through such cases by the average climate of United States Army stations is but 3.5 per thousand. The rarity of acute bronchial and pulmonary inflammations is in striking contrast to the marked progress which is indicated in the development of the phthisical cases, and lends the figures of the latter greater value than they would possess if presented alone.

The immunity from consumption possessed, as a rule, by the inhabitants of elevated lands has led to belief in the curative influence of a residence in such climes, provided the disease be in its incipient stage, or, as the people here say with more unwitting caution, provided the patient is able to stand it. The cases above noted were in the incipient stage, perhaps free from everything but the hereditary predisposition, for it cannot be assumed that these soldiers were doing duty while in the advanced stages, yet they were not able to stand it. Overheating and impure air already spoken of no doubt had an influence on the development of the cases, but these factors do not detract from the value of the figures in the question of causative or curative influence of climate. Bad ventilation and overheating affect more garrisons than that of Fort Bridger, and have their effect expressed in the 3.5 per thousand, while the excess of overheating, with its results, at this post, is reflected back on climate by the cold which originates it.

During the past year among the citizens here, I have seen two cases of consumption. One, very advanced, died within a short time; the other, a tall, young Missourian, with hereditary predisposition, a history of weak lungs and two hemorrhages, came here in hope of benefit in the summer of 1873, and within a few months increased in weight from 130 to 164 pounds. He is still here, in robust health, living most of his waking hours in the open air and on horseback.

Altitude may be preventive of consumption in all cases where the residence is commenced early enough, but in view of the above figures and of other considerations, such as the diminution in the quantity of oxygen through lessened air-pressure, (oxygen in given space at sea-level being to that at Bridger as 100 to 78,) the residence should commence during the period of development—not of the disease, but of the body. As the time for this has passed in the majority of instances, where the question of change of climate comes to be considered, this station must be set down as unsuitable, either from excess of altitude, requiring too great a strain upon the weakened lungs, or from excess or deficiency of some of the other climatic elements, such as temperature and its variations—winds, and moisture, which, though in general terms dependent on altitude, are oftentimes materially modified by local circumstances.

An examination of the above meteorological table, keeping in view the months of prevalence of catarrhs and quinsies, would lead one to infer that a station having an air-pressure of 23.5 inches of mercury is unsuitable to consumptive cases, where the relative humidity is over 60, (saturation being 100,) and where the mean monthly temperature is lower, and its fluctuations greater than 50° Fahrenheit, especially if the variation cause alternate freezing and thaws by its relation to the freezing-point.

On the other hand, in view of the infrequency of bronchial and pulmonary inflammations during the whole year, and of catarrh and quinsy during the months of July, August, and September, one would decide that if such an elevation is to prove beneficial, (if the lungs can accommodate themselves to the rarefied- atmosphere, as in the case of the Missourian, and probably of the three soldiers from the records,) it will be where the humidity is under 50, where the monthly fluctuation of the thermometer does not exceed 50° Fahrenheit, and where the mean monthly temperature is at, or within limits, over, 50° Fahrenheit.

*Meteorological report, Fort Bridger, Wyo., 1870–'74.*

| Month. | 1870–'71. Temperature. Mean. | Max. | Min. | Rain-fall in inches. | 1871–'72. Temperature. Mean. | Max. | Min. | Rain-fall in inches. | 1872–'73. Temperature. Mean. | Max. | Min. | Rain-fall in inches. | 1873–'74. Temperature. Mean. | Max. | Min. | Rain-fall in inches. |
|---|---|---|---|---|---|---|---|---|---|---|---|---|---|---|---|---|
| | ° | ° | ° | | ° | ° | ° | | ° | ° | ° | | ° | ° | ° | |
| July | 67.71 | 87* | 46* | 0.24 | 66.55 | 91* | 36* | 1.04 | 62.54 | 85* | 32* | 0.74 | 66.04 | 87* | 34* | 0.95 |
| August | 61.42 | 87* | 27* | 0.46 | 62.52 | 87* | 26* | 0.06 | 61.76 | 86* | 28* | 1.86 | 63.98 | 92* | 34* | 1.65 |
| September | 51.42 | 80* | 21* | 0.18 | 54.82 | 79* | 24* | 0.00 | 52.51 | 80* | 15* | 0.59 | 54.79 | 79* | 20* | 0.13 |
| October | 41.26 | 70* | 16* | 0.08 | 39.26 | 73* | 12* | 0.82 | 41.29 | 77* | 11* | 0.31 | 39.06 | 79 | —13* | 0.90 |
| November | 34.47 | 56* | 8* | 0.05 | 26.99 | 62* | —27* | 2.80 | 24.37 | 55* | —22* | 0.75 | 34.85 | 63 | 10* | 0.08 |
| December | 18.86 | 48* | —10* | 0.57 | 25.87 | 45* | — 5* | 0.95 | 23.89 | 55* | — 7* | 0.97 | 16.62 | 46 | —13* | 0.60 |
| January | 23.43 | 53* | —12* | 0.45 | 16.25 | 51* | —29* | 0.10 | 22.06 | 43* | —33* | 1.23 | 18.77 | 49 | —20* | 1.51 |
| February | 23.62 | 45* | 3* | 1.15 | 26.33 | 55* | — 3* | 0.20 | 14.62 | 38* | —14* | 1.45 | 13.40 | 35 | —15* | 1.08 |
| March | 29.68 | 49* | 4* | 1.20 | 27.61 | 57* | 0* | 1.00 | 30.34 | 61* | —13* | 0.53 | 19.16 | 44 | —14* | 2.91 |
| April | 38.31 | 67* | 15* | 0.57 | 35.78 | 67* | 11* | 0.70 | 34.27 | 72* | — 0* | 0.92 | 32.92 | 72 | 8* | 1.27 |
| May | 51.81 | 80* | 20* | 0.10 | 49.98 | 81* | 20* | 0.10 | 43.07 | 70* | 17* | 2.14 | 52.04 | 78 | 23* | 1.78 |
| June | 62.93 | 87* | 25* | 0.00 | 58.22 | 82* | 25* | 3.25 | 59.77 | 85* | 24* | 0.25 | 58.39 | 81 | 32* | 0.48 |
| For the year | 42.08 | 87* | —12* | 5.05 | 40.84 | 91* | —29* | 11.02 | 39.23 | 86* | —33* | 11.74 | 39.17 | 92* | —20* | 13.34 |

* These observations are made with self-registering thermometers. The mean is from the standard thermometer.

*Consolidated sick-report, Fort Bridger, Wyo., 1870–'74.*

| Year | | 1870–'71. | | 1871–'72. | | 1872–'73. | | 1873–'74. | |
|---|---|---|---|---|---|---|---|---|---|
| Mean strength { Officers | | 7 | | 5 | | 5 | | 11 | |
| { Enlisted men | | 130 | | 59 | | 96 | | 175 | |
| Diseases. | | Cases. | Deaths. | Cases. | Deaths. | Cases. | Deaths. | Cases. | Deaths. |
| GENERAL DISEASES, A. | | | | | | | | | |
| Typhoid fever | | 1 | | | | | | | |
| Remittent fever | | | | | | | | 6 | |
| Intermittent fever | | 21 | | 8 | | 6 | | 14 | |
| Diphtheria | | | | | | | | 1 | |
| Other diseases of this group | | 15 | | 6 | | 10 | | 26 | |
| GENERAL DISEASES, B. | | | | | | | | | |
| Rheumatism | | 18 | | 9 | | 17 | | 14 | |
| Syphilis | | 2 | | | | | | | |
| Consumption | | 2 | | | | 1 | | 2 | |
| Other diseases of this group | | | | | | | | 1 | |

*Consolidated sick-report, Fort Bridger, Wyo., 1870–'74—Continued.*

| Year | | 1870–'71. | | 1871–'72. | | 1872–'73. | | 1873–'74. | |
|---|---|---|---|---|---|---|---|---|---|
| Mean strength ⎰ Officers | | 7 | | 5 | | 5 | | 11 | |
| ⎱ Enlisted men | | 130 | | 59 | | 96 | | 175 | |
| Diseases. | | Cases. | Deaths. | Cases. | Deaths. | Cases. | Deaths. | Cases. | Deaths. |
| LOCAL DISEASES. | | | | | | | | | |
| Catarrh and bronchitis | | 82 | | 11 | | 50 | | 42 | |
| Pneunomia | | | | | | 1 | | 1 | |
| Pleurisy | | | | | | 1 | | | |
| Diarrhœa and dysentery | | 33 | | 2 | | 3 | | 37 | |
| Hernia | | | | 1 | | | | 1 | |
| Gonorrhœa | | 2 | | | | | | 4 | |
| Other local diseases | | 61 | | 23 | 1 | 58 | | 63 | 1 |
| Alcoholism | | 14 | 1 | 2 | | 1 | | 10 | |
| Total disease | | 251 | 1 | 55 | 1 | 148 | | 222 | 1 |
| VIOLENT DISEASES AND DEATHS. | | | | | | | | | |
| Gunshot wounds | | 3 | | | | 1 | | | |
| Other accidents and injuries | | 36 | | 19 | | 46 | | 32 | |
| Total violence | | 39 | | 19 | | 47 | | 32 | |

# CAMP BROWN, WYOMING TERRITORY.

INFORMATION FURNISHED BY ACTING ASSISTANT SURGEON THOMAS G. MAGHEE, UNITED STATES ARMY.

Camp Brown is situated in the valley of the South Fork of the Little Wind River, Sweetwater County, Wyoming Territory. Latitude, 42° 59′ 33″ north; longitude, 31° 49′ west; altitude, 5,462 feet above the sea; deflection of the needle, 17° 20′. Bryan Station, on the Union Pacific Railroad, one hundred and fifty-four miles distant south of west, is the nearest available point on the railroad. Mails are received by way of Bryan, South Pass City, (the nearest express-office,) and Camp Stambaugh, (the nearest telegraph-office,) about once in five days. Means of access is by the Sweetwater stage, which leaves Bryan Station Mondays, Wednesdays, and Fridays, on the arrival of the train from the East, and remaining over night at McCoy's Ranch, on the Big Sandy, reaches South Pass City early in the afternoon of the second day. The distance is one hundred miles; stage fare $20, and five cents per pound for all baggage in excess of twenty-five pounds. From South Pass City to Camp Stambaugh, (seven miles,) and thence to Camp Brown, (forty-seven miles,) Army transportation is depended on, and it generally requires but one day to reach the latter place. The roads are good, rarely being blocked by snow in the mountains. All supplies are brought in trail-wagons from Bryan, and require twelve to twenty days in transit. The price paid is, during summer $2.25, and after October 1st $3 per hundred-weight.

Wind River Mountains, which, with the Owl Creek Range, surround this point on three sides, are rugged and broken, rising to a height of 10,000 feet above the sea, and are about thirty-five miles through the base. Some of the higher peaks are capped with perpetual snow. Scattered through the range are level plateaus, which are covered in summer with tall grass, wild raspberries, gooseberries, and flowers, and are intersected by crystal brooks, or placid and beautiful lakelets. Some beautiful waterfalls are seen in the courses of the numberless small streams, which, fed by the snow, or cold, clear springs, tumble down the mountains, and, uniting in the valleys on either side, flow respectively into the Gulf of Mexico and the Pacific Ocean. West of the post, at a distance of forty miles, is Frémont's Peak. A little more to the south, and twenty miles nearer, is Chimney Rock, a mass of dark, granitic rock, rising abruptly six hundred feet from its base. The top has an area of seven acres, and attains an altitude of 12,800 feet above the sea. This range has a geological character similar to the Rocky Mountains proper, abounding in outcrops of quartz and having fossils of the Devonian, Silurian, and Carboniferous formations upon the higher portions, while the Triassic and Cretaceous systems are found on the sides and foot-hills. Quartz and gulch mining will doubtless prove remunerative in the range. Sixteen miles north of here is Bull Lake, three miles long and half a mile wide, clear, cold, and sweet, abounding in fish of large size. It empties by Lake Fork into Big Wind River. Eight miles farther north is Crow Hart Butte, a conical mound, rising to a considerable height in a plain, and forming a noted landmark from the south. Five miles southwest, in the foot-hills, is Tesson's Spring. Its temperature is uniformly 50° Fahrenheit, and it contains free sulphydric acid, sulphites and hyposulphites of lime, soda, and magnesia, in quantity, and a trace of carbonate of soda. A sulphurous odor is perceptible at a considerable distance. Two miles east is a large spring, 315 by 250 feet in diameter, of irregular oval shape; sloping to the center, it attains a depth of twenty feet. The edges are clearly defined, being sharp and rocky upon the west side; a deposit of sulphate and carbonate of lime, seamed with silica. The force and temperature of the wind have great influence on the temperature of the spring, which varies from 98° to 115° Fahrenheit. Hot carbonic acid, carbureted and sulphureted hydrogen gases continually bubble up in such quantities in places as to give the spring the appearance of boiling. The water contains in abundance sulphates and carbonates of lime and soda; also chlorate of soda, but no free sulphur; has a pearly-blue appearance, but deposits the carbonates by standing. It discharges into Little Wind River, by an outlet three feet deep, twelve feet wide, and five hundred yards in length. The appearance of the spring and its surroundings would indicate that there was a period of greater activity in bygone years. Used as a bath, the waters have proved decidedly beneficial for rheumatic, neuralgic, syphilitic, and skin diseases; taken internally no perceptible effect is produced. On the north side of the river, nearer the post, is Grimes's oil-well, about twelve feet in diameter, surrounded by a deep layer of asphaltum fifty yards wide, the deposit of the spring. Coal is found in the mountains near here, but it is worthless for fuel. Siliceous limestone is found for building-purposes.

The valley in which the post is located extends about thirty miles to the east, with a uniform width of three miles. The soil is a dark sandy loam, yielding a large return for labor bestowed on it. Although the river is fringed with brush of small growth, no large timber exists. In size, fertility, and timber the valley of Big Wind River far surpasses it. Along the streams the aspen, mountain-birch, choke-cherry, and several varieties of willow are found. A rhizoma grows in some of the cañons, which is gathered in the spring, before it acquires a bitter principle, and having been boiled in several waters, until it resembles cooked tapioca, is seasoned and eaten by the Indians, who have been known to subsist on it alone for three weeks at a time. It is perfectly bland, contains much gluten and starch, and if susceptible of cultivation will doubtless prove a valuable addition to our farinaceous articles of diet.

Game is plentiful, such as the grizzly, brown, and cinnamon bear, mountain lion, white, gray, and prairie wolf, (or coyote,) lynx, red, crossed, and silver-gray fox, wild-cat, beaver, otter, mink, marten, common and white ferret, buffalo, elk, white and black tailed, and red or mule deer, antelope, mountain-sheep, jack and cotton-tailed rabbit, woodchuck, and gopher. Of birds, the wild goose, brant, mallard, teal, and other water-fowl, many kinds of owls and hawks, crows, magpies, whippoorwills, flickers, sage-hens, blue grouse, robins, and many smaller birds are found. Of reptiles, some harmless snakes, lizards, toads, and a few rattlesnakes whose bite is not generally fatal to man, may occasionally be seen.

The post was established in compliance with the terms of a treaty with the Shoshone and Bannock Indians, for their protection against Sioux, Arapahoe, Cheyenne, and other hostile bands. Their agency is a mile and a half south of the post. It contains a stone block-house, steam saw and shingle mill, and several cottages occupied by the agent and employés, and is fearfully filthy. Their chief, Wash-a-kie, has a benevolent and kindly expression of countenance, is well made, strictly honest, and possesses superior intelligence and influence; he is a half-breed Snake and Flathead, brave to a fault, and long the fast friend of the white man. At present about 1,400 rations per diem are issued to them, and they also receive annually large quantities of clothing, &c. A great deal of the clothing and more valuable articles soon become the property of the agency employés and neighboring ranch-men.

This country has been the hunting-ground and winter-quarters for some few white trappers since 1849, and scattered over this and contiguous valleys are burnt ranches, bleaching bones, and rude graves, attesting the success with which hostile Indians have raided them.

The post is on the eastern slope of the Wind River Mountains, on the south or right bank of the river, about 150 yards above its junction with the North Fork. The site is elevated about 50 feet above the river-bed. Originally a sub-post of Fort Bridger, it was built on Big Papoagie River, seventeen miles south of its present site, June, 1869, and named Fort Augur. The name was changed May 28, 1870, to Camp Brown, in honor of Captain Brown, Eighteenth Infantry, killed in the Fort Phil Kearney massacre in 1866. Becoming desirable to be nearer the Indian agency, the present more eligible site was selected June 26, 1871; the old post was dismantled and abandoned, all available material being transported to and used in the construction of the new post.

The parade is 141 by 181 feet, and is surrounded by acequias; its center, occupied by the flag-staff, is also the center of a proposed military reservation, one mile square.

The infantry-barrack is 30 by 75 feet, 10 feet high to the eaves, and, being unceiled, has 28,828 cubic feet of air-space. It contains 27 one-story double wooden bunks, affording to each person 534 cubic feet of space. The bunks have a locker under each. A veranda, 10 feet wide, extends across the front, from each end of which a room, 9½ by 10 feet, is cut off—one for an office, the other for a store-room. The mess-room, kitchen, wash-room, bakery, and store-room are in a separate building. The cavalry-barrack is similar in size and arrangement to that for the infantry, except that 12 feet of the dormitory is cut off at one end for the use of non-commissioned officers, and that the mess-room, kitchen, &c., are in an L adjoining the barrack. The new style of single iron bunk is used, but placed together, two and two, for comfort during cold weather. These buildings are well lighted, excellently ventilated by two small hot-air shafts, which lead through the ridge of the roof in each dormitory, and transoms over the doors, and warmed by wood-burning stoves. They are built of adobes, the outer walls 18 inches thick. The infantry-barrack is roofed with asphaltum and sand on matched plank, and leaks during every storm. The cavalry-barrack is roofed with pine shingles.

The laundresses' quarters are three small log buildings of two rooms each, 20 by 20 by 10 feet, roofed with dirt on poles, and leak badly during every heavy snow. One family occupies each room.

There are three double sets of officers' quarters. Two of these are adobe buildings, 42 by 38 feet, each having a veranda 7 feet wide across the front, and containing two suites of two rooms, 15 by 15 by 10 feet each, separated by a common hall 6 feet wide. The walls are all plastered in hard finish, the wood-work is nicely painted, but neither halls nor rooms have ceilings. To each house is attached an addition, containing three small rooms for kitchen, dining-room, and servant's room. The rooms are well lighted, and warmed by stoves or fire-places. They are roofed with asphaltum and sand, similar to the infantry-barracks. The third building is constructed of hewn pine logs, has a shingle roof, and two halls side by side through the center—one for each set of quarters. The arrangement of the rooms, &c., is similar to the two other buildings.

The guard-house is in a building which also contains the adjutant's office. Although well lighted and warmed, it has no means for ventilation. The cell is above ground; has one window, secured by a board shutter containing a few auger-holes; the ceiling is of logs laid far enough apart to secure good ventilation if the house itself had any provisions for that purpose.

The building used for a hospital is cramped and inconvenient, neither plastered nor ceiled. The ward, 15 feet 2 inches by 22 feet 3 inches, by 10 feet high at the eaves, with the gable, has 4,057 cubic feet of air-space. It contains seven beds, thus giving 579 cubic feet of space to each patient. The dispensary, store-room, and attendant's room, are small, all three occupying but 506 square feet of surface, and are not entirely floored. The odors and noises of one room entering freely all the others, necessitated the removal of the kitchen to a tent in rear of the building. The officer at the time of fitting up the hospital decided that no cellar, kitchen, mess-room, or bath-room, was needed, and that patients should receive their meals from the company kitchen. Ventilation is imperfectly effected by raising the lower sash of the windows, which, however, in the ward are so badly placed as to occasion a draught immediately over some bed, impossible to prevent.

For the use of enlisted men and the hospital but one privy exists. It is large and clean, and being placed in rear of the hospital, over the river, the excreta are carried off by the stream. In rear of the laundresses' quarters is another small privy for their use, which is disinfected when required, by the use of dry earth, lime, or sulphate of iron.　There is a small privy in rear of each set of officers' quarters.

All slop and refuse are carried below camp and dumped into the stream.　The condition and character of the ground are such that natural drainage is all that could be desired.

There are two wells in the post, but except in winter the water brought from South Fork by acequias is used for all purposes, being comparatively soft, at all times cool, limpid, agreeable to the taste, and healthful.

The means of extinguishing fires are two Babcock extingu'shers and buckets, the latter being useless in winter.

East of the building is a garden containing eight acres, which was cultivated by the company stationed here during the summer, affording in their season a plentiful supply of pease, beans, radishes, lettuce, cabbage, onions, and roasting-ears of excellent quality and size.　Beets and potatoes were particularly fine, 70,000 pounds of the latter being raised.　As there is no rain, irrigation is resorted to, this rendering the crops certain.

But one person, the former hospital-matron, having died in four years of occupancy, there is no post cemetery.　She was buried about half a mile east of the post.

The spring is late, and cold weather commences in October, but little snow falls before January. Maximum temperature was 94° Fahrenheit, June 4, 1873; minimum, —28° Fahrenheit, November 20, 1872.　The general direction of wind for seven months, since June 1, 1873, was southwest; average velocity two and two-thirds miles per hour.　The total water-fall from rain and snow for the same time was 3.17 inches.　No records were kept prior to June 1, 1873.　The terrific winds common in surrounding places, are never experienced in this valley, the range of mountains protecting it on every side.

*Meteorological report, Camp Brown, Wyo., 1872-'74.*

| Month. | 1870-'71. | | | | 1871-'72. | | | | 1872-'73. | | | | 1873-'74. | | | |
|---|---|---|---|---|---|---|---|---|---|---|---|---|---|---|---|---|
| | Temperature. | | | Rain-fall in inches. | Temperature. | | | Rain-fall in inches. | Temperature. | | | Rain-fall in inches. | Temperature. | | | Rain-fall in inches. |
| | Mean. | Max. | Min. | | Mean. | Max. | Min. | | Mean. | Max. | Min. | | Mean. | Max. | Min. | |
| | ° | ° | ° | | ° | ° | ° | | ° | ° | ° | | ° | ° | ° | |
| July | | | | | | | | | 70.21 | 94 | 46 | | 70.01 | 93* | 51 | 0.12 |
| August | | | | | | | | | 70.79 | 97 | 56 | | 68.51 | 91* | 51 | 1.41 |
| September | | | | | | | | | 58.63 | 88 | 28 | | 55.43 | 89* | 19 | 0.19 |
| October | | | | | | | | | 49.07 | 88 | 16 | 0.40 | 37.64 | 80* | — 9 | 2.16 |
| November | | | | | | | | | 28.72 | 69 | 10 | 0.40 | 34.78 | 65* | — 3* | 0.15 |
| December | | | | | | | | | | | | | 11.86 | 47 | —17 | 0.15 |
| January | | | | | | | | | | | | | 21.79 | 52 | —12 | 2.34 |
| February | | | | | 29.41 | 58 | —21 | | | | | | 18.48 | 48* | —25* | 0.34 |
| March | | | | | 38.63 | 69 | 12 | | | | | | 25.53 | 59 | —10* | 2.12 |
| April | | | | | 44.01 | 74 | 21 | | | | | | 38.46 | 72 | 6* | 2.92 |
| May | | | | | 57.78 | 85 | 35 | | | | | | 56.04 | 88 | 12* | 1.20 |
| June | | | | | 69.38 | 92 | 47 | | 65.24 | 94* | 33* | 0.42 | 60.67 | 91 | 33* | 0.82 |
| For the year | | | | | | | | | | | | | 41.60 | 93* | —25* | 13.92 |

* These observations are made with self-registering thermometers.　The mean is from the standard thermometer.

*Consolidated sick-report, Camp Brown, Wyo., 1870-'74.*

| | | 1870-'71. | | 1871-'72. | | 1872-'73. | | 1873-'74. | |
|---|---|---|---|---|---|---|---|---|---|
| Year | | | | | | | | | |
| Mean strength | { Officers | 3 | | 2 | | 3 | | 4 | |
| | { Enlisted men | 55 | | 60 | | 54 | | 93 | |
| Diseases. | | Cases. | Deaths. | Cases. | Deaths. | Cases. | Deaths. | Cases. | Deaths. |
| GENERAL DISEASES, A. | | | | | | | | | |
| Typhoid fever | | 1 | | | | | | 10 | |
| Remittent fever | | 2 | | 1 | | | | 11 | |
| Intermittent fever | | 9 | | 2 | | 7 | | 3 | |
| Other diseases of this group | | | | | | | | | |

*Consolidated sick-report, Camp Brown, Wyo., 1870–'74—Continued.*

| Year | | 1870–'71. | | 1871–'72. | | 1872–'73. | | 1873–'74. | |
|---|---|---|---|---|---|---|---|---|---|
| Mean strength ............................. { Officers ........... | | 3 | | 2 | | 3 | | 4 | |
| Enlisted men ...... | | 55 | | 60 | | 54 | | 93 | |
| Diseases. | | Cases. | Deaths. | Cases. | Deaths. | Cases. | Deaths. | Cases. | Deaths. |
| GENERAL DISEASES, B. | | | | | | | | | |
| Rheumatism ........................................................... | | 23 | ...... | 10 | ...... | 4 | ...... | 16 | ...... |
| Syphilis ............................................................... | | 1 | ...... | | ...... | | ...... | | ...... |
| LOCAL DISEASES. | | | | | | | | | |
| Catarrh and bronchitis............................................... | | 12 | ...... | 7 | ...... | 5 | ...... | 25 | ...... |
| Pneumonia............................................................ | | | ...... | | ...... | | ...... | 5 | ...... |
| Pleurisy.............................................................. | | | ...... | 2 | ...... | | ...... | 2 | ...... |
| Diarrhœa and dysentery............................................... | | 10 | ...... | 9 | ...... | 2 | ...... | 20 | ...... |
| Hernia............................................................... | | | ...... | 2 | ...... | | ...... | | ...... |
| Other local diseases.................................................. | | 54 | ...... | 42 | ...... | 23 | ...... | 89 | ...... |
| Total disease ....................................... | | 112 | ...... | 75 | ...... | 41 | ...... | 181 | ...... |
| VIOLENT DISEASES AND DEATHS. | | | | | | | | | |
| Gunshot wounds ...................................................... | | | ...... | 2 | ...... | | ...... | 1 | ...... |
| Other accidents and injuries........................................... | | 22 | ...... | 12 | ...... | 6 | ...... | 44 | ...... |
| Total violence ...................................... | | 22 | ...... | 14 | ...... | 6 | ...... | 45 | ...... |

# POST OF BEAVER, UTAH TERRITORY.

### REPORT OF ASSISTANT SURGEON F. W. ELBREY, UNITED STATES ARMY.

The post of Beaver, in latitude 38° 16′ north, and longitude 34° 50′ 30″ west, about 6,200 feet above the sea, (by barometric measurement,) is situated on the north side of the Beaver River, about one mile from the mouth of Beaver Cañon, in a recess between the foot-hills of the Wahsatch Mountains. It lies two miles east from Beaver City, a Mormon town of about one thousand inhabitants, two hundred miles south from Salt Lake City.

The post was established by four companies of the Eighth Infantry, which were ordered hither for the purpose by Lieutenant-General Sheridan. These companies arrived on May 25, 1872, and were encamped until December 13, 1872, at which time the company barracks were ready for occupation. The building of the officers' quarters, hospital, guard-house, headquarters-building and commissary store-house was commenced in September, 1873. The object in establishing this post seems to have been to further the better maintenance of the laws of the General Government in Southern Utah.

The reservation of the post, declared by the President on May 12, 1873, is of a trapezoidal shape, the sides of which measure, respectively, 1½ miles, 1 mile and 4,970 feet, 1 mile and 2,050 feet, 1 mile and 4,350 feet.

The valley, part of the great Utah Basin, in an inlet of which the post lies, is at this place about ten miles wide, having for its eastern boundary the Wahsatch range of mountains, and the West or Granite range for its western boundary. The scenery is rugged and wild. The materials of the valley, consisting of gravel, sand, and stone, belong to the modified drift formation. Alluvial formations cover a narrow area on both sides of the river. The neighboring mountains are covered with volcanic rocks and lavas. The strata in these mountains lie at all angles to verticality, and in the Wahsatch Mountains they are composed of feldspathic trap, trachyte, and coarse conglomerate; in the western range, of limestone and granite. Silver, gold, copper, bismuth, sulphur, and coal have been discovered in the vicinity, but not in rich deposits. The lowest geological formation noted pertains to the subcarboniferous period. The valley, where not made arable by irrigation, (practicable only along the streams,) grows little else than sage-brush, save here and there a cactus or a yucca, (filimentosa.) Scrub cedar and stunted pine trees cover the sides of the neighboring mountains. Along the water-courses, in the cañons, and further in the mountains, are found the following trees, shrubs, and vines: the cottonwood, the dwarf birch, (*Betula glandulosa*,) the willow, the quaking aspen, the mountain-maple, (*acer spicatum*,) the box-elder, the scrub-oak, (*quercus ilicifolia*,) the white, the yellow, and the red pine, the balsam-fir, (*abies Frasori*,) the common elder, the service-berry, edible, (*amelanchier canadensis*,) the dwarf hawthorn, the sumac, the wild currant, edible, (*Ribesia aureum*,) the bull-berry, edible, (*shepherdi argentea*,) the wild hop, the choke-cherry, edible, the wild rose, and the dwarf sunflower.

In the vicinity are found the following animals: the prairie-wolf or coyote, the gray wolf, the common skunk, the American badger, the porcupine, the wild cat, the jackass-rabbit, the black-tailed deer, the grizzly bear, the black bear, the striped squirrel, (*Tamias striatus*.)

Birds: Sparrow-hawk, sharp-shinned hawk, Lewis's woodpecker, the raven, the yellow-billed magpie, Maximilian's jay, Woodhouse's jay, Brewer's blackbird, ground-robin, long-sparrow, purple finch, grass-finch, Gambel's finch, Wilson's fly-catcher, ruby-crowned wren, water-ouzel, sky-lark, English snipe, winter yellow-legs, spotted sand-piper, great blue heron, bittern, Peale's egret, ground-dove, red-shafted flicker, mallard and green-winged teal, sage-hens, and pine-hens.

Reptiles: The rattlesnake, the common water-snake, the harlequin-snake, and lizards. The two arachnids, the tarantula and scorpion, are found, but are not common.

The atmosphere is remarkably dry. The amount of rain-fall is very small; the number of cloudy days in the year very few. The prevailing winds—and the winds are frequent and of great force, driving before them clouds of dust—blow from the southwest and northwest. Owing to the rapid radiation of the earth's heat, the variation between the temperature of the day and that of the night is always great, often amounting to 40° and rarely to less than 20°. Not often does the thermometer rise higher than 90° in summer or sink to zero in winter. Cool nights are the rule in summer, and cold nights, even to freezing, begin in September and continue till June. Indeed, no month in the year can be counted upon as being surely free from frosts. The climate is healthful. Owing to the diurnal variations in the temperature, catarrhal affections are of comparatively frequent occurrence. Phthisis, when fully established, is not at all benefited by a residence here; but phthisis does not frequently originate here. Acute rheumatism, though not prevalent, yet quite frequently occurs, and usually runs a protracted, subacute course. The various neuralgias are prevalent. No case of malarial disease has originated here. The cases of intermittent fever which have come under treatment were relapses, generally occasioned by colds, the original diseases having been contracted elsewhere.

The water-supply is abundant, and is furnished by the Beaver River, a small but never-failing cold, mountain-stream, having its origin amid the metamorphic and trap rocks of the Wahsatch Mountains. It has the general character of good water, being clear, odorless, tasteless, and soft, and is cool and pleasant to drink. The amount of organic and mineral matters it contains is small. Its main mineral constituents are carbonate of soda, a little lime, and magnesia. The water of the river is conducted, by means of canals, (acequias,) to all parts of the post.

The post is located nearly in the center of the reservation. Its position is not a commanding one, being visible only in its immediate vicinity. Its shape is a rectangular parallelogram, the space inclosed by the buildings measuring, from east to west, seven hundred feet, and from north to south, six hundred and twenty feet. Two company-barracks and the guard-house form the western side of the parade; two company-barracks and the bake-house, its eastern side; the officers' quarters, its southern side, and the hospital, headquarters building, and the commissary store-house, its northern side. All these buildings are stone structures, solid and enduring in appearance, but in appearance only, for the walls are made of rubble-stones, (basaltic lava,) only 18 inches in thickness, except as to the guard-house, of which the walls are 2 feet in thickness. The workmanship and the materials used are very inferior. Nevertheless, considering the general character of the buildings at Army posts, these are pre-eminently good. Around the parade and in front of the four lines of buildings, double rows of cottonwood-trees have been planted, the space (50 feet) between the two ranks of trees being designed for walks and roads. Along each row of trees a small stream of water, derived from the Beaver River, has been made to flow, which furnishes the necessary irrigation to the trees, and a supply of water to all parts of the post.

The post is designed for the accommodation of four companies of infantry.

The company-barracks consist of a main building 100 by 40 feet, and a projection 40 by 30 feet, whereby they become L-shaped. They have shingle roofs; their walls are covered with one coat of rough plastering; the ceilings remain unplastered. The main building is divided into a barrack-room, a first-sergeant's room, and a store-room; the projection, into a mess-room and kitchen. No provision has been made for a bath or wash room and reading-room. A bath-room is all the more an urgent need, since, even in summer, the water of the river is too cold for bathing. With a full company of sixty men, the air-space per man in the barrack-room is 566 cubic feet. For the ventilation of the barracks no special inlets and outlets for the air exist; oppositely-placed windows and doors, open ceilings, and imperfect closure between the roof and the walls, admit and diffuse an abundance of fresh air; but the air causes cold and unpleasant draughts. Sufficient day-light is admitted, and at night artificial light is meagerly obtained from candles. The barracks are warmed by means of wood-burning stoves; the ingress of cold air is, however, so great that thorough warming is impossible. The beds in the dormitories consist of excellent iron bedsteads, (each man having a separate bed,) of bed-sacks filled with hay, which is properly renewed, and of a sufficient number of blankets. The mess-rooms are provided with tables, benches, and all necessary mess-furniture. The kitchens are furnished with large cooking-stoves, and a good supply of kitchen-utensils.

The latrines are placed at a proper distance to the rear of the barracks, and are well constructed.

The new officers' quarters are built according to the plan recommended to the Secretary of War by the board on revision of the Army Regulations, as published in the Report of the Secretary of War for the year 1872. They consist of commanding officer's quarters and five company officers' quarters, each of which contains two sets of captains' quarters. All these buildings are one and a half story houses, with projections to the rear for the kitchens. The half-stories have dormer windows on two sides. They are plastered with two coats of plaster and a coat of hard-finish of plaster of Paris. Ample provision is made for closets, fitted with shelves. The commanding officer's quarters consist of ten rooms with pantry and store-room. The dimensions of the rooms in the main building, eight in number, are 15 by 18 feet each, a hall of 8 feet wide dividing the rooms into sets of two, which communicate with each other, on the first floor, by means of folding-doors. The two rooms in the projection measure 15 by 16 feet. A piazza runs across the front of the main building and on one side of the projection. A captain's quarters consist of two rooms, 15 by 18 feet, on the first floor of the main building, and two attic chambers, of the same dimensions, on the second floor; and of a kitchen-room, with an intervening porch between it and the main building, readily convertible into a dining-room, in the projection. Each set of quarters has a separate hall of 7 feet wide. A piazza runs across the front of the main building.

The headquarters-building is a one-story house, 43 by 34½ feet. It is divided into four rooms, each 16 by 16 feet, and a hall of 8 feet. These rooms serve as commanding officer's office, adjutant's office, quartermaster's office, and court-martial room.

The guard-house is a one-story house, 58½ by 24 feet. Its walls are two feet thick. The interior is divided into a prison and guard-room, each 20 feet square, and officers' room, 12 by 20 feet. The prison-room has special outlets and inlets for its ventilation, loop-holes, namely, above and below. It has one window, with iron grating, and one door. The heating of the room is adequately effected by stoves.

The commissary store-house measures 28 by 100 feet. It is unplastered except as to the office and issuing-room. It is divided into a store-room, 26 by 79½ feet, an office and an issuing-room, each 10½ by 18 feet. Underneath there is a cellar 26 by 96 feet, and 7 feet deep.

The post-hospital is a two-story regulation hospital of twelve beds, as described in Circular No. 2, "Approved Plans and Specification for Post-Hospitals, Surgeon General's Office, Washington, July 27, 1871." A water-tank over the ceiling of the second story, to be filled from the tank-cistern by means of a force-pump, is provided for in the specification, but no provision has been made to distribute thence the water to the various apartments of the building, thus rendering the tank an expensive folly. Attention to this omission was called with the result that the necessary pipes, &c., were authorized to be laid, provided the amount set aside for the building of this post would cover the expenses. The contractor, however, very naturally declines to provide anything not stipulated for in the original specification. An expensive cistern, 15 feet deep and 15 feet in diameter, has been built. Now, it so happens that there is not sufficient rain-fall during the year to make it worth the while to collect it for use. In order to turn the cistern to account the river-water will be made to flow into it, but a smaller and less expensive cistern would have answered the purpose of such a reservoir equally well.

As no provision, in the specifications, was made for a cellar, a separate cellar in the rear of the hospital, 16 by 16 feet, with walled sides and earth roof, was made by a detail of garrison prisoners. The walls of the hospital are only 18 inches thick; indeed the specifications provided for walls of 16 inches only; the contractor, of his own motion, made them 18 inches. Considering the height of the walls, the character of material used, viz, rubble-stones and bad mortar, some apprehension may justly be entertained as to the safety of the building; the more so, as earthquakes are known to occur here. The hospital is well plastered throughout, hard finished with plaster of Paris. The dispensary is fitted with shelves, drawers, and counter; the store-rooms and closets are likewise fitted with shelves. The ventilation of the ward is effected by means of windows, doors, ventilating-shaft, communicating with the ridge-ventilator, and two cold-air pipes laid between the joists and opening under the floor of the piazza, and provided with register-valves. The hospital is a fine one in appearance, and, notwithstanding its faults and defects, will answer its purpose very well.

The post-bakery is a good, plastered, stone building, and has an oven of ample capacity.

The corral and stables are situated to the west of the post, at a distance of about 300 yards. The stables are shingled frame buildings, which provide ample room for the animals at the post.

The laundresses, of whom there are thirteen, are as yet badly provided for. They are housed in tents and shanties, which stand scattered in the neighborhood of the corral.

The post-library is in the adjutant's office and is in charge of the post-treasurer. It is as yet merely a nucleus for future growth; important additions to it are daily expected.

The natural drainage of the post, produced by the gradual inclination of the ground toward the river and by the porousness of the soil, is quite sufficient.

The post is well policed; offal and rubbish are carted away to a distance and there burned.

Company and hospital gardens, which are situated to the east and west of the post, along the river, have been cultivated with signal success, and abundance of potatoes—and this tuber grows to perfection—of turnips, onions, cabbage, carrots, parsnips, lettuce, beans, pease, and radishes were raised. For the cultivation of the hospital garden a detail of one man is made.

The agricultural productiveness of the country is not great, the land adapted for cultivation being limited to the vicinity of mountain-streams. Potatoes, wheat, and barley are the staple productions. Fruit of no kind has been successfully cultivated. Apples and peaches, however, are plentifully brought here from the more northern settlements of the valley; peaches and grapes from settlements in the south, viz, from Saint George and its vicinity. Apples are sold at $3 a bushel, peaches from $3 to $5 a bushel, and grapes at 15 to 20 cents a pound. In the neighboring town of Beaver there is a number of stores, some of which are of considerable size, especially the co-operative store, which is supplied with an extensive stock. Considering the distance from large markets the prices of the goods are very moderate. A number of cows are kept at the post, which are readily obtainable for temporary use from the citizens, some of whom are extensively engaged in stock-raising, for which the mountain-ranges offer some advantages.

The inhabitants of the vicinity are principally Mormons. They are mostly immigrants, of the lowest orders, from England, Scotland, and Wales. Gross ignorance and fanatical subserviency to the priesthood are their chief characteristics. To the priesthood they look for guidance in all the affairs of life, and even for healing in sickness. The gentiles, among them, they look upon as a necessary evil which must needs be tolerated, but contact with them they consider contamination to the latter-day saints.

The mail is served daily, irregularities, however, being of frequent occurrence. Between Beaver City and the nearest railway station, viz, Provo City, fifty miles south of Salt Lake City, the mail is carried by stage-line. As the Utah Southern Railroad is in course of construction, the nearest railroad station will, from time to time, become less distant. Mail communication with the department headquarters at Omaha requires five days; with Washington City, nine days.

*Consolidated sick-report, Beaver City, Utah, 1871–'74.*

| Year | | 1871–'72. | | 1872–'73. | | 1873–'74. | |
|---|---|---|---|---|---|---|---|
| Mean strength { Officers | | 12 | | 12 | | 11 | |
| Enlisted men | | 169 | | 203 | | 195 | |
| Diseases. | | Cases. | Deaths. | Cases. | Deaths. | Cases. | Deaths. |
| GENERAL DISEASES, A. | | | | | | | |
| Typhoid fever | | | | 4 | | 1 | |
| Intermittent fever | | 1 | | 5 | | | |
| Other diseases of this group | | | | 3 | | 25 | |
| GENERAL DISEASES, B. | | | | | | | |
| Rheumatism | | | | 20 | | 19 | |
| Syphilis | | | | 2 | | 2 | |
| Consumption | | 1 | | 4 | 1 | | |
| Other diseases of this group | | | | 2 | | | |
| LOCAL DISEASES. | | | | | | | |
| Catarrh and bronchitis | | | | 55 | | 56 | |
| Pneumonia | | | | 3 | | 1 | |
| Diarrhœa and dysentery | | 2 | | 20 | | 38 | |
| Hernia | | | | | | 2 | |
| Other local diseases | | 3 | | 70 | | 72 | 2 |
| Alcoholism | | | | 8 | | 13 | |
| Total disease | | 7 | | 196 | 1 | 229 | 2 |
| VIOLENT DISEASES AND DEATHS. | | | | | | | |
| Gunshot wounds | | | | | | 1 | |
| Other accidents and injuries | | 1 | | 39 | | 35 | |
| Total violence | | 1 | | 39 | | 36 | |

## CHEYENNE DEPOT, WYOMING TERRITORY.

### INFORMATION FURNISHED BY ACTING ASSISTANT SURGEON A. J. HOGG, UNITED STATES ARMY.

Camp Cheyenne, a *sub-post* of and a mile distant from Fort D. A. Russell, is in the southeastern part of Wyoming Territory, in latitude 41° 8' north and longitude 27° 42' west, near the town of Cheyenne, a station on the Union Pacific Railroad.

The garrison consists of Company B, Twenty-third United States Infantry, a strength of forty-two enlisted men, who are quartered in an excellent barrack-building. Dormitories are well ventilated and warmed; iron bedsteads are used. There is a set of quarters for married soldiers.

Officers' quarters are three sets, and very comfortable. The guard-house is small. There is no hospital. The sick of the command are cared for by the medical officers stationed at Fort D. A. Russell.

Water of a very inferior quality is obtained from a creek which runs near the post. This creek also runs past, and very near to, Fort Russell, and, receiving the drainage of that post, becomes the receptacle of the slops from its laundresses' quarters, as well as the filth from its cavalry stables.

## CAMP DOUGLAS, UTAH TERRITORY.

### REPORT OF SURGEON E. P. VOLLUM, UNITED STATES ARMY.

Camp Douglas is situated on a plateau at the base of the Wahsatch Mountains, two and a half miles east of the business portion of Salt Lake City, at an altitude of 730 feet above it. The altitude of sun-dial is 4,904 feet.* Latitude, 40° 46' 2'' north; longitude, 35° west.

In July, 1862, Col. P. E. Connor, Third California Volunteers, then on duty at Benicia, Cal., received orders to proceed with his command to Utah Territory and establish a military post

---

*Information furnished by Lieut. William L. Marshall, United States Engineers, of Lieutenant Wheeler's exploring expedition.

near Salt Lake City, the object being the protection of the "overland mail-route," then menaced by Indians. Colonel Connor, with six companies of his own regiment and four companies of the Second California Cavalry, numbering some 800 men, arrived at Camp Floyd on the 17th of October, 1862. The command in a day or two took up its line of march to the city, but in consequence of various rumors to the effect that their march would meet with opposition from the Mormon authorities, it halted at the bridge crossing the Jordan River, seven miles from the city. Meantime Colonel Connor, in citizen's dress, had explored the country about Jordan Valley and the foothills on the east and north of the city, and had determined upon the present site of Camp Douglas for his camping-ground, on account of the abundance of good water and the command it would exercise over the city; for while his orders only related to the "overland mail-route," yet the spirit that manifested itself among the Mormons in those days, made it desirable for him to settle upon a site naturally as unassailable as possible. Instead of a hostile demonstration at the Jordan bridge, the command was met by a delegation of Federal and territorial officers and prominent citizens, who welcomed the troops to the country, and on the 20th of the same month they marched through the principal streets of the city, and encamped on the spot where the post cemetery is now located. The officers of the command desired that the camp should be named in honor of their commander, but in the order on the subject he named it after the distinguished Senator, Stephen A. Douglas.

As soon as the command was sufficiently rested preparations were made to go into winter-quarters, which consisted of "dug-outs," and were called "Connor tents" by the troops. They were comfortable, however, and the two following years were spent in them with but little sickness. The first building erected was the present adjutant's office, which was put up shortly after the arrival of the command, and during the summer and fall of 1863 the remaining permanent buildings, all of square logs, were erected, solely by the labor of the troops. The timber necessary was all obtained at a great height upon the Wahsatch range at a point some twelve miles southward.

The reservation was at first declared to be one mile square, but in order to have full command of the stream of water that flowed through the camp, it was enlarged to two miles square, and so remains. In December, 1862, the cemetery was laid out, and in time it was surrounded by a substantial stone fence, inside of which a row of trees was set out and irrigated from a neighboring spring. The gentiles having no cemetery of their own, have always preferred to lay their dead in this place, and their feelings in this particular have generally been gratified by the post-commanders, and even at this date, (January, 1874,) this class of citizens desire to enlarge and ornament it at their own expense for the wants of the future.

The shade-trees at the post, which constitute a great ornament, were presented to Colonel Connor by Mr. Fox, a nurseryman of Salt Lake City, and were planted in the fall of 1863.

In 1864 the building now occupied by the post-commander was erected by General Connor for himself and staff, and he transferred to it the headquarters of the District of Utah, and at the same time re-assumed the command of the post, and so continued till the summer of 1865, when he was assigned to the command of the District of the Plains, leaving Colonel George, of the First Nevada Cavalry, in command. General Connor returned to the command of this post in the fall of 1865, and remained till he was mustered out of the service June 1, 1866.

Maj. William H. Lewis, Thirty-sixth Infantry, relieved Colonel Potter, Fifth United States Infantry, (a short time in command,) in the summer of 1866, and remained till relieved by General John Gibbon, Seventh United States Infantry, who remained about one year, and to him the garrison to-day is indebted for its fine system of water-courses, by which the post is abundantly supplied with good water, flowing at every turn throughout the post, and which, besides being a beautiful and refreshing feature, is essential for irrigating the shade-trees and the gardens. He also conceived the idea of the artificial lake in front of the commanding-officer's quarters, which is a gem in its way, and useful as well as beautiful, as it furnishes abundance of ice for the whole command, and is used during the short skating season as a rink.

In August, 1870, General Gibbon was relieved by General P. R. De Trobriand, Colonel Thirteenth United States Infantry, and in October of the same year he was relieved by Lieut. Col. H. N. Morrow, Thirteenth United States Infantry, who took up the improvements left off by General Gibbon, and has pushed them up to date with zeal and energy. He enlarged the above lake to five times its original size; laid out, graded, and graveled a mile of new road to Salt Lake City; erected the chapel; set out some three hundred trees, and graded and graveled the roads and paths about the garrison.

The camp faces and commands the city on the west. Its general arrangement is shown by Figure 53.

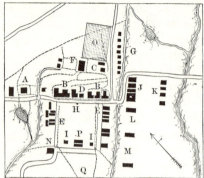

Figure 53.

A, commanding-officer's quarters; B, officers' quarters; C, surgeon's quarters; D, adjutant's office; E, barracks; F, hospital; G, laundresses' quarters; H, flag-staff; I, magazine; J, quartermaster and subsistence store-houses; K, workshops; L, cavalry-stables; M, coal-sheds; N, post-trader; O, hospital garden; P, guard-house; Q, company garden.

Fine dotted lines indicate irrigating streams.

The parade is 375 by 275 feet, and has a stream of water on three sides. There are eleven sets of barracks, nine of which are old buildings of hewn pine and cottonwood, worthless, and rapidly going to decay.

A new barrack has been built, in accordance with drawings of military buildings issued by the War Department, Quartermaster-General's Office, Washington, D. C., September 14, 1870. It is 100 feet long by 30 feet wide in the clear, two stories high, the ceilings being each 10 feet high, and is built of red sandstone, which is found in great abundance on the reservation. The corners and window and door sills are dressed, and the lintels over the doors and windows are flat arches. On the front and rear are triangular pediments in the center, the roof of which reaches nearly to the ridge of the main building. These pediments are provided with circular louvered openings, and the gables have the same in half-circle on each side of the chimney, which communicate with the loft, into which the foul air from the dormitory in the second story can pass, by four openings, 2 feet by 4 feet, left in the ceiling, and furnished with a cover on hinges, with cords for raising and lowering, which arrangement secures ample ventilation. The walls are built of rough-hammered ashlar, the stone coming from the quarry, with good flat beds, easily split and shaped. The porch, 8 feet 4 inches wide, extends along the length of the front on both stories; the windows lower from the top; there is no cellar. The first story is subdivided into a first sergeants' room, 15 by 14 by 9 feet; a non-commissioned officers' room, 15 by 14 by 9 feet; day or reading room, 31 by 17 by 9 feet; armory, 10 by 12 by 9 feet; library, 12 by 12 by 9 feet; wash-room, with trough for basins, 12 by 14 by 9 feet; mess-room well fitted up with tables, benches, &c., 30 by 30 by 9 feet; kitchen, 16 by 18 by 9 feet; cooks' room, 9 by 11 by 6 feet; and store-room, 9 feet by 11 feet 6 inches by 9 feet. The second story or dormitory is ceiled, and plastered on the stone walls, and extends without interruption the whole area of the building, 100 by 30 feet, and has space for 80 bedsteads, which allows 375 cubic feet of air per man; the average occupancy will allow each man about twice that amount. The cost of the building was $7,500, the rock being quarried and hauled by the command.

In 1874, the Lieutenant-General having inspected the post and recommended the erection of another barrack on the same plan and opposite to the one just described, to make the post symmetrical, and also the construction of four other sets, one-story buildings, on the plans of the quarters at Fort Cameron, authority was given to commence the work, the buildings to be erected by the labor of the troops assisted by citizen masons and stone-cutters. The total cost of the five buildings is not to exceed $30,000.

The work commenced in October, 1874. The troops cleared off the old structures, prepared the excavations for the foundations and cellars, quarried all the stone, and supplied the sand for making mortar. All materials used were hauled by Government teams. About one-half the carpentering and all the painting were done by soldiers; skilled mechanics were employed for such work as the troops could not perform.

The season was so far advanced before orders were received to commence operations that it was not thought advisable to undertake the erection of more than two sets of quarters in the year 1874.

The ground on which the new quarters had to be built was occupied as a cantonment in 1862–'63, by the volunteer troops commanded by General Connor. They honeycombed the earth with their "dug-outs," as has been previously explained. On account of the insecure character of the ground, it was necessary to excavate to the bottom of many of these pits in order to reach the subsoil. Some of the foundation-walls were carried down to a depth of 10 feet beneath the natural surface.

One of the one-story barracks authorized is now completed.

The structure consists of a main building and two wings. The main building is 103 feet long and 29 feet wide, and has a veranda, 8 feet wide, extending the entire front. The wings are each 23 feet in width, one being 50 feet long and the other $42\frac{1}{2}$. All ceilings are 12 feet in the clear. In one end of the main building, two rooms are partitioned off, each $12\frac{3}{4}$ feet by $14\frac{1}{2}$ feet; one as orderly-room, and the other as a store-room for company property, surplus arms, &c. The remainder of the main building is occupied as a squad-room, the size of which is 85 by 26 feet in the clear, and contains 26,520 cubic feet of air-space. In practice it is found that in a company of sixty men, and all present, there very seldom, if ever, are more than fifty who at any one time occupy the squad-room night or day. There are certain men of every company, such as the first sergeant, hospital attendants, sick, prisoners, married men, and daily guard-details, who are almost invariably absent from the squad-room; the number so absent usually amounts to one-sixth of the aggregate strength of the company. If fifty men occupy the squad-room, each will have 530 feet of air-space. At present, the average strength of the companies at this post is less than forty men. The longer of the two wings is occupied as the mess-room and kitchen; the former is 28 by 20 feet, and the latter, including the pantry and store-room, is $20\frac{1}{2}$ by 20 feet. A cellar, having an extent equal to that of the entire wing, is excavated beneath the floor to the depth of 8 feet, and accommodates not only the company to which it is attached, but that which occupies the adjoining barrack, which is without a cellar. The foundation-walls of the building are carried down to the bottom of the cellar. Two outside doors and four transom-windows afford sufficient light and ventilation. The other and shorter wing contains three rooms: first, a wash-room, opening out of the main barrack; is 10 by 20 feet, and is fitted with a tray or trough for basins, a water-pipe conducts the waste water under the foundations outside the building; second, a reading-room, 18 by 20 feet, fitted with tables, writing-desk, benches, &c.; third, a room for the company tradesmen, 12 by 20 feet.

All walls below the first floor are 2 feet in thickness, and those above are 18 inches thick. The pipes of heating-stoves, used in the main building, lead to flues 6 by 12 inches in cross-section, which are built in the end-walls and are carried out at the apex of the roof, terminating in chimneys of red brick.

The surface of all walls inside and ceilings are plastered with two coats of lime-mortar, the last coat being hand-floated. Through the ceiling of the main building, and communicating with the loft overhead, are five openings, each 26 inches square, and covered by shutters which are opened and closed at will by means of cords and pulleys. There are two such ventilators in ceiling over the mess-room and kitchen, and one over the reading-room. These openings afford ample means of egress for the foul air. The lofts are ventilated by six half-circle louvered windows in the gables, one in either wing and four in the main building. The area of each of these arches is 2 feet square. Through the foundation-walls, under the floor, openings have been left, 6 by 10 inches, through which can escape any exhalations from the soil under the floors. The floor-joists are 2 by 8 inches, laid 18 inches apart, and securely bridged, all supported in the center by a timber, 8 by 12 inches, which rests on stone piers. The floor is of $1\frac{1}{4}$-inch southern yellow pine, tongued and grooved. The floor of the veranda is of the same material, laid down in white lead. The windows are 10 by 16, 12-light, upper and lower sash sliding. The roof has one-third pitch, and is covered with red-wood shingles. The wood-work is painted with three coats oil-paint.

Another barrack will be a duplicate of the one just described; a third has been begun, but owing to the cold weather it was found necessary to discontinue the laying of stone masonry.

Owing to the very considerable incline in the natural surface, it was thought expedient, as a matter of economy, to dispense with one wing of each of the two remaining barracks, and to place the kitchen and mess-rooms in the basement of each. It was found that there was a falling off in the natural surface in the length of the barrack of 8 feet; very little additional excavation was therefore necessary in order to give the needed space for the rooms above alluded to in the basement.

There are ten sets of officers' quarters in all. The set occupied by the post-commander is situated about one hundred yards to the north of the parade, and is built of adobe bricks, containing twenty rooms, and, as mentioned before, was put up to accommodate the general commanding and staff of the district of Utah. The building consists of a central part and two wings; the former has a hall in the middle, 6 by 10 feet by 10 feet 8 inches; opening to the right is a room 26 by 28 feet by 10 feet 8 inches, divided in the middle by folding doors, making it answer for a parlor and dining-room; to the left is a room 17 by 12 feet by 10 feet 8 inches; in the rear of the hall is a room 9 by 12 feet by 10 feet 8 inches; pantry 13 by 10 feet by 10 feet 8 inches; kitchen 19 by 14½ feet by 9 feet. There are plenty of closets, book-cases, and shelves. The attic is partly finished, and partitioned off for servants' rooms. The wings each contain six rooms, respectively, 15 feet 7 inches by 10 by 9 feet, 11 by 11 by 9 feet, 16 by 8 by 9 feet, 15 feet 7 inches by 10 feet 7 inches by 9 feet, 10 by 9 by 9 feet, and 13 by 13 by 9 feet. In front there is a porch extending the whole length of the main building and wings, 48 feet long by 6 feet wide in front of wings, and 15 feet wide in front of main building. There is a spacious bay-window looking from the front room of the main building, and the porch is deeply shaded by trees. In front and on the north side are spacious gardens, thoroughly irrigated, and the outlook is eastward over a pretty park of trees and lake, and commanding a magnificent view of Salt Lake City, Great Salt Lake itself, with its picturesque mountain-islands, and the ranges bounding the valley on the west. It is well built, commodious, and finished tastefully within by graining and wall-paper. Besides furnishing quarters for the commanding officer, it accommodates two or three subaltern officers in the north wing.

A row of seven sets of officers' quarters faces the parade on the eastern side, and there is a building in the middle of the row occupied as headquarters Thirteenth United States Infantry, with its printing-office and library of 734 books; post headquarters, and library of 635 books, and Western Union telegraph-office. This row of buildings is a humble-looking, one-story, double structure, built of hewn logs, lathed and plastered within, and whitewashed without, and from a short distance presents the appearance of a line of fishermen's huts. As originally put up, each building, comprising quarters for two officers, was 46 feet 6 inches long, 26 feet 6 inches wide, and 9 feet high in the clear. At present the main building of each set has the above dimensions, but the kitchens, which are shed structures of different sizes, and all too small, have been added to the rear, and an extension of a room, 14 feet 6 inches by 14 feet 6 inches wide by 8 feet 6 inches high, has been added to one side of each set, and in one set to both sides. The pitch of each of the several roofs has a different slope, and has been changed from the original angle so as to reach over the kitchens. Put up as these quarters were by unskilled labor, they were only intended to answer a temporary purpose for the accommodation of bachelor officers, but they have been patched up in various ways, by the addition of closets, &c., to adapt them to the necessities of officers' families. Having been built flat on the ground, without any other foundation than the bottom logs, the addition of the kitchens to the rear, so as to keep the same level as the front portion of the building, had to be made in an excavation several feet deep, the consequence of which was that the surface-drainage flowing down-hill from the rear, soaked down the sides of the kitchen, and sometimes it came up under the floors, rendering them sloppy in winter and damp in all seasons of the year. Besides these defects, these quarters have no eave-troughs, and the droppings from the roof passed into the ground underneath and rotted the foundation logs on all sides. As might be supposed, this row of quarters was very unhealthy, and in the winter of 1871-'72 an unprecedented amount of sickness of a febrile and catarrhal character occurred in them, requiring a visit from the medical officer to each quarters at least twice a day, and in some sets every member of the family, servants included, would be found down in bed at the same time. Tracing their sickness to the rotted, wet, and foul condition of the foundation logs and flooring of these buildings, the medical officer repeatedly recommended, in the most urgent manner, that the ground at the rear of them be cut entirely away for some distance to the rear, to let in the rays of the sun, which had never shone on that side, and to replace all the decayed wood of the buildings by new material. This was done, and the excavation was made to slope backwards from the building, with a ditch at the rear side, where a stone wall was put up to sustain the earth. The amount of rotted and water-soaked wood-work that was removed was surprising, but the decaying process had been going on for some years. Eave-troughs were also put up, and the drainage in every respect was made thorough, and the result of all these changes has been an entire disappearance of the diseases that used to be of every day's experience—a happy result that will continue till more decayed wood accumulates, which is certain, as there is no protection of the foundation logs from moisture. A clearer case of cause, effect, and applied remedy in sanitary matters, than the above, never came under the writer's notice. During the past three years, a very considerable amount of repairing has been done to these quarters, yet they are becoming dilapidated rapidly, and the time must soon come when it will be a waste of money to repair them any longer, or it will be better economy to replace them by new ones, as has been recommended by the medical officer several times.

On each side of the hospital stand two other sets of officers' quarters, built of adobes, and each containing six rooms of a fair size, two larger rooms being 18 feet long by 12 feet wide by 9 feet high; the smaller rooms, containing a good amount of closet-room, are of no uniform dimensions. One of these quarters is occupied by the medical officer, and the other is usually assigned to the post quartermaster. At the rear of all the officers' quarters are good-sized yards, divided off by lumber fences, and all the buildings of the post are whitewashed.

The bake-house is built substantially of red sandstone, 20 by 28 by 9½ feet, partitioned off for the baker's room.

The guard-house is built of lumber, with gable-roof and in good style, and sits in front of the old stone building formerly used as such, now converted into a prisoners' room, but connected with it by a covered passage-way 12½ feet by 15 feet by 9 feet. It is 35 feet by 15 feet by 9 feet 2 inches in the clear, subdivided into a guard-room 15 feet by 26 feet by 9 feet 2 inches, not ceiled, heated by a fire-place, and ventilated by a covered opening in the roof-ridge, provided with flaps to close in stormy weather; an officer of the guard's room, 9 feet by 15 feet 8 inches by 9 feet, ceiled, lined with boards, and heated by a fire-place; and a hall leading from the front to the prisoners' room at the rear, 6 by 15 by 9 feet. The time-honored board platforms are provided for the guard to "sleep" upon during the interval of their tours of duty, and until lately, they have worried through the tedious hours, as elsewhere in the Army, in the vain endeavor to snatch a little sleep, in obedience to a cruel custom of the service that requires the guard to find rest in this way. On the recommendation of the medical officer, however, the post-commander has allowed the members of the guard to have bed-ticks filled with straw, and if they are not rendered thereby as comfortable as when in their own quarters, (and there seems to be no sound reason why they should not be equally so, under all possible circumstances,) they, as well as all parties concerned, are well satisfied with the propriety of the change from boards to straw.

Between the guard-house and prisoners' room, on the side of the intervening passage-way, a space has been utilized for a fire-engine house, 15 feet by 9 feet by 9 feet high, and it is occupied by a "Champion Chemical Fire-Engine, No. 1," which is under the exclusive charge of one of the infantry companies. When an alarm of fire is given, every company proceeds to the point of danger with axes, ladders, and buckets, which are always kept filled with water, and the company in charge of the engine works it unmolested by any other parties.

The chapel, used for a school, court-martial room, &c., is built of squared logs, boarded on the outside, lathed and plastered within; is 15½ feet by 26½ feet by 9½ feet high, and is surmounted with a belfry, containing a large plantation-bell.

The hospital has been changed since the issue of Circular No. 4, Surgeon-General's Office, December 5, 1870, by the addition of an extension to the rear, lathed and plastered, making room for a kitchen 13½ feet by 15 feet 3 inches by 9 feet 1 inch high; a knapsack-room, which also serves for a post-mortem room, 13½ feet by 11 feet 9 inches by 9 feet 1 inch high; a hall-way 13½ feet by 7 feet 8 inches by 9 feet 1 inch high; a coal-bin and cellar. Windows have been put in the upper story, which is used as store-rooms. The building has been recently roofed, floored throughout, and thoroughly painted and renovated; but it is rapidly becoming dilapidated, and a new building, to be built of red sandstone, has been estimated for and recommended.

The ice-house is built of logs, with a mud roof, 30 feet by 15 feet by 12 feet; thus far it has preserved the ice very well, on account of the numerous apertures arising from its rude construction, which admitted of free ventilation and the passing off of the moisture arising from the ice.

The post is situated on a broad gravel-bench, at the base of the Wahsatch Range, looking westward. This gravel-bench is one of a series that extend as far as the eye can reach, and rise one above another from the valley up to the base of the mountains surrounding the basin-country, and is a part of the old shore-line of Great Salt Lake as it existed in the glacial period, when the entire basin was filled with water.

Geologists speak familiarly of this ancient lake, which is believed to have extended all the way from the basin-country of Idaho on the north, down to some point in Arizona, throughout the whole of which distance the beach-lines can be easily traced. These well-defined benches slope off, one above another, and are several hundred feet apart, and they are accounted for by the supposition that the rocky barriers that held the water back on the south gave way at different times to the denuding action of the water, and let the level of the lake down several hundred feet at one outburst, till a level was found within the limits of the present Salt Lake Valley. After the mountains surrounding the valley became denuded by the elements, down to a level below the permanent snow-line, the glaciers gradually ceased to form, and the evaporation became greater than the supply of water, and the lake diminished slowly but steadily down to its present limits, which represents the exact balance held between the inflow and the evaporation. The theory of the above periodic outburst of the water southward, finds support in the unparalleled deep cut forming the bed of the Colorado River, it being in places five thousand feet deep, through solid rock.

Looking out, on a winter's morning, from the elevated site of the post, the valley is often seen filled up with floating vapor to the highest level of the old lake-shore, and the valley, with its thriving cities and settlements, and the bases of the surrounding mountains, are submerged, as it were, a thousand feet under water, forming a perfect image of the ancient scene. On the Wahsatch Range, rising on the reservation at the east of the post, the Cretaceous sandstones, and limy and bituminous shales are found; and there are some evidences of the existence of brown coal at the same depth, which doubtless represent the western edge of the zone of coal that crops out 18 miles to the eastward on a grand scale. A few miles to the south of the post the Carboniferous and Devonian ages are well represented around the flanks of the "great dome" of granite, in the celebrated Cottonwood district. The old silurian, quartzite, and crystalline schists are seen in folds, tilted up at high angles. The neighborhood of the post, as well as the whole of Utah, is essentially a mineral country. Her mountain-ranges, covering about two-thirds of her entire area of 84,476 square miles, abound in metallic ores, principally silver and galena, chemically combined; but copper, iron, coal, zinc, gold, and sulphur have also been found in large quantities within her borders.

The extent of the silver-bearing belt of Utah is but partly explored, but as far as the experts and prospectors have made it known, it comes into the Territory at the north from Idaho, following the Wahsatch Range as far south as the marvelous metalliferous deposits in the Cottonwood and American Fork Cañons, where it sends out a branch through the mountains of Parley's Park, and onward to the east along the Uintah Mountains, as far as the Colorado line; another branch continues southward as far as Mount Nebo, where it ends, and the cretaceous sand-rocks overlying the great coal-measures of the southeast commence. It is found again in all of the ranges occupying the western part of the Territory, all the way down to the Arizona line, making an area of not less than 28,158 square miles in extent. This immense silver-bearing region, though believed to exist by the mining world for some years, was quite locked up by the determined opposition of the Mormon authorities, who objected to the working of the precious metals within their borders. It is said that General A. S. Johnston, while at Camp Floyd in 1857, decided upon a similar policy. The man who discovered the mineral-deposits, now so extensively worked in "Camp Floyd district," was a trader connected with Johnston's command; and, seeking a private interview with him, pointed out the extent and value of the minerals buried in the surrounding hills, traversed, more or less, every day by members of his command. Being an excellent mineralogist himself, he readily saw, from the specimens shown him, the truth of the man's statement, and foresaw also the excitement and demoralization that would follow in his command were the presence of the precious metals in the neighborhood of his camp made known. He dismissed his informant, in his peculiar way, with the most solemn threat that his life would be forfeited if he failed to keep his secret; which he held faithfully until recently, when he saw the adventurous prospectors moving about the mountains in the vicinity, like solitary and restless spirits. General Connor, however, in 1863, let loose his California volunteers, largely composed of miners and prospectors, among the mountains, and soon the riches of the "Cottonwoods" were turned up to view. The barriers against the outside world were more effectually overridden by the Pacific Railroad, and the adventurous miners flowed in from the neighboring Territories and California, and brought the treasures to light in all parts of the country; yet the conflict of the jurisdiction of the courts, arising from the antagonism and confusion of religious and political views and interests, between the Mormons and "Gentiles," preventing the settling of questions of law regarding these interests, still keeps out enterprise and capital, and large districts, known to contain extensive deposits of the richest ores, lie undeveloped; in fact, nine-tenths of this great mineral belt may be said to be as yet only scratched over. Notwithstanding these obstacles, Utah, in 1873, rose to the third in rank of the precious-metal-bearing States or Territories, and sent out, exclusive of gold, $11,000,000 in silver bullion, base bullion, and silver-ores.

Iron-ores are found in considerable quantities within eight miles of the post. In Iron County, in the southern part of the Territory, the largest deposits of iron are found that lie between the Mississippi River and the Pacific Ocean, consisting of red and brown hematites, magnetic carbonates, and specular ores. All of these varieties are to be found in immense quantities, near together, in the neighborhood of beds of coal of good quality. So far only one furnace has been put up for the reduction of these ores, but the success has been good.

The coal of Utah comprises several varieties of lignite, of good quality, suitable for all the industrial and domestic uses. The coal-measures are not second in extent to any in the known world. One of them reaches nearly the whole length of the Territory, and is about 300 miles long by 150 miles wide. The beds, varying from 3 to 25 feet thick, generally lie quite horizontal, above the water-line of the country and the plane of the valleys, and are easily reached and worked by the cañons and cuts denuded into them in many places. Several varieties sell in Salt Lake City for from $8 to $11 per ton.

The agricultural portion of the Territory comprises about one-third of the area; consists of strips of valley-land, running generally north and south, between the mountain ranges; are fertile, and under irrigation yield sufficient crops of wheat, barley, oats, Indian corn, and all of the garden vegetables, to enable the people to export these staples in considerable quantities. In 1873, 150 car-loads, of 20,000 pounds each, of barley, and 25 of flour have been shipped to the East; and 300 car-loads of wheat were shipped to San Francisco.

The climate is quite similar to that of Northwestern Texas and New Mexico, and is agreeable most of the year round, excepting for a month or so in winter. The temperature in winter seldom drops to zero, and only two observations below that point have been taken since the post was established. The humidity reaches its maximum in the spring months, when the atmosphere is almost saturated. This arises from the winds at this season passing over Great Salt Lake from the northward, bringing the watery vapors not only from that great body of water, but also from the regions beyond, supplied by the southwesterly currents, that are seen to pass over at a great altitude, most of the winter long. Great Salt Lake, with a shore-line, exclusive of offsets, of 291 miles,* is vast enough to furnish a horizon, in places, like the ocean itself, and being at an altitude of 4,200 feet, some travelers have imagined that on its shore was to be found the most unique and peculiar climate on the face of the globe, combining as it does, the light, pure air of the neighboring snow-capped mountains with that of the briny lake itself, and it is fancied by many that at certain points one may inhale an atmosphere salty and marine, like that found on the shores of the Atlantic, happily combined with a cool, fresh mountain air, like the breath of the Alps themselves. Owing to the absence of marine vegetation about the shores, however, there are none of the pleasant odors to be found as on the sea-shore. For several years past the snow has seldom fallen to a greater depth than a foot, and it soon melts away, while up to 1860 a fall of three feet was not uncommon, with sleighing for a month or so at a time. No tide-gauge observations have ever been made to determine the change in the level of

* Captain Stansbury's Exploration and Survey of the Valley of the Great Salt Lake, 1862, p. 216.

Great Salt Lake, but the inhabitants about the shore estimate that it has risen about one foot a year during the past ten years, which change of level has been caused by the steady increase of the rain-fall of the country, as well as the swelling of the streams flowing into the lake, that drain about one-half of the Territory, most of them flowing from the mining districts, where the tunneling, excavations, blasting, &c., tap the mountains in thousands of places where water never flowed before, for every mine becomes a source of water, sometimes in large amount. The increase in the atmospheric humidity is no doubt in large part caused by the multiplication, of late years, of the irrigating-canals, which expose an immense area of water for evaporation. This is evident in many places by the increased fertility of the lands and greenness of the landscape, and if it continues the necessities of agriculture will soon be met, which in fact is the case at present, were the annual amount, about 20 inches, well distributed throughout the year.

The spring begins about the middle of March, and it is a splendid season. The atmosphere becomes as clear as a diamond, distances vanish as by enchantment, and Great Salt Lake, twenty miles off, appearing like a broad band of indigo, studded with mountain-islands, set on its surface like glittering jewels, seems but an hour's ride away. The city, which is a vast orchard dotted with houses half buried in the foliage, becomes a mass of color, variegated by clumps of the bright blossoms of the peach, pear, apple, plum, and apricot, mingled with the tender colors of the willow, cottonwood, and mulberry. The bright green surface of the valley follows the snow-line as it rises up the mountain sides, leaving a strip of russet color between.

The summer may be said to be hot, dry, and dusty. The mercury seldom rises above 95°, though once, in August, 1871, it reached 105°, and the range is about 30° during the hottest weather, which is necessary to insure the cool breezes found so refreshing at night after the heat of the day. At this season the atmosphere is yellow and brassy, and the flying dust-clouds, from the parched desert surfaces hundreds of miles away, pass over the highest mountains and thicken the air, and while the valley may be regarded as an oasis, yet at this season it furnishes its quota of dust, and the teamsters and road people coming in from a journey suffer from ophthalmia, irritative catarrh, and cough, caused by impalpable particles of alkaline matter that fill the air.

The autumn, on account of the high winds, is the most unpleasant season of the year, and the dust-storms often obscure the noon-day sun, and fill every nook and corner with dirt, from which there is no escape; but as the season advances the aerial movements dwindle down to little spiral dust-whirls, that may be seen in many parts of the valley at the same time, furnishing a curious spectacle. In October, the atmosphere, crisp and bracing, clears up again as in spring, and the landscape softens with the rich browns, russets, and scarlets of the dying vegetation, which reaches high up and mingles with the high rocks at the tops of the mountains, soon to be overlaid, however, in these elevated situations, by the first snows of the season.

The new-comer for a short while feels a difficulty of breathing, arising from the altitude, and the same trouble is often seen with horses, and occasionally travelers speak of feeling giddy and nauseated from the same cause. About once in ten years an epidemic of "mountain-fever" appears to a considerable extent throughout the Rocky Mountain regions, including Utah. Its last appearance was in the fall and winter of 1871–'72. It is a malarial fever commencing as an intermittent, passing on to a remittent, then into a typhoid condition. It may often be cut short by prompt large doses of quinine, but after the typhoid symptoms set in it should be regarded as typhoid fever, and so treated. The mortality is often high, but reduced in proportion to the attention a patient receives in the early stages.

SPECIAL REPORT ON SOME DISEASES OF UTAH, BY SURGEON E. P. VOLLUM, UNITED STATES ARMY.

Regarding the principal diseases of Salt Lake Valley, and the influence of the climate and the altitude on lung troubles especially, I will summarize my views briefly as follows: The adult population are as robust as any within the borders of the United States, and there is a fair number of cases of extreme old age. The weight of sickness falls upon the children, who furnish not less than two-thirds of all the deaths, most of which occur under five years of age. Looking over the register of the undertakers at Salt Lake City, I find the causes of death classified under these headings: "Males, females, adults, children, country, transient, resident, bowels, lungs, brain, fevers, inflammations, child-bed, still-born, old age, polygamy, monogamy, killed accidentally, dropsy, debility, and sundries;" the last heading meaning, unclassified. The following abstract from the undertakers' books shows the percentage of deaths of the diseases mentioned to the whole number of deaths for the years quoted, up to September, 1874:

| Diseases of the— | 1870. | 1871. | 1872. | 1873. | 1874. |
|---|---|---|---|---|---|
| Bowels | 20.10 | 23.36 | 26.44 | 21.15 | 10.87 |
| Lungs | 23.34 | 23.58 | 19.55 | 20.00 | 26.23 |
| Brain | 12.10 | 5.24 | 5.28 | 6.87 | 8.22 |
| Fever | ........ | 11.13 | 10.24 | 13.20 | 12.46 |

The figures of the register show that the male deaths exceed the female in number about 50 per cent. I cannot get the relative proportion. The polygamous children are as healthy as the monogamous, and the proportion of deaths is about the same; the difference is rather in favor of the polygamous children, who are generally, in the city especially, situated more comfortably as to residence, food, air, and clothing, their parents being better off than those in monogamy. It is perhaps too early to express any mature opinions as to the influence of polygamy, as contrasted with monogamy, on the health or constitutional or mental character of the Anglo-Saxon race as seen in Utah; but, as far as the experience has gone, which is long enough to furnish quite a population ranging from twenty-five years downward, no difference can be detected in favor of one or the other. Polygamy in Utah, as far as I can learn, furnishes no idiocy, insanity, rickets, tubercles or struma, or other cachexia, or debasing constitutional condition of any kind. The great mortality in the children here is confined chiefly to the Mormon population, and it may be traced to absence of medical aid, nursing, proper food for sick children, and neglect of all kinds. Among the many mottoes that decorated the Tabernacle on the last anniversary of the advent of the Mormons into Utah was, "Utah's Best Crop: Children." Abundance doubtless cheapens the value of anything, children as well, especially when the issue of several women are begotten in poverty, and all mingled together and contending like birds in a nest for the morsels within reach. The children of Salt Lake City may often be seen in groups insufficiently clad, the lower half of the body bare, playing about in the cold water, that flows directly from the mountains, and down each side of the streets, in front of the residences. The consequence is catarrhs, pneumonia, fevers, and bowel complaints. The nonsensical mummery of the "laying on of hands" is taught and practiced by the priesthood, as a cure for disease, and the faithful and more ignorant resort to it with confidence. Many marvelous cures are narrated as having been brought about by the sacred touch and incantations of the priests; this, with the tea of the sage-brush, and other old woman's slops, constitute the treatment of most of the sick Mormon children, with such consequences as might be expected. A considerable number of cases of necrosis of the tibia in the children occur, and they are attributed to the devitalizing influence of the habit of the children dabbling in the cold mountain-streams, taking effect on the points of bruises and contusions, so common on the legs of children everywhere. Some observers imagine they notice a saddened expression of countenance on the Mormon children; that they have not the cheeriness and laughter common to that age; especially that the young women, who here are robust, ruddy, and well made, lack the amiable, bright and cordial countenance characteristic of young women everywhere, and they attribute this supposed dullness of face to the pre-natal influences of the polygamous relation on the mothers. Certainly at times I have thought that there was some truth in such a notion.

Referring to the undertakers' headings, mentioned above, "bowels" covers chiefly the commoner bowel complaints of children that are caused principally by their exposure to changes of temperature, dabbling in cold water, poor, coarse, and inappropriate food while sick, lime and alkaline drinking-water, and neglect of medical attendance and proper nursing. Under the heading of "lungs" are grouped phthisis, pneumonia, pleurisy, pluro-pneumonia, and bronchitis. Regarding the influence of the altitude and climate of Utah on phthisis, it may be set down as favorable. My experience here with that disease during the past four years has been very small, and my testimony on the subject may therefore be regarded as in favor of the climate. At Camp Douglas my observations have been confined to a few incipient cases among the troops who came from a distance with it and were discharged; to an officer's wife, who inherited it from her father, and who took cold at a ball when far advanced with it, and passed rapidly on to the last stages, returned home and died; and to the case of my assistant, Dr. John E. Spencer, which I will mention. He inherited the disease from his father, developed it by overzeal in hospital and the dissecting-room, and he sought employment in the Army, with a view of getting stationed somewhere in the interior, elevated region of country. Circumstances brought him to this place. When he reported he was pale, thin, and feeble, having some time before had serious hæmoptisis; his pulse was small and rapid, and his respiration hurried and difficult, and a constant harassing cough, that brought up considerable expectoration. A walk of a thousand yards would require him to lie down to recover his wasted strength. His lungs were both consolidated at the top; there was a cavity of some size in the upper lobe of the left lung that gave out a rattling, sibilant sound that could be heard a short distance from him. The bracing weather of the fall coming on soon after his arrival, he commenced to practice a little horseback-riding, and before the winter was well advanced he could ride to Salt Lake City, three miles off, and back, with little fatigue, spending the remainder of the day in comparative quiet. By the following spring, though the winter was open, wet, and changeable, the cavity in his lung was closed up, and gave out no sound to the ear on the chest, and the tubular râles had mostly ceased, and his face took on the color of health; he increased some twenty pounds in weight, and he expressed himself as being as well as he had ever been, his cough having subsided to a minimum condition of a hack, at long intervals, brought on by a bit of food, flying dust, or laughter. During this time he adopted no treatment whatever, and only occasionally took a glass of whisky as a tonic. Having occasion to go to Omaha a year and a half afterward, he contracted measles while there, and returned with his cough re-established and expectorating freely. The cavity in the left lung re-opened, and his general condition nearly as bad as it was when he first reported. Exposure at his door when half-dressed one night, to respond to a patient's call, gave him a chill that was followed the next day by nearly a fatal hæmoptisis. Fearing the influence of the coming winter, he took up his residence at Santa Barbara, Cal., and there regained the good condition he enjoyed at this place; but he allowed his energy to run away with him, he accepted two offices under the corporation, and, after an occasion of overwork and zeal connected with his duties, he had a hemorrhage and died. During my stay here, I have traveled over the length and breadth of the Territory, and have made quite an intimate acquaintance with the people of all classes and degrees, and have yet to learn of a case of phthisis that originated in the country and was unconnected with hereditary transmission. Cases of this kind are sometimes seen in children, the offspring of strumous or consumptive parents. As I have formerly reported, it is the opinion of the local physicians, as well as of the people generally, that if a case comes here in the incipient stage, and is well circumstanced for comforts, that it will get well spontaneously from the beneficial effects of the altitude and the inland dry character of the atmosphere. It is the boast of the people that this is not a consumptive country, which is my opinion decidedly. On the other hand, it is believed that if a patient comes here in the later stages of the disease, that the atmosphere is too rare to give proper support, and that the case will be hastened to a termination more speedily than on the sea-coast.

Altitude is doubtless an important element among the means of relief and cure for phthisis, but it should not be too great. The highest places among the Rocky Mountains have seemed to have a fatal influence on some cases that have been brought indirectly to my attention. The best level has yet to be determined, as the experience of consumptive travelers over the Union Pacific Railroad proves. Patients of this class frequently pass over the road eastward and westward, and they often sink on the way, in consequence of the strain put upon their breathing by the rare atmosphere of the highest places, where they suffer intensely from oppression and difficult breathing. The porters on the sleeping-cars on the road have become accustomed to such cases, and their common remark is, that if such and such a case passes safely over the divide or highest point, at Sherman, which is 8,242 feet above the level of the sea, they will reach the end of their journey, a number of such patients having died near that point.

While at Fort Crook, Cal., in 1849, I saw quite a number of persons in the neighboring country who professed to have been cured of phthisis by crossing the plains on horseback, and from a knowledge of their habits and the conditions of that journey, I then conceived that the best treatment known for consumption was a year of steady daily horseback-riding in a mountainous country, and a diet of corn-bread and bacon, with a moderate quantity of whisky; and I may say, that my experience has taught me nothing better since.

The beneficial influence of this climate on asthma is decided, and deserves a prominent mention. It is also the boast of the people, as well as the physicians, that asthma cannot exist here, excepting under a relieved and modified condition, which I think is the case. I will mention a characteristic case.

Soon after my arrival here in the fall of 1870, I learned from the local physicians that the climate had a beneficial influence on such cases, and I lost no time in informing a young gentleman friend, aged twenty-two years, of the fact. He had no recollection of any period in his life when he had been free from attacks of asthma, and he had spent a good part of every night in his life in inhaling the fumes of niter or stramonium. He spent the year 1869 in quest of some beneficial climate or remedy in all parts of Europe. He arrived here in the fall from Northern New York, where he was born and raised. He was tall, spare, pale, languid, and had never been able to attend business or study to any extent. On his arrival in Salt Lake City he was dispirited, and in a worse condition than he had been for years, his trip to Europe seeming to have made his case worse. He took quarters with me at Camp Douglas, which is 700 hundred feet above Salt Lake City, and 4,800 feet above the sea. I procured him a fine horse and required him to ride with me every day to Salt Lake City, a distance of three miles, to and fro. He would take a good glass of whisky and water, as a regular thing, at each end of the ride. During the following winter, which was often wet, raw, and changeable, I required him to take his ride, in all weathers, and he never omitted it on account of rain, snow, or wind. He braved them all; but having been a house-plant of the most tender raising, he was afraid of taking his death of cold every day, but as the season advanced he began to leave off his mufflers and extra trappings that he had been accustomed to all his life, and he found he could stand a wetting as well as anybody, and began rather to rejoice in the exposure. Before spring a severe catarrhal affection, that required him to use several handkerchiefs a day for several years, began to disappear, and his night attacks of asthma either omitted or were much modified, enabling him to do without his niter-paper. His strength developed to a degree that he had never known before, and he felt so well that he took a trip of pleasure to San Francisco to enjoy the pleasant month of May there, but the effects of the climate brought on his disease again, so badly that he was compelled to return here in a short time, when he found immediate relief, and soon got back to his former state. He found also that when he spent a night in the city, 700 feet below in the valley, his attack would return, though not as badly as before. Before a year was spent here, he found, however, that he could stop in the city with impunity, and he then took up his residence there, and soon afterward went east on a visit to his friends; and so great had the change in his personal appearance been that his father and friends, who awaited his arrival at the depot, failed to recognize him. For the past two years he has visited San Francisco, and lived in New York and Chicago, without any return of his disease.

Another case is that of a middle-aged builder, who has had asthma all of his life. He came to Utah twenty years ago, and enjoyed relief from his ailment the moment he reached the high altitude on the divide of the continent, and he has been free from the severe attacks he used to suffer before coming to this country, but he has never been relieved entirely from them like the above case. He has made occasional visits to friends in Iowa and Missouri, but was always compelled to return on account of a return of his disease in a spasmodic form.

Another case: A middle-aged lady, the mother of several children, was a case of congenital asthma, from which she suffered continually till she came here, three years ago, when the complaint vanished entirely. She has not tried any other climate since her relief.

I could recount some twenty similar cases, all remaining well while they stay here, but some of them suffer a return of the complaint in a modified form by going to the sea-shore. With some of these asthmatics who have enjoyed an absence of their symptoms for some years an attack of catarrh or bronchitis will excite a return of them, but the asthma always subsides on the relief of the complaint that induced its return.

Bronchitis appears in a mild form during the wet and thawing periods of spring and fall, but it always yields to treatment, and I have heard of no deaths from it.

Pneumonia may be regarded as a disease most liable to be produced by the conditions of the climate, and it doubtless makes up the bulk of cases reported as lung diseases on the death-register of the city undertakers. It appears quite commonly in the spring and fall, and it attacks all ages and conditions. It appears frequently in connection with malarial and typhoid fevers, and it sometimes carries off tuberculous children. If taken in time, and is not complicated, however, it yields quite readily to large doses of quinine with opium enough to keep down the pain.

I have the honor to reply to the following queries contained in a letter from your office, dated October 29, 1874:

"First. What is the average pulse and respiration rate at the post?" I had a series of observations taken on twenty-five men believed to be in sound health, with the following results:

| Number. | Age. | Pulse. | Respiration. | Number. | Age. | Pulse. | Respiration. |
|---|---|---|---|---|---|---|---|
| 1 | 21 | 94 | 24 | 14 | 29 | 69 | 27 |
| 2 | 32 | 80 | 29 | 15 | 26 | 81 | 26 |
| 3 | 26 | 81 | 27 | 16 | 27 | 84 | 24 |
| 4 | 27 | 86 | 24 | 17 | 32 | 81 | 26 |
| 5 | 36 | 75 | 23 | 18 | 30 | 84 | 23 |
| 6 | 50 | 88 | 20 | 19 | 22 | 80 | 26 |
| 7 | 34 | 88 | 23 | 20 | 29 | 78 | 27 |
| 8 | 27 | 87 | 25 | 21 | 23 | 76 | 27 |
| 9 | 23 | 80 | 24 | 22 | 23 | 80 | 24 |
| 10 | 27 | 76 | 22 | 23 | 28 | 79 | 26 |
| 11 | 29 | 73 | 25 | 24 | 33 | 84 | 23 |
| 12 | 40 | 80 | 26 | 25 | 22 | 78 | 25 |
| 13 | 30 | 70 | 23 | | | | |

The difference in these rates may be attributed in a measure to the effect of tobacco, which most soldiers use more or less, and which, according to my observations, increases the pulse from ten to twenty and the respiration from three to six per minute. Breathing tobacco-smoke, even by persons who do not use it themselves, will make a perceptible increase over the normal rates; yet these observations correspond very closely to the rates I am in the habit of noting in the examination of applicants for life-insurance. In this class I often make two examinations, and find that a suspiciously-rapid pulse and respiration are caused by the immoderate use of tobacco, especially smoking, and a few days' abstinence will bring them down to the standard required by the insurance-companies.

Second. "How great are the diurnal variations of temperature, at what season are they greatest, and do you attribute any bad effect to them?" The following abstract of monthly mean for 1873, with the greatest diurnal variations, shows that they are greatest in June, July, August, and September, which are the healthiest months here, and I have no reason to attribute any bad effects to these variations, which, however, are far from being great:

| Month. | 7 a. m. | 2 p. m. | 9 p. m. | Diurnal variations. | Percentage of sick. |
|---|---|---|---|---|---|
| January, 1873 | 28 | 35 | 29 | 7 | 33.60 |
| February, 1873 | 23 | 34 | 24 | 11 | 31.30 |
| March, 1873 | 33 | 47 | 39 | 14 | 32.33 |
| April, 1873 | 38 | 50 | 41 | 12 | 26.42 |
| May, 1873 | 45 | 55 | 47 | 10 | 28.74 |
| June, 1873 | 61 | 77 | 65 | 16 | 29.28 |
| July, 1873 | 68 | 85 | 73 | 17 | 23.86 |
| August, 1873 | 65 | 80 | 69 | 15 | 25.38 |
| September, 1873 | 56 | 74 | 62 | 18 | 20.00 |
| October, 1873 | 41 | 56 | 45 | 15 | 21.97 |
| November, 1873 | 38 | 53 | 41 | 15 | 38.68 |
| December, 1873 | 22 | 31 | 24 | 9 | 40.50 |

An opposite state of health is, however, obtained in Salt Lake City during the above months of greatest diurnal variations of temperature, but this difference is attributable to the character of the drinking-water used during these months. The city is situated three miles to the westward, on the bottom of the ancient lake that at one time filled up the Great Salt Lake Valley some thousand feet above its present level. The soil consists of gravel, sand, and cobbles, with a top layer, a few feet thick, of alkaline alluvium. During the months of greatest diurnal variations of temperature, which are hot and dry, the water from wells, which is principally used for drinking and culinary purposes, is at its greatest degree of concentration, with the salts of lime, potash, soda, and magnesia, besides the organic matters that settle down from the surface of the streets, yards, gutters, drains, water-closets, &c., and pass into the soil without any obstruction to their flow either downward or laterally; and, as a consequence, it becomes a purgative mixture, especially to strangers, and the amount of bowel disease, and deaths from its effects, is simply frightful, particularly among the children.

Third. "What is the influence, if any, of adobe habitations on the health of the inmates? Does it predispose to rheumatism, to erysipelas, or to puerperal diseases, &c.?" The experience of the physicians, as well as the population generally of Utah, where this material is very extensively used for building purposes, has established its claims as a most wholesome substance for dwelling-houses. In cases of contagious diseases they attribute disinfectant properties to it, the same as is claimed for powdered earth as used in earth-closets for absorbing emanations from the discharges. Many instances have been narrated to me of cases of scarlet fever, small-pox, and measles, which on being isolated in an adobe house, which here frequently consists of only one room, or in one room of such a house, has failed to communicate the disease to others, and the disease has ceased with the first case. Rheumatism, erysipelas, and puerperal diseases are thought to progress better in buildings of this kind than in any other. In fact, though I have practiced quite extensively among people living in such dwellings, at this writing I do not call to mind any cases of these diseases as occurring in adobe houses, though I have seen them in wooden houses, but no deaths from them, excepting rheumatism in very small percentage. There are many examples of buildings of this kind in Salt Lake City that are upward of twenty-two years old, and the inmates boast of their healthfulness, and profess to esteem them higher than any other kind on this account. An adobe or sun-dried brick is 18 by 9 by 3 inches, and it can be made in this climate in about three weeks during the summer months. The top soil in selected places is taken for this purpose, and the clay is molded without the aid of straw, which is added in California where their brick is made chiefly by Mexicans. In order to construct a durable building of this material the foundation should be laid with stone, and raised about two or three feet above the surface of the ground, so as to prevent soaking upward, by capillary attraction, of the moisture from the ground, and also to prevent the effect of the splashing against the wall of the rain from the eaves. The effect of the rain on the walls is quite superficial; only a thin layer is melted, the water does not soak in, and this layer crumbles off during the next dry season. The adobe is a non-conductor of heat, and on this account it is less liable to condense moisture on the walls, and therefore a building made of this material is less liable to become damp within than one constructed either of brick, stone, or wood. These bricks are made without any pressure, (the mud is simply pounded into the molds,) and they are more or less porous, a quality that favors the absorption of a certain amount of atmosphere into them, and no doubt the organic matters contained therein are more or less oxidized and absorbed in a changed condition. Many of the adobe dwellings hereabouts are whitewashed inside and out, and it is claimed that this wash reduces such a structure, in point of healthfulness, to about the par of a brick house.

*Meteorological report, Camp Douglas, Utah, 1870–'74.*

| Month. | 1870–'71. | | | | 1871–'72. | | | | 1872–'73. | | | | 1873–'74. | | | |
|---|---|---|---|---|---|---|---|---|---|---|---|---|---|---|---|---|
| | Temperature. | | | Rain-fall in inches. | Temperature. | | | Rain-fall in inches. | Temperature. | | | Rain-fall in inches. | Temperature. | | | Rain-fall in inches. |
| | Mean. | Max. | Min. | | Mean. | Max. | Min. | | Mean. | Max. | Min. | | Mean. | Max. | Min. | |
| July ................. | 75.98 | 96* | 54* | 1.48 | 79.09 | 100* | 50* | 0.38 | 73.67* | 91* | 38* | 0.02 | 75.85 | 96* | 56 | 0.12 |
| August ............. | 70.29 | 95* | 44* | 0.45 | 74.99 | 105* | 56* | 0.05 | 73.30* | 91* | 51* | 0.72 | 71.93 | 95* | 57 | 0.94 |
| September ......... | 60.25 | 82* | 45* | 0.45 | 75.24 | 88* | 54* | 0.00 | 61.75* | 88* | 31* | 0.69 | 64.79 | 88* | 37 | 0.42 |
| October ........... | 50.63 | 84* | 30* | 0.85 | 50.34 | 70* | 27* | 0.55 | 53.64 | 78 | 21* | 1.36 | 47.60 | 80* | 21 | 0.84 |
| November .......... | 43.42 | 65* | 28* | 1.39 | 38.04 | 65* | 14* | 0.83 | 32.42 | 55 | 11* | 0.66 | 44.22 | 61* | 30 | 0.38 |
| December .......... | 26.84 | 48* | 4* | 1.85 | 34.99 | 49* | 15* | 1.90 | 32.47 | 51 | 10* | 2.26 | 26.51 | 42* | 9 | 1.20 |
| January ............ | 31.42 | 62* | 8* | 1.60 | 30.50 | 53* | — 2* | 1.30 | 31.07 | 49 | — 3* | 2.18 | 29.43 | 52* | 11 | 1.28 |
| February .......... | 32.53 | 53* | 15* | 2.44 | 36.80 | 62* | 15* | 1.34 | 27.52 | 46 | 0* | 1.89 | 27.33 | 54* | 8 | 1.63 |
| March ............. | 38.59 | 65* | 15* | 3.39 | 40.71 | 66* | 22* | 1.20 | 40.51 | 66 | 13* | 0.90 | 32.54 | 55* | 15 | 2.87 |
| April .............. | 45.43 | 75* | 15* | 3.15 | 44.51 | 65* | 24* | 2.04 | 43.27 | 74 | 26* | 2.00 | 45.71 | 82* | 30 | 0.74 |
| May ............... | 59.66 | 82* | 40* | 5.00 | 58.41 | 87* | 34* | 2.34 | 49.16 | 77 | 19* | 4.10 | 60.69 | 90* | 36 | 2.89 |
| June .............. | 74.68 | 98* | 40* | 0.30 | 68.75 | 90* | 41* | 1.16 | 68.19 | 90* | 45 | 0.24 | 66.79 | 92* | 47 | 0.72 |
| For the year...... | 50.81 | 98* | 4* | 22.35 | 52.69 | 105* | — 2 | 13.09 | 48.91 | 91* | — 3* | 17.02 | 49.45 | 96* | 8 | 13.43 |

* These observations are made with self-registering thermometers. The mean is from the standard thermometer.

44 M P

*Consolidated sick-report, Camp Douglas, Utah, 1870–'74.*

| Year | | 1870–'71. | | 1871–'72. | | 1872–'73. | | 1873–'74. | |
|---|---|---|---|---|---|---|---|---|---|
| Mean strength | Officers | 13 | | 17 | | 16 | | 20 | |
| | Enlisted men | 229 | | 347 | | 313 | | 401 | |
| Diseases. | | Cases. | Deaths. | Cases. | Deaths. | Cases. | Deaths. | Cases. | Deaths. |
| GENERAL DISEASES, A. | | | | | | | | | |
| Typhoid fever | | 2 | 1 | 7 | 5 | 7 | | | |
| Intermittent fever | | 57 | | 209 | | 124 | | 82 | |
| Other diseases of this group | | 54 | 1 | 45 | | 50 | | 20 | |
| GENERAL DISEASES, B. | | | | | | | | | |
| Rheumatism | | 87 | | 54 | | 108 | | 151 | |
| Syphilis | | 5 | | 11 | | 4 | | 8 | |
| Consumption | | 1 | | 1 | 1 | 1 | | | |
| Other diseases of this group | | 11 | | 16 | | 8 | | 5 | |
| LOCAL DISEASES. | | | | | | | | | |
| Catarrh and bronchitis | | 93 | | 101 | | 199 | | 372 | |
| Pleurisy | | 1 | | | | | | | |
| Diarrhœa and dysentery | | 197 | 2 | 230 | | 183 | | 226 | 1 |
| Hernia | | | | | | 2 | | 1 | |
| Gonorrhœa | | 3 | | 10 | | 3 | | 1 | |
| Other local diseases | | 164 | 1 | 165 | | 187 | 1 | 263 | |
| Alcoholism | | 20 | 1 | 22 | 1 | 42 | 1 | 63 | |
| Total disease | | 695 | 6 | 871 | 7 | 918 | 2 | 1,192 | 1 |
| VIOLENT DISEASES AND DEATHS. | | | | | | | | | |
| Gunshot wounds | | 2 | | | | | | 2 | 1 |
| Other accidents and injuries | | 109 | | 147 | | 152 | | 259 | |
| Total violence | | 111 | | 147 | | 152 | | 261 | 1 |

# FORT FETTERMAN, WYOMING TERRITORY.

## REPORT OF ASSISTANT SURGEON J. H. PATZKI, UNITED STATES ARMY.

Fort Fetterman is situated on a plateau on the south bank of the North Platte River, about 800 yards from and 130 feet above the stream; latitude, 42° 8' north; longitude, 28° 4' west; elevation above the Gulf of Mexico, about 5,250 feet. The plateau rises from the river-bottom by steep, almost precipitous, bluffs, and then, rising gradually, merges into the Black Hills, fourteen miles distant.

The nearest post, and the one through which all communication with the East passes, is Fort Laramie, eighty miles to the southeast.

Cheyenne, on the Union Pacific Railroad, is about one hundred and seventy miles to the southeast by the way of Fort Laramie, and one hundred and forty-five miles by a more direct route, not touching that post. Medicine Bow is the nearest station on the Union Pacific Railroad, about ninety miles to the south.

In the spring of 1864 the gold excitement in Montana began to attract emigration. The first train, of about three hundred wagons, guided by "Old Joe," was met at Deer Creek (about twenty miles west) by the Sioux under Red Cloud, who appeared well disposed, but warned the travelers not to go east of the Big Horn Mountains. They followed his advice, and reached Montana unmolested. But other trains preferred the more direct route east of the Big Horn, and the Indians immediately resented this encroachment upon their domains, and began active hostilities. To protect emigration along this "Powder River route," Forts Reno, Phil Kearney, and C. F. Smith were established north of the North Platte River, and finally Fort Fetterman on the south bank, where a ferry was established. The first troops arrived here July 19, 1867, (Companies A, C, H, and I, Fourth Infantry, under Maj. William McE. Dye.) The post received its name in honor of Bvt. Lieut. Col. W. J. Fetterman, captain in the Twenty-seventh Infantry, who, with his whole command, was killed in the Indian massacre near Fort Phil Kearney December 21, 1866.

The carnage among the travelers soon checked emigration, and the completion of the railroad opened less dangerous routes farther west. Still the Indians (Cheyennes, Arapahoes, and Sioux) continued hostilities, attacking detachments and Government trains, and in March, 1868, breaking up all the settlements between here and Fort Laramie, killing most of the inhabitants. The posts north of the Platte were abandoned, the Indians making this one of their conditions in the treaty of 1868, since when they remain on their reservation and appear more peacefully disposed, their young men occasionally harassing small parties or stealing stock. To check such depredations and to protect the railroad is the object of the post at present, which is facilitated by all the posts being in telegraphic communication with each other.

The reservation begins at a point five miles due east of the flagstaff; thence running due north one mile; thence due west ten miles; thence due south six miles; thence due east ten miles; thence due north five miles, to the point of beginning; containing an area of sixty square miles. (General Orders No. 34, series 1867, Headquarters Department of the Platte.) Besides this there are reservations for hay and for wood. The former comprises "the bottom-lands adjacent and pertaining to Deer Creek from its mouth to the foot of the first high range of hills." The latter, "that part of the north range of the Black Hills running almost parallel to and about fourteen miles south of the North Platte River, and that part of said range (including north and south slopes) which lies between Box Elder Creek and its tributary known as Little-Box Elder." (General Orders No. 480, series 1870, Headquarters Department of the Platte.)

The Black Hills furnish fine pine timber, the logs being cut by enlisted men and converted at the post, by two saw-mills, into building-material. Of the value of the hay-reservation, the fact may give some idea that in 1861 Prof. F. V. Hayden, while an assistant to Capt. W. F. Reynolds, United States Engineers, encamped on the creek during a portion of the winter, and that "the stock, nearly two hundred horses and mules, were wintered very nicely in the valley, without a particle of hay or grain, with only the grass which they gathered from day to day." A Mormon settlement occupied this valley until broken up by the expedition of 1854. Fuel and hay are at present furnished under contract.

The lowest geological formation which appears near the post is an outcrop of strata composed of sandstone and clay, of the age of the Rocky Mountain coal or lignite formation of the tertiary period, but to place it in a subdivision has long been the subject of controversy among leading paleontologists of this country. This tertiary coal, as found in the vicinity, contains about 50 per cent. of carbon, is of black color, fractures in cubes, resists poorly the action of the atmosphere and is very friable when exposed. Above this lignite formation is a very hard siliceous sandstone colored with protoxide of iron containing quantities of brown iron-ore; some of the iron-ore is quite rich, but most of it is poor. Just below this stratum is a sand formation which is rich in fossil flora, but being so friable it is impossible to procure good specimens.

A conspicuous feature at the crossing of Spring Creek, about eleven miles southeast from this post, is the bluff wall of tertiary which extends up westward so as to form the high hills on the north side of the valley. "The waters have worn deep into the cream-colored marls so that we have over a restricted area miniature 'bad lands.'" The dome-like hills and the numberless furrows down the sides, the harder layers projecting like verandas, are well shown. "Nearer to the post the predominating constituent in all the rocks, sands, sandstones, clays, &c., is iron, presenting every shade or color that can be derived from that mineral; much of the country on account of its presence has a burnt appearance." (Hayden.) The Black Hills owe to it their somber hue and their name.

A short distance from the post is the Natural Bridge, which Professor Hayden describes in the following terms: "We found it even more wonderful than we anticipated, and it is a matter of surprise that so great a natural curiosity should have failed to attract the attention it deserves. The cañon is about ten miles from the fort, and is formed by the passage of the La Prêle Creek through a long ridge that extends from the La Bonte to Red Buttes. The cañon is one of upheaval and erosion. The ridge is a long, local anticlinical or 'puff,' and the strata incline from each side of the summit. The gorge is very irregular and tortuous, filled with huge masses of rock that have fallen down, obstructing the passage. Where the stream has cut through the rocks direct, we have vertical walls on each side and a narrow gorge; but where the channel passes along a rift, the valley expands out several hundred feet. Where the La Prêle emerges from the cañon it cuts through the limestones and red beds at right angles, forming a regular gorge, with walls 50 to 150 feet high. At the head of this gorge the stream has at some time changed its bed, passing directly through a point of rocks that extend across the channel. The old bed is now overgrown with trees and bushes, but is 50 feet higher than the present one. The little creek must have changed its course slightly, for some reason not apparent now, so that its waters were brought against this point or wall of rock, and finding a fissure or opening through, it gradually wore its present channel. It is certainly as perfect a natural bridge as could be desired. The opening under the bridge is about 150 feet wide and 50 feet high. The old bed is about 300 feet to the northwest. It is also plain that the water flowed over the top of the bridge, which is 50 to 100 feet lower than the top of the gorge, so that we have here some of the intermediate steps which a stream makes in the process of wearing out a gorge or channel. The rocks are mostly limestone, quite pure, arenaceous limestone, and at the base very cherty limestone."

Coal was heretofore obtained by contract for the use of the post at Box Elder Creek, about eighteen miles distant, but a board of survey having found 2,133 pounds of this coal to be equal to 1,600 pounds of coal as prescribed by regulations, its issue was discontinued. Sandstone for foundations, &c., has been extensively quarried in the immediate vicinity; lime is obtained at the Natural Bridge.

The following are the plants and trees observed within a radius of thirty miles, viz:

Violet, buckthorn, sweet-brier, wild plum, wild cherry, wild crabapple, prickly-pear, gooseberry, wild currant, hackberry, whortleberry, sage-brush, pennyroyal, alder, dwarf-willow, cottonwood, common pine, red cedar.

The grazing is good in the valleys, and, in the earlier part of summer, on the hillside. No trees grow near the post except a few cottonwood trees.

Of wild animals, birds, fish, &c., the following are met in the vicinity, viz:

Lynx, wildcat, cougar or mountain-lion, gray wolf, coyote, fox, wolverine, grizzly bear, black and cinnamon bear, badger, weasel, otter, mole, common deer, black-tailed deer, elk, antelope, bighorn, buffalo, jack rabbit, brown rabbit, small prairie squirrel, flying squirrel, prairie-chicken, mountain-grouse, ruffled grouse, sage-chicken, whip-poor-will, cuckoo, bank-swallow, blackbird, oreole, brown thrush, dove, snow-bird, meadow-lark, woodpecker, crane, gray plover, snipe, curlew, wild duck, wild goose, shovel-nosed pike, pike, catfish, buffalo-fish, chub, minnow. Game is abundant within twenty-five miles from the post; buffalo has entirely left the vicinity; an old bull is occasionally seen; elk is often met in very large herds.

The mountain-trout, abundant in the tributaries of the South Platte, is never found in the North Platte, although they head but a few thousand yards apart, (as the Laramie and Cache La Poudre.) Of insects the grasshoppers are the most conspicuous, as they appear in countless numbers, and destroy, often completely, the crops in the post garden.

The North Platte is here about 400 feet wide, and its tributary about 15 feet, almost dry in winter; they are subject to floods in June. There are no ponds or lakes near. Good ice is obtained from the Platte, and stored in a well-constructed ice-house.

The post is built at the confluence of the La Prêle and North Platte. Owing to its elevation it commands an extensive view of the surrounding country. The barracks and officers' quarters are built on the sides of a rectangular parade-ground. A high plank fence used to inclose the whole, but parts of it have been taken down, (to the northwest.)

The hospital, store-houses, and some of the quarters of married soldiers are outside of the inclosure.

The garrison is quartered in four barracks, one of which is a double building. Two are built of boards, lined with adobe, and two of adobe alone, supported by studding. The walls are whitewashed, roofs shingled. They are floored, and have ceilings of canvas. A covered porch runs along the front of the barracks, with a small room, 10 by 15 feet, partitioned off at each corner for orderly sergeant's room and barrack-office. The dimensions are 100 by 24 feet, 14 feet high to eaves. There is a slight variation of the dimensions in the clear in the different buildings on account of the different thickness of their walls. One consists of buildings arranged in a square around a central yard. The air-space per man in the three other barracks is about 550 feet, with the present strength of companies. These buildings are well warmed by stoves, and abundant and good fuel; are well lighted by windows, but badly ventilated, there being no special arrangement for ventilation except in one barrack, where four holes 2 inches square are arranged over each window with slides, but they have been carefully nailed down, and canvas tacked over them, the men complaining of draught. The floors in all the barracks show wide cracks, through which the water used in scrubbing, the sweepings, &c., find their way into the space underneath, which is not ventilated. Candles are used for artificial light. The men sleep on iron bedsteads arranged in pairs so that every two men have the benefit of their combined covering.

The wash-rooms are small rooms, either in the barracks or in the mess-building, warmed and provided with benches. The privies consist of sheds about 150 feet in rear of the barracks, built over deep trenches..

The kitchens and mess-rooms are log buildings, chinked, shingled, floored, without ceilings, with good and sufficient furniture. The dimensions are as follows: Kitchens, 16 by 20 feet, 7 feet high to eaves, 14 feet to ridge; dining-rooms, 27 by 20 feet, 8 feet high to eaves, 14 to ridge.

Besides the rooms (six sets) for laundresses and married soldiers belonging to one of the barracks, there is an adobe building opposite to the hospital, and containing eight rooms, each 10 by 23 feet, 10 feet to ceiling, used for the same purpose, (formerly used for officers' quarters.) These rooms are divided by canvas into two rooms; sheds and tents are used as kitchens. All these rooms are in fair repair, and are rather superior to those at the majority of posts, which is not saying very much.

Seven buildings are used for officers' quarters. All except one are one and a half stories high; most of the attics finished; shingled, plastered, with verandas along front; paling fences in front, and high fences around yards. Buildings are yellow-washed; two are built of logs, one of adobe supported by studding, all others of boards lined with adobe. Three contain each two sets of quarters with separate halls; one contains five sets without halls, two without kitchens. The commanding officer's quarters contain five rooms on the first and two on the upper story; the house is well finished and very comfortable, with pantries, closets, &c., and the necessary out-houses and stable (of adobe) in the yard. One set of quarters contains five rooms, besides hall and kitchen; rather low and small, but quite comfortable. As a whole, these buildings furnish sufficient, most of them fair, some very good, quarters; those contained in the unpromising "log houses" are by no means the worst. The material for adobe is very superior; the thickness of the walls renders the rooms warm in winter. The kitchens are mostly roomy and all furnished with good stoves or ranges and all other necessaries; a root-cellar, shelved, is in each yard. Much of the comfort the officers are enjoying now may be due to the fact that three different sets were successively erected for quarters for the commanding officer. Still the quarters are called fair and good only in comparison with the average quarters on the frontier. Here, as almost everywhere, the results of green lumber and army mechanics are visible in wide cracks in roof, floor, window and door frames, admitting rain, draught, and (worst of all) dust. The chimneys will smoke, the plaster will tumble down, and bed-bugs will defy the house-keeper. Two additional sets of captains' quarters are being built of logs. The water-closets are arranged similarly to those described before.

The offices of the adjutant, post quartermaster, and of the commissary of subsistence, besides quarters for the ordnance sergeant, the telegraph operator, and quartermaster's clerk, are in a new building constructed of boards lined with adobe. They are commodious and comfortable.

The commissary store-house, 100 by 33 feet by 16 feet high, is built of planks lined with adobes. A large cellar underlies the building, but the potatoes last winter and the turnips this winter having been destroyed by frost, the vegetables are kept now in a recently constructed root-cellar of sufficient capacity for storing about 150,000 pounds.

Three buildings for quartermaster's store-houses are adjacent, one of adobe 129 by 33 feet, and two of boards lined with adobe, 118 by 36 and 76 by 13 feet. The buildings appear to answer their purpose. They are built on an elevation about 200 yards north of the parade-ground. The new guard-house is constructed of boards lined with adobe, one story high, shingled roof, 48 by 34 feet by 18 feet to ridge, no ceiling. Owing to the unique interior arrangement, but little benefit from these dimensions accrues to the prisoners. The main building is occupied by the guard. The prisoners occupy separate rooms built of substantial plank within the main building; so as to have a free space around them; they have a plank ceiling; height to ceiling 10 feet. These rooms or cages communicate with the main room by means of a door and two gratings, 3 by 14 inches and 3 by 18 inches, 7 feet from the floor. One such room is at each end of the building; one, 14 by 10 feet, for general prisoners, (average occupancy, 12; greatest, 21;) the other, 18 by 10 feet, for garrison prisoners, (average occupancy, 6; greatest, 10.) In the corner opposite to the general prisoners is the room for the non-commissioned officers of the guard, 11 by 15 feet. Adjacent to the other prisoners' room are three cells, 3 by 6 feet and 7 feet high, with ceilings consisting of grating, used for refractory prisoners and those sentenced to solitary confinement, rarely occupied. There are ten windows (3 by 2½ feet, about 7 feet from the floor) and two doors (6¾ by 2½ feet) in the main building, which is also perforated by numerous loop-holes, (about 2 by 4 inches, now boarded up.) The prisoners sleep on the floor, no bed-sacks or bunks, and but two blankets to each prisoner, being allowed. The guard sleep on a platform along the outer wall of the room for the garrison prisoners. The whole building is well warmed by a wood-stove in the center. No special arrangement for ventilation. The whole is in good repair and kept well policed. This plan is certainly ingenious to prevent the escape of prisoners. Near the guard-house is the magazine, built of logs, 19½ feet square.

The hospital is situated about 150 yards east of the flagstaff, on open, well-drained ground. It is the poorest building at the post. The post-surgeon in 1870 describes it as follows: " It is a second-hand affair, built of logs brought from Fort Casper, (an abandoned post some forty miles west,) in the fall of 1867. For some years it remained a mere shell, with no internal lining of any kind, or ceiling, and without flooring in some of the rooms. Owing to the wretched state of the roof, both light and snow are freely admitted, while the ventilation was more than could be desired." After much waste of ink and paper, the hospital has attained its present condition, which, however poor, would have made the earlier post-surgeons feel quite proud. It is now plastered throughout, floored, and ceiled. The main building is 92 by 20 feet; the L-extensions, the one to the north, 18 by 13 feet, containing the office; the other, 36 by 16 feet, containing mess-room and kitchen. The main building contains: the ward, 20 by 40 feet, and 11½ feet to the ceiling, (the ceiling is about 2 feet 10 inches above the eaves, the intermediate portion of the roof being lathed and plastered;) the dispensary, 14 by 20 feet, sufficiently well furnished with counter, drawers, shelves, &c.; the steward's room, 13½ by 19 feet; the store-room, 14½ by 19¼ feet, (the latter three 8½ feet high.) The store-room is furnished with shelving and liquor-closet. The ward is warmed by two stoves; the steward's room, office, and dispensary, each by one. The mess-room is sufficiently warmed by the range of the adjoining kitchen. The natural illumination of the ward and store room is fair; good in the other rooms. The ward is ventilated by two shafts through ceiling and roof, one foot square in the opening, not capped; no inlet shafts or openings. The number of beds in the ward at present is 10; average occupancy during the year, 8; air-space, 920 cubic feet per man. During the preceding years but few cases required treatment in hospital on account of the immunity of the garrison from serious sickness.

A privy is situated about 100 feet in rear of the hospital, of the kind described heretofore; recently it has been rendered less offensive by means of dry earth. The earth-commode is used without bad effect in the ward by patients too sick to resort to the privy. The yard is inclosed by a high fence; a shed in its rear is used as a stable for a cow kept for the hospital.

In the spring of 1873, two small additions, one to each L-extension, were made. They are now used as steward's room, additional store-room, isolation ward, and bath and ablution room.

The post bakery is built of adobe, 27 by 18 feet; the oven is composed of an iron arch, rounded and based with adobe and sandstone.

There is a commodious building (boards and adobe) near completion, intended to serve the combined purpose of chapel, school, and club-house, and as theater for the dramatic club composed of enlisted men of the post.

The corral lies on the outskirts of the post, to the east; the walls are of adobe, 10 feet high, along which extend sheds built of overlapping slabs, two sides for the horses of a company of cavalry, one for the mules, and the fourth for some ponies and harness-room. Grain-house and ambulance-shed are within, and an old adobe building outside is occupied by a saddler and the stable-guard.

The water used at this post is derived from the North Platte River, and, like all water in this section, is impure and somewhat alkaline. No arrangements have as yet been made for the collection of rain-water or melting snow from the roofs of the buildings. Two imperfect analyses of the water have been made, one in August, when the river was high, and one in December, when it was frozen. Specific gravity, on first occasion, 1004; on the second, 1002. After immersion, red litmus shows a bluish tint; lime tests show a very small quantity of that mineral; but, since the examinations were so imperfectly conducted, little confidence can be placed in them. There is no doubt that large amounts of the sulphates are dissolved. Tests for magnesia exhibit quite a quantity of that substance in the water, though the combination is undetermined. Iron is exhibited in large amount. Sulphur is shown to be present, not only by tests, but also by taste and odor. The organic impurities are not of much amount. Sulphate of soda, which is a very constant impurity in the waters of this section, exists also in the waters of the Platte. Of course, its flavor to one unaccustomed to it is disagreeable; but its influence upon the health of the garrison is not very marked. During 1873, 49 cases of acute diarrhœa and dysentery appeared on the reports, or about 11 per cent. of all cases taken sick. The fact that the season of greatest frequency of these diseases does not correspond to the season of low water, (December, 1872, to May, 1873, 10 cases; June to November, 1873, 39 cases, and similar proportions during preceding years,) does not disprove the effect of the water in their production. Though the water is more impure in winter and early summer, greater quantities of it are consumed in the hot season.

The La Prêle Creek empties into the Platte at the foot of the bench on which the fort is built; its waters are not very different from that of the main river. Near its mouth, and close to the saw-mill, is a spring with sulphurous, cool water, extensively used by the garrison in summer; it is about 700 yards distant from the post.

The slaughter-house is situated on the La Prêle, about 1,200 yards distant. The refuse is carted to the banks of the same creek, about 500 yards above its mouth, and as the water-supply is derived from the Platte, a short distance below, it is sure to be contaminated, and more than ordinarily, during the floods in summer. The water is distributed to the garrison by means of a water-wagon, which is apt to freeze in winter. The water supply is occasionally inadequate; still, no serious inconvenience appears to have arisen, though some medical officers have strenuously advocated the construction of cisterns. Against danger from fire, besides the prescribed buckets kept filled, there are distributed through the post six Babcock extinguishers kept ready for use.

The natural drainage of the grounds is very favorable, and has been improved by grading and trenching. Depressions where pools are apt to accumulate are drained by wooden boxes discharging into the trenches. There are no sewers. The slops and offal are collected in barrels and carted about 500 yards northeast to the banks of the Prêle. Stable-manure is thrown into the ravine close to the corral.

The men bathe in the summer; there are no special arrangements for bathing.

The cemetery is situated on a hill, about 1,000 yards southeast of the hospital, and contains twenty-eight graves, many of them bearing the inscription, "Killed and scalped by Indians."

The post garden, of about four acres, is cultivated by irrigation from the La Prêle, and yields beans, peas, fine potatoes, beets, radishes, and lettuce in sufficient quantity, in favorable seasons, to furnish the companies with about two messes of fresh vegetables in the week; last season was quite favorable. The crops are in some years endangered by grasshoppers. There is no hospital garden. With proper irrigation sufficient ground could be brought under cultivation to furnish abundant and superior vegetables for the whole garrison, with the exception, perhaps, of corn.

There are but few private horses kept at the garrison; cows and chickens by some of the officers and laundresses. They can be bought at Cheyenne at a price of from $45 to $125 for the former, and 75 cents to $1 for the latter, apiece. A few pigs are kept by the companies. A cow is kept for the hospital, bought for $65. The main dependence for food is upon the commissary department, fortunately well supplied with the usual articles, and potatoes, (1½ cents per pound,) onions, (3 cents per pound,) and turnips, (latterly frozen.) The quantities of these fresh vegetables and of the canned articles are sufficient for issue and sale to the companies and officers. The post trader does not keep any necessaries in this line. Nothing can be procured in the country. Fresh vegetables and butter are occasionally procured from Medicine Bow and Cheyenne. A thriving settlement in Colorado, (Greeley,) about thirty miles from Cheyenne, furnishes, occasionally, some articles; but the whole supply, outside of the commissary, is very scanty, expensive, and unreliable. The want of fresh eggs and butter is perhaps the most perceptible. Furniture cannot be procured in this vicinity, and scarcely any nearer than Omaha.

A stage, belonging to the quartermaster's department, capable of carrying about 6 passengers and about 600 pounds of baggage, leaves the quartermaster's depot at Camp Carling, (between Cheyenne and Fort D. A. Russell,) once a week, (on Tuesdays, at present,) for Fort Laramie, which it reaches early in the afternoon of the second day. Fair beds and meals are found in a ranch at the stopping-place of the first day. A "buck-board" leaves Camp Carling every Friday with the mail for Fort Laramie. From that post, Fort Fetterman is reached by Government transportation in three days; two nights camping out, there being no ranches on the road. The post may also be reached from Medicine Bow, (about 100 miles west of Cheyenne,) the post mail-carrier leaving that station on Thursday in a light wagon. But little baggage could be carried in this way. Formerly Indians frequently endangered the road to Fort Laramie; in the latter years they are less troublesome. Snow often interrupts communication. The mail is received from Medicine Bow once a week, (Saturday,) but is, from December to June, apt to be very irregular on account of snow in the passes of the Black Hills, and sometimes the garrison was without a mail for two or three weeks, (in one instance for thirty-two days.) It is sent out Mondays, subject to the mentioned irregularities. A letter may reach department headquarters in four to five and Washington in about eight or nine days.

A telegraph-line connects the posts, and the Associated Press dispatches are received daily at a trifling expense to the officers, (about $2 per month,) an operator, paid by the Government, being stationed here. Otherwise the post is very isolated; no travel interrupts the monotony, there being no posts beyond, and no settlements in the vicinity. The graves of the inhabitants at the crossings of the creeks mark their former location.

Sioux, Arapahoes, and Cheyennes, from their reservation north of the Platte, roam over the vicinity, and visit, at times, the post in small numbers, to trade their furs and robes. They are not allowed to enter the post proper. The Arapahoes rank the lowest among them for cleanliness and fighting qualities. In June, 1868, when going to their reservation, they applied in great numbers at the hospital for treatment for conjunctivitis. Servants cannot be had in the vicinity. Those that could be obtained at Cheyenne are worthless.

The prevailing diseases are affections of the air-passages, (during 1873 nearly 18 per cent. of all cases taken sick,) mostly catarrhs, not always incapacitating the patient for duty. The great amount of ozone in, and the dryness of, the atmosphere, besides the abundance of dust, may account for these affections.

*Meteorological report, Fort Fetterman, Wyo., 1870–'74.*

| Month. | 1870–'71. | | | | 1871–'72. | | | | 1872–'73. | | | | 1873–'74. | | | |
|---|---|---|---|---|---|---|---|---|---|---|---|---|---|---|---|---|
| | Temperature. | | | Rain-fall in inches. | Temperature. | | | Rain-fall in inches. | Temperature. | | | Rain-fall in inches. | Temperature. | | | Rain-fall in inches. |
| | Mean. | Max. | Min. | | Mean. | Max. | Min. | | Mean. | Max. | Min. | | Mean. | Max. | Min. | |
| July | 72.13 | 94 | 54 | 0.62 | 74.39 | 99 | 40 | 3.20 | 67.14 | 93* | 40* | 0.94 | 78.96 | 100* | 42* | 2.17 |
| August | 62.38 | 92 | 34 | 2.46 | 70.35 | 96 | 48 | 0.14 | 67.42 | 96* | 43* | 1.60 | 69.46 | 98* | 28* | 1.02 |
| September | 55.83 | 84 | 32 | 1.36 | 58.89 | 90 | 37 | C.00 | 55.31 | 87* | 17* | 0.00 | 53.37 | 86* | 3* | 0.26 |
| October | 40.75 | 79 | 20 | 0.40 | 43.10 | 75 | 18 | 2.88 | 48.21 | 85* | 13* | 0.60 | 40.78 | 80* | − 6* | 1.04 |
| November | 38.67 | 63 | 2 | 0.02 | 25.53 | 64 | −22 | 2.50 | 27.32 | 57* | −16* | 1.28 | 39.34 | 67* | −18* | 0.50 |
| December | 21.48 | 59 | −25 | 0.46 | 20.17 | 50* | −36* | 3.28 | 17.96 | 54* | −32* | 6.02 | 23.78 | 52* | −14* | 0.24 |
| January | 28.05 | 63 | −15 | 0.36 | 23.58 | 52* | −23* | 0.20 | 20.40 | 53* | −30* | 0.54 | 27.03 | 55* | −18* | 0.30 |
| February | 28.42 | 55 | −25 | 0.46 | 30.07 | 57* | −30* | 1.12 | 20.12 | 59* | −40* | 3.40 | 25.89 | 53* | −13* | 0.26 |
| March | 33.72 | 64 | 5 | 0.58 | 32.17 | 70* | 0* | 0.08 | 39.92 | 70* | 4* | 0.90 | 30.70 | 59 | 4* | 0.64 |
| April | 41.02 | 70 | 17 | 1.44 | 50.97 | 69* | 12* | 1.72 | 37.84 | 74* | 12* | 1.70 | 41.86 | 81 | 18* | 0.88 |
| May | 58.80 | 90 | 35 | 2.06 | 53.94 | 84* | 21* | 4.74 | 49.29 | 85* | 21* | 6.04 | 58.55 | 91 | 23* | 1.02 |
| June | 71.04 | 95 | 55 | 1.14 | 64.14 | 89* | 34* | 1.54 | 75.59 | 99* | 53* | 0.40 | 66.10 | 99 | 29* | 2.58 |
| For the year | 46.02 | 95 | −25 | 11.36 | 45.61 | 99 | −36* | 21.40 | 43.87 | 99* | −40* | 23.42 | 46.32 | 100* | −18* | 10.91 |

* These observations are made with self-registering thermometers. The mean is from the standard thermometer.

*Consolidated sick-report, Fort Fetterman, Wyo., 1870–'74.*

| Diseases. | 1870–'71. Cases. | Deaths. | 1871–'72. Cases. | Deaths. | 1872–'73. Cases. | Deaths. | 1873–'74. Cases. | Deaths. |
|---|---|---|---|---|---|---|---|---|
| Year | 1870–'71. | | 1871–'72. | | 1872–'73. | | 1873–'74. | |
| Mean strength { Officers | 9 | | 10 | | 12 | | 13 | |
| Mean strength { Enlisted men | 190 | | 202 | | 238 | | 259 | |
| **GENERAL DISEASES, A.** | | | | | | | | |
| Typhoid fever | | | | | 1 | | 1 | 1 |
| Typho-malarial fever | 2 | | | | | | | |
| Remittent fever | | | | | 3 | | | |
| Intermittent fever | 14 | | 7 | | 15 | | 17 | |
| Other diseases of this group | 46 | | 10 | | 24 | | 18 | |
| **GENERAL DISEASES, B.** | | | | | | | | |
| Rheumatism | 12 | | 41 | | 66 | | 15 | |
| Syphilis | 3 | | 4 | | 10 | | 2 | |
| Consumption | 1 | | 2 | | 1 | | | 1 |
| Other diseases of this group | 1 | | 1 | | 1 | | 1 | |
| **LOCAL DISEASES.** | | | | | | | | |
| Catarrh and bronchitis | 19 | | 52 | | 108 | | 23 | |
| Pneumonia | 2 | | 1 | | 3 | | 2 | |
| Pleurisy | | | 1 | | | | 4 | |
| Diarrhœa and dysentery | 14 | | 29 | | 51 | | 38 | |
| Hernia | | | 2 | | 4 | | | |
| Gonorrhœa | 7 | | 5 | | 2 | | 1 | |
| Other local diseases | 41 | | 80 | 1 | 135 | | 116 | 1 |
| Alcoholism | 1 | | 10 | | 16 | 1 | 6 | |
| Unclassified | 1 | | | | 1 | | | |
| Total disease | 164 | | 245 | 1 | 441 | 1 | 244 | 3 |
| **VIOLENT DISEASES AND DEATHS.** | | | | | | | | |
| Gunshot wounds | 1 | | 1 | 1 | 3 | | 6 | |
| Drowning | | 1 | | | | | | 1 |
| Other accidents and injuries | 26 | | 57 | | 59 | | 58 | 1 |
| Homicide | | | | | | 1 | | |
| Total violence | 27 | 1 | 58 | 2 | 62 | | 64 | 2 |

# CAMP HARTSUFF, NEBRASKA.

INFORMATION FURNISHED BY ACTING ASSISTANT SURGEON J. R. LAINE, UNITED STATES ARMY.

Camp Hartsuff is situated upon the North Loup River, in the State of Nebraska; latitude, 41° 40′ north; longitude, 21° 59′ west; altitude, 2,600 feet above the sea. It is eighty miles north of the Union Pacific Railroad.

The North Loup is a swift-running stream, about 100 yards wide. It has a treacherous bottom of constantly shifting quicksand, and is only fordable during the summer months.

The valleys in this region are extremely fertile, the soil being a dark vegetable mold over a clay subsoil, producing an abundance of rich grasses, and capable of highly rewarding the agriculturist for his labor. The uplands are exceedingly rough and hilly, cut up by deep cañons. Limestone, unfit for building purposes, is found in large quantities thirty-five miles below the post, upon the North Loup. This stone when burnt makes an inferior quality of lime, which is used in building the concrete quarters. Extensive deposits of marine shell *débris* abound in the hills, and immense beds of gravel, deeply colored with oxide of iron, are found within a convenient distance of the post. Wood is found along the margins of the streams and in the cañons. Cottonwood, white ash, water-elm, red elm, hackberry, box-elder, red willow, cedar, and pine are the principal trees.

The animals indigenous to the country are the elk, black and white tailed deer, antelope, gray wolf, coyote, badger, raccoon, skunk, ground-squirrel, gopher, prairie-dog, beaver, mink, otter, and muskrat. The birds are those peculiar to the whole of these vast plains; flying northward in the spring, and migrating to a more congenial climate as winter approaches. Of reptiles, the rattlesnake is the best represented; the adder and several species of non-venomous serpents are found.

45 M P

The fishes in the streams are the catfish, sucker, white-fish, pike, pickerel, sunfish, gar, and common dace.

The post was located by General E. O. C. Ord, in September, 1874. The object of locating it at this point was to intercept roving bands of Sioux Indians in their descent upon the defenseless settlers in the North, Middle, and South Loup Valleys, and on the Cedar River, and to protect the Pawnee tribe of Indians living upon their reservation.

The immediate location of the post is upon a sloping elevation of 60 feet above the level of the North Loup. A decided slope from this elevation forms a natural and effective drainage for the post. The reservation consists of sections 2 and 10, township 20 north, range 15 west, for the site of the post, and sections 9 and 15 and such parts of sections 10, 11, and 14, township 21 north, range 16 west, as lie south of the Loup River and its tributary, the Calamus River, as a reservation for supplying wood and hay to the post.

The post consists of a rectangle inclosing a parade-ground; quarters for officers and men, and other necessary buildings, being arranged on its several sides. The following buildings are at this time, November, 1874, in process of construction:

The barracks, two in number, each intended for one company, are built of concrete, one story high, with shingle roofs, facing each other from opposite sides of the parade-ground. The infantry barrack is 30 by 80 feet, 12½ feet from floor to ceiling, lighted by twelve windows, four on each side and two at each end, and is ventilated by a shaft at each end of the building. It has two doors in front and two in rear, one of which opens into the mess-room. The mess-room and kitchen are built upon the rear of the barrack, running back at a right angle with it. This building is 24 by 60 feet outside-measurement. The mess-room is 22 by 40 feet, inside, lighted by two windows upon each side, and ventilated by a shaft through the ceiling and roof. The kitchen is 22 by 16 feet, lighted by a window on each side. Mess-room and kitchen floors are of cement. Cleats are nailed upon blocks set into the concrete walls, and the lath nailed upon the cleats; this arrangement will leave an air-space between the wall and the plaster, which is intended to prevent the collection of moisture upon the walls, that would otherwise gather upon a surface colder than the surrounding atmosphere. The dormitory of the cavalry barrack will be 30 by 100 feet; in every other respect the cavalry quarters will be exactly like the other.

The commanding officer's quarters will be a story-and-a-half house, the main part 32 feet square, and an addition in the rear 16 by 20 feet. The house will contain a hall and four rooms upon the ground-floor and five rooms above, and will have a veranda along the entire front. The other officers' quarters, two in number, are double houses, one and a half stories high. The main part of each is 30 by 45 feet, the addition, 27 by 30 feet, containing a hall and four rooms on each side, upon each floor. These quarters will also have a veranda along their entire fronts.

The building to be occupied as headquarters will be a one-story house, 30 by 35 feet, 12 feet from floor to ceiling, to contain a hall and four rooms, each 14 by 15 feet.

The guard-house will be 36 by 50 feet, 9 feet from floor to ceiling, and 11 feet from ceiling to the peak of its hip-roof. The officers' room will be 10 by 13 feet, and the room for casual prisoners 9 by 16 feet. The cells, three in number, 3 by 6 feet 3 inches. The rooms and cells will be surrounded by a banquette. The prison yard will be 50 feet square, surrounded by a stockade inclosing a sink 6½ by 8 feet.

All the above buildings will be made of concrete walls, and will be plastered upon the outside and made to resemble stone.

The quarters of officers and men will all be warmed by wood-burning stoves.

Water will be obtained from wells dug in rear of each set of officer's quarters and of company quarters.

The officers and men now occupy temporary quarters, built of rough lumber. The married men and laundresses occupy log and dirt huts, a little removed from the other quarters.

None of the concrete quarters or other buildings comprising the post as above described are yet completed, (November, 1874;) some of them not yet commenced.

No plan for a hospital has yet been forwarded to the Surgeon-General for approval. The hospital now occupied is a dug-out, 13 by 15 feet, with a dirt roof.

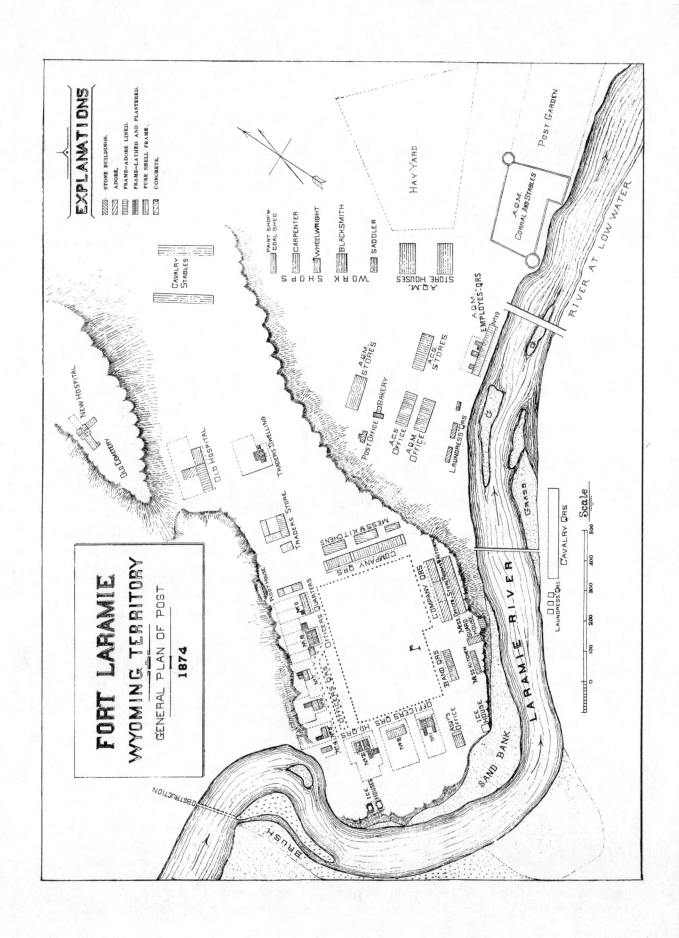

EXPLANATIONS

STONE BUILDINGS.
ADOBE.
FRAME-ADOBE LINED.
FRAME-LATHED AND PLASTERED.
PURE SHELL FRAME.
CONCRETE.

FORT LARAMIE
WYOMING TERRITORY
GENERAL PLAN OF POST
1874

Cavalry Stables

Paint Shop & Coal Shed
Carpenter
Wheelwright
Blacksmith
Saddler
WORK SHOPS

STORE HOUSES
A.Q.M.

New Hospital
Old Cemetery
Old Hospital
Traders Dwelling
Traders Store

A.Q.M. Stores
Post Office
Bakery
A.C.S. Stores
A.C.S. Office
A.Q.M. Office
Laundress Qrs

A.Q.M. Employes-Qrs
Nº10

Post House
Officers Quarters
Nº9
Nº8
Nº7
Officers Qrs
Nº6
Nº5
Nº4

Hd.Qrs.
Adj'ts Office
Nº3
Nº2
Nº1
Officers Qrs

Mess Kitchens
Company Qrs
Band Qrs
Mess Kitchen
Company Qrs
Mess Offic'rs Store Room & Kitchen
Guard House
Ice House
Ice House

Hay Yard

A.Q.M.
Corral and Stables
Post Garden

River at Low Water
Grass
Cavalry Qrs
Laramie River

Sand Bank
Brush
Obstruction

Scale
Laundress Qrs
Cavalry Qrs
0   100   200   300   400   500

Vegetables of all kinds can be purchased at reasonable rates from the settlers in the vicinity. Owing to the short time the post has been established there is no garden under cultivation.

The climate and location may justly be considered healthy. The cases of malarial fever that have been presented for treatment, may be attributed to drinking impure water, and to the extremes of temperature between day and night during the autumnal season. Sudden and extreme changes of temperature are very common. The winds are usually high during spring and autumn. As a rule the winters are not excessively cold, although severe storms of snow and wind frequently occur during the months of February and March.

---

# FORT LARAMIE, WYOMING TERRITORY.

### REPORTS OF ASSISTANT SURGEONS H. S. SCHELL AND R. M. O'REILLY, UNITED STATES ARMY.

Fort Laramie is situated on the west bank of Laramie River, one and a half miles above its junction with the Platte; latitude, 42° 12' 38'' north; longitude, 27° 28' 26'' west; elevation above the sea, 4,519 feet. The reservation, as declared by the President, includes fifty-four square miles.

For history of the post, see Circular No. 4, page 346.

The general plan of the post is shown in the plate opposite. Including the band quarters, there are barracks for seven companies. The barrack on the northeast side contains quarters for three companies. The entire length of the building is 287 feet, but a portion of each set of quarters is occupied by a room for the first sergeants and a baggage-room, so that the net size of each room assigned to a company is 81 feet long, 30 feet wide, and 11 feet high. These rooms are ceiled with half-inch boards, but not plastered. The building is of framed timbers, filled in with adobes, plastered inside and weather-boarded outside. They are one story high, raised about two feet above the ground, but without cellars. Each room contains twelve windows, six on a side. The rooms were constructed when the companies were filled to the maximum. They contain 26,730 cubic feet of air-space each.

Of the two barracks on the southeast side of the parade, the first contains quarters for three companies, the second for one company. These buildings are constructed in every respect like the foregoing, except that the net size of the rooms in the first is 103 by 29 feet, having an air-space of 46,298 cubic feet, and that of the other building 70 by 28 feet, with an air-space of 21,560 cubic feet. The middle set is not occupied. The barracks are all in good repair, heated by means of stoves, well lighted and ventilated, and are furnished with single iron bunks. In the rear of each set of quarters is a commodious kitchen and mess-room. There are but two in rear of the barracks first described. One is divided into two portions. The east end is used as kitchen and mess-room by the company occupying the quarters on the west end of the barracks, and the other is divided between the other two companies. Kitchens for the other sets of quarters are similarly arranged, and all are provided with cooking-stoves, tables, and benches.

There are two new sets of cavalry barracks, built of concrete, two stories high. These are constructed on the general plan recently ordered for barracks, except that the first story is only 10 feet and the second story 9 feet high. This is a very serious error, as it reduces the air space in the dormitories, makes them look low, and not symmetrically proportioned. The ventilation also is defective, there being only two very small shaft-ventilators in each dormitory.

An adobe-lined, shingle-roofed, frame building, 297 by 30 feet, on the south side of the river, was occupied by the two cavalry companies as quarters, until the completion of the new barracks This building is now being changed into quarters for laundresses.

The officers' quarters are, for the most part, fine examples of growth by accretion. They are generally commodious and comfortable. Referring to the plate, No. 1 is a two-story-and-a-half frame, lathed and plastered, 45 by 75 feet, containing two sets of quarters. Each set has a hall, two good-sized rooms, a kitchen and dining-room, and two store-rooms on the first floor. This was originally built for commanding officer's quarters, and has but one staircase to the attic. No. 2 is a frame building, adobe-lined, 65 by 16 feet, with veranda in front. No. 3, the commanding officer's quarters, is a frame building, lathed and plastered, 45 by 35 feet, with an extension for kitchen, &c.   No. 4 is a one-story frame, adobe-lined, 44 by 20, and contains three rooms.   Nos. 5, 6, and 7 are one-story adobe buildings, with verandas in front.   No. 8 is a two-story frame, containing four sets of quarters.   No. 9 is a one-story adobe, 92 by 19 feet, containing two sets of quarters.   No. 10, on the bank of the river, originally intended for quartermaster's employés, is a frame building, adobe-lined, in which seven officers are quartered.

The guard-house is an adobe building, 42 by 18 feet, containing two rooms, one for the officers, the other for enlisted men.   The prison is constructed of stone, 20 by 36 feet, one story high in front, and two stories in rear.   The upper story contains two rooms, plastered and ceiled.   The basement room is of rough stones, whitewashed, has one door and a window toward the river, and on the opposite side, at the top, two small windows for ventilation.   Two cells are partitioned off, on the south side, for refractory prisoners.   The prisoners are kept in the basement room, which contains no furniture.   This room is neither warmed nor lighted.   The situation of the guard-house is badly selected.

The commissary and quartermaster's store-houses are five in number, all wooden buildings, rough boards and battened, excepting the clothing-room, which is frame, and in good condition. Two commissary buildings are each 120 by 30 feet, and 9 feet to eaves.   A similar structure is occupied by the quartermaster as an office and issuing store-house.   The grain-house is 50 by 100 by 20 feet, and has a capacity of 100,000 cubic feet.   In addition to the above, an old frame building, which was formerly used as barracks, is now converted into a store-room for the use of the quartermaster.   The ice-houses for the post, two in number, will hold, together, 386 tons of ice.   The carpenter-shop, wheelwright-shop, blacksmith-shop, saddler-shop, paint-shop, coal-house, &c., are located at the extreme northeast portion of the post, are new, admirably constructed for the purposes for which they were intended, and are kept in good order.

A new hospital, for twelve beds, is in process of construction at this post.   It is on the regulation plan for twenty-four beds, and is built of concrete.   Though still in an unfinished condition, the building was occupied in December, 1874.

The water-supply at this post is ample.   The Laramie River, which bounds one side of the garrison, is a constantly running stream of an average width of 30 feet and depth of 2 feet.   Its gravelly bed is always plainly visible through the clear water except in the time of the spring freshets.   The water used for culinary and household purposes in the garrison is chiefly obtained from the Laramie River above the post, and is hauled around in a large tank on wheels and dispensed as necessity may require.   Good water may be obtained anywhere in the valley of the Laramie by digging 8 or 10 feet, but all the old wells seem to have fallen into disuse, except one in the post garden, which furnishes very cold, clear water in the summer-time.   There is also a spring in the bank of the river, in the rear of the telegraph-office, which furnishes good water.

It is probable that water might be brought directly into the post by means of an acequia a mile and a half long, and the question of its practicability, &c., has been frequently agitated, but as yet no steps have been taken for putting it into execution.

In an examination of the spring-water there was no reaction before boiling, but a slight alkaline reaction afterward, and also a trace of organic matter.   It contained from six to eight grains of chlorine to the gallon; a trace of phosphoric acid, nitric acid, and less nitrous acid than the river-water; no ammonia nor iron.   There was scarcely more than a grain of sediment in twenty-four fluid ounces of the water, and a microscopical examination showed it to be composed of particles of sand, clay, decaying vegetable matter, confervoid vegetation, and five species of infusoria.

There is also a spring in the ravine behind the adjutant's office, which furnishes a perfectly clear, sweet water.   This spring runs about two gallons per minute; the first spring described runs about ten gallons per minute.

The means of extinguishing fire throughout the garrison consist in an ample supply of water-barrels, which are kept standing constantly filled at all the buildings.   About four hundred gallons of water are kept on hand at the hospital, and fire-buckets hung in every room.   Many of the buildings are also provided with fire-ladders as well as buckets.

The post is drained naturally.   It stands on an elevated bench, containing about ten acres, the sides of which slope in all directions, except toward the bluffs back of the hospital, where the soil is gravelly and moisture sinks out of sight immediately. There is no artificial drainage at the post. All refuse, slops, &c., are collected daily and thrown into the river below the post.

The men bathe freely and constantly, in pleasant weather, when off duty, in the stream above the post. There are many places in the river where the water is 10 to 12 feet deep, affording opportunities for swimming. No bath-houses have as yet been erected.

The post cemetery is located about half a mile from the post. There is a post garden, containing about three acres, which is cultivated by enlisted men under the direction of the post chaplain.

*Meteorological report, Fort Laramie, Wyo., 1870–'74.*

| | 1870–'71. | | | | 1871–'72. | | | | 1872–'73. | | | | 1873–'74. | | | |
| | Temperature. | | | Rain-fall in inches. | Temperature. | | | Rain-fall in inches. | Temperature. | | | Rain-fall in inches. | Temperature. | | | Rain-fall in inches. |
| Month. | Mean. | Max. | Min. | | Mean. | Max. | Min. | | Mean. | Max. | Min. | | Mean. | Max. | Min. | |
|---|---|---|---|---|---|---|---|---|---|---|---|---|---|---|---|---|
| July | 75.80 | 100 | 53* | 1.05 | 77.44 | 105 | 55 | 2.00 | 68.17 | 96* | 37* | 3.75 | 72.69 | 96 | 40* | 0.58 |
| August | 64.54 | 97 | 34* | 0.97 | 73.83 | 102 | 52 | 0.80 | 69.31 | 100* | 40* | (?) | 71.81 | 97 | 40* | 0.62 |
| September | 58.21 | 88 | 32* | 2.70 | 62.35 | 94 | 40 | 1.10 | 59.66 | 93* | 27* | 0.50 | 56.21 | 89 | 11* | 0.00 |
| October | 44.29 | 85 | 17* | 2.35 | 46.92 | 86 | 17 | (?) | 48.29 | 90* | 14* | 0.50 | 41.01 | 83 | — 1* | 0.10 |
| November | 41.62 | 66 | 11* | 0.00 | 26.63 | 64 | —18 | (?) | 26.33 | 64* | — 7* | (?) | 35.36 | 67 | —12* | 0.10 |
| December | 22.65 | 56 | —23* | 0.05 | 25.06 | 55* | —33* | (?) | 19.06 | 50* | —23* | 0.80 | 17.93 | 49 | —22* | 2.50 |
| January | 27.95 | 68 | —19* | 0.40 | 26.13 | 57 | —14 | (?) | 21.86 | 55* | —25* | 0.70 | 28.68 | 58 | — 8* | 2.00 |
| February | 30.86 | 59 | — 4* | 0.60 | 33.50 | 63 | —35 | (?) | 20.65 | 49* | —34* | 4.00 | 24.76 | 53 | —29* | 1.25 |
| March | 38.52 | 73 | 9* | (?) | 38.28 | 66 | 5* | (?) | 35.42 | 74* | 2* | 0.50 | 30.87 | 56 | 3* | 0.47 |
| April | 43.23 | 76 | 10* | (?) | 41.56 | 76* | 16* | 2.75 | 37.66 | 85* | 9* | 4.75 | 42.01 | 82 | 7* | 2.25 |
| May | 59.67 | 90 | 34* | (?) | 56.18 | 89* | 24* | 2.00 | 50.82 | 85* | 17* | 3.50 | 59.15 | 90 | 25* | 0.50 |
| June | 73.97 | 97 | 53* | (?) | 65.69 | 96 | 37* | 0.00 | 72.51 | 98* | 40* | 1.00 | 66.89 | 95 | 31* | 1.17 |
| For the year | 48.44 | 100 | —23* | ........ | 47.79 | 105 | —35 | ........ | 44.14 | 100* | —34* | ........ | 45.61 | 97 | —29* | 11.54 |

* These observations are made with self-registering thermometers. The mean is from the standard thermometer.

*Consolidated sick-report, Fort Laramie, Wyo., 1870–'74.*

| | | 1870–'71. | | 1871–'72. | | 1872–'73. | | 1873–'74. | |
|---|---|---|---|---|---|---|---|---|---|
| Year | | 1870–'71. | | 1871–'72. | | 1872–'73. | | 1873–'74. | |
| Mean strength { Officers | | 14 | | 16 | | 25 | | 21 | |
| { Enlisted men | | 301 | | 278 | | 399 | | 418 | |
| Diseases. | | Cases. | Deaths. | Cases. | Deaths. | Cases. | Deaths. | Cases. | Deaths. |
| GENERAL DISEASES, A. | | | | | | | | | |
| Typhoid fever | | 2 | ...... | 6 | 1 | 1 | ...... | 1 | ...... |
| Remittent fever | | 4 | ...... | | | | | 1 | ...... |
| Intermittent fever | | 31 | ...... | 15 | ...... | 10 | ...... | 23 | ...... |
| Other diseases of this group | | 38 | ...... | 4 | ...... | 16 | ...... | 14 | ...... |
| GENERAL DISEASES, B. | | | | | | | | | |
| Rheumatism | | 82 | ...... | 37 | ...... | 24 | ...... | 36 | ...... |
| Syphilis | | 15 | ...... | 9 | ...... | 5 | ...... | 11 | ...... |
| Consumption | | 4 | ...... | 4 | 1 | 1 | ...... | 3 | ...... |
| Other diseases of this group | | 11 | ...... | 4 | ...... | 7 | ...... | 1 | ...... |
| LOCAL DISEASES. | | | | | | | | | |
| Catarrh and bronchitis | | 209 | ...... | 77 | ...... | 99 | ...... | 102 | ...... |
| Pneumonia | | 10 | 2 | | | 7 | ...... | 3 | ...... |
| Pleurisy | | 2 | ...... | 6 | ...... | 1 | ...... | 4 | ...... |
| Diarrhœa and dysentery | | 153 | ...... | 106 | ...... | 178 | ...... | 82 | ...... |
| Hernia | | 3 | ...... | 1 | ...... | 1 | ...... | 1 | ...... |
| Gonorrhœa | | 7 | ...... | 1 | ...... | 2 | ...... | 3 | ...... |
| Other local diseases | | 172 | ...... | 88 | 1 | 52 | 1 | 93 | 2 |
| Alcoholism | | 6 | ...... | 2 | ...... | 12 | ...... | 16 | ...... |
| Unclassified | | | | | | 1 | ...... | | |
| Total disease | | 749 | 2 | 360 | 3 | 417 | 1 | 394 | 2 |
| VIOLENT DISEASES AND DEATHS. | | | | | | | | | |
| Gunshot wounds | | 5 | ...... | 7 | 1 | 5 | ...... | 2 | 3 |
| Drowning | | | | | | | | | 1 |
| Other accidents and injuries | | 90 | ...... | 59 | 1 | 67 | ...... | 66 | 1 |
| Total violence | | 95 | ...... | 66 | 2 | 72 | ...... | 68 | 5 |

# FORT McPHERSON, NEBRASKA.

### REPORT BY ASSISTANT SURGEON C. L. HEIZMANN, UNITED STATES ARMY.

Fort McPherson, Nebr., is situated in latitude 41° 3′ north, longitude 23° 35′ west, at an elevation above the sea of 2,770 feet, on the south bank of the Platte River, twelve miles east of the confluence of the North and South Platte Rivers,* eighteen miles from North Platte City, and five miles southeast from McPherson Station on the Union Pacific Railroad. For history of the post see Circular No. 4, Surgeon-General's Office, 1870, page 334.

The soil being generally sandy is not very successfully tilled, except on the river-bank, and even there, the site of the post-garden, with irrigation by means of a pump, yielding precarious crops of corn, potatoes, and vegetables. On the island, the native grasses are abundant and remarkably nutritious—no other locality in the Platte region comparing with this ; the cottonwood, willow, and wild-plum trees, indigenous here, exist in large quantity.

Three wells, of an average depth of 35 feet, and Cottonwood spring, were once the water-sources, but on account of the accumulation of organic matter and small supply, the river-water alone is now used—distributed daily by a wagon. This water contains considerable lime and magnesia, chlorides, and traces of iron and sulphates. The matters suspended in it, sandy and organic, vary with the season, but at no time are sufficient to render it unpotable.

The little natural drainage, aided by rapid evaporation, is sufficient.

The post commands the section separating the Sioux and Pawnees, as well as the country settled by the whites along the railroad—the Republican and Loup Fork streams. Predatory and hunting bands of the former visit the vicinity ; none, however, reside in the immediate neighborhood. The number of white citizens, traders, contractors' agents, and employés settled on the reservation is 61.

The buildings are arranged about a quadrangle 844 by 560 feet. Two sides are formed by five barracks, three log and two frame ; one (log, shingle-roof) 145 by 27 feet, with wings of 87 by 20 feet ; one (frame, shingle-roof, unoccupied, and out of repair) 108 by 27 feet, with a wing of 69 by 20 feet ; one (log, shingle-roof, unoccupied) 114 by 27 feet, with wing 69 by 20 feet ; one (frame, shingle-roof) 147 by 27 feet, with wing of 69 by 20 feet, and another (log, shingle-roof) 132 by 30 feet, with no wing. Each building contains eighteen windows, and compartments used as dormitories, orderly-rooms, dining and cooking rooms. The dormitories are ceiled. Average air-space per man in two buildings occupied at present is 698 cubic feet. Single iron bedsteads are used. Ventilation is by windows and roof-ventilators.

One side is occupied by officers' quarters—frame, lathed and plastered, with shingle-roofs—in good repair. Three single buildings, 42 by 20 feet ; four double, 54 by 20 feet ; one commanding officer's, 65 by 24 feet. Two single buildings, 40 by 20 feet, are on a line with hospital, in the rear of the main line of officers' quarters. All have kitchens, 24 by 15 feet.

The fourth side is occupied by the adjutant's office, (new,) 41 by 30 feet ; quartermaster's office, (new,) 36 by 30 feet ; the commissary storehouse, (new,) 96 by 25 feet ; and the band quarters, (new,) 52 by 22 feet, with wing 90 by 19 feet.

In the rear of the barracks are the quartermaster's warehouse, (log,) 132 by 30 feet ; the forage building, (log,) 130 by 27 feet ; and six laundresses' houses, (five log and one frame ;) two, 40 by 24 feet ; one, 30 by 15 feet ; one, 40 by 18 feet, with wing 24 by 15 feet ; one, 60 by 18 feet ; one, 30 by 15 feet, with wing 12 by 15 feet ; also, the cavalry stables, log with shingle-roofs ; four, 200 by 30 feet ; and one, 235 by 30 feet.

---

* During high water only. The permanent conjunction takes place eight miles east, at the lower extremity of what is known as Brady's Island.

A new guard-house was erected in 1874. It is built of logs, 42 by 18 feet, and 9 feet high from floor to ceiling, and contains, besides a guard-room, ten single cells, each 6 by 3 feet, and one double cell, 6 by 6 feet. There is no general prison-room. Ventilation is sufficient.

The post-bakery (log) is 45 by 30 feet, with large oven.

The hospital is a log building, well chinked and plastered, with lathed and plastered ceilings and shingle-roof. It consists of a main building 69 by 20 feet, and a wing 56 by 20 feet, forming an "L."

The two ward-rooms, respectively 20 by 38 feet and 20 by 20 feet, will accommodate twenty-four patients, giving to each 466 cubic feet air-space. The dispensary is 20 by 12 feet, the steward's room 10 by 20 feet, and the dining-room and store-room are each 20 feet square. The wash-room, 8½ by 15 feet, adjoins the larger ward. The steward's quarters have a kitchen 14 by 20 feet, adjoining. The hospital kitchen, 16 by 20 feet, communicates with the dining-room in the wing of the building. An addition of a post-mortem room has been made.

There is no post library; but two company libraries, one containing 362 volumes, the other 26 volumes.

The bathing facilities are good in company quarters; the river, however, is preferable in summer. No post or company order for compulsory and systematic bathing has been issued.

Quartermaster and commissary stores are obtained from the depots at Omaha, two hundred and eighty-six miles, by means of the railroad and wagons from McPherson Station. They are in good condition when received and kept so in storehouses as above.

Mails from the east and west are received every morning. No endemic diseases; an epidemic of typhoid fever is recorded in October, November, and December, 1872.

*Meteorological report, Fort McPherson, Nebr., 1870–'74.*

| Year. | 1870–'71. | | | | 1871–'72. | | | | 1872–'73. | | | | 1873–'74. | | | |
|---|---|---|---|---|---|---|---|---|---|---|---|---|---|---|---|---|
| | Temperature. | | | Rain-fall in inches. | Temperature. | | | Rain-fall in inches. | Temperature. | | | Rain-fall in inches. | Temperature. | | | Rain-fall in inches. |
| | Mean. | Max. | Min. | | Mean. | Max. | Min. | | Mean. | Max. | Min. | | Mean. | Max. | Min. | |
| July.................. | 80.85 | 115* | 35* | 1.62 | 77.59 | 100* | 49* | 4.16 | 74.06 | 97* | 48* | 3.09 | 74.99 | 98* | 42* | 0.42 |
| August............. | 71.05 | 110* | 44* | 3.12 | 75.17 | 101* | 40* | 2.01 | 75.42 | 102* | 47* | 1.66 | 77.52 | 103* | 40* | 1.19 |
| September........... | 65.59 | 96* | 36* | 5.48 | 65.04 | 94* | 28* | 1.44 | 64.36 | 102* | 24* | 1.16 | 62.15 | 98* | 19* | 1.16 |
| October............ | 52.58 | 85* | 25* | 0.24 | 54.77 | 102* | 9* | 0.01 | 55.05 | 95* | 14* | 0.36 | 48.77 | 91* | 6* | 0.30 |
| November........... | 46.15 | 80* | 11* | 0.00 | 32.63 | 79* | – 4* | 2.84 | 32.04 | 77* | 1* | 0.06 | 40.67 | 79* | 1* | 0.10 |
| December........... | 28.30 | 60* | –16* | 0.32 | 23.04 | 60* | –11* | 0.28 | 19.21 | 60* | –18* | 0.29 | 24.01 | 58* | – 9* | 0.31 |
| January.......... .... | 32.85 | 78* | – 3* | 0.06 | 25.55 | 63* | –13* | 0.02 | 23.23 | 57* | –20* | 0.68 | 28.47 | 63* | – 4* | 0.10 |
| February........... | 39.05 | 80* | – 8* | 0.32 | 34.23 | 66* | – 6* | 0.53 | 27.35 | 59* | –19* | 0.08 | 26.82 | 57* | –24* | 0.45 |
| March............. | 42.62 | 80* | 3* | 0.42 | 35.95 | 78* | 8* | 0.62 | 41.94 | 86* | 1* | 0.07 | 34.82 | 62* | 10* | 0.78 |
| April............. | 50.09 | 93* | 20* | 2.20 | 51.27 | 89* | 19* | 1.88 | 44.52 | 87* | 10* | 2.90 | 48.32 | 96* | 10* | 0.72 |
| May............. | 62.97 | 95* | 30* | 3.84 | 61.66 | 92* | 28* | 2.94 | 56.73 | 89* | 29* | 8.41 | 65.80 | 96* | 33* | 2.80 |
| June ................. | 75.44 | 104* | 46* | 2.46 | 73.00 | 98* | 46* | 3.46 | 74.43 | 99* | 43* | 3.24 | 74.68 | 103* | 39* | 3.34 |
| For the year....... | 53.96 | 115* | –16* | 20.08 | 50.83 | 102* | –13* | 20.19 | 49.03 | 102* | –20* | 22.00 | 50.58 | 103* | –24* | 11.67 |

\* These observations are made with self-registering thermometers. The mean is from the standard thermometer.

*Consolidated sick-report, Fort McPherson, Nebr., 1870–'74.*

| Year ............................................................................ | | 1870–'71. | | 1871–'72. | | 1872–'73. | | 1873–'74. | |
|---|---|---|---|---|---|---|---|---|---|
| Mean strength ............................................................ { Officers............. | | 12 | | 11 | | 10 | | 9 | |
| { Enlisted men ...... | | 334 | | 264 | | 259 | | 261 | |
| Diseases. | | Cases. | Deaths. | Cases. | Deaths. | Cases. | Deaths. | Cases. | Deaths. |
| GENERAL DISEASES, A. | | | | | | | | | |
| Typhoid fever.................................................................. | | 1 | ....... | 1 | ....... | 4 | 2 | 2 | 1 |
| Remittent fever.............................................................. | | | | | | 10 | | 3 | |
| Intermittent fever .......................................................... | | 13 | | 56 | | 52 | | 26 | |
| Other diseases of this group ........................................ | | 65 | | 10 | | 32 | | 25 | |

*Consolidated sick-report, Fort McPherson, Nebr., 1870–'74—Continued.*

| Year | 1870–'71. | | 1871–'72. | | 1872–'73. | | 1873–'74. | |
|---|---|---|---|---|---|---|---|---|
| Mean strength { Officers | 12 | | 11 | | 10 | | 9 | |
| { Enlisted men | 334 | | 264 | | 259 | | 261 | |
| Diseases. | Cases. | Deaths. | Cases. | Deaths. | Cases. | Deaths. | Cases. | Deaths. |
| GENERAL DISEASES, B. | | | | | | | | |
| Rheumatism | 27 | | 16 | | 43 | | 22 | |
| Syphilis | 13 | | 6 | | 24 | | 17 | |
| Consumption | 1 | | 4 | | 4 | | 3 | |
| Other diseases of this group | 1 | | 1 | | 1 | | 1 | |
| LOCAL DISEASES. | | | | | | | | |
| Catarrh and bronchitis | 48 | | 67 | | 79 | | 46 | |
| Pneumonia | 2 | | 1 | | 3 | | 4 | 1 |
| Pleurisy | 1 | | | | 2 | | 3 | |
| Diarrhœa and dysentery | 68 | | 60 | | 150 | | 100 | |
| Hernia | 2 | | 1 | | | | 4 | |
| Gonorrhœa | 8 | | 8 | | 13 | | 4 | |
| Other local diseases | 199 | | 120 | 1 | 232 | 2 | 221 | |
| Alcoholism | 20 | 1 | 3 | | 12 | | 8 | |
| Unclassified | | | | | | | | 1 |
| Total disease | 469 | 1 | 354 | 1 | 661 | 4 | 489 | 3 |
| VIOLENT DISEASES AND DEATHS. | | | | | | | | |
| Gunshot wounds | 5 | 1 | 1 | | 2 | | 1 | |
| Drowning | | | | | | 6 | | |
| Other accidents and injuries | 197 | 1 | 150 | 2 | 134 | 1 | 154 | |
| Suicide | | 1 | | | | 1 | | |
| Total violence | 202 | 3 | 151 | 2 | 136 | 8 | 155 | |

# MEDICINE BOW, WYOMING TERRITORY.

INFORMATION FURNISHED BY ACTING ASSISTANT SURGEON A. J. HOGG, UNITED STATES ARMY.

The temporary camp of Medicine Bow is situated on the Medicine Bow River, at the crossing of the Union Pacific Railroad, 647 miles west of Omaha; latitude, 41° 46′ north; longitude, 29° 31′ west; altitude, 6,550 feet above the sea.

The Seminole Mountains and Black Hills are about 25 miles to the west and north, and the Medicine Bow Mountains about the same distance to the east and south. The surface of the country in the immediate vicinity is rolling, broken, and somewhat picturesque. The outcropping rocks are shale and sandstone, which doubtless overlie beds of coal. Fossil remains of mollusks are found in the sandstone. The grass in the vicinity is abundant, and of good quality.

About four miles from the camp, and very near the railroad, is a spring of as fine chalybeate water doubtless as there is in the world. There are also several sulphur springs near. Should a permanent post be established at Medicine Bow, these springs, together with the bracing mountain air, would make the locality a desirable summer resort for invalids. Game is abundant. During the months of September and October, hunting parties are from time to time sent out, which keep the command well supplied with the flesh of the elk, black-tailed deer, antelope, mountain-sheep, and bear.

The post was established in 1869, and has been occupied by a company of troops every year since, from the first of May to the first of November, for the purpose of affording protection to the railroad-station, Government stores, and the settlers in the vicinity; and of furnishing escorts for freight-trains, and to officers and their families traveling to and fro between the station and Fort Fetterman, eighty-five miles distant, north.

The troops occupy as quarters either the railroad round-house or tents; more frequently the former, which is spacious and well ventilated.

The sick are either treated in the round-house or sent by rail to hospital at Fort Fred Steele, forty-seven miles west.

Prisoners guilty of trivial offenses are confined in a box railroad-car. Those against whom charges are preferred are sent to Fort Steele for confinement.

Pine wood of good quality is hauled from the low mountains fifteen miles distant. Coal in unlimited quantities can be obtained from the railroad company.

Good water is obtained from the Medicine Bow River, which runs close by.

The locality is a healthy one. The men seldom get sick. Occasionally there is a case of a fever, vaguely called "mountain fever," but which resembles the remittent type more than any other, and is very amenable to treatment.

---

# NORTH PLATTE STATION, NEBRASKA.

INFORMATION FURNISHED BY ASSISTANT SURGEON F. W. ELBREY AND ACTING ASSISTANT SURGEON JOHN RIDGELY, UNITED STATES ARMY.

North Platte Station is situated on the line of the Union Pacific Railroad, three and a half miles from the confluence of the North and South Platte Rivers, and two hundred and ninety-one miles west of Omaha, Nebr. Latitude, 41° 6′ 55″ north; longitude, 24° 22′ 44″ west; altitude, 2,789 feet above the level of the sea.

The post was established in August, 1867, for the protection of the railroad and to serve as a basis of supply for detachments of troops stationed in the vicinity. The ground occupied comprises a little over eight acres adjoining the railroad, and is a portion of an alternate section granted by the General Government to the Union Pacific Railroad. The surface topography of the vicinity is an unbroken prairie, extending seven miles to the east and sixteen miles west, with an average width of six miles, limited by the North and South Platte Rivers. The underlying stratum is of tertiary formation. The soil, being of a rich, alluvial character, is fertile if properly irrigated, irrigation being necessary by reason of the insufficiency of rain-fall and the oft long-continued droughts. The prairie from the South Platte River, being from 40 to 50 feet higher than the North Platte, has an even descent of about 7 feet to the mile toward the latter river, rendering irrigation convenient.

The climate is healthful, and the extremes of temperature, on account of the dry and rarefied atmosphere, are well borne. The rain and snow fall are small. The prevailing winds during the summer are from the southeast, and in winter from the northwest. The winds are frequent, of long continuance, and blow very violently.

The post-grounds, inclosed by a fence, are nearly in the form of a square. The parade occupies a space near the center. All the buildings are constructed of pine wood, the roofs of some being the so-called "composition-roof," consisting of boards covered with tarred-paper secured by means of batting, and of the others common shingles. The barrack-building, accommodating one company, is 127 by 30 feet, and one story high, giving 500 cubic feet air-space per man.

It is warmed in winter by two coal-stoves, lighted and ventilated by six lateral and two end windows placed in opposite sides. Iron bunks are used. The wash-room is partly detached, being 10 by 15 feet, partitioned off from the quarters. The sinks are located about 80 feet in rear of the barracks, and are unexceptionable. The kitchen and mess-room both adjoin the barracks. The kitchen, 14 by 18 feet, is in a bad condition, being open to the weather during storms. The mess-room is a portion of the barracks, made by putting a partition between the two. The post-bakery is 24 by 15 feet, built of wood, and adjoins the rear of the company kitchen.

The quarters of laundresses and married soldiers are contained in a frame building, 32 by 24 feet, divided into four rooms, in bad repair. The interior is lined with tar-paper; during a storm rain and snow enter part of the roof and sides of the building. Two of the rooms are occupied as quarters by the hospital-steward, there being no other provision made for him.

Two one-story buildings are used for officers' quarters, constructed of wood, plastered, covered

46 M P

with shingles, and finished in the plainest style possible. One is divided into two sets of quarters of three rooms each, having attic chambers, and each a kitchen. The other has no attic or kitchen, and contains two rooms each. There are no bath-rooms. Water used for general purposes is supplied from a well located to the rear of these buildings.

The commissary store-house is a one-story building, 20 by 49 feet, covered by a composition-roof in bad repair.

The guard-house previously used, being an old adobe building and perfectly worthless, has been destroyed, and a new building of limestone is in course of erection. This will contain a guard-room, prison-room, and four cells.

The hospital is a frame building, $40\frac{1}{2}$ by $15\frac{1}{2}$ feet, containing a ward, 26 by $14\frac{1}{2}$ feet; dispensary, 13 by 13 feet; kitchen, which forms an L to the main building, $14\frac{1}{2}$ by $11\frac{1}{2}$ feet. Three unfinished rooms on second floor are occupied as quarters by the steward and matron. Two coal-stoves are used. Ventilation and lighting are effected by five windows. The ward contains six beds. An inclosed shed in rear of the ward is used as a bath-room. The stables are of wood, 32 by 150 feet, accommodating about 75 horses.

The North Platte River being distant from the post only 1,741 yards, and the South Platte 2,300 yards, and the soil being very porous, everywhere inexhaustible wells can be dug to a depth not exceeding 10 feet from the surface. The supply for the post is therefore abundant; but the quality of the water is not all that could be desired, on account of its organic impurities, the permanganate of potassa test showing 19 grains to the gallon.

The natural drainage is all-sufficient, the porosity of the soil preventing the collection of stagnant water.

There are no bathing facilities at the post, excepting during the summer months, when the North Platte affords excellent advantages.

The post-garden covers an area of three-fourths of an acre, and is well cultivated, being made productive by irrigation. Cabbage, lettuce, radishes, beets, &c., are raised.

The mails are daily.

The inhabitants of North Platte town are 800 in number, composed of railroad employés, artisans, and small traders.

*Consolidated sick-report, North Platte Station, Nebr., 1870–'74.*

| Year | | 1870–'71. | | 1871–'72. | | 1872–'73. | | 1873–'74. | |
|---|---|---|---|---|---|---|---|---|---|
| Mean strength { Officers | | 5 | | 3 | | 2 | | 2 | |
| { Enlisted men | | 119 | | 72 | | 71 | | 59 | |
| Diseases. | | Cases. | Deaths. | Cases. | Deaths. | Cases. | Deaths. | Cases. | Deaths. |
| GENERAL DISEASES, A. | | | | | | | | | |
| Typho-malarial fever | | | | | | | | 2 | |
| Remittent fever | | | | | | | | 1 | |
| Intermittent fever | | 11 | | 2 | | 4 | | 23 | |
| Other diseases of this group | | 12 | | 18 | | 5 | | 2 | |
| GENERAL DISEASES, B. | | | | | | | | | |
| Rheumatism | | 25 | | 15 | | 12 | | 9 | |
| Syphilis | | 4 | | | | 5 | | | |
| Consumption | | 1 | | | | | | | |
| Other diseases of this group | | 1 | | 1 | | | | 4 | |
| LOCAL DISEASES. | | | | | | | | | |
| Catarrh and bronchitis | | 22 | | 18 | | 18 | | 41 | |
| Diarrhœa and dysentery | | 18 | | 10 | | 9 | | 14 | |
| Hernia | | | | | | | | 1 | |
| Gonorrhœa | | 3 | | 1 | | 2 | | 1 | |
| Other local diseases | | 32 | | 20 | | 23 | | 48 | |
| Alcoholism | | 1 | | 5 | | 3 | | 2 | |
| Total disease | | 130 | | 90 | | 81 | | 148 | |
| VIOLENT DISEASES AND DEATHS. | | | | | | | | | |
| Gunshot wounds | | 3 | | | | 2 | | 1 | |
| Other accidents and injuries | | 31 | | 20 | | 20 | | 46 | |
| Suicide | | | | | | | 1 | | |
| Total violence | | 34 | | 20 | | 22 | 1 | 47 | |

# OMAHA BARRACKS, NEBRASKA.

INFORMATION FURNISHED BY SURGEON CHARLES PAGE AND ASSISTANT SURGEON FRANK MEACHAM, UNITED STATES ARMY.

The post of Omaha Barracks is on the right or west bank of the Missouri River, which is two miles distant at its nearest point. It is four miles northwest from Omaha City, and one and a half miles south from the town of Florence. Latitude, 41° 20′ north; longitude, 18° 57′ west; and altitude, 960 feet above the sea.

To the west is a high rolling prairie; eastward is a level bench extending to the river-bottoms. The soil consists of a rich, black, vegetable mold, from 2 to 5 feet in depth, containing some sand, but entirely free from stones or gravel; the subsoil being a yellowish clay, not impervious to water. Trees are planted around the parade, and where properly set out are growing luxuriantly.

The post was established November 20, 1868. The reservation contains eighty acres, forty of which were contributed by the citizens of Omaha, the balance a purchase by the United States. It is nearly a perfect rectangle in shape, the long axis running north and south. The western side is elevated and overlooks the reservation, the Missouri bottom, and the city of Omaha. The view from the post embraces also the bold hills on the Iowa side of the river, the town of Council Bluffs, and here and there portions of the Missouri River.

The company barracks are ten wooden structures, lined with brick, each 30 by 80 feet, 12 feet high to the eaves, and 24 feet to the ridge, giving a capacity of 43,200 cubic feet. They are wainscoted to the bottom of the windows, and ceiled with half-inch tongued and grooved boards, with three ventilators in the ceiling of each. Each barrack has a porch in front 10 feet wide, from each end of which a room, 10 by 10 feet, is cut off, one for first sergeant's room or office, the other for a store-room, leaving the open porch, 10 by 60 feet.

A building, 21 by 52 feet, 10 feet high, divided into a mess-room, 21 by 40 feet, and a kitchen, 12 by 21 feet, is placed 16 feet in the rear of each barrack, with which it is connected by a covered way, 10 feet wide. The covered ways are used as lavatories. The buildings are well lighted by windows and warmed by coal-stoves.

There are two sinks, each a frame building, 16 by 53 feet, over a pit 11 feet deep. They are located 130 feet to the rear of the mess-rooms of the two middle barracks.

The quarters for laundresses and married soldiers are two frame buildings, each 150 by 30 feet, and divided into nine sets of quarters, each containing two rooms, 15 feet square. Two other buildings, each 30 by 80 feet, and divided into five sets of quarters of two rooms, are occupied by married soldiers.

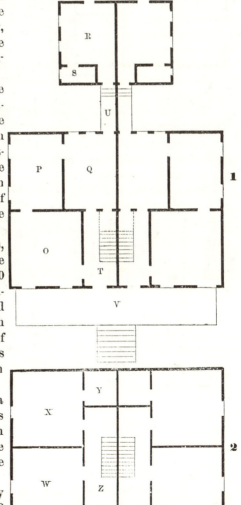
Figure 54.

The officers' quarters are fourteen frame buildings, lined with brick, plain batten finish, and painted a dull yellow color. They are one story high, with attic rooms. There are ten double sets of quarters for line officers, each accommodating a captain and two lieutenants. They are divided into two symmetrical parts, as shown by Figure 54.

1, first floor; 2, second floor; O, parlor, 15 by 14½ feet; P, chamber, 15 by 10½ feet; Q, dining-room, 15 by 10½ feet; R, kitchen, 11 by 12 feet; S, closet, 7½ by 3½ feet; T, hall, 15 by 6½ feet; U, covered way, 10 by 3½ feet; V, veranda, 43 by 8 feet; W and X, chambers, 15 by 15 feet; Y, closet, 5 by 6 feet; Z, hall and stairs.

There are three sets of quarters for the field-officers and the medical officer, the arrangement of which is shown by Figure 55.

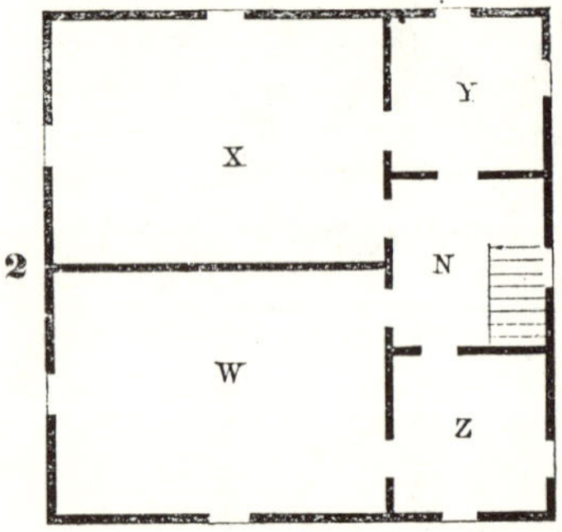

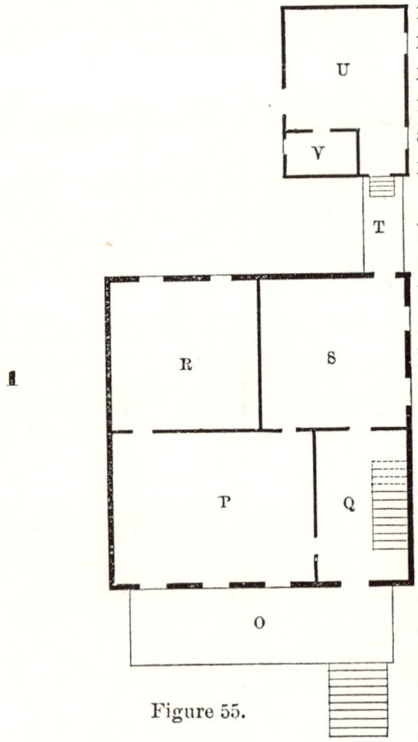

1, first floor; 2, second floor; O, piazza, 28 by 8 feet; P, parlor, 15 by 20 feet; Q, hall, 10 by 15 feet; R, chamber, 15 by 15 feet; S, dining-room, 15 by 15 feet; T, covered way, 10 by 4½ feet; U, kitchen, 13 by 18 feet; V, closet, 4 by 8 feet; W and X, chambers, 20 by 15 feet; Y and Z, rooms 10 feet square; N, hall and stairs.

The commanding officer's quarters is a two-story house, 40 by 50 feet, with a porch, 8 feet wide, in front, and part of each side. There is a hall on the first floor, 40 by 7 feet; on the left is a room, 15 by 36 feet, with a bay-window; on the right are two rooms connected by folding-doors; the front room is 15 by 15½ feet, the back room, 15 by 20 feet; to the rear of these rooms are two smaller rooms, two narrow halls, a cellar-way, and a water-closet; still farther back is the kitchen and laundry. On the upper floor are four rooms, 15 by 15½ feet, with three smaller rooms, a bath-room, and a water-closet.

The commanding officer's quarters are heated by furnaces, burning bituminous coal. All the rest are heated by coal-stoves. They are lighted by coal-oil lamps, and are ventilated by means of the windows, which open from the top as well as at the bottom. There is a privy ten feet to the rear of each kitchen; they consist of small buildings placed over pits. There are no bath-rooms in any of the quarters, except the commanding officer's.

During the summer of 1874, a cistern was built for each set of quarters, thereby affording a good supply of water, which passes through a charcoal and sand filter before it reaches the cistern.

The guard-house is 43¼ by 48½ feet, 12 feet high, with a porch in front, 12 feet wide. The entrance is in front near the center, and leads into a hall, 16 by 4 feet; on the left is a room, 16 by 16 feet, for the officer of the guard; on the right, a room, 22½ by 21 feet, for the guard. The front hall leads into a second, 32 by 4 feet, which is a continuation of the first, separated from it by a strong door; on the left of this passage-way is a room, 18 by 15 feet, in which are confined prisoners of the worst class. At the rear of this room are three cells, 7½ by 4⅓ by 12 feet high. At the rear of the guard-room is a room 24 by 21 feet, in which are confined the lighter cases. All the above rooms are 12 feet high. The guard-house is warmed by stoves burning wood. The prison-rooms are ventilated by three grated windows, 2 feet square, placed 8 feet from the floor. These windows are kept constantly open. There is no ventilation in the cells. The rooms occupied by the prisoners contain 9,088 cubic feet of air-space, and are frequently occupied by 30 men, giving each man 303 cubic feet of air. The cells contain each 390 cubic feet of air. They are seldom used, and only for solitary confinement. With the exception of the want of proper ventilation in these cells, the guard-house is well adapted to its purpose.

Figure 55.

The hospital is located at the north end of the garrison. It is a frame building, lined with brick, batten-finish, painted dull yellow. Its general arrangement is the same as given in Circular No. 4, from the Surgeon-General's Office, 1867, for 48 beds. It is warmed by wood-stoves, and has ridge ventilators. There are 24 beds in each ward, with 990 cubic feet air-space per man. The bath and wash rooms are not well arranged. There are no water-closets in the building. The hospital sink is 80 feet distant. There is no dead-house. The baggage of the patients is stored in one of the small rooms at the end of the wards.

There is a veranda 10 feet wide around the whole hospital, except the kitchen. A bath-room, 10 by 15 feet, is at the end of the veranda. It contains two bath-tubs and a stove with large boilers for heating water in cold weather. A cellar 14 by 35 feet, 8 feet deep, under the main part of the hospital, was constructed in 1871. It is both rat-proof and frost-proof.

The water used at the post is taken from a well north of the north row of barracks, and left at the kitchens each day by the water-wagon. An analysis of the water was made in the winter of 1873, with the following result:

Water ............................................................................................. 999.71
Solid residue, { chlorides ............................................................... .03
{ lime, soda, potash, } carbonates ........................................ .21
Organic matter.......................................................................... .05
                                                                                             ————
   Total................................................................................. 1,000.00

Lime is the principal ingredient of the solid residue.

This water is used almost exclusively by the garrison for drinking purposes, and is considered palatable and wholesome.

As a precaution against fires there are barrels and buckets constantly filled with water in each of the barracks, storehouses, and stables; also at the hospital. In addition, there are one or more patent fire-extinguishers in each of the above-named buildings. A large, double-cylinder, Babcock fire-extinguisher, mounted on wheels, has been added to the means for preventing destruction by fire.

The natural drainage, except at the south end of the grounds, is ample. The artificial drains are simple open ditches, and are used exclusively about the south row of barracks and laundresses quarters. The drains discharge into a small stream that flows in front of the post and empties into the Missouri River. Slops and excreta of the post are hauled away and deposited on the commons northeast of the post.

During the summer the men bathe in the Missouri River, two miles distant. There are no arrangements at the post for bathing in summer or winter.

About 3½ acres are cultivated as post-garden, by men detailed for the duty, under the supervision of the post treasurer.

*Meteorological report, Omaha Barracks, Nebr., 1870-'74.*

| Month. | 1870-'71. | | | | 1871-'72. | | | | 1872-'73. | | | | 1873-'74. | | | |
|---|---|---|---|---|---|---|---|---|---|---|---|---|---|---|---|---|
| | Temperature. | | | Rain-fall in inches. | Temperature. | | | Rain-fall in inches. | Temperature. | | | Rain-fall in inches. | Temperature. | | | Rain-fall in inches. |
| | Mean. | Max. | Min. | | Mean. | Max. | Min. | | Mean. | Max. | Min. | | Mean. | Max. | Min. | |
| July ............... | 79.48 | 100 | 61 | 0.23 | 75.83 | 93 | 60 | 5.34 | 76.69 | 92 | 54* | 6.93 | 79.18 | 95 | 59 | 1.90 |
| August ............ | 70.93 | 95 | 46 | 1.80 | 74.38 | 92 | 56 | 1.90 | 75.47 | 93 | 53* | 1.12 | 81.67 | 101 | 59 | 1.70 |
| September .......... | 65.66 | 80 | 51 | 5.34 | 64.55 | 86 | 39 | 2.28 | 64.15 | 90 | 35* | 2.81 | 66.05 | 93 | 34 | 3.10 |
| October ............ | 51.49 | 78 | 30 | 4.60 | 55.34 | 88 | 33 | 1.75 | 54.65 | 86 | 24* | 2.28 | ...... | ...... | ...... | ...... |
| November............ | 47.65 | 78 | 18 | 0.00 | 32.40 | 70 | — 7* | 2.27 | 30.53 | 64 | — 5* | 0.16 | ...... | ...... | ...... | ...... |
| December ........... | 26.18 | 65 | —18 | 0.00 | 20.36 | 51 | —13* | 1.13 | 18.31 | 58 | —20* | 1.05 | ...... | ...... | ...... | ...... |
| January............. | 28.08 | 58 | — 5 | 0.39 | 20.31 | 45 | —14* | 3.30 | 17.53 | 48 | —21* | (?)15.55 | ...... | ...... | ...... | ...... |
| February............ | 29.29 | 60 | — 8 | 0.24 | 29.31 | 54 | — 8* | 0.10 | 25.31 | 54 | —16* | 1.56 | ...... | ...... | ...... | ...... |
| March............... | 43.73 | 68 | 21 | 0.11 | 32.43 | 67 | 0* | 1.12 | 41.03 | 69 | — 1* | 1.29 | ...... | ...... | ...... | ...... |
| April.............. | 56.37 | 96 | 26 | 2.21 | 52.09 | 85 | 16* | 5.00 | 50.35 | 83 | 31 | 0.95 | ...... | ...... | ...... | ...... |
| May................ | 66.16 | 86 | 36 | 2.65 | 62.57 | 91 | 28* | 9.40 | 60.73 | 84 | 40 | 4.38 | ...... | ...... | ...... | ...... |
| June ............... | 79.47 | 96 | 65 | 2.48 | 73.67 | 90 | 24* | 2.23 | 76.70 | 93 | 56 | 2.80 | ...... | ...... | ...... | ...... |
| For the year ...... | 53.71 | 100 | —18 | 20.05 | 49.43 | 93 | —14* | 35.82 | 49.29 | 93 | —21* | 38.88 | ...... | ...... | ...... | ...... |

* These observations are made with self-registering thermometers. The mean is from the standard thermometer.

*Consolidated sick-report, Omaha Barracks, Nebr., 1870–'74.*

| Year | 1870–'71. | | 1871–'72. | | 1872–'73. | | 1873–'74. | |
|---|---|---|---|---|---|---|---|---|
| Mean strength { Officers<br>{ Enlisted men | 18<br>501 | | 13<br>260 | | 22<br>443 | | 21<br>369 | |
| Diseases. | Cases. | Deaths. | Cases. | Deaths. | Cases. | Deaths. | Cases. | Deaths. |
| GENERAL DISEASES, A. | | | | | | | | |
| Typhoid fever | | 1 | 2 | 2 | 2 | | 1 | 1 |
| Intermittent fever | 27 | | 44 | | 114 | | 99 | |
| Other diseases of this group | 5 | | 8 | | 57 | | 40 | |
| GENERAL DISEASES, B. | | | | | | | | |
| Rheumatism | 31 | | 14 | | 49 | | 49 | |
| Syphilis | 13 | | 10 | | 17 | | 5 | |
| Consumption | | 1 | | | 2 | 1 | | |
| Other diseases of this group | 2 | | | | | | 1 | 1 |
| LOCAL DISEASES. | | | | | | | | |
| Catarrh and bronchitis | 132 | | 59 | | 222 | | 210 | |
| Pneumonia | 3 | | 2 | 1 | 3 | 1 | 3 | 1 |
| Pleurisy | 2 | | 1 | | 4 | | 8 | |
| Diarrhœa and dysentery | 92 | | 27 | | 72 | | 122 | |
| Hernia | | | | | 1 | | 5 | |
| Gonorrhœa | 11 | | 12 | | 27 | | 26 | |
| Other local diseases | 108 | 1 | 51 | | 202 | 1 | 234 | |
| Alcoholism | 13 | | 5 | | 20 | | 37 | |
| Unclassified | | | | | 1 | | | |
| Total disease | 439 | 3 | 235 | 3 | 793 | 3 | 840 | 3 |
| VIOLENT DISEASES AND DEATHS. | | | | | | | | |
| Gunshot wounds | 5 | 1 | 2 | | 4 | | | |
| Other accidents and injuries | 133 | | 96 | 2 | 143 | 1 | 99 | |
| Total violence | 138 | 1 | 98 | 2 | 147 | 1 | 99 | |

# CAMP ROBINSON, NEBRASKA.

### INFORMATION FURNISHED BY SURGEON JOHN F. RANDOLPH, UNITED STATES ARMY.

Camp Robinson, named in memory of First Lieut. Levi H. Robinson, Fourteenth United States Infantry, who was treacherously murdered by Indians in February, 1874, is located in a bend of the White River, on its north or left bank. It is in the northwestern corner of the State of Nebraska, latitude 42° 30′ north, and longitude 26° 21′ west. Cheyenne City is about one hundred and seventy miles distant southwest. Red Cloud Indian agency is one and a half miles east, and on the opposite side of the river. The valley is from five to seven miles wide. The source of White River is not more than twenty miles above this point. All the way down it is fed by small streams and springs, affording excellent camping-places. The soil is a light, sandy loam, formed by washings from the hills. The timber is of an inferior quality, very brittle, and is said to soon decay. The logs for building purposes are hauled from five to seven miles from the hills to the north. The mountains, north and south, are sparsely covered with pine trees. Lime, of bad quality, is found in the vicinity. Indians in the valley are, Ogallala Sioux, Cheyennes, and Arapahoes. The Northern Sioux (Minneconjons) are frequent but unwelcome visitors. Rations, it is said, are issued from the agency every ten days to between eleven and twelve thousand.

The camp is 160 yards square. Officers' quarters are on the north, infantry barracks on the east and west, and cavalry barracks, guard-house, and store-house on the south sides. A small creek runs along its west side, which is dry for most of the year; but in the valley opposite the post are several springs, which afford an ample supply of water of good quality the year round. The plateau, upon which the quarters are being erected, is about 30 feet above the river, which is some 400 yards south, and at this point only 15 or 20 feet wide.

The barracks are built of logs, in panels of 15 feet each. For the infantry they are two in number, each 150 by 24 feet by 9 feet high to eaves, divided in the center to accommodate two companies. They have a shed extension to the rear, 12 feet wide, the length of the building, partitioned off for mess-rooms, kitchens, and wash-rooms. The cavalry barrack is built in the same way, but only 90 feet long, for the accommodation of one company, with mess-room and kitchen like the others. These buildings are unceiled, have shingle roofs, log walls, window-sashes, and are floored. The dormitories afford 685 cubic feet air-space per man. There is no special provision for ventilation. Single iron bunks are furnished.

One building, 142 by 24 feet, 8½ feet to eaves, and from eaves to ridge 7½ feet, is built of logs, with shingle roof, and divided into twelve sets of two rooms each, and occupied as quarters for married soldiers and laundresses.

The officers' quarters are to be all alike, six sets being authorized, each 38 feet long by 32 feet wide and 10 feet high, one for the commanding-officer and five for company officers. They have stone foundations, walls of adobe, and are to be ceiled by boards and plastered. In each building there are to be four rooms, 15 feet square, with a central hall, 4 feet wide. The dining-rooms and kitchens in the rear are to be made of lumber. Only two sets have roofs on yet, (November 3, 1874.) There is no guard-house; wall-tents are used.

The site for the hospital has been selected on a line with the officers' quarters, and a hundred yards west. The plan furnished is that of a provisional hospital, described in Circular No. 2, Surgeon-General's Office, 1871. Some materials, consisting of doors, window-sash, (glazed,) flooring, nails, &c., have been received.

The present accommodations for the sick consist of hospital-tents, four of which are pitched and framed. One is used as a dispensary and for stores—in it the steward sleeps; two for wards, in which are seven beds; the fourth is partially filled with stores, and also furnishes meager quarters for the post-surgeon. They are all grouped on the bluff overlooking the laundresses' quarters. On the side of this bank there has been improvised a kitchen, called in this country a dug-out, consisting of an excavation in the hillside, roofed with slabs and covered with earth. A door is provided on the lower side, and an opening left above to admit light. It is large enough to receive a cooking-stove, and shelving for culinary apparatus. The cook has also reserved space for his bed. The hospital-attendants during the summer dug a well in the creek-bottom, near the kitchen, which affords very good and cold water. The tents are heated by small Sibley stoves, but the warmth afforded is not sufficient in cold weather. Fuel is supplied by contract. It is abundant, but of inferior quality, being soft pine, cut in the neighboring mountains.

---

# FORT D. A. RUSSELL, WYOMING TERRITORY.

REPORTS OF SURGEON C. H. ALDEN AND ASSISTANT SURGEON R. M. REYNOLDS, UNITED STATES ARMY.

Fort David A. Russell is situated in the southeastern part of the Territory of Wyoming; in latitude, 41° 8′ north; and longitude, 27° 42′ west; at an elevation of 6,021 feet above the level of the sea. It lies on the north bank of Crow Creek, a branch of the South Platte, and three miles west of the town of Cheyenne, a station on the Union Pacific Railroad.

The reservation was originally a parallelogram, extending 2 miles east and west, by 3 miles north and south, and containing 3,840 acres. Additions have been made, partly to give increased space for the quartermaster's depot, situated in the southeastern angle. The reservation is about equally divided by Crow Creek, which crosses it from northwest to southeast. This is a small and tortuous but never-failing stream. On either side of the creek are bluffs from 30 to 50 feet high, there being many small bottoms between them. Along the stream the terrace formation can be traced in some places, particularly in the part occupied by the quartermaster's depot, where there are four successive benches rising from the water to the plain. To the north of the creek there is a large level plateau, about a mile wide, beyond which the country is broken. To the south of the stream the country is much broken into low hills for some distance.

The soil on the prairies is barren, nor can the bottom-lands be cultivated except by aid of irrigation. The plains and hills are covered with a low, stunted, scanty grass. Along the creek a few low willows and wild-currant bushes grow. In summer the desolate prairies and bottoms are made brilliant for a short time by a profusion of wild flowers, rich, however, rather in number than variety. The only edible wild plants known are the wild onion, (*Allium stellatum;*) lambs' quarters, (*Chenopodium album;*) and wild currants, (*Ribes aureum.*) The most common wild animals are the coyote, prairie-dog, and striped gopher. Rattlesnakes are occasionally seen. The numerous crania of buffalo testify to their presence in this country at no very distant period, but not probably within eight or ten years. Antelope, and occasionally common deer, can be found at some distance from the post. Of birds the species are numerous. Among game birds are the prairie-chicken, sage-cock, mallard duck, green-winged teal, killdeer, yellow-legged snipe, and Wilson's phalarope.

The weather is at all times subject to sudden and great changes, and the wind blows often with much violence, particularly during the spring and fall. The prevailing wind is northwest, blowing with most severity in February, March, April, September, October, November, and December. Spring opens about May 1, and the first frost comes in September. March is the most inclement month. During all the warm months the temperature is very much lower at night than by day.

The post is located a little to the left of the center of the reservation, its southernmost angle reaching to the edge of the bluff, there about 50 feet above the water, which flows directly beneath. The buildings are entirely of wood; they are arranged around a parade of the diamond form, which is 1,040 feet in its long by 800 feet in its short axis. The long axis is on the magnetic meridian, the variation being 13° 30' east. In the spring of 1870, cottonwood and pine trees were planted around the parade and in other parts of the post. The barracks do not directly face the parade, but are arranged *en echelon*, by which means light and air have free access to all sides of the buildings. Behind the western row of officers' quarters is a "grout" or concrete building, intended for an officers' mess-house, but now used for courts-martial and school. The post is designed to accommodate twelve companies, six each of cavalry and infantry.

The arrangement of the post is shown in the plate opposite.

The general plan of the post was made by Bvt. Brig. Gen. J. D. Stevenson, colonel Thirtieth Infantry, with suggestions by Surgeon C. H. Alden, United States Army. The diamond form of the parade was adopted not only for the sake of appearance, but to avoid the inconvenience of the very large inclosed space, which would have resulted from the ordinary rectangular or square space, owing to the great number of buildings required. There are eleven company barracks, built of rough boards placed upright, with the cracks battened; each is 80 feet long by 30 feet wide, with 11-foot walls, and shingled roof of one-third pitch, and has a porch, 7 feet wide, along the front. Inside there is a lining of adobes, placed on edge, filled in between the timbers to the level of the eaves all around. Each barrack is designed to accommodate eighty men, and allows 480 cubic feet of air-space per man. There is a brick chimney in the center of each barrack. There are but two doors, both in front. The roof and ends above the adobe-lining are so open from the shrinking of the lumber that ventilation is amply sufficient. Some of the barracks have, however, special ventilation-shafts. The water-closet, a small frame building placed over an ordinary sink, is situated about 75 feet in rear of each barrack. At the south end of, and on the line with, the porch of each building is a rough structure of logs placed upright in the earth, about 20 by 50 feet, and shingled. At the south end of this is the company kitchen, about 15 by 20 feet, the remainder of the interior being the mess-hall. Cooking is done by large stoves and caldrons. A wash-room is in somes cases attached to the south end of the kitchen.

The quarters for married soldiers and laundresses now number forty-six sets, scattered to the south and west of the post. The greater part are built of slabs, placed upon end, and consist each of two rooms and a kitchen. Ten of the number are built of adobes, but of the same size and plan as the wooden buildings.

The officers' quarters are chiefly double houses, designed to accommodate the captain of a company on one side and his two lieutenants on the other. There are fourteen of these double houses on the parade, and the commanding officer's quarters, a large two-story building, with four large rooms on each floor and a hall in the center. The quarters for the medical officers is a double house near the hospital. The quartermaster occupies a single set, placed near his warehouse. The officers' quarters, except the commander's, are one-story-and-a-half houses, and are all built of the same materials and in the same style externally as the men's barracks. Inside, the

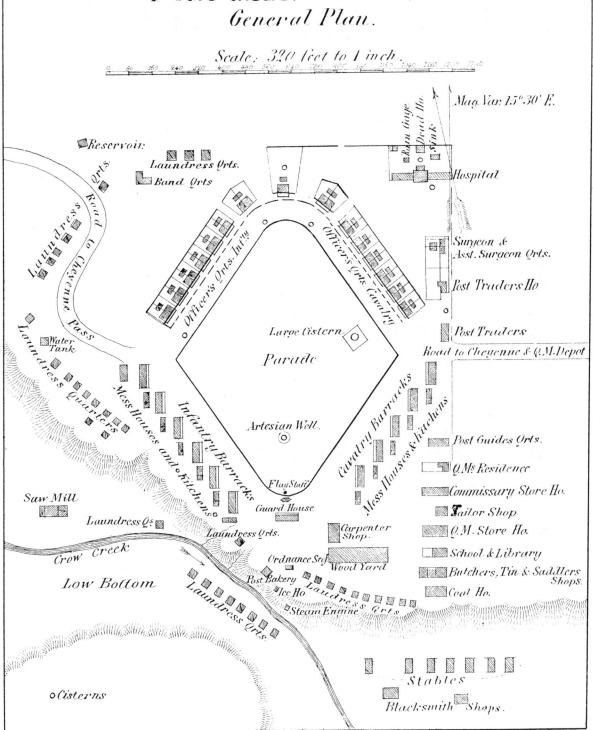

# FORT D.A.RUSSELL, W.T.
## General Plan.

Scale: 320 feet to 1 inch.

0  80  160  240  320  400  480  560  640  720  800  880  960  1040  1120  1200  1280

Mag. Var. 15° 30' E.

Reservoir.

Laundress Qrts.
Band Qrts

Qrts
Road to Cheyenne Pass

Laundress

Hospital

Surgeon & Asst. Surgeon Qrts.

Post Traders Ho.

Post Traders

Water Tank

Road to Cheyenne & Q.M. Depot

Laundress Quarters

Officers Qrts: Infty

Officers Qrts Cavalry

Large Cistern

Parade

Mess Houses and kitchens

Infantry Barracks

Artesian Well.

Cavalry Barracks

Mess Houses & kitchens

Post Guides Qrts.

Q.Ms Residence

Commissary Store Ho.

Saw Mill

Laundress Qs

Laundress Qrts.

Flag Staff

Guard House

Carpenter Shop.

Tailor Shop.

Q.M. Store Ho.

School & Library

Butchers, Tin & Saddlers Shops.

Coal Ho.

Ordnance Srg

Wood Yard

Crow Creek

Low Bottom

Post Bakery

Ice Ho.

Laundress Qrts

Laundress Qrts

Steam Engine

Stables

Cisterns

Blacksmith Shops.

officers' quarters are lined with boards, which are covered with tarred sheathing-paper, and papered. The kitchen and servants' room are in a detached low building in rear of each house. The quarters have no special arrangements for heating, lighting, ventilation, nor supplying water. There are no bath-rooms and no water-closet, except a common sink in the rear.

The adjutant's office is in the set of officers' quarters to the right of the commander's. The commissary and quartermaster's offices are in their storehouses. These latter are two long wooden buildings, about 25 to 100 feet. The style is known as sectional, they having been brought up from Omaha in parts, and put together here.

The guard-house is located at the southern angle of the parade. It is 40 by 40 feet, and constructed in the same manner as the other buildings. It is warmed by two stoves, and ventilated and lighted by windows, of which there are two in rear, two in each end, and one in front. Two doors in front give access to the interior. The building is well adapted for its purpose.

The hospital is located outside and to the northeast of the parade, and is constructed of the same materials and in the same style externally as the barracks. The plan is essentially that laid down in Circular No. 4, 1867, Surgeon-General's Office, but there are some modifications of and deviations from that plan which require notice. In the building the front hall is widened from 5 to 6½ feet. The hall being used as a waiting-room for those presenting themselves at surgeon's call, and the number of these from twelve companies being sometimes large, a greater space than allowed in the plan was required. There are two wards, each accommodating twenty-four beds. The east ward (the most sheltered) is the only one occupied by patients, the other being used as a chapel. Each bed has 66 superficial feet, and since the ward was ceiled 1,011 cubic feet of air-space. One of the little rooms at the end of the ward is fitted up with a bath-tub and as a lavatory. The sink for attendants and convalescents is about 85 feet in rear of the east ward. For the sick in bed two night-chairs are provided, usually kept in the bath-room, each deposit being covered as soon as made with dry earth to disinfect and deodorize it.

The bake-house, a wooden building, built in January, 1874, has an oven with a capacity of six hundred rations. The stables, eight in number, are situated in a bottom near the creek, east of the post. They are long buildings of rough boards, with a row of stalls on each side. There is no post library. Some of the cavalry companies have libraries. There is a hospital library, not medical, of about two hundred volumes. A building, 125 by 25 feet, has been erected by the post-trader, which is divided into a school-room and library and a hall for amusements.

The garrison receives its water-supply chiefly from Crow Creek. Attached to a saw-mill situated in the bottom, west of the post, is a steam-pump which forces the water from the stream up into an elevated wooden tank on the bluff. A water-wagon is filled daily from this tank, and delivers the water for the officers, enlisted men, and laundresses into barrels near their quarters. The water is also made to flow from this tank through a ditch around the parade, thus supplying the trees there planted. There are wells behind the officers' quarters and barracks, but they are not used, because they run dry in summer, and the other plan of supply is at all times more convenient. The commanding officer's residence and hospital have each a well in its inclosure, supplying their occupants with water.

The water from Crow Creek is a little turbid at times in spring when the stream is swollen by heavy rains, but generally the water from both sources is colorless, tasteless, and free from odor. An examination by the soap test gives the following result:

Crow Creek water, hardness (Clark's test) before boiling, 3.5; after 1.75.
Hospital well-water, hardness (Clark's test) before boiling, 5.95; after, 1.75.

An attempt was made to sink an artesian well in the southern angle of the parade, but proved unsuccessful. The boring was commenced early in November, 1872, and reached a depth of 1,420 feet without meeting any other than surface-water.

There being a gradual inclination of the ground on which the post is built toward the creek, the natural drainage is efficient. From this cause, and the gravelly subsoil, water remains but a very short time upon the surface. The kitchen slop and offal are removed daily by persons who raise swine. Dry refuse collected by policing is carried to ravines a short distance below, or east of the post, and burned.

This post has been since its foundation a sort of rendezvous or depot for distribution of troops.

The entire garrison has been changed several times, and the change of commanders is frequent. While there is a large garrison in winter, in early spring, and before the planting season arrives, almost the whole garrison is sent to various points along the railroad, leaving hardly enough men to perform the guard duty and other necessary work for so large a post.

A daily mail is received at the post, it taking about four days for a letter to reach Washington.

Excepting the town of Cheyenne, three miles distant, which has a population probably of about 2,000 persons, the country around is almost uninhabited. There are but very few farms or ranches in the vicinity.

*Meteorological report, Fort D. A. Russell, Wyo., 1870–'74.*

| Month. | 1870–'71. Temperature. Mean. | Max. | Min. | Rain-fall in inches. | 1871–'72. Temperature. Mean. | Max. | Min. | Rain-fall in inches. | 1872–'73. Temperature. Mean. | Max. | Min. | Rain-fall in inches. | 1873–'74. Temperature. Mean. | Max. | Min. | Rain-fall in inches. |
|---|---|---|---|---|---|---|---|---|---|---|---|---|---|---|---|---|
| July | 68.70 | 98* | 40* | 0.30 | 69.13 | 103* | 40 | 0.80 | 63.78 | 91* | 38* | 2.93 | 66.64 | 94* | 43* | 3.68 |
| August | 63.64 | 95* | 30* | 0.07 | 66.09 | 97* | 39* | 0.10 | 64.31 | 97* | 39* | 1.81 | 66.81 | 91* | 46* | 0.94 |
| September | 55.50 | 99* | 20* | 2.14 | 57.60 | 93* | 32* | 0.26 | 57.01 | 88* | 23* | 0.46 | 54.98 | 87* | 26* | 0.18 |
| October | 42.98 | 81* | 8* | 0.44 | 44.37 | 83* | 5* | 0.67 | 46.61 | 85* | 13* | 0.55 | 40.78 | 80* | 0* | 1.05 |
| November | 38.69 | 67* | 1* | 0.34 | 28.32 | 71* | —14* | 2.52 | 29.28 | 63* | —10* | 0.20 | 39.69 | 69* | —12* | 0.33 |
| December | 22.63 | 58* | —29 | 1.18 | 27.06 | 52* | — 7* | 1.38 | 23.83 | 59* | —16* | 0.36 | 27.12 | 62* | —13* | 0.42 |
| January | 28.56 | 61* | —13 | 0.64 | 22.57 | 50* | —23* | 0.85 | 23.89 | 51* | —20* | 0.30 | 26.43 | 59* | — 2* | 0.16 |
| February | 25.87 | 54* | 9 | 0.24 | 30.18 | 56* | —15* | 0.65 | 23.68 | 57* | — 9* | 0.17 | 25.58 | 63* | —26* | 0.34 |
| March | 31.14 | 64* | 2 | 0.58 | 32.10 | 70* | 4* | 1.07 | 37.06 | 68* | — 2* | 0.20 | 25.53 | 56* | — 8* | 1.60 |
| April | 37.29 | 74* | 5 | 1.62 | 39.49 | 71* | 15* | 2.33 | 32.24 | 79* | 1* | 1.42 | 32.38 | 73* | 5* | 1.10 |
| May | 54.19 | 86* | 38 | 1.90 | 51.95 | 81* | 22* | 1.59 | 45.09 | 85* | 21* | 3.61 | 63.90 | 88 | 37 | 1.49 |
| June | 64.90 | 97* | 40 | 1.55 | 61.54 | 90* | 40* | 2.54 | 63.09 | 95* | 36* | 3.13 | 64.93 | 93* | 42 | 1.22 |
| For the year | 44.51 | 99* | —29 | 11.00 | 44.20 | 103* | —23* | 14.76 | 42.49 | 97* | —20* | 15.14 | 44.56 | 94* | —26* | 12.51 |

* These observations are made with self-registering thermometers. The mean is from the standard thermometer.

*Consolidated sick-report, Fort D. A. Russell, Wyo., 1870–'74.*

| Year | | 1870–'71. | 1871–'72. | 1872–'73. | 1873–'74. |
|---|---|---|---|---|---|
| Mean strength | { Officers | 30 | 25 | 28 | 25 |
| | { Enlisted men | 653 | 490 | 548 | 527 |

| Diseases. | Cases. | Deaths. | Cases. | Deaths. | Cases. | Deaths. | Cases. | Deaths. |
|---|---|---|---|---|---|---|---|---|
| GENERAL DISEASES, A. | | | | | | | | |
| Typhoid fever | | 1 | | | | | 1 | |
| Typho-malarial fever | | | 1 | | | | | |
| Remittent fever | 1 | | 10 | | 7 | | 2 | |
| Intermittent fever | 59 | | 27 | | 54 | | 22 | |
| Other diseases of this group | 97 | | 24 | | 220 | | 133 | |
| GENERAL DISEASES, B. | | | | | | | | |
| Rheumatism | 57 | | 33 | | 95 | | 110 | |
| Syphilis | 26 | | 9 | | 28 | | 35 | |
| Consumption | | | 4 | | 6 | | 3 | |
| Other diseases of this group | 4 | | 2 | | 4 | | 6 | |
| LOCAL DISEASES. | | | | | | | | |
| Catarrh and bronchitis | 72 | 1 | 39 | | 297 | | 170 | |
| Pneumonia | 5 | 2 | 9 | | 11 | | 4 | 1 |
| Pleurisy | 2 | | 1 | | | | 1 | |
| Diarrhœa and dysentery | 47 | | 24 | | 114 | 1 | 159 | |
| Hernia | 3 | | 3 | | 4 | | | |
| Gonorrhœa | 6 | | 2 | | 7 | | 17 | |
| Other local diseases | 189 | 1 | 78 | | 376 | 2 | 314 | |
| Alcoholism | 12 | | 21 | | 55 | | 38 | |
| Total disease | 580 | 5 | 287 | | 1,278 | 3 | 1,015 | 1 |
| VIOLENT DISEASES AND DEATHS. | | | | | | | | |
| Gunshot wounds | 11 | 2 | 1 | | 6 | | 3 | 2 |
| Other accidents and injuries | 213 | 2 | 159 | 1 | 315 | 1 | 304 | |
| Homicide | | | | | | | | 2 |
| Suicide | | | | | | | | 1 |
| Total violence | 224 | 4 | 160 | 1 | 321 | 1 | 307 | 5 |

# FORT SANDERS, WYOMING TERRITORY.

REPORTS OF SURGEON J. H. FRANTZ AND ASSISTANT SURGEON GEORGE P. JAQUETT, UNITED STATES ARMY.

Fort Sanders lies on the Union Pacific Railroad, on Laramie Plains, one and three-fourths miles west of Big Laramie River, and about seventeen miles south from its junction with Little Laramie, where the two form the Laramie River; latitude, 41° 13′ 4″ north; longitude, 28° 23′ 22″ west; altitude above the sea, 7,161 feet. Laramie City, situated about three miles north, is the nearest town.

The post was established in July, 1866, pursuant to orders from Major-General Pope, commanding the department, and named Fort John Buford. The name was changed to Fort Sanders in September, 1866, in honor of Brig. Gen. W. P. Sanders, United States Volunteers, captain Second United States Cavalry. The reservation contains an area of eighty-one square miles, lacking about one hundred and forty-five acres on the east bank of the Laramie River, north of the fort, on which is the incorporated town, City of Laramie. It contains good grazing-ground, watered by two streams flowing from springs, and by the Big Laramie River. The surface of the reservation is gently undulating, rolling prairie. The site of the post is slightly elevated above the surrounding plain, and slopes in three directions, affording good natural drainage. The soil, made up of sand and gravel, is quite permeable, and evaporation from it is rapid, owing to its nature and to the winds which prevail almost constantly. A substratum of soft sandstone, apparently 10 or 15 feet in thickness, is found from 3 to 5 feet below the surface of the earth. Limestone abounds in the immediate vicinity of the post, and sandstone, easily quarried, within six miles. The latter, when first taken out, is soft and readily cut, but hardens on exposure, and is a very excellent building-stone.

The City of Laramie is a town of about 1,500 inhabitants.

Spring Creek, which runs by the post, is a living stream, whose source is in several springs rising in a limestone region about three miles east-southeast of the post. A reservoir was constructed by damming the stream about a mile and three-fourths from the post, and the water is brought in ditches through the rear yards of the officers' quarters, the parade-ground in front of the barracks and hospital, and into the post-gardens. The water is hard, but palatable.

A circular artificial pond, about 100 yards in diameter, on which are boats for the use of the garrison in summer, and on which the men are allowed to skate in winter, is kept filled with fresh water from the same reservoir. About eight miles southwest of the fort are four small lakes or large ponds, on which, except when ice-bound, are quantities of aquatic wild fowl.

The post was originally built for four companies, with a parade-ground 223 by 400 feet, two barracks on the north and south sides respectively, officers' quarters on the east, and storehouses on the west. The post has been enlarged so as to accommodate six companies.

The present buildings are located on the four sides of a rectangular parade-ground, 600 feet in its long axis, nearly north and south, and 500 feet wide. Ditches convey streams of water along the north, east, and south sides of the parade, in rear of the buildings, on the east and west, and part of those on the south sides; the water finally emptying into the creek, which runs in a westerly direction at a short distance south of the buildings. On the north side of the parade, beginning at the northwest corner, are the hospital, the headquarters building, (between them the road to Laramie,) and a building containing two sets of officers' quarters; turning south, on the east side, are three buildings, each containing two sets, a building containing a single set, then one containing two sets of officers' quarters; turning west, on the south side, are a building containing two sets of officers' quarters, a barrack containing two sets of company quarters, the post reading-room and library, a set of buildings, of which a part contain two sets of company quarters, adjoining which, and running north on the west line, forming with the first an L, is another part, containing two other sets of company quarters, a cavalry stable, the quartermaster's storehouse, quartermaster's office, commissary storehouse, and commanding officer's quarters at the north end of the west line, at the place of beginning.

The eastern set of barracks is a log building in the form of an L, one leg extending along the line of the parade, the other running south at right angles with the west end of the first. The exterior of each leg is 100 feet in length. This building is divided into three dormitories, with rooms for offices at the east and south extremities. The second set of barracks is also in the form of an L; one leg, 200 feet long and 30 feet wide, extends along the south line of the parade; the other leg, the same length as the first, and adjoining it on the west, runs north 170 feet on the west line, the building thus inclosing the southwest corner of the parade-ground. The east building is divided by a partition in the center into two sets of company quarters. Each set is subdivided into two dormitories, with office-rooms between them. The west building laps across the west end of the other, contains two sets of quarters, each subdivided into one dormitory, with office-rooms next to the center of the building, and a hall at the extremity. There are comfortable mess-rooms, kitchens, &c., in rear of each set of quarters. The last-described barracks are constructed of 2½-inch planks securely nailed to a strong framework; the walls are lathed and plastered inside, but the rooms are not ceiled. Porches extend across the parade sides of all these buildings. The rooms are well lighted, and are warmed by coal-stoves. There is no ridge ventilation.

The quarters for married soldiers and laundresses consist of thirteen sets, of two rooms each.

The commanding officer's quarters consist of a main building and three wings, one at each end, another at the rear, divided into seven rooms, kitchen, servants' room, &c. A veranda extends across the entire front, including the wings. The building is constructed like the barracks last described, and is lathed and plastered throughout. The line-officers' quarters consist of six buildings, each containing two sets, and one building containing a single set. The building at the east end of the north line, containing two sets of officers' quarters, is constructed of planks, in the same manner as the commanding officer's quarters. Each set consists of four rooms, kitchen and servants' room. All these buildings, except the southern two on the east line, are composed of a body with a wing at each end, and, excepting the one described above, are one story high, built substantially of logs, with verandas in front and on the sides. Internally, some are lathed and plastered, others lined with tarred sheathing-board and papered, and a few rooms in two of the houses lined with plain lumber, painted or stained. Each building, comprising two sets of quarters, consists of a main building, with an L in rear, the latter containing kitchen and dining-room. Water is brought from the reservoir through ditches which run through the rear yards of each set of quarters. During cold weather water is hauled in water-carts. These quarters are furnished with the ordinary trench water-closet, placed in rear. There are no bath-rooms. The quarters are heated by stoves, in which coal is used as fuel. They are well lighted, and may be well ventilated by means of the windows, at the option of the occupants.

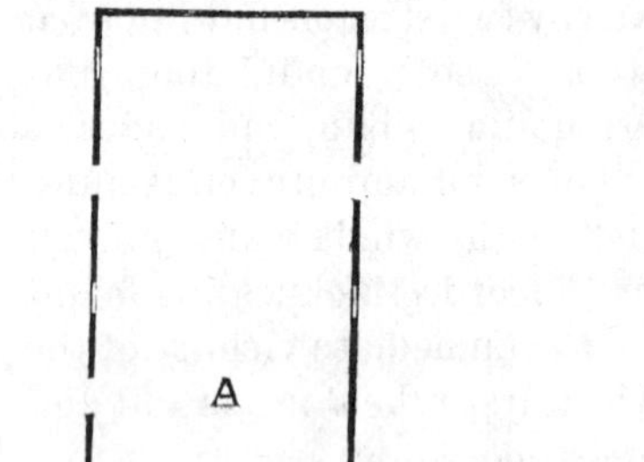

The reading-room and library building is constructed of logs, and was originally built for a company barrack.

The headquarters building, consisting of a main portion and two wings, is built of planks, like the commanding officer's quarters.

There are two quartermaster's storehouses, each 100 by 30 feet, and three commissary storehouses, each 30 by 30 feet and 10 feet high. They are built of logs. The bake-house and magazine, each 30 by 30 feet and 10 feet high, are built of stone.

Figure 56.—Scale, 30 feet to 1 inch.

The guard-house, erected in 1869, is a substantial stone building, divided into guard and prison rooms; dimensions of the former, 16 by 23¼ feet; of the latter, 23¼ by 24 feet; height to ceiling, 11⅙ feet. In the prison-room are two cells, each measuring 4⅔ by 6 feet, occupying adjacent corners. The building is warmed by coal-stoves. The prison-room has four windows, each 1 foot 10 inches by 2 feet 4 inches, and a ventilator, 14 inches square, in the ceiling, extending through the roof, thus affording ample light and ventilation. In the guard-room are three windows, each 2 feet 8 inches by 3 feet 8 inches, and a ventilator, 40 inches square. The average occupancy of the guard house is 13.

The hospital building is constructed of logs, one story high, for the plan of which see Figure 56.

A, ward, 22 by 52 feet; A, ward, 67 by 22 feet; E, bath-room, 6½ by 14 feet. The height of the rooms is 9 feet 9 inches. A veranda, 6 feet wide, extends the length of the building on the southside. The rooms are lathed, plastered, and ceiled, and the whole building is in tolerable repair.

That portion of the figure marked N B represents the ground plan of a two-story log building, 35 by 36 feet, outside measurement, each story 10 feet in height, with a one-story building (N K) attached, the latter measuring 13 by 23 feet, and intended for kitchen purposes.

The wards are warmed by coal-stoves, and are each supplied with ample ventilation and natural light. The wards have a capacity for twelve beds each, giving in the larger 1,135 cubic feet, and in the smaller 950 cubic feet per bed.

The administration building is good, but the wards are sadly in need of repair.

The cavalry stables are two large log buildings; one, on the west side of the parade, is 230 by 32 feet; 12 feet high; the other is south of the principal set of barrack buildings. South of the last building are the quartermaster's stables and corral. The set is 200 feet square. The creek runs through the center from east to west.

The water used at the post is pleasant to the taste, colorless, and free from smell. The permeability of the soil and the infrequency of rain render the surface-drainage all-sufficient. Slops, &c., are hauled away from the post daily.

There are no regular arrangements for bathing. The stream affords facilities during warm weather.

The post garden, under charge of the adjutant, furnishes vegetables to the staff-officers and hospital. Companies are furnished from their respective company gardens.

The general sanitary condition of the post is good. As a class, affections of the more external organs of the respiratory system are most common. The high winds, to which the command is subjected, carry with them quantities of fine particles of dust with which more or less alkali is intermingled, and, by their inhalation, cause irritation of the air-passages.

The post is surrounded by a board fence, which adds to its appearance and keeps out the stock, which is scattered over the plains.

Trees have been planted along the ditches on the sides of the parade in front of the quarters, are growing slowly, and are a relief to the monotony of the treeless plain.

There are many ranches scattered over the valley, chiefly for stock and hay.

*Meteorological report, Fort Sanders, Wyo., 1870–'74.*

| Month. | 1870–'71. | | | | 1871–'72. | | | | 1872–'73. | | | | 1873–'74. | | | |
|---|---|---|---|---|---|---|---|---|---|---|---|---|---|---|---|---|
| | Temperature. | | | Rain-fall in inches. | Temperature. | | | Rain-fall in inches. | Temperature. | | | Rain-fall in inches. | Temperature. | | | Rain-fall in inches. |
| | Mean. | Max. | Min. | | Mean. | Max. | Min. | | Mean. | Max. | Min. | | Mean. | Max. | Min. | |
| July | 66.03 | 85 | 42 | 0.62 | 68.18 | 94 | 49 | 1.62 | 59.96 | 88* | 29* | 2.95 | 65.49 | 93* | 36* | 2.70 |
| August | 60.13 | 90 | 37 | 0.87 | 64.62 | 92 | 44 | 0.00 | 61.78 | 89* | 35* | 3.05 | 53.94 | 88* | 37* | 2.10 |
| September | 52.30 | 76 | 32 | 1.22 | 57.50 | 86 | 36 | 0.40 | 50.93 | 80* | 22* | 1.30 | 53.94 | 84* | 16* | 0.70 |
| October | 41.11 | 71 | 2 | 0.04 | 40.63 | 76 | 9 | 0.68 | 42.52 | 81* | 0* | 0.60 | 38.52 | 77* | −25* | 1.53 |
| November | 37.71 | 61 | − 7 | 0.00 | 26.70 | 60 | −28 | 2.00 | 23.71 | 57* | −32* | 0.60 | 34.83 | 69* | −15* | 0.40 |
| December | 18.52 | 52 | −30 | 0.16 | 24.27 | 49* | − 8* | 0.75 | 23.41 | 60* | −36* | 0.60 | 20.56 | 49* | −24* | 0.90 |
| January | 27.49 | 57 | − 7 | 0.14 | 17.28 | 51* | −45* | 0.50 | 19.07 | 50* | −50* | 0.95 | 24.21 | 47* | −25* | 0.50 |
| February | 23.89 | 54 | 0 | 0.62 | 24.99 | 58* | −25* | 0.70 | 19.41 | 51* | −15* | 0.90 | 18.39 | 46* | −30* | 0.20 |
| March | 30.62 | 56 | 7 | 0.13 | 28.07 | 59* | − 1* | 0.69 | 34.26 | 70* | − 5* | 0.73 | 25.22 | 52* | −12* | 0.85 |
| April | 37.68 | 67 | 13 | 1.22 | 35.09 | 65* | 5* | 2.45 | 30.11 | 66* | −(6)*? | 1.03 | 35.04 | 70* | 2* | 0.45 |
| May | 52.43 | 82 | 31 | 0.55 | 48.40 | 81* | 16* | 2.28 | 43.99 | 74* | 12* | 1.95 | 53.30 | 83* | 14* | 0.87 |
| June | 64.41 | 87 | 40 | 0.00 | 58.24 | 87* | 29* | 2.05 | 61.31 | 86* | 26* | 1.25 | 61.67 | 89* | 23* | 1.76 |
| For the year | 42.69 | 90 | −30 | 5.62 | 41.15 | 94 | −45* | 14.12 | 39.20 | 89* | −50* | 15.91 | 41.29 | 93* | −30* | 12.96 |

* These observations are made with self-registering thermometers. The mean is from the standard thermometer.

*Consolidated sick-report, Fort Sanders, Wyo., 1870–'74.*

| Year | | 1870–'71. | | 1871–'72. | | 1872–'73. | | 1873–'74. | |
|---|---|---|---|---|---|---|---|---|---|
| Mean strength ⟨ Officers............ ⟨ Enlisted men...... | | 9<br>172 | | 8<br>106 | | 15<br>300 | | 23<br>386 | |
| Diseases. | | Cases. | Deaths. | Cases. | Deaths. | Cases. | Deaths. | Cases. | Deaths. |
| GENERAL DISEASES, A. | | | | | | | | | |
| Typhoid fever ...................... | | 1 | ...... | 1 | ...... | ...... | ...... | ...... | 1 |
| Typho-malarial fever.............. | | ...... | ...... | 1 | 1 | ...... | ...... | ...... | ...... |
| Remittent fever ................... | | 1 | ...... | ...... | ...... | 5 | ...... | 1 | 1 |
| Intermittent fever................. | | 7 | ...... | 16 | ...... | 86 | ...... | 75 | ...... |
| Other diseases of this group ...... | | 24 | ...... | 5 | ...... | 72 | 1 | 86 | ...... |
| GENERAL DISEASES, B. | | | | | | | | | |
| Rheumatism ....................... | | 27 | ...... | 12 | ...... | 26 | ...... | 45 | ...... |
| Syphilis ........................... | | 3 | ...... | 3 | ...... | 6 | ...... | 10 | ...... |
| Consumption ...................... | | 3 | ...... | 3 | ...... | ...... | ...... | ...... | ...... |
| Other diseases of this group ...... | | ...... | ...... | ...... | ...... | 6 | ...... | 2 | ...... |
| LOCAL DISEASES. | | | | | | | | | |
| Catarrh and bronchitis ............ | | 37 | ...... | 14 | ...... | 28 | ...... | 40 | ...... |
| Pneumonia ........................ | | 1 | ...... | 2 | 1 | 4 | 3 | 1 | ...... |
| Pleurisy........................... | | ...... | ...... | ...... | ...... | 2 | ...... | 2 | ...... |
| Diarrhœa and dysentery............ | | 48 | ...... | 14 | ...... | 55 | ...... | 76 | ...... |
| Hernia ............................ | | 1 | ...... | 2 | ...... | ...... | ...... | 5 | ...... |
| Gonorrhœa ........................ | | 1 | ...... | ...... | ...... | ...... | ...... | 2 | ...... |
| Other local diseases .............. | | 112 | ...... | 48 | ...... | 115 | ...... | 89 | ...... |
| Alcoholism......................... | | 21 | ...... | 6 | ...... | 8 | ...... | 12 | ...... |
| Total disease ................. | | 287 | ...... | 127 | 2 | 413 | 4 | 446 | 2 |
| VIOLENT DISEASES AND DEATHS. | | | | | | | | | |
| Gunshot wounds ................... | | 3 | 1 | 1 | ...... | 1 | ...... | ...... | ...... |
| Other accidents and injuries....... | | 112 | 2 | 40 | 1 | 118 | ...... | 142 | ...... |
| Homicide.......................... | | ...... | ...... | ...... | 1 | ...... | ...... | ...... | ...... |
| Suicide............................ | | ...... | ...... | ...... | ...... | ...... | 1 | ...... | ...... |
| Total violence ................ | | 115 | 3 | 41 | 2 | 119 | 1 | 142 | ...... |

# CAMP SHERIDAN, (SPOTTED TAIL AGENCY,) NEBRASKA.

## INFORMATION FURNISHED BY ACTING ASSISTANT SURGEON CHAS. V. PETTEYS, UNITED STATES ARMY.

Camp Sheridan is situated in the northwest corner of the State of Nebraska; latitude, about 42° 50' north; longitude, about 25° 37' west. Cheyenne is two hundred and thirteen miles, and Camp Robinson (Red Cloud agency) forty-three miles, distant southwest.

The post was located September 9, 1874, on the east or right bank of the West Fork of Beaver Creek, a tributary of White River, into which it empties about twelve miles farther north. To the east, south, and west is high, rolling ground, intersected by deep cañons, in and on the banks of which are forests of pine, in some of which are also cottonwood, ash, and elm. Looking north, the valley of Beaver Creek opens out; the ground still broken and hilly, with a rapid descent to White River. The camp is near the summit of what seems to have been the shore of a large lake, probably of brackish water, judging by the shells found in the deposits. This ridge, seen from some of the hills in the basin inclosed by it, appears to extend from the Black Hills circularly to the south, east, north, and west to the Black Hills again, with a radius of about forty miles. White River and the South Fork of the Big Cheyenne have their sources and feeders in this ridge, breaking through it. The grass along the streams is rich and nutritious. Hay is obtainable along the bottoms and on the upland, the latter of decidedly the better quality. There is an abundance of pine timber, for building purposes, within three or four miles; also plenty of fuel, consisting of pine, cottonwood, ash, and elm; game comprises black and white tailed deer, bears, and grouse. Ducks and geese also fly over. The climate is good; rather dry. Storms come from every direction, sometimes violent. Ree-corn, potatoes, onions, cabbage, and even tomatoes, can be grown. The season is short. Principal diseases in summer, diarrhœa and dysentery; in winter, catarrhal affections, rheumatism, and neuralgia. Some, but not much, scrofula among the Sioux.

Indians are Spotted Tail's band of Brulé Sioux. In winter the Minneconjons come in from the Black Hills, get their annuities, and return in the spring to the Black Hills, and probably to the Big Horn Mountains.

The post was established for the protection of Spotted Tail's band of Brulé Sioux. The agency buildings are within half a mile of the post, easily overlooked and commanded by it. At the agency are two trading-houses, whose trade is chiefly for furs and beef-hides. Mail is received twice a week, via Cheyenne and Camp Robinson.

The barracks are huts, each 15 feet square, 9 feet to the eaves, built of pine logs chinked with mud, roofed with pine poles covered with gunny-sacks and three or four inches of earth, and having dirt floors. Each hut has a door and window, and is heated by a Sibley stove. In some are double bunks of pine boards; in others two-storied single ones are used. The huts are to contain six or eight men each.

Laundresses' quarters and company kitchens are the same kind of buildings. Cooking is done out of doors, sheltered by paulins.

Officers' quarters are built of logs or split logs, according to choice, are 15 feet square, with board floors, and heated by box-stoves.

The hospital department occupies three huts, of the same character as those for the troops. Two of these, for ward and dispensary, have board floors. The third one, for stores, has a dirt floor.

The guard-house also, is a building similar to the barracks.

Permanent quarters will be commenced as soon as practicable.

Water, excellent at all times, clear and cold, is supplied from perennial springs. It is hauled in barrels, one spring supplying all the wants of the garrison.

*Consolidated sick-report, Camp Sheridan, (Spotted Tail agency,) Nebr., 1874, April 1 to November 1.*

| Year | | 1874. | |
| --- | --- | --- | --- |
| Mean strength | | 243 | |
| Diseases. | | Cases. | Deaths. |
| GENERAL DISEASES, A. | | | |
| Remittent fever | | 3 | |
| Other diseases of this group | | | |
| GENERAL DISEASES, B. | | | |
| Rheumatism | | 36 | |
| Syphilis | | 3 | |
| LOCAL DISEASES. | | | |
| Catarrh and bronchitis | | 45 | |
| Diarrhœa and dysentery | | 140 | |
| Other local diseases | | 3 | |
| Total disease | | 230 | 2 |

# SIDNEY BARRACKS, NEBRASKA.

### REPORT OF ASSISTANT SURGEON A. HARTSUFF, UNITED STATES ARMY.

Sidney Barracks, Cheyenne County, Nebr., is located in latitude 41° north, longitude 26° west, and is 4,326 feet above the level of the sea, and is about 12 feet above Lodge Pole Creek, which flows through the reservation, and on the left bank of which the post is situated.

Troops were first located here in the summer of 1867, and the first buildings were erected on the present site of the post in the autumn of 1869. During the summer and autumn of 1870 the post was enlarged by the addition of several new buildings, since which time only minor changes have occurred, and it remains a two-company post, being garrisoned by one company of cavalry and one of infantry.

The reservation is one mile square, across the northern side of which runs the Union Pacific Railroad, and on the railroad, and immediately contiguous to the post, the little village of Sidney is located. Sidney, an eating-station, is the only town on the railroad between North Platte, about one hundred miles east, and Cheyenne, about one hundred miles west. Its population is about three hundred; has several stores, many saloons, and two hotels, one of which is a first-class house. It is also the county-seat of Cheyenne County. The general appearance of the country is that of a vast, undulating plain. No mountains, rivers, nor trees are visible, and none are to be found within a radius of many miles. The small amount of rain, the want of rivers, and the great altitude of the country render it valueless for agricultural purposes, but especially adapt it for grazing, and many large herds of stock, which thrive throughout the winter by grazing, are kept in this vicinity.

The geological formation and mineral products of this vicinity are, in general, those of the great North American plains, in the midst of which the post is located. This section of the country is all of very late tertiary formation, consisting chiefly of indurated sandy clay. In the bluffs are found ledges of white sandstone, rather friable, but sufficiently strong for building purposes. The soil, though containing but little alluvium, is covered with a short, succulent (buffalo) grass, which is very nutritious, and on which great herds of buffalo in this vicinity live and keep fat.

The wild animals in the vicinity are wild horses, buffaloes, deer, antelope, coyote, rabbit, prairie-dog, gopher, badger, beaver, muskrat, &c. The principal birds are hawk, sage-hen, killdeer, goose, duck, mallard, teal, and blackbird. Fish are found in the Platte Rivers and in Lodge Pole Creek.

Lodge Pole Creek is a small stream running through the great arid plains of Wyoming and Nebraska, a distance of two hundred miles, and emptying into the South Platte River at Julesburgh, about forty-six miles east of here.

The valley of Lodge Pole Creek here is about two miles wide, and bounded on either side by sandstone bluffs about 70 feet high, which limit the regions drained by the South and North Platte Rivers, respectively. The Platte Rivers are each about thirty miles distant.

The plan of the post is that of a parallelogram, measuring 433⅓ yards north and south, by 200 yards east and west, and is inclosed by a neat picket-fence. All the buildings are of frame, well constructed, and for the most part convenient and comfortable. The barracks are three new buildings, one story each, the dimensions of which are, respectively, cavalry quarters, 95 by 29 by 10 feet, and infantry quarters, 85 by 29 by 10 feet, inside measurement. A porch, 8 feet wide, extends the full length in front. The main portion of each building is used as a dormitory, giving an air-space of 525 cubic feet to each man. Ventilation is effected by air-shafts in the center of the roof; windows are ample; single iron bunks are used. The sinks are ordinary holes in the ground, covered, properly disinfected by use of dry earth, lime, and sulphate of iron. Adjoining the dormitories in each barrack building are an ample dining-room, a kitchen, pantry, store-room, and wash-room. Laundresses' quarters are adobe houses, with shingle roofs, comprising seven sets, and are well adapted. The officers' quarters are four double sets, frame buildings, lathed, plastered, and shingle roofs. The buildings are lined between the plastering and weather-boarding with adobes. Size of main buildings, 44 by 30 feet; rear buildings, 24 by 24 feet, and one story high. Each set contains six rooms, four on the first floor, and two on the second; the arrangement of which is shown by Figure 57.

1, first floor. 2, second floor. A, parlor, 14 by 15 feet; B, dining-room, 12 by 15 feet; C, hall, 6½ by 20 feet; D, kitchen, 13 by 14 feet; E, fuel, 10 by 13 feet; F, chamber, 14 by 15 feet; G, chamber, 12 by 15 feet; V, veranda, 6 by 44 feet.

Figure 57.

The buildings are well constructed, spacious, and neat in appearance.

A new building, 73 by 28 by 14 feet, and of the class known as a story and a half, contains two sets of quarters of eight rooms each.

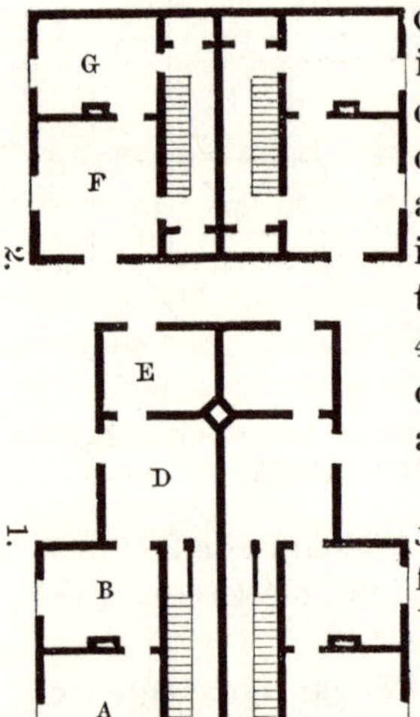

The commanding officer's quarters are two stories high, both main and rear buildings; size, main building, 30 by 35 feet; rear building, 14 by 20 feet. First floor has four rooms, one hall and three closets, viz, parlor 15 by 21½ feet, hall 8 by 15

eet, sitting-room 15 by 14 feet, dining-room 16 by 15 feet, closets 6½ by 5 feet, 5 by 5 feet, and 4, by 5 feet respectively; kitchen 14 by 16 feet. Second floor has six chambers and two closets; size respectively 8 by 11 feet, 15 by 19 feet, 13 by 14 feet, 15 by 16 feet, 9 by 14 feet, 8 by 14 feet. This building has a portico in front 6 feet wide, with balcony on second floor. The store-house is of boards with shingle roof, size 156 by 26 feet, divided into two apartments, which are used by the commissary and quartermaster.

The guard-house is an L-shaped frame building with shingle roof; size of main building 13 by 22 feet, used as a guard-room, is lathed and plastered; size of wing 12 by 16 feet, contains one general prison-room lined with plank, and has but one small grated window. A small room, 8 by 10 feet, in rear of the main building, is used as a "dark cell;" it has no window or means of ventilation excepting the door. A small ventilating-shaft 8 by 8 inches, through the roof, is the only means of ventilating the general prison-room; a similar shaft is used in the guard-room. The guard-house is too small, badly constructed, and badly ventilated. The hospital is an L-shaped frame building, the main portion of which was originally a portable one, size 64 by 24 feet, divided into six apartments, as follows: dispensary, 18 by 13½ feet; steward's room, 14 by 10 feet; ward No. 1, 18 by 24 feet; ward No. 2, 17 by 24 feet; store-room, 11 by 12 feet. In addition to the above apartments there is a small store-room, 4 by 10 feet, located in rear of the steward's room; also a wash-house, 6 by 15 feet, built in rear of ward No. 2. The wing is a permanent building, 30 by 18 feet, containing dining-room, 18 by 16 feet, and kitchen, 18 by 14 feet. A porch, 5 feet wide, is built around the back building and along the southern front of the main building. The rooms are plastered. A ventilator is placed on the top of the hospital between the two wards; trap-doors, 19 inches square, are placed in the ceilings in the center of the wards, and can be opened or closed by the use of a small rope; ventilating-shafts have also been placed under the flooring of either ward; they communicate with the wards by doors in the rear of the stoves. The wards were designed for five beds each, allowing 840 cubic feet air-space per bed. This building stands directly upon the ground, has no space beneath for ventilation, and no elevation for drainage. Owing to a large accumulation of hospital property one of the wards has been appropriated for storage purposes, leaving only one room, 17 by 23 feet, for the sick, and in this the hospital attendant and-cook must sleep. There is no isolation-ward, no dead-house, cellar or cistern. No veranda in front of the ward; no window-blinds, notwithstanding the thermometer occasionally runs above 100°. In but few ways does the building meet the conditions of a well-ordered and well-regulated hospital, and though the monthly sick-report shows that the command is healthy, we could not suitably provide for the ordinary number of sick at a three-company post.

The bakery is also of frame, shingle roof, lathed and plastered, and lined between the weather-boarding and plastered with adobes; divided into two rooms and a hall; the oven is of brick.

The stables are new, ample and commodious; they, with the carpenter and blacksmith shops, stand on the bank of Lodge Pole Creek.

An irrigating-ditch of about one and one-half miles in length, carries an abundant supply of pure, clear water from the creek through the post and through the village of Sidney; trees and shrubbery are planted near the ditch, and it is a very attractive feature of the post.

The post garden, 3½ acres, furnishes nearly all garden vegetables; commissary supplies are abundant and excellent. On the line of the railroad, at towns two hundred miles east of here, vegetables, butter, eggs, poultry, &c., can be obtained and brought here in great abundance and at low rates. Fishing in summer is pretty good, and in the autumn and winter the troops supply the post with buffalo meat, deer, and antelope.

Sanitary condition of the post is excellent. Since the establishment of the post but one soldier has died here.

48 M P

*Meteorological report, Sidney Barracks, Nebr., 1872–'74.*

| Month. | 1870–'71. Temperature. Mean. | Max. | Min. | Rain-fall in inches. | 1871–'72. Temperature. Mean. | Max. | Min. | Rain-fall in inches. | 1872–'73. Temperature. Mean. | Max. | Min. | Rain-fall in inches. | 1873–'74. Temperature. Mean. | Max. | Min. | Rain-fall in inches. |
|---|---|---|---|---|---|---|---|---|---|---|---|---|---|---|---|---|
| July | | | | | | | | | 69.32 | 99* | 39* | 1.84 | 71.80 | 100* | 22* | 1.18 |
| August | | | | | | | | | 71.32 | 104* | 47* | 2.18 | 71.99 | 97* | 46* | 1.82 |
| September | | | | | | | | | 59.81 | 95* | 21* | 0.34 | 59.11 | 89* | 31* | 1.43 |
| October | | | | | | | | | 50.73 | 90* | 12* | 0.18 | 42.60 | 90* | − 2* | 1.08 |
| November | | | | | | | | | 27.71 | 69* | − 8* | 0.04 | 35.41 | 73* | −12* | 0.48 |
| December | | | | | | | | | 17.87 | 57 | −33* | 0.02 | 26.11 | 53* | −22* | 0.26 |
| January | | | | | | | | | 17.13 | 65 | −34* | 0.58 | 26.28 | 61* | − 9* | 0.28 |
| February | | | | | | | | | 19.63 | 50 | −20* | 0.00 | 20.37 | 52* | −34* | 0.46 |
| March | | | | | | | | | 32.24 | 73 | −12* | 0.00 | 30.53 | 60* | 2* | 1.54 |
| April | | | | | | | | | 36.27 | 84* | −10* | 2.39 | 41.37 | 84* | 11* | 0.46 |
| May | | | | | | | | | 50.78 | 85* | 10* | 2.56 | 58.99 | 90* | 25^ | 4.98 |
| June | | | | | 67.30 | 98* | 42* | 1.38 | 69.64 | 100■ | 34* | 0.60 | 67.73 | 96* | 40* | 1.52 |
| For the year | | | | | | | | | 43.54 | 104* | −34* | 10.73 | 45.52 | 100* | −34* | 15.49 |

* These observations are made with self-registering thermometers. The mean is from the standard thermometer.

*Consolidated sick-report, Sidney Barracks, Nebr., 1870–'74.*

| Diseases. | 1870–'71. Cases. | Deaths. | 1871–'72. Cases. | Deaths. | 1872–'73. Cases. | Deaths. | 1873–'74. Cases. | Deaths. |
|---|---|---|---|---|---|---|---|---|
| Year / Mean strength Officers | 6 | | 7 | | 7 | | 7 | |
| Enlisted men | 126 | | 109 | | 111 | | 128 | |
| **GENERAL DISEASES, A.** | | | | | | | | |
| Remittent fever | | | | | | | 2 | |
| Intermittent fever | 9 | | 14 | | 7 | | 10 | |
| Other diseases of this group | 7 | | 5 | | 4 | | 1 | |
| **GENERAL DISEASES, B.** | | | | | | | | |
| Rheumatism | 11 | | 6 | | 14 | | 4 | |
| Syphilis | 7 | | 3 | | 3 | | 1 | |
| Other diseases of this group | 9 | | 4 | | | | | |
| **LOCAL DISEASES.** | | | | | | | | |
| Catarrh and bronchitis | 22 | | 24 | | 43 | | 1 | |
| Pneumonia | | 1 | | | 1 | | 1 | |
| Pleurisy | | | | | 1 | | | |
| Diarrhœa and dysentery | 39 | | 25 | | 22 | | 2 | |
| Hernia | 1 | | | | | | | |
| Gonorrhœa | 1 | | | | | | 1 | |
| Other local diseases | 57 | | 33 | | 50 | | 22 | |
| Alcoholism | 5 | | 10 | | 12 | | 2 | |
| Unclassified | 1 | | | | | | | |
| Total disease | 169 | 1 | 124 | | 157 | | 47 | |
| **VIOLENT DISEASES AND DEATHS.** | | | | | | | | |
| Gunshot wounds | 1 | | 1 | | 1 | | | |
| Other accidents and injuries | 41 | | 60 | | 55 | | 30 | |
| Total violence | 42 | | 61 | | 56 | | 30 | |

# CAMP STAMBAUGH, WYOMING TERRITORY.

### REPORT OF ACTING ASSISTANT SURGEON S. A. GREENWELL, UNITED STATES ARMY.

Camp Stambaugh is situated in Sweetwater County, Wyoming Territory, in latitude 42° 30′ north, longitude 31° 57′ west, about one hundred miles distant from the Union Pacific Railroad, at an altitude of 7,714 feet. It was established as a permanent post in August, 1870.

The post is located upon a plain formed by a natural depression in the country, and which embraces nearly the whole extent of the reservation, which extends one mile either way from the flagstaff.

The boundary of the plain is formed by rough and broken country upon all sides, with the exception of the northwest, where rises a range of the Wind River Mountains to the height of about 600 feet above the post.

The soil being alkaline is unproductive, even with irrigation, which has been practiced for the purpose of making a company garden, but without success.

The only vegetation that flourishes near the post is the wild sage. Distant from the post about sixteen miles, in the sheltered valleys and along the streams, grass of good quality may be found, and also vegetables of an inferior quality are raised, such as potatoes, squashes, and cabbages, but they are frequently destroyed before reaching maturity by the appearance of snow and frost, which may occur in any month of the year.

Timber in the immediate vicinity of the post is very scarce, none other than cottonwood in small quantities being found bordering the streams. In the mountains, about twelve miles distant, pine timber abounds, from which material was obtained for building the post and from which the annual supply of wood is now obtained.

The animals in the vicinity are the gray wolf, coyote, antelope, elk, deer, and the cinnamon and grizzly bears. The smaller game consists of the jack-rabbit, porcupine, beaver, gopher, sage-hens, and a few ducks found in the streams. Fish are found in considerable quantities, though small in size, in the streams which course through the Popoagie valleys, and are generally the mountain trout. The nearest stream from which fish are caught is Twin Creek, nine miles from the post.

The climate is exceedingly dry during the summer, rain seldom falling. The atmosphere is dry and bracing. The fall of snow generally begins early, and may be expected in any month of the year; but usually the winter commences about the 1st of October and continues until June, and is generally very severe, snow falling to a great depth, attended with violent winds and extreme cold. In the winter of 1871 the snow upon the parade-ground was twenty feet deep. The guard-house and adjutant's office were only accessible through tunnels which were cut through the snow. The coldest day observed was January 24, 1871, the mercury falling to 35° below zero.

The post is built of wood, principally pine and cottonwood, obtained from the mountains about twelve miles distant. The buildings were all erected without any special foundation other than ordinary sleepers of hewn logs. The barracks, two in number, built of hewn logs 80 by 32 feet, with an L 48 by 20 feet, are one story high, and were completed in November, 1870. They are shingled and whitewashed, and one set of quarters are ceiled. They are protected upon the outside with boards and battens; one chimney on each end built of bricks; the dormitories, each 60 by 30 feet, affording 418 cubic feet of air to each man. There are five windows, of twelve panes each, in each dormitory. The old wooden bunks, which were formerly used, have been replaced by new iron ones. The space of 20 feet partitioned off from the main part of the building is divided into an orderly-room, store-room, and lavatory. The L part comprises a mess-room 32 by 20 feet, and a kitchen 16 by 20 feet. There is also a cellar under one of the barracks.

The post bakery, 32 by 20 feet, is situated about 35 yards from the hospital, and has a capacity for baking 300 rations at one time.

The married soldiers' quarters are four in number, built of round logs, 20 by 20 feet, and designed for four rooms each. The roofs are shingled. But these quarters are not comfortable, being in bad repair.

There are four buildings for officers' quarters, built of hewn logs, 48 by 36 feet; six rooms, each 16 by 15 feet, with hall through the center 5 feet wide; three rooms on each side of the hall. The houses are all one story high, plastered between logs, ceiled and lined inside with boards and canvas, and papered; protected upon the outside by boards and battens. There are nine rooms which are in an unfinished condition. Each house is intended for two families. The front rooms have each two windows, the other rooms only one. The commanding officer's house has a kitchen attached, and a porch in front; the former 24 by 24 feet, and the latter 36 feet long and 7 feet wide.

The guard-house is of hewn logs, covered with boards and earth, 20 by 20 feet, divided into two rooms; one front room for guard, and the other for prisoners. One end of the prison-room is divided into three cells, each 9 feet high, 6 feet long, and 3 feet wide, ventilated by holes through doors and ceiling; the house ventilated by doors, windows, and grating.

There are two storehouses, one quartermaster and one commissary, each 64 by 16 feet, built of hewn logs, covered with boards and earth, and plastered between logs; protected on the outside by boards and battens. There is a good brick chimney in the commissary building which is warmed by a stove.

The stable is built of round logs, 180 by 30 feet, covered with poles, gunny-sacks, and earth, and plastered between logs with mud. A good well of water is in the stable.

There are six other buildings, used respectively as grain-house, butcher-shop, adjutant's office, quartermaster's office, carpenter-shop, and blacksmith-shop. There is one building, about 300 yards south of the post, used as a slaughter-house. About 50 yards east of the post is a corral for mules.

There are sinks built of lumber in rear of each barrack, officers' quarters, hospital, and two in rear of married soldiers' quarters.

The hospital building is 40 by 36 feet, built of hewn logs, one story high, covered with boards and earth, and protected on the sides by boards and battens, and was erected in the month of October, 1870. It contains five rooms, with a hall 7 feet wide for a distance of 16 feet, thence continued 5 feet wide for 24 feet to the rear of the building, through the center. On one side are the ward, 32 by 16 feet, and kitchen, 14½ by 8 feet. The ward has a capacity for six beds. Upon the opposite side are the office and dispensary, 13 by 16 feet, steward's room, 15 by 16 feet, and mess-room, 14½ by 8 feet. The loft over all these rooms is used as store-room. The office is lined, canvased, and papered, the steward's room canvased and papered, and the other rooms canvased only; all ceiled overhead. It was originally intended that a kitchen should be attached to the hospital, but it has not been built, although a kitchen is needed, as the rooms now occupied for kitchen and mess-room were intended for isolation-wards, and consequently there is no room that can be used as such, which should be the case in all well-regulated hospitals. Several applications have been made to have the hospital building completed according to the original plan, but each has been a failure so far. The hospital is warmed by wood-burning stoves, and is ventilated through doors, windows, and floors, to a greater extent than is necessary for the comfort and protection of the occupants. The ward is lighted by three windows; steward's room, mess-room, and kitchen by one each, and the office by two. There is no bath-room attached to the hospital.

No drainage or sewerage is required other than the natural slope of the ground affords. A stream of water, brought through a ditch from a gulch about one-half mile distant, runs during the summer through the post, thus aiding in the drainage and sewerage, and also affording an abundant supply for all purposes except drinking and cooking, and affording convenient means for extinguishing fires. The water used for cooking and drinking is obtained from two wells, one in front of the married soldiers' quarters and the other in rear of the officers' quarters. The other two are only used for animals, as the water is of an alkaline character. There are no special arrangements for bathing at the post. All refuse matter is transported outside of the post and scattered on the plains.

The inhabitants of the surrounding country, embracing within its limits three towns, number about 100 people, the remnants of a once large mining community. In 1869 and 1870, large numbers of people were attracted to the country by the flattering prospects of gold, which was represented to exist in the Sweetwater mines, in the midst of which the post is located, and for whom it was intended to give protection. The mines were worked in some cases with good success, quartz-mills were erected, and both quartz and placer mining carried on to a considerable extent; but either for the want of sufficient capital, or the mines not affording a very large yield, they were gradually abandoned, and now the only mining that is carried on is placer, and one quartz-mill in operation in the summer-time, but the results are not of such a character as to warrant the investment of much capital or labor. There are three towns, South Pass City, Atlantic City, and Hamilton City, the latter town commonly known as "Miners' Delight," all within a few miles of the post, and were a few years ago in a prosperous condition, but now they are nearly abandoned. South Pass was formerly the county-seat of Sweetwater County, but the county-seat has been lately removed to Green River. The only business represented in South Pass City is one hotel and one billiard-saloon, post-office, and stage station. Atlantic City and Hamilton City will compare favorably with South Pass in point of business.

During the summer there are frequent raids made by the Indians, generally supposed to belong to the Sioux and Arapahoes, who succeed in murdering the settlers and stealing stock. The nearest friendly Indians are the Shoshones and the Bannacks, on their reservation near Camp Brown, about fifty-two miles distant.

The principal route of travel is over the Sweetwater stage-line from Bryan, on the Union Pacific Railroad, over which the mails are brought three times a week.

The prevailing diseases in the post and in the country are catarrh, rheumatism, and erysipelas. Malarial fevers are almost unknown. Two cases of typhoid fever have occurred since the post was established. During the past two and one-half years but very few cases of venereal disease have been treated, most of the cases being brought from other places, but few having been contracted in the vicinity of the post.

*Consolidated sick-report, Camp Stambaugh, Wyo., 1870–'74.*

| Year | 1870–'71. | | 1871–'72. | | 1872–'73. | | 1873–'74. | |
|---|---|---|---|---|---|---|---|---|
| Mean strength { Officers | 5 | | 4 | | 4 | | 5 | |
| { Enlisted men | 128 | | 82 | | 75 | | 66 | |
| Diseases. | Cases. | Deaths. | Cases. | Deaths. | Cases. | Deaths. | Cases. | Deaths. |
| GENERAL DISEASES, A. | | | | | | | | |
| Typhoid fever | | | | | 1 | | 1 | |
| Remittent fever | | | | | | | 2 | |
| Intermittent fever | 6 | | 3 | | 8 | | 4 | |
| Other diseases of this group | 30 | | 6 | | 5 | | 4 | |
| GENERAL DISEASES, B. | | | | | | | | |
| Rheumatism | 31 | | 10 | | 5 | | 8 | |
| Syphilis | 11 | | | | 1 | | 1 | |
| LOCAL DISEASES. | | | | | | | | |
| Catarrh and bronchitis | 16 | | 15 | | 6 | | 15 | |
| Pleurisy | | | | | 1 | | 2 | |
| Diarrhœa and dysentery | 68 | | 9 | | 7 | | 8 | |
| Gonorrhœa | 1 | | 3 | | | | | |
| Other local diseases | 190 | 1 | 33 | | 30 | | 33 | |
| Alcoholism | 6 | | 3 | | 1 | | 2 | |
| Total disease | 359 | 1 | 82 | | 65 | | 80 | |
| VIOLENT DISEASES AND DEATHS. | | | | | | | | |
| Gunshot wounds | 1 | | | | | | | |
| Other accidents and injuries | 41 | | 44 | | 18 | | 16 | 1 |
| Homicide | | 1 | | | | | | |
| Total violence | 42 | 1 | 41 | | 18 | | 16 | 1 |

# FORT FRED STEELE, WYOMING TERRITORY.

INFORMATION FURNISHED BY ASSISTANT SURGEONS J. K. CORSON, J. M. DICKSON, J. H. PATZKI, UNITED STATES ARMY, AND ACTING ASSISTANT SURGEON R. A. CHRISTIAN, UNITED STATES ARMY.

Fort Fred Steele is situated on the west bank of the North Fork of the Platte River, at the point of crossing of the Union Pacific Railroad; latitude 41° 48' north, longitude 30° 6' west; elevation above the sea, about 6,700 feet. The bluff on which the post is placed is about thirty-five feet high, composed of ten feet of loose gravelly alluvium lying on a bed of soft clay slate. Immediately below the railroad-crossing, the river makes an abrupt angle to the west, running along the base of the high, bare bluffs called Rattlesnake Hills. To the south and east are ranges of low sand-hills, above which can be seen Elk Mountain and the Medicine Bow Range. Saint Mary's, the nearest town or settlement, is about twelve miles distant. There are coal-mines at Carbon, forty-one miles distant, and there appear to be numerous beds of coal of varying quality at points more accessible to the post. Near Rawlings's Springs, twenty miles west of this place, coal of good quality is said to exist in large amount. The rocks forming the bluffs directly opposite the post, beyond the Platte, are sandstone of an excellent quality for building purposes, and easily quarried. At some points they appear to be a siliceous sand-rock, the seams stained with iron. Moss and wood agates, carnelians, and jasper are quite plenty in the vicinity.

The soil being alkaline, is unproductive without irrigation, except in some sheltered bottoms along the river, from whence forage for the post is sometimes obtained. Timber, other than cotton-wood, is very scarce nearer than Elk Mountain, twenty-five miles east, where pine is found in abundance. The fuel is an excellent quality of bituminous coal furnished by contractors from mines in Wyoming Territory. Cotton-wood is only used for kindling.

The gray wolf and the coyote abound, the latter coming close to the camp at night in search of offal. Game is abundant; immense herds of antelope and elk are found within a few miles of the fort, and black-tailed deer and mountain-sheep are also plentiful. Among the smaller game are the jack-rabbit and sage-hen.

The climate is exceedingly dry, rain during the fall and winter being almost unknown. The weather is usually mild and bracing during the day, but intensely cold from midnight until day-break. The river, which is very rapid, has been frozen in places almost to solidity.

This post was established in June, 1868. The barracks were occupied by the men before December 1, 1868. They are six in number. Of these, five are built on stone foundations, without cellars, of pine logs squared on three sides, and set in substantial frames, with their interstices filled with mortar. Each company-barrack is 80 by 35 feet, and has a piazza, 10 feet in width, extending along the front, with the exception of the space occupied at each end by rooms, 9 feet square, used by the first sergeant and quartermaster-sergeant as offices.

There is one large room in the interior of each building, the chimneys of which are built of stone. They are warmed by two coal-stoves with drums.

Each dormitory is calculated for the accommodation of one hundred men, with 480 cubic feet of air per man.

There are two excellent ridge-ventilators to each set of quarters, and these are lighted by twelve windows with twelve panes of glass (8 by 12) apiece, and also by glasses placed in the ventilators.

The new Army-pattern single iron bedsteads are in use in all the quarters, except those of Company A, Second Cavalry, where, on account of the number of men, the old double wooden bunks are still retained.

The sinks are vaults 6 by 14 by 10 feet, lie in rear of the company quarters, covered by frame buildings well floored and seated, and with a window and two capped ventilators to each.

A kitchen and mess-room, 15 by 80 by 9 feet, built of rough lumber, in some cases lined with tar-paper, stands in rear of every barrack. The post-bakery, 20 by 40 by 10 feet, is constructed of rough, unhewn lumber. It contains a large stone-inclosed oven, and answers its purpose very well.

For the accommodation of married soldiers there are nine one-story frame houses, 56 by 29 by 9 feet, each divided into two rooms, lathed, plastered, and shingled. These, however, are not sufficient for the number of men requiring them, and several families are living in tents under the bluff.

Besides these there are the quarters for the civilian employés at the post. These are three in number; No. 1, built of rough pine lumber, 50 by 20 by 9 feet in extent; No. 2, of pine slabs, 25 by 30 by 10 feet; and No. 3, of split pine logs, 24 by 14 by 10 feet. All of these are lathed, plastered, and have shingled roofs, and two have inclosed yards in rear. There is a separate mess-house attached to these buildings 30 by 20 by 10 feet large. It is built of rough pine lumber, and has an inclosed yard.

In September, 1873, the building formerly used as a commissary storehouse was converted into quarters for an additional company ordered here. It is a rude affair, 80 by 30 by 12 feet in dimensions, one-half of it built of logs with plastered chinks, the other of boards battened. The walls of the dormitory are covered with tar-paper.

A building of rough boards battened and painted, with a shed-roof, 18 by 25 by 9 feet large, is attached to this barrack as mess and wash room. The kitchen is in the main building, a space 10 by 30 by 12 feet having been partitioned off from the dormitory.

During October, 1873, all of the barracks with their porches were newly floored with grooved and tongued pine boards, and the offices of the commanding officer and post quartermaster and commissary similarly improved.   In November, 1873, the quarters were coated with a drab-colored wash made from a kind of cement found in the neighborhood of the post.   With the exception of some crowding caused by the use of the iron bedstead, there is no objection to make to the barracks.

The commanding officer's quarters is a stone building one and a half stories high, with an additional frame building in rear.   The dimensions of the main part are 44 by 36 feet, containing eight rooms; the back building contains three rooms, and is 28 by 25 feet.   Four frame buildings, one and a half stories high, furnish quarters for officers of the command.   Each is 44 by 34 feet, and is divided into two halls, with rooms on either side, dining-room and kitchen, each 10 by 14 feet.

To these must be added a one-story frame building 36 by 28 by 10 feet in extent, containing four rooms.   A wide hall runs through the house.   It stands alone on the south side of the parade, and is built in the same style as the other officers' quarters, and was used until recently as headquarters.

In general these houses are superior in style, plan, and finish, and are all lathed and plastered. Some have small cellars under the kitchens, and all possess good-sized inclosed yards in rear.   During 1873 their walls were for the most part kalsomined by enlisted men.   Each set is intended to accommodate a captain and two lieutenants.

In place of the former headquarters there has been built a double house, 36 by 28 by 10 feet, of rough pine lumber, lathed and plastered, containing five rooms, for the necessary offices.   The chapel, which is also used as a post library and court-martial room, 20 by 40 by 10 feet, is built of pine boards, battened, lathed, plastered, and shingled.   The books are arranged in suitable closets.

In 1871 the present guard-house was built of stone quarried in the vicinity.   Its dimensions are 50 by 23 by 11 feet.   It is divided into two rooms of equal size, separated by a hall four feet wide.   The guard-room is lighted and ventilated by two large windows, and a door leading into the hall, and the prison by two small windows (barred) on its opposite sides near the ceiling.   Ten prisoners is the average number.

A short distance in rear of the guard-house lies the magazine, an excavation 18 by 20 feet, with a sloping dirt roof.

Two buildings, joined in the shape of the letter L, form the storehouses of the commissary and quartermaster.   One is 130 by 30 by 12 feet; the other 100 by 30 by 12 feet in dimensions.   Both are built of rough boards, battened.   A portion of one end of the building, containing the stores of the commissary, has recently been partitioned off, lathed, plastered, and floored with grooved and tongued boards for an office for the issue and sale of goods by the commissary-sergeant.

The forage-house, which was destroyed by fire in 1872, has been rebuilt with pine lumber; its dimensions are 50 by 20 by 10 feet, and it will contain 800,000 pounds.   The coal-house, also constructed of rough pine, 100 by 30 by 10 feet, has room, when filled to a depth of 6 feet, for 620 tons. Eleven feet of this is partitioned off for a storeroom for lime.   The saw-mill, 80 by 20 by 9 feet, is made of slabs, and contains a steam-engine and all the appliances for cutting heavy logs.

There is a blacksmith-shop, also built of slabs, and well supplied with the necessary tools.   A small rude structure adjoining it serves to store the coal for the forge.   At the same time when the forage-house was burned (August 14, 1872,) the carpenter-shop was also destroyed.   A new one, 60 by 20 by 10 feet, has been erected of pine lumber.

The fire-engine and water-works buildings, one 30 by 20 by 10 feet, with dirt roof, and the other 25 by 15 by 10 feet, with shingled roof, are made out of pine slabs, and situated on the bank of the river.   One of these contains a steam-engine used to pump water in case of fire, to fill the garrison water-cart, and to drive a circular saw for cutting kindling-wood.

An ice-house (in very bad order) is made of undressed cottonwood.   It is 35 by 52 by 12 feet in size, and covers an excavation capable of holding 18,000 cubic feet of ice.   The corral consists of an inclosing fence and sheds of pine slabs, and is 120 by 120 by 8 feet, with room for two hundred and fifty stalls.

Stables for the horses of Company A, Second Cavalry, were built by the soldiers of this command.   They measure 100 by 35 by 18 feet; are constructed of sawed pine logs battened on the side, with ends of battened pine boards.   The roof is shingled and has two ridge ventilators There are forty-eight stalls, each divided by a swinging bar, accommodating ninety-six horses

The stable is situated in the bottom under the bluff, and its refuse matter carted away and dumped into the river. The natural drainage of the post suffices, with good police, for all purposes. There are three buildings occupied by the post-trader, viz, his store, dwelling-house, and saloon. The former measures 66 by 24 by 10 feet, and has a small frame room behind for goods. His house is built of logs, with plastered chinks, and is 48 by 24 by 8 feet. It is placed within a few feet of the store. The saloon, 65 by 40 by 10 feet, is also made of logs, the interstices between which are filled with mortar. The house is lathed, plastered, and shingled, and divided into two rooms; that for the accommodation of officers contains two billiard-tables.

A barrack was used for a hospital until recently. During the years 1873–'74 a new hospital was built on the approved plan for a regulation hospital of twenty-four beds. (Circular No. 2, Surgeon-General's Office, July 27, 1871.) The building fronts due south and is built of pine lumber, inch boarding, machine-dressed, to be battened, lathed and plastered, and is on a stone foundation. On account of the unevenness of the ground the interval between the floor and ground gradually decreases from 3 feet under one ward to a few inches under the other. The cellar under the kitchen is a mere excavation without masonry. The dimensions of the windows were reduced to 34 by 62½ inches, and the pulleys and weights were disallowed. The lower boards to the upper sashes have also been omitted. All the chimneys are built with but one flue. The building being in course of completion work was suspended at the close of the fiscal year, June 30, 1874, for want of funds, but will be resumed again in the spring of 1875.

The following special report on the climate and diseases of this post is furnished by Assistant Surgeon J. H. Patzki, United States Army, dated October, 1874:

The reports of sick and wounded since July, 1868, show the prevailing diseases among the garrison of this post to be catarrhal diseases of the air-passages, disorders of the alimentary canal, and rheumatic and neuralgic affections. These diseases form well-defined natural groups and often blend into each other so that it is difficult to draw the line between them. The disease appears to be called by the generical term catarrh, if no symptoms of localization are predominating, and tonsilitis, laryngitis, or bronchitis, if special parts of the air-passages are prominently attacked. Tonsilitis embraces a large proportion of common sore throat. The irritation very rarely extends to inflammatory diseases of the pulmonary tissue. Diarrhœa, dysentery, and cholera-morbus express but different degrees in the effect of the same cause. At least these diseases have often been simultaneously observed in families in which, soon after their arrival at this post, nearly all the members were attacked with derangement of the alimentary organs. Rheumatism and neuralgia seem closely akin, the former being but rarely of the inflammatory, articular, and commonly of the myalgic variety, accompanied by acute pain and slight elevation of temperature.

The meteorological observations point to some connection between atmospheric influences and the prevalence of these diseases. A prominent feature of this climate is the dryness of the atmosphere, due partly to the elevation and partly to the geographical relations of this place, the prevailing western winds condensing most of their moisture upon the western slope of the Rocky Mountains. The relative humidity reaches its minimum in July; thereafter slowly increasing during August and September, it rises rather suddenly in October, continues to rise during the following month, and reaches its maximum during December, January, February, and March, when it shows but slight variations; it falls rather suddenly in April and continues to do so to July. Thus the season of the greatest frequency of the diseases of the first group coincides with that of the greatest relative humidity, and there is scarcely a doubt that the sudden changes in this regard tend to irritate the respiratory organs which had gradually accommodated themselves to the breathing of comparatively dry air. Even during the summer months an increase of these diseases has been frequently observed during sudden changes in the humidity of the atmosphere. But there must be still other agents active in exciting these diseases, as they often occur throughout the year, without appreciable change in the atmospheric conditions. It would seem that the very dryness of the air produces irritation by rapid evaporation from the mucous membrane of the air-passages; at least an unpleasant sensation of dryness and constant thirst is very perceptible to the new-comer. This irritation is enhanced by the deep, expansive inspirations by which the organism apparently compensates the diminished amount of oxygen in the atmosphere. The rate of respiration is not at all or but slightly increased, and is even apt to be slightly reduced, but the inspirations are deep, and in persons unacclimated, occasionally irregular and of a slightly spasmodic character. Exertion appears to produce some discomfort by increasing the frequency of respiration.

Sufficient observations have not been made to ascertain the influence of ozone on the respiratory organs, but its inertness is very doubtful, and this notwithstanding the fact that it is present in the atmosphere only in a small fraction, and that it can be breathed without perceptible effect when freely diffused through the air of the laboratory; the ozone of the laboratory and that of nature may not be strictly identical.

Another striking peculiarity of this climate is the extreme range of temperature. A daily variation of forty degrees is frequently observed, of fifty degrees not rarely, and of sixty degrees occasionally, (e. g., August 9, 1874, maximum 86°, minimum 26°.) This range of temperature is closely connected with the dryness of atmosphere, as the small amount of aqueous vapor allows the surface of the earth to be rapidly heated by the rays of the sun, and rapidly cooled at night by radiation. This peculiarity no doubt exerts a powerful influence upon the human organism, and is perhaps the most frequent cause of all of the prevailing diseases. But as those of the alimentary canal are most frequent during the season when these sudden fluctuations reach their maximum, it is reasonable to suppose that these phenomena stand to each other in the relation of cause and effect. It has been frequently observed that soldiers were attacked with these disorders after having been on guard-duty during a cool night following a sultry day. During the same season the North Platte, which furnishes the drinking-water, reaches its lowest stage, owing to the absence of snow in the mountains and to the slight rain-fall; its water, though clear and free from organic impurities, is then more alkaline than during any other season, and furnishes thus an additional cause for diseases of the bowels.

Rheumatism and neuralgias are nearly equally distributed over the year, and it would seem that sudden variations of temperature and of relative humidity possess alike the power of producing them.

To all these diseases people become less liable after prolonged sojourn, and the settlers but rarely suffer from them. It is different in this regard with malarial diseases, which affect nearly alike all classes of inhabitants. They are not frequent, (during the last six years 238 cases,) and usually of a mild type. Still, a remittent fever, occasionally very severe, is met with, by the mountaineers called mountain-fever, and much dreaded by them. The most prominent symptoms are headache, severe aching through the whole body, insomnia, furred tongue, frequent full pulse, constipation. Chills are infrequent. The efficacy of large doses of quinine proves the malarial origin; the mountaineers treat it with their panacea, sage-tea, and, as they assert, quite successfully. Men cutting timber along the streams, mostly Danes and Swedes, suffer most from this fever. That persons afflicted with ague rapidly recover in this climate was illustrated in June and July, 1867, when the troops brought from the swamps of Florida, had their systems tainted with this disease. During the two months 96 were rendered unfit for duty out of a mean strength of about 200 men, and many more suffered to a less degree. During the next 4 months but 17 cases occurred, and none during the winter. More than one-half the cases of this class were thus imported.

There is still another disease deserving notice, erysipelas, which undeniably is more frequent here than at frontier posts at lower altitudes, and is apt to complicate the most trivial injuries. Thirty cases occurred among the troops during the last six years, among these Assistant Surgeon Corson, United States Army. They are grouped in small epidemics, which make their appearance during the winter months, only four occurring during the summer.

The exanthemata do not find here conditions favorable to their development. In January, 1869, three cases of measles were imported from Omaha, December, 1871, one case of small-pox by recruits from Newport Barracks, and in January, 1870, two cases of scarlet fever; still, no new case occurred at the post.

Two cases of typhoid fever are recorded since 1868, and two of typho-malarial fever; they probably were all of the latter variety, and identical with the "mountain fever" mentioned before.

The dryness of the atmosphere, though in the beginning unpleasant and irritating, appears at the same time inimical to the development of serious pulmonary diseases. But seven cases of pneumonia and pleurisy occurred during the last six years, and but one case of consumption, (discharged for disability after four months' treatment.)   In one case (Private Taylor, Company G., Thirteenth Infantry) the company commander is of the opinion that the patient owes his life to this climate; he suffered about four years previously with cough, copious expectoration, and great emaciation, and would have been discharged from the service if his condition had not been too low.   He began to improve at Fort Bridger, Wyo., continued to do so at this post, served his full term, and is now following his trade (barber) about forty miles east from here; he still coughs.   The same officer observed great improvement in another soldier, (Private Brady, Company G, Thirteenth Infantry,) who had been afflicted for several years with cough and general impairment of health, but finally recovered in these mountains sufficiently to pass the surgeon for re-enlistment.

No cases of asthma have been observed, but there is no doubt that the lessened atmospheric pressure would tend to ease the distress of asthmatics.   Hay-asthma could certainly be avoided by timely removal to the mountains.

The climate of this vicinity, though possessing certain disadvantages, appears on the whole salubrious.   Only two deaths from disease occurred among the troops within six years, one from disease of the heart and liver, (probably of a syphilitic origin,) and the other from peritonitis in a patient of advanced age and intemperate habits.   The settlers, as a rule, enjoy good health, are of fine physique, with full development of chest, often tall, with florid complexion, and capable of great and prolonged exertion.

In my opinion, patients afflicted with chronic pulmonary diseases, resorting to this climate while still able to resist its unfavorable peculiarities, or, in other words, still capable of acclimation, will be benefited by the improvement of their general condition.   They breathe air free from the noxious elements common to the thickly-settled sections and to the low lands; the increase in the movement of the atmosphere, the greater intensity of light, the lessened atmospheric pressure, have a bracing, exhilarating effect, stimulating the body through the buoyancy of the mind; the cool nights insure sleep and rest, out-door life improves appetite, digestion, and sanguification.   The reduced amount of oxygen provokes fuller inspirations, and thus institutes a gymnastic course for the lungs; the distension of the air-cells seems of importance, if Guéneau de Mussy is correct in his observations, as to the antagonism between emphysema and consumption.   Patients, on the other hand, broken down, in an advanced stage of the disease, with a large portion of the pulmonary tissue obstructed or destroyed, incapable of compensating the diminished amount of oxygen by freer distension of the lungs, find their dyspnœa increased.   The dryness and other irritating properties of the air, as demonstrated by the production of catarrhal diseases in the healthy, the extreme and sudden variations of temperature and moisture, will be greatly to their disadvantage.   They lose all the advantages of out-door life, and enjoy none of the comforts of home.   Thus, they are exposed to the disadvantages of the climate, without reaping any of its advantages.

Though this vicinity appears to share, with other elevated localities, the preventive power in regard to chronic pulmonary diseases, still, the extreme range of temperature peculiar to it must be considered a great disadvantage, as, according to Dr. Charles Th. Williams, "warmth and equability of climate is of greater importance than dryness to patients suffering from phthisis of catarrhal origin."

*Meteorological report, Fort Fred Steele, Wyo., 1870–'74.*

| Month. | 1870–'71. Temperature. Mean. | Max. | Min. | Rain-fall in inches. | 1871–'72. Temperature. Mean. | Max. | Min. | Rain-fall in inches. | 1872–'73. Temperature. Mean. | Max. | Min. | Rain-fall in inches. | 1873–'74. Temperature. Mean. | Max. | Min. | Rain-fall in inches. |
|---|---|---|---|---|---|---|---|---|---|---|---|---|---|---|---|---|
| July | 69.20 | 90 | 50 | ....... | 74.84 | 102 | 50 | 0.35 | 64.18 | 95* | 34* | 0.16 | 69.21 | 96* | 36* | 0.68 |
| August | 63.36 | 90 | 43 | 2.75 | 69.33 | 100 | 40 | 0.22 | 64.37 | 97* | 34* | 0.47 | 66.61 | 93* | 33* | 0.84 |
| September | 58.05 | 81 | 31 | 1.50 | 60.62 | 90 | 35 | 0.82 | 58.41 | 97* | 29* | 0.13 | 55.00 | 83* | 16* | 0.26 |
| October | 46.59 | 80 | 13 | 1.50 | 42.47 | 75 | 5 | 0.98 | 38.64 | 75* | 0* | 0.91 | 37.12 | 75* | − 8* | 1.08 |
| November | 39.62 | 64 | 1 | ....... | 29.10 | 62 | −20 | 2.82 | 26.23 | 56* | 5* | 0.56 | 33.84 | 62* | 2* | 0.10 |
| December | 20.31 | 57 | −22 | 0.34 | 24.36 | 45 | 3 | 1.24 | 23.25 | 50* | 0* | 1.08 | 21.50 | 45* | −20* | 0.56 |
| January | 28.53 | 56 | −10 | 0.44 | 20.61 | 50 | −35 | 0.79 | 19.61 | 41* | −38* | 0.88 | 24.18 | 44* | −17* | 0.07 |
| February | 25.29 | 53 | − 6 | 0.80 | 26.23 | 45* | 0 | 1.38 | 20.22 | 46* | −10* | 1.02 | 18.57 | 42* | −21* | 0.15 |
| March | 31.68 | 61 | 7 | 1.02 | 28.59 | 57* | 8 | 1.12 | 33.34 | 60* | −10* | 0.08 | 25.28 | 50* | − 9* | 0.64 |
| April | 41.52 | 71 | 15 | 1.52 | 35.98 | 65* | 22 | 3.19 | 33.62 | 73* | 5* | 0.36 | 37.69 | 75* | 10* | 1.06 |
| May | 57.36 | 91 | 31 | 1.21 | 49.16 | 88* | 29 | 0.48 | 47.05 | 72* | 19* | 0.62 | 56.34 | 93* | 13* | 0.50 |
| June | 71.83 | 104 | 47 | ....... | 61.35 | 89* | 30* | 1.17 | 66.02 | 96* | 30* | 0.10 | 64.31 | 103* | 27* | 0.29 |
| For the year | 46.11 | 104 | −22 | ....... | 43.55 | 102 | −35 | 14.56 | 41.24 | 97* | −38* | 6.37 | 42.47 | 103* | −21* | 6.23 |

\* These observations are made with self-registering thermometers. The mean is from the standard thermometer.

*Consolidated sick-report, Fort Fred Steele, Wyo., 1870–'74.*

| Year | 1870–'71. | | 1871–'72. | | 1872–'73. | | 1873–'74. | |
|---|---|---|---|---|---|---|---|---|
| Mean strength { Officers / Enlisted men | 14 / 234 | | 8 / 176 | | 10 / 181 | | 13 / 220 | |
| Diseases. | Cases. | Deaths. | Cases. | Deaths. | Cases. | Deaths. | Cases. | Deaths. |
| **GENERAL DISEASES, A.** | | | | | | | | |
| Small-pox and varioloid | | | 1 | | | | | |
| Typhoid fever | 1 | | | | | | | |
| Typho-malarial fever | | | 2 | | | | | |
| Remittent fever | | | | | 5 | | 9 | |
| Intermittent fever | 10 | | 24 | | 8 | | 3 | |
| Other diseases of this group | 14 | | 11 | | 10 | | 28 | |
| **GENERAL DISEASES, B.** | | | | | | | | |
| Rheumatism | 20 | | 9 | | 10 | | 14 | |
| Syphilis | 3 | | | | | | 2 | |
| Consumption | 1 | | | | | | | |
| Other diseases of this group | | | 1 | | | | 1 | 1 |
| **LOCAL DISEASES.** | | | | | | | | |
| Catarrh and bronchitis | 22 | | 23 | | 54 | | 68 | |
| Pneumonia | 1 | | | | | | | |
| Pleurisy | | | | | 1 | | 2 | |
| Diarrhœa and dysentery | 14 | | 24 | | 26 | | 29 | |
| Hernia | | | 1 | | | | | |
| Gonorrhœa | 5 | | | | 1 | | 2 | |
| Other local diseases | 63 | 1 | 50 | | 51 | | 49 | |
| Alcoholism | 8 | 1 | 3 | | 8 | | 6 | |
| Unclassified | | | | | | | 2 | |
| Total disease | 162 | 2 | 149 | | 174 | | 215 | 1 |
| **VIOLENT DISEASES AND DEATHS.** | | | | | | | | |
| Gunshot wounds | 2 | | | | 1 | 1 | 4 | |
| Drowning | | | | 1 | | | | |
| Other accidents and injuries | 84 | 1 | 48 | | 41 | | 45 | |
| Total violence | 86 | 1 | 48 | 1 | 42 | 1 | 49 | |

# DEPARTMENT OF DAKOTA.

(Embracing the State of Minnesota and the Territories of Dakota and Montana.)

## POSTS.

Abercrombie, Fort, Dak.
Abraham Lincoln, Fort, Dak.
Baker, Camp, Mont.
Benton, Fort, Mont.
Buford, Fort, Dak.
Cheyenne Agency, Dak.
Ellis, Fort, Mont.

Grand River Agency, Dak
Hancock, Camp, Dak.
Lower Brulé Agency, Dak.
Pembina, Fort, Dak.
Randall, Fort, Dak.
Rice, Fort, Dak.
Ripley, Fort, Minn.

Seward, Fort, Dak.
Shaw, Fort, Mont.
Snelling, Fort, Minn.
Stevenson, Fort, Dak.
Sully, Fort, Dak.
Totten, Fort, Dak.
Wadsworth, Fort, Dak.

## TABLE OF DISTANCES IN THE DEPARTMENT OF DAKOTA.

| | Chicago | Saint Paul | Fort Abercrombie | Ft. Abraham Lincoln | Camp Baker | Fort Benton | Fort Buford | Cheyenne Agency | Fort Ellis | Grand River Agency | Camp Hancock | Lower Brulé Agency | Fort Pembina | Fort Randall | Fort Rice | Fort Ripley | Fort Seward | Fort Shaw | Fort Snelling | Fort Stevenson | Fort Sully | Fort Totten | Fort Wadsworth |
|---|---|---|---|---|---|---|---|---|---|---|---|---|---|---|---|---|---|---|---|---|---|---|---|
| Chicago | Chicago. | | | | | | | | | | | | | | | | | | | | | | |
| Saint Paul | 409 | Saint Paul. | | | | | | | | | | | | | | | | | | | | | |
| Fort Abercrombie | 640 | 231 | Fort Abercrombie. | | | | | | | | | | | | | | | | | | | | |
| Fort Abraham Lincoln | 872 | 463 | 232 | Ft. Abraham Lincoln. | | | | | | | | | | | | | | | | | | | |
| Camp Baker | 2034 | 1642 | 1411 | 1179 | Camp Baker. | | | | | | | | | | | | | | | | | | |
| Fort Benton | 1859 | 1438 | 1207 | 975 | 204 | Fort Benton. | | | | | | | | | | | | | | | | | |
| Fort Buford | 1117 | 708 | 477 | 245 | 449 | 730 | Fort Buford. | | | | | | | | | | | | | | | | |
| Cheyenne Agency | 889 | 629 | 490 | 245 | 1424 | 1220 | 490 | Cheyenne Agency. | | | | | | | | | | | | | | | |
| Fort Ellis | 1971 | 1688 | 1457 | 1225 | 166 | 250 | 980 | 1470 | Fort Ellis. | | | | | | | | | | | | | | |
| Grand River Agency | 962 | 571 | 340 | 108 | 1287 | 1083 | 353 | 137 | 1333 | Grand River Agency. | | | | | | | | | | | | | |
| Camp Hancock | 868 | 459 | 228 | 4 | 1183 | 979 | 249 | 249 | 1229 | 112 | Camp Hancock. | | | | | | | | | | | | |
| Lower Brulé Agency | 741 | 487 | 589 | 357 | 1536 | 1332 | 602 | 490 | 1582 | 249 | 361 | Lower Brulé Agency. | | | | | | | | | | | |
| Fort Pembina | 826 | 417 | 186 | 350 | 1529 | 1325 | 595 | 595 | 1575 | 458 | 346 | 707 | Fort Pembina. | | | | | | | | | | |
| Fort Randall | 661 | 407 | 552 | 437 | 1616 | 1412 | 682 | 192 | 1575 | 329 | 441 | 80 | 787 | Fort Randall. | | | | | | | | | |
| Fort Rice | 897 | 488 | 257 | 25 | 1204 | 1000 | 270 | 220 | 1250 | 83 | 29 | 361 | 375 | 412 | Fort Rice. | | | | | | | | |
| Fort Ripley | 534 | 125 | 187 | 352 | 1531 | 1327 | 597 | 597 | 1577 | 460 | 348 | 709 | 308 | 532 | 377 | Fort Ripley. | | | | | | | |
| Fort Seward | 772 | 363 | 132 | 104 | 1279 | 1075 | 345 | 345 | 1325 | 212 | 100 | 457 | 246 | 541 | 129 | 252 | Fort Seward. | | | | | | |
| Fort Shaw | 1923 | 1514 | 1271 | 1039 | 140 | 64 | 794 | 1284 | 186 | 1147 | 1043 | 1396 | 1389 | 1476 | 1064 | 1391 | 1143 | Fort Shaw. | | | | | |
| Fort Snelling | 416 | 7 | 233 | 465 | 1644 | 1440 | 710 | 629 | 1690 | 573 | 461 | 591 | 417 | 402 | 490 | 125 | 363 | 1273 | Fort Snelling. | | | | |
| Fort Stevenson | 967 | 558 | 327 | 95 | 1084 | 880 | 150 | 340 | 1130 | 203 | 99 | 452 | 445 | 532 | 115 | 447 | 199 | 944 | 558 | Fort Stevenson. | | | |
| Fort Sully | 846 | 586 | 518 | 252 | 1437 | 1227 | 497 | 7 | 1477 | 144 | 256 | 105 | 604 | 185 | 258 | 604 | 356 | 1291 | 588 | 347 | Fort Sully. | | |
| Fort Totten | 805 | 396 | 156 | 184 | 1363 | 1155 | 429 | 429 | 1409 | 292 | 180 | 541 | 140 | 621 | 209 | 334 | 84 | 1223 | 398 | 126 | 436 | Fort Totten. | |
| Fort Wadsworth | 658 | 249 | 90 | 272 | 1451 | 1247 | 517 | 517 | 1497 | 380 | 268 | 629 | 262 | 656 | 297 | 289 | 234 | 1311 | 249 | 367 | 524 | 240 | Fort Wadsworth. |

# FORT ABERCROMBIE, DAKOTA TERRITORY.

### REPORT OF ASSISTANT SURGEON W. H. GARDNER, UNITED STATES ARMY.

Fort Abercrombie is situated on the west bank of the Red River of the North, twelve miles north of the confluence of its two branches, the Bois de Sioux and the Otter Tail; latitude, 46° 27' north; longitude, 19° 25' west. It is two hundred and thirty miles northwest of Saint Paul, from which place it is easily accessible, the route being by the Saint Paul and Pacific Railroad two hundred and seventeen miles to Breckenridge, thence thirteen miles by ambulance or stage to the fort. Stages run thrice a week from Breckenridge to Forts Abercrombie, Garry, and Pembina, and to Moorehead, distant thirty-five miles on the Northern Pacific Railroad.

The post was located in August, 1858, abandoned in July, 1859, re-occupied in the following July, and the building resumed.

The reservation, although not yet declared, was surveyed in 1867, and contains an area of twenty-two square miles, embracing both sides of the river.

The valley of the Red River of the North at Fort Abercrombie is about 1,700 feet above the level of the sea, and forms a perfectly flat prairie, broken only by the streams which drain it. It commences about fifty miles south of the post, at the divide which separates the waters of Lake Traverse from the waters of Big Stone Lake, and extends eastward into Minnesota to a high range of hills sixty miles distant, called Leaf Mountain; westward in Dakota to the Coteau des Prairies, fifty miles distant, and northward to the débouché of the river in Lake Winnipeg, only contracted at its western side by Pembina Mountain, which is probably the northern abutment of the Coteau des Prairies, once the western shore of the great water that filled this broad Red River Valley. The formation is alluvial; the surface a black, loose soil, deep and fertile, lying upon a horizontal stratum of stiff grayish or bluish clay, with occasional small circumscribed beds of coarse sand and small gravel, while scattered over the prairie, along the banks and in the bed of the streams are granitic, quartzose, and occasionally limestone bowlders of various sizes, from ten pounds to several tons in weight.

The river at its usual stage is about 150 feet broad at Fort Abercrombie, and from two to ten feet in depth, having a swift current, with probably a descent of four inches per mile. From a point three miles above Fort Abercrombie, to Pembina, near the British line, the banks of the stream are heavily wooded, chiefly with oak, ash, and elm, which come almost down to the water's edge to join the red willow and wild rice (*Zizania aquatica*) growing there. Since the Red River flows northward into a colder climate, the snow and ice which form in the water melt on its sources before its outlet is free from ice, and from this cause overflows of its banks frequently take place. The tortuous course of the river also causes in the spring, when the ice breaks up, frequent gorges of ice, and then the country behind the gorge is rapidly flooded, the current seeking new channels and bearing along with crushing force immense fields of ice that sweep away trees, houses, and everything in its path. Georgetown and Pembina, lower down the river, have frequently suffered from these causes, and it is recorded that the waters of the river at one of these spring floods came up into the parade-ground of the fort, at least forty feet above the usual level of the water.

All the cereals and vegetables grow well and abundantly in the valley. The country is excellent for stock-raising, all kinds of prairie-grass being plentiful. Timber is found only along the river bank.

In May, as soon as the ice on the streams breaks up, a large species of fish, called by the Indians and half-breeds "buffalo fish," can be seen in large numbers in the streams, evidently coming from Lake Winnipeg to deposit their spawn. They are not found after June about here. They frequently are caught weighing twenty-five or thirty pounds. Another fish common in the river is the "sheep-head." It is very similar, in general appearance, to the sheep-head caught in Chesapeake Bay, (*Sparis ovis,*) except that the teeth are like the teeth of perch. They are frequently caught weighing twenty-five or thirty pounds, and in taste somewhat resemble their marine namesake.

Fort Abercrombie is a rectangle, 675 by 625 feet, inclosed by a stockade of logs projecting above the ground from 8 to 12 feet, surmounted at the northeast, southeast, and southwest by block-houses of hewn logs, which are pierced with loop-holes for small-arms, and embrasures on the outer side for artillery. The surface inclosed is almost level down to the immediate crest of the bank of the river, and is easily drained by two main drains (uncovered) on the eastern and western sides. The level of the parade-ground is about thirty feet above the usual level of the river.

The company quarters are three buildings, each one story high, boarded outside, and lathed and plastered within, divided into bake-room, store-room, kitchen, dining-room, orderly-room, and two squad-rooms, each 33 by 25 feet, and 9 feet high; each squad-room being intended to accommodate thirty-two men, giving 232 cubic feet of air-space per man. Fortunately these rooms are not very close, for the only ventilation is an air-shaft consisting of a stove-pipe put up alongside the chimney, and opening into it above, nor are they usually occupied by their full complement of men. Deducting those who sleep out of the quarters—perhaps not even twenty men ever sleep in one squad-room at one time—even this, however, will give but 371 cubic feet of air per man.

The quarters for married soldiers are new log shanties, one room, 18 by 16 feet, being allowed for each family. The floor is laid on the ground, and there are but two windows to each set of quarters. No special ventilation.

From the establishment of the post up to the present time it has possessed a remarkable immunity from disease. Scurvy has prevailed to some extent, owing to a want of care in providing the troops here with sufficient vegetable diet.

Phthisis pulmonalis, pneumonia, and most other lung diseases are rare. The only diseases which seem of endemic origin, are a peculiar pharyngitis and tonsilitis, and asthma, which are usually made worse when already existing, and sometimes brought on when not before known to exist. Both of these diseases may have their origin in the fungus of the wild grasses of the prairie surrounding the post, though this view has not been experimentally established.

A small, isolated, frame building is used as quarters by the commanding officer; it contains three small rooms and a kitchen down-stairs. North from this building is a set of captains' quarters, containing three good-sized rooms down-stairs, including the kitchen, and two low attic rooms up-stairs. Next beyond this building is a row of log buildings, 17 by 142 feet, used as quarters by the ordnance sergeant, hospital steward, hospital matron, and containing the post school-room, lieutenants' mess-room, and quartermaster's store-room. There is a large frame building containing five rooms and a kitchen on the lower floor, and two upper attic rooms. It is used for offices by the commanding officer and the adjutant, and contains the quarters of the post surgeon. Adjoining this building is a small frame building containing two rooms, attached to the next set of quarters, which is a frame building lathed and plastered inside. It contains three rooms, including kitchen, on the lower floor, and up-stairs three low attic rooms. Next on the north is another small building but one story high. Adjoining this little building, on the north, is a long one-story frame building, clapboarded, lathed, and plastered, and divided into six rooms for lieutenants' quarters; in the rear of which, and 10 feet distant, is a building, the same length as those quarters, divided into rooms for kitchens for each set of quarters. Opposite the north end of this building is a granary or store-house, 20 by 83 feet, running east and west.

Between two of the company quarters is a small building fronting the parade-ground, 20 by 16 feet, built of hewn logs, which is the guard-house. The interior is divided into one large and two small rooms or cells, about 7 feet square. These are secured by small barred windows, and holes have been made through the logs for ventilation. The average number of prisoners in the guard-house is less than five. The hospital is a two-story frame building, 38 feet square, lathed and plastered within, the interval between the clapboards and plastering being filled in with brick. The lower floor is elevated from 2 to 3 feet above the ground; the height of the lower rooms is 10 feet, the upper 9½. The lower floor is divided into an office, a dispensary, a kitchen, and a dining-room. A hall separates the rooms, and also contains the stairs. Between the kitchen and the dining-room is a pantry, 10 feet long and 4 feet broad. The upper floor is divided by a hall, 8 feet wide, on one side of which is a large room or ward, 28 feet square. Across the hall there are three rooms, two 14 feet square, with a small room, 14 by 10 feet, between them. All the rooms in the hospital are heated with cast-iron stoves, and, except the large ward, have no means of ventilation but the windows and doors. The large ward is ventilated by a shaft passing up by the side of the chimney; it contains five beds, allowing about 800 cubic feet of air-space to each man. This, though hardly half enough in a southern latitude, answers very well here, for the difference between the temperature of internal and external air is so great that diffusion and currents of air occur through the smallest crevices; while the number of patients does not more than average one. The ice-house is a pit, 40 by 20 feet, lined with rough logs, covered with thatch, and well banked around with earth. This ice-house is capable of containing over three hundred tons of ice, this supply usually being ample for three companies during the summer.

The garrison is supplied with water for all purposes from the river. The water is tasteless, inodorous, and colorless, except in summer and when swollen by the spring floods. It contains little oxidizable organic matter, and is a tolerably pure, healthy drinking-water; but, like most river-waters, is hard from the presence of carbonate of lime. There are also at the post six cisterns for the reception of rain-water.

The soil being naturally productive, there is a post-garden cultivated by details of enlisted men, and one belonging to the hospital worked by the attendants and convalescents. During the past year the production of the ordinary culinary vegetables supplied the wants of the garrison and left a sufficient surplus for winter use. A large root-house was in course of construction at the date of the latest information.

*Meteorological report, Fort Abercrombie, Dak., 1870–'74.*

| Months. | 1870–'71. | | | | 1871–'72. | | | | 1872–'73. | | | | 1873–'74. | | | |
|---|---|---|---|---|---|---|---|---|---|---|---|---|---|---|---|---|
| | Temperature. | | | Rain-fall in inches. | Temperature. | | | Rain-fall in inches. | Temperature. | | | Rain-fall in inches. | Temperature. | | | Rain-fall in inches. |
| | Mean. | Max. | Min. | | Mean. | Max. | Min. | | Mean. | Max. | Min. | | Mean. | Max. | Min. | |
| | ° | ° | ° | | ° | ° | ° | | ° | ° | ° | | ° | ° | ° | |
| July | 71.06 | 95 | 44* | 2.70 | 72.95 | 104 | 36* | 1.62 | 72.60 | 95 | 44* | 3.45 | 71.84 | 102* | 34* | 0.92 |
| August | 66.74 | 99 | 32* | 2.80 | 71.83 | 101 | 39* | 0.57 | 68.29 | 96 | 41* | 2.35 | 71.45 | 93* | 43* | 4.03 |
| September | 62.44 | 86 | 32* | 5.10 | 59.91 | 94 | 20* | 1.40 | 58.81 | 85 | 31* | 0.90 | 52.16 | 80 | 20* | 0.44 |
| October | 46.89 | 78 | 19* | 1.10 | 44.79 | 82 | 18* | 0.62 | 49.47 | 81 | 15* | 2.20 | 40.13 | 78 | 10* | 0.26 |
| November | 35.89 | 61 | 10* | 0.10 | 18.72 | 57 | −22* | 0.70 | 20.71 | 49 | −16* | 0.22 | 23.74 | 55* | − 7* | 0.14 |
| December | 16.03 | 50 | −20* | 0.14 | − 0.29 | 34 | −21* | 1.82 | 1.30 | 35 | −32* | 0.55 | 8.49 | 32* | −19* | (?) |
| January | 6.15 | 35 | −20* | 0.60 | 7.22 | 30 | −23* | 0.40 | 1.23 | 29 | −33* | 0.50 | 3.46 | 39* | −29* | (?) |
| February | 10.07 | 33 | −20* | 0.72 | 10.08 | 38 | −27* | 0.41 | 9.56 | 36 | −22* | 0.51 | 6.26 | 31* | −22* | 0.80 |
| March | 21.17 | 47 | −15* | 1.40 | 11.94 | 32 | −20* | 1.50 | 18.69 | 41 | −27* | 0.69 | 14.10 | 42* | −18* | 0.39 |
| April | 39.30 | 70 | 20* | 1.36 | 39.66 | 76 | 4* | 1.50 | 36.00 | 60 | 21* | 2.00 | 32.38 | 80 | 6* | 0.70 |
| May | 63.44 | 96 | 33* | 0.36 | 56.72 | 96 | 29* | 4.20 | 53.06 | 75 | 30* | 2.20 | 67.39 | 102 | 19* | 1.70 |
| June | 69.95 | 96 | 45* | 4.10 | 69.87 | 94 | 40* | 10.15 | 72.65 | 99* | (28)?* | 3.65 | 70.92 | 95 | 35* | 8.16 |
| For the year | 42.43 | 99 | −20* | 20.42 | 36.22 | 104 | −27* | 24.89 | 36.03 | 99* | −33* | 19.22 | 38.52 | 102 | −29* | ........ |

* These observations are made with self-registering thermometers. The mean is from the standard thermometer.

*Consolidated sick-report, Fort Abercrombie, Dak., 1870–'74.*

| Year | | 1870–'71. | | 1871–'72. | | 1872–'73. | | 1873–'74. | |
|---|---|---|---|---|---|---|---|---|---|
| Mean strength | { Officers | 7 | | 7 | | 5 | | 7 | |
| | } Enlisted men | 88 | | 66 | | 53 | | 113 | |
| Diseases. | | Cases. | Deaths. | Cases. | Deaths. | Cases. | Deaths. | Cases. | Deaths. |
| GENERAL DISEASES, A. | | | | | | | | | |
| Remittent fever | | 4 | | | | | | 5 | |
| Intermittent fever | | | | 1 | | | | | |
| Other diseases of this group | | | | 1 | | | | 4 | |
| GENERAL DISEASES, B. | | | | | | | | | |
| Rheumatism | | 15 | | 18 | | 3 | | 2 | |
| Syphilis | | 4 | | | | | | 1 | |
| Consumption | | | | 1 | | 2 | 1 | | |
| Other diseases of this group | | 2 | | | | | | | |

*Consolidated sick-report, Fort Abercrombie, Dak., 1870–'74—Continued.*

| Year | 1870–'71. | | 1871–'72. | | 1872–'73. | | 1873–'74. | |
|---|---|---|---|---|---|---|---|---|
| Mean strength { Officers | 7 | | 7 | | 5 | | 7 | |
| { Enlisted men | 88 | | 66 | | 53 | | 113 | |
| Diseases. | Cases. | Deaths. | Cases. | Deaths. | Cases. | Deaths. | Cases. | Deaths. |
| LOCAL DISEASES. | | | | | | | | |
| Catarrh and bronchitis | 34 | ...... | 35 | ...... | 13 | ...... | 9 | ...... |
| Pneumonia | 4 | ...... | ...... | ...... | ...... | ...... | ...... | ...... |
| Pleurisy | ...... | ...... | 2 | ...... | 1 | ...... | 1 | ...... |
| Diarrhœa and dysentery | 53 | ...... | 35 | ...... | 11 | ...... | 8 | ...... |
| Hernia | ...... | ...... | ...... | ...... | 2 | ...... | ...... | ...... |
| Other local diseases | 38 | ...... | 34 | ...... | 11 | ...... | 18 | ...... |
| Alcoholism | ...... | ...... | ...... | ...... | 1 | ...... | 7 | ...... |
| Total disease | 154 | ...... | 127 | 1 | 43 | 1 | 55 | ...... |
| VIOLENT DISEASES AND DEATHS. | | | | | | | | |
| Gunshot wounds | ...... | ...... | ...... | ...... | 1 | ...... | ...... | ...... |
| Drowning | ...... | ...... | ...... | ...... | ...... | ...... | ...... | 1 |
| Other accidents and injuries | 12 | ...... | 13 | ...... | 11 | ...... | 16 | ...... |
| Total violence | 12 | ...... | 13 | ...... | 12 | ...... | 16 | 1 |

# FORT ABRAHAM LINCOLN, DAKOTA TERRITORY.

INFORMATION FURNISHED BY SURGEON JAMES F. WEEDS, UNITED STATES ARMY, AND BY ACTING ASSISTANT SURGEON J. FRAZER BOUGHTER, UNITED STATES ARMY.

Fort Abraham Lincoln was established June 14, 1872, to protect the engineers and working-parties of the Northern Pacific Railroad. It is situated on the west bank of the Missouri, at the point where the line of the road crosses that river, in latitude 46° 47' north, longitude 23° 47' west. The elevation above the river is 270 feet, and the fort is surrounded on all sides, except the river-front, by ravines, broken and irregular bluffs and hills, and commands an extended view of the surrounding country. Bismarck, the terminus of the eastern section of the Northern Pacific Railroad, is situated on the opposite side of the river. Duluth, the eastern terminus of the road, is 453 miles distant, and Fort Abercrombie 232 miles.

The infantry barrack is 233 by 25 feet; the three cavalry barracks are each 232½ by 24 feet. They are frame buildings. The latter are lined inside with boards and ceiled with plastering. The infantry quarters are lined with the worthless material called "plaster-board." Each dormitory is warmed by two large box-stoves burning wood. Three companies still use the double bunks. The other companies are supplied with single iron bedsteads. Kitchens and mess-rooms are detached buildings in rear of the dormitories.

The barracks afford quarters for nine companies. At the cavalry barracks there are six sets and at the infantry barracks three sets. The dormitories of the former are each 24 by 100 by 12 feet, 28,800 cubic feet air-space; and at the latter, 24 by 64 by 12 feet, 18,432 cubic feet-air space.

The following table will at a glance show the air and floor space of the several dormitories, the number of men who sleep in each, and the floor and air-space per man:

| Companies. | Regiments. | Total air-space of dormitories. | Total floor-space of dormitories. | No. of men who sleep in dormitories. | Air-space per man. | Floor-space per man. |
|---|---|---|---|---|---|---|
| D | Seventeenth Infantry | 18. 432 | 1, 536 | 29 | 635. 51 | 52. 95 |
| A | Sixth Infantry | 18. 432 | 1, 356 | 23 | 801. 39 | 66. 79 |
| H | Seventeenth Infantry | 28. 800 | 2, 400 | 26 | 1, 107. 69 | 92. 30 |
| G | Seventeenth Infantry | 28. 800 | 2, 400 | 40 | 720. 00 | 60. 00 |
| B | Sixth Infantry | 28. 800 | 2, 400 | 24 | 1, 200. 00 | 100. 00 |
| F | Seventh Cavalry | 28. 800 | 2, 400 | 50 | 576. 00 | 48. 00 |
| L | Seventh Cavalry | 28. 800 | 2, 400 | 48 | 600. 00 | 50. 00 |
| Band | Seventh Cavalry | 28. 800 | 2, 400 | 25 | 1, 152. 00 | 96. 00 |

Married soldiers are quartered at the infantry barracks in a log building, 20 by 100 by 8 feet, with dirt floor and roof, which contains seven sets of two rooms each. This building is in bad repair; the roof leaks and the floors are cold and damp. At the cavalry barracks married soldiers occupy a frame building, 186 by 30 feet, which contains twenty-four rooms well ventilated and very comfortable.

Quarters for cavalry officers are seven frame buildings, designed for thirteen sets of quarters; one, a new one-and-a-half-story building, containing ten rooms, eight closets, pantry, kitchen, and an excellent cellar, and occupied by the commanding officer, being a commodious and elegant building; the other six are double, one story, with unfinished attics, each set of quarters containing three rooms and a kitchen, pantry, and cellar. At the infantry barracks there are four one-story frame buildings, each designed for two sets of quarters containing three rooms, kitchen, closet, and cellar. Three of these buildings have the walls lined with "plaster-board," which is a poor substitute for plaster, particularly in cold climates. The cellars of these quarters are small and not frost-proof. A one-story frame building, containing eight rooms, (including two kitchens,) designed for quarters for two officers, was erected at the infantry barracks in 1874. It is plastered and painted inside.

The guard-house at cavalry barracks is 30 by 70 feet; contains a prison-room 29 by 30 feet; guard-room, 18 by 30 feet; sally-port, 10 by 30 feet; five cells, each 10 by 5¼ feet; officers' room, 8 by 10 feet; and a tool-room 8 feet square. Each cell has one window, prison-room two windows, and two ventilators in the floor; the rest of the building is well ventilated. Warming is effected by two open fire-places and three stoves. Average occupancy, 20.56. A block-house with two rooms, each 20 by 20 feet, is used as a guard-house at the infantry barracks. Ventilation is by twenty loop-holes in each room; in winter the loop-holes are closed, when there is no ventilation. The lower room is for the guard, the upper for prisoners.

The hospital is a regulation hospital of twenty-four beds, completed November 8, 1872, but is in several respects very imperfectly constructed and finished. It is a frame building resting on posts of cottonwood, a material which rots rapidly, but logs suitable for the purpose were unobtainable. There is a cistern beneath the administration-building, but no gutters and conductors were provided for filling it, and it was so imperfectly constructed as not to hold water. A material called "aluminous paper-board" was substituted in part for plastering. It is affected by atmospheric damp, is readily permeable by heat, and easily broken and torn. Funds have been furnished during the present year (1874) to complete the cistern and plastering, inclose the hospital-grounds with a board fence, and build a water-closet adequate to the wants of the hospital. The wards are furnished with double windows, rendered necessary by the severity of the winters and the prevalence of violent storms of wind. The wards are 12 feet in internal height. Each room, except the kitchen, has an adjustable ventilator in the chimney near the ceiling. There is a cellar beneath the kitchen, and the entire building, except the kitchen, is surrounded by a veranda 8 feet wide. Earth commodes are kept in closets adjoining the wards for the use of patients too feeble to go out.

*Meteorological report, Fort Abraham Lincoln, Dak., 1873–'74.*

| Month. | 1870–'71. | | | | 1871–'72. | | | | 1872–'73. | | | | 1873–'74. | | | |
| | Temperature. | | | Rain-fall in inches. | Temperature. | | | Rain-fall in inches. | Temperature. | | | Rain-fall in inches. | Temperature. | | | Rain-fall in inches. |
| | Mean. | Max. | Min. | | Mean. | Max. | Min. | | Mean. | Max. | Min. | | Mean. | Max. | Min. | |
| July | | | | | | | | | | | | | 70.32 | 95 | 53 | 0.80 |
| August | | | | | | | | | | | | | 72.75 | 96 | 50 | 1.40 |
| September | | | | | | | | | | | | | 54.96 | 95 | 28 | 0.24 |
| October | | | | | | | | | | | | | 42.42 | 92 | 9 | 0.05 |
| November | | | | | | | | | | | | | 30.54 | 65 | 3 | (?) |
| December | | | | | | | | | | | | | 16.03 | 50 | −16 | 0.00 |
| January | | | | | | | | | | | | | 11.91 | 49 | −33 | 0.30 |
| February | | | | | | | | | | | | | 14.06 | 53 | −18 | 0.00 |
| March | | | | | | | | | | | | | 22.08 | 56 | − 7 | 0.13 |
| April | | | | | | | | | | | | | 38.83 | 92 | 15 | 0.10 |
| May | | | | | | | | | | | | | 59.92 | 98 | 20 | 0.45 |
| June | | | | | | | | | | | | | 68.80 | 98 | 43 | 1.42 |
| For the year | | | | | | | | | | | | | 41.89 | 98 | −33 | |

*Consolidated sick-report, Fort Abraham Lincoln, Dak., 1872–'74.*

| Year | | 1872–'73. | | 1873–'74. | |
|---|---|---|---|---|---|
| Mean strength ...................... { Officers...........<br>{ Enlisted men...... | | 6<br>149 | | 16<br>513 | |
| Diseases. | | Cases. | Deaths. | Cases. | Deaths. |
| GENERAL DISEASES, A. | | | | | |
| Typhoid fever ............... | | ...... | ...... | 2 | ...... |
| Remittent fever............... | | ...... | ...... | 2 | ...... |
| Intermittent fever ............... | | 11 | ...... | 14 | ...... |
| Other diseases of this group............... | | 4 | ...... | 9 | ...... |
| GENERAL DISEASES, B. | | | | | |
| Rheumatism ............... | | 7 | ...... | 21 | ...... |
| Syphilis ............... | | 1 | ...... | 14 | ...... |
| Consumption ............... | | ...... | ...... | 5 | ...... |
| Other diseases of this group ............... | | 1 | ...... | 6 | ...... |
| LOCAL DISEASES. | | | | | |
| Catarrh and bronchitis ............... | | 40 | ...... | 46 | ...... |
| Pneumonia............... | | 1 | ...... | ...... | ...... |
| Pleurisy............... | | ...... | ...... | 3 | 2 |
| Diarrhœa and dysentery............... | | 52 | ...... | 65 | 1 |
| Hernia............... | | 1 | ...... | 6 | ...... |
| Gonorrhœa ............... | | 7 | ...... | 3 | ...... |
| Other local diseases ............... | | 74 | ...... | 120 | ...... |
| Alcoholism............... | | ...... | ...... | 2 | ...... |
| Total disease............... | | 199 | ...... | 318 | 3 |
| VIOLENT DISEASES AND DEATHS. | | | | | |
| Gunshot wounds .... ............... | | 4 | 5 | 5 | ...... |
| Drowning............... | | ...... | 2 | ...... | 3 |
| Other accidents and injuries ............... | | 84 | ...... | 87 | 2 |
| Homicides ............... | | ...... | ...... | ...... | 3 |
| Total violence............... | | 88 | 7 | 92 | 8 |

# CAMP BAKER, MONTANA TERRITORY.

### REPORT OF ACTING ASSISTANT SURGEON GEO. SCOTT OLDMIXON, UNITED STATES ARMY.

Camp Baker is in Smith's River Valley, one mile south of Smith's River; latitude, 46° 39' 48" north; longitude, 34° 7' west; altitude, about 6,000 feet above the sea.

The post was first located on the bank of Smith's River, ten miles farther north, in November, 1869, and was removed to its present site August 18, 1870. The valley of Smith's River (or Deep Creek) is about fifty miles long, with a width varying from three to twenty miles, averaging about five miles. In the immediate vicinity of the post the spurs and foot-hills close in and narrow the valley to a width of barely three miles.

Smith's River, more familiarly known as Deep Creek, a tortuous and tolerably rapid stream, rises in the Bell Mountains, and coursing over a pebbly bottom, with an average breadth of 25 feet and a depth of 3 feet, empties into the Missouri about sixty miles north of the post. A series of hills, running east and west, entirely conceal the river from view on the north side; and after reaching their greatest elevation, at 500 yards from the post, slope in some directions by a gentle decline toward the river, while in others they abruptly terminate in precipitous bluffs, exhibiting sharp angles and a rugged contour, their crevices in more than one instance revealing the bleaching relics of some Indian grave. The opposite banks rise in steep hills of considerable elevation, whose craggy and fantastic summits, presenting scanty patches of verdure and dotted with a stunted growth of pine, stretch away to the southeast and soon present the agreeable contrast of an endless variety of hill and valley. Toward the south and west the land extends in unbroken prairie, presenting at intervals patches of alkaline efflorescence, while a few straggling clumps of willows, fringing the borders of a small lake half a mile distant, is all that meets the eye until, at a distance varying from two to six miles, a low range of hills, running in a westerly direction and ascending to a higher plateau, break the monotonous level.

The rocks in the vicinity apparently belong to the post-tertiary period, and from above downward are a heavy schistose rock, a loose bed of shale, yellow marl, limestone, arenaceous sandstone, and metamorphic sandstone. These beds are broken in every direction and tilted at an angle of about 45°. Granite and syenite are also found in the vicinity.

The valley is covered with a thick growth of bunch-grass, and the mountains clothed to their crests with pine. Along the water-courses is a scanty growth of cottonwood, aspen, and willow.

A good quality of red and yellow pine lumber can be procured at a saw-mill twelve miles distant in a southerly direction.

Water of a good quality is procured from the streams in the vicinity. It is hauled to the post in barrels. Efforts have been made to obtain it from wells; the results, however, were unsatisfactory.

Attempts to establish a post-garden having proved unsuccessful, fresh vegetables are procured from the neighboring ranch-men.

Game of all kinds is abundant, elk, black and white tailed deer, antelope, and mountain-sheep being among the principal varieties; while buffaloes, not observed for many years in the vicinity, were killed during the winter of 1873 a short distance from the post. Mountain-grouse, mallard, wild-goose, hare, curlew, and snipe may also be enumerated as valuable accessories to the table. Black and cinnamon bears are occasionally shot in the vicinity, while the coyote and gray wolf are annually poisoned in large numbers, the sale of their pelts contributing in no small degree to the support of an adventurous population. Otter, beaver, mink, muskrat, ermine, skunk, and prairie-squirrel are also captured. Many of the streams abound in trout, grayling, and white-fish.

There are few cattle-ranches in Smith's River Valley, for which it seems to be much better adapted than to agriculture, as, owing to early frosts, only the more hardy kinds of vegetables can be reared, such as turnips, beets, potatoes, and radishes.

The inhabitants of the surrounding country are chiefly engaged in mining and hunting during the season. The town of Diamond City, eighteen miles distant in a westerly direction, containing a small fluctuating mining population, and Thompson's Gulch, thirteen miles southwest, comprising some scattered cabins connected with hydraulic mining, are the only villages in the neighborhood. The latter village is almost deserted in the winter. There are no Indians in the vicinity.

The line of communication with the east is by way of Diamond City and Helena by stage to Corinne on the Union Pacific Railroad, or from Helena by stage to Benton City, at the head of steamboat navigation on the Missouri. The former route is open at all seasons, the latter only during the summer months.

There is a post-office at the camp, with a regular tri-weekly delivery.

The post is located on a reservation of 2,400 acres, on the left bank of Smith's River.

The quarters for enlisted men consist of one building constructed of squared logs, covered with a shingled roof. It is 100 by 29 feet, divided into a dormitory 77 by 28 feet, a sergeant's room 16 by 14 feet, a property-room of the same size, and a hall, 6 feet wide, between the dormitory and the two other rooms. In rear of this is a building 40 by 16 feet, divided into a mess-room and kitchen, also of logs. The barrack, originally intended for one company, is partitioned by canvas into two rooms and occupied by two companies, giving only 254 cubic feet of air-space per man, and with no special means of ventilation. The rooms are warmed by wood-stoves; iron bedsteads are furnished, with the usual bedding.

There are five small log buildings, two recently erected, for quarters for married soldiers. The size of these ranges from 15 feet square to 24 by 18 feet, and each is about 9 feet high.

The quarters for officers consist of one hewn-log building, containing two sets of quarters, of four rooms each; the front room in each set is 14 by 16 feet, the back room 14 by 9 feet. This building is occupied by the commanding officer and one company officer. The other building is a frame one. It also contains two sets of quarters, of four rooms each, two of which are attic. It is occupied by the medical officer and one company officer, and is extremly cold in winter. These quarters were constructed with open fire-places, but the severity of some seasons necessitates the universal use of stoves. They are ceiled and plastered, and the wood-work is painted. A part of the headquarters building is also used as officers' quarters.

The post-bakery is built of adobes, and is capable of furnishing 120 rations per diem. The oven being defective, material has been procured for the erection of a new bakery.

The post-library is a temporary log building roofed with canvas, 18 by 10 feet.

The guard-house is built of hewn logs, is two stories high, imperfectly lighted by loop-holes. The lower story is occupied by the guard, the upper story by the prisoners.

The hospital is a log structure, built in June, 1871. It contains in the center a ward 29 by 19 feet, with a capacity for six beds, giving to each 918 cubic feet of air-space; lighted by four windows, two on each side. Adjoining one end of the ward are the dispensary and steward's room, each 14 by 11 feet, each lighted by one window. Adjoining the other end of the ward are two other rooms, the same size as the last described, one used as a kitchen, the other as a store-room.

The building was originally intended for hospital purposes; and, although not well adapted, the number of the sick is and has always been so small that it answers the purpose. It is ventilated by trap-doors in the ceiling and by the doors and windows.

The quartermaster storehouse is an adobe building 60 by 30 feet, with a height of 14 feet. Commissary storehouse the same size, built of logs.

The stables are two log buildings. The old stable, 120 by 28 feet, roofed with pine slabs, has been converted into a carpenter and blacksmith shop.

All the buildings are well lighted and ventilated. There are no special means for extinguishing fires.

The drainage is natural, but satisfactory.

*Meteorological report, Camp Baker, Mont., 1872–'74.*

| Month. | 1870–'71. Temperature. Mean. | Max. | Min. | Rain-fall in inches. | 1871–'72. Temperature. Mean. | Max. | Min. | Rain-fall in inches. | 1872–'73. Temperature. Mean. | Max. | Min. | Rain-fall in inches. | 1873–'74. Temperature. Mean. | Max. | Min. | Rain-fall in inches. |
|---|---|---|---|---|---|---|---|---|---|---|---|---|---|---|---|---|
| | ° | ° | ° | | ° | ° | ° | | ° | ° | ° | | ° | ° | ° | |
| July | | | | | | | | | 62.06 | 92 | 40 | | 63.75 | 92* | 48 | 0.88 |
| August | | | | | | | | | 61.38 | 84 | 43 | | 62.49 | 93* | 49 | 0.42 |
| September | | | | | | | | | 50.88 | 78 | 20 | | 50.74 | 82* | 19 | 0.20 |
| October | | | | | | | | | 39.51 | 76 | 8 | | 35.66 | 82* | 0 | 1.10 |
| November | | | | | 19.88 | 58 | −42 | | 20.04 | 58 | −28 | | 32.18 | 69 | −14 | 1.36 |
| December | | | | | 9.43 | 56 | −53 | | 14.55 | 48 | −30 | | 8.76 | 45 | −45 | 0.06 |
| January | | | | | 20.39 | 52 | −30 | | 20.31 | 48 | −32 | 0.84 | 18.83 | 45 | −26 | 0.30 |
| February | | | | | 30.24 | 63 | −36 | | 11.53 | 35 | −43 | 1.22 | 19.89 | 48 | −30 | 0.00 |
| March | | | | | 33.62 | 65 | −2 | | 32.11 | 64* | −12 | 0.32 | 27.65 | 53 | 0 | 0.44 |
| April | | | | | 38.15 | 63 | 21 | | 36.55 | 80* | 14 | 1.20 | 39.91 | 83 | 20 | 0.60 |
| May | | | | | 52.44 | 87 | 31 | | 47.89 | 77* | 31 | 2.04 | 54.83 | 91 | 30 | 2.06 |
| June | | | | | 60.03 | 85 | 44 | | 59.99 | 85* | 42 | 1.10 | 58.52 | 81 | 32 | 1.57 |
| For the year | | | | | | | | | 38.06 | 92 | −43 | | 39.60 | 93* | −45 | 8.39 |

* These observations are made with self-registering thermometers. The mean is from the standard thermometer.
NOTE.—There were no observations of rain-fall taken until January, 1873.

*Consolidated sick-report, Camp Baker, Mont., 1870–'74.*

| Year | 1870–'71. | | 1871–'72. | | 1872–'73. | | 1873–'74. | |
|---|---|---|---|---|---|---|---|---|
| Mean strength { Officers | 3 | | 3 | | 3 | | 3 | |
| { Enlisted men | 64 | | 45 | | 54 | | 54 | |
| Diseases. | Cases. | Deaths. | Cases. | Deaths. | Cases. | Deaths. | Cases. | Deaths. |
| GENERAL DISEASES, A. | | | | | | | | |
| Remittent fever | 1 | | 1 | | | | | |
| Intermittent fever | | | 1 | | 1 | | 2 | |
| Other diseases of this group | 1 | | 5 | | 3 | | 1 | |
| GENERAL DISEASES, B. | | | | | | | | |
| Rheumatism | 3 | | 2 | | 8 | | 6 | |
| Syphilis | 5 | | 2 | | | | | |
| Consumption | 1 | | | | | | | |
| Other diseases of this group | 1 | | | | 1 | | | |
| LOCAL DISEASES. | | | | | | | | |
| Catarrh and bronchitis | 6 | | 5 | | 24 | | 9 | |
| Pneumonia | | | | | 1 | 1 | | |
| Pleurisy | | | | | | | 1 | |
| Diarrhœa and dysentery | 13 | | 4 | | 12 | | 4 | |

*Consolidated sick-report, Camp Baker, Mont., 1870–'74—Continued.*

| Year | 1870–'71. | | 1871–'72. | | 1872–'73. | | 1873–'74. | |
|---|---|---|---|---|---|---|---|---|
| Mean strength   { Officers<br>{ Enlisted men | 3<br>64 | | 3<br>45 | | 3<br>54 | | 3<br>54 | |
| Diseases. | Cases. | Deaths. | Cases. | Deaths. | Cases. | Deaths. | Cases. | Deaths. |
| LOCAL DISEASES—Continued. | | | | | | | | |
| Hernia | | | | | 1 | | | |
| Gonorrhœa | | | 2 | | | | | |
| Other local diseases | 78 | | 35 | | 38 | | 35 | |
| Alcoholism | 4 | | 2 | | 5 | | 1 | |
| Unclassified | 2 | | | | | | | |
| Total disease | 115 | | 59 | | 94 | 1 | 59 | |
| VIOLENT DISEASES AND DEATHS. | | | | | | | | |
| Gunshot wounds | 1 | | | | | | 3 | |
| Other accidents and injuries | 25 | | 27 | | 25 | | 10 | |
| Total violence | 26 | | 27 | | 25 | | 13 | |

# FORT BENTON, MONTANA TERRITORY.

## REPORTED BY ASSISTANT SURGEONS A. B. CAMPBELL AND JOHN D. HALL, UNITED STATES ARMY.

Fort Benton is located on the left bank of the Missouri River, opposite the town of Benton, at the head of navigation, in latitude 47° 45′ north, and longitude 33° 33′ west, approximately. It is sixty-four miles east by north of Fort Shaw, and one hundred and fifty miles northeast of Helena.

The fort was originally built by the American Fur Company in 1846 as an Indian trading-post; was sold in 1864 to the Northwest Fur Company, and was first occupied by United States troops in November, 1869, to receive and forward the freight for Forts Shaw and Ellis. The reservation is one mile wide and three miles long. There are no springs or ponds in the vicinity. A small alkaline spring, eight miles distant, furnishes a camping-place for teams, and another spring, very brackish, twenty-eight miles distant on the same road, gives a point for a stage-station between Benton and Fort Shaw. The wells in town are mostly brackish and inferior to the river-water. One or two, however, furnish excellent water. The river furnishes an unfailing supply, comparatively free from alkali and impurities.

The plain in which the fort and town stand is one of the ordinary bottom-lands of the Missouri, formed by denudation and erosion. The extent of the erosive action of the river is seen in the surrounding bluffs, which rise some 200 feet to the general level of the surrounding prairie. The most common rocky formation in the vicinity is clay-shale, exposed in the bluffs as horizontal coal-black bands. A few miles farther up the river a friable sandstone begins to appear. The strata are uniformly level, and show no evidence of upheaval or disturbance. Extensive treeless prairies are the principal feature of this part of the Territory. There are none of the sage-bush deserts found farther south, but sufficient grass is found in most places to support cattle the year round. Trees and bushes are very scarce, and are only found along the streams. The garden-vegetables which require but a short season can be raised by the help of irrigation. It is believed that wheat and other cereals, except corn, might be produced here abundantly. Fruits, except a few kinds of berries, are entirely wanting. Cottonwood is the principal timber. A tall, hand-some species of fir grows abundantly in the mountains twenty miles south of Benton, and is valu-able for fuel and timber.

The principal animals of this vicinity are as follows: American bison or buffalo, which is common during the winter, but during the remainder of the year does not come so far south; white and black tailed deer, both common; antelope, very abundant; jack-hare and cotton-tail rabbit, both common; beaver, abundant; otter, scarce; black, cinnamon, and grizzly bears; elk and mountain-sheep; gophers and prairie-dogs. Wild swans, ducks, and geese are frequently seen; sage-chickens and curlews are common. Trout are plentiful in some of the creeks. The principal fish found in the Missouri are the pike, sucker, and sturgeon. The latter is much prized by those accustomed to its flavor. Mosquitoes swarm on the prairies, but, fortunately, do not enter the houses to any great extent.

The buildings of the post are constructed of adobes. The barrack is 88 by 20 feet, and 15 feet in height, well propped up inside and out to keep it from falling. It may be called a one and a half story building. The kitchen, mess-room, and offices are on the ground-floor. The dormitories on the second floor are 7½ feet in height, and are respectively 39 and 32 feet in length. The air-space is 245 feet per man. There is a roof-ventilator in good order in each room, but it is found impracticable to keep them properly ventilated in winter. The dormitories are warmed by wood-stoves, lighted by two small windows in each, and by candles. New single iron bunks were received, but were made into double bunks to economize space.

The married soldiers occupy a single building, 53 by 13 by 7 feet; constructed of single adobes laid lengthwise. It is divided into four equal rooms, a single room of only 1,205 cubic feet of air-space for each family.

A new house was built in 1873 for the family of the commanding officer. At latest accounts it was still unfinished, but had two good rooms and a kitchen ready for occupation. Two rooms and a kitchen have also been fitted up temporarily in one of the long buildings on the southwest side of the fort as quarters for the family of one married officer. The other officers occupy hired lodgings in the town.

The guard-house consists of two rooms: one for the guards, 15 by 21 by 21 feet, and one for the prisoners, 16 by 21 by 21 feet. Each room has one rather small window, which is placed very high and cannot be opened. The principal ventilation is by the door. There is but one stove for both rooms. The average occupancy is nine.

The post hospital is a two-story building, 35 by 25 feet, not specially fitted for hospital purposes. The ground-floor contains a ward, 20 by 19¾ by 7½ feet, and kitchen, 20 by 9 feet; the second floor contains the dispensary, 20 by 20 feet; steward's room, 11 by 11 feet, and linen-room, 11 by 9 feet. The ward is poorly lighted by one rather small window. Ventilation is assisted by a ventilating shaft 8 inches square. The room is considered capable of holding six beds, although there is not proper room for more than four. There is an earth-closet placed in the ward, and a good movable privy in rear of the hospital. There is no hospital garden or cow. Ice is collected and stored in the post ice-house. Fresh vegetables can be procured at reasonable prices.

Sudden changes of temperature are very common in winter. The mercury has been known to rise or fall 60° of Fahrenheit within two hours. The most prevalent wind is from the southwest, bringing warm intervals in winter. It often blows with scarcely a lull for twenty days, and brings with it the climate of the Pacific coast. It sometimes rises to a gale, moving fifty or sixty miles an hour.

Authority has been given for renting suitable buildings in the town of Benton, for the accommodation of the command, at a maximum cost of $235 per month.

*Meteorological report, Fort Benton, Mont., 1870–'74.*

| Month. | 1870–'71. | | | | 1871–'72. | | | | 1872–'73. | | | | 1873–'74. | | | |
|---|---|---|---|---|---|---|---|---|---|---|---|---|---|---|---|---|
| | Temperature. | | | Rain-fall in inches. | Temperature. | | | Rain-fall in inches. | Temperature. | | | Rain-fall in inches. | Temperature. | | | Rain-fall in inches. |
| | Mean. | Max. | Min. | | Mean. | Max. | Min. | | Mean. | Max. | Min. | | Mean. | Max. | Min. | |
| | ° | ° | ° | | ° | ° | ° | | ° | ° | ° | | ° | ° | ° | |
| July ................. | 77.60 | 105 | 56* | 0.80 | 72.59 | 98 | 49 | 0.93 | 67.08 | 98 | 40* | 7.56 | 71.69 | 100* | 46* | 1.29 |
| August ............... | 64.19 | 101 | 28* | 0.71 | 69.06 | 96 | 49 | 0.10 | 66.08 | 93 | 38* | 0.80 | 68.82 | 96* | 39* | 2.01 |
| September ........... | 62.20 | 89 | 30* | 0.32 | 63.84 | 92 | 44 | 0.46 | 56.28 | 90 | 29* | 1.82 | 53.75 | 90* | 9* | 0.56 |
| October ............. | 48.15 | 74 | 12* | 0.41 | 49.23 | 76 | 26 | 0.71 | 47.85 | 83 | 16* | 0.19 | 41.59 | 85* | — 4* | 0.19 |
| November ........... | 41.62 | 69 | 8* | 0.14 | 20.42 | 64 | —36 | 0.65 | 24.78 | 59 | —18* | 0.61 | 35.69 | 70* | —17* | 0.86 |
| December............. | 23.14 | 62 | —15* | 0.22 | 6.47 | 50 | —51 | 1.18 | 13.71 | 56 | —39* | 0.55 | 14.38 | 49* | —34* | 0.12 |
| January.............. | 21.51 | 60 | —22* | 0.50 | 19.96 | 47 | —38 | 0.35 | 18.56 | 54 | —29* | 0.60 | 12.12 | 52* | —29* | 0.67 |
| February ........... | 25.81 | 56 | —25* | 0.38 | 27.19 | 60 | —35* | 0.30 | 19.33 | 54 | —34* | 0.65 | 22.58 | 56 | —25* | 0.10 |
| March ............. | 38.35 | 65 | 11* | 0.48 | 36.25 | 62 | —13* | 0.83 | 35.72 | 65 | —22* | 0.22 | 19.81 | 53 | —23* | 0.64 |
| April ............... | 45.31 | 79 | 22* | 1.48 | 44.29 | 72 | 20* | 0.65 | 41.65 | 81* | 11* | 1.12 | 45.44 | 80 | 15* | 0.42 |
| May ................. | 62.18 | 91 | 40 | 1.58 | 55.89 | 84 | 27* | 0.60 | 53.28 | 80* | 27* | 3.03 | 61.49 | 89 | 35* | 2.98 |
| June ................. | 71.53 | 92 | 48 | 0.11 | 64.16 | 91 | 32* | 1.05 | 64.72 | 93* | 34* | 1.65 | 63.69 | 85 | 43* | 2.09 |
| For the year ...... | 48.47 | 105 | —25* | 7.13 | 44.11 | 98 | —51 | 7.81 | 42.42 | 98 | —39* | 18.80 | 42.59 | 100* | —34* | 11.93 |

\* These observations are made with self-registering thermometers. The mean is from the standard thermometer.

*Consolidated sick-report, Fort Benton, Mont., 1870–'74.*

| Diseases. | 1870–'71. | | 1871–'72. | | 1872–'73. | | 1873–'74. | |
|---|---|---|---|---|---|---|---|---|
| Year | | | | | | | | |
| Mean strength { Officers | 3 | | 3 | | 3 | | 4 | |
| { Enlisted men | 59 | | 44 | | 53 | | 55 | |
| | Cases. | Deaths. | Cases. | Deaths. | Cases. | Deaths. | Cases. | Deaths. |
| GENERAL DISEASES, A. | | | | | | | | |
| Typho-malarial fever | 5 | 2 | | | | | | |
| Intermittent fever | 8 | | 3 | | 1 | | | |
| Other diseases of this group | 2 | | | | 2 | | 1 | |
| GENERAL DISEASES, B. | | | | | | | | |
| Rheumatism | 3 | | 13 | | 19 | | 8 | |
| Syphilis | 2 | | 1 | | 1 | | 1 | |
| Consumption | 1 | | 1 | | 1 | | | |
| Other diseases of this group | 4 | | | | | | 1 | |
| LOCAL DISEASES. | | | | | | | | |
| Catarrh and bronchitis | 10 | | 11 | | 74 | | 35 | |
| Pneumonia | | | | | | | 1 | 1 |
| Pleurisy | 4 | | 1 | | | | 1 | |
| Diarrhœa and dysentery | 30 | | 8 | | 33 | | 23 | |
| Gonorrhœa | | | 2 | | 4 | | 1 | |
| Other local diseases | 13 | 1 | 30 | 1 | 64 | | 47 | |
| Alcoholism | 8 | | 7 | | 1 | | 9 | |
| Total disease | 90 | 3 | 77 | 1 | 200 | | 128 | 1 |
| VIOLENT DISEASES AND DEATHS. | | | | | | | | |
| Gunshot wounds | | | 1 | | | | | |
| Other accidents and injuries | 35 | | 39 | 1 | 39 | | 17 | |
| Total violence | 35 | | 40 | 1 | 39 | | 17 | |

# FORT BUFORD, DAKOTA TERRITORY.

REPORTS OF ASSISTANT SURGEONS J. P. KIMBALL AND J. V. D. MIDDLETON, UNITED STATES ARMY.

Fort Buford is situated on the left bank of the Missouri River, two miles below the mouth of the Yellowstone, in latitude 48° north, longitude 26° 57' west. The reservation is thirty miles square.

The Missouri River averages in this vicinity about one-half mile in width in its usual channel. It has a flood-plain which is from forty rods to several miles wide, and which is covered with water in the occasional great floods that occur once in several years. The structure of this plain, as observed in digging wells, consists, for the first eleven feet from the surface, of a porous clay; then, for about three feet, a fine gravel; next is white sand for fifteen feet, and black sand for two feet, below which is a stratum, about twenty-two or twenty-three feet in thickness, of a very tough, grayish-blue clay. As soon as this layer of clay is perforated, water in large quantity rises through the opening and affords an unfailing supply. The average depth of the three wells at the post is 52 feet. The surface of the ground in which they are located is 38 feet above the river at the ordinary stage of water.

The striking feature of this vicinity lies in the "*mauvaises terres*," or "bad lands," which consist of a succession of barren hills, or "buttes," averaging from two to three hundred feet in height. At this point these lands extend back from the plain for five or six miles, beyond which is a rolling prairie.

The only stratified rock that has been observed in the vicinity is a calcareous sandstone tertiary, free from fossils, which crops out abundantly among the clay hills. This stone is valuable for building-purposes, hardening by exposure to the weather. It contains too much carbonate of lime to be used in the construction of ovens, since it crumbles after long-continued exposure to heat.

The country around the post is not arable. The plain just described would produce crops if it could be irrigated.. The country is badly watered. Occasionally, along the river, strips of land are capable of producing corn and vegetables.

The cottonwood forms the bulk of the forests in this vicinity, and is the only wood available in any quantity for fuel or building-purposes. The low bottom-lands are mostly covered with it. The ash-leaved maple, red osiers, dogwood, and green ash are found in the same localities. A few stunted red cedars are found on the hills and in the ravines, along with the wild plum and the choke-cherry. The Missouri currant (*Ribesia aureum*) and smooth wild gooseberry (*Ribes hirtellum*) are also found in the ravines. The buffalo, or bull-berry, (*Shepherdia argentea*,) an edible, acid, red fruit, ripening late in the season, is plentiful in the bottoms. The Indians often subsist on it almost entirely for several weeks in the fall. The pomme blanche, or Indian turnip, (*Psoralea esculenta*,) is abundant in the sandy grounds.

Some of the more important animals are the American bison or buffalo, mountain-sheep, white and black tailed deer, elk, antelope, Canada lynx, wild-cat, American gray wolf, coyote, common red fox, swift fox, prairie-fox, silver-gray fox, Indian dog, grizzly bear, black bear, long-tailed ermine, mink, badger, common skunk, American otter, fisher, American sable, Canada porcupine, jack-hare, gray rabbit, beaver, gopher, and muskrat.

Fort Buford was established in June, 1866, as a one-company post. In the following year the command was increased to five companies, necessitating the erection of a new post, which was built on a rectangular plot of ground, 333 by 200 yards, surrounded by a stockade 12 feet in height. The buildings were, with few exceptions, hurriedly constructed of adobes, without regard to ventilation; and were altogether uncomfortable and inappropriate. In 1871 this stockade was removed, and two sets of officers' quarters, a hospital, guard-house, and storehouses erected outside of the original line of inclosure. In 1872 sixteen sets of officers' quarters were erected, and a number of additions and improvements made in the year following.

The barracks consist of seven adobe buildings with gravel roofs, erected in 1867. Each building is 120 by 21 by 10 feet from the floor to the eaves. The walls are 17 inches thick, but cracked and out of line, and have recently been boarded up on the outside to protect them from the weather. Each barrack is divided into a squad-room, 100 by 21 feet, office, 12 by 21 feet, and store-room, 8 by 21 feet. The floors are laid immediately upon the ground. The squad-room, or dormitory, is lighted by ten windows, and heated by three large wood-stoves. To each barrack there has recently been added a wooden building, containing a mess-room, 25 feet square, and kitchen, 25 by 15 feet. These rooms are lathed and plastered, have the floors raised 18 inches from the ground, are well ventilated and convenient. The old buildings are objectionable as quarters. The ventilation is imperfect, and it is impossible to keep them clean, owing to the constant crumbling of the adobe. There is no day-room for the men, and no bath or wash room. It is extremely difficult at this post for soldiers to keep themselves decently clean, as there are no facilities for bathing, or even for washing the face and hands properly during the winter season.

The married soldiers and laundresses in part occupy the old officers' quarters, while others are lodged in houses built of slabs with earth roofs, in Camptown, on the south side of the post.

The officers' quarters are constructed of wood, and, with the exception of those of the commanding officer, are built in pairs, a double set being under the same roof. The commanding officer's quarters contain in front two rooms, 15 feet square, separated by a hall 5 feet wide, having in rear three smaller rooms and a closet, 7 by 5 feet. There are in addition two rear projections, the one containing dining-room, kitchen, and pantry, and the other a bed-room, 15 by 16 feet, and a servant's room.

The two sets of officers' quarters built in 1871 are one story high with attic. Each contains a hall, 7 feet wide, running the whole length of building, with stairway; a parlor 15 by 16 feet, sitting-room, 15 by 14 feet, connected by folding doors; dining-room, 11 by 15 feet, with closet 3½ by 5 feet, and kitchen in back building. The attic contains two bed-rooms. The sixteen sets of quarters erected in 1872 are one story high without attics. Each contains a hall, 7 by 9½ feet; parlor, 15 feet square; sitting-room, back of parlor, and connected by a small door, 12 by 15 feet; bed-room back of hall, 10 by 15 feet, with closet 7 by 5 feet; dining-room, 12 by 15 feet, with pantry and kitchen, both in back building. The bed-room has no window, and is nearly useless as

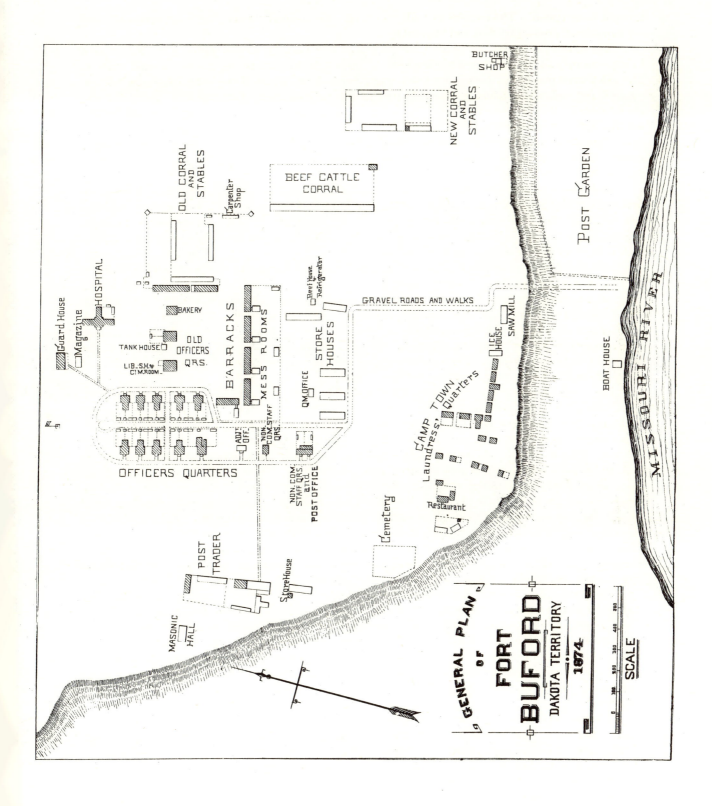

GENERAL PLAN OF FORT BUFORD DAKOTA TERRITORY 1874

SCALE

BUTCHER SHOP

NEW CORRAL AND STABLES

POST GARDEN

MISSOURI RIVER

OLD CORRAL AND STABLES

BEEF CATTLE CORRAL

Carpenter Shop

Beef House & Refrigerator

GRAVEL ROADS AND WALKS

SAW MILL

HOSPITAL

Guard House

Magazine

BAKERY

TANK HOUSE

OLD OFFICERS QRS.

LIB.-S.H.& C.M.ROOM

BARRACKS

MESS ROOMS

STORE HOUSES

QM.OFFICE

ICE HOUSE

CAMP TOWN

Laundress, Quarters

BOAT HOUSE

ADJ.T OFF.

NON.COM.STAFF QRS.

OFFICERS QUARTERS

NON.COM. STAFF QRS. and POST OFFICE

Cemetery

Restaurant

POST TRADER

StoreHouse

MASONIC HALL

a separate room. These quarters are inconvenient in having no passage from the front door to the dining-room and kitchen, and incomplete in having no servant's room. They are hard-finished throughout, the wood-work well painted, and the windows have inside blinds. Twelve of the sets have good cellars.

The quartermaster's and subsistence storehouses consist of six wooden buildings, averaging 124 by 25 feet. There are four of the former and two of the latter, well lighted and ventilated, and kept in good order. Under each commissary storehouse is a cellar for the storage of vegetables, &c. A good supply is kept on hand for issue and for sale to officers. In the fall of 1873 a supply of potatoes was received sufficient to last until the opening of navigation in the spring. In favorable years the post garden affords a valuable accession to the supply of fresh vegetables.

The guard-house is a frame building one story high, erected in 1871, containing a guard-room, 20 by 22 feet; officer's room, 20 by 9 feet; one prison-room, 15 by 35½ feet; and another, 14 by 13 feet; three cells, each 9 by 6½ feet; wash-room, 8½ by 7 feet; and a hall. The height throughout is 11½ feet. There is also a portico for mounting the guard in winter. The ventilation is excellent, the fresh air being brought in by an air-box opening under the stove, and the foul air escaping through registers in the ceiling.

The post hospital is a modification of the plan given in Circular No. 2, Surgeon-General's Office, 1871, for a hospital of twenty-four beds. It is a frame building without veranda, raised 18 inches from the ground upon stone piers. The administration building is two stories high, with the addition of a back building, also two stories high, and contains a hall 7 feet wide, running front to rear, (with stairway,) and intersecting another and similar hall; office and dispensary, each 14 by 15 feet; reading-room, 14 by 17 feet; closet; store-room, 14 by 15 feet, with closet for liquors. The second story contains four rooms, each 14 by 15 feet; a closet, 5 by 6½ feet, and a hall. The back building contains on the lower floor a kitchen, 12 by 16 feet; mess-room, 15 by 16 feet; pantry and hall. On the second floor are the linen-room, 12 by 16 feet; isolation ward of the same dimensions; and a store-room 9 feet square. The wards, arranged as wings, are each 44 by 24 by 12½ feet. Two rooms, 11 by 9 feet, separated by a hall 5 feet wide, are partitioned off from that end of the wing nearest the central building. One is for the attendant and storage of the patients' clothing; the other for bath-room and earth-closet. The ventilation of the wards is imperfect; there are no boxed openings for use in summer, and no ventilating-shafts for winter. Fresh air is brought into the ward by boxes placed under the floor and opening in front of the stoves, the vitiated air escaping by registers in the chimney. Each ward is heated by two large wood-stoves. One of the bath-rooms is furnished with a stove, so as to render it available in winter.

It is difficult to obtain a sufficient amount of water for the hospital. The post is supplied from the river by a water-wagon, and the quantity is necessarily limited. The limited fall of rain would not justify the construction of cisterns for its preservation, but reservoirs of sufficient capacity could be filled with river-water, which would be of great value, especially in case of fire.

The post bakery is a frame building of sufficient capacity to contain two large ovens and all the necessary appurtenances. The bread is sufficient in quantity and excellent in quality.

The post library and court-martial room are in one of the old officers' quarters, conveniently situated. The library contains 366 volumes, principally light reading.

Mail communication is very irregular. During the winter the post is completely isolated. There is no public conveyance, and travel is attended by great danger on account of the excessive cold. The mail is carried between Fargo, on the Northern Pacific Railroad, and this post, via Bismarck and Fort Stevenson, at the expense of the quartermaster's department. It arrives twice a month, except during the most severe part of winter, when the interval will frequently be protracted to a month. The average time required for a letter to go to department headquarters is twenty days.

51 M P

*Meteorological report, Fort Buford, Dak., 1870–'74.*

| Month. | 1870–'71. Temperature. Mean. | Max. | Min. | Rain-fall in inches. | 1871–'72. Temperature. Mean. | Max. | Min. | Rain-fall in inches. | 1872–'73. Temperature. Mean. | Max. | Min. | Rain-fall in inches. | 1873–'74. Temperature. Mean. | Max. | Min. | Rain-fall in inches. |
|---|---|---|---|---|---|---|---|---|---|---|---|---|---|---|---|---|
| July .................. | 73.36 | 99* | 45* | 0.76 | 73.38 | 102* | 40* | 0.55 | 70.20 | 104* | 37* | 2.44 | 67.17 | 100* | 47* | 1.25 |
| August .............. | 61.52 | 97* | 31* | 0.81 | 66.56 | 100* | 34* | 0.10 | 68.51 | 101* | 29* | 1.45 | 66.60 | 102 | 35* | 1.40 |
| September ........... | 60.28 | 90* | (8)?* | 0.45 | 57.03 | 84* | 31* | 0.00 | 53.39 | 97* | 21* | 3.25 | 45.82 | 84 | 16* | 1.10 |
| October ............. | 39.27 | 88* | 11* | 1.25 | 42.15 | 75* | 9* | 0.72 | 41.72 | 85* | 11* | 0.80 | 36.54 | 80* | 5* | 0.45 |
| November............ | 33.39 | 59* | 16* | 0.03 | 14.00 | 53* | −33* | 1.00 | 16.82 | 48* | −28* | 1.04 | 28.21 | 60 | − 2* | 0.69 |
| December ............ | 9.64 | 44 | −25 | 0.25 | 2.38 | 47* | −35* | 1.40 | 1.71 | 48* | −35* | 1.57 | 5.62 | 43* | −27* | 0.01 |
| January ............. | 6.32 | 40 | −35 | 0.21 | 7.47 | 41* | −36* | 1.35 | 2.15 | 45* | −36* | 0.98 | 2.64 | 38* | −28* | 0.15 |
| February ............ | 10.24 | 40* | −31* | 0.19 | 14.90 | 47* | −28* | 0.00 | 6.73 | 40* | −28* | 4.35 | 7.24 | 35 | −25* | 0.20 |
| March................ | 26.62 | 69* | 5* | 0.24 | 22.37 | 46* | −13* | 1.48 | 25.13 | 53* | − 8* | 2.25 | 16.50 | 50 | −22* | 0.25 |
| April ............... | 39.39 | 70* | 18* | 0.45 | 38.06 | 72* | 18* | 1.55 | 37.29 | 69* | 5* | 1.25 | 38.45 | 82 | 7* | 0.19 |
| May ................. | 62.79 | 99* | 31* | 2.43 | 50.93 | 90* | 28* | 1.12 | 48.34 | 74* | 15* | 6.60 | 58.90 | 90 | 25* | 1.80 |
| June ................. | 68.01 | 95* | 40* | 0.90 | 66.33 | 95* | 32* | 1.75 | 65.82 | 91* | 4* | 2.69 | 66.73 | 101 | 40* | 1.02 |
| For the year....... | 40.90 | 99* | −35 | 7.97 | 37.96 | 102* | −36* | 11.02 | 36.48 | 104* | −36* | 28.67 | 36.70 | 102 | −28* | 8.51 |

* These observations are made with self-registering thermometers. The mean is from the standard thermometer.

*Consolidated sick-report, Fort Buford, Dak., 1870–'74.*

| Year .......................................................... | 1870–'71. | | 1871–'72. | | 1872–'73. | | 1873–'74. | |
|---|---|---|---|---|---|---|---|---|
| Mean strength ........... { Officers ............ | 10 | | 9 | | 16 | | 14 | |
| { Enlisted men ...... | 204 | | 178 | | 356 | | 331 | |
| Diseases. | Cases. | Deaths. | Cases. | Deaths. | Cases. | Deaths. | Cases. | Deaths. |
| GENERAL DISEASES, A. | | | | | | | | |
| Typhoid fever........ | 1 | 1 | ...... | ...... | ...... | ...... | 3 | ...... |
| Remittent fever...... | 8 | ...... | 6 | ...... | 3 | ...... | 3 | ...... |
| Intermittent fever ... | | | 9 | ...... | 30 | ...... | 7 | ...... |
| Other diseases of this group........ | 7 | | 1 | ...... | 7 | ...... | 8 | ...... |
| GENERAL DISEASES, B. | | | | | | | | |
| Rheumatism ......... | 27 | | 19 | ...... | 57 | ...... | 100 | ...... |
| Syphilis ............. | 18 | | 12 | ...... | 10 | ...... | 31 | ...... |
| Consumption ......... | | | | ...... | 2 | ...... | | 1 |
| Other diseases of this group........ | 1 | | ...... | ...... | ...... | ...... | ...... | ...... |
| LOCAL DISEASES. | | | | | | | | |
| Catarrh and bronchitis ......... | 68 | | 27 | ...... | 33 | ...... | 28 | ...... |
| Pneumonia.......... | 1 | | 1 | 1 | 1 | ...... | ...... | ...... |
| Pleurisy............ | 3 | | 1 | ...... | 2 | ...... | 1 | ...... |
| Diarrhœa and dysentery ......... | 98 | | 14 | ...... | 29 | ...... | 23 | ...... |
| Hernia ............. | 1 | | 1 | ...... | | | 2 | ...... |
| Gonorrhœa ......... | 2 | | 1 | ...... | 4 | ...... | 3 | ...... |
| Other local diseases........ | 118 | | 77 | 1 | 82 | ...... | 93 | 1 |
| Alcoholism ......... | 3 | | 3 | ...... | 1 | ...... | | |
| Total disease........ | 356 | 1 | 172 | 2 | 261 | ...... | 302 | 2 |
| VIOLENT DISEASES AND DEATHS. | | | | | | | | |
| Gunshot wounds ...... | 5 | ...... | 5 | 1 | 2 | ...... | 1 | ...... |
| Other accidents and injuries........ | 77 | ...... | 51 | ...... | 63 | 1 | 71 | ...... |
| Total violence ........ | 82 | ...... | 56 | 1 | 65 | 1 | 72 | ...... |

# CHEYENNE AGENCY, DAKOTA TERRITORY.

## REPORT OF ACTING ASSISTANT SURGEON G. M. PEASE, UNITED STATES ARMY.

Cheyenne agency is on the west bank of the Missouri River; latitude, 44° 42′ north; longitude, 27° 37′ west, (approximate.)

It is seven miles by land above Fort Sully. Yankton, the present terminus of the Dakota Southern Railroad, is two hundred and thirty-seven miles distant by land and three hundred and fifteen by river below the post. It was established May 17, 1870.

The quarters for enlisted men consist of two buildings, each 115 by 18 feet, 8½ feet in height.

They, as all other buildings at the post, are built of cotton-wood slabs, and roofed with boards of the same timber covered with earth. The interstices in the walls are closed outside by a mixture of lime and mud, and inside by thin battens. Fifteen feet in length is partitioned off for a company office, leaving the dormitories each 100 by 18 feet. Each barrack has five windows, all in the front wall; each window containing twelve panes of 8 by 10 glass; there are also three doors, two in front and one in rear. Each building is warmed by three wood-stoves. There are two ventilators, each 1 by 2 feet, in the roof of each dormitory. Twenty feet in rear of each barrack is a building 78 by 14½ feet, 8½ feet in height, of the same construction as the barrack, divided into a kitchen, 20 feet; a mess-room, 32 feet; a wash-room, 11 feet; and a store-room, 15 feet in length, respectively. The wash-room has two, the kitchen two, and the mess-room three windows. The sinks are 60 feet in rear of the kitchens. These buildings are on opposite sides of the parade-ground, one set facing the north side, the other the south side.

Quarters for married soldiers consist of three small huts, each of one room, containing but 1,368 cubic feet of space, the only opening in which, besides the door, is a window about 2 feet square. They are cramped, unventilated, and unhealthy.

The officers' quarters occupy the west side of the parade-ground, and consist of one building 48 by 28 feet, 9 feet in height, containing five rooms, and having in its rear kitchen and servant's room additional; two buildings, each 40 by 15 feet, 8½ feet in height, containing two rooms and hall, and having in the rear kitchen and servant's room; and one building 70 by 15 feet, 8½ feet in height, containing four rooms and two halls, with two kitchens and two servants' rooms in the rear. The last building was designed for two officers, but is occupied by four. One building similar to this is to be erected. The roofs of these buildings are covered wtih tarred paper and earth, and their walls lined with heavy paper and whitewashed. The rooms are warmed by wood-stoves, and most of them are well lighted.

The guard-house is a temporary structure 30 by 14 feet, with no ventilation, warmed by one wood-stove, and imperfectly lighted through three small windows. Average occupancy, 14.

The hospital consists of one building 30 by 15 feet, 9 feet in height, to which is attached at the rear, in the form of an L, a building 26 by 12 feet, 8 feet in height. The main portion is in one room, being the sick-ward, which is provided with two windows on one side, one window at each end, and two doors on the other side, one of which opens into the wing. This wing is divided into a wash-room 10 by 12 feet, adjoining the ward, and a kitchen 16 by 12 feet. The wash-room has one window, the kitchen two.

There are also belonging to the hospital two other buildings or huts, each 39 by 14 feet, 8 feet in height, one divided into three rooms; steward's room, dispensary, and store-room; the other contains the old ward, 27 by 14 feet, and the old kitchen, 12 by 14 feet.

The stable is on the opposite side of the river.

Fuel consists of cottonwood, furnished by contract.

*Consolidated sick-report, Cheyenne Agency, Dak., 1870–'74.*

| Year | | 1870–'71. | | 1871–'72. | | 1872–'73. | | 1873–'74. | |
|---|---|---|---|---|---|---|---|---|---|
| Mean strength | Officers | 5 | | 5 | | 5 | | 5 | |
| | Enlisted men | 137 | | 90 | | 99 | | 105 | |
| Diseases. | | Cases. | Deaths. | Cases. | Deaths. | Cases. | Deaths. | Cases. | Deaths. |
| GENERAL DISEASES, A. | | | | | | | | | |
| Remittent fever | | 1 | | | | 1 | | 11 | |
| Intermittent fever | | 11 | | 5 | | 16 | | 3 | |
| Other diseases of this group | | | | 2 | | | | | |
| GENERAL DISEASES, B. | | | | | | | | | |
| Rheumatism | | 17 | | 6 | | 19 | | 20 | |
| Syphilis | | 9 | | 9 | | 5 | | 2 | |
| Consumption | | 2 | | 1 | 1 | 2 | | 2 | |
| Other diseases of this group | | 1 | | 2 | | 1 | | | |

*Consolidated sick-report, Cheyenne Agency, Dak., 1870–'74—Continued.*

| Year | | 1870–'71. | | 1871–'72. | | 1872–'73. | | 1873–'74. | |
|---|---|---|---|---|---|---|---|---|---|
| Mean strength {Officers | | 5 | | 5 | | 5 | | 5 | |
| {Enlisted men | | 137 | | 90 | | 99 | | 105 | |
| Diseases. | | Cases. | Deaths. | Cases. | Deaths. | Cases. | Deaths. | Cases. | Deaths. |
| LOCAL DISEASES. | | | | | | | | | |
| Catarrh and bronchitis | | 43 | ...... | 61 | ...... | 54 | ...... | 54 | ...... |
| Pneumonia | | ...... | ...... | ...... | ...... | 1 | ...... | ...... | ...... |
| Pleurisy | | ...... | ...... | 1 | ...... | ...... | ...... | ...... | ...... |
| Diarrhœa and dysentery | | 77 | ...... | 19 | ...... | 59 | ...... | 28 | ...... |
| Hernia | | ...... | ...... | 1 | ...... | 4 | ...... | 1 | ...... |
| Gonorrhœa | | 4 | ...... | 2 | ...... | 2 | ...... | ...... | ...... |
| Other local diseases | | 80 | 2 | 43 | ...... | 71 | ...... | 66 | ...... |
| Alcoholism | | ...... | ...... | 2 | ...... | 1 | ...... | 5 | ...... |
| Total disease | | 245 | 2 | 154 | 1 | 236 | ...... | 192 | ...... |
| VIOLENT DISEASES AND DEATHS. | | | | | | | | | |
| Gunshot wounds | | 2 | ...... | ...... | ...... | 4 | ...... | ...... | ...... |
| Drowning | | ...... | ...... | ...... | ...... | ...... | ...... | ...... | 1 |
| Other accidents and injuries | | 61 | ...... | 38 | ...... | 57 | 1 | 35 | ...... |
| Suicide | | ...... | 1 | ...... | ...... | ...... | ...... | ...... | ...... |
| Total violence | | 63 | 1 | 38 | ...... | 61 | 1 | 35 | 1 |

# FORT ELLIS, MONTANA TERRITORY.

### REPORT OF ASSISTANT SURGEON J. H. KINSMAN, UNITED STATES ARMY.

Fort Ellis is in the southwest part of Montana, at the northeast end of Gallatin Valley, on the East Gallatin River, which, thirty miles to the northwest, joins with the Madison and Jefferson to form the Missouri River. Latitude, 45° 45′ north; longitude, 33° 53′ west; altitude above the sea, 5,800 feet.

This post was established August 27, 1867. The post is on the north side of an elevated prairie, which has high mountains on the north, east, and south, while to the northwest extends the Gallatin Valley. Nearly on the summit of one of these mountains, twelve miles to the south, is Mystic Lake, celebrated for its trout and its flies. About five miles to the east is Bozeman Pass; Bridger Pass is seven miles north of east, and Flathead Pass thirty miles to the north. Virginia City is seventy-three miles distant, in a southwest direction. Gallatin City is thirty-three miles northwest of the post. The post was established for the protection of settlers and miners against the raids of Indians through these mountain avenues, and Flathead Pass, being the most convenient for their incursions, is occupied by a company from the post during the time that the snow is off the ground.

The climate at the post is dry, but snow-storms and severe frosts are not infrequent, even in summer. The ground upon which the post stands, owing to its greater elevation, and being somewhat sheltered from the sun's rays by the adjacent mountains, is colder than the neighboring valley.

Cultivation is confined to the river-bottoms, as the small amount of rain renders irrigation necessary. The soil is very fertile, and large crops of wheat, rye, oats, and barley are raised, and all the more hardy vegetables, such as potatoes, turnips, beets, carrots, &c. The potatoes particularly are of excellent quality, exceedingly farinaceous, and very large.

The river-bottoms are covered with groves of cottonwood and aspen, and thickets of willow. The passes to the Yellowstone River and the country to the south of it open into the valley a few miles from the fort. The neighboring mountains are very broken and precipitous, with huge cliffs of sandstone and limestone, clothed to their summits with vast forests of white pine, red fir, and cedar, and contain immense beds of bituminous coal of good quality. Gold is found in the immediate vicinity of the post, and at Emigrant Gulch, about thirty miles distant, gold-mining is carried on extensively.  Some very rich claims have lately been discovered at this place.  The gold from this locality is much esteemed for the facility with which it can be worked in the manufacture of jewelry.

The rivers and mountain-streams are well stocked with trout and grayling; and elk, black-tailed deer, antelope, mountain-sheep, grizzly and black bear, wolf, mink, ermine, beaver, badgers, and gophers are numerous.

The ground upon which the fort is built slopes gently from the south to the river.  The soil is argillaceous, with a subsoil of gravel.  The buildings of the post are of unhewn pine logs, the interstices are plastered with mortar, and the floors are of pine.  The buildings inclose the parade, 264 by 208 feet.  The plan of the post is shown in Figure 58.

A, headquarters building; B, E, K, barracks; C, old hospital; D, carpenter-shop and bakery; F H, commissary storehouses; I, officers' quarters; J, quartermaster's storehouse; L, post library; M, parade-ground; O, bastion; P, guard-house.

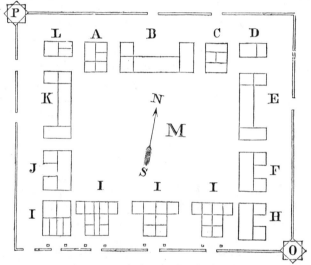

Figure 58.—Scale 151⅓ feet to 1 inch.

There are three sets of company quarters; one for infantry is, 23 by 22 feet, 10 feet high on the sides, and 13 feet in the center, with two wings at the rear, 22 feet long by 20 feet wide.

The cavalry quarters are of same dimensions, with two wings at the rear on each end, 55 by 20 feet, and a center wing, 57 by 40 feet, in one set, and 75 by 40 feet in the other.  These quarters contain mess-rooms, dormitories, kitchens, and other necessary rooms.  Small windows are on the sides; stoves are used for warming; there are no special means of ventilation, the combination of chinks between the logs and high winds affording generally more than the requisite amount of air for comfort during nine or ten months of the year.  The mess-rooms and kitchens are provided with large cellars.  The dormitories are not plastered; they contain the prescribed iron bedsteads, and are occupied, each by one company.  The allotment of air-space to each man is about 600 cubic feet.  The sinks are a short distance from the rear of the barracks.  The laundresses' quarters, seventeen sets, are situated about 300 yards to the north of the post.  They consist of a number of small shanties, but are comfortable quarters.

There are five buildings used for officers' quarters, each of which contains two sets.  These originally consisted of four rooms to each set in three of the buildings, and three to each set in the other.  The old hospital is now used for quarters, and contains three rooms.  All of the buildings have, however, had additions and repairs made to such an extent that some of them have five and some seven rooms.  In most of the quarters two or three rooms are ceiled, the rest being of logs.  The roofs are shingled, of good pitch, and all the quarters are warm and comfortable, considering the material and manner in which they are built.  Some of them have fire-places, some stoves.

The building containing the headquarters offices is 42 feet long and 30 feet wide.  It contains the post commander's, adjutant's, quartermaster's, and commissary's offices, and the sergeant-major's quarters.

The commissary and quartermaster's storehouses are each 62 feet long and 22 feet wide; the former have two wings at the rear 22 by 20 feet; the latter also has two wings, 57 by 20 feet, in one of which is the quartermaster's offices.  Two new frame storehouses, each 120 by 25 feet by 10 feet, have been erected.

About half a mile distant from the post is the saw-mill, newly erected, and which is run by a Leffel turbine-wheel, the water being brought by a ditch from a cañon five miles distant.

The grain-houses belonging to the post are two in number, each about 200 by 25 feet; they are built of lumber, weather-boarded, and will contain together about 2,000,000 pounds of grain.

There are three ice-houses, built of logs, wherein is stored a sufficient quantity of ice for the use of the command.

The guard-house at the fort is in one of the bastions; the lower story used as a guard-room, the upper story as quarters for the prisoners; it is 20 feet square; ceiling, 10 feet high; lighted by two small windows and several small embrasures, warmed by a stove, and furnished with a ventilator in the ceiling; air-space per man, 400 feet. The other bastion is used as a magazine.

The hospital is located five hundred and forty feet southeast of the post. It is a balloon-frame building, weather-boarded on the outside and plastered on the inside, and was first occupied in January, 1871. It consists of a main portion and attic, with a one-story ward attached as a wing. The original plan shows a veranda, 8 feet wide, around the whole building, and a dead-house, 12 by 12 feet, attached to the south side of the building and communicating with the hall, which have not been put up. For general arrangement see Figure 59.

1, first floor; 2, second floor. A, dimensions, 15 by 16 feet; B, dining-room, 15 by 16 feet; C, steward's room, 15 by 16 feet; D, dispensary, 15 by 16 feet; E, dimensions, 15 by 16 feet; F, kitchen, 15 by 16 feet; G, hall, 6 by 36 feet; H, ward, 24 by 40 feet by 12 feet high; I, bath-room, 9 by 6 feet; J, attendant's room, 9 by 6 feet. Second story, K, dimensions, 12 by 15 feet; L, steward's room, 12 by 15 feet; M, store-room, 12 by 14 feet; N, medical supplies, 12 by 14 feet; O, dimensions, 12 by 13 feet; P, store-room, 12 by 24 feet; Q R S, closets; T, hall and stairs.

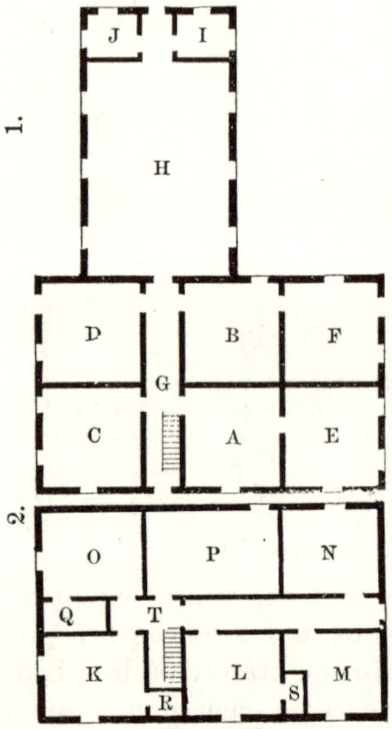

Figure 59.

The rooms on the first floor, excepting the ward, are 9 feet high; those in the second story are each 8 feet high.

On account of the scarcity of quarters, two of the rooms on the ground floor of the main building and two in the attic, namely, A, E, K, and O, are occupied by acting assistant surgeons. The ward was intended for twelve beds, allowing 860 cubic feet air-space to each. It is well lighted by eight windows, placed in opposite sides, and two at the free end, the latter looking out from the bath and clothes rooms. Earth-closets are used in the ward; water-barrels are kept outside the building, filled every morning from the post water-wagon. Means of subduing fires are half a dozen buckets, which in winter are worthless owing to the hard frosts. The privy is about twenty feet from the hospital. There is no dead-house. South of the hospital, two hundred and thirty-three feet, is a frame building, sheathed without and plastered within, containing two sets of quarters, each of three rooms, 15 by 15 feet, with unfinished attic; one of these sets is occupied by the post surgeon. East of this, seventy feet, is another of the same character, partly finished.

Southeast of this three hundred and fifteen feet is the new commissary storehouse, and eighty-five feet south of this the new quartermaster storehouse before referred to. These are framed, sheathed, and measure 120 by 25 by 10 feet. The last four buildings mentioned are the commencement of a new post which was to be erected, but whose construction was stopped by General Order No. 57, War Department, March 28, 1873.

The post bakery was completed in 1871, and is ample for the command.

At a distance of one hundred yards southwest of the post are the cavalry stables, consisting of four log buildings, each 30 feet, with board roofs, and the infantry stables, built in like manner, 90 by 33 feet. They are well lighted and ventilated.

The post library contains about three hundred volumes. Besides this, one of the companies of infantry has a reading-room, belonging to a club, whose library contains about eighty volumes, and who subscribe to eighteen or twenty papers and periodicals. One of the cavalry companies also have a club, who subscribe to many periodicals and papers.

The East Gallatin River, about two hundred yards from and above the post, supplies the command with water, which is brought to the post in tanks. The quality of the water is excellent, and the quantity sufficient for the necessities of the garrison.

The natural drainage of the post is good, the ground sloping to the river.

There are no arrangements for bathing in winter; in summer the men frequently bathe in the river.

The farmers in the vicinity bring in a plentiful supply of potatoes and other vegetables. Game, such as deer, elk, mountain-sheep, and antelopes, is procured by hunters, and sells at ten cents per pound.

Stage connection is had every two days, via Bozeman, with Virginia and with Helena, one hundred and one miles northwest, and the small towns between Bozeman. The nearest settlement is three miles west of the post. Mail arrives and departs daily. A letter requires about fourteen days, depending on the season of the year, to reach department headquarters or Washington.

The Crows occupy the country south of the Yellowstone. They number about three hundred and sixty lodges, including both "River" and "Mountain" Crows. Indians do not often appear about the post. Small parties of Crows visit it occasionally, and the Bannacks, in going to and returning from the Judith, where they hunt buffalo in company with the Crows, generally loiter for a few days about the post and town of Bozeman.

*Meteorological report, Fort Ellis, Mont., 1870–'74.*

| Month. | 1870–'71. Temperature. Mean. | Max. | Min. | Rain-fall in inches. | 1871–'72. Temperature. Mean. | Max. | Min. | Rain-fall in inches. | 1872–'73. Temperature. Mean. | Max. | Min. | Rain-fall in inches. | 1873–'74. Temperature. Mean. | Max. | Min. | Rain-fall in inches. |
|---|---|---|---|---|---|---|---|---|---|---|---|---|---|---|---|---|
| July | 69. 44 | 93 | 52 | ........ | 66. 68 | 95 | 49 | ........ | 60. 36 | 87 | 30* | ........ | 70. 41 | 91* | 34* | ........ |
| August | 59. 42 | 90 | 33 | ........ | 61. 26 | 83 | 35 | ........ | (‡) | (‡) | (‡) | ........ | 65. 84 | 93* | 28* | 1. 21 |
| September | 56. 06 | 86 | 32 | ........ | 56. 89 | 82 | 35 | ........ | (‡) | (‡) | (‡) | ........ | 49. 51 | 83* | 18* | 0. 58 |
| October | 42. 70 | 74 | 9 | ........ | 44. 30 | 68 | 8 | ........ | 44. 09 | 72 | 22 | ........ | 36. 55 | 75* | — 3* | 0. 93 |
| November | 37. 00 | 60 | 10 | ........ | 24. 86 | 55 | —19 | ........ | 25. 40 | 62 | —15 | ........ | 32. 42 | 68* | 2* | 0. 51 |
| December | 29. 79 | 55 | —13 | ........ | 12. 56 | 45 | —45 | ........ | 18. 81 | 59 | —19 | ........ | 11. 99 | 41* | —20* | 0. 86 |
| January | 30. 73 | 60 | —10 | ........ | 18. 23 | 45 | —53 | ........ | 23. 28 | 50 | —40 | ........ | 22. 06 | 46* | —10* | 0. 37 |
| February | 23. 45 | 48 | —22 | ........ | 17. 18 | 54 | —53 | ........ | 15. 91 | 42* | —16* | ........ | 19. 52 | 46* | —19* | 0. 78 |
| March | (†) | (†) | (†) | ........ | 26. 86 | 55 | —10* | ........ | 38. 12 | 62 | 12 | ........ | 24. 56 | 55* | — 3* | 1. 53 |
| April | 40. 46 | 70 | 15 | ........ | 34. 75 | 63 | 10* | ........ | 36. 32 | 72 | 19 | ........ | 39. 71 | 78* | 13* | 0. 54 |
| May | 46. 86 | 85 | 31 | ........ | 48. 38 | 72 | 25* | ........ | 47. 33 | 73 | 31 | ........ | 33. 47 | 82* | 27* | 6. 16 |
| June | 62. 91 | 95 | 37 | ........ | 57. 99 | 80 | 30* | ........ | (§) | (§) | (§) | ........ | 56. 79 | 86* | 28* | 2. 58 |
| For the year | ........ | ..... | ..... | ........ | 39. 16 | 95 | —53 | ........ | ........ | ..... | ..... | ........ | 41. 07 | 93* | —20* | ........ |

* These observations are made with self-registering thermometers. The mean is from the standard thermometer.
† Imperfect.  ‡ No observations taken.  § Incomplete.
NOTE.—Observations for amount of rain-fall were not taken until August, 1873.

*Consolidated sick-report, Fort Ellis, Mont., 1870–'74.*

| Year | 1870–'71. Cases. | Deaths. | 1871–'72. Cases. | Deaths. | 1872–'73. Cases. | Deaths. | 1873–'74. Cases. | Deaths. |
|---|---|---|---|---|---|---|---|---|
| Mean strength { Officers | 11 | | 14 | | 13 | | 13 | |
| { Enlisted men | 279 | | 269 | | 222 | | 273 | |
| **Diseases.** | | | | | | | | |
| GENERAL DISEASES, A. | | | | | | | | |
| Typhoid fever | | | | | | | 1 | ...... |
| Typho-malarial fever | 2 | ...... | 3 | ...... | ..... | ...... | ..... | ...... |
| Remittent fever | | | | | | | 1 | ...... |
| Intermittent fever | 13 | ...... | 19 | ...... | 9 | ...... | 6 | ...... |
| Other diseases of this group | 25 | ...... | 15 | ...... | 26 | ...... | 20 | ...... |
| GENERAL DISEASES, B. | | | | | | | | |
| Rheumatism | 20 | ...... | 10 | ...... | 14 | ...... | 27 | ...... |
| Syphilis | 10 | ...... | 7 | ...... | 11 | ...... | 11 | ...... |
| Consumption | | 1 | | | 1 | | | |
| Other diseases of this group | | | | | 4 | ...... | 2 | ...... |

*Consolidated sick-report, Fort Ellis, Mont., 1870–'74—Continued.*

| Year | | 1870–'71. | | 1871–'72. | | 1873–'73. | | 1873–'74. | |
|---|---|---|---|---|---|---|---|---|---|
| Mean strength { Officers | | 11 | | 14 | | 13 | | 13 | |
| { Enlisted men | | 279 | | 269 | | 222 | | 273 | |
| Diseases. | | Cases. | Deaths. | Cases. | Deaths. | Cases. | Deaths. | Cases. | Deaths. |
| LOCAL DISEASES. | | | | | | | | | |
| Catarrh and bronchitis | | 20 | ...... | 18 | ...... | 42 | ...... | 21 | ...... |
| Pneumonia | | 2 | ...... | ...... | ...... | ...... | ...... | ...... | ...... |
| Pleurisy | | 1 | ...... | 2 | ...... | ...... | ...... | ...... | ...... |
| Diarrhœa and dysentery | | 14 | ...... | 12 | ...... | 14 | ...... | 31 | ...... |
| Hernia | | ...... | ...... | ...... | ...... | 1 | ...... | 1 | ...... |
| Gonorrhœa | | 6 | ...... | 12 | ...... | 3 | ...... | 7 | ...... |
| Other local diseases | | 76 | ...... | 82 | 2 | 65 | ...... | 95 | 2 |
| Alcoholism | | 5 | ...... | 3 | ...... | 2 | ...... | 11 | ...... |
| Total disease | | 194 | 1 | 183 | 2 | 192 | ...... | 234 | 2 |
| VIOLENT DISEASES AND DEATHS. | | | | | | | | | |
| Gunshot wounds | | 4 | ...... | 3 | ...... | 2 | ...... | 4 | 1 |
| Other accidents and injuries | | 85 | ...... | 147 | ...... | 72 | ...... | 108 | ...... |
| Total violence | | 89 | ...... | 150 | ...... | 74 | ...... | 112 | 1 |

# GRAND RIVER AGENCY, DAKOTA TERRITORY.

### REPORT OF ACTING ASSISTANT SURGEON A. H. MANN, UNITED STATES ARMY.

This post is located on the west or right bank of the Missouri River, one hundred and eight miles by land and one hundred and fifty-two miles by the river below Fort Abraham Lincoln, and three hundred and seventy miles by land and four hundred and twenty-three miles by river above Yankton, present terminus of the Dakota Southern Railroad. Latitude, 45° 35′ north; longitude, 23° 21′ west, (approximately.) It was established May 20, 1870.

The quarters for enlisted men consist of two buildings, constructed, like others at the post, of cottonwood logs, chinked with mud, roofed with planks covered with six inches of earth. Each building contains a dormitory, 90 by 20 by 10 feet, lighted by five windows, warmed by two large wood-stoves, and ventilated by an opening 3 by 4 feet in the roof. There is a building containing a kitchen and mess-room in rear of each barrack. There are two frame sinks one hundred yards west of the post.

Quarters for married soldiers consist of six log huts, covered with poles, straw, and earth, situated sixty feet in rear of the barracks.

Officers' quarters consist of seven sets of three rooms each. The rooms are each 15 by 15 feet.

The guard-house is of the same material and style of construction as the other buildings, has three ventilators in the roof, and is kept in good condition.

The post bakery is furnished with a fine large oven.

There are two storehouses, a commissary's and a quartermaster's; also two root-houses.

The hospital-building is constructed of peeled cottonwood logs well chinked with mud and mortar, and roofed like the other buildings. The main portion is 20 by 64 by 12 feet, fronting east. Projecting back from the west side, sixteen feet from the south end of this, is a wing 16 by 32 feet. The main building is divided into a ward, 20 by 32 feet in the center, and two rooms, each 10 by 16 feet, at each end. The front room in the north end is the dispensary; the back one is the steward's room. The front room in the south end is a bath-room; the rear one is a store-room. The wing is divided into two rooms of equal size; the one adjoining the ward being the mess-room, the other the kitchen. The walls and ceiling of the ward are well whitewashed. There are three windows in the ward, two in front, the other in the rear, and one window on each side of the other rooms. Extending along the entire east side or front of the building is a porch 12 feet wide. The ward has a capacity for eight beds, giving 960 cubic feet of air-space to each. The hospital is provided with the usual furniture allowed to a two-company post hospital. The building is well adapted to treatment of the sick, is well ventilated, and satisfactory. There is one sink twenty yards in rear of the hospital.

The fuel used for warming all buildings at the post is oak wood obtained by contract.

The drainage is surface, but satisfactory.

*Consolidated sick-report, Grand River Agency, Dak., 1870–'74.*

| Year | | 1870–'71. | | 1871–'72. | | 1872–'73. | | 1873–'74. | |
|---|---|---|---|---|---|---|---|---|---|
| Mean strength { Officers<br>{ Enlisted men | | 4<br>150 | | 3<br>98 | | 3<br>106 | | 3<br>100 | |
| Diseases. | | Cases. | Deaths. | Cases. | Deaths. | Cases. | Deaths. | Cases. | Deaths. |
| GENERAL DISEASES, A. | | | | | | | | | |
| Typhoid fever | | | | | | 1 | | | |
| Remittent fever | | 2 | | | | | | 4 | |
| Intermittent fever | | 7 | | | | 1 | | | |
| Other diseases of this group | | | | 5 | | 14 | | | |
| GENERAL DISEASES, B. | | | | | | | | | |
| Rheumatism | | 21 | | 25 | | 23 | | 17 | |
| Syphilis | | 3 | | 22 | | 18 | 1 | 2 | |
| Consumption | | | | 1 | | | | | |
| Other diseases of this group | | | | | | | | 1 | |
| LOCAL DISEASES. | | | | | | | | | |
| Catarrh and bronchitis | | 20 | | 31 | | 49 | | 7 | |
| Pneumonia | | | | | | 2 | | | |
| Pleurisy | | | | | | 1 | | | |
| Diarrhœa and dysentery | | 24 | | 35 | | 34 | | 27 | |
| Hernia | | | | | | 1 | | | |
| Gonorrhœa | | | | 2 | | | | | |
| Other local diseases | | 30 | | 52 | | 39 | 1 | 32 | |
| Total disease | | 107 | | 173 | | 183 | 2 | 90 | |
| VIOLENT DISEASES AND DEATHS. | | | | | | | | | |
| Gunshot wounds | | | | 2 | | | | 1 | 1 |
| Drowning | | | | | 1 | | | | |
| Other accidents and injuries | | 34 | | 24 | | 21 | | 11 | |
| Suicide | | | 1 | | | | | | |
| Total violence | | 34 | 1 | 26 | 1 | 21 | | 12 | 1 |

# CAMP HANCOCK, DAKOTA TERRITORY.

REPORTS OF ACTING ASSISTANT SURGEONS B. F. SLAUGHTER AND H. R. PORTER, UNITED STATES ARMY.

This post is on the east bank of the Missouri River, at Bismarck, the point at which the Northern Pacific Railroad crosses the river. It is four hundred and fifty miles west of Duluth, in Minnesota, the eastern terminus of the railroad, and is in latitude 46° 40′ north, longitude 23° 32′ west.

The quarters for enlisted men were erected in the fall of 1872, and consist of one barrack-building constructed of logs and roofed with dirt. It is 100 by 20 feet, 9 feet high, is lighted by six windows, warmed by two stoves, and has no means of proper ventilation. The air-space to the average number of occupants does not exceed 375 cubic feet per man. It is furnished with the double wooden bunks. There is a convenient mess-room warmed by one stove. The kitchen and bakery are in a separate building on the south side of the post.

Married soldiers' quarters consist of two sets, both of which are large and comfortable.

Officers' quarters consist of two sets for captain and first lieutenant; they are good, roomy, and comfortable. There are no quarters for the second lieutenant and surgeon, who have resided in the town.

The guard-house is 20 by 20 feet, lighted by two windows. It is comfortably warmed. There is no separate cell, the prisoners, save for simple offenses, being sent to Fort Abraham Lincoln.

There is one storehouse adjoining the hospital, occupied by the quartermaster's department.

52 M P

The hospital consists of three wall-tents, framed and floored, and is well adapted for the post. It is warmed by two stoves.

There is one stable sufficient to accommodate seven animals. It is warm, roomy, and well ventilated.

The fuel used at this post is ash and cottonwood, furnished by contract.

*Consolidated sick-report, Camp Hancock, Dak., 1872–'74.*

| Year | | 1872–'73.* | | 1873–'74. | |
|---|---|---|---|---|---|
| Mean strength { Officers | | 3 | | 2 | |
| Enlisted men | | 60 | | 48 | |
| Diseases. | | Cases. | Deaths. | Cases. | Deaths. |
| GENERAL DISEASES, A. | | | | | |
| Cerebro-spinal fever | | 1 | 1 | ...... | ...... |
| Typhoid fever | | 2 | ...... | ...... | ...... |
| Remittent fever | | 4 | ...... | 2 | ...... |
| Other diseases of this group | | 4 | ...... | 4 | ...... |
| GENERAL DISEASES, B. | | | | | |
| Rheumatism | | 3 | ...... | 4 | ...... |
| Syphilis | | ...... | ...... | 2 | ...... |
| Other diseases of this group | | ...... | ...... | 1 | ...... |
| LOCAL DISEASES. | | | | | |
| Catarrh and bronchitis | | 6 | ...... | 4 | ...... |
| Pneumonia | | 1 | ...... | 1 | ...... |
| Pleurisy | | 1 | ...... | ...... | ...... |
| Diarrhœa and dysentery | | 23 | ...... | 25 | ...... |
| Gonorrhœa | | 1 | ...... | 2 | ...... |
| Other local diseases | | 14 | ...... | 32 | ...... |
| Alcoholism | | ...... | ...... | 1 | ...... |
| Total disease | | 60 | 1 | 78 | ...... |
| VIOLENT DISEASES AND DEATHS. | | | | | |
| Gunshot wounds | | ...... | ...... | 1 | ...... |
| Other accidents and injuries | | 6 | ...... | 16 | 1 |
| Total violence | | 6 | ...... | 17 | 1 |

\* Eight months only.

---

# LOWER BRULÉ AGENCY, DAKOTA TERRITORY.

### REPORT OF ACTING ASSISTANT SURGEON J. C. BYRNES, UNITED STATES ARMY.

The military station of Lower Brulé Agency, Dakota Territory, is situated on the right bank of the Missouri River, ninety miles by land above Fort Randall, and one hundred and twenty miles below Fort Sully; latitude, 43° 47′ north; longitude, 22° 19′ west; altitude, 1,400 feet above the sea, (approximates.) Yankton, present terminus of the Dakota Southern Railroad, is one hundred and fifty-five miles distant by land, and one hundred and seventy-three miles by river.

The post was located June 8, 1870, at a place about fifteen miles below its present site, and was moved to this place July 21, 1870. This change was effected on the representation of the superintendent of Indian affairs, no doubt induced by the hostile attitude of the Brulé Sioux Indians, who viewed with much dissatisfaction the military occupation of their reservation.

The ground occupied by the post is quadrangular in form, with an area of 1.26 acres. It is situated in the low bottom-land of the Missouri River, about four hundred feet from the declivity of the river-bank. On the west and northwest, and about three hundred feet from the post, is a high ridge which forms the ascent to the high table-lands of Missouri plateau. This ridge, during the long winter, serves as a barrier to the severe north and northwest winds which prevail in this region, and protects the post, in a measure, from their excessive rigor. During the summer this elevated land, so near, acts in an injurious manner by preventing the winds from having free access to the garrison, and thus serving as a disinfectant on the vegetable and other organic matters that undergo decomposition at its base. Altogether the present site is deemed unhealthy for summer occupancy, and seems to have been selected with a view more to winter habitation than permanent occupation.

Water for drinking is obtained from the Missouri River. It is considered very healthy, but during the summer months it is very turbid, and deposits on standing a very large sediment.

The buildings at this post were hastily constructed for winter shelter. They are formed of unhewn cottonwood logs, chinked with mud, and are low and uncouth in appearance.

The barrack is a one-story building, 96 by 22 feet, height 13 feet, lined throughout with cottonwood sheathing. There are two wings running east from the main building, each 60 by 20 feet, of the same height and finish as that building. The barrack is divided into a dormitory 78 by 20 feet clear, and a company-office 15 by 20 feet. The north wing is divided into rooms, a mess-hall adjoining the barrack, and a kitchen; the south wing into three rooms, forming three sets of quarters for married soldiers. These buildings were thoroughly repaired, inside and out, in 1873. Ventilating-shafts were put in the roof of the barrack and mess-room, and the dormitory was furnished with thirty-three iron single bedsteads. The dormitory is lighted by five windows, and warmed by three large box-stoves.

A bath-room, 9 feet 8 inches by 14 feet, was erected in 1874. It is furnished with bath-tub and necessary fixtures to make bathing facilities quite complete. One hundred and sixty gallons of water is furnished daily for bathing purposes.

Married soldiers' quarters are the three sets attached to the barrack, described above, and one log building, 13 by 18 feet, 8 feet high, located in the north wing of the garrison, erected in 1873.

The sink is a log structure, 12 by 10 feet, over a vault, 50 yards from northeast angle of the post.

The post-bakery is in a log building erected in 1873. This building is 65 by 22 feet, 11 feet high, divided into a bakery 20 by 22 feet, and a reading-room 45 by 22 feet. The oven in the bakery has a capacity for 130 rations of bread.

Officers' quarters consist of three log buildings, gable-roofed, each 38 by 32 feet, 12 feet in height, divided into four rooms, with a hall 6 feet wide through the center of the building. There is a kitchen attached to each building. The rooms are lined and ceiled with boards, and the fronts of the buildings are weatherboarded outside. They were thoroughly overhauled and repaired, inside and out, in 1873.

The commissary storehouse is a log building, 64 by 22 feet, 9 feet high, situated on the north end of the garrison. There is an issuing-room, 15 by 20 feet, lined with pine boards, in the west end of the building. There is a large cellar under this storehouse, and a root-house in rear of it.

The quartermaster's storehouse is the same in size as the above, but only 8 feet high. It is located on the south side of the garrison. These buildings were thoroughly repaired in 1873.

The guard-house is a log structure 35 by 18 feet, 7 feet high, divided into a guard-room 18 by 18 feet, and a prison-room 18 by 17 feet. The guard-room is lighted by two windows, the prison-room by one, and each room is provided with a stove for warming.

The hospital is a log structure 65 by 22 feet, outside measurement, fronting east, divided into a steward's room, 10 by 12 feet, in the southeast corner, and a store-room, 10 by 8 feet, in the southwest corner; adjoining these on the north is the dispensary, 15 by 20 feet, then the ward, 25 by 20 feet, and last the kitchen, 13 by 20 feet, which serves also as a mess-room, at the north end. All the rooms are 11 feet in height, and lined throughout with dressed pine boards. The ward has capacity for five beds, giving each 1,100 cubic feet of air-space. Average occupancy, one patient. The ward is provided with a ventilating-shaft through the roof, and is warmed by stoves. The building was thoroughly repaired in the fall of 1874; a piazza was put up along the entire front, the roof was shingled, and the building is now in good condition. The furniture and fixtures are sufficient.

There is no inclosure around the hospital. No drainage, sewerage, or water-closets. One earth-closet commode, and three close-stools. The arrangement of earth-closet and close-stools is satisfactory.

Water is stored in barrels, and kept for immediate use in case of fire.

The stable was erected in 1873, and is 75 by 22 feet, height 10 feet, ventilated by windows and doors; has nine double stalls and a commodious grain-room; building in excellent condition. It stands fifty feet from and facing the river. Refuse is removed in wheelbarrows and cast into the river. Attached to the stable is a cattle-shed, 40 by 12 feet, 7 feet high, containing twelve single stalls.

Fuel is cottonwood, obtained by contract, from groves of timber adjacent to the river-bank, or from islands in the river.

*Consolidated sick-report, Brulé Agency, Dak., 1870–'74.*

| Year | 1870–'71. | | 1871–'72. | | 1872–'73. | | 1873–'74. | |
|---|---|---|---|---|---|---|---|---|
| Mean strength {Officers | 4 | | 3 | | 3 | | 3 | |
| {Enlisted men | 99 | | 56 | | 56 | | 53 | |
| Diseases. | Cases. | Deaths. | Cases. | Deaths. | Cases. | Deaths. | Cases. | Deaths. |
| GENERAL DISEASES, A. | | | | | | | | |
| Typhoid fever | 2 | 1 | | | | | | |
| Typho-malarial fever | | | | | 4 | | 1 | |
| Remittent fever | 19 | | 1 | | 12 | | 3 | |
| Intermittent fever | 7 | | 2 | | 5 | | 7 | |
| Other diseases of this group | 4 | | | | | | | |
| GENERAL DISEASES, B. | | | | | | | | |
| Rheumatism | 20 | | 1 | | 6 | | 6 | |
| Syphilis | 5 | | 7 | | 2 | | 2 | |
| Consumption | 2 | | 1 | | | | | |
| Other diseases of this group | 5 | | | | | | | |
| LOCAL DISEASES. | | | | | | | | |
| Catarrh and bronchitis | 32 | | 6 | | 4 | | 22 | |
| Pneumonia | 3 | | 3 | | 1 | | | |
| Pleurisy | 3 | | | | 1 | | | |
| Diarrhœa and dysentery | 33 | | 11 | | 7 | | 5 | |
| Gonorrhœa | 4 | | 1 | | | | | |
| Other local diseases | 56 | 2 | 14 | | 15 | 1 | 12 | |
| Total disease | 195 | 3 | 47 | | 57 | 1 | 58 | |
| VIOLENT DISEASES AND DEATHS. | | | | | | | | |
| Gunshot wounds | | | | | | | 1 | |
| Drowning | | | | | | 1 | | |
| Other accidents and injuries | 39 | | 8 | | 9 | | 12 | |
| Suicide | | | | | | 1 | | |
| Total violence | 39 | | 8 | 2 | 9 | | 13 | |

# FORT PEMBINA, DAKOTA TERRITORY.

### REPORTED BY ASSISTANT SURGEON EZRA WOODRUFF, UNITED STATES ARMY.

Fort Pembina, Dakota Territory, is located at the extreme northeast point of the Territory; latitude, 48° 56′ 46″. 3 north; longitude, 20° 10′ west. It is about two hundred miles north of the watershed which divides the Mississippi Valley from the valley of the Red River of the North, and is situated on the west or left bank of the river. It is one mile south of the village of Pembina, Dak., and about three and one-half miles south of the boundary-line between the United States and the Dominion of Canada, as established by the International Boundary Commission in September, 1872. Sixty-six miles north of the fort is the town of Winnipeg, (Fort Garry,) a rapidly-growing place, with a population of three thousand. Thirty miles westward is a range of table-land extending irregularly north and south for many miles, with an abrupt front of several hundred feet in height on the eastern border, called the Pembina Mountain. This is the nearest high land to the post. Eastward, in Minnesota, is a prairie region with many swamps, and impassable except during the winter.

There is no mineral formation, no stones or sand in the vicinity. Sand is brought from the base of Pembina Mountain, and limestone is found near Fort Garry. The surface soil consists of a black clayey loam from 1½ to 2½ feet deep, and very fertile. Beneath this is a white clay slightly mixed with marl, but which makes good brick of a cream color, like the Milwaukee brick. This stratum is underlaid by a stiff, moist, blue clay, at least sixty feet in depth.

There are no springs or ponds on the reservation. Water is generally found by digging wells to the depth of 20 to 25 feet, but is not universally distributed at that depth. It seems to flow in veins among the strata of blue clay; and will sometimes be met at a depth of 12 feet, while at no great distance it is not found at the depth of 40 feet.

The site of the fort is 30 feet above low water in the Red River, and is subject to overflow at irregular intervals. In 1826 there was a very destructive flood, which carried away houses and barns, and again in 1852 and 1861 there were great freshets.

The climate is dry and cold, and severe gales of wind are not uncommon. Winter begins in November, and spring in May; and by the 15th of the latter month the grass is fairly started on the prairie.

Planting is done in May and the first ten days of June. The hardy Indian ponies, and even mules, live through the winter without shelter. They reach the dead prairie-grass by pawing away the snow, and quench their thirst by eating the latter.

Cattle cannot endure the exposure, and require to be fed eight months of the year. Sheep thrive well, and are raised in considerable numbers near Fort Garry. The climate is too cold for swine, which are unprofitable except where they have access to oak woods.

The principal indigenous plants of the vicinity are the following: The wild strawberry ripens the second week in June, continues in season three weeks, and is immediately succeeded by the wild raspberry. The wild black currant and high bush blueberry ripen in July; the wild red plum and chokecherry in August. The hazel-nut, wild grape, and bush cranberry ripen in September. These fruits form the principal food of the Indians during the summer.

The chief forest-trees are the oak, ash, elm, basswood, cottonwood, and willow.

The wild animals of this region are the moose, elk, red deer, black bear, wolf, red fox, cross fox, silver fox, raccoon, black marten, prairie gray squirrel, ground-squirrel, flying-squirrel, rabbit, skunk, beaver, otter, mink, and muskrat. The buffalo, which a few years ago roamed in vast herds over the plains of Dakota, has not been seen in this vicinity since 1867. Hunters still start from Pembina to follow them to their retreats; and at Wood Mountain, five hundred miles westward, there is a settlement of nearly one hundred families who live by hunting the buffalo.

Of birds, the bald-headed eagle, kestrel, hawk, shrike, whip-poor-will, woodpecker, chimney-swallow, and martin spend the summer in this region, arriving in April and May, and returning southward in October and November. The crane, loon, cormorant, swan, pelican, wild goose, white brant, ducks, mallard, widgeon, blue and green winged teal, and muganser are also summer visitors. The wild pigeon arrives in April, hatches in July, and departs in September. The prairie-chicken remains all the year. They are hatched in July, and are large enough to kill in the latter part of August.

Sturgeon are caught in the Red River weighing from fifty to two hundred pounds. Their flesh is highly esteemed; and the oil is a favorite domestic remedy for contusions and sprains. The pickerel, wall-eyed pike, (a species of salmon,) the cat-fish, and the gold-eye, (a small species of white-fish,) are also caught in great quantities for food.

Reptiles are few in number, small and harmless. Not so are the insects The horse-fly is extremely numerous and troublesome in July and August. A large fly, called here the "bull-dog," caused great annoyance to the stock of the boundary commission near the Lake of the Woods; but is not very numerous near this post. The mosquitoes swarm in myriads in summer both day and night. They have been known to kill cattle by filling the trachea and causing suffocation. The hardy Canadian voyageurs have been so prostrated by the torture of their bites in crossing the prairies, that they have lain down and wept.

Every year, since the establishment of the post, vast swarms of winged ants have been observed about the 20th of August moving northward. They presented the appearance of dark quivering masses several hundred feet from the ground, were several hours in passing, and the sound of their wings was like the hum of innumerable swarms of bees. They never alighted in the vicinity of Pembina, but occasional stragglers reached the ground. In each instance there was found a large brown female ant one-third of an inch in length, heavy with eggs. Upon her back was mounted a small black male ant, in the act of impregnation.

Grasshoppers have been observed in the Northwest ever since the first settlement of the country, and, although sometimes absent for several years, their re-appearance is only a question of time, and is looked for with dread.

The inhabitants above Saint Joseph's, Dak., and a large portion of the settlers in Manitoba, refrained from planting seed in 1873, fearing that their labor would be in vain. The grasshoppers hatched in immense numbers in Manitoba, and began flying south in July, and on twelve different days were observed at the post in the air. They alighted in the vicinity on several days and destroyed a quantity of growing grain by eating off the stalks near the head; but they soon resumed their flight southward.

On the 25th of March, 1870, a special order (No. 43) was issued from headquarters Department of Dakota, detailing Companies I and K, Twentieth Infantry, to establish a new military post at or near Pembina, Dak. In compliance with this order, Company I, commanded by Capt. Loyd Wheaton, and accompanied by Asst. Surg. Ezra Woodruff, as medical officer, left Fort Abercrombie, then an extreme frontier post, in May, embarking on two flat-boats, to float to their destination by the current of the Red River. The region to be traversed was a wilderness with only three small settlements. Twenty-two miles from Abercrombie was passed the Mission of the Holy Cross, where a few Indians and half-breeds were gathered under the care of a priest. Twenty-eight miles farther appeared Georgetown, a Hudson's Bay trading-post of two or three houses; and thence to Grand Forks, one hundred miles from Abercrombie, there was not a single habitation. Grand Forks, where the principal affluent of the Red River enters, had but a single hut, occupied by one Mick Hoffman, and used by the mail-carriers as a station. The wide prairie, clothed with young grass, showed not a sign of life, except an occasional bird and millions of minute grasshoppers just hatched. Thence to Pembina there was not a single house. At that time the trade of Fort Garry, Pembina, and Saint Joseph's with the United States was carried on in the Red River carts. These singular vehicles were composed entirely of wood, and consisted of two wheels nearly six feet in diameter, with very broad tires, and a small body resting on the axle and shafts. Both ponies and oxen were used to draw them, attached by a peculiar harness of raw-hide. These carts would carry from six hundred to eight hundred pounds, and one man could drive five or six of them in a train. No grease was used, and as a long train crept over the prairie an indescribable noise was made by the creaking of the wheels. It was estimated that three thousand of these carts passed south through Pembina in one season, carrying furs as freight, and returned loaded with various supplies. The broad felloes of the wheels prevented their sinking in the soft ground, and the driver, with only the most primitive tools, could at any time or place repair a broken cart or even construct a new one. When progress was interrupted by a swollen stream, the cart could be taken to pieces and floated across. The irregular mails were transported on these carts during the summer, and through the long winter they were carried by dog-trains, or on the back of a hardy half-breed voyageur.

During the past four years the Red River country has vied with any other portion of the West in the rapidity of its progress. There are now thousands of dwellings where in 1870 there were not more than half a dozen, and every lot of land along the river from Grand Forks to Pembina is said to be taken up by actual settlers. Five steamboats ply upon the Red River, reaching Moorhead, the crossing of the Northern Pacific Railroad, during high water, but are unable to ascend so far during the driest part of summer.

In September, 1871, the Minnesota Stage Company established a line of stages, running thrice a week from Fort Abercrombie to Fort Garry. The Saint Paul and Saint Vincent Railroad was, in the spring of 1874, graded within ten miles of Pembina, but the rails were not then laid beyond the crossing of Red Lake River. A telegraph-line was completed in the autumn of 1872, crossing the parade at Fort Pembina. Thousands of Canadian emigrants have within the last few years passed this place to settle in the bleak regions of the Assinaboine and the Saskatchewan, and are rapidly populating the country between this point and Winnipeg.

Captain Wheaton, with Company I, Twentieth Infantry, arrived at Pembina on the 19th of May. They were joined soon after by Company K from Fort Totten, under command of Capt. A. A. Harbach. The site selected was within the angle formed by the confluence of the Pembina and Red Rivers. The reservation extends three miles along the former and one mile on the latter.

It is a level prairie, except the northwest corner, crossed by the Pembina River, which is skirted with timber.

The fort is four miles south of the boundary-line between the United States and the British possessions, as established by Capt. D. P. Heap, United States Engineers, in May, 1870, and three miles south of the old and still-recognized line surveyed by Major Long in 1823. The fort is located in the northeast angle of the reservation, about two hundred yards from the bank of the Red River, from which it is subject to overflow at irregular intervals.

The buildings are arranged in the form of a rectangle and face the parade-ground, 386 by 280 feet. The whole is surrounded by a wooden palisade fence, and has capacity for two companies of infantry. All the buildings are of wood, except the magazine, which is of brick. The other buildings consist of four double sets of officers' quarters; two company barracks, with separate kitchens; guard-house, hospital, bake-house, storehouse, and stable.

The hospital and the buildings for quarters are constructed in the same manner. Planks three inches thick are laid upon the ground, on which are placed oak posts. Upon these a balloon frame is erected.

The outside is covered with inch boards, tarred felt, and pine sheathing; the inside is lathed and plastered with two coats, the officers' quarters and hospital being also hard-finished. The roofs are covered with inch boards, tarred felt, and shingles; the floors are double, with tarred felt between the courses.

The officers' quarters are four double frame buildings, for the accommodation of eight officers. They are situated on the south side of the parade, and face the north; are one and a half stories high, 46½ by 30 feet, each traversed by a hall in the center from front to rear, 7 feet wide. From this hall the stairway ascends to the attic. The ceiling of the first floor is 11 feet high; of the attic 5½ at the sides and 9 feet in the center. The lower story is divided into parlor, 13 by 16 feet, sitting-room 14 by 15 feet, dining-room 11 by 15 feet, and kitchen 10 by 13 feet. The attic contains two large bed-rooms and two closets.

There is an open fire-place in the parlor; the other rooms have flues for stoves. The rooms are well lighted, and ventilation is secured by registers in the flues.

The company barracks, two in number, built on the plan above described, are located on the north side of the parade. Each building is 178 by 25 feet, and 14 feet from floor to ceiling. Along the south front is a piazza eight feet in width. The center of the building is occupied by two orderly-rooms, 14 by 15 feet. The remainder consists of two dormitories or squad-rooms. Each squad-room is lighted by six windows; ventilated by the chimney-flues and cold-air boxes opening in the floor. It contains one open fire-place and a flue for stove. One 35-inch box heating-stove, with drum, is found sufficient to warm the room. Iron bedsteads are used. There is no wash-room or bath-room. The sinks are in rear of the barracks, and are pits 10 feet deep covered with houses. Fifteen feet in rear of each barrack is a commodious and well-furnished building, 53 by 20 feet, comprising the company kitchen, mess-room, and two pantries.

A substantial log building, 60 by 21 feet, and divided into three equal rooms, is used as quarters for laundresses.

The guard-house is located north of the company kitchens, and consists of a wooden building 38 by 25 feet. A hall, 5 feet wide, passes through the center north and south, from which doors open into the guard-room and prison-rooms. The former is 15 by 24 feet, and of the latter, one is 14 by 16, the other 9½ by 16 feet. The height of the ceiling is 10 feet. In the guard-room is an open fire-place, and in the prison-rooms flues for stoves. The former has two windows, and each of the latter, one. Registers are placed in the flues for ventilation. The average occupancy in 1873 was 10.51.

The hospital, situated in the southwestern corner of the garrison, consists of an administration building and a ward. The former is one and one-half stories high, 37 feet square, with an L on the western side, 21 by 14 feet, for kitchen and pantry. The first floor is crossed by two halls at right angles, having four rooms, viz: dispensary, office, store-room, and dining-room. A stairway with one landing, ascends to the attic; which contains four rooms, entered from a central hall 7 feet wide. One of these rooms is assigned to attendants, one as steward's room, and a third for a dead-room. It has no special fixtures for post-mortem examinations. The ward is one room, 45 by 25 feet, outside measurement. Attached to the southwest corner of the ward, is a room 10 by 13 feet, built for a bath-room and water-closet. It has no furniture save one tin bath-tub. The ward is lighted by ten windows, four on each side and two in the south end. All the windows in the hospital on the first floor are hung with weights. The ventilation of the administration building is by flues containing registers, and is ample. The ward is ventilated by a cold-air box opening in the center of the floor, over which is placed a ventilating-stove. A special ventilating-chimney is built at the south end of the ward, with a register near the ceiling. There are also registers in the chimneys at the north end of the ward. The extreme coldness of the climate renders these provisions sufficient, it being extremely difficult to keep the cold air out. The hospital is warmed entirely by stoves. Two 31-inch box heating-stoves suffice to keep the air in the ward at a proper temperature. The ward is an airy, cheerful-looking apartment, the dispensary neatly fitted up and well furnished. The sink is a double apartment built over a pit 12 feet deep, and is neatly policed. It is in rear of the southern end of the ward, and is reached by a door from the bath-room.

The bakery is in the northeastern portion of the fort, twenty-five feet north and in rear of the company-kitchen. It contains two large ovens and is in good order.

There is no school-room, chapel, or laundry.

The stable is situated about three hundred yards southeast of the fort, near the river-bank. It is a frame building, 140 by 30 feet, raised 2 feet from the ground on posts, and contains stalls for fifty-six horses. It is covered with inch boards and sheeting, and roofed with shingles. No tarred felt is used. The floor is of 2-inch pine plank.

Water is hauled from the river in barrels in winter and in a tank in summer. The supply is ample and the quality good. There are twelve galvanized-iron cisterns, each of a capacity of one hundred and ten barrels. They are sunk in the ground, one at each set of officers' quarters, one at each barrack, one at the hospital, and one at the storehouse. They are useless in winter.

An examination of the Red River water was made in December, 1874, by Asst. Surg. V. Havard, U. S. A., at a time when the river was covered with thick ice. The result showed—

|  | Grains per gallon. |
|---|---|
| Organic matters as obtained by incineration | 4.90 |
| Oxidizable organic matter, as obtained by the permanganate of potassa test | 4.12 |
| Carbonate of lime | 10.09 |
| Chloride of sodium | 1.92 |
| Sulphates, (approximate) | 2. |
| Phosphates | a trace. |
| Magnesia | a comparatively large quantity, not precisely determined. |

The suspended matters, mostly sand and clay, with some organic impurities, estimated from 2 to 4 grains per gallon.

The water when shaken has a reddish-yellow tint, but after settling is, at this season, perfectly clear. It is without taste and no complaint has ever been traced to its use.

There are no facilities for bathing at the post in winter. The river is used in summer.

Slops, offal, and excreta are carted away in barrels and emptied on the bank of the river at a distance from the post.

The cemetery is one-third of a mile south of the post, on the Fort Abercombie road. It is two acres in extent, inclosed by a wooden fence, and thus far contains three graves.

A plat of eight acres in extent, lying southeast of the post, has been inclosed with a rail-fence, and plowed for a post garden. This piece of ground, owing to unskillful management, has yet produced but little. A smaller tract has also been cultivated. The principal products have been potatoes, onions, beets, carrots, parsnips, radishes, green peas, and beans. The supply has never been sufficient for the wants of the garrison. A hospital garden was to be commenced in 1874. There are no officers' gardens. Summer vegetables can be procured in limited quantities from the settlers in the vicinity.

The soldiers have an out-door gymnasium for summer practice, and have started a dramatic association, which furnishes much amusement, and is a source of relaxation to the men.

*Meteorological report, Fort Pembina, Dak., 1871–'74.*

| Month. | 1870–'71. Temperature. Mean. | Max. | Min. | Rain-fall in inches. | 1871–'72. Temperature. Mean. | Max. | Min. | Rain-fall in inches. | 1872–'73. Temperature. Mean. | Max. | Min. | Rain-fall in inches. | 1873–'74. Temperature. Mean. | Max. | Min. | Rain-fall in inches. |
|---|---|---|---|---|---|---|---|---|---|---|---|---|---|---|---|---|
| | ° | ° | ° | | ° | ° | ° | | ° | ° | ° | | ° | ° | ° | |
| July...... | | | | | | | | | 67.66 | 97* | 36* | 3.09 | 67.10 | 89* | 34* | 1.30 |
| August..... | | | | | 63.93 | 100 | 41 | 2.95 | 65.41 | 91* | 34* | 0.82 | 66.43 | 91* | 34* | 2.38 |
| September... | | | | | 53.42 | 82 | 22 | 0.23 | 53.78 | 85* | 25* | 1.67 | 47.78 | 80* | 23* | 2.05 |
| October.... | | | | | 39.35 | 72 | 14 | 1.13 | 43.91 | 77* | 15* | 1.16 | 36.37 | 82* | 3* | 0.56 |
| November.... | | | | | 13.97 | 41* | −33* | 0.54 | 18.28 | 48* | −28* | 0.53 | 15.67 | 45* | −25* | 0.66 |
| December..... | | | | | − 4.43 | 36* | −36* | 0.47 | − 5.72 | 34* | −51* | 2.95 | 6.76 | 35* | −27* | 0.18 |
| January..... | | | | | 3.73 | 31* | −28* | 0.28 | − 4.49 | 31* | −40* | 0.41 | − 3.17 | 37* | −44* | 0.26 |
| February..... | | | | | 5.62 | 39* | −23* | 0.25 | 4.43 | 33* | −31* | 0.75 | 2.99 | 32* | −32* | 0.25 |
| March...... | | | | | 7.73 | 32* | −23* | 0.45 | 12.05 | 43* | −40* | 0.35 | 12.11 | 47* | −29* | 0.35 |
| April...... | | | | | 31.51 | 59* | − 7* | 2.00 | 34.64 | 64* | 16* | 0.39 | 30.32 | 76* | − 4* | 0.20 |
| May...... | | | | | 50.19 | 79* | 28* | 1.90 | 53.76 | 81* | 29* | 2.11 | 57.04 | 98* | 27* | 1.55 |
| June...... | | | | | 64.40 | 94* | 38* | 2.09 | 67.20 | 93* | 38* | 2.91 | 66.29 | 94* | 33* | 3.41 |
| For the year... | | | | | | | | | 34.24 | 97* | −51* | 17.14 | 33.81 | 98* | −44* | 13.15 |

*These observations are made with self-registering thermometers. The mean is from the standard thermometer.

*Consolidated sick-report, Fort Pembina, Dak., 1870–'74.*

| Year ..... | 1870–'71. Cases. | Deaths. | 1871–'72. Cases. | Deaths. | 1872–'73. Cases. | Deaths. | 1873–'74. Cases. | Deaths. |
|---|---|---|---|---|---|---|---|---|
| Mean strength { Officers..... | 6 | | 5 | | 5 | | 6 | |
| { Enlisted men..... | 119 | | 94 | | 80 | | 121 | |
| **GENERAL DISEASES, A.** | | | | | | | | |
| Typhoid fever..... | | | | | 2 | | 1 | |
| Intermittent fever..... | 3 | | 12 | | 2 | | | |
| Other diseases of this group ..... | 16 | | 5 | | 12 | | 32 | |
| **GENERAL DISEASES, B.** | | | | | | | | |
| Rheumatism..... | 7 | 1 | 8 | | 4 | | 7 | |
| Syphilis ..... | | | 1 | | | | | |
| Consumption ..... | | 1 | | | | | | |
| Other diseases of this group ..... | | | | | 2 | | | |
| **LOCAL DISEASES.** | | | | | | | | |
| Catarrh and bronchitis ..... | 66 | | 23 | | 54 | | 78 | 1 |
| Pneumonia ..... | 1 | | | | | | 1 | 1 |
| Diarrhœa and dysentery ..... | 47 | | 54 | | 10 | | 19 | |
| Gonorrhœa ..... | 1 | | 1 | | 1 | | 3 | |
| Other local diseases..... | 68 | | 92 | | 73 | | 93 | |
| Alcoholism ..... | 1 | | 2 | | 4 | | 5 | |
| Total disease..... | 210 | 2 | 200 | | 162 | | 239 | 2 |
| **VIOLENT DISEASES AND DEATHS.** | | | | | | | | |
| Gunshot wounds ..... | | | | | 1 | | | |
| Other accidents and injuries..... | 40 | | 48 | 1 | 28 | | 38 | |
| Total violence..... | 40 | | 48 | 1 | 29 | | 38 | |

# FORT RANDALL, DAKOTA TERRITORY.

## INFORMATION FURNISHED BY SURGEON J. F. WEEDS AND ASSISTANT SURGEON J. P. KIMBALL, UNITED STATES ARMY.

Fort Randall is located on the right bank of the Missouri River; latitude, 43° 1′ north; longitude, 21° 32′ west; altitude above the sea, 1,245 feet; above the river, 56 feet. By land it is seventy-five miles from Yankton, the nearest railroad station. By the river it is two hundred and seventy-seven miles below Fort Sully, the nearest permanent post, and one thousand two hundred and eighty-eight miles above Saint Louis, the main source of supplies. The reservation, as surveyed by Lieut. J. C. Clark, Fourth Artillery, was approved by the President June 14, 1860, and extends on

53 M P

the river from a point eight miles below to sixteen miles above the post, and is eight miles wide, about twenty-five thousand acres being on the left bank of the river.

The post was established by order of General W. S. Harney, U. S. A., as a base of supplies for the posts on the Upper Missouri, and as a protection to settlers against the Indians. The first garrison consisted of Companies C and I, Second Infantry, and Companies D, E, H, and K, Second Dragoons, Col. Francis Lee, Second Infantry, commanding, and the construction of the post was commenced in August, 1856. The post thus commenced, and described in Circular No. 4, Surgeon-General's Office, 1870, p. 386, has been for the most part torn down, and a new post has been built during 1870–'72, under the direction of Lieut. Col. E. S. Otis, Twenty-second Infantry.

The new post was commenced for two companies, but it is now intended for five, and is built on the second terrace above the river, having at the rear a range of hills about 150 feet in height, which, at a level but little below their summits, spread out into the third terrace or rolling prairie.

The post is nearly half a mile from the river, which at this point is about one thousand yards wide and navigable for light-draught steamboats.

The general arrangement of the post is shown in the plate opposite.

The officers' quarters consist of eight buildings. The house occupied by the commanding

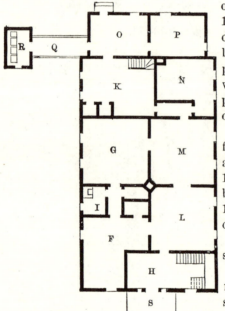

Figure 60.

officer consists of a main building, constructed of logs in 1856–'57, 36 by 60 feet, one and a half stories high, and a one-story frame addition built in 1871, when the original building was repaired and thoroughly renovated. The log portion is weatherboarded and painted outside, and the whole is ceiled with red cedar and painted or lathed and plastered within. The lower story is 10 feet from floor to ceiling. The arrangement of the rooms is shown by Figure 60.

F, chamber, 17 by 18 feet; G, sitting-room, 17 by 17 feet; H, hall, 8½ by 24 feet, with stairs leading to the floor above; I, outside water-closet, 7½ by 10 feet; K, kitchen, 14¼ by 19 feet; L, parlor, 17 by 17 feet; M, dining-room, 17 by 17 feet; N, chamber, 14¼ by 15¼ feet; P, wood-house, 10½ by 14½ feet; Q, summer-kitchen, 10½ by 14½ feet; S, covered porch, 8 by 12 feet.

The rooms on the second floor are low attics, used as sleeping apartments and servants' rooms.

The two buildings, located one on each side of the commanding officer's quarters, are one-and-a-half-story frame structures, in all respects alike. Each consists of a front portion, 47 by 32 feet, and a rear projection, 28 by 28 feet, to the rear of which is attached a one-story frame building with shed-roof, 12 by 34 feet. In front is a veranda, 18 by 8 feet. Each building is divided into two similar and separate sets of quarters. To each set there are on the first floor a parlor, 15¼ by 16 feet, a bed-room, 15¼ by 14 feet, a dining-room, kitchen, and rough room, used as a summer kitchen and laundry. This story is 12 feet high, and has an excellent cellar underneath. The upper portion of each set of quarters contains a hall, four rooms, and two closets. These buildings are substantial, of good material and workmanship. The foundations are of stone, walls filled in with brick, sheathed, weatherboarded, and painted white outside, and lathed and plastered inside. A door opens from the dining-room upon a platform, 5 by 18⅔ feet, leading to a water-closet 6 by 8 feet. The water-closet, like one in rear of the commanding officer's quarters, consists of a walled vault, 12 feet deep, a ventilating-shaft, and suitable superstructure. In the rear are convenient yards and out-houses for keeping cows and poultry.

The two sets of officers' quarters, marked C C in the plan, are similar one-story frame buildings, erected in 1871. Each set contains a hall, 6 by 17 feet, one room 14 feet 8 inches by 17 feet, two rooms of the average dimensions of 13½ by 14 feet, one room 8 feet square, and a pantry. The ceiling is 11 feet high, but part of the rooms are only 7 feet on one side, owing to the slope of the roof. These quarters are built on stone foundations. The walls are lined with brick, plastered

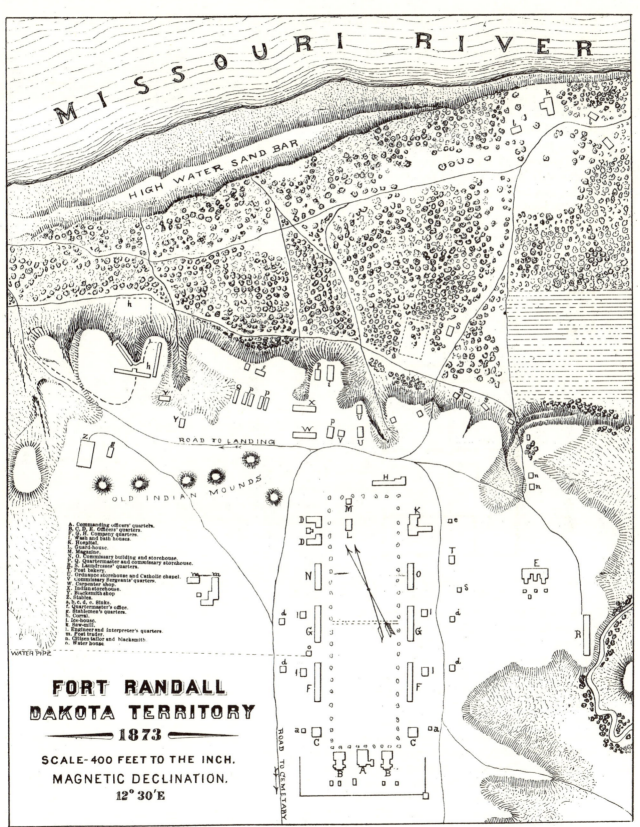

MISSOURI RIVER

HIGH WATER SAND BAR

ROAD TO LANDING

OLD INDIAN MOUNDS

ROAD TO CEMETARY

WATER PIPE

A. Commanding officers' quarters.
B, C, D, E. Officers' quarters.
F, G, H. Company quarters.
I. Wash and bath houses.
K. Hospital.
L. Guard-house.
M. Magazine.
N, O. Commissary building and storehouse.
P, Q. Quartermaster and commissary storehouse.
R, S. Laundresses' quarters.
T. Post bakery.
U. Ordnance storehouse and Catholic chapel.
V. Commissary Sergeants' quarters.
W. Carpenter shop.
X. Indian storehouse.
Y. Blacksmith shop
Z. Stables.
a, b, c, d, e. Sinks.
f. Quartermaster's office.
g. Stablemen's quarters.
h. Corral.
i. Ice-house.
k. Saw-mill.
l. Engineer and interpreter's quarters.
m. Post trader.
n. Citizen tailor and blacksmith.
o. Water house.

# FORT RANDALL
# DAKOTA TERRITORY
## 1873

SCALE—400 FEET TO THE INCH.

MAGNETIC DECLINATION.
12° 30'E

The Graphic Co. Photo-Lith. 39 & 41 Park Place, N.Y.

inside and weatherboarded and painted outside. There are no yards or cellars. There is a neat piazza in front of each, and a sink in rear. The officers' quarters, marked D D in the plan, are one-story frame buildings, erected in 1871–'72. They are L-shaped, having a front portion 21½ by 37½ feet, and a rear projection 21½ by 27½ feet. Each set contains six rooms of good size, a servants' room, pantry, closet, and wood-shed. They are built and finished in the same manner as the preceding, except the brick lining of the walls.

The remaining officers' quarters, marked E on the plate, were constructed in 1872 by altering and enlarging the old hospital. The old portion is of hewn logs; the new additions are framed. The ceilings are 9 feet in height. The building as it now stands is an elongated parallelogram, 100 by 21 feet, with three rear projections, the whole resting upon a stone foundation. The building is divided into three sets of quarters, the arrangement of which is shown by Figure 61.

A, parlor, 15 by 19 feet; B, chamber, 15 by 19 feet; C, (outside tenements,) chambers, 19 by 19 feet; C, (center tenement,) chamber, 13⅔ by 14⅔ feet; D, dining-rooms, 14 by 15 feet; E, kitchen, (E, wood-house, in center building,) 8½ by 9½ feet.

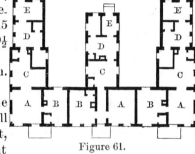

Figure 61.

These quarters have two coats of plaster, with rough finish. There are piazzas in front and sinks in the rear.

The quarters for enlisted men are five buildings, all frame structures, erected since the commencement of 1870. Two, in all respects similar, are each 163 by 24 feet, two stories in height, with verandas 7 feet wide the whole length of both stories, front and rear. They are substantially built of cottonwood, upon stone foundations, the walls being lined with brick, sheathed, weatherboarded, and painted outside, and plastered within. The first story is 10 feet in height, and divided into ten rooms; kitchen, mess-room, reading-room, offices, and store-rooms. The second story is 9 feet 5 inches high in the center and 8 feet 2 inches at the sides, and is divided into two dormitories, 23 by 77½ feet. They are well lighted by fourteen windows in each, and have ridge ventilation. The average occupancy is twenty men to each, allowing each 800 cubic feet of air-space. In winter only one of the dormitories is used, instead of two, when the air-space per man is 400 feet. The heating is by wood-stoves. The men sleep on iron bunks of the latest pattern. Two sets of quarters, built in the same manner as the above, are each 150 by 21 feet, one story high, with a veranda 7 feet wide the whole length in front. They are each 12 feet from floor to ceiling, divided into five rooms; orderly-room, store-room, kitchen, 15 by 20 feet, mess-room, 20 by 39 feet, and dormitory, 20 by 80 feet. The latter has, with the present occupancy, 480 feet of air-space per man, has ridge ventilation, and is well lighted by twelve windows. The remaining set is a one-story frame building, 100 by 17 feet, with an addition adjoining the west end, 25 by 45 feet, and 10 feet from floor to ceiling. The inside is plastered; only the front wall is filled with brick, and painted externally. It contains two dormitories, an orderly-room, and an armory. The dormitories are 16 feet 2 inches by 24 feet 3 inches, and are imperfectly lighted and ventilated by six small windows. A rear projection contains a kitchen, 13 by 23⅛ feet, a mess-room, 23⅛ by 30 feet, and a room for the cook. Thirty feet in rear of the center of this barrack is a frame building, 17 by 30 by 9 feet, used for a wash-room and store-room. It rests upon cedar posts, is sheathed and weatherboarded outside and lined with boards inside, the interspace being filled with sawdust; it is not ceiled. The roof is shingled. It contains a bath-room, 17 by 20 feet, and a store-room, 17 by 10 feet.

A few feet in rear of each of the four sets of quarters first described is a one-story frame building, 20 by 30, designed for lavatory and bath-house. They are finished so far as to be available for the former purpose, but not for the latter. They are well built, with cellars and stone foundations beneath; the walls are lined with grout, sheathed, weatherboarded, and painted externally. About seventy-five yards in the rear of each barrack is a sink, consisting of a trench about 12 feet deep, over which is a rough wooden building. When necessary the trenches are filled up and new ones dug.

At some distance from the post is a one-story frame building, erected in 1871 for laundresses' quarters. It is 156 by 28 feet, and 10 feet from floor to ceiling, weatherboarded and painted externally, and lathed and plastered inside. It is divided into six sets of quarters, each consisting of two rooms, 12½ by 14 feet, and an unplastered wash-room, 12½ by 25 feet. These quarters are neat and comfortable, but insufficient to accommodate all the laundresses, several of whom live in shanties and old log houses about the post.

The ice-house, with a capacity of 400 tons, is old and in bad condition.

The guard-house is constructed in the same general manner with the other buildings at the post. The walls, except of the portion occupied by prisoners, are brick-lined, ceiled to the height of about 5 feet, and the remainder plastered. The prison-room and cells are lined with hard plank,

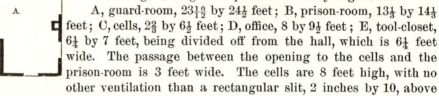

Figure 62.

1½ inches thick. The building is 60 by 25 feet, and 12 feet from floor to ceiling. The ground-plan is shown by Figure 62.

A, guard-room, 23$\frac{10}{12}$ by 24½ feet; B, prison-room, 13⅓ by 14⅓ feet; C, cells, 2⅔ by 6½ feet; D, office, 8 by 9½ feet; E, tool-closet, 6¼ by 7 feet, being divided off from the hall, which is 6¼ feet wide. The passage between the opening to the cells and the prison-room is 3 feet wide. The cells are 8 feet high, with no other ventilation than a rectangular slit, 2 inches by 10, above the door opening into the narrow passage. The prisoners' room is fairly lighted by one window near the ceiling, and a half window at the ordinary height. It is ventilated by these windows and by two shafts, one near the floor, and the other near the ceiling. The ventilation would be good but for the overcrowding of the room. It contains only 2,268 cubic feet of air-space, and the average occupancy during the past two years has been ten. The cells, containing but 132 cubic feet of air-space, are used only to confine for short periods men who have become violent and unmanageable through intoxication.

The post-hospital was built in 1872, in accordance with the plan given in Circular No. 2, Surgeon General's Office, 1871, for a hospital of twenty-four beds, except that one wing for ward has been omitted. It rests upon a stone foundation, 4 feet thick, and well built. There are a few minor deviations from the original plan, the principal of which are that the veranda in front is 8 feet instead of 10 feet wide, and that the window-sashes are not boxed and hung. In rear of the hospital is a sink for the use of convalescents and attendants. The building is sufficiently warmed by a single ventilating fire-place, and a number of box-stoves, burning wood. There are no means of bringing water to the bath-room or removing it other than by hand. There is no hospital inclosure or garden. The average number of sick in hospital is five.

A new post-bakery was built in 1874. It is located a few feet west of the old one shown in plate. The building is a frame, 20 by 28 feet, brick-lined, sheathed, weather-boarded, the walls plastered inside, ceiled with tongued and grooved boards, roof shingled, and rests on a stone foundation. It is painted a light-drab color externally. Within it contains a store-room, 10 by 11½ feet, with a cellar underneath, 6 by 8 by 6 feet, a general working-room, 8⅓ by 28 feet, and two ovens, each 6½ by 8 feet. The ovens are well built, of brick, and have a combined capacity of five hundred rations. The building is well lighted by six windows. The rooms are 9½ feet in height. It is a well-built structure and conveniently arranged.

The post is supplied with water from the Missouri River by a six-horse-power steam-engine The water is pumped from the river through a 2-inch suction-pipe, 25 feet long, and forced through a 1½-inch pipe to the summit of the bluff and 2,700 feet across the plain, to a reservoir of 12,000 gallons capacity inclosed in a water-house. It is then raised by a hand-power force-pump into a water-wagon, in which it is distributed as required. The top of the reservoir is formed of a double floor, five feet below the surface of the ground, and the conducting-pipe is laid below the frost-line. The force-pump by which the water is raised from the reservoir is also designed to serve as a hand fire-engine, and is provided with 850 feet of 1½-inch rubber hose, and has power to throw a stream of water through a half-inch nozzle to the roof of any ordinary two-story building.

*Meteorological report, Fort Randall, Dak., 1870–'74.*

| Month. | 1870–'71. Temperature. Mean. | Max. | Min. | Rain-fall in inches. | 1871–'72. Temperature. Mean. | Max. | Min. | Rain-fall in inches. | 1872–'73. Temperature. Mean. | Max. | Min. | Rain-fall in inches. | 1873–'74. Temperature. Mean. | Max. | Min. | Rain-fall in inches. |
|---|---|---|---|---|---|---|---|---|---|---|---|---|---|---|---|---|
| | ° | ° | ° | | ° | ° | ° | | ° | ° | ° | | ° | ° | ° | |
| July | 81.54 | 107* | 46* | 0.29 | 76.21 | 103* | 51* | 1.53 | 75.31 | 94* | 48* | 2.13 | 75.21 | 100* | 42* | 1.20 |
| August | 70.56 | 100* | 40* | 0.03 | 74.34 | 102* | 43* | 4.44 | 75.55 | 104* | 50* | 2.00 | 77.23 | 103* | 54* | 0.26 |
| September | 64.54 | 92* | 40* | 1.69 | 66.50 | 99* | 19* | 0.48 | 64.99 | 99* | 35* | 0.13 | 60.22 | 99* | 22* | 0.60 |
| October | 49.74 | 80* | 20* | 0.11 | 51.42 | 85* | 16* | 0.41 | 57.73 | 90* | 20* | 1.13 | 47.07 | 84* | 6* | 3.10 |
| November | 43.01 | 73* | 12* | 0.03 | 26.43 | 72* | —14* | 1.28 | 27.91 | 60* | —13* | 0.11 | 36.49 | 75* | 2* | 0.05 |
| December | 23.37 | 67* | —18* | 0.22 | 14.81 | 50* | —17* | 0.21 | 15.79 | 50* | —30* | 0.06 | 19.49 | 48* | —25* | 0.24 |
| January | 22.22 | 61* | —11* | 0.05 | 17.14 | 51* | —21* | 0.10 | 17.98 | 49* | —32* | 0.47 | 18.45 | 56* | —28* | 0.11 |
| February | 28.43 | 61* | —20* | 0.76 | 26.76 | 57* | —11* | 0.22 | 24.38 | 63* | —30* | 1.66 | 22.12 | 58* | —18* | 0.21 |
| March | 38.07 | 76* | 5* | 0.18 | 28.86 | 60* | 3* | 0.85 | 37.18 | 73* | —10* | 0.15 | 31.57 | 66* | — 5* | 0.88 |
| April | | | | | 50.18 | 79* | 20* | 1.06 | 42.24 | 85* | 0* | 2.73 | 44.60 | 95* | 11* | 0.58 |
| May | | | | | 61.50 | 96* | 31* | 1.67 | 55.78 | 83* | 18* | 4.71 | 67.71 | 99* | 10* | 1.76 |
| June | 76.14 | 96* | 46* | 0.48 | 72.99 | 96* | 48* | 1.65 | 75.66 | 97* | 53* | 3.13 | 74.70 | 102* | 43* | 5.70 |
| For the year | | | | | 47.26 | 103* | —21* | 13.90 | 47.54 | 104* | —32* | 18.41 | 47.90 | 103* | —28* | 14.69 |

\* These observations are made with self-registering thermometers. The mean is from the standard thermometer.

*Consolidated sick-report, Fort Randall, Dak., 1870–'74.*

| Year. | | 1870–'71. Cases. | Deaths. | 1871–'72. Cases. | Deaths. | 1872–'73. Cases. | Deaths. | 1873–'74. Cases. | Deaths. |
|---|---|---|---|---|---|---|---|---|---|
| Mean strength { Officers | | 11 | | 9 | | 9 | | 11 | |
| { Enlisted men | | 181 | | 171 | | 197 | | 204 | |
| **Diseases.** | | | | | | | | | |
| GENERAL DISEASES, A. | | | | | | | | | |
| Typhoid fever | | 3 | | 1 | | 2 | | | |
| Remittent fever | | 4 | | | | 8 | | 3 | |
| Intermittent fever | | 14 | | 6 | | 7 | | 19 | |
| Other diseases of this group | | 17 | | 14 | | 6 | | 28 | |
| GENERAL DISEASES, B. | | | | | | | | | |
| Rheumatism | | 30 | | 22 | | 13 | | 29 | |
| Syphilis | | 5 | | 1 | | 4 | | 13 | |
| Consumption | | 3 | | | | 1 | | 1 | |
| Other diseases of this group | | 2 | | 3 | | | | 4 | |
| LOCAL DISEASES. | | | | | | | | | |
| Catarrh and bronchitis | | 58 | | 134 | | 61 | | 92 | |
| Pneumonia | | 3 | | | | | | 2 | 1 |
| Pleurisy | | 2 | | | | 1 | | | |
| Diarrhœa and dysentery | | 51 | | 91 | | 90 | 1 | 60 | |
| Hernia | | | | | | 1 | | 2 | |
| Gonorrhœa | | 1 | | 7 | | 2 | | | |
| Other local diseases | | 165 | | 232 | | 157 | 1 | 100 | |
| Alcoholism | | 9 | | 4 | | | | 2 | |
| Total disease | | 367 | | 515 | | 353 | 2 | 355 | 1 |
| VIOLENT DISEASES AND DEATHS. | | | | | | | | | |
| Gunshot wounds | | | 1 | | | 2 | | | |
| Other accidents and injuries | | 56 | | 102 | | 64 | | 42 | |
| Homicide | | | | | | | 1 | | |
| Suicide | | | 1 | | 1 | | | | |
| Total violence | | 56 | 2 | 102 | 1 | 66 | 1 | 42 | |

# FORT RICE, DAKOTA TERRITORY.

## REPORT OF ASSISTANT SURGEON J. W. WILLIAMS, UNITED STATES ARMY.

Fort Rice is located on the west bank of the Missouri River, ten miles above Cannonball River, and twenty-five miles below Fort Abraham Lincoln; latitude, 46° 40′ north; longitude, 23° 27′ west; altitude above the river, 35 feet; above the sea, 2,200 feet. Fort Sully, the nearest military post below, is distant about two hundred miles. Yankton, distant about five hundred miles, is the nearest railway terminus down the river.

The post is built on the main terrace, a level strip of land about seven miles long by one mile wide. The site of the post is near its southern limit, which is a small creek emptying into the Missouri. West the terrace is bounded by broken country; north by the bluffs of the second terrace; east and northeast by the river and a semicircular strip of bottom-land covered with cottonwood. The reservation has been surveyed, but there is no record at the post of the amount of land held reserved. The geological formation is the middle zone of the Fox Hills group of the cretaceous. A deposit of local drift overlies this group on the hills and ravines to the west of the post. In the vicinity of Cannonball River the Fox Hills group is well marked, and may be easily recognized by the more cheerful appearance that it gives to the surface. On the surface, near the mouth of that river, and embedded in the bluffs, are numerous cannonball-shaped concretions, consisting of brown arenaceous limestone, crowded with molluscous fossils, (Hayden.) No fossils are found near the post. The hills and ravines, overlaid with local drift, are sterile; the main terraces would be productive and yield fair crops could water be applied to them. The bottoms are rich and moist, and produce all the hardier vegetables in seasons when there is a scarcity of grasshoppers. Owing to drought the country is but sparsely timbered, except on the bottoms and along ravines, which are water-courses in the spring. The streams are few, narrow, very tortuous, and traverse a great extent of country. West and northwest dry winds prevail, in consequence of which the annual rain-fall is small and evaporation is in excess of precipitation.

The climate is dry and bracing, but rather too stimulating for consumptives, often causing hemorrhage of the lungs in such cases. The prevailing winds, west and northwest, generally blow with much force; east and south winds bring rain during the warm months. Most of the rain falls in May and the early part of June. A light rain-fall in summer alternates with a heavy snow-fall in winter. Summer extends from June 1 to the end of August. The hot months are June and July; August more resembling September in temperature. The mornings and nights of these months are cool, but are rendered unpleasant by myriads of mosquitoes. September and October are the most pleasant months of the year, the sky being nearly cloudless and the winds from the northwest and west. The winters are long, but not uniformly cold, a rise of temperature often above the freezing-point occurring in January. Winter sets in about the middle of November, and ends about the latter part of April. January is the coldest month.

The timber of the country consists of cottonwood, elm, ash, and oak in limited quantities.

The principal animals of the vicinity are the elk, black-tailed deer, long-tailed deer, mule deer, antelope, beaver, panther, black bear, cinnamon bear, otter, large gray wolf, coyote, red fox, gray or silver fox, crossed fox, wild-cat, badger, common mink, small black mink, white-tailed weasel, rabbit, and hare. The buffalo, once so plentiful about here, is now only to be found in the vicinity of the Yellowstone River.

Of birds the following are the most important: great horned owl, (rare;) great snowy owl, (rare;) bald eagle, gray eagle, war-eagle, prairie-hen, sand-hill crane, blue heron, meadow-lark, wild pigeon, (rare;) jack-snipe, land-snipe, curlew, robin-redbreast, pelican, (rare;) common wild duck, swan, wild goose, and magpie.

Fort Rice was established in 1864. The buildings of the post were erected by the Thirteenth Wisconsin Infantry, and consisted of rude huts of cottonwood logs, with roofs of poles and slabs covered with earth. During the year 1868 the fort was rebuilt, the old quarters demolished, and new buildings erected on the same site. Fort Rice is about three hundred yards from the margin of the river. It has the form of a quadrangle 864 by 544 feet, inclosed on three sides (river side since removed) by a stockade ten feet high. There are two sally-ports and one main entrance fronting the river, and two projecting bastions, two stories high, built of squared and dove-tailed logs; on top is a platform and an octagonal sentry-box. Each story of the bastion is 20 feet 4 inches square, and 7 feet high. The buildings within the stockade are as follows, viz: Four company quarters, (east side;) seven buildings for officers, (west side;) hospital, bakery, two storehouses, and library, (south side;) three storehouses and magazine, (north side.) The guard-house and offices are on each side of the main entrance. These buildings surround the parade-ground; each is parallel to the contiguous wall of the fort. The barrack on the extreme north approaches within twenty-two feet of the north wall of the fort; the most southerly is fifty-eight feet from the south wall, the post-bakery standing between the one and the other. Between the contiguous ends of each pair of the barracks is an alley of 10 feet in width, which is insufficient to admit light to the windows that open upon it, and to retard the progress of fire. These barracks, one story high, have balloon frames of pine lumber; all the rest of the wood-work, except the finishing, is of cottonwood sawed at the post. The frames are sheathed and weatherboarded outside, and well shingled; all of the apartments are ceiled with half-inch boards; the walls are lined between the studding with adobe. The buildings are laid upon good foundations or piers, which are banked with clay in winter to prevent the wind from entering through the floor. Each barrack consists of a main building and two Ls or wings extending at right angles toward the stockade, within fifteen feet of which they terminate. The building thus incloses on three sides a yard of 50 by 60 feet. The main building is divided into dormitory, office, and store-room. The dormitory is 73 feet 3 inches by 29 feet by 9 feet 6 inches, (interior measurement.) The office is 13 by 16 feet; the store-room 13 by 13 feet. Average air-space of dormitory per man is 340 cubic feet. Each wing is 60 by 20 feet, and 10 feet from ceiling to floor. One wing is divided into kitchen and mess-room; the other wing contains four rooms, occupied as laundresses' quarters.

The barracks are well lighted by doors and windows, and warmed in the colder season by stoves. Ventilation is very defective, there being no special arrangement for that purpose. Iron bunks are furnished, two to every three men, or about forty-four bunks to each company. The dormitories are much overcrowded. The company sinks are outside the stockade; no sinks are provided for the laundresses. The barrack kitchens, 20 by 19 feet, are sufficiently commodious. The mess-rooms are each 39 by 19 feet. The officers' quarters are seven frame buildings, elevated upon stone foundations, with verandas in front, and arranged as follows, viz: Commanding-officer's quarters, fronting main entrance, 40 by 30 feet, two stories high, four rooms to the story; two cottages, flanking headquarters, each 30 by 27 feet; four buildings, two on either side of the cottages, each 40 by 30 feet, two stories high, (double sets,) two rooms to the story. The dining-rooms and kitchens are in a rear addition or wing. The rooms are finished with lath and plaster, and floors of planed and matched pine flooring. The cottages are lined between the studding with brick.

The magazine is a substantial stone building, 24 by 23 feet on the outside, and 4 feet from the ground to the eaves. The roof is covered with sods; the floor is two feet below the ground outside.

The guard-house, situated to the right of the main entrance, within the stockade, is a frame building 40 by 20 feet, lined inside with cottonwood planks, roofed with pine shingles; and an addition of squared logs, 32 by 20 feet, with dirt-roof, for a prison-room. The main building is divided into a sergeant's room, 12 by 5 feet 6 inches; a prison-room, 13 by 11 feet 6 inches, (not used;) and three cells, 3 by 3 feet each, (not used.) Two doors and nine windows admit light and air.

The post-hospital is substantially a company barrack, and about as well arranged interiorly for the accommodation of the sick, no bath-room and no means of ventilating the ward having been provided. The building faces the north, and is exposed to the violent winter-storms which invariably come from that direction. Until this year it was roofed with cottonwood shingles, which was very little better than a dirt-roof. In summer, rain poured through it into the ward; in winter, snow drifted through it into the attic, and, melting, kept the ward in dampness, dirt, and confusion. A large amount of property stored in the attic, for want of storage-room, was thus destroyed The body of the hospital is 90 by 24 feet, and the Ls 40 by 20 feet. It is built on stone piers, and constructed of similar materials to those used in the barracks, except the ward, steward's room, office, linen-room, and wash-room, which are floored with dressed pine. The dispensary is 23 by 13 by 10 feet; the ward is 62 by 23 by 10 feet, contains twelve beds, and an air-space of 1,188 cubic feet to each. The wash-room, adjoining the ward, is supplied with bath-tub, mirror, towels, basins, and all other necessary articles. There is no sink for the hospital; a commode is used in the ward. The hospital is warmed by stoves and well lighted.

The post-bakery is a one-story frame house 45 by 20 by 10 feet. The oven has the capacity for baking 1,500 rations of bread in twenty-four hours.

The corral, situated one hundred yards from the south wall of the stockade, is built in the form of a hollow square, four stables, a granary, and storehouse forming the sides. A building for the guard and employés occupies the center, and a cattle-yard adjoins the south side of the corral. Two cavalry stables (double sets) built of pine and cottonwood lumber, with dirt-roofs, were erected this year on a site between the corral and river. They are each 372 by 24 by 10 feet.

There are three ice-houses built of logs, with an aggregate capacity of 1,000 tons. The ice is kept in excellent condition.

The only drinking-water used at the post is obtained from the Missouri River, and is the best to be procured in the country; it is brought around daily by the water-wagon, and allowed to stand in barrels till it settles, when it is tolerably clear and quite pleasant to drink. Many believe the water to be injurious; a large amount of constituents are no doubt held in solution or suspension, as no water can possibly be more turbid, particularly in the spring; but they are nearly all mineral, and almost entirely innocuous. Owing to the barren character of the country through which the Missouri flows, to the rapidity of its current, to the absence of sloughs or lagoons along its course, and to the sparseness of the population upon its banks, the amount of decayed organic matter contained in its waters must be comparatively small. Much stress is laid by some upon the number of so-called "alkali springs" and "alkali creeks," that flow into the Upper Missouri, but the evil nature of these is usually overrated; and, besides, they form but an infinitesimal portion of the waters of the river, the chief source of supply being doubtless the snows and rains of the Rocky Mountains and Black Hills. The small and inconstant water-courses that rise in the plains can add but little. It may be remarked, that among those Indians who have dwelt for generations in permanent villages upon the Upper Missouri, drinking almost exclusively of its waters, bronchocele is very common; while among those who roam at large on the steppes, it is not noticed. We read of similar facts being observed among the permanent dwellers on the Saskatchewan, whose headwaters rise near those of the Missouri.

The fort is at a good elevation above the river, and the soil being dry and porous, no artificial drainage is necessary.

Three hundred yards west of the fort, on a gently sloping hill, is the post-cemetery. It contains one hundred and sixty-three graves. The Government should take some steps to remove the bodies buried in this cemetery to some permanent cemetery, as in case the post were abandoned the graves would be desecrated by Indians.

The nearest supply-depots are at Yankton, five hundred miles, and Saint Louis, one thousand eight hundred and ten miles. The eastern mail leaves the post every Wednesday and Saturday, via Bismarck, Moorhead City, and Northern Pacific Railroad; and every Friday, by the way of Grand River, Fort Sully, and Yankton. A party of Indian scouts are employed in the service.

The post is surrounded by lands of the Sioux nation, from which the reservation is taken. The Sioux, who most frequently visit the post, are tall, muscular, enduring, and healthy. There are comparatively few of these Indians in the surrounding country at present, they having gone to the reservation at Standing Rock.

Fort Rice is eligibly located in a sanitary point of view, no diseases occurring which can be charged to the soil or water, and few to the climate. In summer dysentery and diarrhœa occur, but mostly from imprudence in diet; in winter catarrhal affections prevail to a limited extent. A few cases of consumption have been observed. The complaint set in with hemorrhage in every instance, pursued a more or less rapid course, and resembled successive attacks of catarrahal pneumonia in its progress. Venereal diseases are rare.

The plan of the post is faulty, the site being too small by one-half for a post of four companies. The dormitories, in consequence, afford a sufficient air-space for about thirty men only, while the average of the companies which have occupied them has seldom been less than fifty men to the company. This unavoidable overcrowding of the barracks, and a more or less deprivation of fresh vegetable food in years past, have been the chief causes at work impairing the efficiency of its garrisons. During the first years of occupancy, scurvy was a formidable malady, and destroyed many lives. The scorbutic taint has never been absent until this year, when the daily allowance of vegetables was increased to a little over one pound per man. The intimate relation of the vegetable allowance to the percentage of sick at this post is instructive. In 1871, daily allowance of fresh vegtables per man, 9 ounces; annual per cent. of sick, 261. In 1872, daily allowance of fresh vegetables per man, 12 ounces; annual per cent. of sick, 188. In 1873, daily allowance of fresh vegetables per man, 16 ounces; annual per cent. of sick, 108.

*Meteorological report, Fort Rice, Dak., 1870–'74.*

| Month. | 1870–'71. | | | | 1871–'72. | | | | 1872–'73. | | | | 1873–'74. | | | |
|---|---|---|---|---|---|---|---|---|---|---|---|---|---|---|---|---|
| | Temperature. | | | Rain-fall in inches. | Temperature. | | | Rain-fall in inches. | Temperature. | | | Rain-fall in inches. | Temperature. | | | Rain-fall in inches. |
| | Mean. | Max. | Min. | | Mean. | Max. | Min. | | Mean. | Max. | Min. | | Mean. | Max. | Min. | |
| | ° | ° | ° | | ° | ° | ° | | ° | ° | ° | | ° | ° | ° | |
| July | 72.54 | 102 | 49 | 0.72 | 74.99 | 103 | 59 | 1.10 | 70.16 | 99* | 41* | 1.53 | 71.57 | 104* | 43* | 1.79 |
| August | 61.63 | 98 | 39 | 1.41 | 70.25 | 103 | 42 | 0.51 | 70.43 | 102* | 40* | 1.19 | 72.96 | 98* | 39* | 1.36 |
| September | 60.64 | 82 | 38 | 1.14 | 60.92 | 90 | 34 | 0.00 | 57.01 | 94* | 27* | 0.40 | 54.73 | 96* | 23* | 1.16 |
| October | 42.62 | 80 | 25 | 0.96 | 45.35 | 78 | 14 | 0.38 | 48.25 | 84* | 12 | 0.92 | 41.13 | 89* | 12* | 0.80 |
| November | 37.25 | 68 | 18 | 0.00 | 17.80 | 54* | —28* | 0.34 | 23.83 | 56* | —10 | 0.00 | 33.02 | 70* | — 3* | 0.25 |
| December | 16.70 | 50 | —22 | 0.13 | 1.26 | 46* | —34* | 0.00 | 6.76 | 42* | —27 | 0.34 | 15.54 | 42* | —22* | 0.00 |
| January | 9.57 | 49 | —22 | 0.29 | 9.31 | 40* | —28* | 1.50 | 4.11 | 40 | —30 | 0.72 | 10.66 | 46* | —29* | 1.76 |
| February | 16.43 | 46 | —20 | 0.02 | 14.80 | 45* | —31* | 0.00 | 11.59 | 42 | —19 | 1.66 | 13.59 | 40* | —23* | 0.00 |
| March | 26.24 | 57 | — 5 | 0.44 | 20.29 | 42* | —18* | 0.61 | 27.25 | 54 | — 7 | 0.56 | 24.03 | 64* | — 7* | 0.35 |
| April | 42.13 | 73 | 22 | 2.92 | 34.49 | 78* | 1* | 1.22 | 10.78 | 74 | 24 | 0.10 | 41.13 | 87* | 9* | 0.00 |
| May | 62.74 | 89 | 45 | 0.00 | 49.39 | 79* | 32* | 2.32 | 54.79 | 80 | 38 | 1.90 | 64.47 | 97* | 34* | 1.10 |
| June | 69.96 | 97 | 53 | 3.82 | 67.51 | 101* | 32* | 3.73 | 71.98 | 94* | 48* | 2.25 | 69.98 | 102* | 44* | 5.08 |
| For the year | 43.20 | 102 | —22 | 11.85 | 38.86 | 103 | —34* | 11.71 | 40.58 | 102* | —30 | 11.57 | 42.74 | 104* | —29* | 12.85 |

* These observations are made with self-registering thermometers. The mean is from the standard thermometer.

*Consolidated sick-report, Fort Rice, Dak., 1870–'74.*

| Year | | 1870–'71. | | 1871–'72. | | 1872–'73. | | 1873–'74. | |
|---|---|---|---|---|---|---|---|---|---|
| Mean strength { Officers | | 12 | | 11 | | 13 | | 11 | |
| { Enlisted men | | 243 | | 209 | | 235 | | 2b6 | |
| Diseases. | | Cases. | Deaths. | Cases. | Deaths. | Cases. | Deaths. | Cases. | Deaths. |
| GENERAL DISEASES, A. | | | | | | | | | |
| Typhoid fever | | 1 | | 1 | 1 | 1 | | 1 | |
| Remittent fever | | 7 | | 4 | | 3 | | | |
| Intermittent fever | | 27 | | 20 | | 19 | | 2 | |
| Diphtheria | | | | 1 | | | | | |
| Other diseases of this group | | 23 | | 18 | | 6 | | 8 | |
| GENERAL DISEASES, B. | | | | | | | | | |
| Rheumatism | | 48 | | 53 | | 9 | | 8 | |
| Syphilis | | 17 | | 19 | | 13 | | 3 | |
| Consumption | | | | 3 | | 8 | | 2 | |
| Other diseases of this group | | 5 | | 1 | | 1 | | 2 | |
| LOCAL DISEASES. | | | | | | | | | |
| Catarrh and bronchitis | | 129 | | 75 | | 46 | | 3 | |
| Pneumonia | | 2 | 1 | 1 | | 4 | | 1 | |
| Pleurisy | | 3 | | 22 | | 2 | | 3 | |
| Diarrhœa and dysentery | | 85 | | 110 | 1 | 53 | | 5 | |
| Hernia | | 1 | | 3 | | 1 | | | |
| Gonorrhœa | | 4 | | 7 | | | | | |
| Other local diseases | | 131 | | 202 | | 59 | | 26 | |
| Alcoholism | | 1 | | 2 | | 1 | | 8 | |
| Total disease | | 484 | 1 | 542 | 2 | 226 | | 72 | |
| VIOLENT DISEASES AND DEATHS. | | | | | | | | | |
| Gunshot wounds | | | | 1 | | 5 | | 2 | |
| Drowning | | | | | | | 2 | | |
| Other accidents and injuries | | 86 | | 58 | | 22 | | 28 | |
| Homicide | | | | | | | 1 | | |
| Total violence | | 86 | | 59 | | 27 | 3 | 30 | |

# FORT RIPLEY, MINNESOTA.

INFORMATION FURNISHED BY SURGEON J. F. HEAD, ASSISTANT SURGEON C. K. WINNE, AND ACTING ASSISTANT SURGEON J. J. DE LAMATER, UNITED STATES ARMY.

Fort Ripley, established in 1848 under the name of Fort Gaines, is situated in latitude 46° 10′ 30″ north; longitude, 17° 15′ 45″ west. It stands on the west bank of the Mississippi, seven miles below the confluence of the Crow Wing River. The elevation above the water of the river is about twenty feet. The nearest town or settlement is Crow Wing, distant seven miles, on the east side of the Mississippi. Saint Paul, Minn., is distant one hundred and twenty-five miles, and Brainard, the nearest station on the Northern Pacific Railroad, is seventeen miles.

For further particulars of the history and topography of the post, see Circular No. 4, Surgeon-General's Office, December 5, 1870.

The buildings at the post form three sides of a hollow square, each side being 450 feet, and the river forming the fourth side. The quarters and hospital are frame buildings, lathed and plastered inside, and covered externally with boards, sheathing-paper, and weatherboards painted. The walls are filled with brick. Four buildings, one and a half stories in height, are occupied as officers' quarters, two of which are divided each into two sets. Each of the six sets is essentially the same, and consists of a hall, four rooms, pantry, and store-room in the main building. There is an attachment in the rear, consisting of cellar, kitchen, and two small bed-rooms.

The garrison, consisting of two companies, 103 men, are quartered in the barrack, also one and a half stories high, 263 by 22 feet, with rear additions on the flanks and center. The building upon the main floor is divided into two sections; each section contains two dormitories, 32 by 20 by 11 feet, kitchen, and mess-room. The rear projection at the south end contains a dormitory, 33 by 17 feet, occupied by 12 men, a first-sergeant's room, and a room for a library. The projection at the other end of the barrack contains a similar dormitory, 20 by 17 feet, and a first-sergeant's room. The dormitories are well lighted by windows, and are ventilated by shafts leading into the attic, which is unobstructed by partitions, and communicates with the external air by a roof-ventilator and two openings in the front wall. The heating is by wood-stoves. The bunks are iron frames with wooden slats. There is a veranda 8 feet wide extending along the entire front. The officers' quarters and hospital have similar verandas.

The married soldiers and laundresses are quartered in several buildings and parts of buildings scattered about the post.

The hospital is a modification of that prescribed in Circular No. 4 of 1867. It was erected rather hastily of unseasoned lumber in the fall of 1870, to replace one destroyed by fire. In consequence, the wood-work, especially of the floors, has shrunk to such an extent as to cause serious annoyance and discomfort, and keeps the hospital in an unsightly condition. These defects have been remedied in part by a free use of putty and paint, and by new flooring, which was laid in the lower story in the summer of 1873. Considerable is yet required to remedy the defects in the original construction of the building. In particular no means have yet been provided for warming the bath-room in winter or supplying warm water. There is no water-closet within the hospital. A privy of the ordinary construction is placed on the rear line of the hospital grounds. These grounds are uninclosed, and the soil being a loose sand, unprotected by any fence or vegetation, much dust is blown into the hospital by the winds. The coarse sandy character of the soil has thus far rendered the earth-closets at the hospital unavailable.

The guard-house, fitted up in 1872, stands near the bank of the river, and is 48⅓ by 27¼ feet, entirely surrounded by a platform, 5 feet 10 inches wide. The height of the rooms varies from 8⅛ to 9¾ feet. The center of the building is occupied by the guard-room, 26 by 23 feet, leaving a space of 11½ feet at each end. The space at the south end is divided into a prison-room 19 feet wide, and a wash-room 5½ feet; that at the north end comprises an office 6 feet wide, a dark cell 3½ feet, and a prison-room 14 feet. All the apartments, except the cell, are lighted by windows, and all, with the exception of the office, are furnished with ventilators. The cell has two ventilators, one, a foot square, communicating with the outer air, and the other, 6 by 4 inches, opening into the attic. The prison-rooms have ventilating-shafts extending through the roof. The larger room has also a side ventilator. The guard-room has two ceiling-ventilators, each 1½ feet square. The heating is by wood-stoves.

The water-supply is brought from the river by wagons, but there are also several cisterns at the post. There is one of a capacity of 5,000 gallons adjoining the hospital, and two others similar in the grounds at no great distance.

*Meteorological report, Fort Ripley, Minn., 1870-'74.*

| Month. | 1870-'71. | | | | 1871-'72. | | | | 1872-'73. | | | | 1873-'74. | | | |
|---|---|---|---|---|---|---|---|---|---|---|---|---|---|---|---|---|
| | Temperature. | | | Rain-fall in inches. | Temperature. | | | Rain-fall in inches. | Temperature. | | | Rain-fall in inches. | Temperature. | | | Rain-fall in inches. |
| | Mean. | Max. | Min. | | Mean. | Max. | Min. | | Mean. | Max. | Min. | | Mean. | Max. | Min. | |
| July | | | | | 67.61 | 103* | 26* | 3.07 | 66.94 | 100* | 38* | 6.82 | 67.98 | 102* | 49* | 5.46 |
| August | | | | | 64.69 | 89* | 28* | 4.79 | 63.97 | 85* | 34* | 4.10 | 66.89 | 89* | 43* | 2.18 |
| September | 60.64 | 80* | 43* | 4.22 | 55.37 | 92* | 22* | 2.38 | 50.19 | 80* | 12* | 3.92 | 50.48 | 91* | 21* | 1.94 |
| October | 43.71 | 77* | 15* | 1.11 | 41.41 | 73* | 12* | 1.78 | 38.43 | 71* | 9* | 2.19 | 36.93 | 76* | 8* | 4.71 |
| November | 33.73 | 64* | 0* | 0.34 | 19.97 | 53* | —29* | 4.20 | 16.02 | 50* | —30* | 3.64 | 19.57 | 44* | —10* | 2.19 |
| December | 15.49 | 50* | —23* | 0.54 | —0.13 | 39* | —31* | 3.64 | —1.69 | 36* | —40* | 1.34 | 9.21 | 32* | —38* | 1.08 |
| January | 4.96 | 35* | —35* | 1.01 | 5.67 | 32* | —40* | 1.07 | 1.12 | 32* | —40* | 2.09 | 4.04 | 38* | —38* | 0.83 |
| February | 12.49 | 45* | —34* | 0.94 | 11.66 | 46* | —37* | 0.71 | 8.28 | 38* | —35* | 3.41 | 6.05 | 30* | —30* | 0.80 |
| March | 24.86 | 50* | —8* | 3.49 | 15.17 | 52* | —37* | 1.28 | 21.23 | 48* | —35* | 2.76 | 18.93 | 43* | —20* | 2.00 |
| April | 40.39 | 82* | 19* | 3.30 | 39.64 | 80* | 5* | 1.54 | 37.48 | 64* | 10* | 1.19 | 31.90 | 65* | —5* | 0.63 |
| May | 61.91 | 101* | 26* | 0.51 | 51.16 | 80* | 21* | 4.35 | 52.03 | 74* | 29* | 4.59 | 59.05 | 96* | 20* | 2.31 |
| June | 65.60 | 90* | 32* | 4.91 | 63.76 | 92* | 28* | 3.81 | 68.19 | 93* | 46* | 9.18 | 65.67 | 95* | 34* | 9.30 |
| For the year | | | | | 36.33 | 103* | —40* | 32.62 | 35 18 | 100* | —40* | 45.23 | 36.39 | 102* | —38* | 33.43 |

\* These observations are made with self-registering thermometers. The mean is from the standard thermometer.

*Consolidated sick-report, Fort Ripley, Minn., 1870-'74.*

| Year | 1870-'71. | | 1871-'72. | | 1872-'73. | | 1873-'74. | |
|---|---|---|---|---|---|---|---|---|
| Mean strength { Officers | 3 | | 3 | | 3 | | 5 | |
| { Enlisted men | 76 | | 57 | | 53 | | 83 | |
| Diseases. | Cases. | Deaths. | Cases. | Deaths. | Cases. | Deaths. | Cases. | Deaths. |
| *GENERAL DISEASES, A.* | | | | | | | | |
| Remittent fever | 1 | | 3 | | 3 | | 2 | |
| Intermittent fever | 11 | | 15 | | 3 | | 3 | |
| Other diseases of this group | 7 | | 2 | | 4 | | 8 | |
| *GENERAL DISEASES, B.* | | | | | | | | |
| Rheumatism | 13 | | 18 | | 14 | | 14 | |
| Syphilis | 5 | | 2 | | 3 | | 9 | 1 |
| Consumption | | | 2 | | | | | |
| Other diseases of this group | 1 | | 4 | | 1 | | 6 | |
| *LOCAL DISEASES.* | | | | | | | | |
| Catarrh and bronchitis | 17 | | 26 | | 15 | | 63 | |
| Pneumonia | 1 | 1 | 2 | | 2 | | 11 | |
| Diarrhea and dysentery | 26 | | 21 | | 6 | | 18 | |
| Hernia | | | | | | | 1 | |
| Gonorrhœa | 1 | | 2 | | 1 | | 2 | |
| Other local diseases | 56 | | 69 | | 34 | | 117 | |
| Alcoholism | 1 | | 2 | | 3 | | 8 | 1 |
| Total disease | 140 | 1 | 168 | | 89 | | 262 | 2 |
| *VIOLENT DISEASES AND DEATHS.* | | | | | | | | |
| Gunshot wounds | 1 | 1 | | | 1 | | | |
| Other accidents and injuries | 17 | | 24 | | 22 | | 24 | |
| Total violence | 18 | 1 | 24 | | 23 | | 24 | |

# FORT SEWARD, DAKOTA TERRITORY.

### REPORT OF ACTING ASSISTANT SURGEON E. W. DU BOSE, UNITED STATES ARMY.

Fort Seward, formerly Fort Cross, Dakota Territory, is situated about midway between the Red River of the North and the Missouri River, on the right bank of the James or Dakota River, at the crossing of the Northern Pacific Railroad, and in latitude 46° 52' north, and longitude 21° 35' west; height above the sea, 1,393 feet.

It was established June 3, 1872, by Capt. J. C. Bates, commanding Company B, Twentieth Infantry, U. S. A., pursuant to Special Orders No. 37, headquarters Department of Dakota.

The military reservation is bounded on the south by the Northern Pacific Railroad, and extends due north, and has for its eastern and western boundaries James River and Pipestem Creek, respectively, and contains about one square mile of land. On the bottoms west of the James River, about one-fourth of a mile from the post, a piece of ground, containing about eight acres, has been inclosed for post and hospital gardens. The soil is good, and produces beets, beans, cabbages, corn, lettuce, onions, pease, parsnips, potatoes, and turnips.

The country, for many miles surrounding the post, is a high, gravelly, rolling, dry, and treeless prairie, covered with short grass growing in little tufts or bunches, making good grazing in summer, but not growing in sufficient quantity to pay for harvesting except in little hollows, where the surface-water from the rains and melting snow has collected. There are a few small lakes scattered here and there, the waters of which, almost without exception, are somewhat alkaline; most of them can, however, be used for drinking purposes. The only land which will pay for cultivation is in the bottoms along the streams. The banks of all streams are too high to make it practicable to use the water for purposes of irrigation. The greatest difficulty to overcome in the settlement of this country will be the lack of timber for buildings, fences, and fuel. Practically there is none in all the vast area of country between the Missouri River and the Red River of the North.

There is a slight fringe of timber, chiefly elm, box-elder, willow, and scrub-oak, along the Cheyenne and James Rivers, but even there insufficient for the use of farmers who may settle upon these streams. Coal in any amount or of good quality is as yet undiscovered; nor is stratified rock known to exist. The winters are long and extremely cold, and rapid changes in the temperature are common, sometimes as much as 40° in twenty-four hours. But, on account of the dryness of the atmosphere, these changes seem not to affect the general healthfulness of the country.

The thermometer ranges from 100° in the shade in the summer to —50° in the winter. The snow-fall is not great, but it is not uncommon to have it in May and October, and destructive frosts sometimes occur early in August. The prevailing winds are from the northwest, and, it may be truly said, "are never weary." In winter, severe and blinding storms of wind and snow are of frequent occurrence. Grasshoppers are numerous, and pass over the country in great clouds.

There are but few wild animals in this vicinity.

Fort Totten is eighty miles north; Camp Hancock and Fort A. Lincoln, about one hundred miles west; Forts Wadsworth and Abercrombie, one hundred and twenty-five and one hundred and fifteen miles southeast, respectively. Fargo, Dak., and Moorhead, Minn., are ninety-three miles east, on the Red River of the North.

Saint Paul, Minn., and Saint Louis, Mo., are the principal depots of supply, and the method of transportation is via the Northern Pacific Railroad. The commissariat is well supplied with all articles on the authorized list.

The site of the post is a gravelly plateau, about forty-five feet above the level of the James River, and in the angle formed by the junction of Pipestem Creek and James River. On the east, south, and west sides of this plateau the ground descends very abruptly, affording excellent natural drainage to such extent as to render artificial drainage unnecessary. The principal buildings form a rectangular parallelogram. On the southern side is situated the barrack, which is of sufficient capacity for two companies. It is a large building, 230 by 24 feet, 10 feet in height, divided, commencing at one end, into four sets laundresses' quarters, 15 by 24 feet each, divided into two rooms, 15 by 14 and 15 by 10 feet; company-kitchen, 15 by 24 feet; mess-room, 40 by 24 feet; dormitory, 64½ by 24 feet; vacant room, 35½ by 24 feet; and company-office and store-room, each 16 by 12 feet. All the rooms, except the vacant one, have been ceiled with matched-pine boards. Ventilation has, to some extent, been provided for by arranging two apertures, about two feet square, in the ceiling of the dormitory. A veranda, 8 feet wide, extends along each side of the building. There are seventeen windows and nine doors on each side, and two windows in each end. About forty feet south of the barrack is a small wash-room, furnished with water-barrels, hand-basins, and a heating-stove. It is connected with a wood-shed.

At the southeastern angle, and on the eastern side, is situated the guard-house, 30 by 20 by 10 feet, the guard-room being 18 feet 6 inches by 19 feet, with three windows; the prison-room, 10 by 19 feet, with two windows.

On the north side, and on a ridge slightly above the level of the other buildings, are situated the officers' quarters. These consist of three one-story double cottages, 46 by 31½ feet, containing two sets of quarters of two rooms each, 15 feet square, and connecting by folding doors, and opening into a hall 6½ feet wide and separate to each set of quarters. (See Figure 63.) Over each set of quarters is a room 12 by 15 feet, with dormer-window, which is intended for the use of a servant.

Attached to these cottages is an L, 27 feet 10 inches by 31 feet 6 inches. This is divided into a dining-room and kitchen for each set of quarters. Connected with each dining-room is a pantry 5½ by 7½ feet. There is but one cellar to each building.

At the northwest angle, sixty feet south of a line with the officers' quarters, and on the west side, one hundred feet west of a line with the commissary store-house, is situated the hospital. The building is constructed of lumber, imitative of the plan in Circular No. 2, July 27, 1871, Plate IV, for a provisionary hospital of one story. The site is well adapted to the purpose. On the north and west sides the ground rises to an elevation of twelve or fourteen feet, affording some protection from the cold winds in winter, which usually blow from those directions. Immediately in rear of the hospital the ground descends into a ravine, which gives good drainage into the James River.

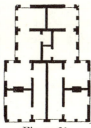

Figure 63.

On the west side is situated the subsistence storehouse, 120 by 25 feet. The southern portion of this building is divided into two small rooms, each 12 feet 6 inches by 20 feet, and used as the office of the assistant commissary of subsistence, and as a store-room for small stores.

At the southwest angle and on the west side is situated the scouts' quarters, 52 by 25 feet, and divided into a kitchen, 11 feet 2 inches by 25 feet, a squad-room, 23 feet 6 inches by 25 feet, and a sergeant's room and store-room, each 12 by 15 feet.

At the foot of the plateau, and between it and the railroad, which is about one hundred yards south of the barracks of the enlisted men, are a small building, erected in the autumn of 1871 as a shelter for a detachment of Company C, Twentieth Infantry, on duty at this place at that time, and before the establishment of the post; a small building used as a temporary storehouse by the Quartermaster's Department; the stable, 125 by 30 feet; the carpenters' shop; the bakery with capacity sufficient for three companies, and the blacksmith and saddlers' shops.

All the foregoing are frame buildings, one story high, and such as are used as quarters have double floors, with tarred paper between; the sides have, first, a layer of inch boards, then one of tarred paper, and over this the clapboards; the interior consists of a layer of inch boards, covered with paper-plastering boards.

The appliances for extinguishing fire are three of Babcock's fire-extinguishers, which are kept properly charged and located in the guard-house, the quartermaster's office, and the office of the assistant commissary of subsistence, respectively, and fire-buckets.

Water at present is obtained from the Pipestem Creek, about three-fourths of a mile distant, and is hauled to the post in a water-wagon. It contains considerable alkaline and vegetable matter, and in summer is rather unpalatable. James River, a tributary of the Missouri, is a small stream about twenty-five feet in width, flowing with a sluggish current in a course almost due south. The water contains a considerable amount of alkaline and vegetable matter, but can be used for drinking purposes, although it is not agreeable to the taste.

*Meteorological report, Fort Seward, Dak., 1873–'74.*

| Month. | 1870–'71. Temperature. | | | Rain-fall in inches. | 1871–'72. Temperature. | | | Rain-fall in inches. | 1872–'73. Temperature. | | | Rain-fall in inches. | 1873–'74. Temperature. | | | Rain-fall in inches. |
|---|---|---|---|---|---|---|---|---|---|---|---|---|---|---|---|---|
| | Mean. | Max. | Min. | | Mean. | Max. | Min. | | Mean. | Max. | Min. | | Mean. | Max. | Min. | |
| | ° | ° | ° | | ° | ° | ° | | ° | ° | ° | | ° | ° | ° | |
| July | | | | | | | | | | | | | | | | |
| August | | | | | | | | | | | | | 67.41 | 96* | 40* | 1.93 |
| September | | | | | | | | | | | | | 67.59 | 99* | 43* | 5.14 |
| October | | | | | | | | | | | | | 48.63 | 84* | 18* | 0.36 |
| November | | | | | | | | | | | | | 36.08 | 83* | 0* | 0.28 |
| December | | | | | | | | | | | | | 23.91 | 64* | −10* | 0.42 |
| January | | | | | | | | | | | | | 10.95 | 41* | −26* | 0.25 |
| February | | | | | | | | | 0.48 | 30 | −35* | 0.34 | 5.14 | 42* | −30* | 0.38 |
| March | | | | | | | | | 5.40 | 37 | −30* | 0.32 | 7.15 | 37* | −25* | 0.20 |
| April | | | | | | | | | 18.83 | 46 | −32* | 0.36 | 14.69 | 58* | −25* | 0.39 |
| May | | | | | | | | | 37.09 | 70* | 18* | 0.22 | 35.60 | 87* | 1* | 0.22 |
| June | | | | | | | | | 51.72 | 76* | 25* | 3.10 | 60.43 | 99* | 28* | 3.10 |
| | | | | | | | | | 70.38 | 98* | 42* | 3.14 | 66.61 | 98* | 37* | 5.83 |
| For the year | | | | | | | | | | | | | 37.01 | 99* | −30* | 18.50 |

* These observations are made with self-registering thermometers. The mean is from the standard thermometer.

*Consolidated sick-report, Fort Seward, Dak., 1871–'74.*

| Year | | 1871–'72.* | | 1872–'73. | | 1873–'74. | |
|---|---|---|---|---|---|---|---|
| Mean strength { Officers | | 2 | | 3 | | 3 | |
| { Enlisted men | | 50 | | 74 | | 50 | |
| Diseases. | | Cases. | Deaths. | Cases. | Deaths. | Cases. | Deaths. |
| GENERAL DISEASES, A. | | | | | | | |
| Intermittent fever | | ...... | ...... | 1 | ...... | ...... | ...... |
| Other diseases of this group | | ...... | ...... | 5 | ...... | 4 | ...... |
| GENERAL DISEASES, B. | | | | | | | |
| Rheumatism | | ...... | ...... | 4 | ...... | 6 | ...... |
| Syphilis | | ...... | ...... | 1 | ...... | 1 | ...... |
| Consumption | | ...... | ...... | 2 | 1 | 2 | ...... |
| LOCAL DISEASES. | | | | | | | |
| Catarrh and bronchitis | | 1 | ...... | 20 | ...... | 6 | ...... |
| Diarrhœa and dysentery | | ...... | ...... | 16 | ...... | 9 | ...... |
| Gonorrhœa | | ...... | ...... | 1 | ...... | ...... | ...... |
| Other local diseases | | 3 | ...... | 21 | ...... | 13 | ...... |
| Alcoholism | | ...... | ...... | 1 | ...... | ...... | ...... |
| Total disease | | 4 | ...... | 72 | 1 | 41 | ...... |
| VIOLENT DISEASES AND DEATHS. | | | | | | | |
| Gunshot wounds | | ...... | ...... | 1 | ...... | 2 | ...... |
| Other accidents and injuries | | ...... | ...... | 27 | ...... | 9 | ...... |
| Total violence | | ...... | ...... | 28 | ...... | 11 | ...... |

\* One month only.

---

# FORT SHAW, MONTANA TERRITORY.

## REPORTS OF SURGEON F. L. TOWN AND ASSISTANT SURGEON J. D. HALL, UNITED STATES ARMY.

Fort Shaw, Montana Territory, is located on Sun River, about twenty miles above its mouth, in latitude 47° 30′ north, longitude 34° 1′ west. The elevation above the sea-level is probably about 3,000 feet. The valley of Sun River is about fifty miles in length, with a variable width of two to five miles, and its general direction is nearly due east and west. Fort Shaw, as a military post, may be said to date from June 30, 1867, when four companies under command of Major William Clinton, Thirteenth Infantry, moved on to the selected site and went into camp. (For history and topography, see report in Circular No. 4, Surgeon-General's Office, 1870, page 409.)

Below the reservation, a good many ranches have been taken up in the valley by settlers, also above the reservation and on the south fork of the river. Several other ranches are located in the hills to the south.

The larger valleys of the Territory, viz, those of the Gallatin, Deer Lodge, Bitter Root, and other rivers, have extensive areas under cultivation. All of them contain much more arable land than Sun River Valley. These valleys produce already large quantities of oats, barley, and wheat, as well as vegetables of nearly all kinds. Grain (with the exception of corn) for the use of the public animals is obtained exclusively in the Territory. Potatoes, onions, turnips, carrots, and cabbages, are generally abundant and cheap. The wheat grown in the Territory is almost entirely of the kind called spring-wheat, owing to the open winters and high winds here prevalent. Prob- ably owing to the lack of winter-wheat, and of first-class mills, the flour is inferior to that brought from the States. The quality of Montana flour seems to be improving, however, and it is found at this post that with the addition of a small proportion of States flour (about one-fifth) to it, this flour makes excellent bread.

Various kinds of large game abound in the country, though not so plentiful in the immediate vicinity of the post. The white-tailed deer frequents the brush along the river; black-tailed deer are found on the higher prairies, and antelopes are quite numerous everywhere. Bands of elk graze along the mountain-slopes, and the mountain-sheep ("big-horns") inhabit the bolder inclines. Hunting these animals affords plenty of sport for those who have much patience and scorn fatigue. Buffaloes approach in winter this side of the Marias and Teton Rivers, and are found in great numbers between here and Fort Benton, sixty-five miles east. Wolves, coyotes, foxes, hares, rabbits, polecats, prairie-dogs, and gophers inhabit the prairies, while grizzly, black, and cinnamon bears, the panther, and lynx are less numerous, and generally confine themselves to the vicinity of the mountains. Wild ducks of various species, such as mallard and teal, likewise wild geese, brant, and wild swans, frequent the rivers and sloughs. Prairie-chickens are found in abundance. The sage-hen, magpie, and the snipe, called Wilson's, are occasionally seen. The curlew, hawk, horned owl, and American eagle are common. The fool-hen and mountain-grouse are also found among the mountains.

The valley is almost destitute of water, aside from the river. A few small springs flow out of the foot-hills along the valley, but generally their feeble rills scarcely more than moisten a few yards or rods of the prairie-bottom, in which they are speedily lost. A large spring or springs come up in the prairie-bottom opposite to and about one and a half miles distant from the post, and form an extensive slough. This slough remains the year round, and is a favorite resort of various species of wild ducks.

The climate of the Territory is exceedingly dry all the year round. At other seasons than the spring and early summer, the showers seem scarcely at all to moisten the exsiccated soil beneath the surface. Snow rarely lies on the ground long after a storm. High westerly winds prevail and drive much of it into drifts; at the same time the current of dry atmosphere moving over the surface melts the snow, and bears away the moisture quite as fast as melted. It is interesting to watch the snow-banks thus mysteriously dwindle away and disappear, perhaps altogether, without leaving the customary puddles of mud and water behind. Snow on the mountains is usually abundant and of great depth. The roads in winter are, as a rule, in fine condition, and the wheeling good. The want of humidity in the atmosphere is to be ascribed partially, perhaps, to the altitude, but is also largely due, probably, to the obstructions of high mountain-chains to the west. The Cascade Range is a formidable obstacle to the passing inland of clouds gathered over the areas of the Pacific. The intervening mountains receive contributions in rains, as the vapors climb to the higher plains and cooler atmosphere beyond, and the main divide of the Rocky Mountains offers the final barrier to the arrival of moisture to the great plains on their eastern slopes. The extremes of mean temperature, although considerable, are not so great, perhaps, between the summer and winter months as one might anticipate, considering the high latitude.

The diurnal oscillations of temperature, however, are usually quite marked at all seasons of the year. The variations in the daily observations, which are registered at 7 o'clock a. m. and 2 o'clock and 9 o'clock p. m., respectively, are frequently from 20° to 30° Fahrenheit. Hence it follows that the nights are generally cool in summer, although the temperature may be high at midday.

The daily oscillation of temperature in July, 1874, was found to average about 35° Fahrenheit. This fact, taken in connection with the fact that no intermittent fever is found here, tends to subvert the theory recently advocated, that intermittent fever is due to excessive diurnal oscillations of temperature.

The heat of summer is quite inconstant; a high temperature rarely obtains for more than three or four days in succession. In winter, likewise, the periods of intense cold are infrequent, and scarcely continue for more than a week at a time. Winds are exceedingly prevalent at all seasons of the year, though they relax somewhat during the summer months. The fact that they attain a monthly mean force of three and four (which is the equivalent of a constant and uniform velocity of 10 to 20 miles an hour) through three-fourths of the months in a year sufficiently indicates this. Their usual direction is down the valley from the west. The location of the post is, however, very favorable to catch the full force of winds. The valley is narrowed slightly here by an encroachment of the bluffs on the south. The air-currents are consequently driven past the post at a somewhat higher velocity than elsewhere.

The post is built around a square of 400 feet side, and very nearly in accordance with plans designed by General Reeve in 1867. The adobe brick was used exclusively in constructing the walls of the buildings. The dimensions of the brick used are 6 inches by 12 inches, with a thickness of 4 inches. All outside walls of buildings are 18 inches in thickness, and the inside walls, likewise of adobes, are 1 foot in thickness. The officers' quarters especially are well finished inside throughout; the walls are plastered, the doors and windows cased, and painted white.

The company quarters are four buildings, each consisting of a main building 102 by 32 feet, with two wings in the rear; one 21 by 60½ feet, divided into a mess-room 18 by 40, and a kitchen 18 by 18 feet, inside measurements; the other, 18 by 64½ feet, divided into four rooms, each 15 by 15 feet inside, for laundresses' quarters. The main building is divided into an orderly-sergeant's room, 15 by 15 feet, with a company store-room in rear, 15 by 14 feet; and four dormitories, each 20 by 30 feet, all inside measurements. The rooms are all 9 feet in height. Each set of buildings incloses three sides of a court. Two of these sets front on the north side of the parade, one at each end of the line; the other two face each other at the north end of the east and west sides of the parade. Each dormitory is well lighted by four windows, 12 square feet of glass to a window, or 48 square feet of glass to a dormitory. A hole 20 inches square is cut through the ceiling of each dormitory, to assist in ventilation. The gables of these buildings, like all others at the post, except the two prison-rooms, are of wood, clapboarded. At present the barracks are occupied by seven companies, crowded into fourteen of the sixteen dormitories. The maximum occupancy in the present reduced state of the companies is not over eighteen men to a dormitory, or 300 cubic feet of air-space per man. Should the companies be filled up to standard, there may be twenty-five men to a dormitory, or only 216 cubic feet to each man.

The laundresses' quarters are generally insufficient. They consist of the above-mentioned sixteen rooms in the wings of the barracks. Only one room is allowed to each, as a rule; the family of each usually numbers from four to six. A small shed or tent has in most cases been put up at the rear of each room, which relieves a little the narrow limits.

The two dormitories not occupied by the troops are used as reading and court-martial rooms.

All the barrack buildings were refloored and reshingled in 1873.

Two buildings for company mess-rooms and kitchens were erected in 1872, some distance in rear of the north barracks. They are balloon-framed, clapboarded; are ample in size, but not so warm nor convenient as the ordinary mess-rooms of adobe attached to the barrack.

The guard-house and band quarters are in a building consisting of a main portion, fronting the east side of the parade, near the center, 68 by 30 feet, with two wings in rear. The building contains the band dormitory, 19 by 30 feet; present occupancy, ten men, giving an air-space of 513 cubic feet per man; sergeant and drum-major's rooms; front room, 15 by 15 feet; back room, 15 by 14 feet; band mess-room, 15 by 15 feet; band kitchen, 15 by 15 feet; one laundress' quarters, 15 by 15 feet; guard-room, 17 by 30 feet, with an alcove 10 by 14 feet added; two prison-rooms of equal size, 22 by 21 feet, built of stone, one built in 1873; and an officer of the guard's room, 10 by 15 feet. The prison-rooms are well lighted by a window in front and rear of each; ventilated by doors and windows; sufficient at present. The present small occupancy of nine men gives air-space 924 cubic feet per man; but with the maximum of thirty, which has existed, the air-space per man would be only 277 feet. All the rooms are 9 feet in height.

The commanding officer's quarters contain a hall, 7 feet wide, with stairway; rooms, each 15 by 15 feet; kitchen, 15 by 12 feet, with pantry and small cellar underneath; servants' room, 15 by 10 feet, and two garret-rooms.

This building is situated on the south side of the parade, fronting on the line, at the center.

The officers' quarters are a double set, under the same roof; hall, 7 feet wide, with stairway; front room, 15 by 15 feet; back room, 13 by 15 feet; small mess-room cut off from hall, 9 by 15 feet; kitchen, 15 by 12 feet, with a pantry and small cellar underneath; servants' room, 15 by 10 feet. Each set of quarters has also a garret-room.

There are six of these buildings—four fronting on the south line of the parade, (two each side of the commanding officer's quarters,) and one on the east, another on the west lines at the south end.

District and post headquarters, on the west side of parade, just north of the center, is 68 feet front. Offices, district headquarters, front rooms, 14 by 15 feet; rear rooms, 14 by 14 feet; offices, post head-quarters, front rooms, 13 by 15 feet; rear rooms, 13 by 14 feet; non-commissioned-staff quarters, each 15 by 15 feet; hall, 7 feet wide, with stairway.

The hospital is 82 feet front. Its arrangement is shown in Figure 64.

A, ward, 24 by 44 feet; B, bath-room, 8½ by 11 feet; G, dead-room, 8½ by 11 feet; C, office, 12 by 18 feet; D, dispensary, 12 by 16 feet; H, main hall; K, kitchen, 12 by 16 feet; L, steward's room, 12 by 15 feet; M, small ward or dining-room, 18 by 30 feet; N, attendants' room, 12 by 18 feet; V, matron's room, 12 by 15 feet. All rooms except the wards are 9 feet high in the clear. The small ward is designed for six beds; mean height, 12 feet; 6,480 cubic feet air-space, or 1,080 cubic feet per bed; habitually used as a dining-room. Main ward, capacity sixteen beds, 24 by 44 feet; mean height, 14

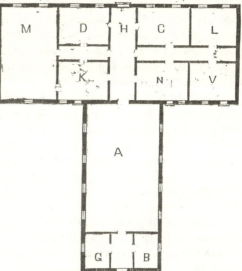

Figure 64.—Scale, 30 feet to 1 inch.

feet; 14,784 cubic feet air-space, or 924 cubic feet air-space per bed. The main hall is 8 feet wide, with stairway side halls, each 4 feet wide; rear hall, 6 feet wide. Shaft-ventilation alone is used in the wards, because of winds and the high latitude. A commodious store-room is finished off under the roof over the surgery, dispensary, &c. The hospital grounds are limited and without shade trees, as the soil is a bed of coarse gravel and pebbles.

This hospital is not built in accordance with the regulation plan, but it seems pretty well suited to this climate. The building seems ample in size, and to be well-conditioned in regard to light, warmth, and ventilation. The grounds have lately been inclosed by a fence, which, by allowing a grass-plot to be kept in front, will add to the appearance of the place. Inside blinds are to be put up at all the windows, with some other needed improvements and repairs. The building stands on the west side of the parade, just south of the headquarters building.

Commissary of subsistence and quartermasters' storehouses are a set of buildings situated on the north side of the parade-ground, in the center of the line, 90 feet front, consisting of two build-ings, each 30 by 90 feet, running north and south, parallel to each other, with a space 30 feet wide between them. These buildings are connected together at the south or front ends by a building 17 by 30 feet. This set of buildings contains office of commissary of subsistence, 16 by 14 feet; clerk's room, 13 by 14 feet; issuing-room, 30 by 15 feet; store-rooms, each 27 by 30 feet; cellar for sub-sistence stores, full size of back store-room; quartermaster's issuing-room, 27 by 30 feet; store-rooms, each 27 by 30 feet. Yard, 30 by 60 feet, inclosed at the rear by a high wall and gate. There is also a storehouse, built in 1872, of sandstone. It is located directly in rear of the old set of store-houses, and between the new frame mess-halls; is 120 by 45 by 10 feet, and runs east and west.

A new post bakery was erected in 1872. It is built of sandstone; is 60 by 20 feet, 9 feet in height, divided into two rooms; one 44½ by 17 feet, (the bakery proper,) the other 12½ by 17 feet, used as a sleeping-room by the bakers, and is located just east of the eastern frame mess-hall. It is well furnished, and ample for all demands of the post.

A stable, on a stone foundation, balloon-frame, clapboarded, 30 by 232½ by 9 feet, divided into a stable proper, with accommodation for 108 animals, with two rooms, one 10 by 9 feet, the other 9 by 9 feet, in east end, used as granary and saddler-shop; and four rooms in west end, two 9 by 12 feet each, one room 8 by 9 feet, and one 9 by 5 feet, used as granary, harness-room, sleeping-room, and sitting-room. This building stands east and west, and is located on the site of the old corral and stables at the northeast corner of the garrison.

The new blacksmith-shop, situated north and west of the stable, is similar in construction to it.

All the buildings above described have permanent shingled roofs.

The privies and out-houses of the officers' quarters are built of adobes, and are in fair condition;

the privies belonging to the hospital are of wood and in satisfactory condition, especially one newly built, which is movable, as it should be; that of the guard-house is similar; those of the laundresses' quarters are insufficient and in bad condition; those of the enlisted men are of wood, and placed on the bank of the river, two hundred to three hundred feet from the barracks—too far off for convenience, but they have the advantage of being pretty sure to be inoffensive.

The temporary wooden storehouse on the east side of the parade, the old stables, hay-ricks, water-tanks, and temporary bakery have been demolished.

The supply of water is obtained at present exclusively from the river, and is distributed to the post by means of a water-cart. The water is comparatively wholesome, except perhaps during rains or the melting of snow, when water which has percolated through the alkaline soil of the valley finds its way into the river. This gives the water a saline taste, and renders it liable to disturb the bowels somewhat. Water may be reached in wells by digging a little below the level of the bed of the river, but it is not suitable for use, for the reason above indicated. The commanding officer has brought a running-stream of water on the parade-ground from the river. A ditch receives the water about six miles above the post, and its entire length is some eight miles. The river at that point is sixty feet or more above the level of the parade. This was an enterprise of great labor and not a little difficulty. The stream is made to run around and within the inclosure of the post, and is very convenient, especially for irrigation. It gives life to the vegetation about the post. Surface drainage only is employed; the slope toward the river is very gentle; water, however, seldom stands on the surface in this dry climate.

The post and company gardens occupy an extensive tract about a quarter of a mile southwest of the post. They are irrigated from the ditch, and produce an ample supply of vegetables for the garrison.

The grasshoppers which annually swarm in myriads in many localities, and are so destructive to vegetation, seldom invade the valley in numbers sufficient to inflict great injury. In 1867 they were quite numerous, and where they prevailed the crops of the settlers suffered.

The cemetery is located about half a mile west of the post.

The prevailing diseases of the post and vicinity are epidemic catarrhs during the fall and winter, and catarrhal inflammations of all mucous membranes; acute diarrhœa, frequently dysenteric, has been especially prevalent at the post; at the same time many cases of febricula occur. Attacks of acute rheumatism are very common notwithstanding the dryness of the climate; probably the sudden transition from a dry to a moist atmosphere, when storms occur, which are often attended with considerable fluctuations of temperature, favors the development of this disease. Remittent and typho-malarial, and probably enteric, fevers are not infrequent in the spring and fall, especially among miners and hunters, or persons who are generally without shelter; these in the parlance of the country are termed "mountain fevers" indiscriminately. Three cases of typho-malarial fever have occurred at the post, two of citizens and one a soldier, and with a fatal termination in each instance. I have known of no cases of intermittent fever that have with certainty originated in the country; neither is phthisis pulmonalis incident to the climate, so far as I have observed; incipient phthisis is frequently apparently arrested in this climate, though but imperfectly if tuberculous exudation has taken place to any extent. Small-pox, when it occurs, makes dreadful ravages among the Indian tribes. A Catholic father, who is laboring with the Blackfeet Indians, gave me the following statement of deaths from small-pox in the Blackfeet Nation alone, from December 2, 1869, to May 1, 1870: Men, 681; women, 378; and of children, 341; this gives a total of 1,400 deaths from small-pox in a population of perhaps 7,000 or 8,000 souls. The younger members of the tribe suffered most, since many of the older members had previously had the disease. A famine fever (relapsing fever probably) also prevailed in connection with small-pox, and increased the mortality. The white population has also suffered from small-pox to some extent the past year.

There is a post-office at Fort Shaw, and a mail-route from Corinne, on the Central Pacific Railroad, via Helena, to Fort Benton, Mont. Coaches pass regularly over the road, and bring the mail three times a week. The distance from the post to Corinne is about five hundred miles. A telegraph-wire extends along the same route, with an office at Fort Shaw.

*Meteorological report, Fort Shaw, Mont., 1870–'74.*

| Month. | 1870–'71. | | | | 1871–'72. | | | | 1872–'73. | | | | 1873–'74. | | | |
|---|---|---|---|---|---|---|---|---|---|---|---|---|---|---|---|---|
| | Temperature. | | | Rain-fall in inches. | Temperature. | | | Rain-fall in inches. | Temperature. | | | Rain-fall in inches. | Temperature. | | | Rain-fall in inches. |
| | Mean. | Max. | Min. | | Mean. | Max. | Min. | | Mean. | Max. | Min. | | Mean. | Max. | Min. | |
| July................... | 72.87 | 101 | 54* | 0.22 | 73.62 | 104 | 45 | 0.00 | 69.06 | 112* | 45 | 1.74 | 72.36 | 100* | 39* | 0.38 |
| August............... | 61.54 | 102* | 24* | 1.64 | 66.49 | 100 | 41 | 0.00 | 66.25 | 88* | 49 | 0.64 | 53.71 | 87* | 34* | 0.36 |
| September........... | 56.42 | 94 | 22 | 0.54 | 56.07 | 83 | 38 | 0.30 | 54.29 | 93* | 26 | 0.92 | 43.21 | 67* | 22* | 0.22 |
| October ............. | 45.56 | 88 | 6 | 0.32 | 48.90 | 83 | 28 | 0.74 | 53.08 | 91* | 21 | 0.18 | 37.06 | 63* | 5* | 0.14 |
| November............ | 40.85 | 62 | 8 | 0.66 | 19.92 | 60 | −37 | 0.79 | 29.01 | 80* | −18 | 0.58 | 31.07 | 60* | − 8* | 0.23 |
| December............ | 25.65 | 54 | −13 | 0.27 | 7.20 | 49* | −37* | 0.96 | 21.53 | 74* | −18 | 0.59 | 21.97 | 52* | −17* | 0.28 |
| January............. | 25.48 | 60 | −20 | 0.32 | 29.12 | 45* | −21 | 0.21 | 25.04 | 67* | −18 | 0.44 | 22.98 | 54 | −17 | 0.29 |
| February............ | 26.92 | 56 | −28 | 0.46 | 34.71 | 70* | −14 | 0.36 | 24.56 | 71* | −18 | 0.67 | 21.39 | 45 | −13 | 0.20 |
| March.............. | 35.53 | 54 | 14 | 0.24 | 37.98 | 81* | 6 | 0.89 | 41.69 | 79* | 1 | 0.04 | 22.18 | 56 | −13* | 0.38 |
| April............... | 41.69 | 72 | 26 | 1.40 | 43.34 | 67* | 27 | 0.41 | 48.87 | 93* | 17 | 0.50 | 44.72 | 78* | 22* | 0.08 |
| May............... | 56.57 | 78 | 37 | 0.48 | 51.71 | 89* | 35 | 0.36 | 57.83 | 98* | 32 | 3.38 | 57.60 | 90* | 30* | 1.06 |
| June ............... | 70.63 | 92 | 48 | 0.26 | 66.19 | 97* | 39* | 0.39 | 66.04 | 98* | 33* | 0.26 | 62.26 | 87* | 40* | 1.14 |
| For the year....... | 46.89 | 102* | −28 | 6.81 | 44.60 | 104 | −37* | 5.41 | 46.43 | 112* | −18 | 9.94 | 40.88 | 100* | −17 | 4.76 |

* These observations are made with self-registering thermometers. The mean is from the standard thermometer.

*Consolidated sick-report, Fort Shaw, Mont., 1870–'74.*

| Year ...................................................... | 1870–'71. | | 1871–'72. | | 1872–'73. | | 1873–'74. | |
|---|---|---|---|---|---|---|---|---|
| Mean strength.................................. { Officers........... | 14 | | 11 | | 15 | | 15 | |
| { Enlisted men...... | 224 | | 197 | | 273 | | 327 | |
| Diseases. | Cases. | Deaths. | Cases. | Deaths. | Cases. | Deaths. | Cases. | Deaths. |
| GENERAL DISEASES, A. | | | | | | | | |
| Typhoid fever............................... | | | 1 | | | | 1 | |
| Remittent fever ............................ | 1 | | | | | | 1 | |
| Intermittent fever.......................... | | | 2 | | 2 | | 15 | |
| Other diseases of this group.............. | 25 | | 18 | | 61 | | 95 | |
| GENERAL DISEASES, B. | | | | | | | | |
| Rheumatism................................ | 11 | | 5 | | 18 | | 54 | |
| Syphilis................................... | 6 | | 5 | | 6 | | 10 | |
| Consumption............................... | 2 | | | | 2 | | 1 | |
| Other diseases of this group.............. | 2 | | | | 2 | | 2 | |
| LOCAL DISEASES. | | | | | | | | |
| Catarrh and bronchitis.................... | 45 | | 16 | | 40 | | 104 | |
| Pneumonia................................. | | | 1 | | 2 | 1 | 4 | |
| Pleurisy................................... | | | 2 | | | | 1 | |
| Diarrhœa and dysentery.................. | 59 | | 20 | | 34 | | 44 | |
| Hernia.................................... | 2 | | | | | | | |
| Gonorrhœa................................ | | | 2 | | 3 | | 4 | |
| Other local diseases....................... | 91 | | 67 | 1 | 114 | 1 | 177 | 1 |
| Alcoholism................................ | 7 | 1 | 2 | | 19 | | 30 | |
| Total disease............................. | 251 | 1 | 141 | 1 | 303 | 2 | 542 | 1 |
| VIOLENT DISEASES AND DEATHS. | | | | | | | | |
| Gunshot wounds........................... | 1 | | 1 | | 3 | | 1 | |
| Drowning................................. | | | | | | | | 1 |
| Other accidents and injuries.............. | 91 | 1 | 102 | | 54 | | 85 | |
| Homicide.................................. | | | | | | 1 | | |
| Total violence............................ | 92 | 1 | 103 | | 57 | 1 | 86 | 1 |

# FORT SNELLING, MINNESOTA.

INFORMATION FURNISHED BY SURGEONS R. H. ALEXANDER AND A. HEGER, UNITED STATES ARMY.

Fort Snelling, originally established in 1819, is situated on a high bluff between the Minnesota and Mississippi Rivers, in latitude 44° 52′ 46″ north, longitude 16° 1′ 54″ west. The altitude above the river is 100 feet; above the sea, 840 feet. Saint Paul, Minn., is six miles distant. On the Mississippi side, the bluff upon which the fort is situated descends abruptly to the water, the river running there almost in a cañon. On the Minnesota side, the slope is more gradual, and ends in low, marshy flats, which extend from one-third to one-half mile on both sides of the river, and are frequently submerged during high water. A stone wall about 9 feet high incloses the fort, and rests on the east side nearly on the edge of the bluff.

The fort is an irregularly-shaped bastioned redoubt. Immediately inside the wall, and running almost entirely about the fort, is a roadway, from which stairs lead at various points to the parade.

The parade at the gorge is eight feet above the roadway, but the latter, by a gradual ascent along the flanks, arrives at the same level at the shoulder angles. It is one hundred feet above the ordinary height of the rivers, and forms nearly a rhombus, inclosed principally by five buildings on its outer edges.

All the principal buildings are of stone, and most of them old and in poor condition.

The arrangement of the post is shown in Figure 65.

A, commanding officer's quarters; B, officers' quarters, (old hospital;) C, band quarters; D,

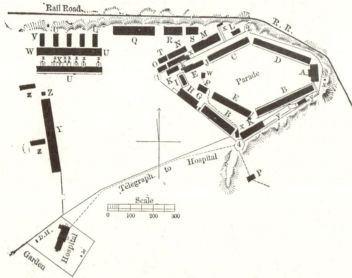

Figure 65.

company quarters; E, offices; F, chapel; G, guard-house; H, butcher-shop; I, magazine; J, post trader; K, K, K, storehouses; L, band kitchen; M, company kitchen; N, ice-house; O, carpenter-shop; P, engine-house; Q, stables; R, carriage-house; S, bakery; T, new granary; U, U, U, U, married men's quarters; V, theater; W, blacksmith-shop; X, wagon-sheds; Y, military storekeeper, (new;) Z, hay-scales; x, sinks, &c.; y, shades; z, cow-stables; 1, 2, 3, 4, towers.

The quarters for officers and men are built of stone. The dimensions of the company quarters are: For basement-rooms, 21½ feet wide and 8 feet high; for sleeping-rooms, each 31 by 21½ by 9 feet. The usual number of occupants is twelve men to one room. Behind the magazine are some frame buildings comparatively new, used as storehouse and offices by the quartermaster.

On the right of the parade is the guard-house, its outer wall being part of the wall which surrounds the fort. It consists of a rectangular stone inclosure, with wooden floor, and roof sloping from the outer to the inner wall, divided by a wooden fence into two rooms, one for the prisoners and one for the guard. It has windows and doors only to the north. The ventilation of the above buildings is entirely natural, and, from the construction, must necessarily be defective. No bad results have been observed recently, as the quarters have not been crowded. The large number of cases of pneumonia in the spring of 1867 seems to have been due to want of ventilation. The fort having been built over forty years ago, with a view of protecting a small garrison from hostile Indians, when it was the aim to place the largest number of soldiers into the least possible space, without any regard to the demands of hygiene, an opinion as to the merits of the construction of buildings is entirely out of the question.

The hospital was completed and first occupied in October, 1874. It is a frame building located about eight hundred feet southwest from the old hospital-building, and built on a plan for a provisionary post hospital of twelve beds given in Circular No. 2, Surgeon-General's Office, Washington, D. C., July 27, 1871.

Figure 66 shows the general arrangement of the rooms.

A, main hall, 7 feet wide; B, side hall, 7 feet wide; C, surgeon's office, 10 by 15½ feet; D and E, steward's quarters, (D, 11 by 15½ feet; E, 14 by 15½ feet;) F, dispensary, 14 by 15½ feet; G,

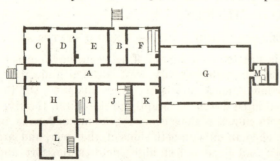

Figure 66.

ward, 24 by 40 feet; H, mess-room, 15½ by 22 feet; I, bath room, 8½ by 15½ feet; J, store-room, 14 by 15½ feet, and stairs leading to attic; K, isolation ward, 12 by 15½ feet; L, kitchen, 16 by 15½ feet, and stairs to cellar; M, earth-closet, 6½ by 7½ feet.

The stable, workshops, ice-house, and other necessary buildings are outside the wall on the bank of the Mississippi, in front of the salient angle of the fort. During the rebellion a number of wooden barracks, storehouses, and stables were erected a short distance above the post, which still remain.

The post was until recently supplied with water from the spring half a mile above by means of water-wagons. This being a great expense to the Government, it was deemed best to supply the post with water from the Minnesota River. This was done in August, 1870. The water is forced by a steam-engine through an inch pipe to a reservoir on the edge of the parade between the chapel and the sutler's store; from the reservoir pipes conduct the water to the quarters, barracks, hospital, stables, &c. Owing to this water being largely impregnated with decaying vegetable matter from the marshes along the river, it is only used for washing purposes, and it is found necessary to still supply the post with drinking-water from the spring by means of a water-wagon.

The means for extinguishing fire are now good, hose having been recently supplied, and reaching to any building in the fort.

The post is drained by ditches leading into the Mississippi, for the most part good. In the early spring, when the snow thaws rapidly, there is some little inconvenience, but not sufficient to interfere with the health of the garrison.

The post garden supplies sufficient fresh vegetables during the summer, and potatoes for the winter.

*Meteorological report, Fort Snelling, Minn., 1870-'74.*

| Month. | 1870-'71. | | | | 1871-'72. | | | | 1872-'73. | | | | 1873-'74. | | | |
|---|---|---|---|---|---|---|---|---|---|---|---|---|---|---|---|---|
| | Temperature. | | | Rain-fall in inches. | Temperature. | | | Rain-fall in inches. | Temperature. | | | Rain-fall in inches. | Temperature. | | | Rain-fall in inches. |
| | Mean. | Max. | Min. | | Mean. | Max. | Min. | | Mean. | Max. | Min. | | Mean. | Max. | Min. | |
| July | 76.49 | 96* | 47* | 2.63 | 72.48 | 94* | 50* | 1.28 | 72.78 | 93* | 51* | 2.24 | 71.09 | 92* | 53* | 2.54 |
| August | 69.40 | 89* | 39* | 5.86 | 69.86 | 91* | 44* | 3.02 | 70.99 | 90* | 46* | 2.77 | 70.87 | 88* | 51* | 1.11 |
| September | 65.30 | 81* | 46* | 2.49 | 58.42 | 87* | 31* | 1.56 | 58.18 | 90* | 60* | 3.01 | 54.11 | 84* | 31* | 1.10 |
| October | 48.60 | 79* | 21* | 1.39 | 49.26 | 78* | 22* | 1.31 | 47.48 | 73* | 24* | 0.20 | 41.74 | 67* | 17* | 0.75 |
| November | 38.08 | 64* | 11* | 1.13 | 25.67 | 54* | —14* | 0.92 | 23.83 | 49* | —21* | 0.50 | 25.96 | 48* | — 7* | 0.76 |
| December | 19.63 | 52* | —15* | 0.35 | 7.72 | 42* | —22* | 0.74 | 3.86 | 36* | —34* | 1.60 | 17.25 | 37* | —18* | 0.31 |
| January | 13.10 | 40* | —16* | 0.79 | 13.77 | 40* | —18* | 0.24 | 4.36 | 31* | —33* | 0.48 | 12.21 | 43* | —23* | 0.49 |
| February | 20.25 | 49* | —17* | 0.30 | 18.40 | 45* | —18* | 0.25 | 11.04 | 40* | —24* | 0.72 | 13.05 | 34* | —26* | 0.63 |
| March | 32.02 | 54* | 6* | 2.11 | 21.80 | 45* | —12* | 1.46 | 25.99 | 49* | —24* | 0.47 | 22.79 | 47* | — 9* | 0.33 |
| April | 47.57 | 82* | 25* | 3.88 | 46.50 | 83* | 25* | 0.97 | 41.84 | 74* | 24* | 2.61 | 37.47 | 69* | 7* | 0.35 |
| May | 66.23 | 91* | 33* | 2.41 | 57.19 | 85* | 34* | 1.80 | 55.36 | 74* | 31* | 4.06 | 61.69 | 92* | 31* | 1.12 |
| June | 70.48 | 91* | 49* | 3.46 | 68.37 | 91* | 48* | 1.98 | 71.74 | 89* | 54* | 3.80 | 68.65 | 89* | 40* | 7.77 |
| For the year | 47.26 | 96* | —17* | 26.80 | 42.45 | 94* | —22* | 15.53 | 40.62 | 93* | —34* | 22.46 | 41.41 | 92* | —26* | 17.26 |

* These observations are made with self-registering thermometers. The mean is from the standard thermometer.

*Consolidated sick-report, Fort Snelling, Minn., 1870-'74.*

| Year | | 1870-'71. | | 1871-'72. | | 1872-'73. | | 1873-'74. | |
|---|---|---|---|---|---|---|---|---|---|
| Mean strength | { Officers | 7 | | 8 | | 9 | | 9 | |
| | { Enlisted men | 104 | | 79 | | 122 | | 129 | |
| Diseases. | | Cases. | Deaths. | Cases. | Deaths. | Cases. | Deaths. | Cases. | Deaths. |
| GENERAL DISEASES, A. | | | | | | | | | |
| Remittent fever | | 15 | | 13 | | 11 | | 18 | |
| Intermittent fever | | 2 | | 3 | | 38 | | 8 | |
| Dipthheria | | 1 | | | | | | | |
| Other diseases of this group | | 6 | | | | 14 | | 2 | 1 |
| GENERAL DISEASES, B. | | | | | | | | | |
| Rheumatism | | 12 | | 11 | | 25 | | 23 | |
| Syphilis | | 1 | | 1 | | 13 | | | |
| Consumption | | | | | | 1 | | 2 | |
| Other diseases of this group | | | | 5 | | 2 | | 2 | |

*Consolidated sick-report, Fort Snelling, Minn., 1870–'74—Continued.*

| Year | 1870–'71. | | 1871–'72. | | 1872–'73. | | 1873–'74. | |
|---|---|---|---|---|---|---|---|---|
| Mean strength { Officers | 7 | | 8 | | 9 | | 9 | |
| { Enlisted men | 104 | | 79 | | 122 | | 129 | |
| Diseases. | Cases. | Deaths. | Cases. | Deaths. | Cases. | Deaths. | Cases. | Deaths. |
| LOCAL DISEASES. | | | | | | | | |
| Catarrh and bronchitis | 33 | | 41 | | 60 | | 63 | |
| Pneumonia | 2 | | 2 | | | | | |
| Pleurisy | | | | | | | 1 | |
| Diarrhœa and dysentery | 25 | | 17 | | 41 | | 44 | |
| Hernia | | | 5 | | 3 | | | |
| Gonorrhœa | 1 | | 1 | | 4 | | 4 | |
| Other local diseases | 79 | 1 | 67 | | 167 | | 157 | 1 |
| Alcoholism | 3 | | 9 | | 24 | | 24 | |
| Total disease | 180 | 1 | 175 | | 403 | | 348 | 2 |
| VIOLENT DISEASES AND DEATHS. | | | | | | | | |
| Accidents and injuries | 35 | | 23 | | 46 | | 27 | |
| Total violence | 35 | | 23 | | 46 | | 27 | |

# FORT STEVENSON, DAKOTA TERRITORY.

### REPORT OF ASSISTANT SURGEON WASHINGTON MATTHEWS, UNITED STATES ARMY.

Fort Stevenson is situated in the northwestern part of Dakota Territory, about eighty-six miles south of the international boundary line, on the left or north bank of the Missouri River, about a quarter of a mile from the river, and half a mile west of the nearest landing-place for steamers. Latitude, 47° 34' north; longitude, 24° 15' west. It is forty yards from the bluff which bounds the bottom-lands, 36 feet above low-water mark of the river, and 12 feet above the flood-mark of 1866. Fort Buford, the nearest post up the river, is distant two hundred and fifty miles by water, and one hundred and fifty by land. Fort Abraham Lincoln is the nearest post down the river, ninety-five miles distant; Bismarck, opposite to it on the river, is the nearest railroad station.

(For history and topography, see Circular No. 4, Surgeon-General's Office, 1870, page 394.)

The general surface is not fertile. The deeper ravines and bottom-lands produce grass sufficiently long to be made into hay, but on the higher ground the grass is too short to be cut. Even on the better soil the second crop of hay is not as abundant as the first. At the present time a wide extent of country must be searched to obtain sufficient hay for the post, and some time hence it will probably be much scarcer. For agricultural purposes only the lower lands seem to be available, but without irrigation none but the hardier vegetables will thrive. In most seasons, and when grasshoppers are not as abundant as usual, careful husbandry may be rewarded by fair produce. At Fort Berthold, and other points in this neighborhood, the Indians have raised on the bottoms of the river, without irrigation, corn, squashes, and beans, with varying success for probably more than a century.

Among the wild animals of the vicinity may be mentioned buffalo, elk, deer, antelope, wolf, gray and red fox, coyote, wild-cat, lynx, skunk, mink, beaver, otter, gopher, prairie-dog, and mice. Birds are: prairie-chicken, duck, plover, snipe, geese, brant, snowbird, crow, gull, sage-hen, crane, pelican, and magpie.

In the Missouri River may be found catfish, perch, shovelnose, and sturgeon.

The post is built in the form of a parallelogram, the sides of which are occupied by neat adobe buildings, one story in height, set up in cottonwood frames, on stone foundations. The parade is 220 feet square, and the general arrangement of the buildings is shown in Figure 67.

Two buildings are used as barracks, one to each company. Their walls are 11 feet from foundation to eaves; are plastered outside with a brown cement, and weather-boarded. On the inside the walls are roughly plastered, and very uneven; they will average 12 to 13 inches in thickness, but when finished they will be about 14 inches thick. The chimneys are of brick, brought from the

States; they pierce the roof about half-way between the eave and ridge-pole, and are built upon the tie-beams; the stove-pipes consequently enter the chimneys above the level of the walls and close to the roof. There are no special means for ventilation. Each of these buildings incloses three sides of a yard, 60 by 68 feet, and may be described as consisting of a body 100 by 22 feet, and two wings or Ls, each measuring 68⅔ by 20 feet. The body of the building is occupied entirely by the dormitory, which is 97⅔ by 19⅔ feet, lighted by six windows, entered by four doors, and warmed by three coal-stoves. The west wing is divided into a dining-room, 42 2/12 by 17⅔ feet, and a kitchen, 24½ by 17⅔ feet. The east wing is divided into an orderly-room, 12¼ by 27⅔ feet; a company store-room, 14 by 17⅔ feet; a company laundry, 13¾ by 17⅔ feet; a room for laundresses' quarters, 13¼ by 17⅔ feet; and a wash-room, 14 2/12 by 7⅔ feet.

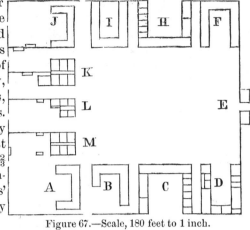

Figure 67.—Scale, 180 feet to 1 inch.

A, B, temporary log houses; C, company barracks; D, hospital; E, sally-port and guard-house; F, officers' quarters; H, company barracks; I, quartermaster's storehouse; J, temporary log house; K, L, M, officers' quarters.

The air-space is 240 cubic feet per man in each dormitory. This does not include the space contained between the roof and the horizontal joists or tie-beams which rest on the walls, for the room may yet be ceiled.

The dormitories are furnished with iron cots.

The wash-room is supplied with a heating-stove, a trough for the basins, a water-barrel, and a slop-barrel. There are also wash-tubs for those who wish to bathe themselves.

Three buildings are now used as officers' quarters. All the floors are of tongued and grooved pine, the chimneys built from the ground, the partitions of lath and plaster, the apartments ceiled, and all the walls plastered on the inside. On the outside they are covered with weather-boards. The walls are 14 inches thick.

The guard-house, situated in the center of the side opposite the commanding officers' quarters, is 60 feet long and 20 feet wide, with a passage, 10 feet wide, across the center, surmounted by a tower, 10 feet square, from which the flagstaff rises. It has sufficient accommodations for the guard, and a prison-room of about 3,800 cubic feet, with three windows. Average occupancy three men; ventilation only by doors and windows.

The hospital, like the barracks, incloses three sides of a rectangular yard. The plan is shown in Figure 68.

A, ward, running between the main buildings, and used as bath and wash room; A, ward, 17⅔ by 44⅔ feet; D, dispensary, 15 10/12 by 17⅔ feet; E, steward's room, 12⅔ by 12 2/12 feet; F, post bakery, 17⅔ by 30¾ feet; K, kitchen, 14 by 17⅔ feet; L, laundresses' quarters, 16 by 17⅔ feet; M, mess-room, 17⅔ by 20 10/12 feet; S, store-room, 13 by 12 2/12 feet; height of rooms, 11 feet.

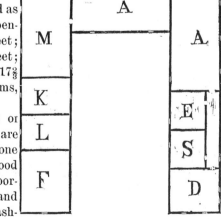

Figure 68.

The yard inclosed is 70 by 38 feet. The outer walls of the hospital form the southeast corner of the fort. They are built of the same material as the barracks, adobe on stone foundation, one story high. There are as yet only cottonwood floors, but it is designed to lay down some matched pine flooring on the ward and dispensary. All the rooms are ceiled and plastered inside, with the exception of the laundry and wash-room, and with one exception the partitions are all about 6 inches thick, of lath and plaster. The description of the roof and windows of the barracks applies to the hospital; the walls are weather-boarded outside.

The post library occupies a room designed as a reading-room for the men, as well as a library, and contains 850 well-selected volumes, including standard works on the physical sciences, travels, history, biography, and the better class of fiction and poetry.

All the water used at this post is brought from the Missouri River by water-wagon. There are streams and springs in the neighborhood, but their water is impregnated with salts, rendering it unpalatable. The Missouri water is the best in the country. It is sweet, and although very muddy, particularly in the spring-time, it becomes clear when allowed to settle. There are no cisterns or reservoirs. The fort is built on sloping ground, and the subsoil consists mostly of gravel. The natural drainage is perfectly efficient, hence there are no artificial drains, and none needed. In winter there is no arrangement for bathing, except the tubs in the wash-rooms already described. In summer the men bathe in the Missouri, and in a stream named Douglas Creek, which flows close by.

On the bottoms, near the mouth of Douglas Creek, about three-quarters of a mile from the post, an irregularly shaped piece of ground, containing between four and five acres, is cultivated as a post garden. Irrigation by hand is practiced during the dry season. Pease, beans, and lettuce grow well; potatoes and onions are produced in quantities sufficient to last the command the greater portion of the year; turnips, beets, cabbages, &c., are raised in less quantities.

The hospital is supplied with vegetables from the post garden.

The nearest railroad point is Bismarck, ninety-five miles distant, down the river.

The only inhabitants of the vicinity are the Indians and whites at Fort Berthold, some seventeen miles distant. The village contains some 2,500 Indians, of the tribes of Arickarees or Rees, Gros Ventres, and Mandans, who eke out a meager subsistence by agriculture, hunting, and the annuities received from the Government.

The present sanitary condition of the post is excellent. Venereal diseases of various forms are the most prevalent throughout the year. In summer we have many cases of acute diarrhœa and acute dysentery of mild types. I do not believe that true malarial disease ever originated here, but it may recur to those who have formerly suffered. Pulmonary disease is almost unknown; we have had, since the post was established, two or three cases of phthisis, supervening on scurvy, or contracted by the patient before he came into the country. The records of this post and Fort Berthold, since June 1, 1865, show but three cases of pneumonia, and these cases were so slight that the diagnosis was made with difficulty.

*Meteorological report, Fort Stevenson, Dak., 1870–'74.*

| Month. | 1870–'71. | | | | 1871–'72. | | | | 1872–'73. | | | | 1873–'74. | | | |
|---|---|---|---|---|---|---|---|---|---|---|---|---|---|---|---|---|
| | Temperature. | | | Rain-fall in inches. | Temperature. | | | Rain-fall in inches. | Temperature. | | | Rain-fall in inches. | Temperature. | | | Rain-fall in inches. |
| | Mean. | Max. | Min. | | Mean. | Max. | Min. | | Mean. | Max. | Min. | | Mean. | Max. | Min. | |
| July | 71.88 | 102 | 52 | 1.65 | 75.97 | 99 | 53 | 3.35 | 69.39 | 103* | 38* | 2.49 | 66.68 | 91* | 41* | 1.80 |
| August | 63.67 | 94 | 40 | 2.42 | 67.81 | 102 | 39 | 0.28 | 69.06 | 101* | 38* | 2.15 | 68.87 | 92* | 33* | 1.95 |
| September | 60.28 | 85 | 34 | 3.00 | 56.69 | 86 | 27 | 0.20 | 56.18 | 86* | 26* | 1.23 | 49.22 | 88* | 16* | 0.97 |
| October | 40.27 | 78 | 16 | 4.15 | 41.99 | 75 | 8 | 0.15 | 45.96 | 81* | 12* | 0.82 | 37.39 | 86* | 4* | 0.00 |
| November | 35.12 | 59 | 16 | 0.09 | 14.66 | 50* | −32* | 1.78 | 18.92 | 50* | −25* | 0.31 | 28.56 | 59* | −5* | 0.03 |
| December | 14.08 | 47 | −28 | 0.37 | −1.66 | 36* | −37* | 0.79 | 0.52 | 40* | −35* | 0.70 | 6.91 | 42* | −27* | 0.04 |
| January | 3.80 | 45 | −35 | 0.76 | 7.97 | 35* | −29* | 1.15 | 1.32 | 37* | −35* | 0.17 | 4.69 | 43* | −29* | 0.02 |
| February | 15.06 | 43 | −28 | 0.80 | 13.28 | 48* | −27* | 0.06 | 7.96 | 43* | −28* | 0.60 | 6.32 | 43* | −32* | 0.00 |
| March | 23.83 | 52 | −2 | 0.80 | 16.99 | 45* | −20* | 0.76 | 22.34 | 51* | −20* | 1.43 | 16.71 | 56* | −24* | 0.42 |
| April | 40.03 | 65 | 20 | 3.50 | 38.01 | 76* | 9* | 0.77 | 37.34 | 69* | 12* | 0.14 | 36.30 | 86* | 3* | 0.04 |
| May | 63.07 | 90 | 45 | 1.58 | 54.42 | 94* | 31* | 0.55 | 50.97 | 75* | 25* | 1.26 | 59.14 | 94* | 32* | 1.10 |
| June | 67.56 | 91 | 51 | 3.00 | 67.55 | 100* | 37* | 1.50 | 66.65 | 91* | 41* | 1.46 | 66.56 | 101* | 38* | 1.51 |
| For the year | 41.55 | 102 | −35 | 22.12 | 37.81 | 102 | −37* | 11.34 | 37.22 | 103* | −35* | 12.76 | 37.28 | 101* | −32* | 7.88 |

* These observations are made with self-registering thermometers. The mean is from the standard thermometer.

*Consolidated sick-report, Fort Stevenson, Dak., 1870–'74.*

| Year | | 1870–'71. | | 1871–'72. | | 1872–'73. | | 1873–'74. | |
|---|---|---|---|---|---|---|---|---|---|
| Mean strength { Officers | | 7 | | 5 | | 5 | | 4 | |
| Mean strength { Enlisted men | | 120 | | 111 | | 111 | | 101 | |
| **Diseases.** | | Cases. | Deaths. | Cases. | Deaths. | Cases. | Deaths. | Cases. | Deaths. |
| GENERAL DISEASES, A. | | | | | | | | | |
| Typhoid fever | | ...... | ...... | 1 | ...... | 1 | 1 | ...... | ...... |
| Intermittent fever | | 11 | ...... | 9 | ...... | ...... | ...... | 10 | ...... |
| Other diseases of this group | | 4 | ...... | 9 | ...... | 2 | ...... | ...... | ...... |
| GENERAL DISEASES, B. | | | | | | | | | |
| Rheumatism | | 7 | ...... | 12 | ...... | 11 | ...... | 21 | ...... |
| Syphilis | | 6 | ...... | 24 | ...... | 5 | ...... | 2 | ...... |
| Consumption | | ...... | ...... | 2 | ...... | 1 | ...... | 2 | 1 |
| Other diseases of this group | | 4 | ...... | 6 | ...... | 1 | ...... | 1 | ...... |
| LOCAL DISEASES. | | | | | | | | | |
| Catarrh and bronchitis | | 23 | ...... | 18 | ...... | 2 | ...... | 23 | ...... |
| Pneumonia | | ...... | ...... | 1 | ...... | ...... | ...... | ...... | ...... |
| Pleurisy | | 1 | ...... | ...... | ...... | ...... | ...... | 1 | ...... |
| Diarrhœa and dysentery | | 17 | ...... | 16 | ...... | 5 | ...... | 23 | ...... |
| Hernia | | ...... | ...... | 1 | ...... | ...... | ...... | ...... | ...... |
| Gonorrhœa | | 6 | ...... | 9 | ...... | 1 | ...... | 3 | ...... |
| Other local diseases | | 57 | ...... | 72 | ...... | 18 | ...... | 27 | ...... |
| Alcoholism | | 3 | ...... | 1 | ...... | ...... | ...... | 1 | ...... |
| **Total disease** | | 139 | ...... | 181 | ...... | 47 | 1 | 114 | 1 |
| VIOLENT DISEASES AND DEATHS. | | | | | | | | | |
| Gunshot wounds | | 2 | 1 | 1 | ...... | ...... | ...... | 1 | ...... |
| Other accidents and injuries | | 19 | ...... | 18 | ...... | 21 | 1 | 19 | ...... |
| **Total violence** | | 21 | 1 | 19 | ...... | 21 | 1 | 20 | ...... |

# FORT SULLY, DAKOTA TERRITORY.

### REPORT OF SURGEON J. P. WRIGHT, UNITED STATES ARMY.

Fort Sully is situated on the east bank of the Missouri River, twenty miles below the mouth of Big Cheyenne River; latitude, 44° 30' north; longitude, 23° 47' west; elevation above sea-level, about 1,660 feet.

There are no towns or settlements in the vicinity. Yankton, the railroad terminus and point of departure, is two hundred and sixty-two miles, by land, southeast; Fort Randall is about one hundred and eighty miles southeast by land.

Fort Sully is about half-way between Fort Benton, the head of navigation, and the mouth of the Missouri. The plateau, on which the post is built, slopes gently toward the south and east, terminating in a deep ravine; to the west a descent less abrupt leads to the first bench, a strip of varying width, on which are the post stables, cattle-yard, and shops. Still farther below is the river bottom, formerly thickly timbered, where the post and hospital gardens are located. The river-channel at this point hugs closely the opposite shore, and there has not been for many years a practicable steamboat-landing nearer than one or two miles below. The original Fort Sully was established in the fall of 1863 by General Alfred Sully, and was situated thirty miles below. The site was undesirable on many accounts, and it was accordingly abandoned for the present one. The construction of the present post was commenced in 1866. The barracks for the men were occupied early in 1867, and soon afterward the post hospital and storehouses were completed. The year subsequently the officers' quarters were completed.

The reservation embraces about 27,000 acres. The geological formation belongs to the cretaceous system. It is overlaid by a sheet of modified drift; bowlders of considerable size, generally of granite, syenite, and limestone, abound. The soil, particularly of the alluvial strips and bottoms skirting the river, is very fertile; but without systematic irrigation crops are uncertain.

56 M P

One of the principal of the "grama" grasses, a term applied to several species of different genera of graminea., the *bouteloua oligostachya* of Torry abounds, and although too short for the scythe, and therefore not available for hay, is a nutritious winter-forage plant. The celebrated buffalo-grass, *buchloe dactyloides*, Engelmann, is among the most nutritious of grasses, but as it never attains the height of over two or three inches, is only available for grazing. Large herds of beef-cattle for the supply of the agencies are grazed hereabouts during the entire winter, and the cattle of the post are partially subsisted in this way during winter, and wholly so in spring and summer. Among the trees and shrubs of this vicinity the cottonwood, elm, rose-elder, red cedar, red osier, dogwood, wild plum, and cherry are common; also the Missouri currant (*ribesia aureum*) and bull-berry (*sheperdia argentea.*) A species of wild grape is among the most abundant of the wild fruits of the vicinity, and a wine of fair quality is made from its juice. The cottonwood is the staple vegetable production of the country, and almost the only reliance for fuel and lumber, serving in the latter case very indifferently. Wild plums of several varieties are extremely abundant in early autumn, and are largely gathered. No cultivated fruits grow here. Efforts have been made to encourage the growth of shade-trees, but the intense heat and dryness of mid-summer have defeated efforts in this direction, excepting in localities shaded during a part of the day by adjacent buildings.

During the latter part of May and the month of June, the plains and hillsides are beautifully green; the low strips skirting the river, the creeks, and the ravines, are decorated with leaf and blossom, and the air pervaded by the delicate but diffusive fragrance of wild grape and honeysuckle, roses and prairie-flowers abounding in profusion and variety. All this vanishes after a few days of intense heat, with sirocco-like wind—the harbinger of mid-summer—and nature returns to her wonted sere and yellow garb. Thus the gladness and exuberance of spring-time seem to merge at once into the imbrowned and withered landscape of November. Flowers from seed obtained in the East attain but a stunted growth when an effort at efflorescence supervenes, soon followed by an abortive fructescence. Even the more common annuals do not thrive, nor can they be grown out of doors without great care.

Of the wild animals several species of wolf and fox are quite numerous, and are hunted with fox and grey hounds, large packs being kept at the post for that purpose. Antelope abound at certain seasons, and are frequently run down and captured by the greyhound. Deer are occasionally seen. Beaver are found within a few miles. Of birds the most interesting to the sportsman are the prairie-fowl, wild goose, plover, snipe, curlew, and duck; of the latter there are several varieties.

In summer the intense heat is sometimes rendered almost insupportable by strong southerly winds, dry and hot as from a furnace; radiation after sundown is, however, wonderfully rapid, and the nights are not usually oppressive; the maximum summer-heat is attained earlier than on the Atlantic slope. A weather-signal station has been in operation at this post since the spring of 1872.

The post is inclosed on its southwestern limits by a heavy stockade, flanked by bastions; the stockade is continued up to and adjoins the storehouses, and these, with the soldiers' barracks, take the place of the stockade on the northeast, thus inclosing the fort. The post is designed for regimental band and four companies of infantry.

The men's quarters consist of two buildings, each 350 by 17 feet, placed end to end, with an interval of 15 feet, forming the sally-port. They are built of cottonwood logs, covered with pine siding, and lathed and plastered. The ceilings are twelve feet high; transverse partitions divide the buildings into squad-rooms, mess-rooms, and kitchens. The squad-rooms measure 20 by 17 feet, and are intended for sixteen men each, allowing about 255 cubic feet of air-space per man; they are provided with iron bedsteads; the ventilation of the barracks is very defective. There are no wash or bath rooms. The privies are ordinary earth latrines, 75 yards in rear. In addition to the above, a building was erected for the regimental band in 1871; length 77 feet, width 29 feet, height of ceiling 18 feet. This barrack is a frame building, and is superior to the quarters of the companies. There are eleven sets of quarters for married soldiers.

The officers' quarters are nine detached frame buildings, built of pine, balloon frames; they rest on brick foundations, with cellars underneath. Each set has a back-building of one story as kitchen. All the rooms are lathed and plastered. Three of the cottages are one and a half stories, and contain each four rooms, a hall, store-room, and pantry. Two of the buildings are one story, and four others one and a half stories, and divided each into two sets of quarters of four rooms. The guard-house and prison-rooms are in the end of the barrack building next the sally-port. The prisoners' room is 15 by 15 feet. The storehouses are five in number; three for quartermaster's and two for commissary stores. There is also a large building for storage of grain.

A building used as chapel was built in 1871. The hospital is located outside the stockade, and near the brink of the ravine, to the south of the post. The dimensions and general arrangement are shown in Figure 69.

A, ward; B, bath-room, 8 by 15½ feet; D, dispensary, 15½ by 16¾ feet; E, steward's room, 15 by 15½ feet; K, kitchen, 14 by 15½ feet; M, mess-room, 14 by 15½ feet; O, office, 15½ by 15½ feet; P, piazza, 8 feet wide; S, store-room, 15½ by 20½ feet. Although there is a bath-room, water cannot be obtained for bathing.

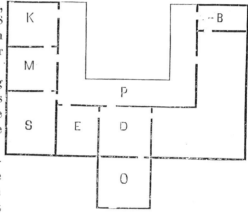

Figure 69.—Scale, 29¼ feet to 1 inch.

The ward is designed for twelve beds, allowing 810 cubic feet of air-space for each; a new room was added for dispensing purposes in 1871, by extending the wing in which is the office, greatly improving the plan.

The post library embraces over two thousand volumes, generally well selected. Water for the use of the post is wholly obtained from the river; as the plain upon which the post is built is one hundred and sixty feet above the river at the lowest stage, the labor thus necessitated is great. Water is dipped by hand from the river into tanks, and two eight-mule teams are employed in hauling it to the post. Well-water in this region is generally strongly impregnated with saline matter. Cisterns properly constructed would be of great service. The drainage of the post is excellent, and requires little artificial aid. The garden inclosure embraces about fifteen acres; crops are uncertain, chiefly from lack of facilities for irrigation; the season is too short to bring many of the later vegetables to maturity. The supply of ice is ample, and it is obtained from the river, and stored in blocks of almost any desired thickness.

A weekly mail reaches the post overland during the entire year, leaving Fort Randall on Monday and due at Fort Sully on Thursday. The mail-wagon is available for passengers, but is always avoided if possible. The river is navigable from April until November. The time from Yankton by boat varies from three days to a week or longer, depending upon the stage of water and the prevalence of calm or windy weather.

A telegraph-line from Yankton to this post was erected in 1871 and completed in March, 1872; since then, for a large part of the time, it has not been in working order. The line stretches over a country frequently swept by winds of great violence, and it is difficult to keep it in repair. Since the completion of the Northern Pacific Railroad to its present terminus, Fort Sully is, with the exception of Forts Buford and Benton, the most inaccessible of the chain of posts along the Missouri River, and can lay claim to the category of desirable frontier posts only on the score of healthfulness.

Endemic malarial disease is unknown here; typhoid fever very rare, and the ordinary diseases of hot weather exceptional. Young children enjoy an immunity to a great extent from many of the more grave disorders common elsewhere. Although the men's quarters are close and ill-ventilated to a degree unexampled, no serious or fatal malady, with possibly a single exception, has resulted. Nevertheless, it cannot be questioned that the effective strength would have averaged higher had these buildings been constructed on sound hygienic principles.

*Meteorological report, Fort Sully, Dak., 1870–'74.*

| Month. | 1870–'71. Temperature. Mean. | Max. | Min. | Rain-fall in inches. | 1871–'72. Temperature. Mean. | Max. | Min. | Rain-fall in inches. | 1872–'73. Temperature. Mean. | Max. | Min. | Rain-fall in inches. | 1873–'74. Temperature. Mean. | Max. | Min. | Rain-fall in inches. |
|---|---|---|---|---|---|---|---|---|---|---|---|---|---|---|---|---|
| July | 80.49 | 107* | 50* | 2.50 | 80.19 | 114 | 48* | 4.50 | 75.46 | 106* | 42* | 4.51 | 74.95 | 108* | 50* | 1.62 |
| August | 71.36 | 105* | 36* | 1.35 | 77.39 | 107 | 41* | 0.25 | 73.41 | 105* | 47* | 1.27 | 76.44 | 104* | 50* | 2.37 |
| September | 66.98 | 92* | 34* | 2.28 | 66.66 | 100 | 24* | 0.00 | 63.59 | 101* | 32* | 1.10 | 57.73 | 100* | 24* | 0.04 |
| October | 49.91 | 87* | 23* | 1.10 | 52.44 | 88 | 15* | 0.20 | 52.98 | 93* | 20* | 0.00 | 43.24 | 87* | 5* | 0.40 |
| November | 43.56 | 71* | 14* | 0.10 | 24.83 | 64* | —11* | 0.30 | 25.83 | 62* | —12* | 0.87 | 35.95 | 69* | 0* | 0.09 |
| December | 29.61 | 64 | —23* | 0.00 | 13.54 | 54* | —19* | 0.11 | 12.09 | 48* | —26* | 0.38 | 14.97 | 45* | —27* | 0.25 |
| January | 18.56 | 61 | —30* | 0.90 | 17.25 | 50* | —22* | 0.00 | 9.38 | 45* | —25* | 0.96 | 16.86 | 52* | —13* | 0.35 |
| February | 23.88 | 59 | —26* | 1.50 | 25.21 | 64* | —14* | 0.10 | 15.05 | 48* | —22* | 0.26 | 20.76 | 60* | —10* | 0.18 |
| March | 33.51 | 70 | 1* | 1.60 | 28.18 | 64* | — 5* | 0.25 | 33.17 | 70* | —11* | 0.44 | 29.11 | 68* | 2* | 0.90 |
| April | 47.53 | 89 | 0* | 2.63 | 44.52 | 77* | 7* | 3.66 | 42.22 | 82* | 15* | 0.95 | 44.44 | 98* | 15* | 0.19 |
| May | 68.38 | 94 | 35* | 2.25 | 59.31 | 96* | 32* | 3.16 | 54.97 | 84* | 32* | 3.12 | 63.68 | 101* | 34* | 4.95 |
| June | 76.14 | 104 | 40* | 1.50 | 72.08 | 108* | 42* | 2.48 | 77.88 | 106* | 48* | 2.09 | 71.01 | 106* | 39* | 5.55 |
| For the year | 50.83 | 107* | —30* | 17.71 | 46.80 | 114 | —22* | 15.01 | 44.67 | 106* | —26* | 15.95 | 45.76 | 108* | —27* | 16.89 |

* These observations are made with self-registering thermometers. The mean is from the standard thermometer.

*Consolidated sick-report, Fort Sully, Dak, 1870–'74.*

| Year | 1870–'71. | | 1871–'72. | | 1872–'73. | | 1873–'74. | |
|---|---|---|---|---|---|---|---|---|
| Mean strength { Officers / Enlisted men | 15 / 217 | | 13 / 232 | | 10 / 214 | | 12 / 213 | |
| Diseases. | Cases. | Deaths. | Cases. | Deaths. | Cases. | Deaths. | Cases. | Deaths. |
| GENERAL DISEASES, A. | | | | | | | | |
| Typhoid fever | | | | | 1 | | 1 | |
| Remittent fever | 2 | | 2 | | 2 | | | |
| Intermittent fever | 8 | | 9 | | 10 | | | |
| Other diseases of this group | 15 | | 17 | | 25 | | 18 | |
| GENERAL DISEASES, B. | | | | | | | | |
| Rheumatism | 47 | | 27 | | 21 | | 31 | |
| Syphilis | 12 | | 1 | | 1 | | 1 | |
| Consumption | 2 | 1 | | | | | 1 | |
| Other diseases of this group | 6 | | 3 | | 3 | | 3 | |
| LOCAL DISEASES. | | | | | | | | |
| Catarrh and bronchitis | 82 | | 47 | | 63 | | 33 | |
| Pneumonia | 2 | | 2 | | | | 1 | |
| Pleurisy | 1 | | 3 | | | | 2 | |
| Diarrhœa and dysentery | 162 | | 54 | | 31 | | 27 | |
| Hernia | | | 1 | | | | 2 | |
| Gonorrhœa | 9 | | | | | | | |
| Other local diseases | 200 | 1 | 130 | | 74 | 1 | 96 | 1 |
| Alcoholism | 5 | | 2 | | 3 | | | |
| Unclassified | 1 | | | | | | | |
| Total disease | 554 | 2 | 298 | | 234 | 1 | 216 | 1 |
| VIOLENT DISEASES AND DEATHS. | | | | | | | | |
| Gunshot wounds | 2 | | | | 1 | | | |
| Other accidents and injuries | 49 | 2 | 45 | | 35 | | 26 | |
| Homicide | | 1 | | | | | | |
| Total violence | 51 | 3 | 45 | | 36 | | 26 | |

# FORT TOTTEN, DAKOTA TERRITORY.

### REPORT OF ACTING ASSISTANT SURGEON JAMES B. FERGUSON, UNITED STATES ARMY.

Fort Totten is situated on the south side of Lake Minniwakan, (commonly called Devil's Lake,) about nine hundred yards from the lake shore. Latitude, 47° 59' 6'' north; longitude, 21° 51' west; and 1,480 feet above the sea. Cheyenne River, the only stream in the vicinity, is six miles south. Turtle Mountain, an isolated group of hills covered with timber, said to be a resort of tribes of hostile Indians, lies about seventy miles northwest of the post, near the British frontier. Fort

Stevenson is distant one hundred and twenty-six miles south of west, and Fort Abercrombie one hundred and sixty-five miles southeast. The nearest towns are Saint Joseph and Pembina, the former one hundred miles distant by road, the latter about one hundred and thirty miles. About ten miles square is held reserved. The country in the vicinity of the post is rolling and well wooded; oak, ash, elm, poplar, and maple being the principal trees. The soil is loam, on a bed of sand and gravel, superimposed on clay, and is suited for cultivation. Many granite bowlders, some of great size, are scattered over the neighboring hills and valleys.

Devil's Lake is about forty-five or fifty miles in length, and from five to fifteen miles in width, dotted with a great number of islands, several of which are more than two miles long, all well timbered. No streams enter or leave the lake; hence the inference that it is fed by springs. Its waters, though salt, are much less so than those of the ocean. Its principal salts appear to be chloride of sodium, and sulphate and carbonate of soda, with lime and magnesium salts. The specific gravity is about 1004.

Of fish, the common pickerel (*Esox reticulatus*) is the only species observed in Lake Minni-wakan.

The climate is very dry. Sudden changes of temperature are common, (a difference of 35° to 40° in twenty-four hours is not unusual,) but do not appear to affect the health as in climates where the atmosphere is more humid. The air is pure and bracing. The contrasts of the seasons are well marked, *i. e.*, the range of temperature between the extremes is very considerable, viz, 132° F.

The prevailing winds during the cold season, and for a greater portion of the year, are from the north and west; south and southwesterly winds prevail during the warm season. Northwest winds in winter bring snow-storms and very cold weather; in summer, sometimes rain and cool weather. The winds at all seasons of the year blow with considerable force. Winter is the longest of the seasons, and may be regarded as commencing November 1, and ending March 31, although light falls of snow occur in both October and April. Vegetation first appears in April, and is killed by the heavy frosts of October.

The site was first occupied as a military post in July, 1867. The original fort was designed to be temporary, the buildings being constructed of rough logs, to be occupied only until suitable structures could be erected for a permanent post. The present fort is situated on a comparatively level tract of prairie, about eight hundred yards south of the old temporary post established by General Terry. As it stands at present, Fort Totten consists of nineteen brick buildings, inclosing a parade-ground 450 by 365 feet.

The arrangement is shown in Figure 70.

A, B, C, D, S, T, officers' quarters; E, hospital; F, magazine; H, quartermaster's storehouse; I, J, J, K, company quarters; L, commissary storehouse; M, bakery; R, adjutant's and quartermaster's offices.

The foundations of the buildings are of bowlders, rocks, &c., found on the lake shore; the brick were made at the post. The exterior walls have an air-chamber of 2½ inches in the clear, making the walls 15½ inches thick. The interior and gable walls are 9 inches thick. This description of the masonry and brick-work is applicable to all the buildings. The company quarters are alike in dimensions, finish, &c. The buildings are 98 feet long by 32 feet wide, two stories high, the first story 11 feet, and the second story 10 feet in the clear from floor to ceiling.

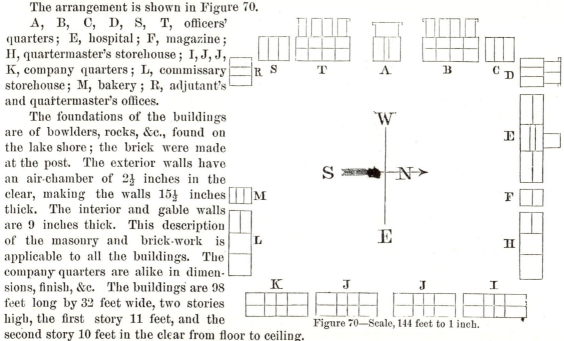

Figure 70—Scale, 144 feet to 1 inch.

Both stories are traversed by two halls, 6 feet wide, extending through the building from front to rear, dividing it into four squad-rooms upon each floor, 30 by 20 feet. A staircase 3 feet wide in each lower hall leads to the story above. Every room is well lighted, and contains four windows. As these windows are placed opposite each other they furnish an excellent means of ventilation in warm weather when they remain open for many hours daily. The only means provided for ventilating these rooms in winter is a small register, about 6 inches square, inserted in the smoke-flue of each room, but this is entirely too small for the purpose intended. Ventiducts to admit cold air were placed beneath the lower compartments, but as no registers have been inserted in the floor over these, they do not assist in ventilating the building in any way.

The rooms are heated by large box-stoves with drums attached, and even in the coldest winter weather they are very comfortable. Single iron bedsteads are used throughout. When constructed each barrack was designed to accommodate one company; as occupied at present, however, the four companies comprising the present garrison are quartered in two and one-half buildings; that is, each company of infantry is allowed four squad-rooms, or half a building, and each cavalry company the remaining half, with two squad-rooms from the adjoining barrack. Two of the lower squad-rooms in each building occupied by the troops are used as orderly-rooms, leaving only six squad-rooms to be used by the enlisted men; this will give about ninety men to a barrack, or fifteen to a room, but as there are always some men absent from each squad, on guard, escort, extra duty, &c., the number of occupants nightly will vary from ten to fifteen in a room, and the air-space from 400, the lowest, to 660 cubic feet, the highest, allowance to each man.

The remainder of the company barracks are used as quarters for the Indian scouts, laundresses, married soldiers, and also as workshops for the company tailors, saddlers, &c.

The company kitchens, &c., are contained in two brick buildings, each building being so placed as to cover the open space between two barracks; thus arranged, nearly one-half of the building is thrown in rear of a company barrack, and this portion contains the kitchen, &c., used by the troops occupying the barrack immediately in its front. Both buildings are exactly alike, being one story high, and 120 by 25 feet, including the walls. They are divided in the center into two parts by a brick wall 12 inches thick; each half contains a kitchen, storeroom, pantry, wash-room, mess-room, and cellar. The kitchen occupies the end of the building, and is 16 by 23½ feet.

The mess-room, 30 by 23½ feet, occupies that portion of the building nearest the center. It contains a fire-place, and is lighted by six windows. The height of the ceiling is 10 feet in the clear throughout.

The cellar, 15 by 21 feet, with a depth of more than 6 feet in the clear, is immediately below the kitchen. It is both dry and warm, for although the mean temperature of some of the winter months falls below zero, yet with a little care vegetables stored here do not freeze. The exterior walls of the building are 9 inches thick, and all the rooms are lathed and plastered.

The commanding officer's quarters is a two-story brick building, 41 feet front by 32 feet deep, with a one-story wing to the rear. The main portion contains two large rooms on the first floor, and four rooms on the second floor, divided on both floors by halls running from front to rear. The wing contains the kitchen and dining-room, a cellar beneath, with a place for a cistern. The floors in this building are laid double, of one-inch boards, and the principal rooms and halls on the first floor have two coats of mortar and hard-finish. The captains' and first lieutenants' quarters consist of two buildings, one each side of the above, each of which is 90 feet long by 32 feet wide, and two stories high. Each set of quarters consists of two rooms on the first floor, and two on the second, with a small hall-room or pantry. The rear wings of this building have each a dining-room and a kitchen, with a cellar beneath. A cistern is to be placed under the dining-room. The water-closets are attached to the wings; they are separated from the cellar under the kitchen only by a wall, 18 inches thick, constructed of stone and lime. The close proximity of the privy to a wall that in time may become permeable appears to be objectionable, as it may at some future day prove a source of annoyance. The rear wings of the center building are under one roof; those of the outer quarters are separate. These buildings are heated by means of stoves, and are well lighted by windows. Their ventilation is effected as described for the company quarters.

The quarters for second lieutenants consists of two buildings, each made up of a main portion 46 by 32½ feet, one story and a half in height, or 17 feet from the eaves to the ground. To this is attached a rear portion, one story high, containing a kitchen and dining-room ; it is 26¼ by 28 feet. The outer walls of the main portion are 12 inches thick ; those of the rear are 9 inches. In the dimensions given above these thicknesses are included. Each building being designed to furnish quarters for two officers, is divided by a brick wall, 9 inches thick, running from front to rear, into two symmetrical halves, each being entirely distinct from the other. The front entrance to each half leads into a hall, 30½ feet long by 6 feet wide and 10 feet high. Doors open from this into two rooms, each 15 feet square and 10 feet high. These rooms connect by folding doors ; the front one contains a fire-place, and each is lighted by two windows. At the farther end of the hall is a door opening into the dining-room. This room, 15 by 11 feet, contains three windows. Adjoining this is a pantry or closet, 7¼ by 3½ feet. The kitchen in rear of the dining-room is 13 by 10 feet. It contains one window. The dining-room, pantry, and kitchen are 9 feet in the clear between the floor and ceiling. A staircase fronting the entrance leads to the upper story, which consists of a passage and two rooms corresponding in area with those immediately beneath. The upper hall is lighted by a small window. The room in front has two windows, and the back room three. The ceiling on this floor is only 4½ feet high at the walls, owing to the slant of the roof. These quarters are not provided with either cistern or cellar.

The office is a small building, 39½ by 28 feet, including walls, and 11 feet from the eaves to the ground. The front entrance leads into an ante-room, 10½ by 7 feet ; from this a door on the left opens into the adjutant's office, which consists of two rooms, connected by a door, the one in front 15 by 14 feet, the one in rear 15 by 12 feet. In the former stand the post library, desks for clerks, &c., while the latter is used as the private office of the commanding officer and post adjutant. A door on the right of the ante-room opens into the rooms used by the quartermaster for his office. These are of the same dimensions, and correspond with those already described. The rooms are all lathed and plastered, and are 9 feet in the clear between floor and ceiling.

The guard-house is a building 38½ by 25½ feet, including the walls, and is situated sixty feet in front of the sally-port on the east side of the fort. It contains a passage, 24 by 5 feet, running across its whole width, dividing it into two parts. On one side is the guard-room, 24 by 15 feet. It is lighted by four windows. On the opposite side of the hall are the prisoners' cells, two in number, one 15 by 13½ feet ; the other 15 by 9 feet. The rooms are all 10 feet high in the clear. One iron-grated window admits light to each cell. The walls of the cells are 12 inches thick, those of the guard-room 8 inches. The smaller cell is rarely used, and the larger only at night. Every room is floored, lathed, and plastered, and both the guard-room and the cell in use are heated by stoves during cold weather. Ventilation is provided for in the guard-room and smaller cell by a small register in each, inserted near the ceiling, over a smoke-flue. The cell most in use, however, has no ventilation whatever, except such fresh air as is admitted by the door and window. The daily average number of prisoners during the last four years has been 3.12, and as the capacity of the larger cell is 2,025 cubic feet, this allows an air-space of about 625 cubic feet to each prisoner, supposing this cell only to have been used.

The bakery is 28 by 20 feet, including walls. It contains a store-room for flour, 10 by 11 feet, and a bake-room, running the whole length of the building, with a width in front of the ovens of 9 feet, and in front of the store-room of 7 feet. This room is furnished with a bread-trough and kneading-table, and is well lighted by four large windows placed on the side. The ovens, two in number, are placed side by side, parallel with the store-room, their doors opening into the bake-room. They each measure 6½ by 8 feet in the clear, and have a capacity together of about 300 loaves.

The magazine is a small building, 18 by 15 feet, on the north side of the parade. The walls are of brick, 18 inches thick, resting on stone foundations.

The hospital is constructed on the plan described in Circular No. 4, Surgeon-General's Office, 1867, having a central administration building, with two wards arranged as wings. The center building is 36 by 37 feet, two stories high. To this is attached a rear building, 21½ by 14 feet, one story high. Both stories of the main building are 12 feet in height from floor to ceiling ; the rear wing is 10 feet in height in the clear. The wings, each 44 by 24 feet, are one story, 15 feet from floor to ceiling in height. Each is divided into a ward, 33 by 24 feet, a bath-room, 11 by 9 feet, a water-closet of the same size, with a passage, 6 by 11 feet, leading to an end door between them.

All the walls and ceilings in the hospital are lathed and plastered. The floors are composed of inch boards, laid double. The wards are each heated by two large box-stoves with drums attached, placed one on each side of the ward; from these the pipes lead to smoke-flues in the wall of the main building. This gives a large surface for radiating heat, and even in winter these rooms are very comfortable. Only one ward has been used for hospital purposes. The west wing was formerly used as a chapel, but has recently been taken by the post quartermaster for a carpenter-shop. The ward in use contains ten beds. The greater number of patients are treated in hospital, few being excused in quarters. The building is well ventilated, the wards being each provided with two registers, side by side, in the center of the ceiling, immediately over which is a louvered opening in the ridge. Beneath the kitchen is a cistern, capable of holding four hundred barrels, and under the mess-room is a large, dry cellar.

The quartermaster's and commissary's storehouses are each 100 by 30 feet, divided into three rooms, with fire-proof walls between the rooms. The rooms can only be entered from the outside. One room in each building has a cellar underneath. These buildings can be driven around and through, and have lofts for storing light and dry articles.

All the buildings described above were built by contract, of bricks made at the post; these, however, were poorly manufactured, the clay containing a large percentage of lime. In order to protect the buildings from the injurious action of the weather, they received two coats of paint externally in 1871.

A strong picket-fence, 6 feet high, placed about one hundred and sixty feet in rear of the back buildings, incloses the whole post.

Beyond the fence, on the south side of the post, are the cavalry and quartermaster's stables. The latter is a large, substantial building, put up by the troops; is well adapted for the purpose intended, and will accommodate sixty animals. The cavalry stable, also built by the troops, is not so substantial as the other, yet it answers very well; is both warm and dry, and is designed for the horses, &c., belonging to companies of cavalry.

There is no reading-room for the use of the enlisted men, the post library being kept at present in the adjutant's office. This library contains but few books adapted to the wants of enlisted men, and is but little patronized by them.

Post-gardens have been cultivated for the past three or four years. Potatoes and other root-crops grow well; also onions, pease, beans, cabbage, corn, &c., and there is no doubt but the cereals could be grown successfully. The only apparent drawback to agriculture in this region, so far as observed, is the destruction caused by countless hordes of grasshoppers, which make their appearance about midsummer every two or three years, and destroy every green thing above ground.

The drinking-water used is supplied by springs in the vicinity, and is very hard, containing a large quantity of carbonate of lime, &c. It is clear and agreeable to the taste, though frequently it acts unpleasantly upon strangers unaccustomed to its use, causing diarrhœa, but this effect soon passes off, or is readily controlled by some mild astringent.

An abundant supply of ice is obtained from the lake during the winter. It is issued daily in summer to both officers and enlisted men. This ice is decidedly alkaline in taste; is very porous, and far inferior to fresh-water ice.

The Indians located on the Indian reservation near here, consist of portions of the Sisseton and Wahpeton bands with a few Cutheads, all belonging to the Sioux Nation. They number about 800, and during the past four years have been quiet, peaceable, and industrious. Many of them live in good log houses erected by themselves with the assistance of the agency mechanics. Some, also, have stables for their ponies and cattle.

Fort Totten is distant eighty-two miles north from Fort Seward, on the line of the Northern Pacific Railroad, and an excellent road connects the two posts, as all supplies for this post now come by this route. Daily trains to Fort Seward usually commence running about the middle of April, and cease some time in the following November. Saint Paul, Minn., distant three hundred and ninety-six miles, is the nearest city from which supplies of clothing or articles required in house-keeping can be obtained. Butter, eggs, fresh vegetables, &c., for winter use, cannot be purchased here, and are usually procured from either Saint Paul or from some of the small towns on the line of the railroad, as Fargo, &c.

There is a weekly mail both summer and winter, between here and Fort Seward. It is carried by contract, and is under the control of the Postmaster-General. The trip from Saint Paul to Seward by rail, via Northern Pacific Railroad, is made in one day and a half, after which a further journey overland of two and one-half days is needed to reach this post. In concluding I would say to all officers and others traveling over the prairie country late in the fall, or during the winter, be careful never to leave a post without being fully prepared to meet extreme cold, no matter how pleasant the weather may be at the time of starting, nor how bright the prospects may appear of the fine weather continuing for several days to come, for there is not a winter but some persons are frozen more or less seriously, and more than one life has been lost, from the neglect of this simple precaution.

*Meteorological report, Fort Totten, Dak., 1870–'74.*

| Month. | 1870–'71. Temperature. Mean. | Max. | Min. | Rain-fall in inches. | 1871–'72. Temperature. Mean. | Max. | Min. | Rain-fall in inches. | 1872–'73. Temperature. Mean. | Max. | Min. | Rain-fall in inches. | 1873–'74. Temperature. Mean. | Max. | Min. | Rain-fall in inches. |
|---|---|---|---|---|---|---|---|---|---|---|---|---|---|---|---|---|
| July | 69.59 | 91 | 50 | 2.33 | 69.04 | 97 | 51 | 0.06 | 68.03 | 99* | 40* | 4.00 | 65.52 | 92* | 43* | 1.03 |
| August | 66.55 | 90 | 43 | 0.82 | 70.84 | 96 | 44 | 1.95 | 66.41 | 100* | 43* | 2.48 | 66.49 | 93* | 42* | 2.34 |
| September | 62.39 | 86 | 40 | 2.04 | 56.11 | 86 | 30 | 0.41 | 53.71 | 86* | 26* | 0.60 | 47.82 | 83* | 25' | 0.70 |
| October | 40.71 | 80 | 19 | 1.32 | 42.01 | 74 | 16 | 0.30 | 45.37 | 77* | 15* | 0.78 | 36.88 | 81* | 2* | 0.06 |
| November | 34.56 | 60 | 6 | 1.10 | 14.83 | 45* | −29* | 0.93 | 16.83 | 40* | −21* | 0.64 | 20.59 | 58* | −10* | 0.77 |
| December | 11.93 | 48 | −26 | 0.24 | −2.24 | 36* | −32* | 1.12 | −2.80 | 36* | −36* | 0.19 | 7.63 | 40* | −26* | 0.05 |
| January | −1.85 | 40 | −34 | 1.80 | 5.79 | 34* | −31* | 0.74 | −5.26 | 29* | −31* | 1.16 | −0.19 | 40* | −33* | 0.38 |
| February | 5.16 | 35 | −34 | 0.74 | 9.55 | 40* | −27* | 0.26 | 4.98 | 38* | −30* | 1.32 | 4.59 | 37* | −25* | 0.03 |
| March | 18.60 | 39 | −8 | 0.90 | 12.08 | 30* | −22* | 3.40 | 15.47 | 39* | −23* | 0.87 | 12.14 | 43* | −19* | 0.49 |
| April | 35.93 | 63 | 20 | 1.87 | 34.41 | 56* | 13* | 3.15 | 33.53 | 60* | 16* | 0.57 | 30.99 | 77* | 0* | 0.62 |
| May | 61.85 | 89 | 34 | 1.04 | 50.95 | 75* | 26* | 1.10 | 50.34 | 74* | 26* | 3.75 | 57.58 | 97* | 29* | 1.43 |
| June | 65.04 | 89 | 50 | 5.91 | 64.63 | 94* | 42* | 1.66 | 66.51 | 93* | 44* | 4.68 | 64.83 | 94* | 35* | 2.52 |
| For the year | 39.20 | 91 | −34 | 20.11 | 35.67 | 97 | 32* | 15.08 | 34.42 | 100* | −36* | 21.04 | 34.57 | 97* | −33* | 10.42 |

* These observations are made with self-registering thermometers. The mean is from the standard thermometer.

*Consolidated sick-report, Fort Totten, Dak., 1870–'74.*

| Year | 1870–'71. | | 1871–'72. | | 1872–'73. | | 1873–'74. | |
|---|---|---|---|---|---|---|---|---|
| Mean strength { Officers | 7 | | 7 | | 5 | | 8 | |
| { Enlisted men | 147 | | 115 | | 108 | | 190 | |
| Diseases. | Cases. | Deaths. | Cases. | Deaths. | Cases. | Deaths. | Cases. | Deaths. |
| GENERAL DISEASES, A. | | | | | | | | |
| Intermittent fever | 1 | | 3 | | | | 6 | |
| Other diseases of this group | 3 | | 5 | | 2 | | 3 | |
| GENERAL DISEASES, B. | | | | | | | | |
| Rheumatism | 11 | | 1 | | 6 | | 9 | |
| Syphilis | 4 | | 3 | | | | 2 | |
| Consumption | 1 | 1 | | | | | 2 | |
| Other diseases of this group | | | | | 1 | | | 1 |
| LOCAL DISEASES. | | | | | | | | |
| Catarrh and bronchitis | 26 | | 14 | | 27 | | 18 | |
| Pneumonia | 2 | | | 1 | 1 | | | |
| Pleurisy | | | 2 | | | | 2 | |
| Diarrhœa and dysentery | 32 | | 3 | | 10 | | 21 | |
| Gonorrhœa | 2 | | 1 | | 1 | | 1 | |
| Other local diseases | 61 | 2 | 26 | | 28 | | 52 | |
| Total disease | 143 | 3 | 58 | 1 | 76 | | 116 | 1 |
| VIOLENT DISEASES AND DEATHS. | | | | | | | | |
| Gunshot wounds | 1 | | 1 | | | | 2 | 1 |
| Other accidents and injuries | 27 | | 18 | | 22 | 1 | 37 | |
| Total violence | 28 | | 19 | | 22 | 1 | 39 | 1 |

57 M P

# FORT WADSWORTH, DAKOTA TERRITORY.

### REPORT OF ASSISTANT SURGEON B. KNICKERBOCKER, UNITED STATES ARMY.

Fort Wadsworth is situated near the head of the Coteau des Prairies, in the eastern part of Dakota Territory; latitude, 45° 43′ 30″ north; longitude, 20° 27′ west; height above the sea, about 2,000 feet. The country consists of high rolling prairie, in the hollows of which are many lakes standing at levels of from forty to eighty feet below the site of the post. A tract of nine by fifteen miles is held reserved. The borders of the lake are sparsely timbered with oak, water elm, lynn, and cottonwood.

The Coteau des Prairies is an extensive deposit of drift on a silurian base, rising about twenty miles north of the post from the bed of an ancient lake, and extending thence about two hundred miles to the southeast. Granite, syenite, sandstone, limestone, feldspar, and clays are mingled with gravel and sand, the more deeply imbedded fragments varying much in size, and having angular projections. A rich vegetable mold, with a slight admixture of sand and clay, light and friable, from one to five feet in depth, forms the surface. A well sunk to the depth of 60 feet revealed, after 40 feet, nothing but sand and coarse gravel, with bowlders. Water was not obtained, and nothing like hard-pan has been found.

The soil is fertile and well suited to cereals and vegetables. Hay made from the Indian and herd grasses is of excellent quality. The yellow and red varieties of the *prunus americana* are found everywhere in profusion, and the gooseberry, raspberry, red and black currants, and grapes also flourish. The extension of the larger trees is prevented by the fires which sweep over the prairie every spring and fall. The waters of the lake are rendered alkaline from surface-drainage of an ash-covered soil; in the larger lakes not so much so as to be unpalatable, but in the smaller it becomes offensive, and in the warm months putrefaction is rapidly set up in their alkaline waters, holding in suspension a large amount of vegetable matter.

Fort Wadsworth was established as a military post in July, 1864, in consequence of the out-break of Indian hostilities on the northwestern frontier. The fort is five hundred feet from and fifty feet above the surface of Rose Lake, which furnishes the water-supply. It incloses about nine and a half acres, has sod-revetted breastworks, and is surrounded by a ditch. The barracks on the east of the parade are two stone buildings, each 200 by 45 feet and one story high, and have a capacity for four companies. The general arrangement is shown in Figure 71.

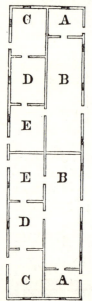

Figure 71—Scale, 60 feet to 1 inch.

A, A, orderly-rooms; B, B, squad-rooms; C, C, kitchens; D, D, mess-rooms; E, E, wash-rooms. They are inconveniently arranged. The flooring is bad, and the ventilation and lighting imperfect. Wood-stoves are used for heating. The dormitories of each company measure 73 feet 8 inches by 14 feet 8 inches by 10 feet, furnishing a cubic capacity of 10,816 feet, or an air-space of 169 cubic feet per man, allowing 64 men to sleep in quarters. Single iron bedsteads are used, furnished with the usual bedding. The sinks, 60 feet distant from the barracks, are pits 30 feet long and 3 feet wide, sheltered by frame-work. The kitchens, 23½ by 19 feet, and the mess-rooms are contiguous to the squad-rooms and dormitories, communicating by a door and window. The laundresses and married soldiers' quarters are nine log-houses, gable-roofed, one story in height, and contain from one to four small rooms, with low ceilings and small doors and windows.

The commanding officer's quarters is a two-story brick building, of that peculiar color resulting from absence of iron from the clay, 38 by 47 feet, containing four rooms, 20 by 18 by 9 feet, on each floor, and four attics under a gable roof. The rooms are divided into pairs by halls, and contain each a fire-place and three windows, which afford the only means of ventilation. The four sets of officers' quarters are constructed of brick, 38 by 95 feet, height to eaves 11 feet, to ridge 25 feet, with a Mansard roof. Attached in rear are two back buildings for kitchens and wood-houses, to which on the same line are smaller double salients of brick for water-closets, all under gable roofs. Half-stories in the former secure servants' rooms. The two middle quarters have a large hall in common, with which the two lower rooms of each set of quarters communicate. From this hall stairs ascend to a like hall, with two attics on either side with similar communication. The lower rooms, 20 by 17 feet, are connected by folding-doors. Attics, 20 by 10 feet, have each a dormer window. The end quarters are the same as the middle, except in possession of a private hall. From all the halls stairs descend to cellars, with dry, gravelly bottoms, under the back rooms.

The adjutant's office is a three-roomed stone building, 19 by 25 by 12 feet, situated on the south side of the parade. Immediately in its rear is the magazine, also a stone structure, 13 by 25 by 8 feet in dimensions, arched with stone and roofed, with small openings for ventilation.

The hospital, a brick structure fronting the parade, is 60 by 32 feet, 12 feet to the eaves, and 25 feet to the ridge. A hall, 6 feet wide, extends through the center of the building, and contains a staircase leading to the upper floor. The plan of the building is shown in Figure 72.

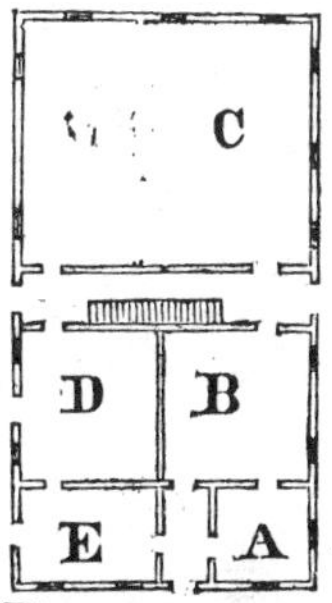

A, office, 10 by 10 feet; B, dispensary, 15 by 15 feet; C, ward, 24 by 30 feet; D, kitchen, 15 by 15 feet; E, wash-room.

All the rooms are ten feet high, plastered and ceiled, warmed by radiating-stoves, and artificially lighted by kerosene-oil.

The ward, dispensary, and kitchen have each a wooden tube three inches square entering at the eaves; in the ward it passes through the ceiling at the center and descends one foot. In the dispensary and kitchen the tubes pass through the ceiling at one side and terminate a few inches below. These are intended for the admission of fresh air.

The ward has a capacity of twelve beds, with an air-space of 600 cubic feet to each.

Figure 72—Scale, 40 feet to 1 inch.

A large store-room is on the second floor, occupying the space over the ward below. Here the baggage of patients is stored. Two rooms, each 7 by 22 feet, are on the opposite side of the hall, and are occupied as dormitories for attendants. The rooms on this floor have sloping sides, corresponding to the pitch of the roof, to within two feet of the floors, from which to the level ceiling is eight feet. The wash-room contains a bath-tub, basins, and other necessary appendages for cleanliness.

Two buildings are appropriated for quartermaster's and commissary's storage: one a stone structure, 200 by 45 feet, originally designed for company quarters; the other, a log building, 145 by 24 feet. The latter is used by the quartermaster, and has a cellar one-third of its extent. The four block-houses, one at each corner of the post, are two stories in height, except the one at the southeast corner, and are now occupied as storehouses.

The guard-house is a one-story brick building, 20 by 50 by 13 feet. It contains two rooms and two cells; the latter, 4 by 8 feet, are damp and dark, with no ventilation except by a small half-circular opening, three inches in diameter, at the top of each cell-door. The rooms are warmed by wood-stoves; have no ventilation, and bad floors. The building has capacity for about twenty men.

The post bakery is a log building, ill ventilated and lighted, having two ovens with a combined capacity for 470 rations of bread.

The stable, situated outside the fort and finely constructed of stone, is 240 by 36 by 15 feet, and contains 78 stalls.

The post library comprises 94 volumes of a miscellaneous character.

There is an abundant supply of water, brought daily in a wagon from the neighboring lake, but unfortunately of poor quality. The heat of summer producing great evaporation, causes extreme shallowness, and the water is filled with animal and vegetable life, in addition to alkaline and earthy ingredients. The water of melted ice is used almost exclusively in summer by a great number of the command in consequence of the unpalatableness of the warm lake water.

The hospital is well supplied with soft water from a galvanized sheet-iron cistern of about 100 barrels capacity.

The drainage is good. There is no system of sewerage. Water from rain and melted snow finds an outlet through excavations made in the embankments, and owing to the sloping nature of the interior of the garrison, it is generally dry and in good condition.

Bathing is freely indulged in during summer, but during the cold season there are no special arrangements for that purpose.

The gardens are three in number, and distant over half a mile from the post.

The commissariat is well supplied. The nearest depot of supplies is at Saint Cloud, Minn., one hundred and ninety-seven miles distant. Twelve months' supplies are usually kept on hand. No eggs or chickens are procurable in the vicinity.

A stage nominally makes one trip a week to Sauk Centre with the mails. It is, however, very irregular, being liable to interruption from snow and floods. The shortest mail time to Saint Paul, department headquarters, is five days; the longest, about thirty days.

From fifteen to thirty miles east of the post are small settlements. The nearest Indians are the Sisseton and Wahpeton bands of Sioux. About 1,200 are settled on Lake Traverse reservation, within seventy miles of the fort. They are chiefly occupied in agricultural pursuits.

On the 29th of July, 1873, a terrific storm of wind, hail, and rain broke over the fort, which seemed to have originated but a few minutes before in a comparatively small, dark cloud. In a few minutes the commanding officer's quarters, one of the company barracks, the guard-house, the adjutant's office, the Government stables, and the old buildings outside the fort, formerly used as quarters for scouts, were either wholly or partially unroofed. Every window exposed to the storm was broken, and the buildings were deluged with water, which caused the plastering to fall. The hospital had one hundred and eighteen panes of glass broken, and the produce of the gardens was destroyed.

*Meteorological report, Fort Wadsworth, Dak., 1870-'74.*

| Month. | 1870-'71. | | | | 1871-'72. | | | | 1872-'73. | | | | 1873-'74. | | | |
|---|---|---|---|---|---|---|---|---|---|---|---|---|---|---|---|---|
| | Temperature. | | | Rain-fall in inches. | Temperature. | | | Rain-fall in inches. | Temperature. | | | Rain-fall in inches. | Temperature. | | | Rain-fall in inches. |
| | Mean. | Max. | Min. | | Mean. | Max. | Min. | | Mean. | Max. | Min. | | Mean. | Max. | Min. | |
| July | 68.63 | 93 | 54 | 2.63 | 70.40 | 102 | 51 | 1.48 | 69.68 | 98* | 43* | 5.04 | 69.19 | 98* | 47* | 3.82 |
| August | 62.74 | 95 | 40 | 0.89 | 68.50 | 94 | 49 | 0.76 | 67.91 | 100* | 44* | 2.56 | 69.13 | 95* | 48* | 2.00 |
| September | 61.61 | 79 | 41 | 0.45 | 56.55 | 93 | 34 | 0.36 | 56.16 | 86* | 29* | 1.34 | 51.18 | 88* | 22* | 1.10 |
| October | 42.79 | 76 | 22 | 1.50 | 42.62 | 75 | 16 | 0.60 | 47.72 | 84* | 15* | 2.46 | 36.42 | 78* | — 9* | 3.26 |
| November | 35.45 | 58 | 11 | 0.20 | 16.62 | 59* | —24* | 0.52 | 17.75 | 42* | —20* | 0.56 | 25.38 | 55* | — 7* | 1.16 |
| December | 16.62 | 55 | —28 | 0.32 | 1.30 | 36* | —30* | 0.20 | 0.79 | 35* | —35* | 0.16 | 9.61 | 33* | —23* | 1.38 |
| January | 5.99 | 35 | —23 | 0.44 | 6.78 | 37 | —29* | 0.20 | 1.38 | 32* | —32* | 2.14 | 4.59 | 40* | —28* | 1.18 |
| February | 13.82 | 42 | —23 | 0.30 | 12.14 | 39 | —26* | 0.22 | 7.33 | 36* | —32* | 1.16 | 8.13 | 32* | —25* | 2.40 |
| March | 22.66 | 48 | 2 | 1.08 | 13.33 | 35* | —20* | 0.64 | 19.81 | 43* | —22* | 1.22 | 18.18 | 51* | —12* | 3.90 |
| April | 40.85 | 84 | 18 | 2.36 | 39.11 | 79* | 4* | 1.78 | 34.78 | 67* | 15* | 2.54 | 35.49 | 80* | 4* | 1.84 |
| May | 61.99 | 84 | 34 | 0.74 | 53.92 | 90* | 29* | 4.38 | 50.88 | 70* | 28* | 4.52 | 60.77 | 93* | 31* | 2.70 |
| June | 66.12 | 88 | 49 | 1.96 | 66.39 | 93* | 41* | 4.02 | 69.55 | 92* | 48* | 2.82 | 66.74 | 96* | 37* | 4.56 |
| For the year | 41.61 | 95 | —28 | 12.87 | 37.30 | 102 | —30* | 15.16 | 36.98 | 100* | —35* | 26.52 | 37.90 | 98* | —28* | 29.30 |

* These observations are made with self-registering thermometers. The mean is from the standard thermometer.

*Consolidated sick-report, Fort Wadsworth, Dak., 1870-'74.*

| Year | | 1870-'71. | | 1871-'72. | | 1872-'73. | | 1873-'74. | |
|---|---|---|---|---|---|---|---|---|---|
| Mean strength { Officers | | 5 | | 5 | | 5 | | 4 | |
| { Enlisted men | | 135 | | 100 | | 82 | | 100 | |
| Diseases. | | Cases. | Deaths. | Cases. | Deaths. | Cases. | Deaths. | Cases. | Deaths. |
| GENERAL DISEASES, A. | | | | | | | | | |
| Cerebro-spinal fever | | | | 1 | 1 | | | | |
| Remittent fever | | 1 | | | | | | | |
| Intermittent fever | | | | 2 | | 3 | | 1 | |
| Other diseases of this group | | 14 | | 5 | | 3 | | 6 | |
| GENERAL DISEASES, B. | | | | | | | | | |
| Rheumatism | | 9 | | 5 | | 22 | | 3 | |
| Syphilis | | | | 2 | | 3 | | | |
| Other diseases of this group | | 7 | | 1 | | 1 | | | |

*Consolidated sick-report, Fort Wadsworth, Dak., 1870–'74—Continued.*

| Year ...... | 1870–'71. | | 1871–'72. | | 1872–'73. | | 1873–'74. | |
|---|---|---|---|---|---|---|---|---|
| Mean strength ...... { Officers ...... Enlisted men ...... | 5 135 | | 5 100 | | 5 82 | | 4 100 | |
| **Diseases.** | Cases. | Deaths. | Cases. | Deaths. | Cases. | Deaths. | Cases. | Deaths. |
| LOCAL DISEASES. | | | | | | | | |
| Catarrh and bronchitis ...... | 35 | ...... | 39 | ...... | 84 | ...... | 14 | ...... |
| Pneumonia ...... | ...... | ...... | ...... | ...... | 1 | 1 | 1 | ...... |
| Pleurisy ...... | 3 | ...... | ...... | ...... | ...... | ...... | 1 | ...... |
| Diarrhœa and dysentery ...... | 11 | ...... | 14 | ...... | 35 | ...... | 5 | ...... |
| Gonorrhœa ...... | 1 | ...... | 2 | ...... | 2 | ...... | ...... | ...... |
| Other local diseases ...... | 69 | ...... | 55 | ...... | 87 | 1 | 10 | ...... |
| Alcoholism ...... | 1 | ...... | 2 | ...... | 3 | ...... | ...... | ...... |
| Total disease ...... | 151 | ...... | 128 | 1 | 244 | 2 | 40 | ...... |
| VIOLENT DISEASES AND DEATHS. | | | | | | | | |
| Gunshot wounds ...... | 2 | ...... | ...... | ...... | ...... | ...... | ...... | ...... |
| Drowning ...... | ...... | 1 | ...... | ...... | ...... | ...... | ...... | ...... |
| Other accidents and injuries ...... | 30 | ...... | 34 | ...... | 26 | ...... | 13 | ...... |
| Total violence ...... | 32 | 1 | 34 | ...... | 26 | ...... | 13 | ...... |

# MILITARY DIVISION OF THE PACIFIC,

### INCLUDING

## DEPARTMENTS OF THE COLUMBIA, OF CALIFORNIA, AND OF ARIZONA.

# DEPARTMENT OF THE COLUMBIA.

(Embracing the State of Oregon and the Territories of Washington, Alaska, and Idaho, excepting Fort Hall.)

## POSTS.

Boisé, Fort, Idaho.  
Canby, Fort, (Cape Disappointment,) Wash.  
Colville, Fort, Wash.  

Harney Camp, Oreg.  
Klamath, Fort, Oreg.  
Lapwai, Fort, Idaho.  
Sitka, Alaska.  

Stevens, Fort, Oreg.  
Townsend, Fort, Wash.  
Vancouver, Fort, Wash.  
Walla Walla, Fort, Wash.  

### TABLE OF DISTANCES IN THE DEPARTMENT OF THE COLUMBIA.

| | San Francisco | Portland | Fort Boisé | Fort Cape Disappointment | Fort Colville | Camp Harney | Fort Klamath | Fort Lapwai | Camp San Juan Island | Sitka | Fort Stevens | Fort Vancouver | Fort Walla Walla | Camp Warner |
|---|---|---|---|---|---|---|---|---|---|---|---|---|---|---|
| San Francisco | San Francisco. | | | | | | | | | | | | | |
| Portland | 679 | Portland. | | | | | | | | | | | | |
| Fort Boisé | 687 | 500 | Fort Boisé. | | | | | | | | | | | |
| Fort Cape Disappointment | 657 | 111 | 611 | Fort Cape Disappointment. | | | | | | | | | | |
| Fort Colville | 1207 | 528 | 524 | 637 | Fort Colville. | | | | | | | | | |
| Camp Harney | 672 | 375 | 225 | 486 | 663 | Camp Harney. | | | | | | | | |
| Fort Klamath | 484 | 395 | 535 | 521 | 923 | 260 | Fort Klamath. | | | | | | | |
| Fort Lapwai | 1051 | 372 | 368 | 483 | 350 | 507 | 765 | Fort Lapwai. | | | | | | |
| Camp San Juan Island | 979 | 300 | 752 | 322 | 818 | 677 | 695 | 675 | Camp San Juan Island. | | | | | |
| Sitka | 1754 | 1075 | 1575 | 960 | 1603 | 1705 | 1470 | 1447 | 1028 | Sitka. | | | | |
| Fort Stevens | 650 | 104 | 604 | 8 | 632 | 479 | 497 | 476 | 329 | 983 | Fort Stevens. | | | |
| Fort Vancouver | 697 | 18 | 432 | 129 | 510 | 357 | 413 | 355 | 278 | 1093 | 122 | Fort Vancouver. | | |
| Fort Walla Walla | 954 | 275 | 271 | 384 | 253 | 405 | 670 | 97 | 535 | 1350 | 349 | 257 | Fort Walla Walla. | |
| Camp Warner | 540 | 505 | 405 | 616 | 793 | 130 | 130 | 637 | 807 | 1580 | 609 | 487 | 538 | Camp Warner. |

## FORT BOISÉ, IDAHO TERRITORY.

REPORTS OF ASSISTANT SURGEONS GEORGE P. JAQUETT AND PETER MOFFATT, UNITED STATES ARMY.

Fort Boisé is located in the Boisé Valley, about half a mile from Boisé City; latitude 43° 37′ north; longitude, 39° west; with an elevation above the sea-level of 2,880 feet. The Boisé range of mountains bounds the post on the north and east, while on the south and west flows the Boisé River. The nearest military posts are Camp Harney, two hundred and fifty-five miles to the west, by way of Canyon City, but by a new route through the Malheur Mountains, passable summer and winter, one hundred and seventy miles, and Fort Lapwai, three hundred and fifty-two miles to the north. Old Fort Boisé, the site of an old Hudson Bay station, is situated about fifty miles to the west, on Snake River. Boisé City, the territorial capital, with a population of about 1,300, adjoins the military reservation on the west.

Fort Boisé was first occupied in July, 1863, for the protection of emigrant trains against the Shoshone Indians of Snake River.

The reservation, rectangular in shape, is one mile in width by two in length. In rear of the garrison the surface is rugged and broken, while the ground occupied by the post and the space extending between it and the Boisé River is level. The valley from a few miles above to the confluence of the Boisé with the Snake River, fifty miles below, is of irregular width and varied surface, and bounded on each side by arid table-lands or broken and barren mountains. The soil for some miles above and below the fort is arable, and by aid of irrigation produces in perfection all the cereals and vegetables appropriate to this latitude.

The soil is a sandy loam, inclining to a mixture of clay and decayed organic matter in the lower portions, on the margins of the streams. The stone used for building-material in the construction of the post is procured in the neighborhood. It is a very soft, coarse, and rather light sandstone. Gold and silver are found; the former, on most of the streams in this section, in the form of placer-diggings; the latter chiefly in the surrounding mountainous regions, and in the form of ledges. Silver City, about sixty miles to the south and west of this point, is surrounded by mountains containing immense deposits of silver-ore. The number of trees indigenous to this region is not large. The only species of hard wood to be found is a stunted tree, which grows in isolated mountain spots, and known as mountain mahogany. The cottonwood and willow grow on the margins of the rivers. The abundance of the cottonwood and its large size first suggested to the French Canadian agents of the Hudson Bay Company, who penetrated the country in early years, the name of Boisé (wood) by which that river is known.

Bears, wolves, coyotes, foxes, beaver, otter, mink, and martens are now rarely seen; mountain-sheep and antelopes are animals of the past. In some valleys the deer is still an inhabitant; but the number of them is gradually growing less. Rabbits and smaller game are still abundant; the former have increased so rapidly as to prove a serious trouble to the agriculturist. Wild geese, ducks, sage-hens, prairie-chickens, pigeons, and many species of smaller and less known birds are met with. Salmon, salmon-trout, mountain trout, and other fish of less importance exist in the streams. Very excellent salmon are taken from those tributaries of the Snake River which have not been rendered turbid by mining.

There are two seasons, the wet and the dry; the former beginning in November and continuing until May, and the latter during the intervening period.

The post is of rectangular form, the quarters, guard-house, and storehouses forming its respective sides. The buildings are principally of stone. Most of them were erected in 1864.

The company quarters are two stone buildings, each 90 by 30 feet, with side walls 10 feet high; only one is at present occupied as quarters. There is a fire-place at each end of the building; windows on either side, and one tier of double bunks. Ventilation is secured by the windows and doors. The dormitory consists of two rooms, and is occupied by one company, giving an air-space of about 800 cubic feet to each man. There are no bath or wash rooms; ablutions are performed in the barrack-room. A stone building, 22 by 50 feet, and about 20 feet to the rear of the company quarters, contains the kitchen and dining-room.

Quarters for married soldiers are seven log houses, containing one room each, heated by fire-places.

The quarters for officers are three stone buildings, one story high, with attic rooms above. They are finished with lath and plaster, have each three rooms and a kitchen on the ground floor, with a hall running from front to rear, and opening into a yard surrounding the house. The one occupied by the commanding officer has an extension, in rear, of 45 by 15 feet, which is separated into dining-room, kitchen, wood-shed, and water-closet. The main building contains four rooms, each about 15 by 15 by 9½ feet, with fire-places looking into each. The remaining buildings have a dining-room, kitchen, wood-shed, and water-closet appended in rear of each lateral half, thus completing two separate and independent sets of quarters under one roof. These quarters contain no bath-rooms.

The quartermaster's and commissary storehouses are also of stone, 100 by 30 feet each, and divided into offices and store-rooms, ample for the storage of all supplies. The commissary building has a cellar for vegetables and other articles.

The guard-house, situated on the north side of the parade-ground, is a stone structure, 40 by 30 feet, and open to the roof. The front room, extending the entire length of the building, is used for the guard, and has a fire-place and two windows. One large room in rear of this is used for general prisoners, and is lighted and ventilated by small openings along the top of the wall. The cell is without light, except that which is admitted through the ventilator. The average occupancy of the guard-house is about four men.

The hospital is a stone building, 56 by 32 feet, with a wing in rear, 40 by 18 feet. The arrangement is shown in Figure 73.

N, hall, 6 feet wide; P, ward, 12 by 22 feet; O and Q, wards, each $17\frac{1}{2}$ by 22 feet; R, dispensary, 12 by $14\frac{1}{2}$ feet; S, store-room, 7 by 12 feet; T, steward's room, 12 by 16 feet; U, mess-room, 11 by 16 feet; V, kitchen, 11 by 16 feet; X, Y, and Z, verandas.

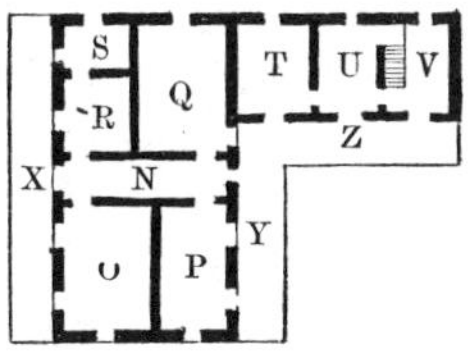

Figure 73.

The front half of the building, containing three wards, a dispensary, and store-room, is the only part of the hospital finished. Only one ward is used as such, containing six beds, with an air-space of about 800 cubic feet to each. It is warmed by open fire-places, and ventilated by doors, windows, and fire-places. An unfinished ward is used as wash and bath room. The office and dispensary are in one room. The wing contains a dining-room, kitchen, and steward's room.

The stables are two large frame buildings situated at the southwest corner of the garrison, and amply isolated.

There is a reading-room in the southwest corner of the unoccupied barrack, where can be found all the prominent newspapers and magazines of the day. These are purchased from the company and post funds.

A small frame building, opposite the quartermaster's storehouse, has been converted into a chapel. The attendance is good, not only from the company but from the town; mostly Catholics.

Southeast of the hospital, some two hundred yards, is the post cemetery; area, one acre; suitably inclosed by a good fence.

A garden, three acres in extent, in the northwest corner of the garrison, supplies the command with all the vegetables of the season. On the Government ranch some thirty thousand pounds of potatoes are raised yearly for the use of the post.

The supply of water for the use of the post is taken from the mountain-stream which flows through the reservation. No reservoir, cistern, or system of water-works is in use, with the exception of a well, sunk upon the margin of the creek, from which the supply may be obtained when the stream is low or the water turbid. A water-wagon delivers a supply to each quarters daily. The quality of the water is good, and the quantity abundant.

In 1873 a ditch was made running irregularly across the southern end of the parade-ground, and back of the company kitchen, which brings water from the creek, above the post. There was also a pond raised on the main creek, some twenty yards east of the stables, from which a good supply of ice, sufficient for the whole command, is obtained in the winter.

Communication is had by a daily stage and mail to and from the Pacific Railroad at Kelton, Utah. The time occupied is from two to three days, according to the season; thence to Washington, from five to seven days. Occasional delays are experienced during the winter from heavy falls of snow, both on the railroad and stage route. Communication with department headquarters at Portland, Oreg., is by stage to Umatilla, on the Columbia River, and thence by water and railway to Portland. Considerable delay in mail communication is frequently experienced on this route, owing to the closing of the Columbia by ice, or to snow or mud on the stage-road, particularly in crossing the Blue Mountains in Oregon.

Immediately around for a few miles, Boisé Valley is occupied by agriculturists; while the sources of Boisé River, and its tributaries and the neighboring streams, afford employment to gold and silver miners. Here and there throughout the country a solitary ranch-man has located in some of the more promising spots, and is occupied in stock-raising and the cultivation of a small domain where water is available.

The post is generally very healthy, there being no diseases of a specific or contagious character ; only a few cases of the common varieties of disease occur, such as acute diarrhœa and rheumatism, with an occasional case of fever, either remittent or intermittent, commonly called in this country mountain or typho-malarial fever. This prevails more especially among the citizens who are occupied in mining or on the farms in the valley along the river.

*Meteorological report, Fort Boisé, Idaho, 1870–'74.*

| Month. | 1870–'71. | | | | 1871–'72. | | | | 1872–'73. | | | | 1873–'74. | | | |
|---|---|---|---|---|---|---|---|---|---|---|---|---|---|---|---|---|
| | Temperature. | | | Rain-fall in inches. | Temperature. | | | Rain-fall in inches. | Temperature. | | | Rain-fall in inches. | Temperature. | | | Rain-fall in inches. |
| | Mean. | Max. | Min. | | Mean. | Max. | Min. | | Mean. | Max. | Min. | | Mean. | Max. | Min. | |
| July | 79.34 | 113 | 55 | 0.44 | 77.34 | 108 | 55 | 0.14 | 76.40 | 107* | 50 | 0.00 | 79.63 | 107* | 55 | 0.15 |
| August | 72.43 | 92 | 47 | 0.09 | 73.93 | 121 | 50 | 0.00 | 74.20 | 102* | 54 | 0.41 | 74.38 | 103* | 54 | 1.65 |
| September | 65.60 | 93 | 38 | 0.00 | 66.80 | 97 | 42 | 0.11 | 62.48 | 95* | 34 | 0.76 | 64.03 | 97* | 32 | 0.45 |
| October | 52.43 | 88 | 25 | 0.24 | 52.41 | 91 | 24 | 0.27 | 56.92 | 95* | 22 | 0.92 | 49.32 | 83* | 20 | 0.24 |
| November | 41.39 | 68 | 25 | 2.13 | 41.37 | 74 | 21 | 1.90 | 34.86 | 74* | 7 | 0.26 | 45.59 | 75* | 20 | 3.95 |
| December | 23.56 | 50 | 0 | 1.26 | 35.23 | 59 | 7 | 5.96 | 33.53 | 67* | 5 | 1.87 | 33.43 | 57* | 2 | 4.19 |
| January | 33.45 | 56 | 13 | 3.54 | 32.50 | 59 | 6 | 4.60 | 33.76 | 52* | 18 | 3.22 | 39.24 | 60* | 9 | 2.35 |
| February | 35.31 | 56 | 23 | 1.29 | 40.03 | 69 | 0 | 6.49 | 31.39 | 54* | 7 | 0.81 | 31.49 | 53* | − 2 | 1.29 |
| March | 38.38 | 61 | 22 | 7.66 | 45.15 | 78 | 24 | 0.83 | 45.69 | 83* | 14 | 0.91 | 40.30 | 64* | 15 | 2.69 |
| April | 46.51 | 76 | 27 | 1.54 | 45.99 | 81* | 33 | 0.84 | 49.73 | 83* | 31 | 1.53 | 50.12 | 81* | 32 | 1.30 |
| May | 59.94 | 91 | 36 | 2.75 | 59.87 | 91* | 37 | 0.73 | 57.70 | 88* | 41 | 0.49 | 63.54 | 95* | 36 | 1.35 |
| June | 74.29 | 106 | 41 | 0.64 | 71.26 | 104* | 52 | 0.22 | 70.16 | 100* | 47 | 0.15 | 68.25 | 98* | 48 | 0.63 |
| For the year | 51.89 | 113 | 0 | 21.49 | 53.49 | 121 | 0 | 22.09 | 52.24 | 107* | 5 | 11.33 | 53.28 | 107* | − 2 | 20.24 |

* These observations are made with self-registering thermometers. The mean is from the standard thermometer.

*Consolidated sick-report, Fort Boisé, Idaho, 1870–'74.*

| Year | 1870–'71. | | 1871–'72. | | 1872–'73. | | 1873–'74. | |
|---|---|---|---|---|---|---|---|---|
| Mean strength. { Officers | 4 | | 3 | | 3 | | 3 | |
| { Enlisted men | 60 | | 25 | | 41 | | 43 | |
| Diseases. | Cases. | Deaths. | Cases. | Deaths. | Cases. | Deaths. | Cases. | Deaths. |
| GENERAL DISEASES, A. | | | | | | | | |
| Remittent fever | 2 | | 3 | | 4 | | | |
| Intermittent fever | 5 | | 1 | | 1 | | 17 | |
| Other diseases of this group | 1 | | 3 | | 3 | | | |
| GENERAL DISEASES, B. | | | | | | | | |
| Rheumatism | 6 | | 1 | | 6 | | 2 | |
| Syphilis | 5 | | 3 | | 4 | | | |
| LOCAL DISEASES. | | | | | | | | |
| Catarrh and bronchitis | 11 | | 1 | | 2 | | 5 | |
| Pleurisy | | | | | | | 1 | |
| Diarrhœa and dysentery | 4 | | | | 5 | | 9 | |
| Gonorrhœa | 9 | | | | 3 | | 2 | |
| Other local diseases | 24 | 1 | 12 | | 12 | | 16 | |
| Alcoholism | 15 | | | | 2 | | 1 | |
| Total disease | 82 | 1 | 24 | | 42 | | 53 | |
| VIOLENT DISEASES AND DEATHS. | | | | | | | | |
| Gunshot wounds | 1 | | | | | | | |
| Other accidents and injuries | 20 | | 4 | | 4 | | 4 | |
| Homicide | | | | | | | | 1 |
| Total violence | 21 | | 4 | | 4 | | 4 | 1 |

# FORT CANBY, (CAPE DISAPPOINTMENT,) WASHINGTON TERRITORY.

REPORTS OF ASSISTANT SURGEON W. E. WHITEHEAD, AND ACTING ASSISTANT SURGEON F. S. STIRLING, UNITED STATES ARMY.

Fort Canby is situated on the north side of the mouth of the Columbia River, in Pacific County, Washington Territory; latitude, 46° 16′ 13″ north; longitude, 47° 0′ 13″ west.

This post has been occupied since April 5, 1864, and was called Fort Cape Disappointment until January 28, 1875, when the name was changed to Fort Canby in compliance with General Order No. 5, Adjutant-General's Office, Washington, D. C., dated January 28, 1875, in honor of the late Brig. and Bvt. Maj. Gen. Edward R. S. Canby, United States Army, who was murdered by Modoc Indians April 11, 1873.

The promontory on the north side of the mouth of the Columbia River, known as Cape Disappointment, runs out to the southeast as a long, narrow point, two miles in length, with an average width of a half mile, partly inclosing the south and west sides of a body of water known as Baker's Bay. This point rises into a high, rocky ridge; in some places, densely wooded.

The post is located on this point; the fortifications being on the south, or Columbia River side, and elevated some 200 feet above the garrison buildings, which are situated at the water's edge on Baker's Bay.

The rocks in the vicinity are of volcanic origin. Trees are spruce, fir, hemlock, sugar-pine, alder, crab-apple, &c. There are many fruit-bearing shrubs, such as raspberries, currants, gooseberries, &c., in many places forming dense thickets of undergrowth.

The principal animals in the region are elk, black-tailed deer, black and brown bears, sea and land otters, beavers, and minks. The birds are principally aquatic, geese, ducks, &c. There are some pheasants, woodcock, grouse, and smaller birds. The fish are salmon, halibut, herring, &c.

The reservation contains about one square mile. All the buildings, with the exception of the officers' quarters and the house occupied by the ordnance-sergeant, are located about forty feet from high-tide line, or, rather, from the bulkhead of logs, set into the sand and filled in behind with stones and earth, and are only four or five feet above high-water mark. The strip of comparatively level ground upon which the buildings are placed, is only seventy-five to one hundred feet in width from the water-line to the foot of the bluff. This strip at the northwest end of the garrison widens out so that a small parade-ground has been laid out, graded, and sown with grass. The buildings mostly face the bay, and are located as follows: Commencing at the east end, the first building is an unoccupied storehouse; fifteen feet west of it is the quartermaster and commissary storehouse; twenty feet west is the blacksmith-shop; twelve feet north of it, and facing east, is the stable; ten feet north of the stable is an ordnance storehouse; about sixty feet northwest from this, is the guard-house, built on piles over the water; one hundred and twenty-five feet south of west of the guard-house is a building containing two sets of laundresses' quarters; twenty feet northwest of this is the post bakery; twenty-five feet northwest of it are the company-quarters; sixty feet northwest of these is a building containing two sets of laundresses' quarters; twenty-five feet northwest is a small building used as a school-house; thirty-five feet northwest of it is the carpenter-shop; twenty feet northwest is the adjutant's office; twenty-five feet northwest of which, on the same line, but about six feet higher, is the hospital; about three hundred feet northwest from the hospital, on the summit of a ridge, some fifty feet above the sea-beach, and separated about fifty feet from each other, are three cottages comprising the officers' quarters. About a quarter of a mile northeast from the easternmost building, on a point jutting out to the northeast, is the wharf, with a small storehouse upon it. This wharf is so sheltered that small vessels can make a landing in any weather.

The quarters for enlisted men consist of a two-story frame barrack, 80 by 30 feet, 28 feet in height, clapboarded and lined; the lower story, divided into a squad-room, 56 by 30 feet, and a kitchen, 24 by 30 feet; the upper story is in one room, the dormitory. Attached to the rear is a one-story addition, 18 by 80 feet, used as a mess-room. A porch runs along the entire front of the building, under which the stairs leading to the upper story are placed. The dormitory is well lighted, ventilated by ridge ventilator, but is not warmed artificially. It is furnished with iron single bedsteads, and with the present occupancy affords about 680 cubic feet air-space per man. The other rooms are well lighted and provided with necessary furniture and fixtures. The sink is located over the water.

Married soldiers' and laundresses' quarters are four frame buildings, each containing two sets; the ordnance sergeant's quarters are near the batteries. The hospital steward's quarters are in a small frame building, damp and uncomfortable, near the hospital.

Officers' quarters are three frame double cottages, each containing two sets of quarters, consisting of three rooms and a kitchen on the lower floor, and two attic rooms above to a set. Each set has a bath-room attached, which is furnished, through wooden pipes, with water from a mountain-spring; and is also furnished with a cellar, and a cistern with filter for rain-water. The rooms are large, the buildings are in fair condition, and comfortable. The privies are common pits, housed over, in rear of the quarters.

The guard-house is 36½ by 34 feet outside. The lower story is built of hewn logs, the walls being very thick. It is 10 feet in height, and is divided into fourteen cells, two small rooms, and two narrow halls or passages. Cell No. 1 contains 719 cubic feet of space, the only ventilation being by the door leading into a narrow hall, and two openings, each 3 by 16 inches, in the rear wall; has four wooden bunks, two on a side, and is intended for four men, giving to each 18 feet superficial area, and 179 cubic feet of air-space. Cell No. 2, for four men, giving each 175 cubic feet space. Cell No. 3, for four men, air-space 201½ cubic feet each. The last two cells have each a single opening in the rear wall 16 by 3 inches. There are three front cells west of the main hall, opening into a room 15 by 8 feet; dimensions of these cells 6 feet 1 inch by 5 feet 1 inch; each occupied by one man. They have no ventilation except by cracks in the doors. There is a large heating-stove on the lower floor, which tends still further to vitiate the air. Add to the very insufficient air-space the bedding in the cells, and in winter the damp clothing of the prisoners, and it will give some idea of the hygienic condition. There are four windows in this story, but the door of the prison is tight, and so shuts off much ventilation. This prison is used for general prisoners sent from other posts. Average number of prisoners in 1874 was 19.77.

The upper story is built of planks, is 10 feet 4 inches in height, and divided into a guard-room 26 by 33 feet, an office, a cell for garrison-prisoners, and a tool-room. It is warmed by a large heating-stove. The ventilation is ample.

The hospital is a neat one-story frame building, clapboarded outside, and lathed and plastered within. It contains two wards, each 15 by 18 feet, intended for four beds, giving to each bed an air-space of 945 cubic feet. It also contains a dispensary, kitchen, mess-room, store-room, and bath-room. The wards and principal rooms are 14 feet in height. There is a brick cistern, holding 6,000 gallons of water. The building is in good repair, has some defects, but on the whole is well adapted for its purpose. It is well lighted; the wards are warmed by fire-places, the other rooms by stoves. A neat fence surrounds the building and a small garden. The privy is an ordinary housed pit in rear of the building. One earth-closet is in use. The furniture and fixtures are sufficient.

The quartermaster and commissary occupy jointly a long frame building, with a large store-room at each end, and office-rooms in the center.

The post-garden has an area of three acres. It furnishes a sufficient supply of vegetables during the summer and autumn, but not enough for winter.

The water-supply is derived from a spring near the top of the promontory, directly behind the company quarters. The water is conveyed by wooden pipes and filtered through a box containing charcoal and sand; from this it is carried by wooden pipes to the company-kitchen and to the rear of the hospital.

The means of extinguishing fire are buckets. At the hospital is a force-pump, connected with the cistern.

There is a regular tri-weekly mail, by steamer, to Portland, Oreg.; time to Portland, two days.

*Meteorological report, Fort Canby, Wash., 1870–'74.*

| Month. | 1870–'71. Temperature. Mean. | Max. | Min. | Rain-fall in inches. | 1871–'72. Temperature. Mean. | Max. | Min. | Rain-fall in inches. | 1872–'73. Temperature. Mean. | Max. | Min. | Rain-fall in inches. | 1873–'74. Temperature. Mean. | Max. | Min. | Rain-fall in inches. |
|---|---|---|---|---|---|---|---|---|---|---|---|---|---|---|---|---|
| July | | | | | 59.96 | 70 | 52* | 0.50 | 59.88 | 93* | 49* | 0.98 | 57.57 | 87* | 49 | 0.81 |
| August | | | | | 61.83 | 79 | 46* | 0.10 | 56.31 | 66 | 46* | (?) | 58.09 | 70 | 50 | 0.30 |
| September | | | | | 58.10 | 86 | 40* | 2.50 | 54.49 | 68* | 46* | (?) | 53.94 | 61 | 43 | 0.64 |
| October | | | | | 54.79 | 66 | 39* | 2.10 | 50.17 | 68* | 36* | (?) | 47.06 | 68 | 32 | 2.80 |
| November | | | | | 47.79 | 59 | 34* | 5.03 | 42.13 | 75* | 30* | (?) | 45.00 | 60 | 27 | 2.25 |
| December | | | | | 42.75 | 54* | 17* | 11.11 | 42.07 | 57* | 28 | 1.44 | 34.55 | 49 | 23 | 7.10 |
| January | | | | | 44.39 | 55* | 29* | 7.54 | 41.90 | 52* | 30 | 5.61 | 37.61 | 48 | 21 | 14.54 |
| February | | | | | 45.80 | 56* | 28* | 12.75 | 36.21 | 56* | 28 | 6.81 | 36.38 | 48 | 26 | 10.82 |
| March | | | | | 47.79 | 66* | 37* | 8.20 | 42.96 | 70* | 35 | 9.27 | 38.54 | 56 | 29 | 4.12 |
| April | | | | | 49.56 | 66* | 35* | 6.64 | 46.87 | 64* | 34 | 1.07 | 47.88 | 69* | 33* | 3.55 |
| May | 52.71 | 64 | 44* | 0.76 | 55.12 | 72* | 40* | 1.46 | 49.78 | 93*(?) | 38 | 0.70 | | | | |
| June | 58.58 | 70 | 42* | (?) | 59.24 | 82* | 46* | 1.17 | 53.05 | 78* | 44 | 1.99 | 54.25 | 72* | 38* | 6.25 |
| For the year | | | | | 52.26 | 86 | 17* | 59.10 | 47.98 | 93* | 28 | (?) | | | | |

\* These observations are made with self-registering thermometers. The mean is from the standard thermometer.

*Consolidated sick-report, Fort Canby, Wash., 1870–'74.*

| Year | 1870–'71. | | 1871–'72. | | 1872–'73. | | 1873–'74. | |
|---|---|---|---|---|---|---|---|---|
| Mean strength { Officers | 3 | | 3 | | 2 | | 2 | |
| { Enlisted men | 70 | | 44 | | 29 | | 52 | |
| Diseases. | Cases. | Deaths. | Cases. | Deaths. | Cases. | Deaths. | Cases. | Deaths. |
| **GENERAL DISEASES, A.** | | | | | | | | |
| Typho-malarial fever | 2 | | | | | | | |
| Intermittent fever | 14 | | 1 | | 2 | | 5 | |
| Other diseases of this group | | | | | | | | |
| **GENERAL DISEASES, B.** | | | | | | | | |
| Rheumatism | 20 | | 6 | | 1 | | 13 | |
| Syphilis | 9 | | | | 2 | | 4 | |
| Other diseases of this group | 1 | | | | | | | |
| **LOCAL DISEASES.** | | | | | | | | |
| Catarrh and bronchitis | 19 | | 3 | | 2 | | 5 | |
| Pneumonia | | | | | | | 3 | |
| Pleurisy | | | 1 | | | | | |
| Diarrhœa and dysentery | 13 | | 14 | | 1 | | 6 | |
| Hernia | 1 | | | | | | | |
| Gonorrhœa | 4 | | 1 | | 3 | | | |
| Other local diseases | 53 | 1 | 25 | 1 | 7 | | 24 | |
| Alcoholism | 2 | | 3 | | | | 13 | |
| Total disease | 138 | 1 | 54 | 1 | 18 | | 73 | |
| **VIOLENT DISEASES AND DEATHS.** | | | | | | | | |
| Gunshot wounds | | | | | 1 | | | |
| Other accidents and injuries | 24 | | 12 | | 4 | | 22 | |
| Total violence | 24 | | 12 | | 5 | | 22 | |

# FORT COLVILLE, WASHINGTON TERRITORY.

REPORT OF ACTING ASSISTANT SURGEONS E. Y. CHASE AND WILLIAM D. BAKER, UNITED STATES ARMY.

Fort Colville is situated in Washington Territory, in latitude 48° 41′ north, longitude 40° 52′ west; altitude above the sea, 2,800 feet. It is about thirty-five miles south of the dividing-line between the United States and British Columbia, and fourteen miles east of the Columbia River. The Cascade range of mountains is about one hundred and fifty miles west. Fort Lapwai is the nearest United States military post.

The post was established June 30, 1859, to guard against the Indians, who were very hostile, having defeated Colonel Steptoe near the Spokane River the previous year, in June. The Government reserve consists of about one square mile of land of a very irregular form. On the north side it is bounded by Mill Creek, a small stream of water, which runs the Government saw-mill; on the east and west sides by hills ranging in height from 200 feet on the east side to 800 or 900 feet on the west. On the south side the reserve is an open valley. The town of Colville is north of the post about one-half mile.

The soil of the valley is very fertile, producing in abundance all the cereals, except Indian corn, for which the nights of the summer are too cold. Much of the land in the vicinity is too dry for any farming purposes, except where it can be irrigated, when any of it will produce fine crops of wheat and oats.

The geological formation is limestone, interspersed with granite, quartz, and slate. Of mineral productions, gold in minute quantities is found in the sands of all the mountain-streams. Galena is also occasionally found in small quantities. Iron is generally diffused. But a small portion of the soil upon the reservation is tillable. It is mostly an elevated terrace, composed of gravel, but on the north side, near the creek, the soil is a rich loam, containing considerable alkali; and this is the location of the post-garden. Clay of good quality for making brick is found in abundance in the vicinity. Pine and fir grow in great abundance, suitable for rough building and agricultural purposes, especially valuable for fire-wood; also white cedar, tamarack, cottonwood, wild-cherry, vine-maple, thorn, hazel, and willow.

White and black tailed deer are seldom seen in this vicinity; black and brown bears are in abundance; cougar, lynx, coyote, red fox, wolverine, beaver, otter, marten, mink, fisher, and badger are found. Of birds, there are ruffed grouse, wood or blue grouse, caper-cailzie, or cock of the mountain, prairie-grouse, curlew, pigeon, dove, ducks, and geese, and other varieties of water-fowl in great abundance. Of fishes there are the salmon and salmon-trout, in the Columbia River and all its large tributaries not too much obstructed by falls. Trout are in great abundance in all streams.

Snow sometimes falls during the first week in November, and in rare instances, as early as the middle of October, but in these cases melts soon, and begins to fall steadily about Christmas, when it lies on the ground until the 1st of March. The cold is extreme, the atmosphere dry, crisp, and bracing.

The fort is located very near the center of the reservation, upon an elevated and level gravelly plain, containing about one hundred and fifty acres of ground. It is distant from the creek, bounding the reserve on the north side, about five hundred yards, and elevated above it about sixty feet. The post is built of hewn logs, the buildings being arranged on four sides of a square parade, laid out on the magnetic meridian, which here varies 22° 40′ to the east.

On the east side are four sets of company-quarters, only one set of which is now occupied as such. Each set comprises a barrack-building 88 by 28½ feet, inside measurement, 10½ feet high from floor to ceiling. The occupied barrack is well ceiled with rough boards, and against its north end is a frame building, 15 by 16 feet, and 9 feet high, used as a first sergeant's room. Each of the barrack-buildings is intended to accommodate a full company. Of the other three buildings, the middle one is used as a theater, with a room, 20 feet wide, partitioned off for ablution-room; one as a drill-room during wet or inclement weather; the fourth has never been finished, and at present is the quartermaster's storehouse. The barracks are warmed by two immense fire-places, one at each end of the room, and lighted by two windows in front and four in the rear, and ventilated by a large opening in the ceiling, in the middle of the room, communicating with openings at the ridge of the roof, protected by boxes perforated for exit of the air. The fire-places also are very efficient ventilators. When the quarters are full the air-space per man is 572 cubic feet, but as it is never completely full the real space per man is much greater. The room contains 23 wooden bunks, 3½ feet wide, each occupied by two men. The only wash and bath room for the soldiers is the room before mentioned, as a portion of the middle barrack-building; it has a large fire-place and sinks, but no bath-tub. Each barrack-building has its kitchen and mess-room in a long building with one large room, situated sixty feet back, with its long diameter perpendicular to the barrack; it is 60 by 20 feet, and 10½ feet high.

The one now in use has two windows on each long side; one door in front and two in the rear. Three small rooms are partitioned off the rear end of the room for a pantry, wash-room, and wood storage; it has a large fire-place and fine range. There are eleven sets of laundresses' quarters, built of logs. Two buildings are used as officers' quarters; five more built for that purpose, are now used as offices, post-library rooms, hospital and store-rooms. All are built of hewn logs, and well finished in a plain, substantial manner, are lathed and plastered, and well painted inside. Two of them have been hung with paper, at the expense of officers living in them. They are one and a half stories high, the rooms above having never been finished. Each set contains four rooms with hall between, in the building proper, and kitchen and pantries in the rear. In the set of quarters occupied by the commanding officer, (middle set in the row,) the main building contains four rooms, with a hall, 7 feet wide, running between from front to rear; the rooms are 16 by 16 by 9 feet, the upper half-story not having been finished. In the rear are the pantry, 9 by 9½ by 8 feet, and the kitchen, 14 by 14½ by 8 feet; then a porch, 6 feet wide, running back 51 feet, and in front of the wood-shed and kitchen; the wood-shed is next to the kitchen, and is 25 feet long; in the rear of the wood-shed is the privy. The two sets of quarters, which are on the east and west sides of the commanding officers' quarters, were originally intended as double quarters, but in dividing the rooms for that purpose they were made entirely too small for comfort, the largest room in the building having been only 12 by 13½ feet in size; the fault was remedied by removing the partition separating one of the halls, and closing one front door, thus giving a large parlor, 12 by 21 feet in size; the height of the ceilings in both buildings is 9 feet; they have a porch, 6 feet wide and 47 feet long; a hall, 7 feet wide, runs from front to rear, the depth of the front rooms. At the end of the hall is a small room, 9 by 12 feet; on the left of this room is a bed-room, 9 by 12 feet, and in front, left side, is a room, 12 by 13½ feet. All the buildings are heated by open fire-places, supplied with water by an iron pipe which runs through the kitchens from the reservoir, and have no bath-rooms.

The commissary storehouse is a building 101 by 30 by 13 feet; it has a cellar, 7 feet deep, under its whole length. The quartermaster's storehouse is an old set of barracks, the old kitchen in its rear being used as a granary for oats.

The guard-house is a building of hewn logs, 40½ by 30½ feet; it has two large rooms front, 16½ by 15⅜ feet, divided by a hall, 6 feet wide, and four rooms back, of various dimensions, for cells. It is warmed by two large fire-places, and has no special arrangement for ventilation. It is abundantly large, and sufficiently secure and gloomy; it has but one window, and that is in the guard-room.

The hospital is built of hewn logs, well lathed and plastered, and is whitewashed within and without; it is 42 by 30 feet, the part forming the kitchen, mess-room, and linen-room joining the main building at right angles; this portion is 45 by 18 feet, and has an uncovered porch, 6 feet wide, running its whole length. The plan is similar to that of the quartermaster's office; four rooms, with hall, 7 feet wide, between; the room on the left of the front door is 14 by 16 feet; the surgery, in the rear of this room, 14 by 16 feet. The room on the right of the front door is 13 by 15 feet; the room back of that, 15 by 16½ feet. A porch, 6 feet wide, runs the whole length of the building on the west side or front. Behind the surgery, and in the addition, is the linen-room, 10 by 12 feet, with shelving all around, and a small room, 7 by 12 feet, used as a sleeping-room for the steward. Back of these rooms is the mess-room, 16 by 16 feet, and back of that the kitchen, 16 by 18 feet. A small addition, back of the kitchen, made of rough boards, is used as a wood-shed. The height of the ceilings, in the main buildings, is 9 feet; of the mess-room and kitchen, 8 feet. The main building is lighted by six windows. There is no arrangement for ventilation, except by letting down the top sash a few inches. Three rooms are used as wards; each has three beds; the air-space per man is from 585 to 720 cubic feet. No bath nor wash room; patients wash out of doors when able; otherwise in the wards. The privy is a small building, 75 feet to the rear of the hospital. The hospital is in very poor condition, but authority has been granted to have it put in good repair. It is unoccupied at present. A building originally intended for officers' quarters is temporarily used as a hospital. A room 17 feet long by 13 feet wide and 9 feet high is used as a ward. It is occupied by three beds, giving an air-space of 663 cubic feet to each, is warmed by a fire-place, but has no special means of ventilation.

59 M P

The Government stable is 117 by 31¼ feet; it is built of unhewn logs; is 9 feet high from floor to loft, and divided in the middle into two portions, by a passage, 13 feet 4 inches wide, running from side to side. On each side of each division are rows of stalls against the walls. The whole building has but one window, and that in the east end; is rough, dark, and poorly ventilated.

The library contains about 50 volumes.

The post is supplied with water from the creek; it is raised about 50 feet, by means of a water-ram, furnishing 1,080 gallons per day. The water is received in a reservoir of 50 barrels capacity, and is distributed throughout the garrison by means of iron pipes; the supply being insufficient, daily use of the water-cart is necessary. The water contains a small quantity of lime, and is of excellent quality. The natural drainage is excellent. There is no bath-house. For bathing the men go to the creek.

The post garden is situated in a bend of the creek, and contains about eight acres of ground. All the ordinary vegetables do well here, excepting melons, tomatoes, cucumbers, corn, beans, and squashes, for which the nights are too cold in summer, and the frosts too early and hard for them to mature. There are no hospital nor officers' gardens.

The mail is received once a week, is regular in summer, but not in winter. It requires ten days for a letter to reach department headquarters at Portland.

Attached to the Colville agency are about 3,000 Indians, in various localities, and of the following tribes, viz: Colvilles, Spokanes, Pend d'Oreilles, Okinakanes, Cœur d'Alenes, Sanpoils, Lakes, Isle de Pierres, and Methows.

The general health of this post and vicinity is unusually good; there was no prevailing disease during the past year. Malarial diseases are entirely unknown in the country. Not one case of phthisis originated at this place; but two or three cases, which were imported, rapidly improved under treatment; phthisis, however, is very prevalent and very fatal among the Indians.

*Meteorological report, Fort Colville, Wash., 1870–'74.*

| Month. | 1870–'71. | | | | 1871–'72. | | | | 1872–'73. | | | | 1873–'74. | | | |
|---|---|---|---|---|---|---|---|---|---|---|---|---|---|---|---|---|
| | Temperature. | | | Rain-fall in inches. | Temperature. | | | Rain-fall in inches. | Temperature. | | | Rain-fall in inches. | Temperature. | | | Rain-fall in inches. |
| | Mean. | Max. | Min. | | Mean. | Max. | Min. | | Mean. | Max. | Min. | | Mean. | Max. | Min. | |
| | ° | ° | ° | | ° | ° | ° | | ° | ° | ° | | ° | ° | ° | |
| July.................. | 71.31 | 96 | 51 | 1.50 | 71.18 | 91 | 56 | 1.06 | 71.39 | 103* | 30* | 0.50 | 68.83 | 95* | 36* | 0.40 |
| August.............. | 67.71 | 92 | 44 | 0.54 | 68.03 | 84 | 51 | 1.16 | 66.73 | 96* | 35* | 0.90 | 67.69 | 96* | 35* | 0.60 |
| September .......... | 58.74 | 86 | 36 | 0.24 | 60.69 | 77 | 37 | 0.56 | 55.19 | 89* | 22* | 0.85 | 57.76 | 83* | 12* | 0.07 |
| October ............ | 45.52 | 72 | 25 | 0.78 | 47.78 | 73 | 17 | 0.36 | 43.51 | 74* | 9* | 0.33 | 42.37 | 76* | 10* | 0.16 |
| November.......... | 35.36 | 57 | 31 | 1.90 | 33.86 | 49 | 13 | 4.24 | 25.81 | 59* | — 8* | 0.41 | 35.47 | 63* | — 2* | 0.51 |
| December........... | 22.27 | 46 | 4 | 2.46 | 22.69 | 48 | —22 | 4.00 | 20.83 | 50* | —20* | 2.32 | 20.27 | 59* | —22* | 0.47 |
| January............ | 27.66 | 43 | — 8 | 2.48 | 22.94 | 46* | —18* | 5.52 | 25.21 | 48* | —10* | 0.97 | 25.24 | 48* | —13 | 0.31 |
| February ...... .... | 25.83 | 45 | — 9 | 2.08 | 30.93 | 46* | —20 | 3.67 | 25.39 | 50* | —20* | 1.25 | 28.29 | 43* | 0 | 0.44 |
| March............. | 36.22 | 52 | 16 | 2.40 | 38.76 | 61* | 14* | 1.55 | 37.42 | 64* | 15* | 1.47 | 32.52 | 63* | 8 | 0.98 |
| April.............. | 49.07 | 68 | 34 | 1.52 | 43.76 | 64* | 15* | 0.24 | 46.58 | 75* | 20* | 1.24 | 45.61 | 78* | 24 | 0.56 |
| May............... | 60.68 | 77 | 42 | 2.54 | 56.29 | 79* | 20* | 0.86 | 52.96 | 79* | 20* | 1.08 | 57.53 | 91* | 34 | 4.22 |
| June .............. | 68.95 | 90 | 48 | 1.96 | 64.22 | 85* | 30* | 0.28 | 60.07 | 82* | 30* | 0.62 | 58.17 | 85* | 41 | 3.49 |
| For the year....... | 47.44 | 96 | — 9 | 20.40 | 46.76 | 91 | —22 | 23.50 | 44.25 | 103* | —20* | 11.94 | 44.98 | 96* | —22* | 12.21 |

* These observations are made with self-registering thermometers. The mean is from the standard thermometer.

*Consolidated sick-report, Fort Colville, Wash., 1870–'74.*

| Year ....... | | 1870–'71. | | 1871–'72. | | 1872–'73. | | 1873–'74. | |
|---|---|---|---|---|---|---|---|---|---|
| Mean strength................. | { Officers............. | 3 | | 4 | | 3 | | 3 | |
| | { Enlisted men...... | 55 | | 54 | | 48 | | 54 | |
| Diseases. | | Cases. | Deaths. | Cases. | Deaths. | Cases. | Deaths. | Cases. | Deaths. |
| GENERAL DISEASES, A. | | | | | | | | | |
| Remittent fever.................................................. | | 5 | ...... | 2 | ...... | 3 | ...... | 1 | ...... |
| Intermittent fever................................................ | | 3 | ...... | 8 | ...... | 9 | ...... | | ...... |
| Other diseases of this group ...................................... | | 7 | ...... | | ...... | 2 | ...... | 4 | ...... |

*Consolidated sick-report, Fort Colville, Wash., 1870-'1874—Continued.*

| Year | | 1870-'71. | | 1871-'72. | | 1872-'73. | | 1873-'74. | |
|---|---|---|---|---|---|---|---|---|---|
| Mean strength { Officers | | 4 | | 3 | | 3 | | 3 | |
| { Enlisted men | | 55 | | 54 | | 48 | | 54 | |
| Diseases. | | Cases. | Deaths. | Cases. | Deaths. | Cases. | Deaths. | Cases. | Deaths. |
| GENERAL DISEASES, B. | | | | | | | | | |
| Rheumatism | | | | 1 | | 5 | | 14 | |
| Syphilis | | 1 | | 1 | | 4 | | 1 | |
| Consumption | | | | 1 | | | | | |
| Other diseases of this group | | | | | | | | | |
| LOCAL DISEASES. | | | | | | | | | |
| Catarrh and bronchitis | | 10 | | 8 | | 9 | | 12 | |
| Pneumonia | | | | | | 1 | 1 | | |
| Pleurisy | | | | | | | | 3 | |
| Diarrhœa and dysentery | | 5 | | | | 16 | | 13 | |
| Hernia | | 1 | | 1 | | 1 | | 1 | |
| Other local diseases | | 13 | | 11 | | 16 | | 12 | |
| Alcoholism | | 5 | | 5 | | | | 4 | |
| Total disease | | 50 | | 38 | | 66 | 1 | 65 | |
| VIOLENT DISEASES AND DEATHS. | | | | | | | | | |
| Accidents and injuries | | 12 | | 7 | | 9 | | 23 | |
| Suicide | | | 1 | | | | | | |
| Total violence | | 12 | 1 | 7 | | 9 | | 23 | |

# CAMP HARNEY, OREGON.

## INFORMATION FURNISHED BY ASSISTANT SURGEONS CHARLES STYER, B. KNICKERBOCKER, AND C. B. BYRNE, UNITED STATES ARMY.

Camp Harney is situated at the mouth of Rattlesnake Creek, in a cañon of the same name, opening into Harney Lake Valley, in Grant County, Oregon. Latitude, 43° 30' north; longitude, 41° 27' west; and about 4,200 feet above the level of the sea.

The cañon is about a mile long, with precipitous walls of dark volcanic rock from four to six hundred feet in height. Its breadth at the post is about three hundred yards. The reservation is six miles square, and, extending into Harney Valley, includes about fifteen square miles of level and serviceable land.

Harney Lake Valley, formerly known as "Big Meadows," is about 50 miles long by 30 wide and contains two lakes of considerable size, known as Malheur and Harney Lakes, which have no outlets, the water of each being somewhat brackish.

Rattlesnake Creek, from which the post derives its supply of water, rises about ten miles north of this place in the mountains. The water is of good quality, clear, sparkling, and perennial. In summer the stream is maintained by springs, and the water remains cold throughout, except during the heat of the day.

The character of the country to the north, east, and west of this place is broken, rugged, and mountainous. Just at this point, where the mountains lower down and give place to the valley or flat, all vestige of timber disappears; and to the south, southeast, and southwest nothing but sage and a few stunted junipers are to be found. In the opposite direction, however, as the mountains recede from this point, they become wooded with juniper, fir, and pine. The geological formation of this section of country is singular. The flat already alluded to, adjacent on the south, is composed of alluvium, and in places the soil is impregnated with saline matter. The hills immediately bounding the valley present in many places bold, continuous cliffs, of probably five hundred feet in height, resembling a line of coast-rocks. The face of the rocks near the creek, where not crumbled away or concealed by *débris*, has well-defined marks of having at some time formed the limit to a body of water, being washed and worn as is usual in such situations. The face of the rock furthermore presents evidence of its aqueous origin, exhibiting well-marked strata. These remarks apply only to the comparatively low range of hills immediately circumscribing the valley. At the foot-hills below the cliffs are large detached rocks of volcanic origin, in many of which are imbedded specimens of petrified pine. No mineral products of value have been discovered in the vicinity.

The following-named animals and birds are found in the vicinity: Grizzly, black, brown, cinnamon, and fox bear, (the last-named animal has a head resembling a fox, the other portions of the body those of a bear;) California lion; panther; wildcat; gray, timber, and prairie wolf (or coyote;) lynx; red, silver-gray, and cross fox; beaver; otter; pine and stone martens; mink; fisher; weasel; badger; skunk; muskrat; elk; white-tailed, black-tailed, and mule deer; antelope; jack and cotton-tailed rabbit; gray and ground squirrel; chipmunk; black, gray, and bald eagle; black, yellow, mouse, and mottled or snake hawk; hooting and snowy owl; sage-hen; pintail; pine and prairie grouse; pheasant; wild geese; brant; canvas-back, spike, mallard, teal, and widgeon duck; swan; English or jack and common American snipe; plover; curlew; sand-hill and swamp crane; variegated blackbird; robin; yellow-hammer; sap-sucker; bluebird; titmouse; magpie; white-breast snowbird; yellowbird. Immense flocks of wild geese and ducks remain in the low marshy lands during the spring and summer.

Private conveyance is the only means of communication with the nearest railroad station, Winnemucca, Nev., distant two hundred and eighty miles. Portland, Oreg., the nearest city of any magnitude, is reached from Canyon City by a weekly line of stages to the Dalles, thence by steamboat and railroad down the Columbia River. The only obstacle to travel during the year is occasioned by snow, which usually falls to such a depth in winter as to preclude the possibility of passage from camp except on snow-shoes. This causes in the season mentioned great irregularity in the transmission of mail-matter. When there is no interruption, the usual time occupied in the transit of mails to department headquarters is from ten to fourteen days, and to Washington one month.

The only inhabitants at the post or in its vicinity are roving bands of Pi-Utes or Snake Indians.

The post was first located in August, 1867, as a base of operations against the Indians occupying the Malheur and Stein's Mountain section of country in the south and east of Oregon. It was first known as Camp on Rattlesnake Creek, then as Camp Steel, then Camp Crook.

The quarters for enlisted men consist of three buildings, standing in a line on the east side of the parade, with a space of two hundred and fifty feet between them, each 30 by 100 feet, built of unhewn logs, with shingled roofs, and divided into two dormitories, one at each end of the building, with an orderly's room, and a store-room between them. Each dormitory has an air-space of 11,056 cubic feet, is lighted by two windows in front, and one in rear, and warmed by a large stove. The only ventilation is by the doors and windows and a hole in the gable. The roofs and floors are in a dilapidated condition. The mess-rooms and kitchens are in three buildings, each 25 by 61 feet, one in rear of each barrack.

Laundresses and married soldiers occupy four log buildings, each 16 by 24 feet, containing a single set, and two frame buildings, boarded and battened, each containing two sets. The roofs are leaky, and the floors decayed and broken.

There is a post bakery in rear of the mess-room of the middle barrack. It is a frame, boarded and battened, very cold in winter, and the floor is very much decayed and broken through.

The sinks for the enlisted men (one to each set of quarters) are located about one hundred and fifty yards in rear of and across the creek from the barracks.

The officers' quarters are in a row facing the west side of the parade, and consist of four log and two frame buildings. The commanding officer occupies a log building, 32 by 42 feet, divided into four rooms and a hall, which runs through the center of the building from front to rear. The line officers occupy three log and two frame buildings, the latter covered with upright boards, the joints battened. Each building is 33 by 48 feet, divided, by a double hall running through the center, into two sets of quarters, of two rooms each. Each set of quarters has an addition in the rear, containing two small rooms, one used as a kitchen. These buildings are all one story high, with unfinished attics; all have verandas running across the fronts, and were originally neatly finished, but have become very much out of repair; the frame buildings, especially, being very cold in winter.

The adjutant's office, or headquarters building, is a log building, 32 by 43 feet, one story high, divided into four rooms and a hall. A veranda extends across the front.

The guard-house is 32 by 42 feet. Inside, 29 by 40 feet. Large cells, 14 by 29 feet. Small cells, each 7 feet 10 inches by 3 feet 6 inches. Height of ceiling, 11 feet. It is warmed by a stove placed in the center of the guard-room, and is ventilated by doors and windows. The average occupancy during the past year has been five.

All timber used in the building of the post was procured from the timbered hills to the north, a distance of three miles. In a cañon beyond is situated the saw-mill. All the buildings were built of green lumber, and the consequent contraction, gives ample ventilation, without exposing the health of the inmates.

The commissary-storehouse is 30 by 100 feet, and the quartermaster's storehouse is 30 by 80 feet; both built of logs, one and a half stories high, are substantial and secure, and of suitable capacity, but are badly roofed, causing much damage to Government property.

There are two cavalry stables, each 30 by 190 feet, frame buildings in good condition, with a capacity for seventy-five horses each.

The hospital was built in 1867. The site is well chosen, on a knoll, fifty yards northwest from any other post buildings, where the nature of the soil and position of the building are such as to render sewerage unnecessary. The hospital faces east, and consists of a building 34 by 43 feet, one story and an attic high, divided below into a ward 16 by 30 feet, a hall 6 by 30 feet, a dispensary 16 by 16 feet, and a steward's room 14 by 16 feet, all 10 feet high; and above into a hall, store-room, and attendant's room. At right angles with, and eight feet in rear of, the main building, with which it is connected by a rough boarded space, (part of which is used as a lavatory,) is a one-story log building, 17 by 33 feet, divided into two rooms, a kitchen and mess-room. The main building has a deep veranda across the east and south sides. The inside of this building on the lower floor is wainscoted. There is a small yard around the east and south of this building, inclosed by a post and rail fence, used for raising such vegetables as lettuce, radishes, &c., but owing to the dryness of the climate is of little practical value. The ward is heated by a stove, the other apartments by open fire-places. There are no provisions for ventilation except by the doors and windows. The wash-room adjoins the rear of the large ward. It contains a trough running the width of it, with a waste-pipe leading to a subterranean drain. It is used also as a bath-room, and contains one bath-tub. The privy is fifty feet in rear of the hospital. There is no dead-house. The baggage of patients is stored in a closet underneath the stairs leading to the attic.

There is no laundry, chapel, nor school-house.

The stables are two in number, one hundred and fifty feet apart, built of boards and divided into single stalls, with a capacity for seventy-five horses each.

Water is obtained from Rattlesnake Creek, a small stream running through camp from a spring half a mile above camp, and from wells in rear of each set of barracks. The quantity is unlimited, and by proper police being enforced the quality is excellent.

The soil being very porous, moderate amounts of rain and snow are rapidly absorbed. This, during the greater part of the year, is all that is needed for proper drainage.

There are as yet no general arrangements made for bathing.

Owing to the occurrence of severe frosts during each month of the year, together with immense swarms of crickets and grasshoppers, it has been found impossible to cultivate a garden with any surety of success. For two seasons the attempt was made, and the result proved but a total loss.

*Meteorological report, Camp Harney, Oreg., 1870–'74.*

| Months. | 1870–'71. | | | | 1871–'72. | | | | 1872–'73. | | | | 1873–'74. | | | |
|---|---|---|---|---|---|---|---|---|---|---|---|---|---|---|---|---|
| | Temperature. | | | Rain-fall in inches. | Temperature. | | | Rain-fall in inches. | Temperature. | | | Rain-fall in inches. | Temperature. | | | Rain-fall in inches. |
| | Mean. | Max. | Min. | | Mean. | Max. | Min. | | Mean. | Max. | Min. | | Mean. | Max. | Min. | |
| July | 77.19 | 95 | 55 | 0.00 | 77.68 | 100 | 58 | 0.64 | 71.60 | 97* | 30* | 0.00 | 70.03 | 93* | 41* | 0.96 |
| August | 72.32 | 98 | 52 | 0.05 | 73.91 | 99 | 54 | 0.12 | 67.65 | 95* | 34* | 0.01 | 66.89 | 96* | 33* | 0.37 |
| September | 64.14 | 89 | 45 | 0.00 | 65.05 | 90 | 40 | 0.11 | 54.91 | 87* | 25* | 0.63 | 59.69 | 93* | 18* | 0.34 |
| October | 50.52 | 82 | 23 | 0.00 | 49.62 | 80 | 21 | 0.03 | 48.90 | 83* | 17* | 0.82 | 44.69 | 79* | 9* | 0.25 |
| November | 40.64 | 63 | 20 | 0.09 | 36.87 | 62 | 10 | 1.05 | 27.61 | 65* | 4* | 0.25 | 40.44 | 66* | 13* | 1.08 |
| December | 24.62 | 52 | – 6 | 0.57 | 32.56 | 53* | 1* | 2.83 | 29.74 | 49* | – 2* | 0.53 | 22.89 | 40 | 6* | 2.41 |
| January | 33.63 | 50 | 14 | 1.37 | 27.75 | 48* | 1* | 1.69 | 30.44 | 45* | 3* | 3.15 | | | | |
| February | 33.27 | 48 | 11 | 0.48 | 35.78 | 57* | – 8* | 1.68 | 24.48 | 44* | – 3* | 1.24 | | | | |
| March | 37.80 | 58 | 18 | 2.20 | 41.21 | 69* | 19* | 0.35 | 37.79 | 68* | 5* | 0.30 | | | | |
| April | 45.63 | 80 | 33 | 0.66 | 41.69 | 67* | 20* | 0.10 | 40.39 | 69* | 10* | 1.00 | | | | |
| May | 53.30 | 82 | 35 | 1.09 | 58.69 | 80* | 33* | 0.14 | 49.46 | 75* | 21* | 0.27 | | | | |
| June | 70.43 | 100 | 36 | 0.00 | 67.37 | 90* | 33* | 0.11 | 59.37 | 84* | 25* | 0.53 | | | | |
| For the year | 50.29 | 100 | – 6 | 6.51 | 50.68 | 100 | – 8* | 8.85 | 45.19 | 97* | 3* | 8.73 | | | | |

* These observations are made with self-registering thermometers. The mean is from the standard thermometer.

*Consolidated sick-report, Camp Harney, Oreg., 1870–'74.*

| Year | 1870–'71. | | 1871–'72. | | 1872–'73. | | 1873–'74. | |
|---|---|---|---|---|---|---|---|---|
| Mean strength { Officers | 7 | | 7 | | 4 | | 7 | |
| { Enlisted men | 185 | | 99 | | 85 | | 112 | |
| Diseases. | Cases. | Deaths. | Cases. | Deaths. | Cases. | Deaths. | Cases. | Deaths. |
| GENERAL DISEASES, A. | | | | | | | | |
| Typhoid fever | 2 | | | | | | 1 | 1 |
| Remittent fever | | | | | | | 3 | |
| Intermittent fever | 45 | | 9 | | 30 | | 7 | |
| Other diseases of this group | 70 | | 20 | | 14 | | 5 | |
| GENERAL DISEASES, B. | | | | | | | | |
| Rheumatism | 35 | | 11 | | 13 | | 5 | |
| Syphilis | 2 | | 3 | | 4 | | 2 | |
| Consumption | 1 | | | | 1 | | 1 | |
| Other diseases of this group | 2 | | | | | | 3 | |
| LOCAL DISEASES. | | | | | | | | |
| Catarrh and bronchitis | 40 | | 24 | | 31 | | 5 | |
| Pneumonia | | | 1 | | | | | |
| Pleurisy | | | 1 | | 2 | | | |
| Diarrhœa and dysentery | 3C | | 19 | | 24 | | 11 | |
| Hernia | 4 | | | | | | | |
| Gonorrhœa | 2 | | | | 1 | | 3 | |
| Other local diseases | 201 | | 72 | | 46 | | 19 | |
| Alcoholism | 6 | | | | 2 | | 2 | |
| Unclassified | | | | | | | 1 | |
| Total disease | 440 | | 160 | | 168 | | 68 | 1 |
| VIOLENT DISEASES AND DEATHS. | | | | | | | | |
| Gunshot wounds | 2 | | | | 1 | | | |
| Drowning | | 1 | | | | | | |
| Other accidents and injuries | 109 | | 21 | | 33 | | 10 | 1 |
| Total violence | 111 | 1 | 21 | | 34 | | 10 | 1 |

# FORT KLAMATH, OREGON.

### REPORT OF ASSISTANT SURGEON HENRY MCELDERRY, UNITED STATES ARMY.

Fort Klamath is situated in Jackson County, in Southwestern Oregon. Latitude, 42° 39′ 4″ north; longitude, 44° 40′ west; altitude, 4,200 feet above the sea.

It is on the eastern margin of a valley in the Cascade Mountains. The valley runs north and south; is about twenty miles long and seven miles wide at the point where the post is located. Toward the south it widens somewhat, and extends to Upper Klamath Lake, about seven miles distant. High hills and mountains wall in the valley on the north, east, and west. Among the peaks, Scott's Peak is the most prominent to the north, Mount Pitt in the range to the west, and farther south, in the same range, is seen, far in the distance, the perpetually snow-clad summit of Mount Shasta. The range of hills bordering the valley on the east, near the foot of which the post is located, extends south to the Klamath Indian agency, five miles from the post; there the range becomes broken, and, a few miles further on, is cut by the valley of Williamson's River, which flowing from the northeastward, empties into Upper Klamath Lake at a point about twelve miles from the post.

The site of the post, and the ground immediately about it, is somewhat above the general level of the valley, and is tolerably well drained. Between the post and Wood River, however, the ground is low in places, and in the spring and summer is marshy. It is not until the latter part of July, or the beginning of August, that the marshy places become dry. During those two months the mosquitoes are generally very troublesome at the post, and the prevailing wind, blowing over these flats toward the post, brings with it the germs of miasmatic diseases, which affect the garrison more or less at that season of the year.

The rocks about the post are mostly of volcanic origin. At least a layer, more or less thick, of lava-rock seems to overlie the older formations, pumice abounding in the forest and on the hills. A good arable alluvium covers the general surface of the valley. A superior quality of sandstone, suitable for building purposes, is quarried in the hills to the southeast of the Klamath Indian agency.

There is considerable game about the post. The black, cinnamon, and grizzly bear; red and black-tailed deer, and antelope, are found in the mountains and higher table-land; ducks, geese, and other water-fowl abound upon the lake and marshes in the neighborhood of the mouth of Wood River, at all seasons of the year; pinnated, a species of ruffed and a dusky grouse, plover, curlew, and snipe, are found in season, but none of them in abundance.

Six streams, the waters of which are all, excepting that of one, of crystal clearness, flow through the valley within a short distance of the post; one of these, Linn Creek, runs a few rods in rear of the officers' quarters; another, Wood River, meanders through the valley about a mile to the westward. All these streams, as well as Williamson's River and Klamath Lake, abound in a very superior quality of salmon-trout, ranging from a few ounces to fifteen pounds in weight. These fish take the fly greedily, and are very gamy; their capture affording excellent sport from the middle of May until the latter part of September.

Fort Klamath is thirty-six miles distant from Linkville, the nearest post-office, and ninety-eight miles from Jacksonville by the shorter route, and one hundred and twenty-five miles by way of Linkville and Ashland. The shorter route is blockaded by snow, and practically impassable from about the 1st of December to the 1st of July. The longer route is also practically impassable for teams in the winter, on account of snow, which does not disappear till about the middle of May. A horse-trail is kept open by the mail-carrier. It is about one hundred and twenty miles from the post to Yreka. The two ends of the railroad are connected by the "California and Oregon daily line of stage-coaches," which pass through Jacksonville and Ashland. From these points passengers can only reach the post by means of military, hired, or private conveyances, there being no line of public stages. The mail now comes from Linkville twice a week; the military mail is brought from there on Wednesdays and Saturdays by a quartermaster's employé. It takes a letter about six days to come from department headquarters at Portland, and about fifteen days to come from Washington. The nearest military post is Camp Warren, one hundred and hirty miles distant.

The barracks for the men are situated along the southern border of the parade-ground. The dormitories, for two companies, are in one long building running east and west, 197 feet long and 30 feet wide, raised 18 inches from the ground, with verandas along its entire front and rear. It is built of one-inch pine lumber and roofed with shingles. A large double fire-place and a board partition across the middle of the building divide it into two dormitories. On each end of the building three small rooms are partitioned off for company offices, sergeants' rooms, and store-rooms. The rooms are all 10 feet 2 inches high in the clear, and are ceiled with rough pine boards. Each dormitory is lighted by ten windows, five on each side, opposite each other; and each has two doors, one on each side, near the partition dividing the building, and is also provided with two ventilators, 2½ by 2½ feet, in the ceiling. The east dormitory is heated by a large stove placed in the center of the room, and by the fire-place in the center of the building. The stove-pipes of this and nearly all other buildings at the post pass through the ceiling and roof, the wood-work being only protected by zinc. This has been found to be very unsafe, as many fires have been caused about the post by this arrangement of the stove-pipes. The west dormitory is heated by two stoves and the fire-place. Running back south from the center of the main building, at right angles to and connected with it by a board walk, is a building 100 by 38 feet, raised 1 foot from the ground, and built of the same materials as the building above described. It is divided by a board partition running its entire length. The east part of the building is divided into a mess-room, 53 by 18 feet; a kitchen, 17 feet 6 inches by 18 feet; a quartermaster-sergeant's room, 14 by 18 feet; and a first sergeant's room or company office, 15 by 18 feet. The west part is divided into a mess-room, 47 feet 6 inches by 20 feet; a kitchen, 26 by 20 feet; the balance being divided into two rooms, one used as a cobbler-shop, the other as a company store-room. All the rooms, except the last two, are 13 feet 5 inches to the ceiling; the last two are only 11 feet high. Adjoining the kitchen of the east set, is a small company bath-room, 9 feet 4 inches by 12 feet, 8 feet high to ridge. The bath-room for the western set is a detached building 10 feet 5 inches by 13 feet 7 inches, 7 feet 8 inches high to ceiling, situated near the mess-room, furnished with a bath-tub and wash-sink, and is heated by a small stove. Each company has constructed a root-house near its kitchen for preserving the winter store of vegetables.

The laundresses' quarters are situated along Linn Creek, to the southeast of the line of officers' quarters. They consist of two frame buildings, each 60 by 29 feet, raised 18 inches from the ground, with verandas 8 feet wide in front. Each building is divided into four sets of quarters, consisting of two rooms to a set. The front rooms are 15 feet 6 inches by 15 feet, and 11 feet to the ceiling; the back rooms are 13 feet 6 inches by 15 feet, 7 feet to the ceiling. Each set is lighted by a window in the front, and one in the rear room; has a door in front, one in rear, and one between the rooms.

The ordnance-sergeant's quarters, situated a little farther up the creek, contains two rooms; one is 15 by 15 feet, 8 feet to ceiling, lighted by two windows, and has two doors; the other is 9 feet 10 inches by 5 feet, 7 feet 6 inches to the ceiling, has one window and one door.

The post bakery is situated on Linn Creek. The building is 25 by 20 feet, 8 feet to ceiling, has three windows and two doors. Both the building and the oven are new.

The line of officers' quarters extends along the east side of the parade-ground, facing west. They consist at present of four sets, one set having been burned down several years ago. Authority has been granted to build a new set of officers' quarters, and it is expected that it will be done during the coming spring. Each set is raised two feet from the ground, is built of one-inch pine lumber, walls and floors double, and was originally a building 40 by 29 feet, with a veranda 8 feet wide extending entirely around it. Each building has a hall 6 feet 6 inches, running through the center from front to rear, on each side of which are two rooms, each 14 feet 6 inches by 16 feet 6 inches, 10 feet 6 inches to the ceiling in height. The walls and ceilings are all painted. The rooms in all the quarters, except the commanding officers', are heated with stoves. By boarding in the rear verandas, other rooms have been added to the officers' quarters. The commanding officer's quarters has two rooms each, on the north and south sides, formed by boarding up the end verandas. These rooms are 8 feet high in the clear, the front ones being 8 by 17 feet in size. In this set of quarters the hall has been partitioned across, and four fire-places have been built. In the three other sets, kitchens and servants' rooms have been formed by boarding up the rear verandas, and in one set a room 8 by 17 feet, 8 feet to the ceiling, has been formed in like manner on the north side. The commanding officer's and one other set of quarters have cellars attached. There is a stable for two horses in rear of one set of quarters, a cow-house in rear of another, chicken-houses in rear of three of them, and a sink in rear of each set.

The adjutant's office is contained in a building of the same dimensions and style as, and on a line with, the officers' quarters. It is located at the southeast corner of the parade-ground. A large room on the east side of the hall in this building is used as a post library and school-room. The room is 17 by 29 feet, 10 feet 8 inches to the ceiling.

The post hospital is situated at the northeast corner of the parade-ground, on a line with the officers' quarters, one hundred and forty feet distant from the last one, and the main building was originally of the same dimensions and style, and built of the same materials as those buildings. It faces the south. The front room on the west side of the hall is used as an office and steward's room, and is lighted by three windows. Adjoining this room at the rear is the dispensary, lighted by one window and furnished with suitable fixtures, &c. These rooms are each 14 feet 6 inches by 17 feet, 10 feet 8 inches in height. On the east side of the hall is the store-room, 16 feet 6 inches by 29 feet, same height as the other rooms, is lighted by five windows, each of which is furnished with outside shutters, and has proper shelving, a closet for linen and cupboard for knapsacks. In rear, three rooms have been formed by boarding up the veranda; a kitchen adjoining the store-room, a mess-room adjoining the dispensary, and a wash-room between the kitchen and mess-room. A wood-shed has been built over the steps in rear of the wash-room. In rear of this building there is a log building formerly used as a stable; this has been partitioned off and fixed up, one side as a root-house, the other as a chicken-house. A temporary ward 45 feet 6 inches by 24 feet 2 inches, 7 feet 9 inches high at the eaves and 16 feet 3 inches at the ridge, to contain ten beds, giving each 1,293 cubic feet of air-space, was constructed in 1873. It is a short distance from the hospital building, runs east and west, and was constructed by strengthening the frame-work of one of the canvas wards used during the summer, weather-boarding it with rough slabs, shingling the roof and putting a veranda in front. It is raised eight inches from the ground, has a single board floor, and is not ceiled. It has six windows, three on each side, the upper sashes of which can be lowered six inches with a slanting louver-board to direct the air toward the top of the room. The ward is heated by two stoves, under each of which is an opening one foot square for entrance of fresh air; there is also a ventilator in the roof around each stove-pipe. There is a door at each end of the room. There are three small rooms in rear of the ward; one used as a bath and wash house, heated by a small stove; another used as a wood-house; and the third, where the earth-closet commode is placed. The building is whitewashed inside. There is a detached sink in rear of this ward. A new hospital for twelve beds is now (January, 1875) in process of construction.

The guard-house is situated on the southwest corner of the parade-ground. It is a log building, 32 feet square, shingle roof; is raised two feet from the ground, with a veranda in front, 8 feet wide. It is divided into a room for the guard and four cells; the former 19 by 31 feet; the rooms, 10 feet 6 inches in height to the ceiling. The guard-room is lighted by two windows; the two larger cells by one window each. The two smaller cells are each provided with an aperture, 8 inches square, for the entrance of fresh air. The building is heated by one large stove. There is a sink in rear of the guard-house for the use of the prisoners.

The quartermaster and commissary storehouses are situated on the north side of the parade-ground, facing the company quarters. They consist of two structures: one, a log building, 74 by 36 feet, 12 feet to the eaves, raised two feet from the ground, divided in the center by a partition, half of the building being used as a quartermaster storehouse and office, the other half as a commissary storehouse and office; the other, a temporary structure, boarded up on the sides with rough slabs, covered with canvas, and used for protecting quartermaster stores; it is 43 by 24 feet, 10 feet to eaves. There is also a frame building in rear of and a short distance from the line of officers' quarters, which is used as a commissary and ordnance storehouse; it is 30 by 28 feet, 20 feet to ridge.

The magazine is situated not many feet from the guard-house; it is built of logs, and is 18 feet square.

The stables are situated immediately south of the adjutant's office, and run north and south. They are built of inch lumber, balloon frame, with shingle roof. The cavalry stables are 256 by 31 feet 9 inches, 23 feet from ground to ridge. The quartermaster's stable and granary are in one building, 263 by 32 feet 9 inches, 23 feet from ground to ridge. This latter building and the cavalry stables are connected by a shed, 100 feet long. Each stable has a ventilator in the ridge, 17 feet 8 inches long, with louver shutters.

In the vicinity of the stables are the wheelwright and cavalry blacksmith shops.

The post trader's store is located upon Linn Creek, about three hundred yards in rear of the line of officers' quarters. The building is 44 by 19 feet 6 inches, 10 feet 4 inches to ceiling. There is a room on the south end of this building used as an officers' billiard-room. The post trader keeps on hand a good supply of general merchandise.

There is a very good restaurant at the post, in which there is a room set apart as an officers' mess-room.

There are but two or three ranches in the neighborhood.

The water-supply for the garrison is obtained from Linn Creek, which heads in a spring at the foot of the hills, a short distance above the post. It is distributed by the water-wagon about the garrison once or twice a day. The water of this stream has a constant temperature of about 40° Fahrenheit and furnishes the garrison with an excellent quality of drinking-water.

The present contract price of beef at the post is eight and one-half cents per pound; mutton is supplied at any time in lieu of beef, and at the same price. During the spring and summer the supply of beef and mutton is ample, and of excellent quality; but during the winter the quality is generally inferior, owing to the impossibility of obtaining proper pasturage for the animals in the vicinity of the post at that season.

In consequence of the frosty nights that are liable to occur at all seasons of the year, only a very few vegetables can be raised; lettuce, radishes, and turnips are grown in the company and

60 M P

hospital gardens. During the fall the post teams are sent into Rogue River Valley, and a winter supply of vegetables, chickens, eggs, &c., are brought out for the use of the garrison. They are obtained in the valley at that season of the year at very reasonable prices. The Klamath Indians bring a considerable quantity of game and fish into the post.

Fuel consists of soft pine wood. The last contract price of fuel was $3.47 per cord.

*Meteorological report, Fort Klamath, Oreg., 1873–'74.*

| Month. | 1870–'71. | | | | 1871–'72. | | | | 1872–'73. | | | | 1873–'74. | | | |
|---|---|---|---|---|---|---|---|---|---|---|---|---|---|---|---|---|
| | Temperature. | | | Rain-fall in inches. | Temperature. | | | Rain-fall in inches. | Temperature. | | | Rain-fall in inches. | Temperature. | | | Rain-fall in inches. |
| | Mean. | Max. | Min. | | Mean. | Max. | Min. | | Mean. | Max. | Min. | | Mean. | Max. | Min. | |
| | ° | ° | ° | | ° | ° | ° | | ° | ° | ° | | ° | ° | ° | |
| July | | | | | | | | | | | | | 64.16 | 96* | 31* | |
| August | | | | | | | | | | | | | 63.33 | 94* | 29* | 0.00 |
| September | | | | | | | | | | | | | 57.91 | 97* | 15* | 2.30 |
| October | | | | | | | | | | | | | 44.79 | 90* | 7* | 0.02 |
| November | | | | | | | | | | | | | 39.86 | 75° | 15* | 1.20 |
| December | | | | | | | | | | | | | 26.34 | 45* | −12* | 3.89 |
| January | | | | | | | | | | | | | 26.92 | 49* | 0* | 2.60 |
| February | | | | | | | | | 27.83 | 52 | − 4 | | 26.09 | 56* | − 5* | 1.88 |
| March | | | | | | | | | 38.78 | 72 | 15 | | 29.97 | 62* | − 4* | 2.57 |
| April | | | | | | | | | 39.76 | 72 | 14 | | 42.20 | 72* | 6* | 0.99 |
| May | | | | | | | | | 47.19 | 77 | 29 | | 52.55 | 80* | 28* | 0.51 |
| June | | | | | | | | | 53.28 | 85* | 30* | | 54.62 | 83* | 27* | 0.67 |
| For the year | | | | | | | | | | | | | 44.06 | 97* | −12* | |

\* These observations are made with self-registering thermometers. The mean is from the standard thermometer.

*Consolidated sick-report, Fort Klamath, Oreg., 1870–'74.*

| Year | 1870–'71. | | 1871–'72. | | 1872–'73. | | 1873–'74. | |
|---|---|---|---|---|---|---|---|---|
| Mean strength { Officers | 2 | | 4 | | 3 | | 7 | |
| { Enlisted men | 62 | | 85 | | 78 | | 169 | |
| Diseases. | Cases. | Deaths. | Cases. | Deaths. | Cases. | Deaths. | Cases. | Deaths. |
| GENERAL DISEASES, A. | | | | | | | | |
| Typhoid fever | | | | | | | 12 | 2 |
| Typho-malarial fever | 5 | | 1 | | | | | |
| Remittent fever | | | | | 1 | | 2 | |
| Intermittent fever | 3 | | 3 | | 19 | | 21 | |
| Other diseases of this group | 1 | | 3 | | 1 | | 8 | |
| GENERAL DISEASES, B. | | | | | | | | |
| Rheumatism | 26 | | 7 | | 9 | | 20 | |
| Syphilis | 4 | | 3 | | 11 | | 15 | |
| Consumption | 4 | | 1 | | 3 | | 6 | |
| Other diseases of this group | | | | | 1 | | 4 | |
| LOCAL DISEASES. | | | | | | | | |
| Catarrh and bronchitis | 1 | | 15 | | 5 | | 31 | |
| Pneumonia | 1 | | 1 | | 2 | | 1 | |
| Pleurisy | 2 | | | | | | | |
| Diarrhœa and dysentery | 28 | | 22 | | 14 | | 46 | |
| Hernia | | | 2 | | | | 3 | |
| Gonorrhœa | 7 | | 1 | | 7 | | 11 | |
| Other local diseases | 41 | | 76 | 1 | 30 | | 105 | 1 |
| Alcoholism | | | 3 | | 1 | | 6 | |
| Unclassified | | | | | | | 3 | |
| Total disease | 123 | | 138 | 1 | 104 | | 294 | 3 |
| VIOLENT DISEASES AND DEATHS. | | | | | | | | |
| Gunshot wounds | | | 1 | | 55 | 2 | 1 | |
| Arrow wounds | | | | | 2 | | | |
| Other accidents and injuries | 15 | | 29 | | 33 | | 24 | |
| Homicide | | | | | | 1 | | |
| Total violence | 15 | | 30 | 1 | 90 | 2 | 25 | |

# FORT LAPWAI, IDAHO TERRITORY.

REPORTED BY ASSISTANT SURGEON C. R. GREENLEAF AND ACTING ASSISTANT SURGEON GEORGE C. DOUGLAS, UNITED STATES ARMY.

The post of Fort Lapwai is situated in latitude 46° 32′ north, longitude, 40° west, on the right bank of a stream of the same name, three miles from its confluence with the Clearwater. The latter is itself a tributary of the Snake River. The Blue Mountains are distant about twenty-five miles to the west. Lewiston, a town of about five hundred inhabitants, situated at the junction of the Clearwater and Snake Rivers, is twelve miles to the northwest. Fort Walla Walla, ninety-six miles southwest, is the nearest occupied military post.

The geological character of the country is volcanic and glacial, with terraces of basaltic trap cropping out. Lapwai Valley contains about four square miles of land, admirably fitted for agricultural purposes. The cereals and tubers of the temperate zone yield abundantly and mature well.

The trees and plants indigenous to the soil are the cottonwood, willow, birch, cedar, and pine trees; the sumac, alder, wild cherry, with strawberry and huckleberry, in the mountains. A bulbous root, called by the Indians "camas," and a favorite article of food with them, grows quite luxuriantly on the prairies south of us. It resembles somewhat the common onion, and is gathered in the month of August, at which time nearly the whole tribe (Nez Percés) move to the camas prairie, dig and prepare the root for winter use, by first drying and then powdering it between stones.

Of wild animals there are the grizzly, cinnamon, and black bears, cougar, gray and black wolf, coyote, red and gray fox, moose, common red and black-tailed deer.

Of birds there are bald and gray eagles, falcons, owls, prairie-chickens, grouse, and ducks, (teal and mallard.)

Of fish there are the brook and salmon trout and the salmon.

The nearest river, Clearwater, is a mountain-stream, navigable for steamboats about four months in the year, when raised by the melting of the snow in the spring. Its waters are of great purity. The Lapwai has a pebbly bottom, with cottonwood trees and willows fringing its banks.

The climate of this region is pleasant, and while there are wide ranges in the temperature they do not appear to have any detrimental effect upon the health of the inhabitants. The prevailing winds are from the north, and are mild in the winter and spring, but in the summer and fall blow occasionally with great violence. A wind, called by the natives "chinook," is prevalent in this region at all times of the year. It comes suddenly with great violence, and is always attended with a very great rise in the temperature. In winter one of these winds has been known to commence blowing in the evening at a time when there were three or four inches of snow on the ground, and by morning not a trace of snow could be seen. In summer the heat attending them is like that from a furnace, and vegetation withers before the hot blast.

The post was first established in November, 1863, and its construction completed in the fall of 1864. It was intended to accommodate one company of cavalry and one of infantry, and quarters for the men and stabling for the horses were erected. In July, 1867, the post was abandoned, and remained unoccupied until the following November. The reason for stationing troops at this point was to protect the settlers from the Indians. The military reserve embraces a square mile, within which is an inclosed space of ten acres occupied by the post.

The post-buildings occupy the four sides of a square, inclosing the parade-ground. The barracks are two frame buildings, on the east side. They rest upon stone foundations, raised about two and a half feet from the ground. Both are battened without and lined within with boards and are 10 feet in height to the eaves. The north barrack is 112 by 30 feet. A porch 8 feet wide runs along the western face of the building. In the north end is the orderly-room, 21 by 30 feet, leaving a dormitory 91 by 30 feet. This room had originally a fire-place at each end, but these being out of repair it is now warmed by three box-stoves. It is lighted by five windows, 3 by 4 feet, on its western side, and four on its eastern. Four doors open upon its west and three upon its east side.   There is no ceiling, and, the roof being leaky, the room is very uncomfortable in stormy weather.   The present occupancy is 38, which allows an air-space of 1,000 cubic feet per man.   The north barrack differs in no material respect except size, being 91 by 30 feet.   The occupancy is 34; air-space, 897 feet.   Iron bunks of the new pattern are used.   In rear of each barrack is a kitchen and mess-room, in one log building, 44 by 19, with lavatory and bath-room attached.   Latrines have been built at some distance from the company quarters, on the edge of the Lapwai.   When occasion requires they are filled with earth, and the sheds over them removed.

The laundresses' quarters are rooms built of slabs, 16 by 14 feet, and 10 feet high to the eaves. The interstices are filled with mortar, and the walls lined within with boards.   Each room has an open fire-place and an attached shed.   These quarters are very uncomfortable.   A frame building has recently been erected as a set of laundresses' quarters, consisting of two rooms and a kitchen attached.

The quarters for officers are two double frame buildings, each 46 by 54 feet, one story and a half high, lathed and plastered throughout, containing eight rooms upon the ground-floor and two garret-rooms.   The front rooms measure 14 feet by 14 feet 9 inches by 12 feet; rear rooms, 11 feet by 14 feet 9 inches; the dining-room, 13 by 11 by 9 feet, and the kitchens 18 by 12 feet.   A hall 7 feet wide extends from front to rear, dividing the buildings into two sets of quarters each.   They are in bad repair.

The commissary storehouse is one frame building, shingled and lined with boards; 50 by 22 feet by 20 feet high.   It has a cellar 20 by 12 by 8 feet, in fair condition.   The quartermaster's store-house is a log building, 81 by 20 by 17 feet, with shingled roof.   It is in poor condition.

The adjutant's office is a frame building, 30 by 20 feet, shingled, battened outside, lathed and plastered within, with a porch on the north side.

The bake-house is a log building, 29 by 21 feet, with shingled roof.   It has recently been provided with a new brick oven, which is well adapted to its purpose.

The guard-house is a one-story frame building, with shingled roof, board-lined, 40 by 30 feet, containing a prison-room, 16 by 16 feet, and three cells, each 4 by 8 feet, which are ventilated by grated openings in the doors and ceilings.   The guard-room, occupying the whole front of the building, with a porch, is 17 feet deep, heated by a stove, and lighted by two windows in front and one in the west end.   The ventilation is deficient.

The hospital stands upon a natural slope which terminates in the Lapwai.   It is a frame building, one story and a half high, upon a stone foundation which is three feet high in front, decreasing to the level of the ground in the rear.   There is a front porch on the east side.   The building is in fair condition, but the arrangement is objectionable, and accommodation insufficient.   It is 41 feet in front, with an L extending in rear, lathed and plastered throughout, and contains four rooms upon the ground-floor, with bath-room and wood-shed attached.   A hall, 6 by 15 feet, divides the main building into two rooms, used as ward and dispensary, with a small store-room in rear of the latter.   The ward, 20 by 15 by 12 feet, contains four beds, giving to each an air-space of 900 cubic feet.   The dispensary is 15 feet square.   The kitchen and mess-room, in rear of the ward, are each 12 by 12 by 10 feet.   The bath-room is 12 by 8 feet, and provided with bath-tub and conveniences for washing.   Above the ward and dispensary are two garret-rooms, lathed and plastered, with two windows to each.   That over the dispensatory is occupied by the hospital attendants; the other is used as a store-room.   Beneath the hall and ward is a cellar, 10 by 8 by 8 feet, without artificial walls or floor, or access of light.   The hospital is warmed by stoves, and imperfectly ventilated by doors and windows.   The privy is located thirty feet distant from the building.

An abundant supply of excellent water is obtained from two wells, one midway between the company quarters, and the other in the southeast corner of the parade.   Water for cleansing purposes is brought from the Lapwai.   Buckets are kept constantly filled with water as a precaution against fire.   There are also at the post two Babcock's fire-extinguishers, and a number of hand force-pumps, with a supply of hose.

The natural drainage is found sufficient.   A post-garden of about twenty acres is cultivated, and produces abundantly the vegetables common to this latitude.

The nearest large city is Portland, Oreg., which is reached by steamboat in the summer months from Lewiston, and during the fall and spring by stage to Wallula, thirty-two miles from Walla

Walla, on the Columbia River, where a steamer starts for Portland; and in the winter by stage to the Dalles on the Columbia River, where steamer is taken. The only serious interruption to travel occurs during the winter from snow on the Blue Mountains, but the weekly mails are seldom detained. A letter going to department headquarters requires seven days.

The nearest Indians are the Nez Percés, numbering about 3,000, who are peaceable and well disposed. Their agency is situated at the confluence of the Lapwai and Clearwater, about three miles north of the post.

The only mineral yet discovered is gold. The most important mining camps are Oro Fino, seventy-five miles in an easterly direction, Elk City, ninety miles, Florence, one hundred miles, and Warruns, one hundred and fifty miles distant, with Lewiston as their base of supplies.

*Meteorological report, Fort Lapwai, Idaho, 1870–'74.*

| Month. | 1870–'71. Temperature. Mean. | Max. | Min. | Rain-fall in inches. | 1871–'72. Temperature. Mean. | Max. | Min. | Rain-fall in inches. | 1872–'73. Temperature. Mean. | Max. | Min. | Rain-fall in inches. | 1873–'74. Temperature. Mean. | Max. | Min. | Rain-fall in inches. |
|---|---|---|---|---|---|---|---|---|---|---|---|---|---|---|---|---|
| July | 76.62 | 103 | 65 | 0.00 | 76.45 | 99 | 57 | 0.55 | 75.63 | 104* | 39* | 0.21 | 72.95 | 99* | 45* | 0.74 |
| August | 70.00 | 99 | 46 | 1.00 | 73.54 | 101 | 51 | 0.27 | 70.92 | 96* | 41* | 0.20 | 72.25 | 100* | 40* | 0.15 |
| September | 63.80 | 93 | 41 | 0.30 | 64.77 | 89 | 40 | 0.35 | 59.61 | 88* | 29* | 0.98 | 60.90 | 94* | 20* | 0.49 |
| October | 50.52 | 82 | 27 | 0.45 | 52.40 | 80 | 21 | 0.20 | 50.97 | 79* | 18* | 0.63 | 47.77 | 83* | 17* | 0.18 |
| November | 44.41 | 62 | 27 | 1.27 | 41.98 | 63 | 29 | 3.59 | 32.96 | 64* | 0* | 4.03 | 43.73 | 72* | 11* | 0.79 |
| December | 34.14 | 64 | 13 | 0.20 | 32.14 | 50 | 4 | 1.46 | 34.48 | 52* | 6* | 3.04 | 28.41 | 48* | − 5* | 1.05 |
| January | 41.35 | 57 | 17 | 3.09 | 40.09 | 65 | 11 | 1.02 | 37.59 | 51 | 8* | 1.88 | 37.05 | 54* | 5* | 2.12 |
| February | 39.79 | 61 | 15 | 1.12 | 42.28 | 57 | 16 | 3.12 | 34.04 | 48 | 11* | 0.60 | 36.49 | 52* | 10* | 0.94 |
| March | 45.64 | 60 | 33 | 4.25 | 46.81 | 66 | 33 | 1.85 | 47.08 | 68 | 26* | 1.22 | 43.23 | 65* | 21* | 0.85 |
| April | 52.97 | 72 | 42 | 1.35 | 49.42 | 70* | 24* | 0.34 | 51.19 | 75 | 27* | 1.30 | 53.82 | 79* | 30* | 0.85 |
| May | 60.05 | 83 | 45 | 3.26 | 61.25 | 92* | 29* | 0.48 | 57.05 | 77 | 32* | 1.14 | 63.76 | 97* | 40* | 0.95 |
| June | 70.32 | 91 | 49 | 1.50 | 69.78 | 96* | 38* | 0.21 | 64.19 | 84* | 39* | 0.79 | 66.41 | 92* | 42* | 2.14 |
| For the year | 54.13 | 103 | 13 | 17.79 | 54.21 | 101 | 4 | 13.44 | 51.31 | 104* | 0* | 15.72 | 52.23 | 100* | − 5* | 11.25 |

* These observations are made with self-registering thermometers. The mean is from the standard thermometer.

*Consolidated sick-report, Fort Lapwai, Idaho, 1870–'74.*

| Year | | 1870–'71. | | 1871–'72. | | 1872–'73. | | 1873–'74. | |
|---|---|---|---|---|---|---|---|---|---|
| Mean strength { Officers / Enlisted men | | 3 / 75 | | 4 / 79 | | 4 / 84 | | 4 / 105 | |
| Diseases. | | Cases. | Deaths. | Cases. | Deaths. | Cases. | Deaths. | Cases. | Deaths. |
| GENERAL DISEASES, A. | | | | | | | | | |
| Typhoid fever | | | | | | | | 1 | |
| Intermittent fever | | 1 | | 4 | | 1 | | 13 | |
| Other diseases of this group | | 3 | | 5 | | 8 | | 6 | |
| GENERAL DISEASES, B. | | | | | | | | | |
| Rheumatism | | 10 | | 13 | | 9 | | 21 | |
| Syphilis | | | | 6 | | 3 | | 5 | |
| Consumption | | 1 | | | | | | | |
| Other diseases of this group | | | | | | 1 | | 2 | |
| LOCAL DISEASES. | | | | | | | | | |
| Catarrh and bronchitis | | 10 | | 15 | | 7 | | 35 | |
| Pneumonia | | | | | | 2 | | | |
| Pleurisy | | | | | | 1 | | | |
| Diarrhœa and dysentery | | 6 | | 7 | | 12 | | 17 | |
| Gonorrhœa | | 3 | | 3 | | 3 | | 2 | |
| Other local diseases | | 27 | | 50 | 1 | 60 | | 87 | |
| Alcoholism | | | | 1 | | 2 | | 6 | |
| Total disease | | 61 | | 104 | 1 | 109 | | 195 | |
| VIOLENT DISEASES AND DEATHS. | | | | | | | | | |
| Gunshot wounds | | 1 | | 1 | | 1 | | | |
| Other accidents and injuries | | 11 | | 23 | | 23 | | 31 | |
| Total violence | | 12 | | 24 | | 24 | | 31 | |

# SITKA, ALASKA.

### REPORT OF ASSISTANT SURGEON JOHN BROOKE, UNITED STATES ARMY.

The town of Sitka, including the military post of the same name, is located on the western side of Baranoff Island, in latitude 57° 3′ north, and longitude 58° 36′ west. It is built upon the shore of Sitka Bay, about ten miles from the open ocean, and upon a point of the island where the bay divides into two arms, one of which runs about ten miles into the island and terminates in Silver Bay, while the other passes round the northern end of the island to join the inland waters.

In the year 1799 the old Russian Fur Company was re-organized under the name of the Russian-American Fur Company, and the new company was granted control of all the American Pacific coast north of latitude 55°. The directorship of the company was given to Alexander Baranoff, who established his headquarters at Kodiak Island.

In the same year (1799) one of the company's vessels explored the Alexandrian Archipelago, and carried back a considerable number of valuable furs; and in consequence of the report made by the explorers, Baranoff himself visited Sitka Bay, and commenced the construction of a fortified factory at or near the place where Sitka now stands. This he completed the following spring, named it Fort Archangel Gabriel, and took formal possession of the territory in the name of Russia.

In May of 1802 the Sitka Indians attacked the new settlement, killing all of the officers and thirty of the men. The remainder escaped to the woods, where most of them were hunted down and slain by the savages. In the spring of 1804, Baranoff again sailed from Kodiak for Sitka, taking with him this time four vessels, and a number of Aleutian Kyaks, and nearly a thousand Russians and Aleuts. He attempted to take the place by storm, but was repulsed with considerable loss; but after a short siege the savages abandoned it in the night, first killing all their young children to prevent them from giving the alarm. Baranoff burned the old fort, and soon after commenced a new one, which he named Fort Archangel Michael, while the settlement was known as New Archangel. A ship-yard was established, and a number of vessels were built in the course of a few years.

In 1836, the small-pox appeared at Sitka; vaccination was practiced by the Russians, but it was discouraged by the Indian shamans, and the disease spread with frightful ravages for a number of years among the native tribes along the coast.

During the later years of the Russian-American Fur Company's occupation of Sitka a number of measures were introduced tending to improve the condition of the people. It had become the company's headquarters, and a colonial school was established, where pupils were educated for its service; a large hospital was built in the town, and another, for skin diseases, was established at the mineral springs, some ten miles distant.

The negotiations for the purchase of Russian America by the United States were opened in the year 1866, and the purchase was concluded by a treaty which was signed at Washington on the 30th of March, 1867. This treaty was ratified on the 20th of the following June, and promulgated by proclamation of the President on the same date.

Commissioners were appointed by the two governments to arrange the formal transfer of the Territory. They met in the town of Sitka, " and on the eighteenth day of October, in the year 1867, at the governor's house in that town, Captain Pistchanroff, as such commissioner for and in the name of His Imperial Majesty the Emperor of Russia, formally transferred and delivered to Lovell H. Rousseau, as commissioner aforesaid, who received the same for and in behalf of the United States, the territory, dominion, property, dependencies, and appurtenances ceded to the United States of America by treaty above referred to, and as bounded and described in that treaty. The transfer was made under mutual salutes of artillery, the United States taking the lead, and in strict accordance with our instructions in that behalf."*

The Territory was attached to the Department of California, as the military district of Alaska, and Bvt. Maj. Gen. J. C. Davis was assigned to the command by instructions under date of Sep-

---

* From the report of the commissioners.

tember 6, 1867. One company of the Second Artillery and one of the Ninth Infantry were ordered at the same time to proceed to New Archangel or Sitka, and, on the formal transfer of the Territory by the commissioners, General Davis landed his troops and established the military post. It has continued to be garrisoned by two companies since that time.

On the 11th of April, 1868, the Territory was made a military department, with the headquarters at Sitka, and posts were established at Kodiak, Kenay, Tongass, and Wrangell; but the garrisons were subsequently withdrawn from these places, and Sitka remained, as it is now, the only garrisoned post in the Territory.

In July, 1870, the Department of Alaska was discontinued, and the Territory attached to the Military Department of the Columbia.

The parade and most of the buildings belonging to the military post are located in that part of the town which is nearest the harbor and wharf. The parade is partially inclosed on the northwest and northeast sides by officers' quarters, on the southeast side by the building used as post headquarters and custom-house office, and by private stores, and on the southwest side by the quartermaster's storehouse and the beach.

The barrack-building is situated at the southern angle of the parade, and in its immediate vicinity are the subsistence storehouse, the bakery, an old building used as married soldiers' quarters, and a large building known as the Governor's House, or Castle.

It may be premised that nearly all of the buildings constituting the post are constructed of squared logs, which are generally of large size. They were public buildings at the time of the cession of the Territory, and became the property of the United States by virtue of the second article of the treaty. They are entered numerically on the official list of public buildings, and such of them as are described in this article will be designated in accordance with that list.

No. 1 stands on the northwest side of the parade, and was erected by the Russians for a school-house in 1833. It was roofed, floored, and weather-boarded by the Quartermaster's Department in 1868–'69; is of one story with attic; is 56 feet long and 36 feet wide; contains six rooms, and is quite comfortable and in good repair. There are porches in front and in the rear, and also yards of sufficient size. The building is occupied as quarters by the post-commander.

Nos. 2, 3, 4, and 5 are all connected, and form a continuous row along the northeast side of the parade.

The building is one story in height, with roomy attics; was erected by the Russians for officers' quarters, and is still used for that purpose; but was reroofed, lined, and otherwise repaired after the transfer of the Territory. It is 88 feet long, 43 feet wide, and is divided into four sets of quarters; two of the sets containing three rooms each, the others containing four rooms each, exclusive of the kitchens and attics.

In the rear of each set is a kitchen, wood-shed, and water-closet; and beneath these a sewer runs the entire length of the building, and finally empties into the bay. Sinks from the kitchens empty into this sewer, and through it a stream of water runs during a great portion of the year, so that the water-closets are generally clean and inodorous. A small yard is inclosed in front and rear of each set of quarters.

The quarters are quite neat and comfortable, and in fair repair, almost the only imperfection being occasional leakages during heavy storms, the comparative lowness of the ceilings, and the want of sufficient ventilation beneath the floors. The rooms are warmed by either open fire-places or stoves.

No. 16, known as the "Governor's House," was built by the Russians in 1836, and stands close to the water's edge upon a hill of such height that it overlooks the entire town. It is 50 by 87 feet, two stories high, and divided into commodious rooms, and has been furnished in a very creditable manner. One of the largest rooms has been arranged as a theater, with a very good stage and scenery, and it is occasionally used by a local minstrel troupe. The remainder of the building is used when required as officers' quarters.

No. 14 is the barrack-building. It is a large log structure, weather-boarded, three stories high on the front, 66 feet wide and 70 feet long, and was built by the Russians in 1854 for the purpose for which it is now used. The front of the lowest story is used as a guard-house, and contains a guard-room, 28 by 44 feet, with an air-space of about 9,570 cubic feet; a prison-room, 15 by 27 feet, with an air-space of 3,037 cubic feet; and five cells, each 4 by 8 feet, and with an air-space of 224 cubic feet. The entire guard-house is fairly lighted by windows, but there is no special arrangement for ventilation; and, as the windows are on one side only, they answer that purpose in a very imperfect manner.

The second and third stories furnish quarters for one company each. They are arranged in almost precisely the same manner, a hall passing through the middle of the building its entire length, with the barrack-room, orderly-room, and store-room on the northwest side, and on the opposite side the wash-room, mess-hall, and kitchen. The latter rooms are of sufficient size, and very fairly answer the purposes for which they are used. The barrack-room of the second floor is 54 by $25\frac{1}{2}$ feet, and $8\frac{10}{12}$ feet in height, giving an air-space of 12,163 feet. That of the third story is $26\frac{3}{12}$ by $56\frac{2}{12}$ by $8\frac{1}{2}$ feet, giving an air-space of 11,914 cubic feet. The bunks in use are of wood, single, but arranged in two tiers, thus retaining one of the evil features of the old "relics of barbarism."

The barrack-rooms are both heated by stoves; they are lighted by windows on one side and end only, the other end being cut off by the orderly-room, while the other side is a blank wall, except for an entrance-door near each end. There are no means of ventilating the rooms excepting by the doors and windows; the latter have the advantage of movable upper sashes. The building is surrounded on three sides by other buildings, while the fourth side, that on which the barrack-rooms are, has an exposure toward the northwest, and consequently does not receive a ray of sunlight during the gloomiest months of the year.

A plan for a ventilating-shaft to pass through both rooms was proposed by the writer several months ago, but the absence of sufficient material and proper workmen at the post has so far prevented the execution of the plan.

Fortunately for the soldiers themselves the companies now garrisoning the post are not full, and several of the bunks are therefore but singly occupied. After deducting the space occupied by the beds and the bodies of the men, the room of the second floor gives, as now occupied, 350 cubic feet of air per man; and that of the upper floor 470 feet per man. When the companies are filled, all of the bunks will necessarily be occupied; the actual air-space will then be 276 feet per man, and this in rooms with no special arrangement for ventilation, in a cold and wet climate, and where, during a considerable portion of the year, a gleam of sunshine is but rarely seen. The water-closet for the use of the men is just behind the quarters, and over the bay at high water.

No. 17, standing at the southeast side of the parade, is a handsome two-story building, and was built by the Russians in 1857. The lower floor is used as post headquarters and custom-house, the rooms on the upper floor are occupied as post library, reading-room, printing-room, &c.

No. 23 is the post hospital. It stands upon the shore of the bay, about 8 feet above the sea level, fronting toward the southeast, and at a distance of 630 yards from the barracks. It is built of square logs, is weather-boarded on the outside, and lined inside either with dressed boards or canvas; the rear of the building is on a level with the ground, while the front is raised about two feet on a rough stone wall. It was erected by the Russians in 1843, and was intended for a hospital with forty beds. The main building is 85 by 41 feet, and 20 feet to the square. The chief entrance is by a double door in the front, which opens into a wide hall, and from this hall an open staircase leads to the second story, while in rear of the staircase is a room which serves as a *post-mortem* room. The portion of the first floor which is on the east side of the hall is divided into five rooms of reasonable size, and is used as quarters by the medical officer resident at the hospital. On the opposite side of the hall are also five rooms, one 14 by $13\frac{1}{2}$ feet, used as an office; one $13\frac{1}{2}$ by $7\frac{3}{4}$ feet, which is suitable for steward's quarters; a dispensary, $14\frac{3}{4}$ by $13\frac{1}{2}$ feet; a mess-room, 20 by $13\frac{1}{2}$ feet; and a kitchen, 20 by 23 feet. The dispensary is fitted up with a counter, shelves, and drawers; in the kitchen a pump connects with a cistern outside, and a sink for washing dishes, &c., connects with a sewer beneath the building.

The height of the lower story is 7 feet 9 inches in the clear.

The staircase opens on the second floor into a wide hall, which extends from the rear half way across the building; and from the back end of this hall a door opens upon an outside stairway leading to the ground below, and giving access from the second floor to the wood-shed, water-closet, &c.

At the other end of this hall is a room 12 by 12½ feet, which has frequently been used for Indian patients. The second floor is a trifle over 8 feet high in the clear.

The east end is 40 by 36 feet, has five windows in front, and the same number in the rear, and probably was originally but one room, but is now divided.

The smaller room has no special use; the larger is used as a store-room, and contains only open shelves and a closet for liquors and small-stores.

The west end of the second floor is divided into a ward, attendants' room, and laboratory.

The ward is an L-shaped room, the long arm extending across the entire end of the building and the short arm running along the front. The room is lined and ceiled with boards, painted, is lighted by five windows in front, one in the end, and three in the rear, and has an air-space of a little over 9,000 cubic feet. The average number of patients in the ward during the year 1872 was six, which, including one attendant, would give an air-space of at least 1,300 feet per man. A brick chimney passes up at the angle of the room, and is inclosed by a wooden casing which opens beneath a board on the roof. Into this casing there are openings from the ward, and, as there is more or less fire kept up almost the year round, the arrangement answers the purpose of a ventilating-shaft quite well. The middle upper light of most of the windows is fixed in a separate frame, which frame is hung upon hinges, so that it can be opened or closed at will. In this way plenty of fresh air can be introduced into the ward, and thorough ventilation secured, the only objection being that the fresh air is necessarily admitted cold.

The ward is heated by means of a wood-stove. Adjoining the ward, and opening into it, is the attendants' room, 10 by 13½ feet; and adjoining this, but opening directly into the ward, and also into the hall, is the bath-room and lavatory.

It contains a fixed bath-tub, wash-sink, and water-closet, (the latter not being now used,) all of which communicate by means of lead pipes with the sewer beneath the building.

The sewer commences at the rear of the hospital, and opens into the bay just below high-water mark.

There are two commodes for use in the hospital, and an ordinary pit, housed over, a few yards behind the building.

At each end of the main hospital building is a wing 11½ by 30 feet, and two stories high, but they are of little real use.

The hospital is rather dilapidated in some of its parts, but it is nevertheless quite comfortable and serviceable. A considerable space is inclosed both in front and in rear of the building; part of this is cultivated, and yields a moderate supply of potatoes, cabbage, radishes, and lettuce.

There are several other buildings which belong to the post, and which are used as quartermaster's and subsistence storehouses, married soldiers' quarters, shops, engine-house, &c. A good fire-engine is kept ready for immediate use.

Wood for the use of the post is obtained, originally, by Indians, and generally consists of yellow cedar, though sometimes mixed with Sitka spruce, (abies Sitkensis.) The former makes excellent fuel; the latter burns well when dry, but when wet it can scarcely be burned at all.

Water is obtained from Indian River, a pure and limpid stream which empties into the bay about a mile distant. It is brought and distributed by means of water-carts, although the cost of maintaining these for a few years would suffice to bring the water in pipes from the river, and have it running at the doors of the quarters and barracks.

A stream of some size empties into the bay, between the barracks and hospital, but the water consists largely of surface-drainage from swampy land, and generally is so impregnated with vegetable matter as to be unfit for drinking or culinary purposes. A large lake, which is on this stream just behind the town, furnishes an ample supply of ice.

Subsistence supplies for the post are brought from Portland, Oregon. Fresh beef is generally issued weekly. The cattle are usually kept some time after being landed before they are killed; but, partly from want of sufficient range and partly from the injurious effects of the climate, they rarely improve by being kept; and the meat is lean, pale, dry, and devoid of the peculiar flavor of good fresh beef.

Venison in abundance and of good quality; grouse, ducks, halibut, salmon, clams, &c., can

61 M P

usually be purchased of the Indians when in season; but their edibility is rather impaired by the filthy habits of the venders. Native potatoes can occasionally be purchased in small quantities, and are quite good when freshly taken from the ground, but soon become impaired by keeping; but the greater part of the fresh vegetables used have to be brought from Portland. They are consequently scarce and expensive.

Milk is scarce and sells for twenty cents a quart in coin.

The only regular communication is by means of a steamer which plies monthly between Sitka and Portland, and which carries the mail. When the trip is made by running outside it can be accomplished in four or five days, but it is ordinarily made on the inside waters, and occupies eight or ten days, and sometimes even more. A letter may reach Washington from Sitka in eighteen days.

The town of Sitka lies close to and back of the military post, and contains about three hundred inhabitants, five-sixths of whom constitute what is known as the Russian population. This This is composed of native Russians, creole Russians, and various mixtures of Russians, Aleuts, and Indians. The remaining population consists chiefly of traders and saloon-keepers.

There is a church of the Greek Oriental persuasion, and a resident missionary priest. There is also a small chapel, which was fitted up by members of the Lutheran church some years since.

Commencing quite close to the post, and extending directly along the shore of the bay, is the village of the Sitka Indians. It contains some twelve hundred inhabitants, and is separated from the post and town by a stockade, in which are two small block-houses. These Indians are quite industrious, and are the only catchers of fur-bearing animals in the vicinity, deriving considerable revenue from the sale of marten, mink, otter, fox, wolverine, and bear skins. They also bring in deer-skins in large numbers, amounting to many thousands in the course of the year. They have substantial houses, which, for Indian habitations, are quite comfortable.

These Indians are, in many respects, in advance of most of the uncivilized North American tribes, although they are not provided with revolvers and breech-loading rifles, their chief arm being still the old flint-lock musket, such as were formerly sold from the Hudson Bay Company's stores.

The physical appearance of the country around Sitka has been likened to the first picture in the common-school atlas, of the comparative height of mountains. A chain of mountain-peaks, of various heights, encompass the place on every side, except that toward the open sea, while the narrow strip of level country which lies between the town and the mountain-base is so covered with moss and rotten timber that its surface resembles water-soaked sponge. Several small glaciers can be seen on the mountain-sides during the middle of summer; in winter, they are entirely covered with snow. Some ten or fifteen miles westward from the town is Mount Edgecombe, an extinct volcano, with the furrowed tufa near the top and the remains of the crater still plainly visible. It forms an important landmark for mariners entering the bay.

Gold exists in quartz ledges at Silver Bay, some six or eight miles distant. These ledges have lately been prospected to a considerable extent, and some rich specimens found.

The climate of Sitka is execrable. The tops of the mountains, which almost encompass the place, are more or less covered with snow and ice during the entire year, and consequently act as condensers to the moisture contained in the warmer air which comes in from the ocean. Rain is, therefore, an almost daily feature of the place. During the winter, snow sometimes takes the place of rain, lying last winter to the depth of over three feet at one time. During the year 1873 the rain-fall was 74.64 inches. In one month of this year (October) it amounted to 17.98 inches. The cold is never very intense, the thermometer seldom, if ever, getting as low as zero, while, on the other hand, it rarely reaches 70° in the warmest summer weather, and fires are lighted almost every day in the year. During the shortest days, there are but six hours of sunlight, and, as the sun only attains an elevation of about 10°, it follows that on cloudy days, which are the rule, it is dark and gloomy at midday, while during the months of June and July it never grows entirely dark, the nights being rather a prolonged twilight.

It might naturally be supposed that, in such a climate, acute rheumatism and acute pulmonary inflammations would be very common; but such is not the case. During a tour of nearly fifteen months, I have seen but one case of typical acute rheumatism, and not a single case of uncomplicated pneumonia or pleuritis. Cases of subacute rheumatism, however, and pains and aches of a few days' duration, are quite frequent. Pulmonary phthisis is not uncommon, and forms a large percentage of the cases of diseases even among the native Indians. Venereal diseases figure largely in the list, comprising fifteen per cent. of the entire number taken on the sick-report during the year 1873.

Cases of sickness not infrequently occur in which there is a general adynamic condition of the system, without definable disease, a condition which is doubtless due to the depressing influences of almost continuous wet, and cool, and cloudy weather; a monotonous diet, in which fresh fruits and vegetables play an insignificant part; the almost entire absence of out-door amusements; and the want of opportunities for sufficient exercise in the open air.

### Meteorological report, Sitka, Alaska, 1870–'74.

| Month. | 1870–'71. | | | | 1871–'72. | | | | 1872–'73. | | | | 1873–'74. | | | |
|---|---|---|---|---|---|---|---|---|---|---|---|---|---|---|---|---|
| | Temperature. | | | Rain-fall in inches. | Temperature. | | | Rain-fall in inches. | Temperature. | | | Rain-fall in inches. | Temperature. | | | Rain-fall in inches. |
| | Mean. | Max. | Min. | | Mean. | Max. | Min. | | Mean. | Max. | Min. | | Mean. | Max. | Min. | |
| July | 57.83 | 79* | 51 | 2.44 | 53.53 | 64 | 47 | 2.79 | 57.12 | 74* | 34* | 2.51 | 54.63 | 74* | 37* | 1.54 |
| August | 60.18 | 82* | 51 | 6.39 | 53.88 | 72 | 47 | 13.33 | 57.15 | 68* | 38* | 2.65 | 54.97 | 65* | 30* | 7.64 |
| September | 55.02 | 67* | 42 | 9.16 | 50.72 | 67 | 40 | 7.70 | 51.13 | 67* | 37* | 6.13 | 51.83 | 70* | 28* | 4.09 |
| October | 47.55 | 64^A | 28* | 9.46 | 46.41 | 60 | 32 | 14.54 | 45.17 | 60* | 28* | 8.85 | 46.56 | 55* | 31* | 13.98 |
| November | 39.15 | 53* | 13* | 11.58 | 32.77 | 50* | 4* | 5.36 | 36.74 | 55* | 19* | 6.58 | 38.63 | 57* | 14* | 8.02 |
| December | 36.12 | 48 | 25 | 7.55 | 31.81 | 50* | 7* | 3.54 | 36.42 | 60* | 16* | 5.97 | 33.91 | 48* | 14* | 5.77 |
| January | 28.27 | 46 | 5 | 3.00 | 37.03 | 55* | 25* | 4.84 | 29.18 | 48* | 9* | 8.40 | 23.94 | 43* | — 4* | 2.74 |
| February | 34.47 | 48 | 25 | 3.22 | 31.88 | 54* | 2* | 2.07 | 33.59 | 48* | 14* | 7.96 | 31.23 | 46* | 11* | 5.87 |
| March | 36.34 | 50 | 25 | 4.74 | 40.61 | 50* | 27* | 8.59 | 35.87 | 45* | 23* | 3.87 | 32.80 | 64* | 9* | 2.27 |
| April | 39.76 | 51 | 31 | 4.00 | 39.87 | 58* | 25* | 3.14 | 41.56 | 66* | 22* | 2.83 | 45.63 | 70* | 25* | 2.23 |
| May | 46.75 | 60 | 37 | 1.90 | 47.72 | 74* | 28* | 3.18 | 47.29 | 72* | 29* | 1.67 | 52.48 | 75* | 32* | 2.01 |
| June | 49.12 | 63 | 42 | 6.00 | 49.92 | 68* | 36* | 3.70 | 52.39 | 72* | 30* | 3.27 | 55.59 | 82* | 34* | 3.46 |
| For the year | 44.21 | 82* | 5 | 69.44 | 43.01 | 74* | 2* | 72.78 | 43.63 | 74* | 9* | 60.67 | 43.52 | 82* | — 4* | 59.62 |

* These observations are made with self-registering thermometers. The mean is from the standard thermometer.

### Consolidated sick-report, Sitka, Alaska, 1870–'74.

| Year | 1870–'71. | | 1871–'72. | | 1872–'73. | | 1873–'74. | |
|---|---|---|---|---|---|---|---|---|
| Mean strength { Officers<br>{ Enlisted men | 7<br>122 | | 9<br>107 | | 8<br>106 | | 8<br>88 | |
| Diseases. | Cases. | Deaths. | Cases. | Deaths. | Cases. | Deaths. | Cases. | Deaths. |
| GENERAL DISEASES, A. | | | | | | | | |
| Typhoid fever | | | | | 1 | | | |
| Remittent fever | | | 5 | | 1 | | | |
| Intermittent fever | 10 | | 3 | | 3 | | 1 | |
| Other diseases of this group | 3 | | 4 | | 2 | | | |
| GENERAL DISEASES, B. | | | | | | | | |
| Rheumatism | 35 | | 28 | | 39 | | 28 | |
| Syphilis | 24 | | 37 | | 27 | | 17 | |
| Consumption | | | | | 1 | | 1 | |
| Other diseases of this group | 2 | | 1 | | | | 2 | |
| LOCAL DISEASES. | | | | | | | | |
| Catarrh and bronchitis | 15 | | 12 | | 33 | | 46 | |
| Pneumonia | | | | | 1 | | 1 | |
| Pleurisy | 2 | | 3 | | 2 | | 2 | |
| Diarrhœa and dysentery | 13 | | 12 | | 5 | | 8 | |
| Hernia | 5 | | 1 | | | | | |
| Gonorrhœa | 10 | | 3 | | 4 | | 9 | |
| Other local diseases | 53 | 1 | 58 | | 65 | 1 | 70 | |
| Alcoholism | 4 | | | | | | | |
| Total disease | 176 | 1 | 167 | | 184 | 1 | 185 | |
| VIOLENT DISEASES AND DEATHS. | | | | | | | | |
| Drowning | | | | | | 1 | | |
| Other accidents and injuries | 48 | | 26 | | 31 | | 19 | |
| Suicide | | | | | | 1 | | |
| Total violence | 48 | | 26 | 2 | 31 | | 19 | |

# FORT STEVENS, OREGON.

## REPORT OF ASSISTANT SURGEON D. L. HUNTINGTON, UNITED STATES ARMY.

Fort Stevens, latitude, 46° 31′ north; longitude, 47° 58′ west, is located upon the extremity of Point Adams, at the mouth of the Columbia River, and guards the south channel of that river.

The point itself is a low, sandy spit, formed by the deposits of the river modified by the action of the sea. The soil is light and sandy, supporting, however, a heavy growth of spruce and hemlock; but, for agricultural purposes, is poor, and not to be relied upon.

For several years the western shore has suffered much erosion from the sea, and unless timely precautions are taken, it is probable that, in time, the invasion of the sea will render the point untenable.

The flora of this region is limited chiefly to trees of the genera *Pinus* and *Abies*, some few vines, and shrubs, but is particularly rich in ferns, mosses, and lichens, as well as in all the fungous growths peculiar to mild temperature and great humidity.

The animal kingdom presents a wide range. The elk, deer, black bear, cougar, and wolf are not unfrequently found; the marten, otter, mink, and beaver are common; the rabbit, squirrel, skunk, and smaller animals, abound.

Of birds, there are the wild goose, duck, swan, pelican, gull, crane, eagle, hawk, woodpecker, bluejay, swallow, wren, robbin, and pigeon.

Of fishes, we have the salmons, salmon-trout, sole, flounder, sturgeon, perch, porgy, smelt, and others; of shell-fish, oysters, clams, and crabs. The oysters are small and inferior, and unpalatable by reason of a coppery taste.

The climate is equable, much more so than on the same isothermal line of the Atlantic coast. The year is practically divided into a dry and wet season. The former embraces the months of May, June, July, August, and September, during which but little rain falls. The rains commence, usually, in October, and continue, almost without intermission, until May.

Sudden or excessive changes of temperature are very uncommon. During the year 1873 the highest recorded temperature is 86°; the lowest, 24°. The average mean temperature of several years is about 54°.

Snow and ice are not common, and generally, during the winters, vegetation is not entirely suspended.

The annual rain-fall is excessive, and is confined to the wet season. During 1873, 77.80 inches fell, which is about the average of years.

The prevailing winds of winter are southeast and southwest, occasionally northeast. The former are warm and humid; the latter, dry and cold. During summer, the prevailing wind is from the northwest.

The post and works were built under the supervision of the United States engineers, and were first occupied by a company of the Eighth California Volunteers, April 25, 1865.

The present garrison is Company E, Fourth United States Artillery. The fort itself is an irregular bastioned earthwork surrounded by a moat, and mounted with an armament of heavy ordnance. No repairs of importance have been made upon it for several years, and it is consequently at the present time in a most dilapidated condition.

The post is built directly in the rear of the work, and the several buildings comprising it are substantial wooden structures, well adapted to their purposes. The barrack, erected in 1866, is a one-story building, with porch running along its entire front. It is divided into two squad-rooms, each 38 by 30 feet; height, 14 feet; lighted by windows of ordinary size. Ventilation is effected by means of these windows, and by transoms over the doors, which are placed opposite to each other. The rooms are heated by large box-stoves. During the past year these dormitories have been well ceiled and finished, adding both to their comfort and appearance. Light iron single bedsteads have been substituted for the cumbrous double wooden bunks formerly in use. Between these squad-rooms are two rooms used as a company office and first sergeant's room, each 17 by 10 feet, and a hall, 20 by 13. The company mess-room and kitchen are removed from the main building about seventy yards. The mess-room is of good size and commodious, measuring 35 by 22 feet. The kitchen adjoins the mess-room, and measures 16 by 16 feet. The laundresses' quarters are two buildings one and a half stories high, accommodating two families each, containing each two rooms, 16 by 16 feet. They have lately been repaired and ceiled, and are now quite comfortable quarters.

Four houses, cottage style, are used as quarters for officers; three of them are built on the same plan, the fourth slightly modified. They are built of wood, one and a half stories high, with an L. On the ground-floor they are divided into a parlor, 16 by 14 feet; a bed-room adjoining, 12 by $12\frac{1}{2}$ feet; a dining-room, 13 by 12 feet; a kitchen, 12 by 12 feet, with good sized pantry adjoining, and a store-room or wash-room, 12 by 10 feet. On the upper story is a bed-room, 15 by $15\frac{1}{2}$ feet, 9 feet high; a second bed-room, 13 by $13\frac{1}{2}$ feet, and two smaller rooms suitable for store-rooms or closets; over the kitchen and wash-room is a loft divided into two good sized rooms, suitable for servants. Under the kitchen is a small cellar, and in the rear of the building a good woodshed. The houses are in good repair, with walls and ceilings hard finished and painted. The larger rooms below are heated by fire-places, the upper rooms by stoves.

A large rain-water tank is built in the rear of each house, and communicates with the inside by pipes. Each house is surrounded by a large piece of land, well fenced, suitable for garden or lawn.

There are three storehouses at the post; that belonging to the quartermaster's and commissary departments is a large and spacious building of one and a half stories, $112\frac{1}{3}$ feet in length, and $30\frac{1}{3}$ in breadth, with a porch running its entire length. Internally it is conveniently divided into offices and store-rooms for the different departments.

The ordnance building, 81 feet 2 inches by 22 feet 3 inches, is exclusively used for the storage of ordnance property. The engineer storehouse is a much smaller building, and much out of repair.

The guard-house is situated on the north edge of the parade-ground, and is thoroughly constructed of solid planking. The foundation is brick; the floors are double, and the intervening space filled with cement. The building is T-shaped; the extreme length of the cross part is 67 feet 8 inches; the width, 32 feet 10 inches. The length of the other portion is 28 feet, and its width, 24 feet 3 inches. It has a height of 10 feet in the clear.

The transverse portion of the building contains the cells, ranged on either side of a hall 12 feet 2 inches wide. The cellars are 7 by 12 feet, and open by a door into cell-halls, 9 by 12 feet, which halls communicate by grated doors with the main hall. The cells are 9 feet 5 inches high, and are ventilated by grated apertures near the ceiling; four of these apertures are 12 by 16 inches; the remainder, 8 by 12 inches. The guard-room in the main portion of the building is 15 by 24 feet. The building is heated by stoves; lighted by windows at the ends of the main and transverse halls. A trap or skylight 2 feet square is placed at the point of juncture of the two halls. The cell-doors are solid without openings, while those closing the cell-halls have a grated aperture 5 feet by 8 inches.

The cells are arranged for three bunks in each, but crowding to this extent is never necessary, as there are rarely more than two or three prisoners in confinement at a time. Allowing one prisoner to each cell, the arrangement for ventilation seems to be good, as by the general arrangement of the building a good current of air is in continual motion.

Laying aside the consideration of several minor defects, which could be easily remedied, this guard-house is the best building of the kind I have seen in the Army.

The hospital building is placed upon a sandy knoll, and a little elevated above the general level. It consists of a main building and addition or L. The main structure measures 25 feet 6 inches by 46 feet 10 inches; the addition 22 feet 5 inches by 24 feet 2 inches. At either end of the main building are the wards, each 24 feet 11 inches by 15 feet 8 inches, and open to the roof, with a ridge opening for ventilation, 9 feet by 12 inches. The air-space in each ward is 1,234 cubic feet per bed. Five beds are placed in each ward. The wards are lighted by five windows each, and ventilation is further secured by transoms over the doors.

Between the wards, and opening upon the hall connecting them, is the dispensary, 14 by 12 feet, well furnished with counter and shelves, and warmed by a stove. To the rear of this room, and also opening upon the hall, is the steward's room, 14 by 10 feet.

In the addition is the kitchen, 16 by 12 feet, and beyond this a large closet and bath-room, 7 by 7½ feet, with bath-tub and water-sink.

Outside the house is a water-closet and urinal, conveniently reached by a covered porch.

A small garden is attached to the hospital, which produces a small amount of vegetables.

The convenience of the building would be increased by carrying out the addition sufficiently to admit of a new kitchen and a more spacious bath-room, using the present kitchen as a mess-room.

A tank for rain-water is much needed for the supply of the hospital, and to provide sufficient water for bathing purposes; at present all the water used is brought by buckets from a well, fifty yards distant.

During the past year the knoll upon which the hospital, is built has been regraded, and it is hoped that the building will soon be inclosed by a neat fence.

As protection against fire, buckets kept filled are relied upon.

A post bakery is in operation at the post, and can supply bread daily for two hundred men.

The public stable contains stalls for fifteen animals, is well lighted and ventilated.

The post library contains two hundred and thirty-two books, principally novels and general literature; such periodicals and papers are taken as the post-fund will admit of from time to time

The post derives its supply of water from wells and from cisterns or tanks. The wells are distributed as follows: one in the cellar of each officers' quarters, one near the stables, one at the company mess-room, one in the fort, and two on or near the parade. They are only used during the dry season, and the water from them is limited in quantity and inferior in quality. During the rainy season a plentiful supply of wholesome rain-water is obtained from wooden tanks or cisterns placed at nearly the same points as indicated above in the mention of the wells. Their capacity is not sufficient to insure a supply long after the discontinuance of the rains. In view of the limited quantity of inferior water during the dry season of the year, it is most desirable that large tanks should be built for the storage of rain-water, insuring a constant supply of good water for drinking and cooking purposes, and, in case of fire, the means of preventing the destruction of valuable property.

The natural position of the post and the character of the soil both favor a ready and easy drainage, which is materially assisted by two large and deep drains, which run the length of the post and are connected with lateral branches, by which the surplus water is discharged upon the beach.

The especial drainage and sewerage of the several quarters is fair, and is mainly under the care of the general police, and is well attended to.

The poverty of the soil, the shifting sand, and the dry season, all interfere with the successful culture of post or hospital gardens; yet, by perseverance and industry, the current wants of the summer are met by a fair supply of vegetables, but enough for a winter's demand are not raised. Vegetables can be purchased in the surrounding country at reasonable rates.

The nearest town of any importance is Astoria, distant seven miles, the oldest American settlement on the coast, having been established in 1811, by John Jacob Astor, as a trading-post, and now numbering about 1,200 inhabitants. This town furnishes a market for all supplies needed for domestic purposes and which are not furnished by Government.

A chartered steam-tug conveys the mail from Astoria to the post twice a week, and is the only means of communicating with the mainland, the town being inaccessible by roads, owing to the broad swamp-lands which separate Point Adams from the interior. During the stormy season of the year the communication is liable to be very irregular.

From Astoria a tri-weekly steamboat runs to Portland, a distance of one hundred and eleven miles, and the steamships of the Oregon Steamship Company leave for San Francisco weekly.

A letter for the headquarters of the department requires from one to four days for its transmittal, and from twelve to eighteen days to Washington, D. C.

The country in the vicinity of the post is mainly of the same character as the reservation, flat and sandy, and in places densely wooded. The soil is generally poor, but on some farms well cultivated and productive. The grazing seems to be excellent, and considerable attention is paid to raising horses, cattle, and sheep. Passing inland from the coast the surface soon becomes rough and broken by the foot-hills of the Coast range of mountains, the strip of arable land along the shore rarely exceeding from twelve to fifteen miles in width.

A few individuals of the Clatsop tribe of Indians reside in this vicinity. They are industrious and well-behaved.

It can hardly be said that there are any prevalent diseases at this post; certainly none which can be attributed to local causes, except that in the spring-time catarrhal and rheumatic affections are somewhat common.

The influence of epidemics is rarely felt, and the general health of the command is excellent.

*Meteorological report, Fort Stevens, Oreg., 1871–'74.*

| Month. | 1870–'71. | | | | 1871–'72. | | | | 1872–'73. | | | | 1873–'74. | | | |
|---|---|---|---|---|---|---|---|---|---|---|---|---|---|---|---|---|
| | Temperature. | | | Rain-fall in inches. | Temperature. | | | Rain-fall in inches. | Temperature. | | | Rain-fall in inches. | Temperature. | | | Rain-fall in inches. |
| | Mean. | Max. | Min. | | Mean. | Max. | Min. | | Mean. | Max. | Min. | | Mean. | Max. | Min. | |
| | ° | ° | ° | | ° | ° | ° | | ° | ° | ° | | ° | ° | ° | |
| July | | | | | 60.64 | 82* | 49* | 0.81 | 61.38 | 79* | 44* | 3.60 | 59.96 | 75* | 49* | 1.55 |
| August | | | | | 61.55 | 80* | 48* | 0.16 | 60.04 | 75* | 50* | 6.25 | 61.21 | 86* | 49* | 2.75 |
| September | | | | | 58.25 | 75* | 44* | 1.82 | 56.51 | 75* | 37* | 5.35 | 57.06 | 70* | 44* | 0.95 |
| October | | | | | 54.21 | 66* | 39* | 1.76 | 54.65 | 67* | 36* | 3.27 | 50.21 | 70* | 35* | 3.91 |
| November | | | | | 46.09 | 55* | 32* | 12.03 | 42.32 | 57* | 31* | 9.78 | 45.95* | 56* | 31* | 6.96 |
| December | | | | | 39.43 | 52* | 21* | 13.90 | 42.27 | 54* | 30* | 10.90 | 38.33* | 52* | 24* | 6.33 |
| January | | | | | 41.60 | 53* | 30* | 6.50 | 44.71 | 52* | 30* | 14.75 | 40.90* | 54* | 27* | 18.08 |
| February | | | | | 45.51 | 54* | 30* | 15.28 | 39.56 | 50* | 30* | 10.28 | 40.73* | 50* | 30* | 12.69 |
| March | | | | | 49.54 | 59* | 40* | 6.57 | 46.56 | 66* | 34* | 20.76 | 43.00* | 57* | 32* | 6.05 |
| April | | | | | 48.82 | 65* | 34* | 5.00 | 49.84 | 72* | 36* | 3.40 | 50.88* | 70* | 39* | 5.66 |
| May | | | | | 54.29 | 71* | 31* | 4.60 | 53.24 | 77* | 39* | 1.87 | 55.37* | 69* | 44* | 4.04 |
| June | | | | | 58.69 | 84* | 44* | 6.90 | 57.98 | 71* | 45* | 5.52 | 56.80* | 67* | 47* | 5.90 |
| For the year | | | | | 51.55 | 84* | 21* | 75.33 | 50.75 | 79* | 30* | 95.73 | 50.03 | 86* | 24* | 74.87 |

NOTE.—The mean temperatures with the mark (*) have been derived from the registering thermometers, there being no standard during the period at the post.

*Consolidated sick-report, Fort Stevens, Oreg., 1870–74.*

| Year | 1870–'71. | | 1871–'72. | | 1872–'73. | | 1873–'74. | |
|---|---|---|---|---|---|---|---|---|
| Mean strength { Officers | 3 | | 2 | | 2 | | 3 | |
| { Enlisted men | 74 | | 46 | | 31 | | 54 | |
| Diseases. | Cases. | Deaths. | Cases. | Deaths. | Cases. | Deaths. | Cases. | Deaths. |
| GENERAL DISEASES, A. | | | | | | | | |
| Intermittent fever | 10 | | 1 | | | | | |
| Other diseases of this group | 35 | | | | | | 1 | |
| GENERAL DISEASES, B. | | | | | | | | |
| Rheumatism | 8 | | 3 | | 6 | | 9 | |
| Syphilis | 8 | | 3 | | 3 | | | |
| Consumption | | | | | 1 | | 1 | |
| Other diseases of this group | | | 2 | | | | | |
| LOCAL DISEASES. | | | | | | | | |
| Catarrh and bronchitis | 6 | | 3 | | 2 | | 13 | 1 |
| Diarrhœa and dysentery | 4 | | 2 | | | | 4 | |
| Hernia | 1 | | | | | | | |
| Gonorrhœa | 3 | | 1 | | 1 | | | |
| Other local diseases | 35 | | 24 | | 5 | | 15 | |
| Alcoholism | 4 | | | | 1 | | 1 | |
| Total disease | 114 | | 39 | | 19 | | 44 | 1 |
| VIOLENT DISEASES AND DEATHS. | | | | | | | | |
| Gunshot wounds | 1 | | | | 1 | | | |
| Drowning | | | | | | 2 | | |
| Other accidents and injuries | 12 | | 12 | | 6 | | 12 | |
| Total violence | 13 | | 12 | | 2 | 7 | 12 | |

## FORT TOWNSEND, WASHINGTON TERRITORY.

Fort Townsend is situated on Port Townsend Bay, about four miles southwest of the town of Port Townsend, the county-seat of Jefferson County, Washington Territory, in latitude 48° 10′ north, longitude 45° 40′ west, approximate.

The reservation contains $621\frac{97}{100}$ acres, fronting about three-fourths of a mile on the western shore of the bay. Large vessels can come directly to the wharf.

The post was re-established July 17, 1874; having been unoccupied for more than twelve years.

The buildings are ten in number, consisting of one company barrack, three sets of officers' quarters, and one hospital-building, all frame; one guard-house, one bakery, one office-building, and one storehouse, of logs, battened in part; also one stable, which is simply two log pens.

The barrack is a large frame building, two stories high, with a veranda in front. The lower story contains a mess-room, kitchen, and two store-rooms. The upper story, 12 feet in height, contains two dormitories, each 47 by 31 feet, and a small room for the first sergeant.

The quarters for married soldiers consist of four sets. The guard-house is undergoing repairs. It is warmed by a fire-place; the ventilation is good.

The hospital is a large building, and is undergoing repairs. It is well lighted and well ventilated; is a one-story and attic building, the story being 12 feet in height. It contains two wards, each 26 by 15 feet, a dispensary 12 feet square, a kitchen 12 feet square, and a mess-room, not in use at present.

The stables are located five hundred yards in rear of camp.

The post is supplied with water from a never-failing and excellent spring, which is about one thousand feet in a direct line from the company quarters, at the foot of a steep hill, on the road to the landing.

The fuel used at the post is pine; is of an excellent quality, and is obtained by contract.

There are a few Chinook Indians in the vicinity.

The means of subduing fire is a Johnson's patent hand-pump. In case of a fire, the difficulty would be to obtain water. A reservoir to catch the rain-fall ought to be constructed.

---

## FORT VANCOUVER, WASHINGTON TERRITORY.

INFORMATION FURNISHED BY SURGEON-GENERAL J. K. BARNES AND SURGEONS J. H. BILL AND R. H. ALEXANDER, UNITED STATES ARMY.

Fort Vancouver is situated on the north bank of the Columbia River, one hundred and twenty miles from its mouth and five miles east of the confluence of the Willamette River, on the Oregon side; latitude, 45° 40′ north; longitude, 48° 27′ west. It is directly east of the old town of Vancouver, once the principal Pacific trading-post of the Hudson's Bay Company, and is eight miles, by water, from the city of Portland, Oregon. The reservation has a frontage of one thousand two hundred yards along the Columbia River, and extends back about a mile and a half. The post buildings commence about two thousand feet from the river, a tract of low ground, subject to overflow, and used as a pasture, intervening. Immediately north of the post the forests of red fir commence, and extend to the foot-hills of the Cascade Range, interspersed with prairies, varying from one to six miles across. These prairies are now occupied with farms. The strips of land lying between the Columbia and Willamette Rivers, through which the road to Portland passes, is a thickly-timbered bottom-land, which is frequently overflowed from river to river. The ground occupied by the post is a gravel-bank, commencing four hundred or five hundred yards from the river. It rises twenty feet above the low ground, and extends back many miles, and more than ten miles up the river. In all this extent there is not a rock to be seen. The soil is sterile. Here and there are depressions in the gravel, rendered fertile by the accumulation of vegetable detritus.

Fir, cedar, ash, and alder are the principal trees; oak, hazel, and dogwood are mere bushes. The Oregon grape is plentiful, and giant ferns abound in the greatest variety.

Salmon, salmon-trout, smelts, and suckers are found in the streams. Bears, cougars, foxes wolves, deer, and elk are found in the mountains, and otters and beavers along the rivers.

There are neither springs nor ponds near the post. Water has been found by boring to a depth of one hundred feet. The post is supplied with the muddy and impure water of the Columbia, which is brought in a wagon and emptied into barrels; also with drinking-water from the main of the Vancouver Water Company.

Snow is infrequent, and is occasionally observed deeply colored, red, blue or purple, by infusoria.

The post was established in 1849; was intended for six companies, and occupies about 1,100 yards square. For the general arrangement see Figure 74.

A, officers' quarters; B, C, barracks; D, adjutant's office; E, guard-house; F, stables; G, bakery; H, hospital; I and J, latrine; K and L, barns; M, hospital garden; N, squatter; O, engine and shop; P, grain-house; Q, quartermaster's department stables; R, corral; S, garden; T, U, V, W, storehouses; X, mission-house; Z, grave-yard.

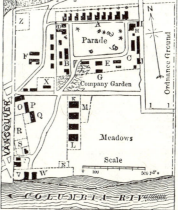

Figure 74.

The company quarters are two frame buildings, two stories in height, on the east and west sides of the parade. The east barrack is 80 by 30 feet; has windows on opposite sides; detached kitchen and mess-room in the rear, and is intended for one hundred and forty men, but is not now occupied. The west barrack is 90 by 30 feet. The kitchen and mess-room in the rear were last year connected with the main building by a hall 31 by 14 feet, in which a bath-room has been fitted up, supplied from the pipes of the water company. Iron bedsteads are used in the dormitories. The latrines are earth-pits, kept disinfected for a time, and at last they are filled up and new ones dug. The quarters for married soldiers and laundresses are log huts, scattered about all parts of the post and greatly out of repair.

Seven log buildings and four frame buildings, fronting the north side of the parade, are occupied as quarters for officers. The log houses were built of carefully-selected logs of red fir, underpinned, the crevices chinked and plastered, and the walls and ceilings lined with dressed lumber. They are of the pattern known as " four pens and a passage," giving four rooms and two attics, with kitchen and servants' room in the rear. The usual size is 30 by 36, with rear extension, 15 by 30, and piazzas in front. They are heated by fire-places, and were once commodious dwellings, but are now old and much out of repair. The frame cottages are similar in plan and dimensions to the log houses, but are inferior in comfort, having been built by contract and in a careless manner. The pipes of the water company have been introduced into all the kitchens, and, indeed, have been brought to all the inhabited buildings at the post except the band quarters.

The guard-house is a two-story frame building, having on the lower floor a prisoners' room, 18½ by 30½ by 10 feet, and nine cells, each 6½ by 4½ by 10 feet. The guard-room is in the second story. The building was thoroughly repaired in 1874, and the ventilation improved. The average occupancy during the past year was 5⅔.

The present hospital building was constructed in 1859, and has accommodations for thirty patients. It is a fir frame, weather-boarded with cedar, the interior lathed and plastered throughout. The plan and dimensions are given in Circular No. 4 of 1870. The three wards contain twenty-eight beds. The average occupancy last year was 1¼.

The natural drainage at the post is excellent. Water sinks into the deep, porous gravel, or runs down the steep declivity, rendering artificial drainage unnecessary.

Patches of fertile ground are found in the vicinity capable of producing in abundance all the principal vegetables of the Northern and Middle States. Some of these are cultivated as post and hospital gardens with a success varying from year to year according to the skill and labor bestowed.

62 M P

*Consolidated sick-report, Fort Vancouver, Wash., 1870–'74.*

| Year ................................................ | | 1870–'71. | | 1871–'72. | | 1872–'73. | | 1873–'74. | |
|---|---|---|---|---|---|---|---|---|---|
| Mean strength ............................... { Officers ............ | | 6 | | 9 | | 7 | | 8 | |
| { Enlisted men ...... | | 145 | | 136 | | 98 | | 170 | |
| Diseases. | | Cases. | Deaths. | Cases. | Deaths. | Cases. | Deaths. | Cases. | Deaths. |
| GENERAL DISEASES, A. | | | | | | | | | |
| Remittent fever ..................................... | | ...... | ...... | 31 | ...... | ...... | ...... | 1 | ...... |
| Intermittent fever................................... | | 44 | ...... | 31 | ...... | 8 | ...... | 18 | ...... |
| Other diseases of this group ................ | | 24 | ...... | 4 | 1 | 3 | ...... | 20 | ...... |
| GENERAL DISEASES, B. | | | | | | | | | |
| Rheumatism .......................................... | | 29 | ...... | 39 | ...... | 10 | ...... | 20 | ...... |
| Syphilis ................................................ | | 37 | ...... | 15 | ...... | 4 | ...... | 8 | ...... |
| Consumption ........................................ | | 1 | ...... | ...... | ...... | ...... | 1 | 2 | ...... |
| Other diseases of this group ................ | | 7 | ...... | 3 | ...... | | | | |
| LOCAL DISEASES. | | | | | | | | | |
| Catarrh and bronchitis .......................... | | 57 | ...... | 76 | ...... | 31 | ...... | 59 | ...... |
| Pneumonia ........................................... | | | | 2 | | | | | |
| Diarrhœa and dysentery ....................... | | 31 | ...... | 34 | ...... | 19 | ...... | 23 | ...... |
| Hernia .................................................. | | 3 | ...... | 1 | ...... | 1 | ...... | 1 | ...... |
| Gonorrhœa ........................................... | | 9 | ...... | 9 | ...... | 2 | ...... | 9 | ...... |
| Other local diseases ............................ | | 96 | 1 | 132 | ...... | 54 | 1 | 53 | ...... |
| Alcoholism ........................................... | | 22 | ...... | 18 | ...... | 9 | ...... | 4 | ...... |
| Unclassified ......................................... | | ...... | ...... | 8 | ...... | ...... | ...... | ...... | ...... |
| Total disease........................... | | 360 | 1 | 372 | 1 | 141 | 2 | 218 | ...... |
| VIOLENT DISEASES AND DEATHS. | | | | | | | | | |
| Accidents and injuries .......................... | | 26 | ...... | 21 | ...... | 20 | ...... | 44 | ...... |
| Homicide ...... | | ...... | ...... | ...... | ...... | ...... | 1 | ...... | ...... |
| Suicide .................................................. | | ...... | 1 | ...... | 1 | ...... | ...... | ...... | ...... |
| Total violence........................... | | 26 | 1 | 21 | 1 | 20 | 1 | 44 | ...... |

# FORT WALLA WALLA, WASHINGTON TERRITORY.

### REPORTED BY SURGEON C. H. ALDEN, UNITED STATES ARMY.

Fort Walla Walla is situated in the southeastern part of Washington Territory, and about half a mile south of the town of Walla Walla. The latitude is 46° 4' north; longitude, 41° 21' west. The elevation above the sea is 865 feet. Wallula, the nearest point on the Columbia River, is thirty miles distant. Portland, Oreg., is two hundred and seventy miles west, and Fort Lapwai, Idaho Territory, the nearest military post, is distant ninety-seven miles.

There appears to have been an old trading-post called Fort Walla Walla, located at Wallula on the Columbia, but it was long since abandoned. The present post was established in the fall of 1856, the troops, four companies of the First Dragoons and two of the Ninth Infantry, Colonel Steptoe in command, occupying a log cantonment just east of the town of Walla Walla, until the spring of 1858, when the permanent buildings were commenced on the present site. The garrison remained the same, one company of dragoons only being relieved until the summer and fall of 1861, when it was relieved by California volunteers. Oregon and Washington volunteers successively occupied the post until the summer of 1867, when it was abandoned and the buildings placed in charge of a quartermaster's agent. In August, 1873, after the close of the Modoc war, the post was re-established, and is now occupied by three companies of the First Cavalry and two of the Twenty-first Infantry.

The reservation is one mile square, the post itself being situated on a small plateau near its center. The valley of Walla Walla is remarkably fertile and is intersected by many small watercourses, two of which run near the post, all branches of the Walla Walla, which empties into the Columbia at Wallula.

There are many fine ranches in the valley and along the base of the Blue Mountains, which lie eight to ten miles east of the post. The soil in this vicinity is extremely light in character, making the roads deep with dust in summer.

Too short a time has elapsed since the writer's arrival for any study of the geology, flora, and fauna of this region, and but few general facts can be given.

Cottonwood, willow, birch, pine, red and white fir, tamarack, alder, and wild cherry are the principal woods, coming chiefly from the nearest mountains.

Of wild animals, there are black and cinnamon bears, coyotes, black-tailed deer, &c.

Of game birds, there are blue grouse, prairie-chickens, and ducks, teal and mallard; and of fish, trout, salmon-trout, and salmon.

From an old meteorological register, the only record of any kind found at the post, the following summaries are obtained. The mean temperature for eight years from 1857 to 1864, inclusive, was 51° 5'. The extremes were lowest January 15 and 16, 1862, when the thermometer went down to 24°. The highest, 107°, on the 7th of August, 1860. The winters of 1856–'57 and of 1861–'62 were very severe.

The mean annual rain-fall for these eight years was 22.3 inches, but the fall was very irregular in amount, 50.66 inches having fallen in 1862, and but 4.06 inches in 1863. Little rain falls in June, July, August, and September. The prevailing winds are southwest and southeast. The changes in the temperature are very sudden. The effects of the warm wind from the southeast, called the "chinook," are here very apparent, removing a heavy fall of snow in a few hours.

The buildings forming the post are arranged around a rectangular parade-ground 325 by 915 feet. The officers' quarters and the barracks are situated opposite to each other on the long sides of the parade. The adjutant's office and commissary storehouse occupy one of the short sides, opposite to the court-martial room; guard-house and post-trader's store on the other.

The hospital and quartermaster storehouse are detached, lying to the west and southwest of the parade.

The cavalry and quartermaster's stables, granary, and workshops are still farther west. The buildings are all constructed of the same materials and in the same general manner, being of wood, the outside covered with rough boards placed upright with the cracks battened and the roofs shingled.

The officers' quarters are composed of five one-story-and-a-half cottages, each building being double, and containing two separate sets. The sets are all alike, and each set has below a hall, two rooms about 15 feet square, and in the attached back-building a small dining-room and kitchen. Up-stairs there are two attic-rooms. A porch runs along the entire front of the building, the rooms are lined with boards and papered, and the ceilings plastered. There are fire-places in all the rooms but one. The buildings are comfortable but not in good repair, the floors being uneven from the decay of the posts supporting them; and the roofs leak.

There are six barracks, five only being now occupied as such, the sixth being used as a reading-room and carpenter-shop. They are of the same construction as the officers' quarters. Each barrack is 95 by 31 feet 6 inches, having a porch along the front, and divided within into two dormitories, each 30 by 41 feet 8 inches, and in the middle between them a first-sergeant's office 10 by 18 feet 6 inches. The interior shows the adobe lining, and some of the dormitories are ceiled with rough boards or muslin. Each dormitory contains eighteen or twenty single bedsteads, and each occupant has an average of 664 cubic feet of air-space. The rooms have each six windows, and are warmed by a large wood-stove in the center. A large fire-place and the numerous cracks afford ample ventilation. In fact, the buildings are too open to be comfortable in cold weather, and need repair.

About forty feet in rear of each barrack is a small wooden building, containing, on the right, a kitchen 15 feet square, and on the left, a mess-room 15 by 30 feet.

The guard-house is the only two-story building at the post. It contains below a prison-room 21 by 19 feet 8 inches, and eight cells opening into a center hall between them. The walls of this lower story are lined with logs. Outside stairs in front give access to the second story, which is divided into two rooms for the guard and its officer. There is a porch in front of the building above and below.

The hospital consists of a story and a half main building with a one-story L. The building is not well arranged nor well adapted to its purpose, and is not in good repair. A porch runs along the front, and from the front entrance an 8-foot hall runs across the building.

To the right of this hall lie the dispensary and office; to the left, the largest ward, containing six beds. A smaller ward opens from this, containing four beds. The larger room is heated by a stove, the other by a fire-place. Each bed has an average of 65 feet superficial area and 600 feet cubic air-space. There are shafts intended for ventilation extending from the ceilings of the ward up into the space under the roof, but such violent down-draughts are produced by them in winter when fires are lighted that they have to be closed. Renewal of air is provided for as far as possible by the fire-places and stove, and frequently opened windows and doors. The one-story L-wing contains the mess-room, kitchen, and store-room. There is a small cellar under the latter. The upper rooms, three in number, are occupied by the steward and attendants, and one of them is used occasionally as a ward. All the rooms of the hospital are plastered. Many improvements in the hospital are needed, especially more perfect arrangements for ventilating the wards, a lavatory, bath-room, water-closet, laundry, and more store-rooms.

An appropriation has been made for the erection of an additional ward and for extensive general repairs.

There are earth-commodes in the wards and a common sink in the rear of the hospital. Sinks of the same kind are provided for officers and men. There are a few trees in front of the building.

The married soldiers' quarters are two long, low buildings, each divided into seven single rooms, situated in bottoms on the creeks to the east and west of the garrison.

The remaining buildings, commissary and quartermaster storehouses, adjutant's office, stables, and workshops, scarcely demand special description.

There is no post bakery.

Produce of all kinds can be obtained very cheaply, flour $1\frac{95}{100}$ cents per pound and beef $4\frac{1}{2}$ cents per pound. Cost of the ration at this post is $14\frac{60}{100}$ cents.

The post is supplied with good water from the creek by a water-wagon, which delivers it daily to the quarters and barracks.

Owing to the location of the post, the natural surface-drainage is good.

Communication with department headquarters is, when the river is open, by stage to Wallula, thence by boat to Portland. In winter by stage to the Dalles and thence by boat. When the Columbia is frozen below the Dalles, communication is almost cut off, only a scanty letter-mail being sent between that place and Portland by the trail over the Cascade Mountains. It takes three days in summer and from five to eight days in winter for a letter to reach department headquarters. Eastern mails come daily overland by rail to Kelton, on the Union Pacific, and thence by stage via Boisé.

In summer it takes about ten days for a letter to come from Washington; in winter four to six days longer, owing to detention by snow on the mountains.

The town of Walla Walla contains about three thousand inhabitants, about two hundred of whom are Chinese.

The nearest Indians are on the Umatilla reservation, about forty miles distant.

The prevalent diseases in this vicinity are malarial and rheumatic affections. Venereal affections are also very common among the troops.

*Consolidated sick-report, Fort Walla Walla, Wash., 1873–'74.*

| Year | | 1873–'74. | |
|---|---|---|---|
| Mean strength | { Officers ........... | 12 | |
| | { Enlisted men ...... | 235 | |
| Diseases. | | Cases. | Deaths. |
| GENERAL DISEASES, A. | | | |
| Typhoid fever | | 1 | 1 |
| Remittent fever | | 5 | ...... |
| Intermittent fever | | 35 | ...... |
| Other diseases of this group | | 20 | ...... |
| GENERAL DISEASES, B. | | | |
| Rheumatism | | 28 | ...... |
| Syphilis | | 6 | ...... |
| Other diseases of this group | | 5 | ...... |

*Consolidated sick-report, Fort Walla Walla, Wash., 1873-'74—Continued.*

| Year | 1873-'74. | |
|---|---|---|

| Mean strength { Officers | 12 | |
| Enlisted men | 255 | |

| Diseases. | Cases. | Deaths. |
|---|---|---|
| LOCAL DISEASES. | | |
| Catarrh and bronchitis | 30 | ..... |
| Pleurisy | 3 | ..... |
| Diarrhœa and dysentery | 35 | ..... |
| Hernia | 1 | ..... |
| Gonorrhœa | 8 | ..... |
| Other local diseases | 101 | 1 |
| Alcoholism | 10 | ..... |
| Total disease | 288 | 2 |
| VIOLENT DISEASES AND DEATHS. | | |
| Gunshot wounds | 4 | ..... |
| Other accidents and injuries | 74 | 1 |
| Total violence | 78 | 1 |

# DEPARTMENT OF CALIFORNIA.

(Embracing the State of Nevada, the post of Fort Hall, Idaho, and so much of the State of California as lies north of line from the northwest corner of Arizona Territory, to Point Conception, Cal.)

## POSTS.

Alcatraz Island, Cal.
Angel Island, Cal.
Benecia Barracks, Cal.
Bidwell, Camp, Cal.
Gaston, Camp, Cal.

Hall, Fort, Idaho.
Halleck, Camp, Nev.
Independence, Camp, Cal.
McDermit, Camp, Nev.
Point San José, Cal.

Presidio, Cal.
Wright, Camp, Cal.
Yerba Buena Island, Cal.

## TABLE OF DISTANCES IN THE DEPARTMENT OF CALIFORNIA.

| Post | Chicago | San Francisco | Alcatraz Island | Angel Island | Benicia Arsenal | Camp Bidwell | Fort at Fort Point | Camp Gaston | Fort Hall | Camp Halleck | Camp Independence | Fort at Lime Point | Camp McDermit | Point San José | Camp Wright | Yerba Buena Island |
|---|---|---|---|---|---|---|---|---|---|---|---|---|---|---|---|---|
| Chicago | Chicago. | | | | | | | | | | | | | | | |
| San Francisco | 2347 | San Francisco. | | | | | | | | | | | | | | |
| Alcatraz Island | 2345 | 2 | Alcatraz Island. | | | | | | | | | | | | | |
| Angel Island | 2342 | 5 | 4 | Angel Island. | | | | | | | | | | | | |
| Benicia Arsenal | 2336 | 28 | 26 | 23 | Benicia Arsenal. | | | | | | | | | | | |
| Camp Bidwell | 2363 | 395 | 393 | 390 | 371 | Camp Bidwell. | | | | | | | | | | |
| Fort at Fort Point | 2347 | 7 | 5 | 7 | 35 | 398 | Fort at Fort Point. | | | | | | | | | |
| Camp Gaston | 2539 | 334 | 332 | 329 | 350 | 551 | 341 | Camp Gaston. | | | | | | | | |
| Fort Hall | 1685 | 942 | 940 | 937 | 918 | 958 | 949 | 1130 | Fort Hall. | | | | | | | |
| Camp Halleck | 1826 | 581 | 579 | 576 | 557 | 597 | 588 | 769 | 421 | Camp Halleck. | | | | | | |
| Camp Independence | 2397 | 524 | 522 | 529 | 530 | 540 | 531 | 712 | 992 | 631 | Camp Independence. | | | | | |
| Fort at Lime Point | 2345 | 8 | 4 | 5 | 22 | 395 | 12 | 331 | 938 | 581 | 532 | Fort at Lime Point. | | | | |
| Camp McDermit | 2020 | 487 | 485 | 482 | 464 | 503 | 494 | 675 | 611 | 254 | 537 | 484 | Camp McDermit. | | | |
| Point San José | 2350 | 3 | 5 | 8 | 31 | 398 | 10 | 337 | 945 | 584 | 521 | 11 | 490 | Point San José. | | |
| Camp Wright | 2546 | 195 | 193 | 190 | 197 | 685 | 192 | 265 | 856 | 776 | 719 | 190 | 678 | 198 | Camp Wright. | |
| Yerba Buena Island | 2344 | 3 | 3 | 5 | 28 | 395 | 10 | 334 | 942 | 581 | 524 | 10 | 487 | 5 | 198 | Yerba Buena Island. |

# ALCATRAZ ISLAND, CALIFORNIA.

### REPORT OF ASSISTANT SURGEON EDWIN BENTLEY, UNITED STATES ARMY.

Alcatraz Island is situated in the bay of San Francisco; latitude, 37° 49′ 33″ north; longitude, 45° 21′ 19″ west.

Lime Point is three and one-fourth miles distant due west, Fort Point three and one-half miles south of west, Point San José one and one-fourth miles south, and the water-front of the city of San Francisco one and three-fourths miles east of south.

The island is an irregular oblong in shape, is rocky and precipitous on all sides, rises to a height of 136 feet above tide-water, and has an area of about nineteen acres. It is composed of a fine-grained sandstone, and is almost destitute of vegetation. The temperature is mild and equable, but from the situation of the island in the middle of the bay of San Francisco, and three miles from the Golden Gate, the entrance to the harbor, it is exposed to the violence of the winds from every quarter, and in the spring and autumn is enveloped in dense fogs during a great part of the time. From the conformation and rocky character of the island the drainage is naturally perfect. A Government steamer calls twice daily for communication with San Francisco and the different posts in the harbor.

The buildings at present occupied by the garrison are as follows:

The citadel on the summit of the island, built of brick, is 200 by 100 feet, two stories high above the basement, with bastion fronts facing to the northwest and southeast. It is well ventilated by the main hall, passages, and windows. It is used as officers' quarters, quartermaster's and subsistence offices, and store-rooms, and two rooms on the first floor of the northwestern bastion, one as a dispensary, the other as a store-room for medical supplies. The set for each officer consists of two large and comfortable rooms, with dining-room, kitchen, bath-room, and water-closet attached.

A small frame building, 15 by 28 feet, containing the offices of the commanding officer and adjutant, is near the citadel.

On the northern declivity of the island are three double cottages, occupied by married soldiers and their families; they are each 30 by 22½ feet.

On the southern slope is a frame building containing three sets of laundresses' quarters; two of these contain three rooms each; one set contains two rooms. Each set is 30 by 22½ feet. A small cottage building, with office and room for the ordnance sergeant, and a stable with a capacity for stabling twelve horses, are also situated on this side of the island.

On the northeastern declivity are the prison buildings, blacksmith-shop, carpenter and paint shop, shoe and barber shop, the wharf, and two boat-houses. The center of the collection of buildings comprising the prison is an old caponniére, which is regarded as useless at the present time for the defense of the post. It contains in the basement a wash-room and bath-room for the prisoners; on the first floor the guard-room, and on the opposite side ten single cells, and four dungeons occasionally employed for the punishment of refractory prisoners. On the top of the caponniére a strong frame-building has been erected, containing fifty-six cells in two tiers, twenty-eight on each side. A second building is of brick, with forty-five cells arranged in three tiers, a room for the non-commissioned officers of the guard, and one room, formerly used as a reading-room, but at present containing the printing-office. A third building is constructed of strong planks, and contains forty-eight single and four double cells, in two tiers. Galleries run along the tiers and connect the different buildings. The average size of the cells is 8¼ by 6 by 3¼ feet, giving to each an air-space of 161 cubic feet. They are ventilated by air-tubes in the walls, and by leaving open spaces 2 inches wide at the top and bottom of the door of each cell. All these buildings are lighted by skylights and warmed by iron stoves. Adjoining these buildings are the kitchen and mess-room for prisoners, and a chapel serving also as the reading-room and library for prisoners. In the loft of the chapel building are located a temporary hospital and a tailor-shop.

Of the two barrack buildings formerly occupied by the troops, one was torn down by the engineers in December, 1873, to make room for the erection of batteries; the other was destroyed by fire April 19, 1874. There being on the island no other buildings for the reception of troops, the two companies stationed at the post are encamped on the top of an unfinished fort on the north-eastern extremity of the island. Each company occupies five regulation hospital-tents and two wall-tent . The tents are floored. Two frame buildings, each 20 by 35 feet, one for each company, serve as reading and sitting room during the day. Kitchens and mess-rooms are fitted up in the casemates of the fort. The bakery is also established in a casemate, and has a capacity for turning out four hundred rations per day.

The hospital was removed from the citadel in 1871, and established in the barrack building, which was destroyed by fire in April, 1874. On the demolition of the lower barrack by the engineers, the company which had occupied it was placed in the hospital. The school-room, reading-room, and gymnasium were then fitted up as dispensary, ward, and store-room for medical supplies; and a ward for sick prisoners and two store-rooms were established over the chapel of the prison buildings.

The hospital in the barrack-building was destroyed by fire April 19, 1874. Since that time the building formerly used as a bakery has been repaired and fitted up as a hospital for the sick of the garrison. It contains a ward with a capacity for six beds, giving an air-space of 1,200 cubic feet to each; one store-room, and one attendant's room. A porch extends along the southern side of the building. An adjoining building, of smaller dimensions, contains the mess-room and kitchen.

For recreation and improvement the garrison and prisoners have a large library, containing over one thousand volumes of standard literature, religious works, and works of fiction, at their disposal; the leading eastern and western daily papers are also subscribed for.

The garden on Angel Island, formerly cultivated, was given up, as it cost more to raise vegetables at that place than to purchase them in the markets of San Francisco.

The water used on the island is taken from the Spring Valley Water-Works, San Francisco, and is brought over in the steamer. For the storage of this water a system of twenty-one cisterns, with a capacity of two hundred and forty-one thousand five hundred and forty-three gallons, is excavated on the summit of the island, equal to a supply for five hundred men for eight months, allowing two gallons per day as the ration of water. Pipes conduct the water to some of the buildings; to others it is daily conveyed in the water-cart.

*Meteorological report, Alcatraz Island, Cal., 1870–'74.*

| Month. | 1870–'71. | | | | 1871–'72. | | | | 1872–'73. | | | | 1873–'74. | | | |
|---|---|---|---|---|---|---|---|---|---|---|---|---|---|---|---|---|
| | Temperature. | | | Rain-fall in inches. | Temperature. | | | Rain-fall in inches. | Temperature. | | | Rain-fall in inches. | Temperature. | | | Rain-fall in inches. |
| | Mean. | Max. | Min. | | Mean. | Max. | Min. | | Mean. | Max. | Min. | | Mean. | Max. | Min. | |
| | ° | ° | ° | | ° | ° | ° | | ° | ° | ° | | ° | ° | ° | |
| July .................. | 60.88 | 69 | 57 | 0.00 | 55.37 | 61 | 50 | 0.00 | 55.35 | 66* | 46* | 0.00 | 55.34 | 69* | 47* | 0.00 |
| August ............... | 62.42 | 70 | 58 | 0.00 | 56.19 | 62 | 52 | 0.00 | 57.38 | 69* | 50* | 0.00 | 57.56 | 75* | 48* | 0.00 |
| September............. | 61.29 | 70 | 55 | 0.03 | 57.95 | 73 | 55 | 0.00 | 57.78 | 90* | 50* | 0.04 | 56.29 | 70* | 48* | 0.00 |
| October .............. | 62.29 | 83 | 55 | 0.00 | 60.60 | 78 | 54 | 0.00 | 57.38 | 89* | 45* | 0.10 | 59.28 | 85* | 46* | 0.74 |
| November............. | 60.33 | 76 | 53 | 0.61 | 56.50 | 84 | 46 | 2.02 | 56.45 | 81* | 43* | 2.84 | 57.41 | 80* | 45* | 0.93 |
| December ............ | 54.38 | 65 | 49 | 2.94 | 53.38 | 87 (?)* | 40* | 10.82 | 51.92 | 71* | 38* | 7.33 | 50.15 | 60* | 40* | 9.15 |
| January ............. | 53.39 | 68 | 45 | 2.39 | 52.88 | 71* | 41* | 3.05 | 54.95 | 78* | 42* | 2.34 | 49.17 | 62* | 37* | 5.11 |
| February............. | 52.57 | 64 | 44 | 2.34 | 53.31 | 67* | 40* | 7.07 | ........ | ........ | ........ | ........ | 51.14 | 68* | 40* | 1.68 |
| March............... | 54.56 | 71 | 48 | 0.52 | 53.44 | 71* | 42* | 1.46 | 53.49 | 78* | 43* | 0.84 | 50.91 | 67* | 39* | 2.43 |
| April................ | 53.90 | 75 | 49 | 1.49 | 54.16 | 81* | 41* | 0.65 | 54.18 | 82* | 41* | 0.30 | ........ | ........ | ........ | ........ |
| May ................. | 54.50 | 62 | 49 | 0.12 | 54.22 | 86* | 43* | 0.14 | 54.48 | 74* | 45* | 0.00 | ........ | ........ | ........ | ........ |
| June ................ | 54.56 | 62 | 50 | 0.00 | 57.07 | 88* | 48* | 0.00 | 55.63 | 76* | 46* | 0.00 | 57.65 | 78* | 48* | 0.00 |
| For the year....... | 57.09 | 83 | 44 | 10.44 | 55.42 | 88* | 40* | 25.21 | ........ | ........ | ........ | ........ | ........ | ........ | ........ | ........ |

* These observations are made with self-registering thermometers. The mean is from the standard thermometer.

*Consolidated sick-report, Alcatraz Island, Cal., 1870–'74.*

| Year | 1870–'71. | | 1871–'72. | | 1872–'73. | | 1873–'74. | |
|---|---|---|---|---|---|---|---|---|
| Mean strength   { Officers <br> { Enlisted men | 5 <br> 254 | | 7 <br> 259 | | 6 <br> 258 | | 6 <br> 229 | |
| Diseases. | Cases. | Deaths. | Cases. | Deaths. | Cases. | Deaths. | Cases. | Deaths. |
| GENERAL DISEASES, A. | | | | | | | | |
| Remittent fever | 11 | ...... | 1 | ...... | 1 | ...... | 6 | ...... |
| Intermittent fever | 35 | ...... | 19 | ...... | 40 | ...... | 32 | ...... |
| Other diseases of this group | 19 | ...... | ...... | ...... | 13 | ...... | 6 | ...... |
| GENERAL DISEASES, B. | | | | | | | | |
| Rheumatism | 42 | ...... | 53 | ...... | 57 | ...... | 31 | ...... |
| Syphilis | 22 | ...... | 23 | ...... | 21 | ...... | 3 | ...... |
| Consumption | 4 | ...... | 2 | ...... | ...... | ...... | ...... | ...... |
| Other diseases of this group | 1 | ...... | 1 | ...... | 2 | ...... | 1 | ...... |
| LOCAL DISEASES. | | | | | | | | |
| Catarrh and bronchitis | 67 | ...... | 54 | ...... | 37 | ...... | 59 | ...... |
| Pneumonia | 1 | 1 | ...... | ...... | ...... | ...... | ...... | ...... |
| Pleurisy | 1 | ...... | 14 | ...... | 6 | ...... | 5 | ...... |
| Diarrhœa and dysentery | 108 | ...... | 39 | ...... | 43 | ...... | 63 | ...... |
| Hernia | 5 | ...... | 1 | ...... | ...... | ...... | 5 | ...... |
| Gonorrhœa | 5 | ...... | 1 | ...... | 2 | ...... | 3 | ...... |
| Other local diseases | 142 | 1 | 134 | ...... | 146 | ...... | 75 | 1 |
| Alcoholism | 12 | ...... | 9 | ...... | 3 | ...... | 6 | ...... |
| Unclassified | 1 | ...... | 1 | ...... | 1 | ...... | ...... | ...... |
| Total disease | 476 | 2 | 357 | ...... | 372 | ...... | 295 | 1 |
| VIOLENT DISEASES AND DEATHS. | | | | | | | | |
| Accidents and injuries | 59 | ...... | 83 | ...... | 69 | ...... | 83 | 1 |
| Total violence | 59 | ...... | 83 | ...... | 69 | ...... | 83 | 1 |

# ANGEL ISLAND, (CAMP REYNOLDS,) CALIFORNIA.

REPORTS OF ASSISTANT SURGEONS A. H. HOFF AND D. L. HUNTINGTON, UNITED STATES ARMY.

This post, formerly called Camp Reynolds, is on Angel Island, in the bay of San Francisco, about five miles distant west of north from the city of San Francisco, and is in latitude 37° 51′ 20″ north; longitude, 45° 22′ 18″ west.

The island is irregular in outline, with bold abrupt shores in most places, and rises at the center to a height of 820 feet above the sea. Its area is about one square mile. The surface is cut up by ravines or cañons, which widen as they approach the shore, furnishing several large plateaus for cultivation. Most of these cañons are supplied with water from springs well up on the hillsides. The rocks are cretaceous sandstone, with dikes of trap and serpentine. The island is covered with a deep rich soil, teeming with verdure. The only level ground is a small portion of the eastern extremity near Point Blunt. At this point there is a quarry of soft sandstone, used for building purposes. The climate is mild and pleasant; the prevailing winds westerly, but the mountains which run north from the mouth of the harbor, about five miles west of here, protect the island from the violent winds and from the fogs, which are of such frequent occurrence about the harbor and bay. The reservation includes the whole island.

The camp is situated on the western extremity of the island, facing the Golden Gate, in an irregular depression formed by three hills; the water-front being a pretty sand-beach about 1,000 feet in length. It is the only available building-ground near. The site is about 1,000 by 800 feet in dimensions, is elevated in the center, and has the officers' quarters on one slope, those of the enlisted men on the other. The drainage is naturally good. The post is supplied with water from springs on the hill-sides, conducted by pipes to the buildings; the quality is good, but the supply in summer is insufficient. The post was first occupied September 12, 1863.

The barracks consist of two frame buildings, each 90 by 30 feet, and 13 feet in height to the eaves; erected in 1864. These buildings are divided each into a dormitory, an office, and a store-room; are well lighted by windows, and warmed by stoves; the dormitories are ventilated by ridge

63 M P

ventilators, and afford about 700 cubic feet of air-space to each occupant, as usually occupied. They are furnished with iron single bedsteads of the new pattern. Mess-rooms, kitchens, and wash-rooms are in rear of the main buildings. The sinks that are used in the night are in the rear of these buildings, placed over and connecting with the main drains, and are drenched each morning; those used in the day-time are placed over the water, and are flushed by the tide.

Married soldiers' quarters are two double cottages, with two rooms and attic in each set. They are comfortable, but insufficient for the number frequently at the post.

The quarters for officers comprise four plain, substantially built frame houses. The commanding officers' quarters are contained in a one-story and attic building, and consist of four rooms, each 14 by 16 feet. One set of quarters is a two-story building, containing three rooms and kitchen downstairs, and one room upstairs; two of the rooms being 14 by 16 feet, the others averaging about 8 by 10 feet. One building, one story and attic, contains two sets of three rooms 14 by 16 feet, and an attic, each. One two-story building contains two sets, three rooms 14 by 16 feet each; and two sets, two rooms 12 by 14 feet each.

The adjutant's office is one of the sets of officers' quarters. The commanding officer's house is furnished with a bath-room, the others are not.

The post bakery is 49 by 17 feet, has an oven capable of baking 1,600 rations of bread per day, and is in every way well adapted and sufficient for its purpose.

The guard-house is of wood, 18 by 56 feet. It has four cells cut off from the main building and is well ventilated.

The quartermaster's storehouses, 25 by 60 feet, built of wood, one story, are located near the wharf.

The stables, built of wood, are situated on the eastern slope of the triangle, opposite the hospital, some distance above, and in the rear of the officers' quarters.

The hospital is situated on the western slope, 100 feet above the level of the sea, in a fine, airy position. It has been recently erected in accordance with the plan in Circular No. 4. It has one ward for twelve beds, with bath-room and water-closets attached. The grounds around it are graded and completed, and make one of the most beautiful spots on the island.

The old hospital is at present used as a chapel, and the surgeon's quarters are assigned to the chaplain. It is about three-quarters of a mile from the post, and should be moved over to the camp to be used for school, library, chapel, &c., there being no suitable buildings at the post for such purposes. The grounds near it are cultivated as a garden.

The post is a depot for recruits, the average number of which is about 250.

There are three gardens cultivated. The supply of vegetables is abundant.

The post is to be enlarged to a four-company one, and it is expected that the necessary additional buildings will be erected during the present year, 1875.

*Meteorological report, Angel Island, Cal., 1870-'74.*

| Month. | 1870-'71. | | | | 1871-'72. | | | | 1872-'73. | | | | 1873-'74. | | | |
|---|---|---|---|---|---|---|---|---|---|---|---|---|---|---|---|---|
| | Temperature. | | | Rain-fall in inches. | Temperature. | | | Rain-fall in inches. | Temperature. | | | Rain-fall in inches. | Temperature. | | | Rain-fall in inches. |
| | Mean. | Max. | Min. | | Mean. | Max. | Min. | | Mean. | Max. | Min. | | Mean. | Max. | Min. | |
| July | 66.43 | 93 | 37 | 0.00 | | | | | 60.94 | 76* | 52* | 0.00 | 58.89 | 83* | 48* | 0.00 |
| August | 67.16 | 85 | 54 | 0.00 | | | | | 60.61 | 76* | 51* | 0.01 | 62.01 | 85* | 49* | 0.00 |
| September | 63.12 | 78 | 54 | 0.00 | | | | | 62.46 | 84* | 53* | 0.00 | 59.38 | 73* | 49* | 0.00 |
| October | 59.51 | 74 | 53 | 0.00 | | | | | 59.52 | 82* | 48* | 0.10 | 60.02 | 85* | 44* | 0.71 |
| November | 58.22 | 73 | 48 | 0.70 | | | | | 56.40 | 72* | 38* | 1.81 | 55.74* | 74* | 41* | 0.29 |
| December | 51.21 | 65 | 40 | 1.70 | | | | | 50.79 | 64ₓ | 36* | 10.14 | 47.58* | 57* | 37* | 6.59 |
| January | 52.52 | 62 | 43 | 1.38 | | | | | 54.67 | 72* | 34* | 1.42 | 46.53* | 62* | 34* | 2.29 |
| February | 50.71 | 62 | 41 | 2.96 | | | | | 49.73 | 68* | 34* | 4.01 | 49.27* | 64* | 34* | 0.74 |
| March | 53.87 | 74 | 46 | 0.77 | | | | | 54.36 | 75* | 39* | 0.60 | 49.19* | 64* | 35* | 1.29 |
| April | 55.67 | 74 | 44 | 1.55 | | | | | 56.30 | 83* | 37* | 0.24 | 55.25* | 80* | 44* | 0.26 |
| May | | | | | | | | | 59.42 | 80* | 45* | 0.00 | 58.96* | 93* | 46* | 0.33 |
| June | | | | | | | | | 62.04 | 88* | 46* | 0.00 | 61.58* | 88* | 47* | 0.00 |
| For the year | | | | | | | | | 57.27 | 88* | 34* | 18.33 | 55.37 | 93* | 34* | 12.50 |

* These observations are made with self-registering thermometers. The mean is from the standard thermometer.

*Consolidated sick-report, Angel Island, Cal., 1870–'74.*

| Year. | | 1870–'71. | | 1871–'72. | | 1872–'73. | | 1873–'74. | |
|---|---|---|---|---|---|---|---|---|---|
| Mean strength ........................ { Officers ............ | | 7 | | 8 | | 5 | | 5 | |
| { Enlisted men ...... | | 212 | | 153 | | 106 | | 106 | |
| Diseases. | | Cases. | Deaths. | Cases. | Deaths. | Cases. | Deaths. | Cases. | Deaths. |
| GENERAL DISEASES, A. | | | | | | | | | |
| Remittent fever ..................... | | | | 1 | | | | 3 | |
| Intermittent fever ................... | | 49 | | 44 | | 17 | | 18 | |
| Other diseases of this group ......... | | 14 | | 7 | | 8 | 1 | 9 | |
| GENERAL DISEASES, B. | | | | | | | | | |
| Rheumatism ......................... | | 39 | | 20 | | 22 | | 17 | |
| Syphilis ............................ | | 45 | | 11 | | 20 | | 12 | |
| Consumption ........................ | | 1 | 1 | | | 1 | | | |
| Other diseases of this group ......... | | | | 1 | | 2 | | | |
| LOCAL DISEASES. | | | | | | | | | |
| Catarrh and bronchitis .............. | | 118 | | 23 | | 12 | | 35 | 1 |
| Pneumonia .......................... | | 2 | | 2 | 1 | | | | |
| Pleurisy ............................ | | | | 1 | | | | 1 | |
| Diarrhœa and dysentery ............. | | 72 | | 65 | | 29 | | 22 | |
| Hernia .............................. | | 3 | | | | | | | |
| Gonorrhœa .......................... | | 52 | | 9 | | 2 | | 2 | |
| Other local diseases ................. | | 180 | 1 | 93 | | 76 | | 93 | |
| Alcoholism .......................... | | 9 | | 3 | | 4 | | 14 | |
| Unclassified ........................ | | 1 | | | | | | | |
| Total disease ....................... | | 585 | 2 | 280 | 1 | 193 | 1 | 226 | 1 |
| VIOLENT DISEASES AND DEATHS. | | | | | | | | | |
| Gunshot wounds ..................... | | | | | | 1 | | 3 | |
| Drowning ........................... | | | 1 | | | | | | |
| Other accidents and injuries ......... | | 53 | | 35 | | 31 | | 43 | |
| Suicide ............................. | | | | | 1 | | | | |
| Total violence ...................... | | 53 | 1 | 35 | 1 | 32 | | 46 | |

# BENICIA BARRACKS, CALIFORNIA.

## REPORT OF ACTING ASSISTANT SURGEON D. WALKER, UNITED STATES ARMY.

The post of Benicia Barracks is situated on a point of land on the western end of Suisun Bay, at the place where the bay contracts to form the straits of Carquinez, which connect Suisun and San Pablo Bays. It is in latitude 38° 2′ 1″ north; longitude, 45° 5′ west.

The reservation contains $99\frac{78}{100}$ acres and was ceded to the United States in 1849. Suisun Bay is on the east, and Carquinez Straits on the south. The confluence of the Sacramento and San Joaquin Rivers is to the east of and in plain view of the post. The post is one mile east of the town of Benicia, and is twenty-eight miles by water from San Francisco, with which there is daily communication by steamers. The surrounding country is rolling and devoid of timber. There are many outcroppings of rocks, their trend being invariably from northeast to southwest, and dip of strata about 80°. The rocks are metamorphic and limestone. From the latter the celebrated Benicia cement is manufactured. East of the quartermaster's stables is a quarry of sandstone, excellent for building purposes. Selenite is also found in the vicinity. The soil is argillaceous, of the kind known as adobe clay, cracking to a depth of over four feet in summer, and extremely tenacious in winter. The surface is so rolling that water does not lie for any length of time in winter. Late in the summer and autumn there is an absence of all vegetation, but in the latter end of February and the beginning of March the entire country presents the appearance of an immense flower-garden.

The post was first established in April, 1849; it was abandoned August 9, 1866, and re-established November 17, 1866. It is the headquarters of the First Cavalry, and a receiving-depot for cavalry recruits, and is also occupied by two companies of cavalry. The buildings are located on a comparatively level piece of ground, about 64 feet above the sea.

The quarters for enlisted men consist of six sets, each composed of a building 77 by 30 feet, occupied as a dormitory, adjoining the rear of which is a building, 49 by 18 feet, divided into a mess-room, 34 by 18 feet, and a kitchen, 15 by 18 feet. The dormitories are well lighted by windows, are warmed by wood-burning stoves, and ventilated at the ridge. They are furnished with the new pattern iron, single bedsteads. The buildings are all frame, and afford comfortable housing for the soldiers. At a distance of one hundred feet in rear of each set of quarters is a latrine, which is daily policed, and, when necessary, filled with earth; the drainage is in a direction away from any dwellings.

The married soldiers occupy one frame building, 117 by 22 feet, divided into eight sets of two rooms each. These quarters are rude in construction and most uncomfortable, giving but poor protection from the weather, and are productive of much infantile sickness. The married non-commissioned officers are housed in a frame building, 60 by 24 feet, containing four sets of two rooms each. Attached are two kitchens and two mess-rooms; these are much more comfortable than the general laundresses' quarters.

The commanding officer's quarters consist of a frame building, 30 by 80 feet, with an addition 25 by 45 feet; it is located southwest from the hospital.

The other officers' quarters are situated on the eastern side of the parade-ground, and consist of three two-story frame buildings, each 35 by 48½ feet, and containing eight rooms, comprising two sets of quarters. At the rear of each building is a kitchen, 19½ by 25 feet, the one belonging to the middle building being a frame structure; the other two are stone. A cottage, 25 by 40 feet, containing four rooms, with a kitchen attached, has also been repaired for officers' use.

The adjutant's office, 30 by 50 feet, faces the south side of the parade-ground, and contains a billiard-room and the post library.

The guard-house is on a line with the adjutant's office; is 30 by 26 feet, containing a guard-room, a large room for prisoners, and four cells. It is well ventilated. The guard-room is warmed by a wood-stove.

The post bakery is nearly new, and has a capacity for baking 2,000 rations daily.

The commissary storehouse is a frame building, 25 by 80 feet, one and a half stories high.

The quartermaster's storehouse is also a frame building, 15 by 30 feet, 16 feet in height.

The hospital consists of a main building, 74 by 24 feet, one and a half stories high, built of sandstone in 1854; adjoining this on the west is a one-story stone building, 36 by 45 feet, containing the dispensary, store-room, prisoners' ward, and two rooms for steward's quarters; in rear of and adjoining this latter building is a frame addition, 29 by 16 feet, containing the kitchen and mess-room. The lower floor of the main building contains two wards, each 30 by 22 feet in the clear, 15 feet high from floor to ceiling, and having each a capacity for eight beds, giving 1,235 cubic feet air-space to a bed. The upper floor also contains two wards with a capacity for four beds each. The main building fronts east and has a hall 9 feet wide through the center, leaving a ward on each side; this hall is continued through the entire length of the addition. The hospital is located about one hundred and twenty yards outside of the parade-ground. It is well lighted, is warmed by wood-fire-places, and is well ventilated. The latrines are in the rear, drainage is good and falls away from the building. In rear of the hospital is a small frame building used as a wood-shed, in one end of which is a room, 12 by 12 feet, containing a fire-place, and intended to serve as a bath-room; it is very inconvenient, and useless except as a mere lavatory. There is a cistern under the hospital with a capacity of 37,000 gallons. There is no danger of fire external to the building itself, as it is isolated. The only means of subduing a fire is by buckets.

The quartermaster's stable is on a slope some one hundred and sixty yards south of the commissary storehouse; it is 160 by 36 feet, 22 feet in height.

The cavalry stables consist of two buildings on the south line of the parade, being two of the eight buildings originally used as company quarters. They have been converted into stables by taking out the floors, and filling the space underneath solidly with earth.

There are no gardens cultivated at the post. With the small garrison and the facility for obtaining vegetables of all kinds, it would not be an economy to attempt gardening.

The water-supply is limited in summer, though without stint in winter. Two wind-mills, pumping from a depth of 30 feet, produce a large amount of water, and the cisterns scattered over the post have a capacity of over 200,000 gallons. Water-wagons are sent around each morning. The water is hard but otherwise good. Rain-water to a considerable extent is collected in the cisterns and used for drinking-purposes. There are no available means for bathing by the men.

The fuel used at the post is hard wood.

The drainage is surface and good, the natural conformation of the ground rendering it easy and efficient.

### Meteorological report, Benicia Barracks, Cal., 1870–'74.

| Month. | 1870–'71. | | | | 1871–'72. | | | | 1872–'73. | | | | 1873–'74. | | | |
|---|---|---|---|---|---|---|---|---|---|---|---|---|---|---|---|---|
| | Temperature. | | | Rain-fall in inches. | Temperature. | | | Rain-fall in inches. | Temperature. | | | Rain-fall in inches. | Temperature. | | | Rain-fall in inches. |
| | Mean. | Max. | Min. | | Mean. | Max. | Min. | | Mean. | Max. | Min. | | Mean. | Max. | Min. | |
| | ° | ° | ° | | ° | ° | ° | | ° | ° | ° | | ° | ° | ° | |
| July | | | | | 67.03 | 84* | 52* | 0.00 | 68.32 | 91 | 47* | 0.00 | 71.43 | 102 | 57 | 0.00 |
| August | | | | | 67.96 | 93* | 53* | 0.00 | 69.35 | 96 | 46* | 0.00 | 69.42 | 94 | 51 | 0.00 |
| September | | | | | 67.22 | 92* | 53* | 0.00 | 66.85 | 89 | 46* | 0.00 | 67.69 | 92 | 55 | 0.00 |
| October | | | | | 66.35 | 89 | 46* | 0.16 | 62.58 | 84 | 45* | 0.02 | 64.27 | 89 | 50 | 0.11 |
| November | 57.00 | 80 | 42 | (?) | 55.31 | 81 | 36* | 1.47 | 54.76 | 68 | 27* | 1.25 | 59.26 | 74 | 49 | 0.70 |
| December | 45.24 | 65 | 31 | 1.74 | 49.02 | 60 | 30* | 11.11 | 48.85 | 61 | 25ᶜ | (‡) | 48.28 | 60 | 36 | 8.03 |
| January | (†) | (†) | (†) | (†) | 48.37 | 59 | 33* | 2.14 | 51.87 | 66 | 21* | (‡) | 47.31 | 60 | 35 | 4.38 |
| February | 48.51 | 64 | 34 | 2.61 | 51.49 | 62 | 39* | 5.00 | 47.71 | 62 | 21* | (‡) | 51.93 | 67 | 40 | 1.09 |
| March | 54.69 | 78 | 42 | 0.44 | 53.00 | 65 | 46* | 1.24 | 55.61 | 73 | 26* | (‡) | 54.18 | 69 | 42 | 2.47 |
| April | 59.13 | 76 | 46 | 0.45 | 56.51 | 75 | 37* | 0.78 | 58.87 | 76 | 39* | 0.22 | 60.39 | 78 | 49 | 0.66 |
| May | 61.74 | 85* | 43 | 0.00 | 63.76 | 83 | 44* | 0.32 | 65.16 | 90 | 49* | 0.00 | 63.48 | 86 | 50 | 0.46 |
| June | 68.86 | 95* | 55 | 0.00 | 69.25 | 99 | 47* | 0.08 | 69.32 | 88 | 59* | 0.00 | 70.47 | 94 | 57 | 0.00 |
| For the year | | | | | 59.61 | 99 | 30* | 22.30 | 59.94 | 96 | 21ᴬ | | 60.67 | 102 | 35 | 17.90 |

\* These observations are made with self-registering thermometers. The mean is from the standard thermometer.
† Incomplete.　　‡ Rain-gauge broken.

### Consolidated sick-report, Benicia Barracks, Cal., 1870–'74.

| Year | 1870–'71. | | 1871–'72. | | 1872–'73. | | 1873–'74. | |
|---|---|---|---|---|---|---|---|---|
| Mean strength { Officers | 8 | | 10 | | 9 | | 12 | |
| { Enlisted men | 149 | | 174 | | 115 | | 269 | |
| Diseases. | Cases. | Deaths. | Cases. | Deaths. | Cases. | Deaths. | Cases. | Deaths. |
| GENERAL DISEASES, A. | | | | | | | | |
| Typhoid fever | | | 1 | | | | 1 | |
| Typho-malarial fever | | | | | | | 2 | |
| Remittent fever | | | 1 | | | | | |
| Intermittent fever | 51 | | 60 | | 45 | | 111 | |
| Diphtheria | | | 1 | 1 | | | | |
| Other diseases of this group | 12 | | 4 | | 2 | | 20 | |
| GENERAL DISEASES, B. | | | | | | | | |
| Rheumatism | 18 | | 11 | | 29 | | 108 | |
| Syphilis | 10 | | 22 | | 15 | | 44 | |
| Consumption | | | 5 | | | | 2 | |
| Other diseases of this group | | | 2 | | | | 1 | |
| LOCAL DISEASES. | | | | | | | | |
| Catarrh and bronchitis | 29 | | 39 | | 46 | | 81 | |
| Pneumonia | 4 | | 3 | | 1 | | 5 | 1 |
| Pleurisy | 1 | | | | | | 2 | |
| Diarrhœa and dysentery | 45 | | 47 | | 36 | | 84 | |
| Hernia | | | | | | | 4 | |
| Gonorrhœa | 1 | | 8 | | 6 | | 14 | |
| Other local diseases | 69 | 1 | 42 | | 113 | | 198 | 1 |
| Alcoholism | 10 | | 10 | | 22 | | 38 | |
| Total disease | 250 | 1 | 256 | 1 | 315 | | 715 | 2 |
| VIOLENT DISEASES AND DEATHS. | | | | | | | | |
| Gunshot wounds | 2 | | | | 1 | | | |
| Other accidents and injuries | 31 | | 31 | | 54 | | 148 | |
| Suicide | | 1 | | | | | | |
| Total violence | 33 | 1 | 31 | | 55 | | 148 | |

# CAMP BIDWELL, CALIFORNIA.

INFORMATION FURNISHED BY ASSISTANT SURGEONS D. G. CALDWELL AND CHARLES SMART, UNITED STATES ARMY.

Camp Bidwell is situated in Surprise Valley, on the eastern slope of the Warner Mountains, eight miles from the southern boundary of Oregon, and the same distance from Nevada; latitude 42° 10′ north; longitude, 43° 12′ west; elevation above the sea-level, 4,680 feet. The post was established in August, 1865. The reservation is three miles long, by one and three-eighths miles in width, and ascends gradually from Willow Creek on the east for about one-half mile, after which the ascent is abrupt to the summit of the mountain. The Warner Mountains, like the great Sierra Nevadas, of which they are really a portion, have a slate base, and superimposed are strata of quartz. Sandstone also abounds near the surface, and forms the greater portion of the lower range of hills. Gold, silver, and copper are found in various portions of these mountains. The ravines traversing their surface contain vast forests of pine and cedar.

Surprise Valley, sixty miles long and six miles wide, although destitute of timber, is very fertile and well adapted for grazing and agriculture. It contains three lakes of about equal size, their combined area being about one hundred square miles. These lakes have no outlet, and are strongly saline.

The post is situated near the northeast corner of the reservation. All the buildings except two are constructed of pine logs, one story high, with shingle roofs. They are warmed by open fire-places, well lighted, and with apertures for ventilation at the eaves.

The men's barracks, two in number, measure 110 by 26 feet each, divided by log partitions into three squad-rooms and a hall. These buildings were lined, ceiled, and floored throughout in the fall of 1872, and are now in fair condition. The mess-rooms and kitchens are two log buildings containing two rooms each, furnished with cooking-stoves and dining-tables. These buildings have been improved in the same manner as the barracks. The sinks are wooden structures placed over a small stream in rear of the barracks.

The officers' quarters consist of four buildings, each 31 by 42 feet, lined and floored throughout. Two of the buildings have bath-rooms.

Two log buildings occupied as quarters of married soldiers were destroyed last year by fire.

The guard-house, divided into guard-room and prison-room, is 24 by 35 feet. It is warmed by stoves. The ventilation is by the windows and chimney; and in addition the prison-room has two small openings in the walls.

The hospital is a building of hewn logs, erected in 1865, badly arranged and very much decayed. Authority was given, November 30, 1874, for the erection of a new frame hospital of twelve beds. The plan is a modification of that given for a provisionary hospital on Plate 4 of Circular No. 2 of the Surgeon General's Office, July 27, 1871. The main building is to be two stories high; the ward, kitchen, and mess-room, one story. The whole to rest upon a stone foundation.

The company stables are contained in a frame building, 225 by 30 feet, weather-boarded and shingled. It was erected in the fall of 1872, and is in good condition. The commissary and quartermaster's storehouse is a frame building, 100 by 31 feet, constructed of rough boards, battened on the outside and roofed with shingles. It is in fair condition.

A fair supply of potatoes, turnips, cabbage, beets, onions, &c., is usually obtained from a post-garden of eight acres. The more tender vegetables and fruits are liable to be killed by the frosts of spring and fall.

Surprise Valley contains a scattered population of about 800, engaged in agriculture and stock-raising.

Communication is by semi-weekly mail to Reno, on the Central Pacific Railroad; liable, however, to be interrupted by snow in winter.

*Meteorological report, Camp Bidwell, Cal., 1870–'74.*

| Month. | 1870–'71. | | | | 1871–'72. | | | | 1872–'73. | | | | 1873–'74. | | | |
|---|---|---|---|---|---|---|---|---|---|---|---|---|---|---|---|---|
| | Temperature. | | | Rain-fall in inches. | Temperature. | | | Rain-fall in inches. | Temperature. | | | Rain-fall in inches. | Temperature. | | | Rain-fall in inches. |
| | Mean. | Max. | Min. | | Mean. | Max. | Min. | | Mean. | Max. | Min. | | Mean. | Max. | Min. | |
| July | 76.31 | 96* | 44* | 0.76 | 73.37 | 92* | 43* | 0.38 | 74.19 | 93* | 39* | 0.00 | 75.25 | 96* | 43* | 0.14 |
| August | 74.11 | 99* | 38* | 0.05 | 73.44 | 93* | 39* | 0.02 | 69.53 | 92* | 45* | 0.26 | 70.89 | 94* | 38* | 0.21 |
| September | 64.84 | 88* | 33* | 0.00 | 62.01 | 84* | 28* | 0.20 | 57.47 | 83* | 29* | 1.18 | 62.03 | 85* | 24* | 0.40 |
| October | 49.09 | 79* | 22* | 0.03 | 49.56 | 79* | 22* | 0.20 | 51.23 | 77* | 27* | 0.46 | 45.11 | 76* | 12* | 0.63 |
| November | 39.10 | 67* | 21* | 2.29 | 35.82 | 61* | 15* | 0.79 | 32.41 | 52* | 9* | 1.69 | 40.15 | 55* | 20* | 1.14 |
| December | 21.82 | 47* | — 8* | 9.10 | 35.39 | 53* | 12* | 3.25 | 32.34 | 46* | 7* | 1.94 | 25.21 | 41* | —10* | 3.29 |
| January | 31.34 | 48* | 5* | 1.23 | 31.63 | 50* | 7* | 1.16 | 35.64 | 50* | 35* | 2.22 | 27.72 | 48* | 5* | 1.51 |
| February | 34.13 | 52* | 17* | 3.26 | 37.55 | 56* | 7* | 3.97 | 28.23 | 42* | 4* | 1.66 | 25.33 | 49* | 1* | 1.08 |
| March | 37.30 | 60* | 42* | 3.21 | 40.69 | 60* | 21* | 1.32 | 41.62 | 67* | 13* | 0.60 | 31.20 | 50* | 9* | 1.05 |
| April | 45.19 | 72* | 9* | 0.00 | 40.49 | 68* | 19* | 0.77 | 43.97 | 72* | 15* | 2.06 | 43.93 | 67* | 25* | 1.12 |
| May | 54.34 | 84* | 22* | 0.97 | 58.06 | 82* | 28* | 1.82 | 51.89 | 80* | 27* | 0.78 | 55.47 | 80* | 30* | 0.64 |
| June | 70.62 | 94* | 31* | 0.16 | 67.99 | 89* | 40* | 0.06 | 64.39 | 85* | 32* | 0.10 | 60.54 | 86* | 34* | 1.06 |
| For the year | 49.84 | 99* | — 8* | 21.06 | 50.50 | 93* | 7* | 13.94 | 49.07 | 93* | 4* | 12.95 | 46.90 | 96* | —10* | 12.27 |

\* These observations are made with self-registering thermometers. The mean is from the standard thermometer.

*Consolidated sick-report, Camp Bidwell, Cal., 1870–'74.*

| Year | | 1870–'71. | | 1871–'72. | | 1872–'73. | | 1873–'74. | |
|---|---|---|---|---|---|---|---|---|---|
| Mean strength { Officers | | 3 | | 3 | | 3 | | 4 | |
| { Enlisted men | | 64 | | 76 | | 40 | | 61 | |
| Diseases. | | Cases. | Deaths. | Cases. | Deaths. | Cases. | Deaths. | Cases. | Deaths. |
| GENERAL DISEASES, A. | | | | | | | | | |
| Typho-malarial fever | | | | | | | | 1 | 1 |
| Intermittent fever | | 14 | | 9 | | 9 | | 6 | |
| Other diseases of this group | | 7 | | 1 | | 2 | | | |
| GENERAL DISEASES, B. | | | | | | | | | |
| Rheumatism | | 4 | | 18 | | 3 | | 16 | |
| Syphilis | | 1 | | 1 | | | | 1 | |
| Consumption | | 1 | 1 | 1 | | | | | |
| Other diseases of this group | | | | | | 1 | | 2 | |
| LOCAL DISEASES. | | | | | | | | | |
| Catarrh and bronchitis | | 2 | 1 | 3 | | 11 | | 5 | |
| Pleurisy | | 1 | | 1 | | 1 | | | |
| Diarrhœa and dysentery | | 4 | | 20 | 2 | 19 | | 30 | |
| Hernia | | 1 | | | | | | | |
| Gonorrhœa | | 1 | | 2 | | 1 | | 1 | |
| Other local diseases | | 16 | 1 | 18 | | 24 | | 40 | |
| Alcoholism | | | | 1 | | | | 2 | |
| Total disease | | 52 | 3 | 75 | 2 | 71 | | 104 | 1 |
| VIOLENT DISEASES AND DEATHS. | | | | | | | | | |
| Gunshot wounds | | | | | | 1 | | 3 | |
| Other accidents and injuries | | 21 | | 22 | | 9 | | 16 | |
| Homicide | | | | | | | | | 1 |
| Total violence | | 21 | | 22 | | 10 | | 19 | 1 |

# CAMP GASTON, CALIFORNIA.

### REPORT OF ASSISTANT SURGEON THOMAS F. AZPELL, UNITED STATES ARMY.

Camp Gaston is situated in Hoopa Valley, Klamath County, California, in latitude 41° 3′ 56″ north; longitude, 46° 12′ west; altitude, 397 feet above the level of the sea.

The camp is located on the west bank of the Trinity River, fourteen miles above its junction with the Klamath, and between the Trinity and Redwood chains of mountains, which belong to the Coast range of the Sierra Nevadas. Distant from the village of Arcata, forty miles; from the town of Eureka, fifty-three miles; from the town of Orleans, thirty-three miles south by trail across the Trinity range; from Camp Wright, one hundred and five miles north by trail and wagon road.

Fort Gaston, as it was formerly called, was established in December, 1858, by Capt. E. Underwood, Fourth United States Infantry, in consequence of Indian depredations in the vicinity, and was named in memory of Second Lieut. William Gaston, First United States Dragoons, who was killed in an engagement with Indians in Washington Territory, on the 17th of May, 1858. The military reservation is an irregular square, containing 451.5 acres. Hoopa Indian reservation, near the center of which the camp is located, is about ten miles square. Hoopa Valley is about seven miles in length by an average of two in breadth, with the Trinity River winding from south to north midway between the two mountain-ranges.

The geological formation of Hoopa Valley is for the most part alluvial, with large deposits of auriferous and micaceous sand along the bed and banks of the river, thickly covered in many places with medium-sized bowlders of azoic rock, worn smooth by the action of the water. About two-thirds of the ground occupied by the military reservation is a thick bed of broken shale. This forms excellent paths and roads when beaten hard by usage. The bed-rock of the valley, to judge by its outcroppings, is principally an upheaval of slate, with the laminæ now lying at various angles with the plane of the river, generally about 45 degrees. Placer mining is carried on to some extent both above and below Hoopa reservation.

The soil of the military reservation is principally barren and unproductive, and covered with patches of poison oak, lupine, and stunted grass. About twenty acres, however, along the river-bank can be advantageously cultivated, the most fertile portion of which is now used as the post garden. Indigenous forest-trees and ornamental plants are in great variety.

Wild animals and game of every description are rapidly disappearing from the immediate vicinity of the post. A few deer and an occasional black bear are still to be found within the limits of the Indian reservation, and are yet numerous in the mountains beyond. The same may be said of the wild cat, and the large panther called " the California lion." Cinnamon and grizzly bears are still to be found, it is said, in the mountain-ranges in sight of the camp, but they are rarely hunted, as the Indians are afraid to attack them. A peculiar ruffed grouse is plentiful, and much hunted; quail also abound in season; wild ducks appear in numbers on the Klamath. A few snipe and pheasants are occasionally found, and the migratory pigeon arrives in the fall in large numbers.

The fish of the Trinity and Klamath Rivers are of few varieties, but in considerable numbers. They seem only to comprise salmon, sturgeon, and eels; a few brook-trout are caught in the neighboring streams.

The water-supply of the camp is obtained from the lower creek, and at a distance of about a mile and a half from the flagstaff. The water is of good quality; it is conducted in ditches along the side of the western hills, and thence distributed throughout the camp. The quantity is ample, and the numerous small divergent streams are rapid and well filled through the whole of the dry season. For purity and convenience of distribution the water-supply of the garrison is hardly to be surpassed.

The camp consists mainly of a parade-ground, about 600 feet square, bounded on the four sides by barracks, officers' quarters, &c. The buildings are chiefly of logs, sawn timber, and adobes, and many of them are much dilapidated. The capacity of the camp is for two companies of infantry. The garrison, on the 31st of December, 1874, was two officers and fifty-two enlisted men.

It has been decided to abandon the post in the spring.

*Meteorological report, Camp Gaston, Cal., 1870–'74.*

| Month. | 1870–'71. | | | | 1871–'72. | | | | 1872–'73. | | | | 1873–'74. | | | |
|---|---|---|---|---|---|---|---|---|---|---|---|---|---|---|---|---|
| | Temperature. | | | Rain-fall in inches. | Temperature. | | | Rain-fall in inches. | Temperature. | | | Rain-fall in inches. | Temperature. | | | Rain-fall in inches. |
| | Mean. | Max. | Min. | | Mean. | Max. | Min. | | Mean. | Max. | Min. | | Mean. | Max. | Min. | |
| | ° | ° | ° | | ° | ° | ° | | ° | ° | ° | | ° | ° | ° | |
| July................ | 77.32 | 110 | 55 | 0.00 | 72.79 | 103 | 47 | 0.32 | 73.10 | 107* | 49* | 0.00 | 73.14 | 108 | 49 | 0.63 |
| August............ | 79.01 | 114 | 48 | 0.00 | 75.49 | 109 | 52 | 0.00 | 73.77 | 104 | 51 | 0.00 | 73.28 | 108 | 49 | 0.00 |
| September.......... | 64.85 | 95 | 45 | 0.41 | 63.71 | 91 | 43 | 2.10 | 65.86 | 97 | 43 | 0.31 | 69.69 | 99 | 45 | 0.00 |
| October........... | 54.53 | 85 | 30 | 0.07 | 55.16 | 85 | 33 | 0.70 | 57.44 | 92 | 40 | 1.28 | 56.83 | 82 | 35 | 1.90 |
| November.......... | 48.48 | 63 | 27 | 7.77 | 46.74 | 67 | 32 | 5.94 | 46.45 | 68 | 21 | 3.13 | 53.63 | 68 | 38 | 2.21 |
| December.......... | 41.12 | 56 | 24 | 5.22 | 46.56 | 60 | 31 | 11.14 | 44.50 | 70 | 19 | 5.05 | 42.85 | 56 | 27 | 8.70 |
| January........... | 42.76 | 57 | 27 | 5.62 | 45.07 | 65 | 24 | 7.37 | 48.81 | 64 | 34 | 6.03 | 41.99 | 57 | 28 | 15.40 |
| February.......... | 45.51 | 59 | 35 | 4.44 | 48.83 | 69 | 34 | 13.07 | 43.27 | 63 | 30 | 8.35 | 42.99 | 62 | 28 | 5.70 |
| March............. | 48.48 | 76 | 29 | 7.54 | 52.56 | 76 | 37 | 5.49 | 52.66 | 83 | 32 | 3.06 | 45.33 | 73 | 30 | 9.35 |
| April............. | 54.71 | 81 | 42 | 4.40 | 51.95 | 86 | 36 | 4.94 | 56.89 | 85 | 38 | 2.40 | 53.74 | 83 | 35 | 3.95 |
| May............... | 57.92 | 86 | 40 | 2.71 | 61.27 | 92 | 42 | 0.47 | 61.38 | 93 | 29 | 0.39 | 62.31 | 94 | 45 | 2.06 |
| June.............. | 70.52 | 106 | 48 | 1.10 | 69.16 | 105 | 50 | 0.67 | 67.17 | 97 | 54 | 1.09 | 65.64 | 100 | 49 | 0.40 |
| For the year...... | 54.10 | 114 | 24 | 39.28 | 57.42 | 109 | 24 | 52.21 | 57.61 | 107* | 19 | 31.09 | 56.31 | 108 | 27 | 50.30 |

\* These observations are made with self-registering thermometers. The mean is from the standard thermometer.

*Consolidated sick-report, Camp Gaston, Cal., 1870–'74.*

| Year ......................................................... | | 1870–'71. | | 1871–'72. | | 1872–'73. | | 1873–'74. | |
|---|---|---|---|---|---|---|---|---|---|
| Mean strength.................................... { Officers.......... | | 6 | | 7 | | 5 | | 4 | |
| { Enlisted men...... | | 115 | | 95 | | 65 | | 80 | |
| Diseases. | | Cases. | Deaths. | Cases. | Deaths. | Cases. | Deaths. | Cases. | Deaths. |
| GENERAL DISEASES, A. | | | | | | | | | |
| Remittent fever......................... | | 3 | ...... | 3 | ...... | 1 | ...... | | ...... |
| Intermittent fever...................... | | 18 | ...... | 8 | ...... | 1 | ...... | 2 | ...... |
| Diphtheria.............................. | | 1 | ...... | | ...... | | ...... | | ...... |
| Other diseases of this group............. | | 1 | ...... | 2 | ...... | 5 | ...... | 6 | ...... |
| GENERAL DISEASES, B. | | | | | | | | | |
| Rheumatism............................. | | 21 | ...... | 29 | ...... | 17 | ...... | 22 | ...... |
| Syphilis................................ | | 9 | ...... | 34 | ...... | 7 | ...... | 3 | ...... |
| Consumption............................ | | | ...... | | ...... | | ...... | 1 | ...... |
| Other diseases of this group............. | | 1 | ...... | | ...... | | ...... | | ...... |
| LOCAL DISEASES. | | | | | | | | | |
| Catarrh and bronchitis.................. | | 9 | ...... | 8 | ...... | 4 | ...... | 30 | ...... |
| Pneumonia.............................. | | | ...... | | ...... | | ...... | 2 | 1 |
| Pleurisy................................ | | 2 | ...... | | ...... | | ...... | 2 | ...... |
| Diarrhœa and dysentery................. | | 11 | ...... | 25 | ...... | 28 | ...... | 25 | ...... |
| Gonorrhœa.............................. | | | ...... | | ...... | 1 | ...... | 6 | ...... |
| Other local diseases.................... | | 41 | ...... | 49 | ...... | 57 | ...... | 74 | 1 |
| Alcoholism.............................. | | 1 | ...... | | ...... | | ...... | 1 | ...... |
| Total disease...................... | | 118 | ...... | 158 | ...... | 121 | ...... | 174 | 2 |
| VIOLENT DISEASES AND DEATHS. | | | | | | | | | |
| Gunshot wounds......................... | | | ...... | | ...... | | ...... | 3 | ...... |
| Drowning............................... | | | ...... | | 1 | | ...... | | ...... |
| Other accidents and injuries............. | | 31 | ...... | 23 | ...... | 13 | ...... | 36 | ...... |
| Total violence..................... | | 31 | ...... | 23 | 1 | 13 | ...... | 39 | ...... |

# FORT HALL, IDAHO TERRITORY.

### REPORT OF ACTING ASSISTANT SURGEON J. T. PINDELL, UNITED STATES ARMY.

Fort Hall is located in Lincoln Valley, Oneida County, Idaho Territory, on the northeastern portion of the Shoshone and Bannack Indian reservation, forty miles east of old Fort Hall, on Snake River; latitude, 43° 7′ north; longitude, 35° 12′ west; altitude, as ascertained by barometrical observation, 4,700 feet above the sea.

The post was established in May, 1870, in compliance with Special Order No. 47, headquarters

64 M P

Military Division of the Pacific, March 15, 1870, by Capt. J. E. Putnam, Twelfth United States Infantry, for the purpose of maintaining proper control over the Shoshone and Bannack Indians, numbering about 1,200, placed upon the reservation.

The Indian reservation, as also the military, was surveyed by Lieutenant Sears, United States Engineers, in June, 1870, and declared such by the President in October, 1870; the former reserve contains about three thousand square miles, the latter six hundred and forty acres.

The nearest military posts are the following: Fort Bridger, one hundred and fifty miles southeast; Camp Douglas, at Salt Lake, one hundred and sixty miles south; Fort Boise, two hundred and fifty miles west, and Fort Ellis, the same distance north. Corinne, Utah, the nearest station on the Central Pacific Railroad, is one hundred and forty miles due south. The nearest settlements of any importance are the Indian agency at Ross Fork, seventeen miles, and Malade City, the county-seat, ninety miles distant.

To the southeast, fifty-eight miles, are a number of soda-springs, which, located in a valley of great beauty, and possessing valuable medicinal properties, are frequented by a few pleasure-seekers and invalids.

In the distance, toward the northwest, can be seen the great Snake River Basin. This is an open, nearly level plain, about one hundred miles in width and two hundred in length, surrounded by a series of lofty mountain-ranges, and covered with sand and sage-brush, with here and there exposures of basaltic rock.

Lincoln Valley lies among the foot-hills bordering the Snake River Basin on the east, and measures in its course from north to south about five miles long, and in immediate vicinity of post one-half mile wide. It is well sheltered from the cold winds by the surrounding hills, is fertile and grassy, affording excellent grazing, and, with irrigation, yielding good crops of cereals, vegetables. &c. At the head of the valley, about two miles southeast of the post, are a number of warm springs, strongly impregnated with lime and alumina, and varying in temperature from 70° to 80°. These springs form the source of Lincoln Creek, which follows the course of the valley, and finally reaches the Blackfoot River (a tributary of Snake River) some five miles to the north. In this valley, as also in others of the Snake River and its branches, evidences of basaltic overflow exist. The regularly-stratified rocks in immediate vicinity, and which form the bases of the surrounding mountain-ranges, consist chiefly of limestones, sandstones, and quartzites.

A fine-grained red sandstone, of free quality, and considered suitable for building-material, is found a mile east of the post.

Timber for mechanical purposes is very scarce throughout this region of country. Most of the lumber used in erecting the buildings was procured from Truckee River, California, and the balance of the other sawed lumber from Corinne, Utah.

A stunted growth of pine and cedar is found in isolated spots on the foot-hills, as also sage-brush and a few other shrubs.

As the country is, to a great degree, ranged over by the Shoshone and Bannack Indians, wild animals and game of every description seem to be rapidly disappearing. Bears, antelopes, badgers, and coyotes are occasionally seen.

The variety of fish is limited; brook-trout are caught in the neighboring streams.

The climate of this region is generally pleasant, though subject to wide ranges in temperature.

The winter begins early in December and lasts until April.

The prevailing winds during the summer are from the south and west; during the winter from the south and southwest.

The camp is an unfortified one, having accommodations for one company of infantry. The most important buildings were completed during the year 1871; the others were added subsequently by Capt. J. L. Viven and Lieut. James S. King, Twelfth United States Infantry. They are constructed substantially of wood, and arranged around a parade measuring 750 feet long and 250 feet wide.

The company barrack is on the south side of the parade, sixty feet from the southeast angle. This is a single-story frame building, 26 by 90 feet, with shingle roof and a porch 6 feet wide in front. The dormitory (only room) is ceiled, plastered, and painted, the cubic measurement of which is sufficient to give about 616 cubic feet of air-space per man at the average occupancy. This room is warmed by two stoves, well ventilated, and lighted by ten windows and two doors; a trapdoor in the ceiling also admits of some escape of air to attic and roof.

The objectionable double wooden bunk was used until quite recently, when the iron bedstead was substituted.

A log building, 20 by 30 feet, with shingle roof, and twelve feet in rear of company barrack, is used as kitchen and mess-room. In this locality was also constructed, during the past summer, another log house, containing barber-shop and bath-room; prior to this the facilities for washing or bathing were such as the streams of water, flowing in ditches by the door, afforded. The sinks are placed at suitable distances in rear, and consist of pits covered with frame buildings.

The officers' quarters occupy the east side of the parade, and consist of two frame buildings, with shingle roofs, the distances between being thirty-seven and one-half feet. These are each 29 by 34 feet, and 11 feet high to eaves, and divided by a hall in the center into two sets of quarters of two rooms each. They are ceiled, plastered, and painted, and have porches 6 feet wide in front. Each building has kitchen and dining-room in rear, and under the same roof. On a line with the officers' quarters, thirty-seven and a half feet south, stands a frame building of the same dimensions, divided into four rooms, and used for office purposes.

The guard-house, a single-story log building, with shingle roof and board floor, is situated on the same side with and fifty feet west of the company barrack. It is divided into a guard-room, 16 by 16 feet and 8 feet high; prison-room, 9 by 12 feet, and cell, 4 by 9 feet. The guard-room is warmed by a stove and lighted by a window. The ventilation of the prison-room and cell is imperfect.

The married soldiers have quarters sixty feet west of and on a line with the guard-house. This building is partly frame, partly log, 26 by 64 feet, and divided into four sets of quarters of two rooms each. It is ceiled, plastered, and painted.

The building for quartermaster and commissary stores is a frame one, 30 by 100 feet, with shingle roof, and a porch 6 feet wide in front. It is situated on the north side of the parade, forty feet from its northeast angle, and is divided into two rooms, 30 by 50 feet each, with a capacity for six months' supply for one company. Extending in a line with and fifty feet west of the storehouse, is the post hospital, a frame building constructed in accordance with "plan of a provisionary hospital" of one story, Circular No. 2, Surgeon-General's Office, July 27, 1871. It is shingled, ceiled, plastered, and painted; also well built, and suitably and neatly furnished.

The post bakery, 16 by 26 feet, stands forty feet west of and on a line with hospital building, and is well adapted for the purpose.

The blacksmith-shop, 16 by 26 feet, is built of logs, with shingle roof, and stands at the northwest corner outside of the inclosure.

The carpenter-shop has the same dimensions, and is one hundred feet west of the blacksmith-shop.

A log building, 18 by 24 feet, and about three hundred yards north of the workshops, is occupied by the post-trader.

Standing outside of the parade, near the southwest angle, is the corral. This is a parallelogram in shape, 100 by 150 feet, and has its buildings so arranged as to form part of the walls of the inclosure. These comprise two stables, two granaries, wagon-shed, harness-shop and saddler's room; the whole built of logs, except the granaries and saddler-shop, which are of lumber. A fine stream of water flows through the yard.

In rear of the officers' quarters, and at a suitable distance, is a stable used for private animals. In this locality is also a cellar or root-house, 16 by 20 feet, for the storage of seeds, vegetables, &c., in winter.

An ice-house, 14 by 17 feet, with a capacity for 40 tons, is located on the hill-side two hundred yards from the southeast angle of the parade.

In the construction of the post none of the buildings were provided with chimneys; stoves are in general use, the pipes passing out through the roofs.

The numerous streams of water, conveyed in artificial channels about the camp, buckets and axes kept in readiness, and a few Babcock fire-extinguishers in the quartermaster's department, constitute the means of subduing fire.

The company garden covers an area of about ten acres, is well cultivated, and made productive by irrigation. Vegetables in abundance, and of great variety, are raised for the summer and winter use of the entire command.

The commissary department is liberally supplied, and the quality of stores good. Fresh beef is delivered by contract, in such quantities and at such times as required.

Pine wood is used for fuel, furnished by contract, and hauled a distance of eighteen miles.

The water-supply for purposes of irrigation and police is conveyed from Lincoln Creek, on the southeast side of the valley, by a ditch two and a half miles long, and thence distributed throughout the garrison. This water, coming from the warm springs, is too much impregnated with earthy matters to be suitable for domestic use. The water used for drinking and cooling purposes is supplied by a pretty mountain-stream flowing on the east side of the camp. It is of good quality and unlimited in quantity.

The ice for summer use is obtained from the Blackfoot River, a distance of five miles.

The company library comprises 200 volumes of a miscellaneous character.

The drainage of the camp is natural and sufficient; the soil being porous, all water is quickly absorbed.

There seem to be no prevailing diseases peculiar to this climate, as the general health of the command since the establishment of the post has been excellent.

The cemetery on the hill-side, five hundred yards from the camp, contains but one grave, that of a sergeant who perished from exposure to extreme cold.

The subsistence and other stores are transported over a good wagon-road connecting Corinne with the post; this road is open eight or nine months in the year.

The mails leave daily for Corbett Station, twelve miles distant, letters reaching San Francisco in about five, and Washington in nine days.

Communication is by stage or wagon from Corinne to Ross Fork, or Corbett Station, and thence by ambulance or horseback to the post.

*Meteorological report, Fort Hall, Idaho, 1871–'74.*

| Month. | 1870–'71. | | | | 1871–'72. | | | | 1872–'73. | | | | 1873–'74. | | | |
|---|---|---|---|---|---|---|---|---|---|---|---|---|---|---|---|---|
| | Temperature. | | | Rain-fall in inches. | Temperature. | | | Rain-fall in inches. | Temperature. | | | Rain-fall in inches | Temperature. | | | Rain-fall in inches. |
| | Mean. | Max. | Min. | | Mean. | Max. | Min. | | Mean. | Max. | Min. | | Mean. | Max. | Min. | |
| July | | | | | 77.35 | 102 | 55 | 0.13 | 69.39 | 91 | 40 | 0.15 | 73.58 | 97 | 44* | 0.10 |
| August | | | | | 74.73 | 101 | 56 | 0.09 | 69.50 | 94* | 30* | (?) | 69.28 | 92 | 38* | 1.76 |
| September | | | | | 67.81 | 97 | 40 | 0.80 | 57.75 | 90* | 27* | (?) | 57.80 | 85 | 18* | 0.00 |
| October | | | | | 50.07 | 90 | 23 | (?) | 50.81 | 82 | 18* | 0.20 | 43.37 | 80 | 7* | 1.10 |
| November | | | | | 36.85 | 68 | 6 | 0.59 | 29.51 | 63 | —12* | 0.75 | 39.44 | 60 | 15* | 0.70 |
| December | | | | | 31.79 | 60 | 3* | (?) | 31.00 | 60 | — 6* | 0.45 | 23.10 | 48 | — 4* | (?) |
| January | 31.95 | 54 | — 3 | (?) | 25.20 | 44 | — 8* | (?) | 28.43 | 44 | —12* | 0.20 | 27.84 | 48 | — 4* | (?) |
| February | 30.51 | 46 | 16 | (?) | 33.28 | 53 | —11* | 0.61 | 24.57 | 50 | —11* | 1.05 | 21.45 | 43 | — 6* | (?) |
| March | 37.14 | 65 | 19 | 1.13 | 38.13 | 66 | 23 | (?) | 38.21 | 70 | — 1* | (?) | 28.79 | 52 | 2* | (?) |
| April | 48.72 | 76 | 30 | 0.63 | 42.49 | 74 | 26 | 0.60 | 42.10 | 78 | 12* | (?) | 42.43 | 78 | 22* | 0.00 |
| May | 60.31 | 92 | 37 | 0.94 | 57.81 | 85 | 34 | 0.48 | 48.36 | 77 | 25* | 2.57 | 57.84 | 86 | 31* | 3.00 |
| June | 71.63 | 99 | 33 | 0.33 | 65.07 | 89 | 42 | 2.20 | 65.14 | 87 | 34* | 0.20 | 63.32 | 87 | 37* | 0.40 |
| For the year | | | | | 50.05 | 102 | —11* | | 46.23 | 94 | —12* | | 45.96 | 97 | — 6* | |

* These observations are made with self-registering thermometers. The mean is from the standard thermometer.

*Consolidated sick-report, Fort Hall, Idaho, 1870–'74.*

| | 1870–'71. | | 1871–'72. | | 1872–'73. | | 1873–'74. | |
|---|---|---|---|---|---|---|---|---|
| Year | Cases. | Deaths. | Cases. | Deaths. | Cases. | Deaths. | Cases. | Deaths. |
| Mean strength { Officers | 2 | | 2 | | 3 | | 2 | |
| { Enlisted men | 77 | | 43 | | 37 | | 52 | |
| **Diseases.** | | | | | | | | |
| GENERAL DISEASES, A. | | | | | | | | |
| Remittent fever | | | 2 | | | | | |
| Intermittent fever | 4 | | 2 | | | | | |
| Other diseases of this group | 2 | | 2 | | | | | |
| GENERAL DISEASES, B. | | | | | | | | |
| Rheumatism | 6 | | 8 | | 3 | | | |
| Syphilis | 2 | | | | 2 | | | |
| Consumption | | | | | 1 | | | |
| Other diseases of this group | 1 | | | | | | | |
| LOCAL DISEASES. | | | | | | | | |
| Catarrh and bronchitis | 1 | | | | 3 | | 7 | |
| Pleurisy | 2 | | | | | | | |
| Diarrhœa and dysentery | 7 | | 4 | | 1 | | 2 | |
| Gonorrhœa | 3 | | | | 2 | | 1 | |
| Other local diseases | 31 | | 14 | | 10 | | 21 | |
| Alcoholism | | | | | 3 | | 1 | |
| Total disease | 59 | | 32 | | 25 | | 32 | |
| VIOLENT DISEASES AND DEATHS. | | | | | | | | |
| Gunshot wounds | 2 | | | | | | | |
| Other accidents and injuries | 23 | | 6 | | 3 | | 4 | |
| Total violence | 25 | | 6 | | 3 | | 4 | |

# CAMP HALLECK, NEVADA.

## REPORTS OF ACTING ASSISTANT SURGEONS L. H. PATTY AND C. B. BRIERLY, UNITED STATES ARMY.

Camp Halleck is situated at the foot of the. western slope of the East Humboldt Mountains, in Elko County, Nevada; latitude, 40° 48' 45'' north; longitude, 38° 16' 34'' west; altitude, about 6,000 feet above the sea.

Halleck, on the Central Pacific Railroad, twelve miles north, is the nearest railroad station. Elko, the county-seat and nearest important town, is thirty miles distant northwest.

The reservation contains nine square miles, includes some good grass-land, and abundance of timber. The mountains are composed of granite, with quartz and limestone. The soil in the immediate vicinity is a fine rich loam, which is very fertile if irrigated. There are several fine streams in the reservation, which at some seasons of the year are filled with trout. There is one of these immediately south of the post, and another at the north. Along the border of the latter is a fine growth of cottonwood and poplar trees, which stretches up into a large mountain cañon, where fuel and timber are cut. The atmosphere is dry and bracing, but very rare, on account of the great elevation; violent exercise causing considerable dyspnœa. The camp is well sheltered from cold winds by mountains which inclose it on the north, east, and west, and, except for a southern breeze, the air is at all times singularly calm. The winter snows are very heavy.

The post was established in July, 1867. The buildings are arranged on the sides of a rectangular parade-ground; all are shingle-roofed.

The quarters for enlisted men consist of two barrack-buildings, each 87 by 25 feet, fronting the south side of parade; one built of logs, stockade-fashion; the other of adobes. These buildings contain the dormitories, which are not ceiled, are open at the eaves, and are provided with ridge-ventilators, but are very imperfectly lighted by four small windows on one side only of each. Adjoining the dormitory of each set is an orderly-room, 15 by 15 feet, and a store-room, 15 by 10 feet. In rear of these are two other buildings, one of adobe, the other stockade, each 45 by 20 feet, divided into mess-room and kitchen.   There are no wash-rooms nor bath-rooms.   The sinks are 200 feet in rear of the quarters.

Married soldiers are quartered in a frame building, 84 by 24 feet, 9 feet in height, divided into seven sets, of two rooms each.   The building is located at the southwest of the garrison.

The post-bakery is an adobe building, located immediately in the rear of the kitchens, and has an oven capable of baking two hundred loaves.

Officers' quarters consist of four one-story houses, built of adobes, each 32 by 36 feet, divided into two sets of two rooms, on either side of a central hall; each set having a "lean-to" kitchen. These buildings occupy the east side of the parade.   A frame building, on the east end of the north line of the parade, built in 1870 for quarters for the commanding officer, was destroyed by fire in October, 1873.   Another frame building, just west of the one burned, built also in 1870 for an adjutant's office, has been converted into officers' quarters.   The building is 30 by 40 feet.

The guard-house is on the west side of the parade; is a stockade building, 30 by 44 feet.   It is divided into a guard-room, prison-room, and three cells.   The guard-room is warmed by a large fire-place, and is moderately well ventilated.   The prison-room and cells are insufficiently lighted, and very imperfectly ventilated.

The hospital is located north of and on a line with the row of officers' quarters on the east side of the parade.   It consists of an adobe building one story high, 30 by 40 feet in size.   It fronts west, and contains at the north end a steward's room 14 by 15 feet, another 8 by 9 feet, a store room, 7 by 8 feet, and a mess-room, 8 by 15 feet.   Separated from these, by a hall, are a dispensary, 20 by 20 feet, and an attendants' room, 8 by 20 feet.   Attached to the south end of this building is a frame building, 24 by 30 feet, containing the ward, having a capacity for ten beds.   Adjoining the main building on the east, and on a line with the north end, is a kitchen, 10½ by 10 feet, built of adobes; on the south of this is a porch, 10 by 8 feet.   The principal rooms are 10 feet in height. The ward is boarded and battened outside, lined and ceiled with tongued and grooved boards inside.   The larger rooms are warmed by fire-places.   Water for daily use, and resource in case of fire, is collected in a reservoir twenty yards from the hospital.

There are two storehouses on the north line of the parade, one 60 by 25 feet, the other 60 by 30 feet.

There are two stables situated in rear of the west side of parade; they are each 180 by 34 feet.

Water is supplied from a small mountain-stream running along the south end of the camp, and by a ditch which brings a supply from another stream about a mile distant north.   The supply is abundant, quality clear, pure, and cold.

Each company cultivates a garden.   They produce an abundant supply of vegetables.

The drainage of the post is good.

*Meteorological report, Camp Halleck, Nev., 1870–'74.*

| Month. | 1870–'71. | | | | 1871–'72. | | | | 1872–'73. | | | | 1873–'74. | | | |
| | Temperature. | | | Rain-fall in inches. | Temperature. | | | Rain-fall in inches. | Temperature. | | | Rain-fall in inches. | Temperature. | | | Rain-fall in inches. |
| | Mean. | Max. | Min. | | Mean. | Max. | Min. | | Mean. | Max. | Min. | | Mean. | Max. | Min. | |
| July | 70.50 | 86* | 48* | 0.00 | 71.48 | 107* | 39* | (?) | 70.79 | 88 | 42 | 0.20 | 69.61 | 102* | 23* | 0.20 |
| August | 69.05 | 82 | 49* | 0.00 | 70.25 | 94* | 55* | (?) | 69.09 | 89 | 52 | 0.00 | 69.32 | 100* | 24* | 0.00 |
| September | 56.05 | 79* | 30* | 0.00 | 62.69 | 88 | 38 | 0.00 | 57.88 | 82 | 30 | (?) | 57.88 | 82* | 19* | 0.00 |
| October | 46.01 | 70* | 26* | 0.00 | 43.64 | 78 | 18 | 0.35 | 48.23 | 77 | 30 | (?) | 44.47 | (?)93 | 3 | 0.04 |
| November | 38.32 | 55* | 12* | 0.34 | 31.81 | 60* | —12* | 2.10 | 32.07 | 68 | 4 | (?) | 40.44 | 66* | 20* | 0.15 |
| December | 24.47 | 46* | 4* | 0.29 | 28.59 | 48* | — 6* | 0.85 | 28.62 | 60 | 4 | (?) | 21.46 | 48* | —13* | 2.40 |
| January | 27.69 | 50* | — 1* | 0.29 | 25.59 | 47* | — 4* | 0.02 | 27.99 | 56 | 8 | 0.09 | 24.71 | 50* | — 4* | (?) |
| February | 29.73 | 55* | 11* | 0.38 | 31.36 | 57* | — 3* | 2.70 | 22.80 | 39 | 5 | (?) | 21.41 | 48* | —18* | (?) |
| March | 35.79 | 62* | 15* | 0.57 | 35.46 | 65* | 10* | 0.06 | 30.43 | 64 | — 8 | (?) | 29.43 | 69* | 1* | (?) |
| April | 42.36 | 84* | 18* | 1.01 | 39.43 | 72* | 13* | 1.50 | 41.41 | 80* | 7* | (?) | 39.70 | 84* | 12* | 0.05 |
| May | 55.57 | 78* | 22* | 3.90 | 52.86 | 91* | 24* | 1.60 | 47.19 | 85* | 13* | (?) | 54.65 | 104* | 28* | 0.25 |
| June | 65.48 | 111* | 25* | 0.46 | 61.45 | 102* | 26* | (?) | 65.57 | 103* | 25* | 0.00 | 60.75 | 108* | 31* | 1.08 |
| For the year | 46.75 | 111* | — 1* | 7.24 | 46.21 | 107 | —12* | ........ | 45.17 | 103 | — 8 | ........ | 44.49 | 108* | —18* | ........ |

* These observations are made with self-registering thermometers.   The mean is from the standard thermometer.

*Consolidated sick-report, Camp Halleck, Nev., 1870–'74.*

| Year | 1870–'71. | | 1871–'72. | | 1872–'73. | | 1873–'74. | |
|---|---|---|---|---|---|---|---|---|
| Mean strength { Officers | 6 | | 6 | | 4 | | 5 | |
| { Enlisted men | 142 | | 95 | | 70 | | 90 | |
| Diseases. | Cases. | Deaths. | Cases. | Deaths. | Cases. | Deaths. | Cases. | Deaths. |
| GENERAL DISEASES, A. | | | | | | | | |
| Typhoid fever | | | 1 | | | | | |
| Remittent fever | 1 | | 2 | | | | | |
| Intermittent fever | 62 | | 11 | | 3 | | 16 | |
| Other diseases of this group | 8 | | 2 | | 1 | | | |
| GENERAL DISEASES, B. | | | | | | | | |
| Rheumatism | 16 | | 18 | | 8 | | 12 | |
| Syphilis | 8 | | 3 | | 2 | | 2 | |
| Consumption | 4 | | | | 1 | | | |
| Other diseases of this group | | | | | | | 5 | |
| LOCAL DISEASES. | | | | | | | | |
| Catarrh and bronchitis | 48 | | 10 | | 5 | | 23 | |
| Pneumonia | | | 1 | | | | | |
| Pleurisy | | | 3 | | 1 | | 1 | |
| Diarrhœa and dysentery | 44 | | 11 | | 5 | | 41 | |
| Hernia | | | | | | | 2 | |
| Gonorrhœa | 3 | | 7 | | 2 | | 3 | |
| Other local diseases | 69 | | 39 | | 41 | | 65 | 1 |
| Alcoholism | 15 | | 2 | | 3 | | 11 | |
| Total disease | 278 | | 110 | | 72 | | 181 | 1 |
| VIOLENT DISEASES AND DEATHS. | | | | | | | | |
| Gunshot wounds | 1 | | 1 | | | | | |
| Other accidents and injuries | 42 | | 42 | | 37 | | 31 | |
| Total violence | 43 | | 43 | | 37 | | 31 | |

# CAMP INDEPENDENCE, CALIFORNIA.

### REPORT OF ASSISTANT SURGEON C. B. WHITE, UNITED STATES ARMY.

Camp Independence is situated in Owen's River Valley, on the eastern slope of the Sierra Nevada, three miles west of Owen's River, in Inyo County, California; latitude, 36° 55' north; longitude, 41° 7' west, (approximates;) altitude, 4,958 feet above the sea.

Owen's Valley at this point is about twelve miles wide, having the Sierra Nevada on the west, and the Inyo or Monache range on the east. The highest peaks of the Sierra in this region reach an altitude of 15,000 feet, and are snow-covered during the entire year. The Inyo range is about 8,000 feet high. The bottom-lands on either side of the river are very fertile, but the higher grounds of the valley are dry, and bear only patches of bunch-grass, artemisia, and valueless shrubs. Pine timber is abundant in the Sierras.

The climate is dry, little rain or snow falling, except on the mountains, so that for cultivation irrigation is necessary. Prevailing winds, north and southeast.

The town of Independence, the county-seat of Inyo County, is two and a half miles south of the post. The nearest railway-station is Tipton, on the Visalia Branch of the Central Pacific Railroad. Carson City is about the same distance, but for two hundred and forty miles in any direction dependence must be placed upon stages, wagons, or horseback for communication with the outside world. There are tri-weekly mails both with Tipton and Carson City.

The post was first occupied in March, 1862, to protect some quartz-mills and miners from Indian depredations, was abandoned in 1864, and re-occupied in March, 1865, on account of renewed hostilities on the part of the savages. It is located on Oak Creek, which rises in the Sierra, and is a large and constant tributary of Owen's River. The reservation is three-fourths of a mile long by one-fourth of a mile wide, with a fall of one foot in thirty from west to east. The soil is light and sandy. In addition there is a wood reservation of two miles square in the Sierra, four miles west of the post, and a grazing reserve three miles square one mile east of the post. A short distance above the post a dam has been constructed on the creek, and the water led in three streams through the camp. One supplies the quarters of the men and officers; a second, the hospital ; and the third, the quarters of the married soldiers. After passing through the post these streams irrigate the post garden. The drainage is excellent.

Most of the original buildings, which were constructed of adobes, were destroyed by an earthquake March 26, 1872. The present buildings are located on the four sides of a parallelogram, forming the parade-ground and lawns in front of the officers' quarters. These grounds are set out with trees, and covered with grass. A live hedge forms the westerly bound of the camp.

The barrack is a frame building 164 by 30 feet, 17 feet high to the eaves, with a high-peaked shingle roof. This building, like most others at the post, is constructed of boards set upright and nailed to a strong frame-work, battened externally at the joints, and the frame-work lined with boards internally. A porch 8 feet wide extends entirely around the quarters. The building is located at the east end of the parade, upon which it fronts. An addition 20 feet wide adjoins the center of the main building in the rear, and extends east 50 feet; it is 12 feet high at the eaves, is built in the same manner as the former, and is divided into a mess-room and kitchen. These buildings are abundantly lighted by windows, and well warmed by stoves. The ventilation is excellent; the air-space per man, for average occupancy, is 1,200 cubic feet. In these, and all the other new buildings, except the officers' quarters, galvanized iron flues do duty as chimneys.

Married soldiers' quarters consist of four buildings located near the northeast corner of the parade, each building being 48 by 12 by 11 feet, with a porch 6 feet wide along the front. They are frame buildings, the living-rooms board-lined, the kitchens lined with canvas. There is attached to each set a shed about 8 by 10 feet, for wood and lumber room.

Officers' quarters comprise four frame houses, with hipped roofs, shingled; the commanding officer's, 42 by $33\frac{1}{2}$ feet in size, is located on the west line of the grounds; the first lieutenant's stands north of it, on the same line; the second lieutenant's is near the west end of the north line, and the surgeon's near the west end of the south line, the last three being 37 by 31 feet. Each house has a hall through the center from front to rear, with two rooms on each side. A rough board building, for kitchen, pantry, and servants' room, adjoins the rear of each house; there is also a porch 8 feet wide surrounding the front and ends of each. The rooms are all $11\frac{1}{2}$ feet in height. They are lined and ceiled with $\frac{3}{8}$-inch red-wood lumber, well lighted by windows, warmed by stoves, and are, altogether, very handsome, commodious, and convenient quarters. Chimneys of adobes are built in each house, but have to be carefully braced with wood, and extended above the roof by galvanized iron flues, to prevent accidents from earthquakes.

The guard-house is a frame building 28 by 14 by 12 feet, with a porch 8 feet wide along the front. It has one cell constructed of heavy timber well bolted with iron. It stands on the south side of the parade, is ventilated by windows and doors, and warmed by a stove.

The post-bakery, 20 by 20 feet, is located in rear of the north end of the barracks. It is a frame building, in good order and well adapted to its use.

The hospital, located on the north side of the parade, is a frame building 40 by 34 feet, with a kitchen 14 by 16 feet, a pantry 11 by 6 feet, and a cook's room 14 by 8 feet in an adjoining building in rear. It is built of red-wood lumber, outside and within, with valley lumber for frame, roof, and floors, and has a porch 8 feet wide across the front and ends of the main building. The main building has a hall $6\frac{5}{12}$ feet wide in the center, running back $23\frac{9}{12}$ feet to a bath-room $9\frac{3}{12}$ by $6\frac{5}{12}$ feet. On the east side of the hall are a dispensary $16\frac{3}{12}$ by $13\frac{9}{12}$ feet, with a store-room $16\frac{3}{12}$ by $5\frac{1}{2}$ feet, between it and the mess-room, which is $16\frac{3}{12}$ by $13\frac{2}{12}$ feet; the kitchen adjoins and communicates with the mess-room. On the east side of the hall are, in front, the steward's room, $16\frac{1}{2}$ by 12 feet, and in rear of it the ward, $16\frac{1}{2}$ by $20\frac{3}{4}$ feet. The rooms in the main building are all $11\frac{1}{2}$ feet in height; the kitchen is 9 feet high. The building is well lighted by windows; the ward has a ventilator in the ceiling, and is intended for five beds, affording 787 cubic feet of air-space to each. The hospital is complete, in good repair, and is commodious and handsome. A building 14 by 32 by 11 feet stands some forty feet in rear of the hospital. It is a frame structure, and contains a dead-room 14 by 16 feet in the west end, a privy 14 by 8 feet in the east end, with a passage between them. The dead-room is lighted by three windows and a sky-light. The privy is over a deep pit.

All the sinks at the post are placed over deep vaults to avoid contaminating the water running in ditches.

The hospital grounds are about 150 feet front by 200 feet deep, set out with shade-trees, and covered with grass, and with a small flower-garden in front.

The storehouses are an old adobe building 95 by 27 feet, which was formerly the company quarters, and a new frame building of the same size, both located on the south side of the parade.

The stable, or shed for animals, stands some distance southeast from the post, is an open shed 150 by 15 feet, 12 feet in height, fronts south, and forms the north side of the corral, which is 150 feet square, inclosed on the three other sides by a fence 6 feet high, and has a stream of water running through it.

A contract has been let to bring water in pipes to the various houses and kitchens at the post from a point on the creek considerably elevated above it; a hydraulic ram of one hundred feet force is to make the delivery in large quantity, sure at all times, by means of large tanks of reserve water. This will materially add to the convenience of the people in camp, as well as make a most valuable provision against conflagrations.

The post-garden is at the east of the camp. It is very productive, furnishing an abundance of vegetables for the whole command.

The cemetery is about one-eighth of a mile northwest from the camp; it is 200 feet square, inclosed by a fence. There is a stream of water on the north, and one on the south sides, which are fringed with weeping-willows. The ground has been laid off into roads, paths, and grave-spaces; the existing graves having been renumbered recently.

*Meteorological report, Camp Independence, Cal., 1870–'74.*

| Month. | 1870–'71. | | | | 1871–'72. | | | | 1872–'73. | | | | 1873–'74. | | | |
|---|---|---|---|---|---|---|---|---|---|---|---|---|---|---|---|---|
| | Temperature. | | | Rain-fall in inches. | Temperature. | | | Rain-fall in inches. | Temperature. | | | Rain-fall in inches. | Temperature. | | | Rain-fall in inches. |
| | Mean. | Max. | Min. | | Mean. | Max. | Min. | | Mean. | Max. | Min. | | Mean. | Max. | Min. | |
| July | 79.97 | 102* | 53* | 0.35 | 78.40 | 104* | 49* | 0.00 | 75.57 | 100* | 48* | 0.28 | 79.94 | 106* | 51* | 0.00 |
| August | 77.18 | 107* | 49* | 0.10 | 78.29 | 101* | 51* | 0.00 | 78.27 | 104* | 31?* | 0.12 | 75.67 | 100* | 44* | 0.05 |
| September | 68.69 | 95* | 43* | 0.00 | 70.59 | 100* | 37* | 0.00 | 67.74 | 92* | 47 | 0.00 | 70.14 | 92* | 43* | 0.10 |
| October | 59.06 | 90* | 28* | 1.10 | 57.29 | 89* | 28* | 0.00 | 59.74 | 88* | 21 | 0.00 | 56.15 | 86* | 29* | 0.00 |
| November | 47.21 | 75* | 25* | 0.00 | 46.66 | 75* | 26* | 0.65 | 43.27 | 77* | 12* | 0.00 | 52.34 | 75* | 26* | 0.00 |
| December | 36.56 | 62* | 14* | 1.00 | 43.43 | 66* | 18* | 4.70 | 40.40 | 73* | 8* | 1.18 | 27.42 | 60* | — 2* | 3.40 |
| January | 38.52 | 68* | 17* | 0.00 | 39.08 | 64* | 17* | 0.00 | 43.84 | 73* | 19* | 0.00 | 33.33 | 55* | 16* | 2.40 |
| February | 39.68 | 69* | 11* | 1.28 | 44.07 | 78* | 23* | 0.30 | 40.03 | 65* | 12* | 0.40 | 40.05 | 64* | 20* | 1.00 |
| March | 50.26 | 77* | 26* | 0.00 | 48.62 | 77* | 26* | 0.28 | 53.50 | 86* | 14* | 0.00 | 44.24 | 72* | 23* | 0.00 |
| April | 55.33 | 84* | 26* | 0.00 | 51.47 | 89* | 22* | 0.55 | 54.46 | 91* | 21* | 0.00 | 54.58 | 84* | 28* | 0.00 |
| May | 64.84 | 93* | 40* | 0.00 | 65.66 | 95* | 37* | 0.18 | 61.00 | 92* | 29* | 0.00 | 64.03 | 95* | 29* | 0.00 |
| June | 74.13 | 105* | 41* | 0.30 | 73.70 | 100* | 38* | 0.00 | 74.01 | 100* | 44* | 0.00 | 73.56 | 100* | 43* | 0.01 |
| For the year | 57.62 | 107* | 11* | 4.13 | 58.11 | 104* | 17* | 6.66 | 57.65 | 104* | 8* | 1.98 | 58.04 | 106* | — 2* | 6.96 |

* These observations are made with self-registering thermometers. The mean is from the standard thermometer.

*Consolidated sick-report, Camp Independence, Cal., 1870–'74.*

| Year | | 1870–'71. | | 1871–'72. | | 1872–'73. | | 1873–'74. | |
|---|---|---|---|---|---|---|---|---|---|
| Mean strength { Officers<br>{ Enlisted men | | 3<br>59 | | 4<br>55 | | 4<br>45 | | 3<br>45 | |
| Diseases. | | Cases. | Deaths. | Cases. | Deaths. | Cases. | Deaths. | Cases. | Deaths. |
| GENERAL DISEASES, A. | | | | | | | | | |
| Remittent fever | | 1 | | 1 | | | | | |
| Intermittent fever | | 10 | | 2 | | 5 | | 6 | |
| Other diseases of this group | | 5 | | 1 | | 4 | | 2 | |
| GENERAL DISEASES, B. | | | | | | | | | |
| Rheumatism | | 20 | | 12 | | 1 | | 7 | |
| Syphilis | | | | 3 | | | | 5 | |
| Consumption | | 1 | 1 | | | | | | |
| Other diseases of this group | | | | | | | | | |

65 M P

*Consolidated sick-report, Camp Independence, Cal., 1870-'74—Continued.*

| Year | | 1870-'71. | | 1871-'72. | | 1872-'73. | | 1873-'74. | |
|---|---|---|---|---|---|---|---|---|---|
| Mean strength { Officers | | 3 | | 4 | | 4 | | 3 | |
| { Enlisted men | | 59 | | 55 | | 45 | | 45 | |
| Diseases. | | Cases. | Deaths. | Cases. | Deaths. | Cases. | Deaths. | Cases. | Deaths. |
| LOCAL DISEASES. | | | | | | | | | |
| Catarrh and bronchitis | | 11 | ...... | 1 | ...... | 1 | ...... | 6 | ...... |
| Diarrhœa and dysentery | | 1 | ...... | 1 | ...... | 4 | ...... | 23 | ...... |
| Hernia | | 1 | | | | | | | |
| Gonorrhœa | | | | 2 | | | | | |
| Other local diseases | | 13 | ...... | 18 | 1 | 10 | ...... | 15 | ...... |
| Alcoholism | | 11 | | 10 | | 3 | | 3 | |
| Total disease | | 74 | 1 | 51 | 1 | 28 | ...... | 67 | |
| VIOLENT DISEASES AND DEATHS. | | | | | | | | | |
| Accidents and injuries | | 15 | ...... | 6 | | 3 | ...... | 16 | |
| Total violence | | 15 | ...... | 6 | | 3 | ...... | 16 | |

# CAMP McDERMITT, NEVADA.

INFORMATION FURNISHED BY ACTING ASSISTANT SURGEONS GEORGE GWYTHER, WILLIAM H. CORBUSIER, AND GEORGE M. KOBER, UNITED STATES ARMY.

Camp McDermitt is situated in Humboldt County, Nevada; latitude, 42° 58' north; longitude, 40° 37' west; altitude, 4,700 feet. Winnemucca, the nearest town, is eighty miles south by west, on the Union Pacific Railroad.

The post was established in 1865, and named after Lieut. Col. C. McDermitt, Second California Cavalry. In 1866-'67 the post was built. It is near the mouth of a cañon formed by a break in the Santa Rosa Mountains, through which runs a very clear and pure stream, known as the east branch of Quinn's River. Wood is very scarce. A few antelopes, deer, and mountain-sheep are found in the vicinity. Prairie and sage chickens and ducks are plentiful. The streams abound in mountain and salmon trout. The post is built around a parade 660 by 285 feet. The men's quarters are two stone buildings, each 104 by 24 feet. As at present occupied, the dormitory gives 763 cubic feet air-space per man. Single iron bedsteads are used. Warming is effected by wood-stoves. Ventilation is by two shafts reaching from the ceiling into the chimneys, aided by cracks and crevices near the windows and doors. The mess-room, and the kitchen communicating, are in a separate building. There are three sets of married soldiers' quarters, of two rooms each.

Officers' quarters are three sets, one of stone, the remaining two of adobe. The guard-house is a stone building, 23 by 23 feet, with no flooring or ceiling. Has three cells; one lighted by a window, the others by openings in the doors.

The hospital is a stone building, 30 by 28 feet, divided in two parts, one of which is a ward, 24 by 17 by 8 feet; the other is subdivided, and used as dispensary and kitchen. The ward is well heated, lighted, and ventilated, and contains four beds, giving to each 816 cubic feet of air-space. There is no wash-room or dead-house. There are two stables; one of stone, 184 by 28 feet; the other frame, 147 by 32 feet. The storehouse is a stone building, 75 by 34 feet, partitioned off into three rooms.

All the water used at this post is obtained from the river. It is very good until the snow on the mountains is melted. When the river becomes low and filled with vegetable matter, casks are sunk near the river so that the water may filter through the gravel into them. There are neither sewers nor drains. Slops, offal, &c., are carted half a mile below the post, and there thrown out.

A post garden is within one mile of the post, in which a good variety of vegetables are raised, but nearly all of its products are annually consumed by the grasshoppers; vegetables for the hospital and troops are also procured from citizens at a distance.

The only communication with Winnemucca, the nearest railroad station, is by stage. It takes a letter from ten to twelve days to reach here from Washington, and from five to six days from San Francisco, Cal. The country is sparsely settled. Attached to the post, under protection of the military, and living on the opposite bank of the creek close by, are a number of Pah-Ute Indians, about one hundred and fifty persons. They are fed and protected by the post, and some of them are found useful as herders of stock, being competent and trustworthy.

The register of sick since the establishment of the post in 1865 shows conclusively the healthiness of the locality. No epidemic and but little endemic disease has presented itself. No sickness has been observed among the Indians.

*Meteorological report, Camp McDermitt, Nev., 1870–'74.*

| Month. | 1870-'71. Temperature. Mean. | Max. | Min. | Rain-fall in inches. | 1871-'72. Temperature. Mean. | Max. | Min. | Rain-fall in inches. | 1872-'73. Temperature. Mean. | Max. | Min. | Rain-fall in inches. | 1873-'74. Temperature. Mean. | Max. | Min. | Rain-fall in inches. |
|---|---|---|---|---|---|---|---|---|---|---|---|---|---|---|---|---|
| July | 76.72 | 98 | 50 | 0.30 | 74.87 | 100 | 51 | 0.37 | 73.46 | 100* | 40* | 0.00 | 75.50 | 99 | 43 | 0.23 |
| August | 71.64 | 104 | 47 | 0.00 | 74.61 | 102 | 56 | 0.00 | 72.15 | 101* | 43* | 0.01 | 70.94 | 97 | 35 | 0.28 |
| September | 61.25 | 90 | 40 | 0.00 | 63.66 | 92 | 43 | 0.00 | 58.27 | 91* | 26* | 0.15 | 63.52 | 92 | 24 | 0.42 |
| October | 49.10 | 81 | 26 | 0.06 | 48.58 | 78 | 17 | 0.54 | 52.73 | 88* | 20* | 0.10 | 47.05 | 86 | 11 | 0.66 |
| November | 40.25 | 67 | 19 | 0.34 | 34.12 | 65 | 8 | 0.76 | 31.28 | 59* | 5* | 0.30 | 43.51 | 72 | 16 | 0.74 |
| December | 24.08 | 50 | −4 | 0.35 | 34.67 | 55* | 10 | 2.68 | 32.98 | 54* | 4* | 1.30 | | | | |
| January | 30.46 | 55 | 2 | 1.69 | 30.36 | 53* | 7 | 0.54 | 36.04 | 56* | 6* | 0.69 | | | | |
| February | 30.52 | 50 | 10 | 0.60 | 36.85 | 65* | 7 | 1.06 | 28.88 | 53* | 0* | 2.99 | | | | |
| March | 35.21 | 65 | 20 | 1.20 | 39.69 | 69* | 17 | 0.21 | 41.86 | 72* | 10* | 0.28 | | | | |
| April | 45.08 | 76 | 25 | 1.30 | 40.78 | 70* | 27 | 0.48 | 42.35 | 85* | 11* | 0.40 | | | | |
| May | 55.64 | 86 | 35 | 0.77 | 55.89 | 85* | 27* | 0.39 | 49.51 | 81* | 23* | 2.73 | | | | |
| June | 71.25 | 100 | 32 | 0.10 | 65.72 | 94* | 29* | 0.00 | 63.37 | 85* | 29* | 0.00 | | | | |
| For the year | 49.11 | 104 | −4 | 5.71 | 49.98 | 102 | 7 | 7.03 | 48.57 | 101* | 0* | 8.95 | | | | |

* These observations are made with self-registering thermometers. The mean is from the standard thermometer.

*Consolidated sick-report, Camp McDermitt, Nev., 1870–'74.*

| Year | | 1870-'71. | | 1871-'72. | | 1872-'73. | | 1873-'74. | |
|---|---|---|---|---|---|---|---|---|---|
| Mean strength { Officers / Enlisted men | | 2 / 52 | | 3 / 68 | | 2 / 60 | | 3 / 65 | |
| Diseases. | | Cases. | Deaths. | Cases. | Deaths. | Cases. | Deaths. | Cases. | Deaths. |
| GENERAL DISEASES, A. | | | | | | | | | |
| Remittent fever | | 1 | | 2 | | 1 | | | |
| Intermittent fever | | 33 | | 36 | | 13 | | 7 | |
| Other diseases of this group | | 1 | | 2 | | | | 7 | |
| GENERAL DISEASES, B. | | | | | | | | | |
| Rheumatism | | 4 | | 9 | | 5 | | 2 | |
| Syphilis | | 6 | | 6 | | 4 | | 2 | |
| Consumption | | 1 | | | | | | | |
| Other diseases of this group | | | | 1 | | | | | |
| LOCAL DISEASES. | | | | | | | | | |
| Catarrh and bronchitis | | 7 | | 17 | | 9 | | 4 | |
| Pneumonia | | | | 2 | 1 | 2 | | 1 | |
| Pleurisy | | 1 | | 1 | | | | | |
| Diarrhœa and dysentery | | 29 | | 26 | 1 | 18 | | 15 | |
| Gonorrhœa | | 2 | | 2 | | 1 | | 2 | |
| Other local diseases | | 18 | | 20 | | 7 | | 10 | |
| Alcoholism | | 4 | | | | 3 | | | |
| Unclassified | | | | | | | | 1 | |
| Total disease | | 107 | | 124 | 2 | 63 | | 51 | |
| VIOLENT DISEASES AND DEATHS. | | | | | | | | | |
| Gunshot wounds | | 2 | 1 | | | | | 1 | |
| Other accidents and injuries | | 19 | | 29 | | 14 | | 9 | |
| Suicide | | | 1 | | | | | | |
| Total violence | | 21 | 2 | 29 | | 14 | | 10 | |

# POINT SAN JOSÉ, SAN FRANCISCO HARBOR, CALIFORNIA.

INFORMATION FURNISHED BY ASSISTANT SURGEONS W. A. BRADLEY, E. J. MARSH, AND EDWIN BENTLEY, UNITED STATES ARMY.

This post is built upon the point of that name, or, as it is more commonly called, "Black Point." It is in latitude 37° 48′ 12″ north, longitude 45° 21′ 18″ west. It is on the southern margin of the Bay of San Francisco, and lies on the outside, and distant to the northwest half a mile from the city wharves. To the westward, about a mile, along the curvature of the shore, is the Presidio of San Francisco, and beyond that, at the harbor mouth, the fortification of Fort Point; over against it, in the center of the harbor channel, is the island of Alcatraz. The post is three-quarters of a mile distant from the terminus of the nearest street-cars.

San José is a rocky point which, with an elevation of 80 feet, projects into the bay northward. It is steep and bare on its western face, less so on its eastern or sheltered face; and on both sides it falls away into low sand-mounds. Back from the bay it is continuous with the sand-hills, on which the western portion of the city is built.

The climate is similar to that of the Presidio; but on account of the sand-hills which lie between the point and that post, and the prevailing direction of the wind, it is much more exposed to sand-storms during the summer and autumn. Its elevation is insufficient to prevent it from being wrapped up in the fog-banks that creep in from the ocean.

There is very little vegetation in the neighborhood, as all the ledges that otherwise would afford a footing to vegetable growth are buried in the shifting sands. On the brow of the less exposed eastern face a small space around the officers' quarters, under cultivation, yields a large show of flowers during the greater portion of the year. Immediately on the landward side of the post buildings is a deep excavation in the rock which is sheltered from sand-drift, and always contains more or less stagnant water, but no evil effects on the health of the post can be traced to its presence. With this exception the ground requires no artificial drainage.

In the small cove on the sheltered side of the point a wharf has been built, at which a Government steamer calls twice daily for communication with the city; but the post supplies are generally brought out by wagons, as, with the exception of a quarter of a mile of sand-hill, the road to the paved streets of the city is good.

The battery is placed on the western face of the point, and well on the brow of the hill; above it are built two sets of company quarters, of which one only at the present time is occupied. They are each of wood, 90 by 30½ by 13 feet. Thirteen feet of this length is partitioned off at one end, and divided into two rooms—one an office, the other a company store-room. The barrack is furnished with iron single bedsteads, and affords 560 cubic feet per man of its average occupancy. It is heated by one stove in the center of the building, lighted by seven windows, and ventilated by the ridge. Two tables and four benches complete its furniture. The kitchens and mess-rooms, in two buildings, each 60 by 20 feet, are in rear of the barrack buildings, as is also the bakery, which is 38 by 16 feet.

The married soldiers' quarters are in the rear, or on the landward side of the company barracks, and consist of two frame buildings, 32 by 24 feet, each divided into two sets of quarters, and a third building, 25 by 16 feet, forming another set. Near these are the stables for the few quartermaster's horses and mules and officers' stock at the post.

Between these buildings on the western brow and the officers' quarters on the east, the crown of the point is occupied by a small parade-ground facing the bay, and backed by certain of the other buildings of the post. The guard-house is a frame building, 34 feet 9 inches by 18 feet 6 inches, divided into a guard-room, with a stove and three windows, a prison-room with two windows, and four cells, with a small window or ventilator each.

The hospital is a one-story frame building, consisting of a main portion 32½ by 17¼ feet, divided into a ward 16¼ by 13 10/12, a dispensary, 16¼ by 12 10/12 feet in the clear, with a double fire-place with a small closet each side between them; adjoining this in the rear is another portion, 19¼ by 17¼ feet, divided into a mess-room, 16¼ by 10 1/2 feet, and a kitchen, 16¼ by 8 1/6 feet, in the clear. The whole building is under one hipped roof, and a porch 6 feet wide extends along the front and across the end of the main portion, and the side of addition. The ward is furnished with four iron single bedsteads, giving an air-space of 900 cubic feet to each bed; it is well lighted and ventilated. The building is warmed by coal-fires in open grates. A small building near the hospital is occupied for steward's quarters and store-room.

Serious cases of sickness are not treated here. When such occur at the post they are sent for treatment to the hospital at the Presidio. There is a large building for quartermaster and subsistence, and two smaller for ordnance stores.

The officers' quarters are five frame cottages of different size and plan, but all are comfortable and pleasantly situated on the sheltered brow, with a luxuriant flower-garden around them. They were cottages of citizens before the point was taken up as a Government post.

The sinks of the men are open trenches, which are closed over with earth when filled. The water-closets of officers' quarters discharge into the bay, into, which, also, all post refuse is thrown.

The water supply is unlimited, and of good quality. It is furnished by the water company free of charge, as the works are situated on the Government reservation.

Along the back of the officers' quarters, separating them from the parade-ground, is a high sheltered fence or lattice wall of laths, as a protection against the violent winds and sand-drift. The western limit of the post is similarly protected. The area thus sheltered includes the sites of the buildings above mentioned, and measures about five acres.

There are no special means of recreation at the post, except a company library of 125 volumes, but the city is so near that they are unnecessary.

There is a garden containing one acre at the post, and another of two acres at Presidio. These are cultivated by enlisted men, and furnish vegetables in sufficient quantity.

*Meteorological report, Point San José, Cal., 1870–'74.*

| Month. | 1870–'71. | | | | 1871–'72. | | | | 1872–'73. | | | | 1873–'74. | | | |
|---|---|---|---|---|---|---|---|---|---|---|---|---|---|---|---|---|
| | Temperature. | | | Rain-fall in inches. | Temperature. | | | Rain-fall in inches. | Temperature. | | | Rain-fall in inches. | Temperature. | | | Rain-fall in inches. |
| | Mean. | Max. | Min. | | Mean. | Max. | Min. | | Mean. | Max. | Min. | | Mean. | Max. | Min. | |
| July............ | *62.36 | 80† | 48† | ..... | 60.11 | 87† | 39† | 0.00 | 56.06 | 78 | 43 | 0.00 | 60.39 | 78 | 50 | 0.00 |
| August......... | | | | 0.00 | 52.51 | 78† | 32†? | 0.00 | 61.15 | 79 | 52 | 0.02 | 50.31 | 72 | 35 | 0.00 |
| September...... | 61.56 | 76† | 34† | 0.00 | 55.30 | 80† | 34† | 0.00 | 59.84 | 69 | 54 | 0.00 | 57.37 | 68 | 52 | 0.00 |
| October........ | 60.16 | 85† | 30† | 0.00 | 54.37 | 90† | 34† | 0.00 | 59.30 | 80 | 48 | 0.25 | 58.09 | 78 | 48 | 0.57 |
| November....... | 56.10 | 71† | 37† | 0.04 | 47.64 | 70† | 33† | 3.20 | 57.38 | 71 | 48 | 2.03 | 55.56 | 69 | 46 | 1.24 |
| December....... | 50.90 | 62† | 29† | 2.42 | 51.29 | 68† | 31† | 10.82 | 52.18 | 71 | 35 | 5.80 | 48.48 | 57 | 41 | 4.19 |
| January........ | 48.99 | 65† | 23† | 2.24 | 48.66 | 65 | 35 | 2.20 | 49.22 | 63 | 39 | 0.84 | 47.25 | 61 | 39 | 2.60 |
| February....... | 48.40 | 63† | 32† | 1.90 | 49.48 | 75 | 34 | 4.44 | 49.67 | 68 | 40 | 5.18 | 49.33 | 62 | 42 | 1.00 |
| March.......... | 51.86 | 78† | 35† | 1.40 | 50.03 | 71 | 37 | 1.41 | 52.95 | 69 | 40 | 0.56 | 49.83 | 63 | 41 | 1.91 |
| April.......... | 55.39 | 74† | 36† | 0.40 | 58.85 | 90 | 49 | 0.83 | 54.80 | 82 | 40 | 0.00 | 54.69 | 70 | 48 | 0.70 |
| May............ | 53.98 | 73† | 34† | 1.02 | 54.22 | 70 | 43 | 0.00 | 62.26 | 75 | 55 | 0.00 | 57.94 | 81 | 50 | 0.22 |
| June........... | 54.20 | 78† | 34† | 0.00 | 58.81 | 87 | 48 | 0.13 | 61.07 | 84 | 52 | 0.00 | 58.81 | 82 | 51 | 0.08 |
| For the year... | ........ | ..... | ..... | ..... | 53.44 | 90† | 31† | 23.03 | 56.32 | 84 | 35 | 14.68 | 54.00 | 82 | 39 | 12.51 |

* No former observations.   † These observations are made with self-registering thermometers.   The mean is from the standard thermometer.

*Consolidated sick-report, Point San José, Cal., 1870–'74.*

| Year | 1870–'71. | | 1871–'72. | | 1872–'73. | | 1873–'74. | |
|---|---|---|---|---|---|---|---|---|
| Mean strength { Officers<br>{ Enlisted men | 3<br>88 | | 3<br>46 | | 3<br>35 | | 4<br>59 | |
| Diseases. | Cases. | Deaths. | Cases. | Deaths. | Cases. | Deaths. | Cases. | Deaths. |
| GENERAL DISEASES, A. | | | | | | | | |
| Remittent fever | 1 | | 1 | | | | 2 | |
| Intermittent fever | 7 | | 2 | | 5 | | 4 | |
| Other diseases of this group | 1 | | | | 2 | | 1 | |
| GENERAL DISEASES, B. | | | | | | | | |
| Rheumatism | 9 | | 12 | | 2 | | 6 | |
| Syphilis | 23 | | 3 | | 2 | | 1 | |
| Consumption | | | | | 2 | 1 | | |
| Other diseases of this group | | | | | | | | |
| LOCAL DISEASES. | | | | | | | | |
| Catarrh and bronchitis | 5 | | 5 | | 6 | | 7 | |
| Pneumonia | | | | | 2 | | | |
| Pleurisy | | | | | | | 2 | |
| Diarrhœa and dysentery | 4 | | 3 | | 1 | | 5 | |
| Gonorrhœa | 3 | | 1 | | | | 2 | |
| Other local diseases | 20 | | 14 | | 14 | | 31 | |
| Alcoholism | 6 | | 1 | | 1 | | 4 | |
| Total disease | 79 | | 42 | | 37 | 1 | 65 | |
| VIOLENT DISEASES AND DEATHS. | | | | | | | | |
| Gunshot wounds | 2 | 1 | 1 | | | | | |
| Other accidents and injuries | 3 | | 5 | | 3 | | 24 | |
| Total violence | 5 | 1 | 6 | | 3 | | 24 | |

# THE PRESIDIO OF SAN FRANCISCO, CALIFORNIA.

INFORMATION FURNISHED BY SURGEONS J. C. BAILY AND J. C. M'KEE, UNITED STATES ARMY.

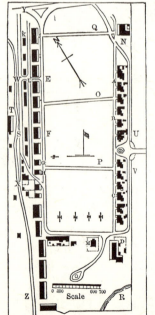

Figure 75.

The Presidio of San Francisco, Cal., is situated in the northwest suburbs of the town, on a gravelly slope which ascends gradually from the sands and salt-water marshes on the southern margin of the harbor of San Francisco. It overlooks the bay, and has in view the posts of Fort Point, a mile to the northwest, near the harbor-mouth, that of Alcatraz Island to the north and eastward, and that of Point San José to the east.

The reservation contains about 1,540 acres, and has a frontage on the bay of about a mile and a half. Back from the post the ground rises more rapidly into grass-covered hills. There are no shade-trees in the vicinity. The climate is varied and variable; oftentimes mild and pleasant during the early part of the day, and chilly and damp toward its close. Strong winds frequently prevail toward the end of summer and autumn, while in winter there is much moisture in the atmosphere, either falling as a heavy rain or enveloping the post in a thick, penetrating mist, which creeps in from the ocean and spreads itself over the lower-lying portions of the harbor boundaries.

The site of the post is well drained naturally, by a fall of one foot in twenty, but this is aided by shallow ditches around the various buildings, so that even immediately after heavy rains there are no standing pools. The parade-ground is grassy during the whole year.

The post is built on three sides of a parallelogram, 550 by 150 yards, which is open to the bay or northeast side. The general arrangement is shown in Figure 75.

A, B, C, D, officers' quarters; E, F, barracks; G, guard-house; H, adjutant's office; I, wagon-shop; J, quartermaster; K, bakery; L, storehouse; M, chapel; N, hospital; O, P, Q, plank walks; R, small stream, (sometimes dry;) S, gate in rear of barracks; T, sutler; U, V, picket fence in rear (east) of officers' quarters; W, X, picket fence in rear (west) of barracks; Y, road to Presidio wharf and beach; Z, road to mountain-lake.

Thirty-six feet in front of the row of officers' buildings, and extending along their whole length, is a wind-fence or lattice screen of lath, 12 feet high, with branches extending at right angles from it to the buildings. This has recently been built to shelter these quarters from the strong winds that sometimes blow from the ocean. Trees, pine and acacias, have been planted at 18-foot intervals between the main fence, and the buildings. All the buildings, with the exceptions noted below are of wood, and well lighted and ventilated by the windows and ridge.

The men's quarters consist of one building, 80 by 18 feet, one 95 by 18 feet, and four, each 51 by 18 feet, each one story and accommodating one company, with kitchens and mess-rooms adjoining; kitchens furnished with monitor ranges; one building, 117 by 25 feet, two story, for two companies, with kitchen and mess-room in an adjoining building, 117 by 16 feet; four buildings, 120 by 30 feet, each for two companies, with kitchens and mess-rooms in basements.

The officers' quarters consist of one building, 114 by 32 feet, three story, with a wing, 40 by 30 feet, thirty-nine rooms, for bachelor officers' quarters; twelve one-and-a-half-story cottages, 31 by 18 feet, with water-closets and bath-rooms attached, comfortable and neat, for married officers.

The laundresses' quarters consist of one building, 90 by 28 feet, one story, twelve rooms; one, 45 by 37 feet, two story, twelve rooms; eight, 60 by 27 feet, one story, eight rooms each; one, 160 by 29 feet, with eighteen rooms; one, 87 by 55 feet, with fourteen rooms; one, 45 by 26 feet, with three rooms; one, 60 by 23 feet, with three rooms—one story, adobe, occupied by seven families.

The post-buildings consist of one building, 36 by 30 feet, one story, four rooms, adjutant's office; one, 40 by 30 feet, two stories, with porch in front; upper story a guard-room; lower divided into a main prison-room, 35 by 20 by 12 feet, and cells, each 10 by 5 by 12 feet; chapel, 45 by 30 feet; school-house, 30 by 18 feet; bake-house, 42 by 18 feet—oven turns out a batch of 412 rations; hospital, 80 by 40 feet.

The workshops consist of a wheelwright-shop, 80 by 30 feet; blacksmith-shop, 50 by 20 feet.

The storehouses consist of a magazine, 28 by 23 feet; quartermaster's and subsistence storehouse, 110 by 30 feet, one story, brick foundation; storehouse for hay and grain, 66 by 24 feet; storehouse for hard-wood lumber, 51 by 18 feet; gun-sheds, 175 by 30 feet, with ordnance stores in loft.

The stables consist of two buildings for battery horses, 215 by 30 feet, with eighty-seven stalls each, well ventilated; forage-loft overhead; mule-shed, 430 by 16 feet.

The hospital at the eastern angle of the parade-ground, in line with the officers' quarters, is a two-story building, 80 by 40 feet, with a wing, 35 by 22 feet, on brick basement, with porch in front, and small inclosure behind. It is arranged for fifty beds, to each of which it gives an area of 76 feet, or 1,025 cubic feet. Its average occupancy is nine. It is divided into four wards, 40 by 22 by 14 feet, a smaller ward for prisoners, 20 by 10 by 13 feet, and an attendants' room, 20 by 18 by 13 feet; each is furnished with water-pipes and marble basin, wardrobe, bedside tables, and chairs. They are well warmed by grated fire-places for coal, and lighted and ventilated by the windows. In addition to these, there is a dispensary, furnished with hot and cold water and the necessary fixtures; a library containing a large and very good selection of books; a post-mortem room with table, and two well-fitted up bath-rooms. The kitchen is likewise furnished with hot and cold water, has a good range, and an adjoining pantry and store-room. The mess-room, 30 by 20 by 10½ feet, is fitted up with the necessary tables and benches, and cupboards for crockery. In the basement, besides the kitchen and pantries, are two store-rooms for medical supplies, and a coal-cellar. On the upper floor are two water-closets, which empty through the main sink in the inclosure into the sewer.

The hospital library contains five hundred volumes, comprising travels, biography, history, fiction, and books of a religious character.

The water-supply of this post is derived from the flume of the Spring Valley Water Company. It is forced by a windmill and mule-power into a reservoir at the southern or higher end of the post, whence it is supplied by pipes to the different buildings. The supply is abundant, and the quality excellent. The waste-water pipes and latrines empty into a large covered sewer, which runs on either side of the post, and discharges into tide-water.

A cow is kept for hospital use. A small garden yields all the vegetables necessary for the hospital, and is cultivated by one of the attendants.

The post is arranged for sixteen companies, but during the greater portion of the year 1874 its garrison consisted only of the field, staff, band, and four companies of the Fourth Artillery, giving a mean strength of nineteen officers and one hundred and sixty-two men. The quarters occupied by these troops are fitted up with iron bedsteads, and 1,500 cubic feet of air-space is allowed per bed. Their diet has been of good quality and variety. Large company gardens, well cultivated, render the post almost independent of other sources of vegetable supplies.

*Meteorological report, Presidio of San Francisco, Cal., 1870–'74.*

| Month. | 1870–'71. | | | | 1871–'72. | | | | 1872–'73. | | | | 1873–'74. | | | |
|---|---|---|---|---|---|---|---|---|---|---|---|---|---|---|---|---|
| | Temperature. | | | Rain-fall in inches. | Temperature. | | | Rain-fall in inches. | Temperature. | | | Rain-fall in inches. | Temperature. | | | Rain-fall in inches. |
| | Mean. | Max. | Min. | | Mean. | Max. | Min. | | Mean. | Max. | Min. | | Mean. | Max. | Min. | |
| July | 60.97 | 83 | 54* | 0.00 | 55.68 | 63 | 46* | 0.00 | 77.25 | 95* | 58* | 3.58 | 56.54 | 76* | 48* | 0.02 |
| August | 61.61 | 71 | 53* | 0.00 | 56.41 | 65 | 48* | 0.00 | 58.30 | 70* | 48* | 0.03 | 58.71 | 77* | 41* | 0.00 |
| September | 60.01 | 71 | 51* | 0.04 | 59.50 | 74 | 48* | 0.00 | 58.44 | 80* | 49* | 0.07 | 56.98 | 69* | 50* | 0.00 |
| October | 60.10 | 85 | 45* | 0.00 | 61.43 | 92* | 45* | 0.04 | 57.25 | 79* | 46* | 0.14 | 58.77 | 77* | 45* | 0.56 |
| November | 56.20 | 71 | 43* | 0.50 | 54.30 | 78* | 39* | 2.41 | 54.42 | 67* | 41* | 2.93 | 56.91 | 71* | 44* | 0.80 |
| December | 48.33 | 63 | 35* | 3.22 | 52.31 | 63* | 36* | 9.96 | 51.13 | 61* | 37* | 8.58 | 49.71 | 58* | 38* | 9.57 |
| January | 49.26 | 63 | 37* | 2.19 | 51.85 | 61* | 42* | 5.03 | 53.41 | 67* | 40* | 4.25 | 48.11 | 62* | 37* | 3.96 |
| February | 49.03 | 58 | 36* | 3.30 | 54.00 | 63* | 42* | 10.50 | 49.71 | 66* | 38* | 7.39 | 49.50 | 60* | 36* | 1.31 |
| March | 52.41 | 72 | 39* | 0.61 | 53.33 | 60* | 42* | 2.61 | 53.39 | 77* | 40* | 0.58 | 49.56 | 66* | 35* | 2.57 |
| April | 52.63 | 71 | 41* | 1.81 | 52.51 | 73* | 38* | 1.08 | 52.95 | 78* | 38* | 0.46 | 54.03 | 74* | 42* | 0.67 |
| May | 53.98 | 67 | 40* | 0.38 | 54.52 | 85* | 45* | 0.00 | 53.92 | 73* | 45* | 0.11 | 56.87 | 86* | 44* | 0.18 |
| June | 55.42 | 64 | 50* | 0.00 | 58.25 | 89* | 48* | 0.07 | 55.59 | 66* | 47* | 0.06 | 57.99 | 81* | 45* | 0.00 |
| For the year | 51.93 | 85 | 35* | 12.05 | 55.34 | 92* | 36* | 22.70 | 56.31 | 95* | 37* | 28.18 | 54.47 | 86* | 35* | 19.64 |

\* These observations are made with self-registering thermometers. The mean is from the standard thermometer.

*Consolidated sick-report, Presidio of San Francisco, Cal., 1870–'74.*

| Year | 1870–'71. | | 1871–'72. | | 1872–'73. | | 1873–'74. | |
|---|---|---|---|---|---|---|---|---|
| Mean strength { Officers | 15 | | 20 | | 10 | | 13 | |
| { Enlisted men | 294 | | 252 | | 150 | | 216 | |
| Diseases. | Cases. | Deaths. | Cases. | Deaths. | Cases. | Deaths. | Cases. | Deaths. |
| GENERAL DISEASES, A. | | | | | | | | |
| Small-pox and varioloid | | | 1 | | 1 | | | |
| Remittent fever | | | | | 1 | | | |
| Intermittent fever | 71 | | 44 | | 27 | | 25 | |
| Diphtheria | | | | | | | 1 | |
| Other diseases of this group | 2 | 1 | 1 | | 9 | | 17 | |
| GENERAL DISEASES, B. | | | | | | | | |
| Rheumatism | 91 | | 53 | | 26 | | 41 | |
| Syphilis | 102 | | 24 | | 43 | | 40 | |
| Consumption | 2 | 2 | 3 | 1 | 3 | | 2 | 1 |
| Other diseases of this group | 1 | | | | | | 12 | |
| LOCAL DISEASES. | | | | | | | | |
| Catarrh and bronchitis | 137 | | 42 | | 16 | | 82 | |
| Pneumonia | 6 | 2 | 1 | 1 | 1 | 1 | 1 | |
| Pleurisy | | | 1 | | 2 | | | |
| Diarrhœa and dysentery | 72 | | 27 | | 30 | | 48 | |
| Hernia | 3 | | | | | | 3 | |
| Gonorrhœa | 30 | | 12 | | 5 | | 21 | |
| Other local diseases | 148 | | 85 | | 82 | | 141 | 1 |
| Alcoholism | 26 | | 28 | | 27 | | 24 | |
| Total disease | 691 | 5 | 322 | 2 | 273 | 1 | 458 | 2 |
| VIOLENT DISEASES AND DEATHS. | | | | | | | | |
| Gunshot wounds | 1 | | | | 1 | | 1 | |
| Drowning | | | | | | | | 1 |
| Other accidents and injuries | 95 | | 68 | | 59 | | 99 | |
| Homicide | | | | 1 | | | | 1 |
| Suicide | | | | | | | | 1 |
| Total violence | 96 | | 68 | 1 | 60 | | 100 | 3 |

# CAMP WRIGHT, CALIFORNIA.

INFORMATION FURNISHED BY ASSISTANT SURGEON E. J. MARSH AND ACTING ASSISTANT SURGEON
L. H. PATTY, UNITED STATES ARMY.

Camp Wright is situated in Mendocino County, California. Latitude, 39° 55′ north; longitude, 45° 45′ west; altitude, about 1,800 feet. Round Valley, in which the post is placed, is in the Coast range of mountains, by the high ridges of which it is surrounded, and is about eight miles in diameter. No roads enter it, but there are several trails. The nearest town of any note is Ukiah, distant sixty-five miles. Capto, in Long Valley, twenty-five miles south, is the nearest post-office, from which a tri-weekly mail is brought to the post. Owing to the steepness of the trails all supplies are packed into the valley on mules.

An Indian reservation, upon which about twelve hundred Indians of various tribes have been gathered, is established two and a half miles from the post, and about five hundred whites are settled in the vicinity. The soil is fertile, producing large crops of cereals and all kinds of vegetables. Round Valley was first occupied by troops in the latter part of 1858, was abandoned in 1861, and re-occupied in December, 1862, when the present post was established, and named in honor of the department commander. The military reservation is one mile square.

The post is situated about one-half mile from the dividing ridge, on the western side of the valley, on a slightly undulating, gravelly bottom, which in summer becomes parched.

The supply of water is deficient in the vicinity of the post during the dry season. Two wells supply the garrison during winter and spring, but from July to October these become nearly dry, and water is hauled from a creek about two miles distant. Eel River nearly surrounds the valley, is fordable in summer, but in winter swells to a rapid and dangerous stream.

The climate is very dry, except during the rainy season, and there is scarcely any dew. The rainy season varies greatly, from November to July, or from January to May. Little or no snow falls here. The drainage is good, and all the quarters are shaded by fine oak trees.

The company barrack is a frame building, 120 by 30 feet, 11 feet high to ceiling, and 23 feet to ridge, with a veranda, 8 feet wide, around it. It was erected in 1874, and stands on the south side of the parade. It is divided into a dormitory, 100 by 30 feet, in west end of building, and an adjutant's office, a first sergeant's office, and a small store-room, occupying the east twenty feet. The dormitory is warmed by two stoves, ventilated by the doors and windows, and is furnished with iron bedsteads. The mess-room and kitchen occupy sixty feet of the old adobe quarters. This building was formerly 200 by 30 feet, but one hundred feet in length of the west end of it was torn down in December, 1874, the balance being used as mess-room and kitchen in the west end, and woodhouse and store-room in the east forty feet.

Married soldiers' and laundresses' quarters are in two frame buildings located some distance west of the parade, each containing two sets. One set is occupied as a tailor-shop.

The post bakery is a frame building, 26 by 16 feet, situated west of the parade; is ample for the post, and in good condition.

Officers' quarters consist of one brick building, 38 by 38 feet, containing six rooms, with a frame kitchen attached, being the commanding officer's quarters; one log building, 50 by 22 feet, four rooms, the post surgeon's quarters; and one log building, 38 by 36 feet, six rooms, the post quartermaster's quarters.

The guard-house is a new frame building, erected in 1874, faces the west side of the parade, is 30 by 20 feet, and contains a guard-room, 14 by 20 feet, a prison-room, 9 by 20 feet, and five cells, each 4 by 7 feet; the rooms are 10 feet in height. It is ventilated by the doors and windows, and warmed by a stove.

The storehouse is a frame building, 88 by 26 feet, 12 feet high to eaves, and 20 feet to ridge, was erected in 1873, and faces the west side of the parade south of the guard-house. In 1874, a room, 13 by 8 feet, was added at the north end, to be used as quarters for the commissary sergeant.

Stables are sheds, sufficient for thirteen animals, and are located one hundred and twenty yards south of the barracks.

The hospital, situated two hundred yards east of the camp, is a one-story frame building, 54 by 16 feet, with an addition, 12 by 20 feet, adjoining the rear. The building fronts southwest. The main portion is divided into a ward, 20 by 16 feet, in the southerly end; then, in succession, northerly, an office, 8 by 13 feet, with a passage, 3 feet wide, in the rear; a hall, 4 feet wide, running across the building; a dispensary, 8 by 16 feet, and a store-room, 14 by 16 feet. The addition in rear is used as a kitchen and mess-room; it is in one room. All the rooms are 10 feet in height at the eaves. The ward and store-room are the only rooms ceiled.

All the sinks at the post are mere pits, or trenches, covered over when filled, and new ones dug.

The post garden comprises about one-fourth acre of the parade-ground, producing some onions, lettuce, &c.

*Meteorological report, Camp Wright, Cal., 1870–'74.*

| Month. | 1870–'71. Temperature. Mean. | Max. | Min. | Rain-fall in inches. | 1871–'72. Temperature. Mean. | Max. | Min. | Rain-fall in inches. | 1872–'73. Temperature. Mean. | Max. | Min. | Rain-fall in inches. | 1873–'74. Temperature. Mean. | Max. | Min. | Rain-fall in inches. |
|---|---|---|---|---|---|---|---|---|---|---|---|---|---|---|---|---|
| July | 80.54 | 108 | 53* | 0.00 | 76.55 | 105 | 46* | 0.00 | 78.44 | 104* | 46* | 0.00 | 78.67 | 110* | 35* | 0.10 |
| August | 78.65 | 110 | 55* | 0.00 | 79.35 | 108 | 46* | 0.00 | 77.28 | 109* | 46* | 0.20 | 75.59 | 104* | 39* | 0.00 |
| September | 68.15 | 97 | 42* | 0.00 | 67.55 | 95 | 46* | 0.50 | 67.97 | 108* | 34* | 0.00 | 73.48 | 103* | 39* | 0.05 |
| October | 60.36 | 93 | 25* | 0.00 | 60.13 | 93 | 29* | 0.31 | 66.23 | 103* | 31* | 0.36 | 60.24 | 98* | 26* | 0.34 |
| November | 49.80 | 72 | 25* | 1.28 | 46.53 | 72* | 23* | 4.03 | 52.19 | 85* | 18* | 5.20 | 56.42 | 86* | 27* | 4.98 |
| December | 38.91 | 57 | 20* | 1.19 | 44.58 | 64* | 21* | 16.64 | 46.26 | 76* | 16* | 7.24 | 43.55 | 62* | 22* | 15.50 |
| January | 43.06 | 63 | 20* | 2.66 | 44.45 | 62* | 27* | 11.52 | 48.91 | 77* | 28* | 3.55 | 43.60 | 74* | 21* | 12.94 |
| February | 42.60 | 60 | 24* | 4.60 | 47.29 | 60* | 30* | 19.78 | 45.11 | 81* | 27* | 6.92 | 45.46 | 74* | 26* | 5.46 |
| March | 49.00 | 79 | 30* | 7.10 | 52.50 | 75* | 30* | 5.34 | 54.69 | 89* | 26* | 2.91 | 46.89 | 78* | 24* | 7.26 |
| April | 54.37 | 80 | 39* | 1.07 | 51.20 | 81* | 27* | 0.66 | 55.75 | 83* | 26* | 1.13 | 55.26 | 85* | 32* | 3.72 |
| May | 57.79 | 86 | 33* | 1.96 | 63.25 | 88* | 35* | 0.12 | 62.14 | 90* | 38* | 0.04 | 61.56 | 92* | 36* | 1.16 |
| June | 73.42 | 107 | 40* | 0.00 | 71.93 | 102* | 43* | 0.04 | 67.24 | 93* | 32* | 0.30 | 68.02 | 98* | 35* | 0.26 |
| For the year | 58.05 | 110 | 20* | 19.86 | 58.77 | 108 | 21* | 58.94 | 60.18 | 109* | 16* | 27.85 | 59.07 | 110* | 21* | 51.77 |

* These observations are made with self-registering thermometers. The mean is from the standard thermometer.

*Consolidated sick-report, Camp Wright, Cal., 1870–'74.*

| | | 1870–'71. | | 1871–'72. | | 1872–'73. | | 1873–'74. | |
|---|---|---|---|---|---|---|---|---|---|
| Year | | | | | | | | | |
| Mean strength { Officers | | 4 | | 4 | | 3 | | 4 | |
| { Enlisted men | | 53 | | 46 | | 38 | | 45 | |
| Diseases. | | Cases. | Deaths. | Cases. | Deaths. | Cases. | Deaths. | Cases. | Deaths. |
| GENERAL DISEASES, A. | | | | | | | | | |
| Remittent fever | | | | 1 | | | | | |
| Intermittent fever | | 4 | | 7 | | 1 | | | |
| Other diseases of this group | | | | | | | | 1 | |
| GENERAL DISEASES, B. | | | | | | | | | |
| Rheumatism | | 1 | | 5 | | 3 | | 12 | |
| Syphilis | | 2 | | 3 | | | | | |
| Consumption | | 2 | 1 | | | | | | |
| Other diseases of this group | | | | | | 1 | | | |
| LOCAL DISEASES. | | | | | | | | | |
| Catarrh and bronchitis | | 3 | | 1 | | 12 | | 7 | |
| Pneumonia | | | | 1 | | | | | |
| Pleurisy | | | | 1 | | | | | |
| Diarrhœa and dysentery | | | | 4 | | 1 | | 4 | |
| Gonorrhœa | | 22 | 1 | 5 | | 4 | 2 | 1 | |
| Other local diseases | | | | | | | | 18 | |
| Alcoholism | | 3 | | 1 | | 1 | | 2 | |
| Total disease | | 37 | 2 | 29 | | 23 | 2 | 45 | |
| VIOLENT DISEASES AND DEATHS. | | | | | | | | | |
| Accidents and injuries | | 10 | | 9 | | 7 | | 7 | |
| Total violence | | 10 | | 9 | | 7 | | 7 | |

# YERBA BUENA ISLAND, SAN FRANCISCO, CALIFORNIA.

## REPORT OF ACTING ASSISTANT SURGEON DAVID WALKER, UNITED STATES ARMY.

This island, in latitude 37° 48′ 45″ north, and longitude 45° 17′ 45″ west, is situated in the Bay of San Francisco, California, some two and a half miles northeast of the city, with an altitude from 35 to 75 feet above sea-level. It is of irregular shape, hilly outline, and contains one hundred and sixteen acres. The only part of its surface fitted for a camp is the small plateau on which the post is located, which is flanked northeast and southwest by hills, and open to the southeast and northwest. The climate is mild but moist, complete saturation frequently occurring at night. The prevailing winds are westerly from the ocean.

The surface-drainage of the island is satisfactory. Its water-supply is of excellent quality and is derived from a well and a tank, filled by exudation from seams in the rock.

The post was established in 1868, and is still in an unfinished condition.

It was discontinued as a station for troops, and turned over to the Ordnance Department October 20, 1873, and is at present in charge of an ordnance sergeant.

*Meteorological report, Yerba Buena Island, Cal., 1870–'74.*

| Month. | 1870–'71. | | | | 1871–'72. | | | | 1872–'73. | | | | 1873–'74. | | | |
|---|---|---|---|---|---|---|---|---|---|---|---|---|---|---|---|---|
| | Temperature. | | | Rain-fall in inches. | Temperature. | | | Rain-fall in inches. | Temperature. | | | Rain-fall in inches. | Temperature. | | | Rain-fall in inches. |
| | Mean. | Max. | Min. | | Mean. | Max. | Min. | | Mean. | Max. | Min. | | Mean. | Max. | Min. | |
| | ° | ° | ° | | ° | ° | ° | | ° | ° | ° | | ° | ° | ° | |
| July | 62.78 | 90 | 56 | 0.00 | ........ | ........ | ........ | ........ | 59.84 | 74* | 50* | ........ | 60.37 | 82* | 48* | 0.00 |
| August | 62.87 | 76 | 56 | 0.00 | ........ | ........ | ........ | ........ | 61.53 | 76° | 50* | ........ | 60.36 | 78* | 50* | 0.00 |
| September | 60.73 | 70 | 54 | 0.00 | 61.84 | 80 | 56 | ........ | 60.86 | 82* | 50* | ........ | 59.97 | 74* | 50* | 0.00 |
| October | 62.39 | 92 | 54 | 0.00 | 61.36 | 82* | 50* | ........ | 60.17 | 82* | 48* | ........ | 59.76 | 75* | 44* | 0.00 |
| November | 57.43 | 72 | 50 | 0.04 | 55.42 | 73* | 41* | ........ | 55.97 | 72* | 41* | ........ | ........ | ........ | ........ | .... |
| December | 50.30 | 64 | 40 | 1.57 | 52.23 | 66* | 40* | ........ | 52.12 | 62* | 34* | ........ | ........ | ........ | ........ | .... |
| January | 49.20 | 64 | 38 | 1.27 | 52.21 | 70* | 40* | ........ | 54.21 | 65* | 40° | ........ | ........ | ........ | ........ | .... |
| February | ........ | ........ | ........ | ........ | 53.86 | 64* | 43* | ........ | 50.84 | 74* | 40* | ........ | ........ | ........ | ........ | .... |
| March | ........ | ........ | ........ | ........ | 54.76 | 70* | 45* | ........ | 54.29 | 83* | 40* | ........ | ........ | ........ | ........ | .... |
| April | ........ | ........ | ........ | ........ | 55.51 | 80* | 40* | ........ | 56.26 | 74* | 40* | ........ | ........ | ........ | ........ | .... |
| May | ........ | ........ | ........ | ........ | 57.61 | 84* | 42* | ........ | 58.34 | 76* | 44* | ........ | ........ | ........ | ........ | .... |
| June | ........ | ........ | ........ | ........ | 59.43 | 90* | 46* | ........ | 60.87 | 78* | 54* | ........ | ........ | ........ | ........ | .... |
| For the year | ........ | ........ | ........ | ........ | ........ | ........ | ........ | ........ | 57.10 | 83* | 34* | ........ | ........ | ........ | ........ | .... |

* These observations are made with self-registering thermometers. The mean is from the standard thermometer.

# DEPARTMENT OF ARIZONA.

(Embracing the Territory of Arizona and so much of the State of California as lies south of a line from the northwest corner of Arizona Territory to Point Conception, California.)

Apache, Camp, Ariz.
Bowie, Camp, Ariz.
rant, Camp, Ariz.
La Paz, Camp, Ariz.

Lowell, Camp, Ariz.
McDowell, Camp, Ariz.
Mojave, Camp, Ariz.
Rio Verde Indian Reservation, Ariz.

San Carlos Indian Reservation, Ariz.
Verde, Camp, Ariz.
Whipple, Fort, Ariz.
Yuma, Fort, Cal.

## TABLE OF DISTANCES IN THE DEPARTMENT OF ARIZONA.

| | SF | Pres | Apache | Bowie | Grant | La Paz | Lowell | McDowell | Mojave | NSDB | Rio Verde | San Carlos | Ft San Diego | Verde | Whipple |
|---|---|---|---|---|---|---|---|---|---|---|---|---|---|---|---|
| San Francisco | | | | | | | | | | | | | | | |
| Prescott | 882 | | | | | | | | | | | | | | |
| Camp Apache | 1229 | 210 | | | | | | | | | | | | | |
| Camp Bowie | 1118 | 364 | 197 | | | | | | | | | | | | |
| Camp Grant | 1129 | 375 | 117 | 49 | | | | | | | | | | | |
| Camp La Paz | 885 | 197 | 407 | 435 | 446 | | | | | | | | | | |
| Camp Lowell | 1025 | 221 | 222 | 111 | 122 | 356 | | | | | | | | | |
| Camp McDowell | 960 | 109 | 285 | 236 | 247 | 217 | 123 | | | | | | | | |
| Camp Mojave | 717 | 168 | 378 | 532 | 543 | 168 | 433 | 277 | | | | | | | |
| New San Diego Barracks | 552 | 535 | 689 | 578 | 589 | 345 | 479 | 420 | 513 | | | | | | |
| Rio Verde Indian Reservation | 916 | 34 | 186 | 398 | 378 | 231 | 254 | 131 | 202 | 569 | | | | | |
| San Carlos Indian Reservation | 1209 | 284 | 74 | 162 | 80 | 481 | 202 | 327 | 452 | 669 | 260 | | | | |
| Fort at San Diego | 546 | 529 | 683 | 572 | 583 | 339 | 473 | 414 | 507 | 6 | 563 | 663 | | | |
| Camp Verde | 928 | 46 | 170 | 410 | 362 | 243 | 252 | 115 | 214 | 581 | 16 | 244 | 575 | | |
| Fort Whipple | 883 | 1 | 211 | 365 | 376 | 198 | 222 | 110 | 169 | 536 | 35 | 285 | 530 | 47 | |
| Fort Yuma | 738 | 332 | 491 | 380 | 391 | 147 | 281 | 222 | 315 | 198 | 366 | 471 | 192 | 243 | 333 |

# CAMP APACHE, ARIZONA TERRITORY.

REPORT OF ASSISTANT SURGEONS J. B. GIRARD AND L. Y. LORING, UNITED STATES ARMY.

Camp Apache is situated on the south bank of the East Fork of White Mountain River, a short distance above and within view of its junction with the North Fork, in latitude 33° 40' north ; longitude, 32° 52' west; altitude, nearly 6,000 feet above the sea.

Previous to the year 1870 the country, in the heart of which Camp Apache now stands, was only known as the home of the Coyotero Apaches, a warlike and untamed tribe of Indians, whose relations with the white and Mexican populations of the surrounding districts had always been marked by a decided hostility. In order to check the inroads of the savages on the settlements south of the Gila River, a military station had been established at old Camp Goodwin, which for several years was one of the links in the chain of outposts designed for the protection of the white settlers. That place proved to be one of the most malarial stations in Arizona, and owing to this defect it was finally decided to abandon it and transfer the garrison to a more favorable locality. Major John Green, of the First Cavalry, then commanding officer of that post, having selected this spot as the most eligible and affording the best facilities for controlling the hostile bands of the neighborhood, occupied it with two companies, L and M, of his regiment, in May, 1870. A few months later Camp Goodwin was totally broken up, and the infantry company, (B Company, Twenty-first Infantry,) heretofore left in charge of the post, moved out and joined the cavalry command. The new camp was designed at first as a temporary station, but the experience of the following two years demonstrated so forcibly the necessity of keeping an armed force in this region that during the summer of 1872 steps were taken to make it a permanent post. It was named successively Camp Ord, Camp Mogollon, Camp Thomas, and finally the present name of Camp Apache was settled upon.

The White Mountains or Sierra Blanca, on the southwestern slope of which the post is situated, consist of a cluster of rounded summits, from ten to twelve thousand feet in height, which constitute the most elevated range of Eastern Arizona, their tops being covered with snow during a great portion of the year. To the eastward they extend into New Mexico, and connect with other chains; on the Arizona side they are prolonged in a northwesterly direction by a somewhat lower range, known as the Mogollon, which gradually merges in the so-called Black Mesa, an extensive system of volcanic plateaus, extending to the Grand Cañon of the Colorado. The Black Mesa terminates abruptly on the south by a long line of cliffs or bold escarpments. These cliffs and the ranges above described form the divide between the streams running north into the Colorado Chiquito and those flowing southward into the Gila. Chief among the latter is the Rio Salado or Salt River, which, with its tributaries, rises in the Sierra Blanca itself, and their waters during the course of past ages have deepened their beds so as to cut profound cañons into the flanks of the mountains, and hollow out extensive valleys wherever the nature of the underlying rocks was favorable to that process. In one of these valleys, near the junction of the two forks of the White Mountain River, stands Camp Apache, in full view of the main summits of the Sierra Blanca, which loom high up in the eastern horizon, as dark masses during the warm season, and snowy crests in winter. North of the post the country gradually rises as far as the top of the Mogollon range, beyond which stretches the broad plain of the Colorado Chiquito ; southward a rapid descent of nearly 4,000 feet leads to the Gila River, sixty miles distant. Westward the valley of the White Mountain River slopes by easy degrees down to the Tonto Basin, a broken and hilly region between the Black Mesa and the Rio Salado.

The mountain-ranges described under the names of Sierra Blanca, Mogollon, and Black Mesa present one and the same geological character. They consist of the original sedimentary beds, fractured and uplifted by the action of subterranean forces, and of extensive outflows of lava, which, issuing from various outlets, once overspread the country, covering it with a sheet of molten matter, the remains of which are now seen in the shape of more or less isolated basaltic tables, usually connected with extinct volcanic craters and cones. The uplifting force acting on the sedimentary strata operated in such a uniform and equable manner as not to cause any foldings of the beds, but simply to make them dip at a moderate angle to the northeast. In consequence of this, the geologist who ascends these mountains on the southern side meets with a succession of terraces or benches bounded by high and steep cliffs, while from the opposite side the summits are reached by a very gradual and easy slope. In many places the erosive action of running water has been exerted to the extent of totally destroying the former appearance of the country, leaving nothing in view save isolated table-mountains covered with basaltic caps; closer research, however, discloses the fact that all these buttes and basaltic sheets were originally connected and united in one system. As mentioned before, extensive valleys and deep cañons have been formed on the flanks of the mountains by the many streams which have their origin in the abundant snows of the summits. Their waters have gradually washed away the softer strata, when these were exposed on the surface, but where the sedimentary beds were protected by a hard and resisting shell of basaltic lava, the action of water has been to undermine the whole structure and cause the sudden fall of immense masses of rock down to the level of the streams, leaving on each side walls or escarpments almost perpendicular. In some cases, after a valley was excavated by either of these processes, later outflows of lava were poured from the hillsides, partly filling the excavation. These new deposits were in their turn also acted upon by running water, and deep cañons cut through them; a striking instance of this phenomenon is met with on the very site of Camp Apache. The basaltic rock found in the vicinity of the post is rusty colored to black, very heavy and massive, and breaks off in hexagonal prismatic columns. The period of activity of the igneous forces by which the outflows of lava have been produced is evidently posterior to the cretaceous, and as none but post-tertiary beds have been found overlying the trap-rocks, it is highly probable that the eruptions took place in very recent geological times. Owing to the peculiar structural features of this country, and the frequency of high, precipitous cliffs, the faces of which are but sparingly covered with vegetation, the sedimentary strata can be examined without difficulty and artificial sections made with the greatest ease. Those observed in the immediate vicinity of the post belong exclusively to the upper carboniferous series. There is much uniformity in the character and sequence of the beds; the great mass of them consist of arenaceous shales, colored red by oxide of iron. Among the argillaceous beds, and alternating with them, are strata of more or less compact grayish sandstone, sometimes containing fossils. This stone is used at the post for building purposes, and, though soft when quarried, hardens rapidly on exposure to the air. A soft laminated sandstone of a drab color is also found among the upper strata, and seams of gypsum are observed in various places between the clays. By following the course of the river westward, deeper beds are seen coming to the surface; they conform essentially in lithological character to those already described, but the fossils found in them assimilate their age to the lower carboniferous. Half-way between the post and the summit of the Mogollon range, Mr. G. K. Gilbert, chief geologist of Lieutenant Wheeler's expedition, has met with organic remains in soft sandstone, which enable him to refer the beds to the Jurassic period, immediately above the carboniferous. A bluish limestone has recently been discovered a few miles up the river, and is now being quarried and burned for use at the post; it apparently does not contain fossils. Beds of bituminous coal are said to exist in the neighborhood, but their location is unknown, and their existence somewhat problematical.

The climate of Camp Apache, owing to the elevation above the sea-level, is much colder than its latitude would lead one to infer. As a rule, the winters are severe. Snow-storms are frequent from December to April. Spring opens in April, the vernal months are warm and dry, and vegetation does not fairly start before the advent of the rainy season, which extends from the latter part of June to September. During that period, few days pass without heavy showers and thunderstorms, and the heat of the atmosphere, which would otherwise be unendurable, is always tempered to a remarkable degree by the all-pervading dampness, and never becomes excessive. With the cessation of the rains, hot weather returns for a few weeks, and the autumn months are marked by disagreeably warm days alternating with cold and chilly nights. Even during the hottest part of the year the nights are wonderfully cool and pleasant.

The cool and moist nature of this climate, as compared with that of the lower districts of Arizona, entails a corresponding difference in the character of the vegetation, which partakes here of a northern and Alpine type. The plateaus and river-bottoms are covered during the rainy season with a rich growth of grama-grass, and afford unlimited grazing of an excellent quality. The banks of the streams are lined with groves of shady trees, whose dark foliage in summer contrasts with the general red hue of the soil. Chief among them are the ever-recurring cottonwood, the ash, walnut, box-elder, various willows, and, in cañons where moisture and shade are plentiful, the beech, and a handsome species of oak, (*quercus acrifolia*.)

The hills and table-lands are the home of the evergreen oak, the juniper, red cedar, and several species of pine, two of which, the nut-pine and the yellow pine, are very abundant. The latter species is highly valuable, as it furnishes all the timber necessary for the construction of the post.

Shrubs and herbaceous plants are abundant, and the variety of species found growing within any circumscribed space is surprisingly great. The most conspicuous among them are the western locust, (*Robinia Neo Mexicana*,) wild grape, woodbine, dogbane, hop, currant, gooseberry, wild tea, sweet sumac, &c., all early-flowering species. Later in the season the country becomes covered with a profusion of coarse, yellow-flowered compositæ, many of them of gigantic size.

The soil of the river-bottoms is very fertile, and eminently adapted to agricultural purposes; most cereals, wheat, oats, barley, and especially corn, grow to perfection with a moderate amount of labor. A few acres of ground near the post have been placed under cultivation as company-gardens, and the success met with has fully equaled the most sanguine expectations. Almost every variety of culinary vegetable has been produced without any difficulty whatever, and scurvy, caused by lack of vegetable food, can never attack troops garrisoned here, without the grossest kind of negligence.

Panthers, wild-cats, (*lynx rufus*,) and cinnamon bears haunt the pine forests of the mountains, and their skins are occasionally brought into the post by Indians. Coyotes are abundant. Gray wolves and foxes are often seen. A few deer are occasionally shot, and herds of elk are said to roam over the wildest portions of the White Mountains.

Few birds are permanent residents of this district. The wild turkey is quite abundant, mountain-quails are less numerous, and a few ducks and snipes frequent the streams.

The mountain streams contain many species of fish, among which a variety of speckled trout is highly esteemed.

Reptiles are very scarce; a few small lizards, harmless snakes, and frogs are the only representatives of this class. What is said of reptiles may apply also to venomous insects. During the rainy season tarantulas are often met with prowling about buildings, and a few centipedes crawl out of their holes, but at other times they are hardly ever to be seen.

The post itself is built on a basaltic plateau of seventy or eighty acres in area, elevated about 100 feet above the level of the East Fork of the White Mountain River, which here flows through a narrow and abrupt cañon. The surface-soil is composed of coarse sand and gravel mixed with rounded and water-worn pebbles, and underlaid at variable depths by compact volcanic rock. The natural drainage of the place cannot be excelled; from the flag-staff, in the center of the parade, the ground slopes gently in all directions, and, where the plateau proper terminates, a steep descent forms the boundary on all sides except the south, where a long gully or ravine separates the post from the neighboring hill. Even after the most profuse rains, not a pool of water can be seen on the parade-ground, as it all runs off rapidly or is absorbed by the porous, gravelly soil.

The labor of building the post has been performed entirely by troops, and, owing to the former belief that the camp would only be temporary, the older buildings are all of a rough and primitive character. Rough-hewn pine logs were for a long time the only procurable material, and, as lumber had to be sent from Tucson, two hundred and thirty miles distant, boards were used with great economy. During the summer of 1872 a steam saw-mill arrived at the post, lumber was fabricated, and much labor expended on repairing and enlarging the officers' quarters, without improving, however, the appearance of the camp. A small appropriation of money having been granted for further improvements, it is the understanding that most of the houses will be rebuilt.

The post is laid out in a peculiar and exceptional manner. The center of the area is occupied by the men's quarters, three parallel rows of squad-rooms running north and south. Two of these rows, for the cavalry companies, consist each of eight buildings; a space of twelve feet separates the houses from one another, and a company parade-ground, two hundred feet wide, extends between the two rows. The infantry row contains only five buildings, and stands three hundred feet west from the cavalry. Each building is constructed of rough-hewn logs, chinked with mud and roofed with boards, and measures 20 by 18 feet, outside-measurement, with a height of 9 feet to the eaves. There are neither floors nor ceilings. One door in front and a small window in the rear admit light and air, and a large fire-place serves to warm the house in winter. The furniture consists of a number of old-fashioned two-story bunks and a few benches and tables, all manufactured by the men out of rough lumber. If all the enlisted men at the post (more than two hundred) were lodged in these twenty-one rooms, five of them being already reserved as company storehouses and first-sergeants' rooms, the overcrowding that would necessarily result could not fail to be highly injurious to the health of the inmates; but this evil is prevented by at least one-half of the command being constantly on detached service or scouting duty, away from the post, so that the occupancy of any building at no time exceeds seven or eight men; furthermore, the chinks and cracks in the walls are sufficiently numerous to admit all the air necessary for respiration and for carrying off the exhalations from pulmonary and cutaneous surfaces. In summer most of the men prefer to sleep in the open air, so as to avoid the persecutions of the numberless bed-bugs which infest the quarters. One company of infantry occupies a large stockade building, 100 by 24 feet, shingle-roofed, situated at the southern side of the garrison, and formerly used as a quartermaster's storehouse. At right angles to the three rows of squad-rooms, and on the south side, are three buildings, containing the company kitchens and mess-rooms. Each building is 65 by 20 feet, with a height of 9 feet to the eaves, is built of logs, except the company mess-room, which is frame, and has a shingle roof and board floor. The kitchen, at one end, is 20 feet square, and the mess-room measures 45 feet in length.

Back of the company mess-houses, near the ravine which constitutes the southern boundary of the plateau, is a line of nine small houses, built of slabs and rough boards. They are occupied by laundresses, and do not conform to any special plan. The ravine itself conveniently conceals the men's sinks, which occupy the lowest part of the gully, and consist of deep trenches, surrounded by stockades and covered with brush.

On the west side of the post, just beyond the mess-houses and on the same line, is a new bakery, erected in 1873. It is a neat, cottage-like frame house, consisting of a main building, 32 by 16 feet, divided equally in two rooms, and a small wing, 12 by 14 feet, occupied as quarters by the baker. The oven is built of adobes, and is sufficiently capacious to bake four hundred rations. The house is floored, shingle-roofed, and ornamented with a porch.

Stretching from east to west, on the north side of the parade, is a row of eight sets of officers' quarters, so far apart from each other that a distance of fully one-quarter of a mile separates the end houses. Each set consisted originally of one room, 18 by 20 feet, on the same general plan and of the same material as the men's squad-rooms, but with a shingle roof, and of a kitchen of the same size, forty feet in rear of the main building. Six sets have since been enlarged by the addition of a new room, also 18 by 20 feet, separated from the old one by a hallway, 10 feet wide. All these quarters are roughly floored, and the walls are lined internally with old canvas and shelter-tents; they are hot in summer and cold in winter, leak badly in rainy weather, are poorly lighted, more than sufficiently ventilated, and altogether afford a miserable kind of shelter. As a general thing they are supplied with badly-constructed fire-places, which render them almost uninhabitable. Many of the rooms occupied by the officers remind the writer of the old-fashioned log cabins used by the negroes in the South and West, only requiring the horizontal iron bar and pot-hooks in the fire-place to make the resemblance complete. A one-and-a-half-story frame house was constructed during the summer and fall of 1874, for the commanding officer. This house contains, on the first floor, a hall running from front to rear, on either side of which are two rooms, each about 18 by 20 feet, lined with planed boards. There is a like arrangement of rooms on the second floor; they are, however, encroached upon by the roof. A small kitchen adjoins the main building in the rear.

On the east side of the post is a row of five buildings, disposed in the following order from north to south, viz: Adjutant's office, commissary storehouse, quartermaster's storehouse, guard-house, and infantry barrack, (old quartermaster's storehouse,) parallel with the rows of men's squad-rooms.

The adjutant's office is a log building, 18 by 20 feet, with a board floor and shingled roof.

The commissary storehouse was built in 1874, is 130 by 23 feet, 12 feet high to the eaves, and 20 feet to the ridge, and is a good, substantial building, having a deep cellar, with good solid stone foundation. An office and room for canned goods is partitioned off from the main room, at the east end. The inside is plastered throughout, and furnished with ventilators, consisting of round holes in the walls just below the eaves.

The quartermaster's storehouse is a stockade-building, 100 by 24 feet, is weather-boarded, and has a shingled roof.

The guard-house is built of rough logs, is 28 by 18 feet, and 9 feet high. It is divided into two apartments of equal size, the guard-room and the prison, the first of which has a fire-place, a window, and bunks for the guard. A small stockade addition, 12 by 18 feet, on the northern end of the building is divided into cells for special prisoners. The prison-rooms are without windows, and their only means of ventilation are the numerous cracks in the walls and roof.

Some two hundred and fifty yards from the row of infantry squad-rooms, on an isolated spur which constitutes the extreme western limit of the plateau, stands the post hospital. The construction of this building dates only from the spring of 1872. The sick men of the post were kept in tents, in this by no means mild climate, until every one else was housed, and, in spite of the strong and repeated demands and protests of the medical officers then on duty, a peremptory order from department headquarters became necessary, in order to compel the post commander finally to comply with requests which the dictates of humanity alone ought to have transformed into law. In April, 1872, nearly two years after the first occupation of this locality by troops, the sick were transferred from their canvas wards to the present building.

The main portion of the hospital consists of a building 40 feet long and 20 wide, 10 feet high to the eaves and 17 feet to the ridge. It is made of rough-hewn logs, plastered with mud, shingle-roofed, and floored, but without ceiling. The ventilation is effected by an air-box 3 feet square, placed in the center of the ridge and provided with windows on two sides, which swing on pivots and can be easily opened and closed by means of a pulley and rope. The crevices between the logs are imperfectly chinked, and, as the building is unlined and unceiled, except by pieces of old canvas tacked to the logs, it is found almost impossible to keep it warm in cold weather. At times the roof leaks so badly that the beds have to be moved. A door opens at each end of the building, and the sides are pierced by six small windows, the sashes of which revolve on hinges. A thin defective partition made of roughly split clap-boards, which renders sounds and odors produced in one room common to both, divides the building into two rooms, one, the dispensary, being 10 feet by the width of the house, the other, the ward, occupying the balance of the building. A building standing fifty feet in rear of the above was erected in November, 1873. It is 28 by 14 feet, is constructed of slabs nailed to a framework, the joints broken by strips nailed on from the inside, rooted with boards, and divided by a board partition into two rooms, one 12 by 14 feet, used as steward's quarters; the other, 16 by 14 feet, is a store-room. A rough shed, constructed of slabs by the hospital attendants, adjoins this. It is 26 by 13½ feet, and is divided by a partition into a kitchen 16½ feet long and a dining-room 9½ feet long. A hospital tent standing in rear of the hospital is used alternately as a convalescent ward and a dead-house. A small root-house and a small frame privy, two hundred feet from the hospital, complete the hospital-buildings.

The location of the post-hospital is excellent and the drainage perfect. A few steps from the buildings the ground slopes abruptly down to the cañons and river-bottom, so that in wet weather water cannot remain in the neighborhood longer than a few minutes. The spot is adorned by a few pines and cedars which grow on the edge of the plateau, and from the door of the dispensary a fine view is obtained of the two forks of the White Mountain River, which effect their junction a few hundred yards below, after emerging from their respective cañons; this is probably the most picturesque piece of scenery about Camp Apache.

On a piece of rising ground, which forms the southeastern extremity of the post, are located

67 M P

the quartermaster's corral, cavalry stables, grain-house, and shops. The corral, a frame inclosure, 150 by 200 feet, contains sheds for the quartermaster's stock, a quartermaster's and commissary's offices, a saddler-shop, and a few other small apartments. The cavalry stables, also frame, are 200 by 30 feet, corral-shape, that is with sheds on each side and a space in the middle open to the air; they are two in number. The grain-house is built of frame very strongly put together, shingle-roofed, and measures 60 by 20 feet. The carpenter, wheelwright, blacksmith, and paint shops are still farther in the rear, and consist of slab buildings very roughly constructed.

The garrison is supplied with water from the East Fork, a short distance above the post This water is palatable and clear, except during the rainy season, when it carries with it much fine sediment. The stream, though small, never dries up, and the supply of water is always abundant. No chemical analysis of it has ever been made, but as the stream flows through strata of limestone and gypsum, it doubtless is impregnated with calcareous salts.

Camp Apache being situated in the center of the White Mountain Indian reservation, no white men are allowed to settle in the neighborhood, and the only inhabitants of the country are the Coyotero or Sierra Blanca Apaches, numbering 1,650 persons. This tribe is divided into about fifteen subtribes or bands. The reservation contains about eight thousand square miles of territory, situated in the northeastern part of Arizona. This tract contains a large part of the White Mountains, which render it extremely rugged and picturesque. These Indians, from their long residence here, have all the instincts and habits of a mountain people. They, in connection with the Loshe-Apaches and Co-ni-nas, are the hereditary enemies of the Indians to the east and north of this, chief among which are the Navajo, Moquis, and Pueblos. The valley of the Little Colorado, which is a boundary between their respective lands, is considered neutral ground. Here, should parties of the hostile tribes meet, no fight ensues.

These Indians have been more or less friendly to the whites for a number of years. They are encamped in the immediate vicinity, within hearing distance of the post, with an agency near by, where they report every ten days to draw rations of meat and flour. Many of them have become sufficiently civilized to appreciate the advantage of supporting themselves by agricultural labor, and have accordingly commenced to cultivate several pieces of ground, and to raise corn and barley.

The physique of these Indians, to a casual observer, does not appear at all to be a striking or unusual one, either as regards size or development, but on closer inspection it will be observed that they are compactly built, and are generally well muscled and sinewy. Their chests are generally deep and square, the sternum and clavicles standing forward prominently and well up, indicating great chest capacity. Their hands and feet, of both men and women, are remarkably small and delicately formed, the ankles and wrists remarkably so. The women are more heavily muscled than the men, owing to the constant drudgery they undergo. They carry readily two and three hundred pounds upon their backs. The physiognomy of these people in repose is very mild, and as pleasant as their coarse features will permit of, but during excitement it lights up, and every feature, particularly the eyes, betoken deviltry and blood-thirstiness. This ferocity of countenance has even been observed by the writer during the excitement attendant on witnessing a dance by a masked figure. Their morality as regards truth and honesty is found to be high. A liar is contemned and tabooed among them, debts are scrupulously paid, both among themselves and when dealing with the whites; still it must be said that many of them will steal when opportunity offers.

Camp Apache is two hundred and thirty miles distant from Tucson, the capital of the Territory, and about equally distant from Prescott, the military headquarters of the department. The roads to this place, except the one to New Mexico, are but little better than trails, which lead over mountains and valleys with little regard, it might almost be said, to the laws of gravitation. The Camp Grant road from here to the Gila River may be called simply terrific, oftentimes causing the traveler to look back with fear and trembling over the places that he has passed. For this reason pack-mules take the place generally of other means of transportation, especially in the case of small parties traveling to and fro. On account of the excessive isolation from other points of civilization, by long distances and almost impassable roads, officers and men suffer many discomforts and inconveniences, both physical and mental.

The mail arrives and departs once a week, but sometimes, on account of high water in the mountain-streams, there is no mail received for several weeks at a time. A letter from Washington is generally three or four weeks old when received here, it having generally to take the following circuitous route: From Washington, via San Francisco, to San Diego, Cal.; from there to Tucson, thence to Camp Bowie, the nearest post-office to this place; from Bowie it is sent by cavalry couriers to New Camp Grant, then to the San Carlos reservation, on the Gila River, and from there here. This could be greatly improved by having a mail-route from Fort Wingate, N. Mex., which is about one hundred and sixty miles from this place.

*Meteorological report, Camp Apache, Ariz., 1872–'74.*

| Month. | 1870–'71. Temperature. | | | Rain-fall in inches. | 1871–'72. Temperature. | | | Rain-fall in inches. | 1872–'73. Temperature. | | | Rain-fall in inches. | 1873–'74. Temperature. | | | Rain-fall in inches. |
|---|---|---|---|---|---|---|---|---|---|---|---|---|---|---|---|---|
| | Mean. | Max. | Min. | | Mean. | Max. | Min. | | Mean. | Max. | Min. | | Mean. | Max. | Min. | |
| July | | | | | | | | | 73.05 | 96 | 62 | ...... | 79.39 | 104 | 60 | ...... |
| August | | | | | | | | | 71.48 | 95 | 61 | ...... | 70.62 | 88 | 66 | ...... |
| September | | | | | | | | | 65.21 | 89 | 38 | ...... | 69.96 | 92 | 52 | ...... |
| October | | | | | | | | | 55.50 | 86 | 11 | ...... | 58.90 | 92 | 28 | ...... |
| November | | | | | 38.60 | 64 | 16 | ...... | 40.14 | 70 | 6 | ...... | 48.13 | 81 | 25 | ...... |
| December | | | | | 37.17 | 69 | 16 | ...... | 39.74 | 70 | 11 | ...... | 34.02 | 62 | 6 | ...... |
| January | | | | | 33.77 | 69 | 1 | ...... | 37.13 | 68 | 3 | ...... | 27.38 | 68 | 6 | ...... |
| February | | | | | 40.29 | 82 | 18 | ...... | 38.15 | 65 | 12 | ...... | 35.71 | 65 | 10 | ...... |
| March | | | | | 45.10 | 81 | 20 | ...... | 49.57 | 81 | 21 | ...... | 43.35 | 72 | 18 | ...... |
| April | | | | | 50.32 | 83 | 23 | ...... | 52.66 | 84 | 28 | ...... | 49.87 | 88 | 31 | ...... |
| May | | | | | 64.74 | 97 | 39 | ...... | 62.26 | 87 | 39 | ...... | 64.31 | 94 | 38 | ...... |
| June | | | | | 73.14 | 98 | 55 | ...... | 74.34 | 104 | 51 | ...... | 74.79 | 101 | 57 | ...... |
| For the year | | | | | | | | | 54.93 | 104 | 3 | ...... | 54.70 | 104 | 6 | ...... |

NOTE.—The above observations have been taken with the dry-bulb thermometer, there being no instruments except the dry and wet bulb thermometers at the post.

*Consolidated sick-report, Camp Apache, Ariz., 1870–'74.*

| Year | | 1870–'71. | | 1871–'72. | | 1872–'73. | | 1873–'74. | |
|---|---|---|---|---|---|---|---|---|---|
| Mean strength, { Officers | | 4 | | 6 | | 4 | | 5 | |
| { Enlisted men | | 168 | | 150 | | 126 | | 150 | |
| Diseases. | | Cases. | Deaths. | Cases. | Deaths. | Cases. | Deaths. | Cases. | Deaths. |
| GENERAL DISEASES, A. | | | | | | | | | |
| Cerebro-spinal fever | | | | 1 | | | | | |
| Remittent fever | | | | | | 2 | | 1 | |
| Intermittent fever | | 446 | | 133 | | 68 | | 13 | |
| Other diseases of this group | | 5 | | 9 | | 9 | | 1 | |
| GENERAL DISEASES, B. | | | | | | | | | |
| Rheumatism | | 23 | 1 | 29 | | 22 | | 12 | |
| Syphilis | | 3 | | 4 | | 5 | | 4 | |
| Consumption | | | | | | 1 | | | |
| Other diseases of this group | | 1 | | 3 | | | | | |
| LOCAL DISEASES. | | | | | | | | | |
| Catarrh and bronchitis | | 17 | | 59 | | 75 | | 3 | |
| Pneumonia | | 1 | | 1 | | | | 1 | 1 |
| Pleurisy | | 6 | | 5 | | 1 | | | |
| Diarrhœa and dysentery | | 87 | | 157 | 1 | 61 | 1 | 34 | |
| Hernia | | 3 | | 1 | | | | | |
| Gonorrhœa | | 2 | | 9 | | 4 | | 4 | |
| Other local diseases | | 63 | | 235 | 1 | 83 | 2 | 61 | |
| Alcoholism | | | | | | 1 | | 2 | |
| Total disease | | 657 | 1 | 646 | 2 | 332 | 3 | 136 | 1 |
| VIOLENT DISEASES AND DEATHS. | | | | | | | | | |
| Gunshot wounds | | 1 | | 3 | | 1 | | 1 | |
| Arrow-wounds | | | 1 | | | | | | |
| Other accidents and injuries | | 23 | | 51 | | 73 | | 36 | 1 |
| Suicide | | | 1 | | 1 | | 1 | | |
| Total violence | | 24 | 2 | 54 | 1 | 74 | | 37 | 1 |

# FORT BOWIE, ARIZONA TERRITORY.

INFORMATION DERIVED FROM REPORTS OF ASSISTANT SURGEON CHARLES SMART AND ACTING
ASSISTANT SURGEON S. A. FREEMAN, UNITED STATES ARMY, 1870.

Camp Bowie is situated in a pass in the Chiricahua Mountains, known as Apache Pass, through which the road from Tucson to Mesilla penetrates, about one hundred miles east of the former town. It is in latitude 32° 40′ north, longitude 32° 27′ west, and elevated about 4,826 feet above the sea. The post was established under the name of Fort Bowie, in August, 1862, by Company G, Fifth California Volunteer Infantry, as a protection to the road at this dangerous point, and as a guard to the important springs found here. It was placed on the summit of a hill overlooking the water-supply, having high mountains on the north and south, and the broken rocky country constituting the pass on the east and west, beyond which, in these directions, the view becomes more open, and the scrub-oak growth of the highlands gives place to grass.

Up to 1868 the post was a most irregular one, the houses, or rather huts, being built on and under the ridges of land on the hill summit and slope; but at that time a new post was commenced on an adjoining hill which afforded a better site.

The reservation includes about one square mile, and is in every part well drained by the irregularity of the surface.

Large game, as turkeys, deer, and bears are found in the mountains. All the buildings at the post are constructed of adobes, with dirt roofs, and many of them with dirt floors. They are arranged on the sides of a rectangular parade in the following order: On the south side are three sets of officers' quarters; on the east side, going north, are a set of officers' quarters, adjoining which, on the north, is the adjutant's office; then a building containing the post library and school-room, the post bakery, a set of company quarters; on the north side, going west, are a set of company quarters, (unoccupied,) and two large storehouses; on the west side, adjoining the last storehouse at the rear of the west end, and forming with it an L, which incloses the northwest corner of the parade, is the post hospital. At a short distance in rear of the south end of the hospital is the guard-house.

The company quarters on the east side of the parade comprise a building, 156 by 30 feet, 12 feet in height, divided as follows: A portion of the south end is partitioned into two rooms, a tailor-shop in front and a barber-shop in rear, joined on the north by two squad-rooms, each 50 feet long, then a store-room, and at the north end an orderly's room. In the rear of this building, at a short distance, is a smaller building, 56 by 20 feet, containing a mess-room, 40 feet long, and a kitchen. South of, and on a line with, this is a building 25 by 12 feet, 10 feet high, containing a bath-room and lavatory.

The company quarters on the north side of parade consist of a barrack building, 80 by 24 feet, 12 feet high, divided into two equal-sized squad-rooms; adjoining the rear of this, at the east end, is a wing 66 by 16 feet, containing a mess-room and kitchen. Adjoining the main building on the west end is another wing, containing an orderly's room in front and a store-room in the rear. There is, in rear of this set, a building containing a bath-room and lavatory, similar to the one connected with the east set of quarters. Each set of company quarters is supplied with a sink built of adobes. The buildings are well lighted and ventilated, and are warmed by stoves and fireplaces. The dormitories are furnished with iron single bedsteads.

Married soldiers' quarters are at the old post; they are comfortable and sufficient.

The officers' quarters consist essentially of a main part, containing two rooms, 15 by 15 feet, 12 feet in height, separated by a hall, with a wing in the rear, containing a dining-room and kitchen to each set. They were refloored and reroofed in 1874. The set for the commanding officer was built in that year. They are now much more comfortable than the average of officers' quarters in Arizona.

The guard-house is 36 by 16 feet, divided into two rooms, one for a guard-room, the other for a prison, is warmed by fire-places, and is well lighted and ventilated.

The building for the library and school was built in 1874, is 35 by 18 feet, 14 feet in height, and is divided into two equal-sized rooms, separated by a hall 5 feet wide.

The hospital building was erected in 1865. It was originally built for and used as quartermaster's store-rooms, was afterward occupied as barracks for an infantry company, and finally as a hospital. Although the building is in tolerable repair it is poorly adapted for hospital purposes. Beginning at the north end, the building is divided into a store-room, 12 by 18 feet; a ward, 48 by 18 feet; a dispensary, 12 by 18 feet, used also as quarters by the hospital steward; and a kitchen, 12 by 18 feet. All the rooms are 10 feet in height, and all, except the ward, have dirt floors. The ward is floored with boards, is provided with two doors and four windows, (which are the only means of ventilation,) is warmed by a stove, and has a capacity for nine beds, giving an air-space to each of 960 cubic feet.

The storehouses are ample, dry, and in good condition, the westerly one, used for commissary stores, being provided with a cellar, 50 by 20 feet, 12 feet deep, with a hard cement floor, well ventilated, and used for storing perishable articles.

The shops, and stables and corral in rear of them, are at the north of the garrison, with the road from Tucson to La Mesilla between.

The post garden is about one-fourth of a mile distant. It produces a small supply of vegetables. Vegetables are also purchased from ranch-men living on the Gila and San Pedro Rivers.

Communication from San Francisco is by way of San Diego, Fort Yuma, and Tucson. Mails arrive from the east on Tuesdays, Thursdays, and Saturdays, and from the west on Mondays, Wednesdays, and Fridays.

The inhabitants in the vicinity are mostly Apache Indians, settled on their reservation since October, 1872. Their physical condition is good. Some Mexicans and a very few Americans are settled along the Gila and San Pedro Rivers.

*Meteorological report, Camp Bowie, Ariz., 1870–'74.*

| Month. | 1870–'71. | | | | 1871–'72. | | | | 1872–'73. | | | | 1873–'74. | | | |
|---|---|---|---|---|---|---|---|---|---|---|---|---|---|---|---|---|
| | Temperature. | | | Rain-fall in inches. | Temperature. | | | Rain-fall in inches. | Temperature. | | | Rain-fall in inches. | Temperature. | | | Rain-fall in inches. |
| | Mean. | Max. | Min. | | Mean. | Max. | Min. | | Mean. | Max. | Min. | | Mean. | Max. | Min. | |
| | ° | ° | ° | | ° | ° | ° | | ° | ° | ° | | ° | ° | ° | |
| July ............... | 76.85 | 91 | 68 | 4.50 | 80.62 | 96 | 68 | 7.90 | 77.58 | 96 | 62 | 1.67 | 85.10 | 103* | 71 | 0.50 |
| August ............ | 76.89 | 92 | 67 | 5.42 | 79.86 | 93 | 69 | 2.30 | 75.61 | 94 | 58 | 3.36 | 75.90 | 97* | 64 | 1.34 |
| September .......... | 75.36 | 93 | 56 | 1.00 | 75.02 | 93 | 56 | 1.00 | 72.27 | 92* | 60 | 0.77 | 78.81 | 99* | 67 | 0.01 |
| October ............ | 65.84 | 85 | 45 | 0.00 | 65.09 | 87 | 40 | 0.70 | 62.15 | 90* | 31 | 0.00 | 64.78 | 96* | 42 | 0.03 |
| November........... | 57.54 | 70 | 42 | 0.00 | 53.34 | 73 | 39 | (?) | 48.83 | 78* | 22 | 0.15 | 53.57 | 85* | 33 | 1.12 |
| December .......... | 44.49 | 68 | 30 | (?) | 49.86 | 70 | 25 | (?) | 48.88 | 80* | 30 | 2.95 | 43.43 | 70* | 20 | 2.02 |
| January ............ | 46.07 | 66 | 30 | (?) | 44.67 | 67 | 22 | (?) | 44.47 | 68* | 0 | 0.00 | 45.18 | 67* | 21 | 2.33 |
| February............ | 49.93 | 70 | 32 | (?) | 50.50 | 72 | 34 | (?) | 45.50 | 65* | 26 | 1.16 | 41.36 | 67* | 20 | 5.40 |
| March.............. | 56.16 | 75 | 35 | (?) | 56.21 | 77 | 35 | 0.00 | 56.71 | 87* | 32 | 2.22 | 47.99 | 79* | 32 | 1.50 |
| April............... | 61.13 | 85 | 34 | (?) | 56.50 | 87 | 34 | 0.25 | 61.53 | 85* | 32 | 0.00 | 54.51 | 82* | 32 | 0.35 |
| May ............... | 72.79 | 93 | 55 | 0.18 | 71.06 | 98 | 48 | 0.20 | 70.61 | 95* | 57 | 1.09 | 72.02 | 100* | 48 | 0.00 |
| June ............... | 82.77 | 98 | 66 | 0.60 | 78.84 | 100 | 60 | 1.04 | 81.91 | 105* | 64 | 0.14 | 83.89 | 100* | 67 | 0.00 |
| For the year....... | 63.82 | 98 | 30 | ........ | 63.46 | 100 | 22 | ........ | 62.17 | 105* | 0 | 13.51 | 62.21 | 103* | 20 | 14.60 |

* These observations are made with self-registering thermometers. The mean is from the standard thermometer.

*Consolidated sick-report, Camp Bowie, Ariz., 1870–'74.*

| Year | 1870–'71 | | 1871–'72 | | 1872–'73 | | 1873–'74 | |
|---|---|---|---|---|---|---|---|---|
| Mean strength { Officers | 5 | | 4 | | 4 | | 3 | |
| { Enlisted men | 141 | | 100 | | 100 | | 119 | |
| **Diseases.** | Cases. | Deaths. | Cases. | Deaths. | Cases. | Deaths. | Cases. | Deaths. |
| GENERAL DISEASES, A. | | | | | | | | |
| Typho-malarial fever | | | | | 9 | 1 | | |
| Remittent fever | 2 | | | | | | | |
| Intermittent fever | 79 | | 43 | | 155 | | 34 | |
| Other diseases of this group | 3 | | 1 | | 5 | | 16 | |
| GENERAL DISEASES, B. | | | | | | | | |
| Rheumatism | 36 | | 12 | | 32 | | 56 | |
| Syphilis | 11 | | 6 | | 4 | | 3 | |
| Consumption | 2 | | | | | | | |
| Other diseases of this group | 1 | | | | 8 | | 7 | |
| LOCAL DISEASES. | | | | | | | | |
| Catarrh and bronchitis | 43 | | 20 | | 24 | | 35 | |
| Pneumonia | | | | | | 1 | | |
| Pleurisy | 4 | | | | | | | |
| Diarrhœa and dysentery | 80 | | 54 | 1 | 96 | 1 | 75 | |
| Hernia | | | 2 | | | | | |
| Gonorrhœa | 2 | | | | 2 | | | |
| Other local diseases | 148 | | 64 | | 137 | | 81 | |
| Alcoholism | 2 | | | | 8 | | 4 | |
| Total disease | 413 | | 202 | 1 | 480 | 3 | 311 | |
| VIOLENT DISEASES AND DEATHS. | | | | | | | | |
| Gunshot wounds | 5 | | 6 | | | | | |
| Other accidents and injuries | 30 | | 33 | | 44 | | 41 | |
| Total violence | 35 | | 39 | | 44 | | 41 | |

# CAMP GRANT, ARIZONA TERRITORY.

### REPORT OF ASSISTANT SURGEON GEORGE M'C. MILLER, UNITED STATES ARMY.

Camp Grant is in Pima County, in the southeastern part of Arizona, in latitude 32° 25′ north; longitude, 32° 23′ 10″ west; altitude, 3,985 feet above the sea.

Old Camp Grant, of which the present post is the successor, was located at the confluence of the Arivaipa and San Pedro Rivers, about sixty miles northwest of here. The locality of the old camp was so extremely malarious and unhealthy that it was found absolutely necessary to abandon the post, which was done, and the new post established in January, 1873.

The post is located about two miles from Mount Graham, at its southwestern base, upon a sort of mesa, which is about four miles wide, and has a decided slope toward an extensive plain in a southwesterly direction. The plain is about fifteen miles wide, and over a hundred miles long, with a general direction from northwest to southeast. Mount Graham is a part of the Sierra Bonita, the latter constituting a portion of the Pinaleno system of mountains, which form the northeastern boundary of the plain, while the Oak Grove Mountains lie to the south and west. The Chiricahua Mountains are visible to the southeast, and the Santa Catarina range at a great distance to the south and southwest; in fact, Camp Grant may be said to be located in a vast amphitheater, surrounded by mountains. There is a pass to the eastward, an outlook toward the south, and also toward the northwest along the direction of the plain. The highest point of Mount Graham is 10,375 feet above the level of the sea.

No metals have as yet been discovered near the post. Metallic copper has, however, been found at Mount Turnbull, sixty miles distant, northwest.

The most conspicuous and abundant tree in the vicinity is the mesquite. It grows near the base of the mountains, on the foot-hills, on the mountains themselves up to a certain altitude, and sparsely on the mesas. It furnishes an excellent fuel, and is so abundant—forming complete forests in some places—that the supply of wood for the post will probably prove practically inexhaustible.

Various species of pines and firs grow on the tops of the mountains, particularly the white and yellow pines and the white and yellow firs. The pines have furnished nearly all the lumber used in building the post. The quantity of these trees is unlimited. They grow to a considerable height, and their trunks are in some instances five feet in diameter. The juniper-tree grows likewise on the mountains. The berries of this tree are often used as food by the Indians. The cottonwood, two species of oak, one species of sycamore, and a narrow-leaved species of willow grow along the margins of the streams, though not very abundantly.

The principal grasses found in the neighborhood are the sacaton and three varieties of the grama. The grama is an excellent pasture for horses and cattle, and furnishes the hay used at the post. It is cut up by the roots with a hoe, and stacked at convenient points.

The country abounds in game; deer, antelope, wolf, wild turkey, duck, and quail are in easy reach from the camp. Many species of birds are found in the region, mostly migratory, and insects are numerous and of many kinds. The musquito is unknown at the post.

The climate of Southeastern Arizona is an eminently disagreeable one. The warm season is very protracted and the days very hot. The nights, however, are comparatively cool; otherwise the heat would be absolutely insupportable. The winters are mild, almost as much so as those of Florida; but violent winds, frequent at all seasons, are particularly prevalent during the cool portion of the year, and very heavy rains are also then frequent, especially during the months of January and February. There are, however, occasional periods of pleasant and even charming weather, especially during the autumnal months. The mildness of the winters is fortunate for the military, preventing much discomfort to imperfectly sheltered officers and men. The climate lacks equability at all seasons. The thermometer may indicate, in winter, a point below freezing at day-break, and the cold may be very uncomfortable, while at 2 o'clock p. m. of the same day a thin coat may prove unpleasantly warm to the wearer. Notwithstanding the mildness of the winters, the frequent and great variations of temperature will always render the climate an unsuitable one for phthisical invalids. Catarrhal affections, of every grade of severity, are exceedingly common.

The nearest town is Tucson, one hundred and sixteen miles distant, southwest. Camp Bowie, the nearest military post, is forty-nine miles distant, southeast. The distance from Prescott, on an air-line, is about two hundred miles, but as it is reached only by way of Tucson, the distance is practically more than three hundred and fifty miles. Passable roads connect Camp Grant with the places mentioned, as well as with the San Carlos Indian Agency, eighty miles distant, north.

Should a person desire to reach Camp Grant from the Atlantic States, his first step would be to proceed by rail to San Francisco. His next objective point will be the town of Yuma, on the Colorado River, opposite Fort Yuma. In order to reach this point the traveler may elect between the route by steamer via the Gulf of California and the Colorado River, occupying about twelve days from San Francisco, or he may go by steamer to San Diego, and thence take the stage to Yuma, traveling a distance of about two hundred miles over the barren mountains and deserts of Southern California. The trip over the latter route is made in six days. From Yuma to Tucson, a distance of two hundred and seventy-five miles, the journey is made by stage in three days and nights; and from Tucson to Camp Grant, by Government or private conveyance. Baggage is usually left at Yuma, in care of the depot-quartermaster, who sends it by train to Camp Grant. Trains leave Yuma with Government supplies several times in the course of each month, and occupy a month, and often more time, in making the trip. The journey is tedious, rough, and fatiguing, and the traveler will find himself, long before he reaches his destination, thoroughly shaken up, contused, and excoriated.

No post-office has yet been established at Camp Grant. The mail is conveyed by a mail-party of soldiers, three times a week, to Camp Bowie, which is situated on the regular mail-route from Tucson to Santa Fé and Pueblo, N. Mex., at the latter point reaching railroad communication. Letters reach Washington in about twenty-one days, and Prescott, the headquarters of the Department, in ten days.

The military reservation upon which the post is located is six miles square.

The parade-ground is 800 feet square. A roadway, 75 feet wide from the line of buildings, is fenced off on each side, leaving a central inclosure 650 feet square. The surface of the parade has a very decided slope toward the south.

The south line of the parade is occupied by four sets of company quarters. Each set comprises a barrack, containing a dormitory, company offices, and store-rooms, and a detached building for mess-room and kitchen. The barrack consists of a main portion, 120 by 20 feet, with a wing, 40 by 20 feet, in rear of each end. Three of the dormitories, occupied by cavalry companies, afford an average air-space of 500 cubic feet per man; the fourth, occupied by an infantry company, gives an average of 650 cubic feet per man. The dormitories are warmed by fire-places and stoves; the lighting and ventilation are fair, and they are furnished with iron bunks. On a line with the rear ends of the wings of each barrack, and directly back of its central part, is a building 40 by 20 feet, containing the mess-room, adjoining the rear of which is an addition, 20 feet square, for the kitchen.

In rear of each barrack, six hundred feet from the line of the parade, is a house facing south, containing two sets of laundresses' quarters, each set consisting of three rooms. Half way between each of these buildings and the kitchen of the company to which it belongs, is a double sink, covered by a frame building, one compartment of the building being used by the company, the other by the laundresses. All these quarters are built with adobe walls upon stone foundations, and all are shingle-roofed. The adobe walls are carried up as high as the eaves all around, the gables being covered with upright boards battened. The laundresses' quarters are not all finished yet, and at this time hospital and wall tents, and wooden frames covered with paulins, are in use. Some of these are quite comfortable, while others are much dilapidated and unfit for occupancy.

Officers' quarters are located on the north line of the parade. The commanding officer's house is in the center of the row, and is 50 by 90 feet. It is traversed by a hall from front to rear, and by one from side to side, cutting it into four portions, each containing two rooms. Ten feet in rear of this, but under the same roof, is another portion, containing a dining-room and kitchen. The whole structure is surrounded by a veranda. There are rooms in the attic for the use of servants, and for store-rooms. On each side of this building are two double houses, each containing two sets of quarters. Each house is 50 by 68 feet, divided by a partition running from front to rear. On each side of this partition is a hall running back two-thirds of the length of the building, and intersecting a transverse hall. The portion in front, cut off by these two halls, is divided into two rooms; the portion in rear of the transverse hall is in one room. There is the same arrangement of detached kitchen and dining-room as in the commanding officer's quarters, except that the kitchen adjoins the rear of the dining-room. There are also attic rooms for servants, &c. A veranda surrounds the whole building except the rear of the kitchens. These buildings are all constructed with stone walls, and are shingle-roofed. Only two of the above-described houses are entirely completed; the others are in various stages of progress.

At the center of the east side of the parade is the hospital. It consists essentially of two buildings, each 22 feet on the parade, and running back to the east 64 feet. These buildings are placed forty feet apart, and are connected by a central building, 40 by 22 feet, with a veranda on each side of it, front and rear. One of the side buildings is used as a ward, with a capacity for twelve beds, giving an air-space to each of 1,525 cubic feet. The other side building is in part used as an isolation ward, containing three beds, with an air-space of 3,000 cubic feet to each. A building, directly in rear of the hospital, is 20 feet wide, and runs east 35 feet, containing the mess-room, 20 feet square, in front, and the kitchen, 15 by 20 feet, in the rear. The dead-house and sink are in a building, 20 by 15 feet, situated two hundred and fifty feet east of the kitchen. This building is not yet completed. These buildings are all on stone foundations, adobe walls and shingle roofs. The hospital is well lighted and ventilated, and is well furnished with all necessary furniture and fixtures. There is an excellent office and dispensary in separate rooms. There is no bath-room nor laundry. A bath-house is to be erected as soon as possible, but the hospital washing is done by the matron at her quarters.

The adjutant's office, a building 20 by 45 feet, is north of, and on a line with, the hospital. It is built with adobe walls, on a stone foundation, and is shingle-roofed.

To the west of, and on a line with, the officers' quarters is the chapel and school-building.

The center of the west line is occupied by the storehouses. These are contained in a building 200 feet long by 25 feet wide, with a wing at the rear of each end, 25 by 50 feet. There is a shed in rear of the main building between the two wings, which is continued along the inner side of the wings, forming a porch 15 feet wide. This building is divided into two equal portions; one occupied by the commissary, the other by the quartermaster.

The guard-house is located twenty-five feet south of the storehouses. It is 55 feet long and 40 feet wide, 12 feet high to the eaves and 22 feet to the ridge; is built of stone up to the level of the eaves, the gables being closed with upright boards battened. The roof is shingled. The ventilation is at the ridge. There are two doors and three grated windows in front, two grated windows in the north wall; in the south and west walls three windows each, and a slat window in each gable. There is a fire-place and chimney at the western side of the building. The chimney is of stone up to the level of the eaves; above this it is of adobes. The building has no internal divisions or compartments. It is rather dark, but is well ventilated.

A building, located north of the storehouses, near the north end of the west line, is 45 by 22 feet, 11 feet high to the eaves and 17 feet to the ridge, and is used as offices. It is built of stone to the eaves, the gables are boarded and battened, and the roof shingled. There are one door and two windows in both the front and rear walls. It is not ceiled overhead, being open to the roof. It has an adobe fire-place and chimney at each end, is quite well lighted and ventilated, and is a very commodious building.

Eighty feet south of the guard-house, and receding sixty feet from the western side of the parade, is the bakery. It is 36 by 20 feet, 11 feet high to the eaves, and 17 feet to the gable. It is built of stone to the eaves, boarded and battened gables, and is shingle-roofed. It has a door and two windows in front and two windows in the rear. There is an adobe fire-place and chimney at the southern end. The oven, built of adobes, projects from the southern end, and is inclosed by a stone structure, 12 by 12 feet, 11 feet high. The oven is provided with an adobe chimney, and has a capacity sufficient to supply bread for four companies.

The corral is situated some distance south of the garrison.

The water-supply is nearly everything that could be desired, being derived from brooks which have their sources at high altitudes on the neighboring mountains, in numerous springs fed by rains and melting snows. There are three of these streams in the neighborhood of the post, which are conveniently available. One flows on the western side of the camp, and is immediately contiguous. This stream is the principal source of supply. It is dammed at a convenient point above, and from the reservoir thus formed the water is drawn and distributed by water-wagons. Iron pumps also are sunk in the stream at several points below the dam. Of the two other available streams, one is distant a mile to the west, the other a mile and a half to the east of the post. The water is very pure and palatable. The qualitative analysis made with various reagents furnishes negative results, showing the absence of mineral impurities, at least in any appreciable quantities. The test with the permanganate of potash, however, indicates the presence of organic matter, though in a very slight degree. The water is unobjectionable as a beverage, and satisfactory for all detergent purposes. Efforts are made to preserve it from contamination; nothing is allowed to be thrown into the streams above the points where the water is taken out.

These mountain-streams run out but a short distance in the valley where they sink, apparently lost, but re-appear many miles below. There is no visible water in the plain, but one would scarcely believe it, for, looking far in the distance appears a tranquil lake with vessels floating on its quiet bosom, a mere phantom, however, which vanishes as it is approached, the alluring mirage which has so frequently cheered the weary travelers of desert countries, and as often doomed them to disappointment and sorrow.

The means of subduing fire at the hospital are four large barrels in rear, and twenty-two leather fire-buckets distributed through the buildings, all kept constantly filled with water.

68 M P

*Meteorological report, Camp Grant, Ariz., 1870–'74.*

| Month. | 1870–'71. Temperature. Mean. | Max. | Min. | Rain-fall in inches. | 1871–'72. Temperature. Mean. | Max. | Min. | Rain-fall in inches. | 1872–'73. Temperature. Mean. | Max. | Min. | Rain-fall in inches. | 1873–'74. Temperature. Mean. | Max. | Min. | Rain-fall in inches. |
|---|---|---|---|---|---|---|---|---|---|---|---|---|---|---|---|---|
| | ° | ° | ° | | ° | ° | ° | | ° | ° | ° | | ° | ° | ° | |
| July | 87.60 | 108 | 70 | 2.32 | 87.05 | 116 | 72 | (?) | 86.13 | 104* | 72 | 4.10 | 87.96 | 109* | 58* | 1.70 |
| August | 84.58 | 102 | 70 | 2.98 | 90.14 | 106 | 73 | (?) | 84.31 | 102* | 72 | 4.20 | 78.39 | 102* | 55* | 5.20 |
| September | 79.12 | 99 | 56 | 0.09 | 86.93 | 106 | 65 | (?) | 78.38 | 95* | 61 | 1.10 | 75.52 | 99* | 53* | 2.50 |
| October | 68.80 | 98 | 46 | 0.00 | 72.56 | 99 | 36 | 0.10 | 70.33 | 95* | 36 | 0.30 | 63.76 | 100* | 35* | 0.46 |
| November | 57.29 | 84 | 30 | 0.10 | 58.01 | 86 | 29 | 2.00 | 54.90 | 78* | 26 | 0.00 | 51.30 | 81* | 31* | 3.38 |
| December | 42.69 | 75 | 22 | 1.90 | 51.21 | 73 | 30 | 1.50 | 52.66 | 74* | 32 | 1.18 | 47.41 | 82* | 21* | 1.75 |
| January | 45.88 | 74 | 20 | 0.06 | 47.57 | 74* | 29 | 1.50 | 49.73 | 69* | 21 | 0.00 | 47.20 | 85* | 20* | 1.58 |
| February | 48.59 | 79 | 26 | 1.20 | 55.91 | 82* | 36 | 0.30 | 51.94 | 72* | 36 | 0.10 | 43.61 | 80* | 16* | 2.87 |
| March | 57.83 | 83 | 30 | 0.40 | 61.03 | 85* | 36 | 0.00 | 62.26 | 89* | 44 | 1.00 | 52.49 | 86* | 28* | 2.45 |
| April | 63.32 | 98 | 39 | 3.11 | 66.05 | 95* | 46 | 0.70 | 61.92 | 97* | 24* | 0.00 | 58.55 | 93* | 30* | 0.58 |
| May | 76.75 | 104 | 55 | 0.20 | 78.72 | 108* | 57 | 0.40 | 70.42 | 94* | 35* | 0.50 | 71.84 | 101* | 30* | 0.07 |
| June | 86.91 | 110 | 65 | ?1.90 | 87.19 | 108* | 66 | 0.90 | 81.56 | 110* | 50* | 1.40 | 84.13 | 105* | 54* | 0.00 |
| For the year | 66.61 | 110 | 20 | 14.26 | 70.19 | 116 | 29 | ........ | 67.04 | 110* | 21 | 13.88 | 63.51 | 109* | 16* | 22.54 |

\* These observations are made with self-registering thermometers.  The mean is from the standard thermometer.

*Consolidated sick-report, Camp Grant, Ariz., 1870–'74.*

| Year | 1870–'71. | 1871–'72. | 1872–'73. | 1873–'74. |
|---|---|---|---|---|
| Mean strength { Officers | 4 | 5 | 6 | 4 |
| { Enlisted men | 135 | 124 | 198 | 135 |

| Diseases. | 1870–'71. Cases. | Deaths. | 1871–'72. Cases. | Deaths. | 1872–'73. Cases. | Deaths. | 1873–'74. Cases. | Deaths. |
|---|---|---|---|---|---|---|---|---|
| GENERAL DISEASES, A. | | | | | | | | |
| Typhoid fever | 2 | | | | | | | |
| Typho-malarial fever | | | 3 | | 26 | 1 | 6 | 2 |
| Remittent fever | 1 | | 3 | | 3 | | | |
| Intermittent fever | 446 | 1 | 155 | 1 | 380 | | 72 | |
| Other diseases of this group | 12 | | 5 | | 1 | 1 | 3 | |
| GENERAL DISEASES, B. | | | | | | | | |
| Rheumatism | 11 | | 10 | | 18 | | 8 | |
| Syphilis | 14 | | 4 | | 5 | | 12 | |
| Consumption | | | 2 | | 2 | | | |
| Other diseases of this group | 2 | | 12 | | 5 | 1 | 1 | |
| LOCAL DISEASES. | | | | | | | | |
| Catarrh and bronchitis | 46 | | 11 | | 5 | | 11 | |
| Pneumonia | 1 | | | | | | | |
| Pleurisy | 16 | 1 | 6 | | 6 | | | |
| Diarrhœa and dysentery | 65 | | 49 | | 93 | 3 | 41 | |
| Hernia | 3 | | | | | | | |
| Gonorrhœa | 10 | | 2 | | 2 | | 2 | |
| Other local diseases | 90 | | 68 | | 79 | 1 | 129 | |
| Alcoholism | | | 1 | | 2 | | 12 | |
| Total disease | 719 | 2 | 331 | 1 | 627 | 7 | 297 | 2 |
| VIOLENT DISEASES AND DEATHS. | | | | | | | | |
| Gunshot wounds | 2 | 1 | 3 | | | | 5 | |
| Drowning | | | | | | | | 1 |
| Other accidents and injuries | 72 | | 44 | | 44 | 1 | 67 | |
| Suicide | | | | | | 1 | | |
| Total violence | 74 | 1 | 47 | | 44 | 2 | 72 | 1 |

# CAMP LA PAZ, ARIZONA TERRITORY.

### REPORT OF ACTING ASSISTANT SURGEON L. N. CLARK, UNITED STATES ARMY.

Camp La Paz is situated on the left bank of the Colorado River in Yuma County, Arizona Territory; is in latitude 33° 38′ north, longitude 37° 30′ west, (approximate,) and was established April 20, 1874.

The garrison occupies the buildings of the town of La Paz, a deserted Mexican town, which was formerly the county-seat of Yuma County, and is seven miles above the town of Ehrenberg, one hundred and forty-seven miles above Fort Yuma, and one hundred and sixty-eight miles below Camp Mojave.

The buildings are adobe structures, with dirt roofs. They have received the repairs necessary to make them habitable. The dormitories of the enlisted men afford an average air-space of 1,578 cubic feet per man; they are ventilated by doors and windows, are warmed by stoves, and are furnished with iron bedsteads and the usual fixtures and furniture. The company kitchen is 12 by 18 feet, and has one door and one window. The mess-room is 15 by 57 feet, and has three doors and three windows.

Officers' quarters, as well as married soldiers' quarters, are in buildings similar to those occupied by the company.

The guard-house contains a guard-room, 18 feet square, and a cell 13 by 18 feet.

The hospital occupies the former court-house. It is an adobe building, in good preservation, and is now undergoing extensive repairs.

The fuel used at the post is mesquite and cottonwood, furnished by contract.

The water-supply is obtained from the river. The only means for subduing fires are buckets filled with water.

---

# CAMP LOWELL, ARIZONA TERRITORY.

REPORTS OF ASSISTANT SURGEONS HENRY LIPPINCOTT AND J. B. GIRARD, UNITED STATES ARMY.

Camp Lowell is situated on the Rillito, about eight miles south of the highest peak of the Santa Catarina Mountains, and seven miles east of Tucson, in Pima County, Arizona Territory. Latitude, 32° 12' north; longitude, 33° 49' west; altitude, about 2,530 feet above the sea.

The plain or mesa on which the post is located is bounded on the north by the Rillito River and Santa Catarina Mountains, on the east by a continuation of those mountains, on the south by the Santa Rita Mountains, and on the west by the Santa Cruz River and a low range of mountains which have not received a name. It is part of the vast extent of rolling ground which stretches from the Rio Grande westward beyond the Colorado into Southern California, interrupted at irregular intervals by abrupt and very rugged sierras, and by water-courses which, with few exceptions, are dry during the greater part of the year.

This portion of Arizona is somewhat similar in appearance and geological formation to that part of the Territory stretching northwest toward the Colorado. The mountains in this vicinity differ, however, from those in the belt of country just referred to, in that they are more regular, and have not that forbidding aspect which characterizes the bowlder-covered upheavals skirting the Maricopa desert.

Regular and symmetrical as the Santa Catarina and other mountain ranges which surround this plain appear in the distance to be, yet they are by no means without inequalities. In them are deep clefts, uninviting passes or gaps, and long, tortuous, and precipitous cañons, some of them only accessible to the Indian and the soldier who pursues him. These mountains belong to the latest Tertiary period. Limestone, sandstone, and silver-bearing quartz enter largely into their formation. The alluvial deposit at this camp is about two feet deep, resting on a layer of calcareous sedimentary deposit from two to four feet in thickness; underneath this is a layer of gravelly earth about fifteen feet thick, and below that a stratum of clay from one to two feet thick, when a bed of gravel of unknown thickness is reached, in which, at a depth of from five to ten feet, living water is obtained.

The Rillito River takes its rise by three distinct streams in the Santa Catarina Mountains. This river, or rivulet, and the branches which unite to form it, like the majority of the streams in the Territory, sink in many places, and running under ground for some distance, rise again. It is insignificant in size at this point, but its bed enlarges as it descends to join the Santa Cruz, nine miles north of Tucson. Its waters cease to run above ground about a mile below the camp, and do not rise again until they join the Santa Cruz. The Rillito also receives an underground tributary near the post, its waters coming from the cienaga or swamp in the southeastern portion of the mesa, and about twenty-three miles distant from this camp.

The cottonwood grows at intervals on the banks of the Rillito and Santa Cruz, and in some places attains considerable proportions. There are forests of excellent white pine, interspersed with a few pitch-pines, in the Santa Catarina and Santa Rita Mountains, but they are difficult of access. The white ash and white oak attain considerable size in the foot-hills in the western part of the reservation, and on the borders of the stream the alder and sycamore grow quite large. There are two varieties of the mesquite tree, a species of acacia. With few exceptions these trees are very small and stunted in the mesa, but in the valley of the Rillito, and in that part of the Santa Cruz Valley north of the San Xavier Mission and south of Tucson, they grow quite large; would make excellent lumber for some purposes, and are unsurpassed for fuel. From the larger tree a gum, closely resembling gum-arabic, exudes, which has been collected in large quantities for the market. These trees produce beans which are very nutritious, and enter largely into the diet of the Indians, and are also eaten by horses and cattle. The varieties are distinguished by the pods, the larger being from four to six inches in length; the smaller, known as the screw-bean, is two to four inches. The beans of each resemble the ordinary bean. They are gathered by the Indians in the fall, and when dried are converted into a kind of meal, which is made into porridge.

Wheat and barley are the principal cereals raised in this part of the Territory. There are several farms on the Santa Cruz near Tucson, which produce these grains in fair quantities; but the finest and best producing farms are on the river near the Sonora line. The San Pedro Valley also produces wheat and barley. Pease, beans, radishes, carrots, beets, turnips, okra, egg-plant, cucumbers, squashes, melons, &c., are successfully raised, and it is here "par excellence" that the tomato attains perfection. It is very doubtful if a finer quality of this vegetable can be produced in the United States than can be seen in the Camp Lowell post garden at the proper season. Irish potatoes fail here on account of too great richness of the soil, and cabbages cannot be raised successfully on account of insects. These vegetables grow well in the San Pedro and Sonsita Valleys, which lie on the other side of the Santa Catarina Mountains. Irrigation is universally practiced wherever farming or gardening is carried on; without it nothing desirable would grow.

Black and cinnamon bears, black and white tailed deer, antelopes, yellow foxes, raccoons, and cotton-tailed rabbits, are all found within thirty miles of the post. Among the birds in this neighborhood are the wild turkey, sand-hill crane, canvas-back, large gray, mallard, and teal ducks, curlew, common snipe, woodcock, mountain quail, wild pigeon, meadow-lark, and in winter the wild goose. Among the reptiles are several species of lizard, the most prominent of which is the "Gila monster;" the rattlesnake, black snake, water-snake, and water-moccasin are also numerous; the land-terrapin, bull-frog, horned frog, and a large species of toad are also seen; among the insects are the centipede, (some of which are of enormous size,) the tarantula, and the scorpion. These are to be found everywhere in Southern Arizona.

Tucson, the capital of the Territory, the nearest town, according to the last census, had a population of 3,200. Seven-eighths of the people are Mexican, and the Spanish language is more spoken than the English. It has been a town of some importance for a century. The Mexican government had a military post there before the country was ceded to the United States, and it is now the principal place for the exchange of commodities between Arizona and Sonora. In Tucson there are a number of heavy mercantile houses, a tin-shop, blacksmith and wagon shops, two flour-mills, and restaurants, but no hospitals. The stores are good, and almost anything essential to comfort, except furniture, can be procured, although at higher prices than in the East.

The Indians inhabiting this portion of Arizona are the Papagoes, a half-civilized tribe. They are peaceable and self-supporting. As late as 1871 the Apaches infested this part of the Territory, thus rendering communication with other parts almost impossible. Now, however, people can travel with safety in any part of Arizona.

The reservation extends five miles north, five miles south, eleven miles east, and four miles west from the center of the camp, embracing a sufficient area of territory for grazing purposes, as well as securing control of the water-course. This tract of land, like the mesa of which it forms a part, has a dry, sandy soil, and is studded with mesquite-trees, sage-brush, and several varieties of cacti. It also affords excellent grama and sacatone grasses, which are utilized for the cavalry horses and stock pertaining to the post.

A military post of the same name as this was established near Tucson during the war of the rebellion, and was garrisoned until March 19, 1873, when the troops were removed to this point, with a view to the establishment of a permanent station. This camp is important as a military station, because of its proximity to the Mexican border, the Sonora line being only about eighty miles distant.

The only buildings completed are two sets of officers' quarters, the guard-house, and the store-house. There are in process of construction two sets of infantry and one of cavalry quarters, one set of quarters for the band, and a hospital. All these buildings are constructed of adobes, with mud roofs. The barracks are not yet roofed, (December 31, 1874.)

The infantry barracks will be each 145 by 18 feet. The cavalry barrack will be 155 by 18 feet. The quarters for the band will be 95 by 18 feet.

The commanding officer's quarters consist of a main building, 46 by 46 feet, external measurement. Two halls, each 9 feet 8 inches wide, pass at right angles to each other through the center of the house, dividing it into four equal-sized rooms. The walls are 10 feet high, and the rooms are well ventilated at the eaves. In rear of this house is a detached building, $33\frac{1}{4}$ by $18\frac{1}{4}$ feet, with an addition $27\frac{1}{3}$ by $15\frac{1}{2}$ feet, external measurements. This building contains a dining-room, $21\frac{2}{3}$ feet long, a kitchen, two rooms for servants, and a pantry. There is a cellar under part of this building.

The other set of officers' quarters consists of a main building, containing two rooms, each 18 by 15 feet, one 15 by 15, one 15 by 13, and one 15 by 7 feet. A rear building with addition, contains a mess-room, 18 by 15, a kitchen, 15 by 15, a servants' room, 12 by 12, and a pantry, $5\frac{1}{2}$ by 12 feet.

The guard-house, probably one of the best in the Territory, is 52 feet square, external measurement, to which is attached a corral, or inclosed yard, 28 by 48 feet, interior measurement. This inclosure is for the use of the prisoners when not at labor. The building has two halls at right angles to each other, cutting it each way nearly through the center. It is divided into a general prisoners' room, (with stone walls,) $20\frac{1}{6}$ by $19\frac{3}{4}$ feet, a guard-room, $19\frac{3}{4}$ by $18\frac{1}{2}$, room for garrison prisoners, $18\frac{1}{2}$ by 11, room for officer of the guard, 16 by 11, room for sergeant of the guard, 8 by 11 feet, a wash-room and tool-room. All the rooms are 10 feet high, lighted by windows with iron gratings, and are excellently ventilated at the eaves. There are, in addition, four cells, each $7\frac{1}{6}$ by $4\frac{1}{4}$ feet, 10 feet in height, like the general prisoners' room, built of stone, all the rest of the building being constructed of adobes. Only the cells are used for prisoners, the balance of the building being used as adjutant's office, library, and quarters for the non-commissioned staff. Prisoners are kept in tents.

The hospital, under course of erection, when finished will be, it is believed, almost unexceptionable in all its appointments. An effort has been made to comply with the instructions in Circular No. 2, Surgeon-General's Office, July, 1871. The roof is made of mud, therefore ventilation will be at the eaves instead of at the ridge. A comparatively cool place can always be found in the building, in consequence of the arrangement of the halls. The ward will be heated in the winter by stoves, the rooms by fire-places. The ward is 50 by 24 feet, and, like all the rooms, is 15 feet in height, thus allowing 1,200 cubic feet of air-space to each bed, if the number is restricted to twelve, and 1,125 feet to each, if four additional ones are required. The rooms are to be 15 by 15 feet, and will be very convenient and ample. The building containing the kitchen and mess-room is separated by a distance of thirty feet from the main building. In this hot climate this separation is absolutely necessary, for if the kitchen and ward were under one roof, the flies in summer would be unendurable. The ward and rooms will be sufficiently lighted.

The storehouse for the quartermaster and commissary contains five rooms, each 18 by 18 feet, 12 feet in height.

The post bakery measures $31\frac{1}{6}$ by $15\frac{1}{4}$ feet, and has an addition for the ovens; this extension is $13\frac{1}{3}$ by $18\frac{1}{6}$ feet, external measurement. The building is divided into three rooms; one, the bake-room, is 12 by $15\frac{7}{12}$ feet; another is $11\frac{5}{12}$ by $4\frac{7}{12}$ feet; the third, $11\frac{5}{12}$ by $6\frac{7}{12}$ feet, is used as a sleeping-room by the baker. The walls of this house are 10 feet high; the ventilation is at the eaves. Capacity of the ovens, two hundred rations.

The garrison has been and still is quartered in tents. Before leaving the subject of quarters it is proper to add that the beds of the men are in wooden bunks, elevated about 18 inches above the floors of their tents.

There are no adequate facilities for bathing, but these are contemplated in the erection of the new quarters.

So far, it has not been decided to build a chapel or school-house at the post, but it is very desirable that the latter, especially, should be built.

The cemetery is located just without the limits of the town of Tucson. It has a wall around it, and a considerable amount of care has been taken in preserving it.

The locality of this camp is favorable, so far as the supply of vegetables is concerned. Situated as it is in the valley of the Rillito, the garrison has been and can be liberally supplied with these products, without an extraordinary amount of labor or a great expenditure of money.

The post garden, comprising about five acres of excellent land, is located northwest of the camp, and about six hundred yards distant from it. The garden is irrigated by means of an acequia, or ditch, which taps the river about a mile and a half above the post, and extends for some distance below it, furnishing water not only for the garden but for the "ranches" or farms below the camp.

The supply of water for the garrison is obtained from wells and the acequia. That obtained from the wells is somewhat hard; its solid contents being principally sulphate and carbonate of lime, some magnesia and iron being also found in it. In it, also, hydrochloric acid is detected by a solution of nitrate of silver. The water from the ditch is, in the winter season, much purer than the well-water. It is devoid of odor, contains less earthy matter, a precipitation does not result from the addition of nitrate of silver, and, although it doubtless contains much organic matter in the summer and fall months, still the permanganate detects very little in it in the winter.

There are several warm springs in that portion of the mesa stretching to the east, but their chemical constituents are unknown. Evidences of the presence of the salts of sodium, magnesium, and potassium, are seen in the soil to the southwest. It is said that some of the waters in the neighborhood of Tucson contain so much lime as to be the cause of a certain amount of renal calculi, and that it is a common thing for the people using said water to keep by them a weak solution of nitric acid, which they add to that used for drinking purposes. So far, in this camp, bad effects of any kind, from the use of the well or ditch water, have not been observed, or at least not directly traced.

Throughout the Territory it is customary to cool the drinking-water by means of porous ollas. These, when filled, are suspended in a current of air, and protected from the direct and indirect rays of the sun; evaporation takes place readily, and thus the temperature of the water is reduced.

The drainage of the post is natural; the ground being somewhat rolling, that portion of the water which is not absorbed by the soil passes off rapidly to the stream.

Mails are received from the East, via San Francisco, three times in each week; from Santa Fé and Prescott, twice a week, returning as often; time from this camp to San Francisco, ten days; to Saint Louis, via Santa Fé, about fifteen days. The stage carrying the mails to and from San Diego and Yuma, Prescott, and Tucson, also carries passengers.

The annual medical supplies are received from San Francisco; are brought thence by steamer to Yuma, from which point they are conveyed in citizen trains to this place; time occupied in coming here, from date of requisition, generally about four months. Medical supplies are also obtained from the sub-depot at Yuma, and were it not for the slow means of transportation for all kinds of stores passing through the Territory, that point would be invaluable in emergencies as a base of supplies to the distant posts.

Many valuable ledges of silver and copper ores have been discovered in this portion of Arizona; some of them, it is thought, were worked as long ago as the time when the San Xavier church was in course of erection, and it is supposed that the remnants of arastras, found in some of the mountains of Southern Arizona, belonged to a people who occupied this region long before the Jesuit fathers came here. The Cañon de Oro, in the Santa Catarina range, situated northwest from Tucson, is noted for its placer gold diggings, but the scarcity of water for sluicing purposes, together with the constant dread of the Apaches, caused an early abandonment of them.

*Meteorological report, Camp Lowell, Ariz., 1870–'74.*

| Month. | 1870–'71. Mean. | Max. | Min. | Rain-fall in inches. | 1871–'72. Mean. | Max. | Min. | Rain-fall in inches. | 1872–'73. Mean. | Max. | Min. | Rain-fall in inches. | 1873–'74. Mean. | Max. | Min. | Rain-fall in inches. |
|---|---|---|---|---|---|---|---|---|---|---|---|---|---|---|---|---|
| July | 83.74 | 101 | 72 | 2.82 | 87.48 | 114 | 70 | 1.02 | 86.00 | 114 | 59* | 3.94 | 90.89 | 113* | 39* | 0.08 |
| August | 83.06 | 98 | 73 | 2.04 | 86.63 | 112 | 71 | 3.70 | 85.36 | 107 | 63 | 3.81 | 81.89 | 104* | 46* | 2.73 |
| September | 77.72 | 94 | 66 | 0.00 | 85.12 | 112 | 62 | 2.00 | 79.87 | 106 | 48 | 3.06 | 80.14 | 103* | 32* | 0.62 |
| October | 69.90 | 93 | 40 | 0.00 | 72.37 | 102 | 35 | 0.00 | 73.52 | 104 | 23 | 0.40 | 70.78 | 101* | 21* | 0.00 |
| November | 59.56 | 79 | 42 | 0.00 | 58.05 | 90 | 28 | 0.29 | 55.46 | 84 | 17* | 0.00 | 59.94 | 91* | 30* | 1.32 |
| December | 45.89 | 74 | 28 | 0.94 | 55.26 | 87 | 30 | 0.35 | 54.92 | 85 | 24* | 1.39 | 48.92 | 78* | 25* | 0.97 |
| January | 51.83 | 80 | 18 | 0.52 | 49.31 | 80 | 13* | 0.54 | 51.80 | 80 | 19* | 0.00 | 53.08 | 78* | 19* | 1.76 |
| February | 51.11 | 86 | 29 | 0.64 | 55.63 | 94 | 27* | 0.12 | 53.00 | 82 | 30* | 0.69 | 47.99 | 75* | 21* | 1.66 |
| March | 57.95 | 94 | 29 | 0.06 | 61.71 | 98 | 23* | 0.00 | 65.14 | 96 | 27* | 1.01 | 54.15 | 79* | 30* | 1.19 |
| April | 62.34 | 108 | 35 | 0.04 | 64.02 | 107 | 24* | 0.05 | 68.13 | 106* | 37 | 0.00 | 60.50 | 97* | 34* | 0.43 |
| May | 78.34 | 113 | 52 | 0.00 | 78.63 | 116 | 39* | 0.01 | 77.06 | 110* | 48 | 0.00 | 74.58 | 103* | 42* | 0.07 |
| June | 89.33 | 116 | 65 | 0.40 | 88.19 | 115 | 52* | 0.26 | 87.69 | 118* | 39* | 0.00 | 84.77 | 108* | 44* | 0.00 |
| For the year | 67.56 | 116 | 18 | 7.46 | 70.20 | 116 | 13* | 8.26 | 69.83 | 118* | 17* | 14.30 | 67.30 | 113* | 19* | 10.83 |

* These observations are made with self-registering thermometers. The mean is from the standard thermometer.

*Consolidated sick-report, Camp Lowell, Ariz., 1870–'74.*

| Year | 1870–'71. Cases. | Deaths. | 1871–'72. Cases. | Deaths. | 1872–'73. Cases. | Deaths. | 1873–'74. Cases. | Deaths. |
|---|---|---|---|---|---|---|---|---|
| Mean strength { Officers | 5 | | 6 | | 5 | | 9 | |
| { Enlisted men | 72 | | 133 | | 127 | | 180 | |
| **GENERAL DISEASES, A.** | | | | | | | | |
| Typho-malarial fever | | | 1 | | 7 | | | |
| Remittent fever | | | 4 | | 3 | | 4 | 1 |
| Intermittent fever | 70 | | 91 | | 137 | | 63 | |
| Other diseases of this group | 6 | | 4 | | 2 | | 4 | |
| **GENERAL DISEASES, B.** | | | | | | | | |
| Rheumatism | 6 | | 7 | | 8 | | 4 | |
| Syphilis | 2 | | 7 | | 8 | | 17 | |
| Consumption | | | 1 | | 1 | | | 1 |
| Other diseases of this group | 2 | | 3 | 1 | 4 | | 1 | |
| **LOCAL DISEASES.** | | | | | | | | |
| Catarrh and bronchitis | 3 | | 2 | | 20 | 1 | 7 | |
| Pneumonia | 1 | | 2 | | 2 | 1 | 1 | |
| Pleurisy | 4 | 1 | 2 | | 2 | | | |
| Diarrhœa and dysentery | 20 | 2 | 28 | | 39 | 1 | 34 | |
| Hernia | 1 | | | | 1 | | 1 | |
| Gonorrhœa | 6 | | 6 | | 7 | | 18 | |
| Other local diseases | 22 | | 34 | | 62 | | 78 | |
| Alcoholism | 2 | | 1 | | 10 | | 13 | |
| Total disease | 145 | 3 | 193 | 1 | 313 | 3 | 245 | 2 |
| **VIOLENT DISEASES AND DEATHS.** | | | | | | | | |
| Gunshot wounds | 3 | | 2 | 1 | 1 | 1 | 1 | |
| Other accidents and injuries | 22 | | 26 | | 31 | 1 | 44 | |
| Suicide | | 1 | | | 1 | | | |
| Total violence | 25 | 1 | 28 | 3 | 32 | 3 | 45 | |

# CAMP McDOWELL, ARIZONA TERRITORY.

INFORMATION FURNISHED BY ASSISTANT SURGEONS CHARLES SMART AND C. DEWITT, AND ACTING
ASSISTANT SURGEON JAMES REAGLES, UNITED STATES ARMY.

This post is situated on the west bank of the Rio Verde, about eight miles above its junction with the Salt River, in latitude 33° 40′ north, and longitude 34° 37′ west, at an elevation of 1,800 feet above the sea-level. It is forty-five miles north of the Maricopa and Pimo villages, and the same distance southwest of Camp Reno. It is reached by steamer from San Francisco to San Diego, Cal., thence by mail stage via Yuma and to Maricopa Wells, from which place a weekly mail is carried north to the post. The Indians have seldom interfered with this mail-route, but the rising of the Colorado in Southern California frequently delays the transmission of the mails, and the floods of the Gila and Salt River have cut the post off from communication with the outside world for three and four weeks at a time. Letters usually reach San Francisco in fifteen days, and Washington, by the eastern route, in twenty-five days. This part of the Rio Verde basin is surrounded by mountains : the high line of the Mazatsal peaks on the east, twenty miles distant ; a lower range, to which no name has been applied, fifteen miles distant on the west ; the numerous low peaks from which the river issues on the north, and the grotesquely abrupt mountains of the Salt River country on the south. On both sides of the Verde, near the post, the mesa rises almost from the water's edge, becoming more and more broken by deep and narrow ravines, until it blends with the foot-hills of the mountain-ranges on the east and west. The river is thus well confined, and its bottom-lands free from marshes. The strip of easily irrigated bottom-land is very narrow, yet much good soil could be reclaimed by irrigation from large acequias. Cotton-wood, willow, and alder grow along its banks, tangled frequently by grape-vines, which yield a small acid fruit. Mesquite, ironwood, palo-verde, artemisia, and species of *opuntia* and *cereus* cover the mesa, in some parts even rendering it impassable ; the more open parts furnish indifferent grazing. Scrub and live oak and pine of large growth are found on the Mazatsal, but the building-timber is almost all in inaccessible situations. Quail and rabbits are abundant on the mesa, and deer are found in the mountains, but less frequently than in the more northern portion of the Territory. Coyotes, rattlesnakes, scorpions, lizards, centipedes, and tarantulas are to be met with here as in other parts. The soil is dry and porous, and well drained by its decided slope toward the ravines.

The post was established in 1865, by five companies of California volunteers, as a point from which to operate against, or treat with, the Indians of the neighboring mountains. The reservation taken up measured, from the center of the parade-ground, three miles north and south and two miles east and west. This included the greater part of the arable land in the immediate neighborhood. Building was immediately commenced and continued until early in 1866, when the essential part of the post was finished. One hundred and fifty acres of the bottom-land were then cleared for cultivation, water being brought to it by an acequia from a point four miles up the river.

The climate is warm and dry. Although the thermometer in the day-time in summer may show a high degree of heat, the nights are commonly not oppressive. Thunder-clouds from the mountains drop a heavy passing shower once or twice a month. In winter the rains are lighter, though of much longer duration. Snow falls on the mountains, but not on the mesa. The winds are variable and light, except when immediately preceding a thunder-storm.

The post as planned and built in 1865 consisted of a parade-ground, 525 by 435 feet, with its center one-third of a mile from the margin of the river, and 50 feet higher than its level. This height, attained by gradual rise of the ground, gives, with the aid of some shallow trenching, a very efficient surface-drainage. The buildings were arranged along the sides of the parade-ground as follows : On the west and farthest from the river the quarters of the commanding officer, a comparatively large square building, with a hall and two rooms on either side. On the south a line of quarters for officers ; four houses facing the parade, each divided into four rather small rooms.

A kitchen was afterward attached to the rear of each of these buildings. On the north, immediately opposite the officers' quarters, four sets of company barracks, with their gables toward the parade, each 187 by 24 feet, divided by transverse partitions into two dormitories and four smaller rooms, for use respectively as kitchen, mess-hall, office, and store-room for company property. The hospital was placed on the west, and the quartermaster's store, bakery, and sutler's store on the east of this column of barrack buildings, and separated from them by broad streets. On the east the guard-house, ordnance storehouse, and house for the preservation of fresh meat for issue. Outside of these lines of buildings were the corrals, of high, close-set upright posts, on the southeast, and the laundresses' quarters, of primitive-looking adobe huts, on the north. The sinks, still farther north, were deep trenches, inclosed by a thick wall of willow and cottonwood branches. At its establishment this post was intended to be the largest and most solidly built in the Territory. For ornaments and future shade a line of cottonwood saplings were planted at short intervals along the sides of the parade-ground, and were watered assiduously for two years, during which time they flourished and promised well, but after this they showed signs of decline, in spite of the attention paid to them, and so came to be neglected. All the buildings were of adobe, with earthen floors, mud roofs, and open fire-places. The roofs were flat, and had mud, sand, and lime cement laid over seguara ribs, which in turn were supported by cottonwood timbers. These timbers, or *vigas*, raised the roof from 8 to 10 inches above the wall, and so left ample space for ventilation. But, however carefully built by the California troops, the buildings proved unequal to the heavy washing showers of the summer, and the penetrating rains of the winter months. The roofs leaked almost from their first exposure, and the walls cracked and washed away in place after place, until, in spite of constant repairs, many of the houses became almost untenantable.

The present company quarters consist of two adobe buildings, each 150 by 20 feet, with a wing, 12 by 65 feet, extending across one end, and reaching, 45 feet, to the rear of the building, and another, 12 by 45 feet, extending from the rear of the other end of the building. These buildings are used as dormitories, company offices, store-rooms, shops, &c. The dormitories are each lighted by twenty windows, warmed by stoves and fire-places, are well ventilated, and afford an air-space of 900 cubic feet per man of average occupancy. They are furnished with iron bunks and the usual fixtures, and are very comfortable. In rear of each barrack is an adobe building, 15 by 50 feet, for a mess-room, having an addition adjoining the rear, 15 by 21 feet, for a kitchen. The walls of all these buildings are 12 feet high, and the roofs are shingled. One set of these quarters is located near the east end of the south line of the post; the other set is at the southeast angle, and extends along the east line.

Married soldiers' quarters are adobe huts, covered and surrounded with brush. They are located some distance to the east of the men's quarters. They are the miserable tumble-down hovels that were constructed when the post was first established, and are unfit to live in.

Officers' quarters comprise ten sets: the commanding officer's house on the west of the parade, mentioned above, and nine sets on the south line, built in 1872 and 1873. They are adobe structures, with shingle roofs, are plastered and in good condition.

A building originally erected for and occupied as headquarters District of Arizona, situated half-way between the post and the river, and nearly on a line with the north side of the parade, is used as officers' quarters. It is built after the plan of the commanding officer's quarters.

The guard-house consists of a guard-room and a prison-room; the former, 16 by 28 feet; the latter, 30 by 28 feet. It is well ventilated, is warmed by fire-places, but the dirt roof is in a leaky condition, making it very uncomfortable.

The storehouses are three good adobe buildings erected in 1872.

A new bakery was erected in 1872. It is an adobe structure with shingle roof, and contains two brick ovens in good order.

The hospital, recently completed, is shingle-roofed, surrounded by a veranda, and is well adapted to its purpose. The principal ward is 33 by 12 feet, 12 feet in height. It contains eight beds, affording an air-space of 594 cubic feet to each. The office and dispensary are in one room. The kitchen and mess-room are convenient. The rear veranda is used as a lavatory; there is a small store-room, and an attic, which is used for storing surplus articles.

The post garden furnishes a liberal supply of fresh vegetables.

69 M P

The water-supply has been wagoned in barrels from the Rio Verde since the post was estab-lished. It is of excellent quality. An attempt was made to sink a well on the parade-ground, but no water was struck. Cases of malarial disease did not occur among the troops until scouting was commenced, and the command exposed in malarious districts.

Although the Rio Verde contains an abundance of fish, they are soft and flavorless.

The cemetery is distant about a quarter of a mile northwest from the buildings. It measures 75 by 60 feet, is surrounded by a temporary fence, and contains the graves of twenty-six soldiers and seven citizens.

The means of subduing fire are buckets and barrels, kept constantly filled.

*Meteorological report, Camp McDowell, Ariz., 1870–'74.*

| Month. | 1870–'71. Temperature. Mean. | Max. | Min. | Rain-fall in inches. | 1871–'72. Temperature. Mean. | Max. | Min. | Rain-fall in inches. | 1872–'73. Temperature. Mean. | Max. | Min. | Rain-fall in inches. | 1873–'74. Temperature. Mean. | Max. | Min. | Rain-fall in inches. |
|---|---|---|---|---|---|---|---|---|---|---|---|---|---|---|---|---|
| July | 90.21 | 109 | 74 | 0.90 | 93.12 | 108 | 74 | 0.16 | 86.38 | 107* | 62* | 9.16 | 84.98 | 113* | 72* | 0.00 |
| August | 89.49 | 104 | 71 | 1.98 | 91.41 | 107 | 76 | 2.03 | 83.49 | 101* | 66* | 7.17 | 88.31 | 108* | 65* | 0.56 |
| September | 83.35 | 104 | 65 | 0.22 | 85.76 | 104 | 72 | 0.20 | 77.60 | 96* | 51* | 0.08 | 84.96 | 110* | 54* | 0.00 |
| October | 73.02 | 101 | 53 | 0.40 | 73.44 | 101 | 55 | 0.00 | 69.17 | 98* | 20* | 0.00 | 71.48 | 108* | 33* | 0.00 |
| November | 62.01 | 85 | 44 | 0.00 | 58.79 | 86 | 37 | 1.24 | 53.72 | 85* | 17* | 0.00 | 64.80 | 99 | 33* | 0.21 |
| December | 47.54 | 74 | 25 | 0.00 | 52.17 | 75 | 32 | 0.20 | 53.02 | 89* | 21* | 1.56 | 52.36 | 83 | 27* | 4.70 |
| January | 51.22 | 75 | 30 | 0.25 | 46.00 | 90* | 24* | 0.50 | 50.57 | 83* | 16* | 0.00 | 55.93 | 83 | 24* | 3.10 |
| February | 52.74 | 71 | 34 | 0.40 | 53.22 | 82* | 31* | 0.40 | 50.10 | 80* | 20* | 1.60 | 51.62 | 78 | 18* | 2.86 |
| March | 59.38 | 79 | 40 | 0.00 | 60.57 | 83* | 32* | 0.00 | 61.72 | 95* | 30* | 0.90 | 57.55 | 79 | 31* | 1.06 |
| April | 67.76 | 92 | 48 | 0.40 | 64.97 | 94* | 32* | 0.53 | 64.06 | 100 | 29* | 0.00 | 63.22 | 97 | 43* | 1.30 |
| May | 83.22 | 102 | 70 | 0.00 | 77.31 | 105* | 49* | 0.30 | 76.44 | 101 | 45* | 0.16 | 78.39 | 105 | 43* | 0.30 |
| June | 91.46 | 107 | 69 | 0.00 | 87.24 | 107* | 56* | 0.31 | 88.69 | 113* | 49* | 0.00 | 89.71 | 114 | 54* | 0.00 |
| For the year | 70.95 | 109 | 25 | 4.54 | 70.33 | 108 | 24* | 5.88 | 67.91 | 113* | 16* | 20.63 | 71.11 | 114 | 18* | 14.09 |

* These observations are made with self-registering thermometers. The mean is from the standard thermometer.

*Consolidated sick-report, Camp McDowell, Ariz., 1870–'74.*

| | 1870–'71. | | 1871–'72. | | 1872–'73. | | 1873–'74. | |
|---|---|---|---|---|---|---|---|---|
| Year | | | | | | | | |
| Mean strength { Officers | 5 | | 10 | | 6 | | 3 | |
| { Enlisted men | 147 | | 221 | | 219 | | 111 | |
| Diseases. | Cases. | Deaths. | Cases. | Deaths. | Cases. | Deaths. | Cases. | Deaths. |
| **GENERAL DISEASES, A.** | | | | | | | | |
| Typhoid fever | 1 | | 2 | | | | | |
| Typho-malarial fever | | | | | 1 | | | |
| Remittent fever | 7 | | 2 | | | | | |
| Intermittent fever | 93 | | 36 | | 68 | | 7 | |
| Other diseases of this group | | | 11 | | 2 | | | |
| **GENERAL DISEASES, B.** | | | | | | | | |
| Rheumatism | 17 | | 11 | | 13 | | 5 | |
| Syphilis | 5 | | 12 | | 12 | | 6 | |
| Consumption | | | 1 | 1 | 1 | 1 | | |
| Other diseases of this group | | | | | 1 | | | |
| **LOCAL DISEASES.** | | | | | | | | |
| Catarrh and bronchitis | 35 | | 29 | | 11 | | 5 | |
| Pneumonia | | | 1 | 1 | | | | |
| Pleurisy | 1 | | 3 | | | | | |
| Diarrhœa and dysentery | 69 | 1 | 101 | 2 | 34 | | 5 | |
| Hernia | 1 | | 1 | | | | | |
| Gonorrhœa | 3 | | 2 | | 1 | | 4 | |
| Other local diseases | 88 | | 96 | 3 | 97 | 1 | 42 | |
| Alcoholism | | | 1 | | 11 | | 2 | |
| Total disease | 320 | 1 | 309 | 7 | 252 | 2 | 76 | |
| **VIOLENT DISEASES AND DEATHS.** | | | | | | | | |
| Gunshot wounds | 3 | | 2 | | 1 | | | |
| Arrow wounds | 1 | | | | | | | |
| Other accidents and injuries | 78 | | 77 | | 53 | | 33 | 1 |
| Homicide | | | | | | 1 | | |
| Total violence | 82 | | 79 | | 54 | 1 | 33 | 1 |

## CAMP MOJAVE, ARIZONA TERRITORY.

REPORT OF ACTING ASSISTANT SURGEONS F. S. STIRLING AND JAMES B. LAURENCE, UNITED STATES ARMY.

This camp is situated on a gravel bluff on the east bank of the Colorado River, near the head of Mojave Valley; latitude, 35° 6′ north; longitude, 37° 28′ west; altitude, 600 feet above sea-level, and 75 feet above the river. It was established in 1858 for the protection of emigration over the Southern Overland Route to California, the Mojave and other Indian tribes being then hostile, and having in the summer of 1857 committed depredations on parties of emigrants. The Indians remained hostile until severely defeated by the troops under Major Armistead, who encountered them in the valley below the fort and drove them back with great loss. They then sued for peace.

The Indians now occupying this region of country number about two thousand five hundred souls; they have never lived on a reservation, are peaceful, and, strange to say, industrious, cultivating the low lands bordering the river. Pumpkins, watermelons, corn, and wheat are the chief products of the Indian gardens.

The post was abandoned in May, 1861, and re-garrisoned in May, 1863, by two companies of the Fourth Regiment California Volunteer Infantry.

The plateau extends north and south about forty miles, with an average width of ten or twelve miles. There are two reservations, each three miles square. The camp is built on the upper one. The lower reservation is on the low bottom-land, about six miles south of the post. Part of it is subject to overflow; the soil is fertile, and is covered with coarse grass, cottonwood and mesquite trees, with a dense undergrowth of willows and arrow-weed. With this exception the country is a waste. The elevated plains are covered sparsely with a growth of greasewood bush, interspersed with varieties of the cactus family.

Rabbits and quails are found in large numbers; ducks and geese abound in the sloughs, and the river affords an abundance of fish of the salmon species. Deer, mountain-sheep, and antelope are found in the hills. The mountains, on either side of the river, are barren and destitute of timber. But few springs of water are found in the adjacent mountains, and the country may be described as a sterile plain, broken by arroyos or dry gulches.

The climate is healthy, the winters pleasant, but the summers extremely hot. There is no rainy season, though thunder-showers are frequent in July and August. The annual rise of the Colorado takes place in June. The prevailing winds in the summer are from the south, and passing over the arid plains, the air is so heated that it scorches like that from an oven. The nights are as hot as the days, the temperature not varying in the slightest degree for hours—so hot that no one can sleep in a house, the whole garrison lying on the open plain, endeavoring to catch the faintest breeze, the walls of the houses becoming so heated as to render the barracks unendurable.

The post buildings consist of one-story adobe structures, arranged on the sides of a rectangular parade situated on a level plain.

The barracks consist of two buildings located on the north side of the parade, one having a shingle roof, the other a dirt one, both having dirt floors. Each building is 90 by 35 by 16 feet, is well ventilated by openings under the eaves, and by windows and doors. The building with shingle roof is occupied as a dormitory. It is warmed by two open fire-places and two stoves, affords about nine hundred cubic feet of air-space per man, for average occupancy, and is very comfortable. It is furnished with iron single bedsteads.

Kitchen and mess-room are in a building situated a few feet from the barrack. This buildin is 80 by 35 feet, and was originally intended for two companies. It was floored in 1874. The barrack-office and store-room are in the western end of the barrack. They were floored in 1874, and are commodious and comfortable.    A small root-house, in rear of the mess-rooms, answers its purpose admirably.

Married soldiers' quarters are comfortable adobe buildings, situated from two to four hundred yards north of the parade.   These buildings were erected and formerly occupied by citizens, and formed part of the town of Mojave City.

Officers' quarters, situated on the south side of the parade, comprise two adobe buildings, well finished, roomy, and comfortable.   One of these, occupied by the commanding officer, was built in 1873, is 51 by 15 feet, divided into three rooms; the other is an adobe set, divided by an adobe partition, having three rooms on each side.   Each room in these buildings is 14 feet in height, is ceiled and floored, has two doors and four windows, and is provided with an open fire-place.   A comfortable stockade building, containing four rooms, each 16 by 12 feet, floored, ceiled with canvas, and dirt-roofed, is also used by officers as quarters.

The guard-house is on the east side of the parade, is 20 by 35 feet, 12-foot walls, containing a guard-room, 20 by 20 feet, and two cells, each 10 by 15 feet.   It is well ventilated by openings at the eaves, by windows, and an open fire-place.

The post bakery, on the north side of the parade, is in very good repair, and has a capacity of one hundred and twenty rations.

Storehouses are two fine and abundantly capacious buildings, shingle-roofed, well ventilated, and in good repair, situated, one on the east, the other on the north side of parade.   The one on the east side was erected in 1873, and is 85 by 35 feet.

The hospital was completed in 1873, is in excellent condition, and well adapted for its purpose. It is located about two hundred yards north of the barracks, and faces south.   It is built of adobes, is floored and ceiled, has a shingle roof, with a ventilator at the ridge the whole length of the building.   A porch, 10 feet wide, surrounds the entire building.   Commencing at the west end, there is a ward, 40 by 20 feet, having a capacity for eight beds, giving to each an air-space of 1,200 cubic feet; next to the ward is a hall, 5 feet wide, running across the building; then, an isolation ward, 10 by 20 feet; adjoining this is a store-room, 9 by 20 feet; and at the east end of the building, a dispensary, 10 by 20 feet.   The rooms are all 12 feet high in the clear.   There are seven large windows and two doors in the large ward; the isolation ward has two large windows and two doors, and the dispensary has four large windows and two doors.   Immediately in rear of the main building, and thirty-five feet distant, is the building containing the kitchen and mess-hall.   The walls are adobe, 18 inches thick and 12 feet high.   The kitchen is 15 by 17 feet; the mess-hall, 15 by 12 feet.   These rooms are floored with boards, but are not ceiled.   The building is shingle-roofed, is well lighted and ventilated, and well furnished with fixtures and furniture.   The dead-house is situated directly west of the main building, one hundred and sixty feet distant from it, is built of adobes, has a shingle roof, and is 10 feet square, inside measurement.   The walls are 10 feet high.   Water is introduced into the dead-house, which is also used as a bath-room.   This building has two large windows and one door.   To the left of the mess-hall, and forty-five feet distant, is the sink, an adobe structure, 13 by 6 feet, with walls 10 feet high, and a shingle roof.   It is built over a pit, 15 feet deep, and has a ventilating shaft extending four feet above the roof.   There is a hydrant between the main building and the kitchen.   The dead-house contains an excellent shower-bath and conveniences for bathing.   Shade-trees were set out in 1874 on the east and south sides of the hospital; they are in a thriving condition, and already add greatly to the comfort and appearance of the hospital grounds.

The stables are frame buildings, open at the sides, shingle-roofed, with stalls for fifty-two animals, and situated in a corral with high adobe walls.   All are nearly new and in fine condition.

The post is bountifully supplied with water from the Colorado River, by means of a six-horse-power steam-engine.   The water is pumped into a tank capable of holding six thousand gallons, from which it is conducted by pipes to all parts of the post.

The post being situated so near to, and from sixty to seventy-five feet above the river, on a gravelly bluff, the drainage is naturally perfect.

The sinks for the men are trenches covered by frame buildings, situated in a ravine; those for the officers are deep pits covered by adobe buildings.

There is no post garden; few vegetables can be obtained in the vicinity of the post, and these are held at too exorbitant rates for purchase. The troops have an abundance of potatoes, onions, cracked wheat, buckwheat, flour, &c., procured through the Subsistence Department from San Francisco, and paid for from the company fund.

The means of communication are by wagon or horseback, over fair and, at present, safe roads. There is also a steamer, monthly, from Fort Yuma, Cal., by means of which most of the supplies are brought to the post. The river is easily navigable from April to November; but during the remainder of the year with more or less difficulty, owing to sand-bars and shifting channels. There is a semi-weekly mail to and from San Francisco and the East, via Ehrenberg, brought from the latter place on horseback, and a weekly mail to and from Prescott, Ariz.

*Meteorological report, Camp Mojave, Ariz., 1870-'74.*

| Month. | 1870-'71. Temperature. | | | Rain-fall in inches. | 1871-'72. Temperature. | | | Rain-fall in inches. | 1872-'73. Temperature. | | | Rain-fall in inches. | 1873-'74. Temperature. | | | Rain-fall in inches. |
|---|---|---|---|---|---|---|---|---|---|---|---|---|---|---|---|---|
| | Mean. | Max. | Min. | | Mean. | Max. | Min. | | Mean. | Max. | Min. | | Mean. | Max. | Min. | |
| | ° | ° | ° | | ° | ° | ° | | ° | ° | ° | | ° | ° | ° | |
| July | 95.81 | 118 | 82 | 0.71 | 96.75 | 115 | 81 | 0.66 | 91.69 | 112* | 61* | 0.00 | 100.11 | 118* | 47* | 0.00 |
| August | 92.97 | 115 | 76 | 1.90 | 95.87 | 110 | 79 | 0.00 | 90.92 | 113* | 68* | 0.90 | 91.78 | 116* | 52* | 3.80 |
| September | 82.95 | 105 | 63 | 0.00 | 87.71 | 105 | 59 | 0.00 | 83.74 | 109* | 55* | 0.00 | 89.72 | 108* | 45* | 0.00 |
| October | 72.57 | 103 | 50 | 0.78 | 73.59 | 98 | 52 | 0.10 | 73.09 | 98* | 37* | 0.00 | 75.14 | 105* | 27* | 0.00 |
| November | 63.77 | 83 | 42 | 0.00 | 58.57 | 81 | 36 | 0.00 | 55.45 | 81* | 29* | 0.00 | 66.21 | 89* | 36* | 0.50 |
| December | 49.57 | 72 | 29 | 0.27 | 55.27 | 73 | 34 | 0.03 | 51.45 | 75* | 23* | 0.10 | 51.97 | 67* | 29* | 2.80 |
| January | 55.06 | 78 | 34 | 0.00 | 50.24 | 75* | 21* | 0.00 | 74.70 | 78 | 28* | 0.00 | 56.39 | 70* | 27* | 0.10 |
| February | 55.35 | 74 | 37 | 0.02 | 56.75 | 83* | 33* | 0.10 | 54.53 | 73* | 14* | 0.80 | 53.29 | 69* | 29* | 5.00 |
| March | 64.68 | 82 | 42 | 0.00 | 61.29* | 85* | 36* | 0.00 | 69.66 | 92 | 41 | 0.10 | 62.09 | 80* | 39* | 0.20 |
| April | 68.79 | 96 | 47 | 4.05 | 66.15 | 92* | 40* | 0.20 | 72.29 | 99 | 49 | 0.10 | 72.22 | 96* | 54* | 0.10 |
| May | 81.41 | 105 | 62 | 0.00 | 80.53 | 110* | 47* | 0.00 | 78.27 | 102* | 64 | 1.20 | 83.43 | 107* | 63* | 0.90 |
| June | 92.86 | 117 | 65 | 0.00 | 88.53 | 114* | 59* | 1.00 | 91.75 | 112* | 39 (?)* | 0.00 | 92.35 | 111* | 75* | 0.00 |
| For the year | 72.98 | 118 | 29 | 7.73 | 72.60 | 115 | 21* | 2.09 | 72.29 | 113* | 14* | 3.20 | 74.56 | 118* | 27* | 13.40 |

* These observations are made with self-registering thermometers. The mean is from the standard thermometer.

*Consolidated sick-report, Camp Mojave, Ariz., 1870-'74.*

| Year | | 1870-'71. | | 1871-'72. | | 1872-'73. | | 1873-'74. | |
|---|---|---|---|---|---|---|---|---|---|
| Mean strength | Officers | 3 | | 2 | | 2 | | 2 | |
| | Enlisted men | 73 | | 46 | | 26 | | 44 | |
| Diseases. | | Cases. | Deaths. | Cases. | Deaths. | Cases. | Deaths. | Cases. | Deaths. |
| GENERAL DISEASES, A. | | | | | | | | | |
| Intermittent fever | | 17 | | 4 | | | | 1 | |
| Other diseases of this group | | | | 1 | | | | 3 | |
| GENERAL DISEASES, B. | | | | | | | | | |
| Rheumatism | | 10 | | 3 | | 5 | | 14 | |
| Syphilis | | 18 | | 17 | | 11 | | 15 | |
| Consumption | | 2 | | 1 | | 2 | | | |
| Other diseases of this group | | | | | | | | 4 | |
| LOCAL DISEASES. | | | | | | | | | |
| Catarrh and bronchitis | | 8 | 1 | | | 6 | | 3 | |
| Pleurisy | | | | | | 1 | | | |
| Diarrhœa and dysentery | | 20 | | 3 | | 7 | | 10 | |
| Gonorrhœa | | 2 | | 2 | | 1 | | 4 | |
| Other local diseases | | 54 | 3 | 19 | 1 | 18 | | 30 | |
| Alcoholism | | 12 | | 5 | | 1 | | 1 | |
| Total disease | | 143 | 4 | 55 | 1 | 52 | | 85 | |
| VIOLENT DISEASES AND DEATHS. | | | | | | | | | |
| Gunshot wounds | | 1 | 1 | 1 | | | | | |
| Drowning | | | | | 1 | | | | |
| Other accidents and injuries | | 36 | | 6 | | 6 | | 11 | |
| Total violence | | 37 | 1 | 7 | 1 | 6 | | 11 | |

# RIO VERDE INDIAN RESERVATION, ARIZONA TERRITORY.

REPORT OF ACTING ASSISTANT SURGEON WILLIAM H. CORBUSIER, UNITED STATES ARMY.

This is a temporary camp at the Rio Verde Indian agency; situated two and one-half miles west of the Rio Verde and sixteen miles north of Camp Verde. It is located on a small stream, which comes out of the rocks about one hundred and fifty yards west of the camp, and is a continuation of a stream which comes down the mountains, sinks in a cañon about two and one-half miles west of this place, runs through limestone, and makes its appearance again near the camp. The water has lime in solution, and is warmer at its place of exit than it is below, and has received from the Indians the name Hok-e-roo-ya, (hot water.) All the water for the use of the post is taken from this stream.

Since the commencement of the year 1874, from fifteen to thirty men of Company K, Fifth Cavalry, and from thirty to one hundred and twenty Indian scouts, under Second Lieut. W. S. Schuyler, Fifth Cavalry, have been stationed here. At this time (December 31, 1874,) there are eighteen soldiers and forty scouts at the post. The soldiers have occasionally been changed, but the detail has always been from Company K.

Until the 2d of June last the camp was near the Rio Verde, and the men suffered very much from intermittent fever. The Indian agency being there the troops could not leave, and the agent could not be prevailed upon to move. In June, Lieutenant Schuyler took charge of the agency, and immediately moved out of the river-bottom to the present location, at the foot of the mountains, 300 feet higher than the river.

There are about one thousand five hundred Indians on the reservation, composed of Apache Yumas and Apache-Mojaves—two tribes, speaking two different languages. These Indians are under three head chiefs, and are divided into fourteen bands, under petty chiefs. The Apache-Yumas and Apache-Mojaves are tall, well-built men. The Apache-Tontos are short, but tough and wiry, and more able to endure hardships than the others. Scouts are selected from the Indians, and enlisted for six months. For a time they lived in shelter-tents, and were camped two hundred yards back of the soldiers; but they now live with their people in brush-shelters of their own make. Soldiers' clothing is issued to them. In general they are dirty in their habits, but are slowly improving.

Until December the men lived in old A-tents or in shelter-tents, but at that time they completed an adobe house, in which they now live altogether. The small stream spoken of runs about one hundred and twenty-five feet north of the camp. There are many acres of a calcareous deposit from this stream, covered by one or two feet of clayey soil, and on this, where there is a slope of one foot in fifteen, the quarters are built.

The barrack faces the east, is 39½ by 21½ feet, with walls 6 feet high and 18 inches thick; has a canvas roof and dirt floor, and has a door and two small windows in each of the walls, front and rear. The doors and windows are canvas. There is a large chimney at the south end, which heats the room and makes it quite comfortable. The men sleep on rough, wooden single bedsteads, provided with ticks filled with grass, and plenty of blankets. The beds are arranged around the rooms with the heads toward the walls.

North of this house eighteen feet is an adobe kitchen and dining-room in one, 23 by 16½ feet, with walls 8 inches thick. It is also covered with canvas, and contains a stove and cooking-utensils, a table, benches, &c. Outside at the north end is an oven in which the bread is baked.

Officers' quarters consist of hospital-tents framed and floored, and provided with adobe fire-places and chimneys.

The guard-house is a wall-tent. The place of confinement for Indian prisoners is a hole sixteen feet square, dug in the side of a steep hill. A stone wall ten feet high is built on each side, and it is covered with a dirt roof. Although it is not to be commended, it is warm, well ventilated, and secure, and is the best that could be devised for a temporary guard-house.

As there are no hospital accommodations here, this being but a temporary camp, men sick enough to go to hospital are usually sent to Camp Verde. A wall-tent is used as a dispensary.

There are no stables for the horses; they are kept one hundred feet in rear of the quarters. Back still farther is the sink; a new one is dug every two months. The Indian prisoners are constantly cleaning up; the refuse is burned, so the camp is kept very clean.

There is a heavy growth of cedar on the hills all around, and this is the wood furnished by the contractors for fuel.

The duties while here are light, but in the mountains a great deal of the scouting is done on foot; three or four days' rations have to be carried, besides a blanket, carbine, and cartridges, and the duties are very arduous. High mountains have to be climbed, and deep, rocky cañons crossed under a broiling sun or through the snow, in order to find hostile Indians. The rarified air frequently adds greatly to the fatigue, causing palpitation of the heart, dyspnœa, and often exhaustion.

*Consolidated sick-report, Rio Verde Indian Reservation, Ariz., 1873–'74.*

| Year | | 1873–'74.* | |
|---|---|---|---|
| Mean strength | { Officers | 1 | |
| | { Enlisted men | 21 | |
| Diseases. | | Cases. | Deaths. |
| GENERAL DISEASES, A. | | | |
| Intermittent fever | | 26 | ...... |
| LOCAL DISEASES. | | | |
| Gonorrhœa | | 2 | ...... |
| Other local diseases | | 3 | ...... |
| Total disease | | 31 | ...... |

\* 10 months only.

# SAN CARLOS INDIAN RESERVATION, ARIZONA TERRITORY.

REPORT OF ACTING ASSISTANT SURGEON H. M. MATTHEWS, UNITED STATES ARMY.

The camp at the San Carlos Indian agency is a subpost of Camp Apache, is situated on the San Carlos River, and is distant seventy-four miles west of south from that post.

The garrison is quartered in tents. The enlisted men have one adobe building, 50 by 30 feet, which is used as a kitchen and mess-room.

A rough log building, lighted and ventilated through the crevices between the logs, and warmed by an open fire-place, is used as a guard-house. Its principal occupants are refractory Indians from the agency.

There is one storehouse built of adobes, used by both the commissary and quartermaster. It is 72 by 24 feet, with a dirt roof.

Mesquite and cottonwood, obtained by contract, are used for fuel.

A small room added to the storehouse is used as a dispensary and store-room for medical supplies.

## CAMP VERDE, ARIZONA TERRITORY.

REPORTED BY ACTING ASSISTANT SURGEON L. SANDERSON, UNITED STATES ARMY.

Camp Verde is situated in Yavapai County, Arizona, in latitude 34° 33' north; longitude, 34° 57' west; at an elevation of 3,500 feet above the level of the sea, and about 80 feet above the water of the Rio Verde, upon its right or western bank, and from the nearest point of which it is distant about a mile. It is about forty miles east of Prescott, the nearest town and post-office, from which the mails are brought at irregular intervals by a person from the camp for that purt pose. Camp McDowell is ninety miles south by trail along the Verde, through a country extremely rough and broken.

The valley of the Rio Verde, through the greater portion of its course from north to south, is very narrow, being little else than a cañon, with bare and rugged hills on each side; but in this locality it is about seven miles wide, with a rich alluvial bottom, which produces a rank vegetation, with a luxuriant growth of cottonwood, willow, and alder, and which, when irrigated, yields excellent crops of corn, barley, and vegetables. The Mogollon range of mountains bounds this valley on the east, the Black Mountains on the west. The latter rise to an elevation of about 3,000 feet above the river, and furnish pine timber suitable for building. Deer, antelope, and wild turkeys abound. Gold has long been known to exist in the vicinity, but has not been mined until recently, on account of the hostility of the Indians. Diggings commenced last summer have been found to pay liberally.

Old Camp Verde, formerly Camp Lincoln, was originally established by Arizona volunteers mostly Mexicans, during the war of 1861, as an outpost from Fort Whipple, to protect Prescott County and admit of its settlement. It was first occupied by regular troops in 1866. The first shelters erected were of the most primitive character, and the more permanent quarters, commenced in 1868, were never completed. The location was considered unhealthy and unsuitable; and in the spring of 1871 the present site was selected, and the building of a new post commenced. The location is a mesa, about one mile south of the old post, and half a mile south of the confluence of Beaver Creek with the Verde. In September of the same year work was abandoned from the discharge of citizen employés. Three sets of company quarters, the guard-house, and two sets of officers' quarters had then been finished, and the frame of a third set had been put up. Nothing further was done until September, 1873, except what could be accomplished by the labor of the troops. By their labor alone the third set of officers' quarters was rendered habitable, and a building similar to the company quarters, (now used as store-house for the quartermaster and commissary stores,) provisionary hospital, a temporary corral, and three stables were built. Work was resumed in the early part of September, 1873, and continued through the succeeding year.

The present garrison consists of two companies of cavalry and two of infantry. The buildings of the post are arranged on three sides of a rectangular parade, 692 by 481 feet. The south side is occupied by a building of "pice," 100 by 20 feet, with a piazza 6 feet wide. It is divided into offices for the adjutant, quartermaster, and commissary, a school-room, and three sets of laundresses' quarters. Adjacent to this is an adobe building, 130 by 20 feet, with a piazza 6 feet wide, occupied as quarters for married soldiers. It is divided by transverse partitions into ten sets of quarters. Each set is again divided into two rooms, 12 by 13 feet and 12 by 7. Upon the east side are the three sets of officers' quarters—frame buildings lined with adobes. They are one story high, 50 by 18 feet, with each a wing 34 by 18 feet. The main building is surrounded by a piazza 12 feet wide. Each set contains, besides the first floor, attics for store-rooms and servants' rooms. The west side contains four sets of company quarters, three frame buildings, and one of "pice." Each consists of a one-story building, 100 by 24 feet, with L 76 by 24. The main building contains dormitory, office, and store-room; the wing, saddle-room, kitchen, and mess-room. The dormitories are 72 by 24 feet, and 12 feet to the eaves, furnished with double wooden bunks in single tiers. They are ventilated by doors, windows, open fire-places, and latticed windows at the gable ends. Each dormitory is lighted by six windows. The kitchens are 25 by 24 feet; the mess-rooms 42 by 24. In the infantry quarters, a tailor-shop takes the place of the saddle-room.

The guard-house is a frame building, 51 by 32 feet, by 12 feet to the eaves, and is divided into a guard-room, 16 by 21 feet, warmed by stoves, two prison-rooms of the same size, and five cells,

8 by 3 feet, lighted and ventilated by long, narrow apertures near the ceiling. The average number of prisoners is eleven. It stands on the west side of the parade.

The provisionary hospital, built by the troops, is a frame structure, 80 by 24 feet, and 12 feet to the eaves, unceiled and unlined, except the ward, which is ceiled and lined with old canvas. The south end is occupied by the ward, 28 by 24 feet. It contains eight beds, with an air-space of 8,064 feet. The dispensary and dining-room, each 12 by 18 feet, communicate with the ward. These rooms communicate with store-rooms, each 12 by 15½ feet. The steward's quarters and laundry occupy the north end of the building, and are each 12 by 16 feet, without communicating with the other parts of the building. There is a separate kitchen, 12 by 16 feet, a few yards in rear of the mess-room. The hospital is in the same line with those buildings which form the west side of the parade. It contains no post-mortem room, bath-room, or water-closet. A bath is occasionally extemporized in the dining-room, and an earth-closet is used in the ward. The building is quite unsuited to the purpose for which it is used. The average number of patients in the hospital is two.

The magazine is a stone building, about one hundred and fifty feet to the rear of the west line of buildings. The bakery is built of adobes, 20 by 30 feet, and contains two ovens, with a capacity of one hundred and fifty loaves each. Two sets of officers' quarters, uniform in size with the others, and a commissary store-house of " pice," were erected in 1874.

The cemetery is about two miles northeast of the post, and is inclosed by a substantial fence, 154 by 50 feet, and contains the graves of eighteen soldiers and six citizens, most of whom fell victims to hostile Apaches. The graves are covered with stones, to protect them from the coyotes.

No trees of any kind grow upon the mesa, and the buildings are exposed to the full glare of the sun's rays, which at times are very intense. Should water, however, be brought upon the parade-ground, as is expected, a luxuriant shade could be quickly produced from cuttings of cottonwood.

The supply of water for the post is brought by water-carts from a spring on Beaver Creek, one mile distant, for drinking purposes, and from the river for other uses. The spring-water is cold, even in summer, and holds but little inorganic matter in solution. Other methods of obtaining a more abundant supply of water are in contemplation.

Company-gardens are cultivated along the river, about a mile and a half above the camp, which furnish to the garrison a supply of vegetables, excellent, varied, and abundant. There is no garden set apart specially for the hospital.

The Rio Verde Indian reservation extends from about three miles above Camp Verde for forty miles along the river, and ten miles on each side. On this reservation are about two thousand Indians, consisting of the Mojave, Yuma, and Tonto bands of Apaches, who, until the spring of 1863, were roaming the mountains, committing depredations, but who now, for the most part, seem disposed to remain on their reservation, and even to adopt some of the customs of civilized life.

*Meteorological report, Camp Verde, Ariz., 1870–'74.*

| Month. | 1870-'71. Temperature. | | | 1870-'71. Rain-fall in inches. | 1871-'72. Temperature. | | | 1871-'72. Rain-fall in inches. | 1872-'73. Temperature. | | | 1872-'73. Rain-fall in inches. | 1873-'74. Temperature. | | | 1873-'74. Rain-fall in inches. |
|---|---|---|---|---|---|---|---|---|---|---|---|---|---|---|---|---|
| | Mean. | Max. | Min. | | Mean. | Max. | Min. | | Mean. | Max. | Min. | | Mean. | Max. | Min. | |
| July | 85.15 | 108 | 69 | 3.06 | 89.21 | 109 | 74 | 0.84 | 85.12 | 104 | 64 | 2.22 | 86.75 | 113 | 48* | 0.14 |
| August | 80.49 | 100 | 59 | 0.89 | 86.94 | 105 | 70 | 0.26 | 80.62 | 102* | 50* | 4.35 | 81.17 | 102 | 58* | 2.52 |
| September | 74.19 | 101 | 48 | 0.00 | 76.93 | 100 | 50 | 1.09 | 74.78 | 100* | 36* | 1.12 | 75.68 | 97 | 41* | 0.26 |
| October | 63.29 | 99 | 35 | 0.60 | 60.79 | 87 | 33 | 1.10 | 64.13 | 93* | 16* | 0.10 | 62.00 | 95 | 21* | 0.00 |
| November | 54.08 | 84 | 30 | 0.10 | 47.23 | 68 | 32 | 0.39 | 46.20 | 72* | 6* | 0.00 | 49.78 | 74 | 20* | 0.74 |
| December | 38.77 | 75 | 8 | 0.58 | 44.04 | 64 | 23 | 0.26 | 43.53 | 69 | 16 | 0.83 | 29.33 | 57 | 6* | 3.26 |
| January | 45.14 | 68 | 28 | 0.20 | 39.83 | 66 | 22 | 0.47 | 42.22 | 69 | 10 | 0.00 | 40.80 | 59 | 5* | 2.65 |
| February | 45.32 | 69 | 26 | 0.00 | 48.34 | 79 | 34 | 1.12 | 43.46 | 63 | 20 | 1.16 | 40.37 | 60 | 12* | 2.05 |
| March | 53.89 | 80 | 33 | 0.02 | 58.72 | 80 | 31 | 0.16 | 59.12 | 82 | 38 | 0.00 | 51.24 | 72 | 19* | 1.05 |
| April | 65.28 | 87 | 37 | 0.73 | 63.91 | 94 | 37 | 1.56 | 61.58 | 90 | 31 | 0.00 | 57.50 | .87 | 27* | 1.48 |
| May | 71.90 | 97 | 50 | 0.00 | 75.25 | 111 | 49 | 0.54 | 69.90 | 95 | 45 | 0.15 | 70.23 | 102 | 34* | 0.08 |
| June | 85.87 | 109 | 64 | 0.00 | 80.57 | 110 | 54 | 0.66 | 80.15 | 112 | 47* | 0.20 | 81.14 | 107 | 43* | 0.00 |
| For the year | 63.61 | 109 | 8 | 6.18 | 64.31 | 111 | 22 | 8.36 | 62.56 | 112 | 6* | 10.13 | 60.49 | 113 | 5* | 14.19 |

* These observations are made with self-registering thermometers. The mean is from the standard thermometer.

*Consolidated sick-report, Camp Verde, Ariz., 1870–'74.*

| Year | | 1870–'71. | | 1871–'72. | | 1872–'73. | | 1873–'74. | |
|---|---|---|---|---|---|---|---|---|---|
| Mean strength { Officers | | 7 | | 6 | | 5 | | 4 | |
| { Enlisted men | | 212 | | 141 | | 131 | | 152 | |
| Diseases. | | Cases. | Deaths. | Cases. | Deaths. | Cases. | Deaths. | Cases. | Deaths. |
| GENERAL DISEASES, A. | | | | | | | | | |
| Remittent fever | | | | 2 | | 1 | | | |
| Intermittent fever | | 206 | | 136 | | 187 | | 110 | |
| Other diseases of this group | | 2 | | | | 3 | | 11 | |
| GENERAL DISEASES, B. | | | | | | | | | |
| Rheumatism | | 11 | | 7 | | 12 | | 14 | |
| Syphilis | | 3 | | 1 | | 1 | | 4 | |
| Consumption | | | | 2 | | | | | |
| Other diseases of this group | | 1 | | 1 | | 1 | | 3 | |
| LOCAL DISEASES. | | | | | | | | | |
| Catarrh and bronchitis | | 6 | | 25 | | 24 | | 13 | |
| Pneumonia | | | | | | 1 | | | |
| Pleurisy | | 3 | | | | | | | |
| Diarrhœa and dysentery | | 19 | | 15 | | 42 | | 35 | 1 |
| Hernia | | | | | | | | 1 | |
| Gonorrhœa | | | | | | 3 | | 5 | |
| Other local diseases | | 47 | | 56 | 1 | 76 | 1 | 84 | |
| Alcoholism | | | | 3 | | 7 | | 5 | 1 |
| Total disease | | 298 | | 248 | 1 | 358 | 1 | 285 | 1 |
| VIOLENT DISEASES AND DEATHS. | | | | | | | | | |
| Gunshot wounds | | 2 | 1 | 1 | 2 | 4 | | 3 | |
| Other accidents and injuries | | 38 | 1 | 39 | | 63 | | 59 | |
| Total violence | | 40 | 2 | 40 | 2 | 67 | | 62 | |

# FORT WHIPPLE, ARIZONA TERRITORY.

REPORTS OF ASSISTANT SURGEONS P. MIDDLETON AND HENRY LIPPINCOTT, UNITED STATES ARMY.

This post is on the left bank of Granite Creek, a small stream, one of the sources of the Rio Verde, and is one mile northeast from the town of Prescott, the county-seat of Yavapai County, and headquarters of the Department of Arizona; latitude, 34° 29′ 6″ north; longitude, 35° 27′ 30″ west.

The valley of Granite Creek is one of the many to be found around the base of Granite Mountain, the northern extremity of the Sierra Prieta. Its whole extent is covered with pine timber and as the small plateau on which the post and town are built is receded from, the ground, stil timbered, becomes much broken by ravines, and finally rises to the bare mountain-peaks of grayish granite. But on the northwest, beyond the immediately surrounding hills, the country is open and rolling, covered with bunch-grass and dotted with spreading juniper, until the Bill Williams and San Francisco Mountains break through and interrupt its undulations. Prescott, formerly the capital of the Territory, is a small town, the center and supply-depot of a large but sparsely settled mining and agricultural district. The numerous valleys within a radius of thirty miles have rich but limited bottom-lands, many of which are cultivated, and yield all the produce of temperate climates; the mountains are rich in free gold and gold sulphurets. It is reached from San Francisco by way of Los Angeles to Fort Mojave and Willow Grove, which lies west from it about one hundred miles, or along the southern road from Los Angeles and San Bernardino, by way of La Paz, on the Colorado River.

The post was first located December 23, 1863, near Postal's Ranch, twenty-four miles northeast of Prescott. The location was changed and the present post established May 18, 1864, as the then headquarters of the District of Arizona. The site selected was on a small plateau, a mile above the town, and seventy feet above the level of the creek, to which it inclines, yielding a good natural drainage. It originally consisted of a rectangular stockade, the wall of which formed the outer wall of the various buildings inclosed in it. It was built of strong undressed pine logs, the crevices being filled in with mud, and the roofs of all the buildings shingled. Ventilation was imperfectly effected, as most of the doors and windows opened on the inclosed parade-ground. The men's quarters, kitchen, and bakery occupied one side, with the officers' quarters opposite; the store-rooms another, with the guard-house, adjutant's office, and laundresses' quarters opposite.

The present buildings were all erected during and since the year 1872, except the guard-house.

The quarters for enlisted men consist of the following buildings: One frame barrack, 140 by 30 feet, 12 feet in height, shingle roofed, with a wing, 30 by 15 feet, in rear of each end. The main portion is divided into two dormitories, each 65 by 30 feet, with a hall 10 feet wide between them. The wings are each divided into two rooms of equal size, one used as an orderly's room, the room adjoining it is a store-room; in the other wing one room is used as a tailor-shop, the adjoining one as a bath-room. A porch 10 feet wide extends around the whole building. There is another barrack building, similar in all respects to the above, except that the main portion is only 110 feet long by 24 feet wide. In rear of, and fifty feet distant from, the barrack buildings are the kitchens and mess-rooms. The set belonging to the larger barrack is in a building 75 by 24 by 12 feet, divided into a mess-room, 45 by 24 feet, a kitchen, 20 by 24, and a store-room, 10 by 24 feet. The set belonging to the other barrack is in a building 70 by 20 feet, divided similarly to the other. The band is quartered with the infantry soldiers in the smaller barrack, but occupies an old shed as a kitchen and mess-room. The dormitories afford an air-space of 780 cubic feet per man of average occupancy. Each of the dormitories in the larger barrack has eleven large windows; those in the smaller have eight each; these, in connection with the doors and open fire-places, furnish excellent ventilation. The rooms are warmed by stoves and fire-places, and are furnished with single bedsteads and other necessary furniture and fixtures.

Married soldiers' quarters consist of a frame building divided into twelve sets, each set comprising a front room, 15 by 14, and a back room, 12 by 14 feet. All the rooms are 12 feet from floor to ceiling, and are comfortable. A porch, 8 feet wide, extends along the whole front of the building.

Officers' quarters consist of eight sets, all frame buildings one and a half stories in height. One set contains four rooms, 15 by 15 feet each, two of these on each side of a hall 8 feet wide, running from front to rear. In rear of, and adjoining these rooms, is a kitchen, 12 by 12 feet, a pantry bath-room, cellar and usual out-houses. The attic is finished for servants' rooms, &c. The other sets are all built on the same general plan. They each contain two rooms, each 15 by 15 feet, communicating with a hall running from front to rear; have a kitchen 9 feet square, with adjoining rooms similar to the set first described. The attics are also similarly finished; the rooms on the first floor of each building are all 9 feet in height, and in all respects they are excellent quarters.

The guard-house, used at present, is the old stockade one. An excellent stone building for this purpose is in course of construction; its dimensions are 61 by 33 feet, 12 feet in height. It will contain a guard-room, 14 by 22 feet; a prison, 13½ by 22 feet; 6 cells, each 7 by 3 feet, and a hall 17 by 4 feet; will be warmed by stoves, lighted by windows, and ventilated by grated windows and doors.

The commissary storehouse, built in 1872, is an adobe building with shingle roof. It is 125 by 24 feet, divided into a store-room 86 feet long, in the central part, with a smaller-sized room at each end. The quartermaster's storehouse, just completed, is 119 by 24 feet.

The stables afford room for 84 horses; connected with them are a saddle-room, quarters for the commissary-sergeant of cavalry, saddler's and farrier's room, and forage-room. The corral, inclosed by a board fence which includes the stables, &c., is 150 by 120 feet.

The old hospital building, located between the post and the town of Prescott, was burned down November 23, 1874. A new hospital built of adobe is in process of construction, and nearly completed at this time, (December 31, 1874.) It will consist of an administration building, crossed by two halls 8 feet in width, running at right angles to each other, and will contain six rooms, each 15 feet square, intended for dispensary, isolation-ward, steward's room, nurse's room, store-room, and a spare room. A ward, 50 by 24 feet, in the form of a wing, adjoins one end of this building; a piazza 10 feet wide surrounds the whole. At the farther rear corner of the ward, a portion of the piazza is inclosed, forming a room 9 feet square, inside, for the earth-closet. The ward is to be heated by two stoves.

About twenty yards in the rear of the above is an adobe building containing a dining-room 15 feet square; a kitchen and laundry, each 12 by 15 feet; a pantry and bath-room, each 8 by 15 feet. A piazza 8 feet wide entirely surrounds this building, and a covered way 6 feet wide connects it with the hospital building. A dead-house and privy are about thirty yards in rear of the hospital.

The water supply of the post is derived from wells, and is of excellent quality, cold and pure. It is raised by a force-pump, and distributed to the buildings by pipes.

The post garden is on the creek, just east of the garrison; potatoes, cabbages, turnips, corn, beets, tomatoes, melons, and cucumbers are successfully cultivated.

Neither game nor fish is found within a reasonable distance. There are no Indians nearer than the Rio Verde reservation.

The climate of this district is mild during the spring and summer months, there being none of the long-continued and scorching heats which, in the southern portion of the Territory, kill all vegetation except that on the margin of the streams. Frequent rains fall in the autumn, and during the winter the mountains are covered with snow, which, in severe seasons, may lie even in the valleys for two or three weeks at a time.

*Meteorological report, Fort Whipple, Ariz., 1870–'74.*

| Month. | 1870–'71. | | | | 1871–'72. | | | | 1872–'73. | | | | 1873–'74. | | | |
|---|---|---|---|---|---|---|---|---|---|---|---|---|---|---|---|---|
| | Temperature. | | | Rain-fall in inches. | Temperature. | | | Rain-fall in inches. | Temperature. | | | Rain-fall in inches. | Temperature. | | | Rain-fall in inches. |
| | Mean. | Max. | Min. | | Mean. | Max. | Min. | | Mean. | Max. | Min. | | Mean. | Max. | Min. | |
| July | 72.92 | 89 | 57 | 7.98 | 77.13 | 92 | 66 | 4.00 | 74.97 | 86 | 31* | 3.74 | 79.11 | 91 | 65 | 1.56 |
| August | 69.08 | 83 | 57 | 3.49 | 76.38 | 91 | 64 | 1.80 | 72.51 | 87 | 48* | 6.25 | 73.14 | 85 | 64 | 4.78 |
| September | 61.40 | 82 | 45 | 0.00 | 68.16 | 88 | 47 | 1.51 | 68.73 | 80 | 32* | 0.04 | 68.97 | 82 | 50 | 0.30 |
| October | 52.91 | 77 | 30 | 1.59 | 56.16 | 74 | 37 | 1.40 | 57.56 | 78 | 12* | 0.24 | 55.68 | 81 | 33 | 0.00 |
| November | 46.88 | 67 | 42 | 0.30 | 43.82 | 62 | 19 | 0.52 | 44.96 | 68 | – 1* | 0.00 | 46.73 | 72 | 29 | 0.80 |
| December | 33.19 | 62 | 4 | 0.53 | 41.80 | 60 | 17 | 0.00 | 40.25 | 66 | 12 | 0.64 | 35.09 | 65 | 10 | 2.55 |
| January | 40.73 | 70 | 15 | 0.70 | 35.77 | 60 | – 1 | 0.50 | 39.09 | 60 | 11 | 0.00 | 38.57 | 67 | 17 | 5.51 |
| February | 43.50 | 68 | 21 | 1.20 | 42.68 | 66 | 10* | 0.80 | 36.35 | 55 | 13 | (?) | 35.46 | 55 | 10 | 5.68 |
| March | 50.12 | 75 | 34 | 0.10 | 47.19 | 63 | 12* | 0.12 | 51.22 | 73 | 25 | 0.23 | 41.50 | 65 | 20 | 3.56 |
| April | 50.48 | 71 | 33 | 1.92 | 49.56 | 75 | 13* | 1.62 | 53.62 | 77 | 29 | 0.17 | 49.48 | 75 | 34 | 1.70 |
| May | 62.73 | 81 | 44 | 0.47 | 63.83 | 86 | 31* | 1.47 | 60.26 | 74 | 45 | 0.40 | 60.91 | 82 | 41 | 0.65 |
| June | 71.79 | 92 | 50 | 0.00 | 72.80 | 88 | 36* | 1.24 | 72.93 | 92 | 50 | 0.42 | 71.97 | 88 | 55 | 0.00 |
| For the year | 54.64 | 92 | 4 | 18.28 | 56.27 | 92 | – 1 | 14.98 | 56.04 | 92 | – 1* | ........ | 54.72 | 91 | 10 | 27.09 |

* These observations are made with self-registering thermometers. The mean is from the standard thermometer,

*Consolidated sick-report, Fort Whipple, Ariz., 1870–'74.*

| Year | 1870–'71. | | 1871–'72. | | 1872–'73. | | 1873–'74. | |
|---|---|---|---|---|---|---|---|---|
| Mean strength { Officers / Enlisted men | 6 / 98 | | 4 / 68 | | 6 / 145 | | 5 / 132 | |
| Diseases. | Cases. | Deaths. | Cases. | Deaths. | Cases. | Deaths. | Cases. | Deaths. |
| GENERAL DISEASES, A. | | | | | | | | |
| Typho-malarial fever | | | | | | | 1 | 1 |
| Remittent fever | | | 1 | | 7 | | | |
| Intermittent fever | 68 | | 3 | | 4 | | 27 | |
| Other diseases of this group | 3 | | | | 11 | | 12 | |
| GENERAL DISEASES, B. | | | | | | | | |
| Rheumatism | 10 | | 3 | | 7 | | 34 | |
| Syphilis | 5 | | 7 | | 4 | | 3 | |
| Consumption | | | | | | | 1 | |
| Other diseases of this group | 4 | | 1 | | 3 | | | |
| LOCAL DISEASES. | | | | | | | | |
| Catarrh and bronchitis | 22 | | 10 | | 12 | | 67 | |
| Pneumonia | 3 | | 1 | | | | | |
| Pleurisy | | | | | 1 | | 4 | |

*Consolidated sick-report, Fort Whipple, Ariz., 1870–'74—Continued.*

| Year | | 1870–'71. | | 1871–'72. | | 1872–'73. | | 1873–'74. | |
|---|---|---|---|---|---|---|---|---|---|
| Mean strength ............................................. ⎰ Officers............⎱ Enlisted men...... | | 6<br>98 | | 4<br>68 | | 6<br>145 | | 5<br>132 | |
| Diseases. | | Cases. | Deaths. | Cases. | Deaths. | Cases. | Deaths. | Cases. | Deaths. |
| LOCAL DISEASES, CONTINUED. | | | | | | | | | |
| Diarrhœa and dysentery........................... | | 30 | ...... | 4 | ...... | 19 | ...... | 40 | ...... |
| Gonorrhœa ............................................. | | 2 | ...... | 1 | ...... | 3 | ...... | 2 | ...... |
| Other local diseases ............................... | | 43 | 1 | 16 | 1 | 36 | 1 | 70 | 1 |
| Alcoholism........................................... | | 8 | ...... | 1 | ...... | 3 | ...... | 58 | ...... |
| Total disease................................. | | 198 | 1 | 48 | 1 | 110 | 1 | 319 | 2 |
| VIOLENT DISEASES AND DEATHS. | | | | | | | | | |
| Gunshot wounds ..................................... | | 6 | 1 | 3 | 1 | 2 | ...... | 1 | ...... |
| Other accidents and injuries ................... | | 51 | ...... | 24 | ...... | 29 | ...... | 102 | ...... |
| Homicide ............................................. | | ...... | ...... | ...... | ...... | ...... | 1 | ...... | ...... |
| Suicide................................................. | | ...... | ...... | ...... | ...... | ...... | ...... | ...... | 2 |
| Total violence.............................. | | 57 | 1 | 27 | 1 | 31 | 1 | 103 | 2 |

# FORT YUMA, CALIFORNIA.

REPORTS OF ASSISTANT SURGEONS J. V. LAUDERDALE AND GEORGE S. ROSE, UNITED STATES ARMY.

To protect the emigrants of Southern California from the attacks of hostile Indians, it became necessary in the year 1850 to establish a military post from which assistance could be promptly extended when required. With this object in view, on November 27th of that year, Bvt. Maj. S. T. Heintzelman, captain Second Infantry, received instructions from headquarters of the tenth military district, Monterey, California, to establish a post somewhere near the junction of the Gila with the Colorado. The camp was first established on the "bottom," near what was known as "the old ferry crossing," about a half mile below the junction of the two rivers, but was subsequently moved in March, 1851, to the top of the bluff, on the site of an old "Spanish mission," said to have been in operation in the year 1700. Owing to the scarcity of supplies, and the difficulty of obtaining provisions, the camp was abandoned in June, 1851. On the 29th of February, 1852, Major Heintzelman returned and re-established a permanent garrison.

Fort Yuma is located in latitude 32° 23' 3'' north; longitude, 37° 33' 9'' west; altitude, 267 feet above tide-water. The rocky bluff on which the fort is built is, at its highest point, just 110 feet above the bank of the river.

After receiving the Gila at a point one hundred and eighty miles from its mouth, the Colorado River turns suddenly westward and forces its way through a rocky defile, 70 feet high, 350 yards long, and 200 yards wide, thus cutting off a narrow rocky bluff and leaving it as an isolated eminence on the California side of the river. On this rocky eminence, which has been shifted not many ages since from the Arizona to the California side of the ever-varying stream, (and during high water it is hard to tell which side it is on, as the water flows freely all around it,) stands Fort Yuma, rising gray and somber above the broad sea of green as it is approached on the emigrant road from Pilot Knob. At this point the bottom-lands adjacent to the river average seven miles in width, and are covered with a dense growth of cottonwood and mesquite. Chains of low serrated hills and mountains limit the view on nearly every side, all bare and gray, save when painted by the sun with delicate tints of blue and purple.

The river at the fort is two hundred yards wide, shallow, except in its channel, and impeded by sand-bars. The first successful effort to navigate the Colorado was made in December, 1852. A small side-wheel steamer, the Uncle Sam, made the first voyage, consuming fourteen days from the mouth of the river; the delay, however, was chiefly owing to an accident to the boiler. In the spring of 1854 Mr. George A. Johnson built and equipped a new steamer, the General Jesup, capable of carrying sixty tons of freight. She was succeeded by other stern-wheel steamers of increased size and capacity. At present five large and commodious vessels are engaged in the carrying-trade on the river.

The mountains in the vicinity are small spurs of the Sierra Nevada. According to Dr. J. Newberry, geologist of Lieutenant Ives's Colorado River expedition, "these ranges belong to the great Rocky Mountain series, and are much older than the Coast range, from which they differ in many respects. Their nucleus consists of granite and gneissoid rocks. The granite is a coarse variety, with a predominance of the feldspathic element, and an almost total absence of hornblende; many large crystals of albite are seen; these are loosened from their matrix by atmospheric agencies, and are readily detached, so that the surfaces of granite are uneven, full of cavities, and have a look of friability. The general hue of the granite in this vicinity, when exposed for any length of time to the elements, is of the reddish tint characteristic of the Rocky Mountain series. Disintegration of surface is continually going on. But very few plants find any soil among the *débris* of these rocks, and the mountains and hills present no appearance of vegetation."

Valuable minerals are found in the slopes of the foot-hills north of the post, but, owing to the scarcity of water, the development of these mines has been very limited; granular gold is, however, brought in in considerable quantities. Silver, in combination with lead, is also found in the Castle Dome range, fourteen miles north of Yuma. One mine has been scientifically worked there recently, and the yield is said to have been such as to warrant a continuance of the work. No smelting-works have as yet been established in this vicinity; the ore is all shipped to San Francisco for reduction.

Beyond the bottoms, on either side of the river, arises an elevated plain or mesa, which extends to the mountain-range. Nothing can be conceived more desolate than this vast plain; not a blade of grass exists, and, except here and there a scattered cactus, not a green thing is seen to relieve the eye from the light ash color, so trying to the sight.

The bottom-land surrounding the fort, and forming the right bank of the river, is covered with a heavy growth of arrow-weed, mesquite, and willow, and is intersected by a number of sloughs and lagoons, former beds of the river. The soil is alluvial, overlying a stratum of sand, and is exceedingly productive. On these lands the Indians plant in the month of July, or as soon as the annual overflow subsides. They cultivate corn, beans, pumpkins, water-melons, and musk-melons. No system of artificial irrigation has been attempted, but there is no doubt that if a practical effort was made much of the land on both the Gila and Colorado could be cultivated with success. There can also be no doubt that on many of the sloughs wheat, cotton, and sugar-cane will grow. The soil and climate are also well adapted to the cultivation of the vine, fig, and tropical plants.

The principal wild animals of the vicinity are the American fox, the coyote, raccoon, skunk, beaver, weasel, jack rabbit, cotton-tail rabbit, squirrel, and gopher. The birds are the buzzard, owl, (three varieties,) whippoorwill, swallow, lark, robin, mocking-bird, thrush, sparrow, linnet, quail, plover, sand-hill crane, blue heron, white heron, Colorado turkey, (wood ibis,) snipe, curlew, water hen, duck, (four varieties,) goose, (two varieties,) pelican, &c. Reptiles comprise the turtle, toad, lizard, rattlesnake, black-snake, and water-snake. Of insects the greatest pest is the small red ant. The hill on which the fort stands may be said to be an immense ant-hill. During the summer they invade the closet, pantry, trunk, and bed, and frequently attack the body. They are particularly fond of oleaginous compounds; the various kinds of pomades are always selected, and the individual who indulges in hair tonics is apt to suffer for it. The mosquito is only troublesome in July, during the annual overflow.

The tribe of Indians occupying the reserve lying on this section of the Colorado, is known as the Cu-cha-no or Yuma. They hold a middle place on the river, between the Co-co-pahs and Mojaves, the former of whom claim the first hundred miles, extending north from the mouth of the river, the Yumas the second, and the Mojaves the third. All are known as River Indians, to distinguish them from Mountain Indians. The Yumas, since September, 1852, when they were subdued by General (then Captain) Heintzelman, have been on friendly terms with the whites, and there seems to be no record of a violation of the treaty made at that time. Physically, this tribe is a superb specimen of the race. Their chief dependence for food is on the mesquite bean and the products of their agriculture. The river and lagoons abound with several varieties of fish; all, however, have a muddy taste, are full of small bones, and of most inferior quality.

The winter may be said to commence about November. During this season the days are usually warm, and the nights cold, the difference in temperature being very great. In the low lands ice sometimes forms. The atmosphere is exceedingly dry, and very little rain falls during the winter. When the coast rains prevail in California sometimes a few drops fall here. The climate is rendered somewhat disagreeable by occasional violent sand-storms, usually from the northwest. They can be seen approaching for some hours, gradually obscuring the sun; finally they burst with sudden fury, filling the air and everything around with a fine dust. These sand-storms sometimes last three days; in the intervals between them no more delightful climate could be desired. Fires are necessary during these months, November to March, and heavy under-clothing is required to protect the body from the sudden change of temperature which takes place after sundown.

Spring commences about the last of February, and is without rain. The cottonwoods and willows put forth new leaves, but owing to the continued cold nights, the leaves do not mature before the middle of April. Fires are still required in the evenings and early mornings.

The heat rapidly increases from the latter part of May, and in June, July, August, and September may be said to be intense. In the months of July and August (the rainy season in Sonora) clouds are seen passing to the northeast accompanied with rain, thunder, and lightning; occasionally they reach the vicinity of Yuma, and are most refreshing. During the months of April, May, and June no rain falls; then, with the thermometer at 105°, the perspiration is scarcely seen upon the skin, and it becomes dry and harsh, and the hair crispy. Furniture put together at the North and brought here falls to pieces; traveling-chests gape at their seams, and a sole-leather trunk contracts so that with difficulty the tray can be lifted. Furniture to hold together must be made of the very driest timber. The extreme dryness of the atmosphere is observed in the ink that dries so rapidly upon the pen that it requires washing off every few minutes. A No. 2 "Faber" leaves no more trace on paper than a piece of anthracite, and it is necessary to keep one immersed in water while using one that has been standing in water some time. Newspapers require to be unfolded with care; if rudely handled they break. I was called to inspect some commissary stores a short time ago, and the loss they had sustained was remarkable. Twelve-pound boxes of soap weighed ten pounds. Hams had lost 12 per cent., and rice 2 per cent. of their original weight Eggs that have been on hand for a few weeks lose their watery contents by evaporation; the remainder is thick and tough; this has probably led to the story that our hens lay hard-boiled eggs.

The mercury gained the highest point last summer, on the 2d day of July, when, for two hours, it stood at 113° in the shade. All metallic bodies were hot to the touch; my watch felt like a hot boiled egg in my pocket; the cords of my grass hammock were like heated wires. At such times, if the wind is from the south, the air is like that from the mouth of a furnace, hot and ovenish.

The effort to cool one's self with an ordinary fan would be vain, because the surrounding atmosphere is of a higher temperature than the body. The earth under foot is dry and powdery, and hot as flour just ground, while the rocks are so hot that the hands cannot be borne upon them. The parade is always hot at midday, and the story told of a dog that ran on three legs across it, barking with pain at every step, may be correct, though I have never seen it tried.

This post, although not the most southerly, is the hottest military post in the United States; the highest temperature recorded in our books since 1850, when the post was established, is 119°, observed at 2.25 p. m., June 16, 1859. A temperature of 100° may exist at Fort Yuma for weeks in succession, and there will be no additional cases of sickness in consequence.

The dress must be of the lightest, suitable to the temperature. The lightest woolen fabrics that are made should be worn next to the skin, or, if woolen is not borne well, cotton. The dress of the natives is very simple. The heavily fringed kilt, made of the bark of the cottonwood, or woolen yarn, in two divisions which hardly come together at the hips, and worn about the loins, is the fashion which obtains among the Yuma women, while the men of this tribe encumber themselves with about two yards of muslin, and a belt or strap.

Ice is never seen, not even on the coldest day in winter. I do not think it would be desirable

to have the article in summer if it could be furnished. The water we drink is relatively cool at 60°
to 75°, and is very refreshing.

We have none of the malarial diseases incident to the cities of the Gulf of Mexico, or along
the eastern seaboard. The heat depresses the already debilitated, and we miss the tonic effect of
cold weather; but those who come here in good health, and observe the ordinary rules for preserving it, will have nothing to fear from the high temperature.

The influence of the great "Colorado Desert" on the climate is more or less felt in all the
counties comprising the southern half of the State. The desert is an immense oven, where a hot
and rarefied air is generated, which rages in hot blasts from time to time over these counties. The
rain which waters the northern portion of Mexico, does not travel across this desert, the moisture
being taken up by the hot, dry air. These dry and desiccating currents exhaust also the moisture
which comes down from the north in winter, so that there is a large rainless area on the southern
border of the State, which is year after year robbed of its moisture by the proximity of this desert.
Geologists affirm that at one time the greater part of this desert was covered by the waters of the
Gulf of California, and the theory is maintained that if the greater part were again submerged,
hot winds would cease to rage over these southern counties, and as much rain would fall there as
on the northern part of the State. The climate would then become cooler and more equable.
Much of the land comprising the desert has been found to be below the level of the low tides of the
Gulf, and practical engineers maintain that, at comparatively small expense, this great desert
furnace can be cooled by covering it with water. The theory is, that were the desert a sea it would
send up a column of atmosphere charged with moisture, which meeting the colder currents from
the ocean, would precipitate frequent showers, and thus change large tracts of the country from
barrenness to fertility.

The nearest city is San Diego, Cal., two hundred miles distant, nearly due west, across the
great Colorado Desert.

The town of Yuma, numbering one thousand three hundred inhabitants, chiefly Mexicans,
occupies the left bank of the Colorado, on the lower point of land at the junction of the Gila with
it, and directly opposite the fort. All freights for the supply of troops, and merchandise for the
inhabitants of Arizona, are shipped by steamer from San Francisco to the mouth of the Colorado,
where it is transshipped on barges and steamers of light draught to Yuma, whence it is distributed
to all parts of the Territory.

The usual mode of entrance for travelers is also by this route. The commodious steamships
engaged in the trade, and the pleasure and comfort of the sea voyage, are so much to be preferred
to the overland desert trip, that few select the latter route. Passengers and freight are landed at
Yuma in fourteen days from date of sailing from San Francisco. By steamer to San Diego, and
stage thence to Yuma, the journey may be accomplished in half the time.

Three mails are received weekly from the East by way of San Francisco and San Diego; three
weekly from Tucson and the southern portion of the Territory, and two from Prescott, the headquarters of the department.

The completion of the United States military telegraph marks an epoch in this section of the
country. Fort Yuma is not only in electric connection with the outside world, but also with the
more important towns of Arizona. Business in all departments of the service is conducted with a
dispatch, and movements against Indians can be controlled with a precision that could not be
effected under the old *régime*.

The limits of the reservation and the boundaries of the same were restricted in January, 1867,
and declared to be as follows:

*Reserve on the north side of the river.*—On the north by an east and west line through a point
three miles due north of the flag-staff; on the west by a north and south line through a point one
mile due west from the flag-staff; on the east and south by the left bank of the Colorado River.

*Reserve on the south side of the Colorado.*—So much of the land between the river and the line
of the "Gadsden Purchase" as lies between two north and south lines, one drawn through a point
passing through the middle of the mouth of a slough running into the river on the north side,
and just below the depot; and one passing through a point equidistant from the east wall of the

quartermaster's depot and the mast of the ferry on the south side of the river; and, in addition thereto, so much of the same tract bordering on the south bank of the Colorado, next below its confluence with the Gila, as is comprised between the Colorado and a line commencing at a point on the south bank of the river, one hundred feet below the line of the cable of the ferry, and running due south three hundred feet, and thence due east to the Gila River.

Before reaching the fort the road leads the traveler through a long avenue, shaded by young cottonwoods and mesquite, with an impenetrable growth of arrow-bush and cane; at length he arrives at the bend of the river, and the water no longer bears the *colorado* or ruddy tint which gives it its name, but appears of a muddy color, the red being due to reflected light. What appeared in the distance to be a heavy fortification resolves itself into a collection of substantial adobe houses, inclosed by deep verandas, which shut out every direct ray of sunlight, and exhibit an air of privacy unsurpassed by the surroundings of a Mormon harem. Shade-trees are an impossibility, and "grassed surfaces" unknown. Paragraphs 42 and 43, Revised Regulations, do not apply to Fort Yuma.

Leaving the flat land along the river, the rocky hill toward the fort is ascended by an easy winding roadway, cut out of the side of the bluff, and the hollow square called the parade is reached. Not one single blade of grass, or vine, or tree, worthy of the name, is seen; all is rock and the *débris* of rock, and in many places the abraded faces of the crumbling feldspathic granite form the substantial but gritty pathway.

All the buildings at the post are of sun-dried brick, and neatly plastered within and without. They are constructed one story high, with lofty ceilings, large rooms, with double sash doors extending from floors nearly to ceiling, and affording the freest ventilation. The roofs are made double like the walls, inclosing an air-chamber, and over all a metal sheathing. Each house is surrounded on all sides by a veranda.

The claim of Yuma to the designation of fort rests on certain unpretentious intrenchments scattered along the slopes of the bluff, which command the river and the bottom-lands adjacent; they are not visible from the river, and the spectator is not aware of their existence until he steps to the edge of the bluff and looks down upon their gabion revetments. They were constructed for barbette guns, but are now dismantled.

This not being a point for offensive operations, the garrison is small and chiefly engaged in guard duty at the large quartermaster's depot across the river, and in escorting supply trains to the interior of Arizona.

The parade is a stony lawn—the rocky hill roughly dressed and made smooth by filling in with fine stone, and inclosing a space two hundred by six hundred feet in extent, with a gentle slope toward the river. This hill consists of a mass of granite, which rises abruptly from the bed of the river, runs northwest, and terminates as abruptly as it commences about one thousand yards from the bank.

The arrangement of the post is shown in Figure 76.

Three sets of company quarters are located on the northeastern side of the parade. Each set comprises a barrack-building, 78 by 68 feet, and in rear of it, twelve feet distant, a kitchen 20 feet square, having a small store-room adjoining. Like all the buildings at the post, the walls are three feet thick, being composed of double adobe walls, with a space between, and all the rooms are 12 feet high from floor to ceiling.

The barrack-building is surrounded on all sides by a veranda 12 feet wide, and is divided into a dormitory, mess-room, orderly's room, and store-room. The dormitory occupies the front of the building, is 72 by 39 feet, lighted by eight large windows, and warmed by two fire-places, one at each end. It gives an air-space of seven hundred cubic feet per man, of average occupancy. The mess-room is in rear of the dormitory, and is 51 by 21 feet; the orderly's room and the store-room adjoin one end of the mess-room, and are each 20 by 10 feet, the orderly's room being at the rear and opening upon the rear veranda. The dormitories are furnished with iron single bedsteads, the kitchens with excellent stoves and ranges, and all the rooms with furniture and fixtures sufficient to make them comfortable and convenient. No provision has been made for wash-rooms or bath-rooms for the men; during the summer, however, the men usually bathe in the river every

71 M P

evening about sundown. The privies are situated in rear of each set of quarters, distant about one hundred feet, and consist simply of covered trenches. They are covered from time to time with dry earth or lime. Only two of the above-described sets of quarters are occupied by troops at present; the third set is used as a quartermaster's and commissary's store-room, and a medical purveying sub-depot.

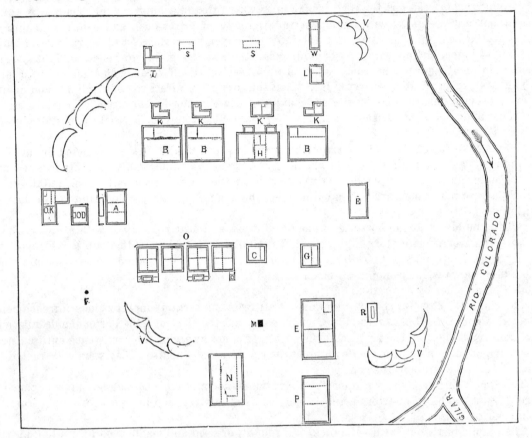

Figure 76—Scale, 160 feet to 1 inch.

A, commanding officer's quarters; B, company quarters; C, quartermaster and adjutant's offices; E, storehouses; F, flag-staff; G, guard-house; H, hospital; K, kitchen; L, ordnance office; MN, corral; O, officers' quarters; OD, dining-room; OK, kitchen; P, shops; R, reservoir; S, sinks; T, sutler's store; V, bastions; W, bakery.

The quarters for laundresses and married soldiers consist of adobe huts, arranged about the garrison without regard to system. They are unworthy the name of buildings, and utterly unfit for the purposes for which they are used. Three of the laundresses have been assigned quarters in the "officers' row," because no suitable buildings could be found anywhere else about the post.

The commanding officer's set of quarters is an isolated building, and forms the northwest boundary of the parade. Its dimensions are 51 feet front by 33 feet deep. It contains four rooms, each 15 by 13 feet, two of them on each side of a hall 12 feet wide, which runs through the center of the house. The building is entirely surrounded by a veranda 12 feet wide, is well ventilated and commodious. A kitchen 20 feet square is separated from the rear of the house, by the veranda, with which it communicates.

The other officers' quarters form the southwestern boundary of the parade, and consist of one double house, 33 feet front, by 53 feet deep, divided by a partition running lengthwise from front to rear, into two sets of three rooms each. Separated from the rear of this building by the veranda, 12 feet wide, is a building 20 by 32 feet, divided into two kitchens. This building was intended for captains' quarters. The quarters for lieutenants are three double houses, each 40 feet front by

36 feet deep, divided into two sets of two rooms each, with a building containing two kitchens in the rear. Each house is surrounded by a veranda, and adjacent houses have their verandas meet, so that the inmates may pass from one house to another without exposing themselves to the sun. The addition of Venetian blinds to each window and door would afford more privacy than can now be obtained, owing to the close proximity to each other of the officers' quarters, and the necessity of keeping windows and doors open during the hot weather.

The adjutant's office is a commodious, well-constructed building, situated on a line with the officers' quarters, and 50 feet from the lower set. The dimensions are 37 by 20 feet. A compartment has been partitioned off, which is used as a post library. The building is surrounded on all sides by a veranda 12 feet wide.

The guard-house is 25 feet front by 37 feet deep, and situated on a line with the officers' quarters, at the extreme southern corner of the parade. It has a basement under it, a portion of which has been partitioned off into four cells, each 5 by 9 feet, 6 feet in height. These cells are badly ventilated, and have no means of warming in winter; they are not floored, and are therefore kept clean with difficulty. A room over the cells, 15 by 12 feet, is used as a general prison-room, is deficient in ventilation, and altogether too small for the purpose for which it is used. From twelve to twenty persons lie huddled together on the floor every night; and if there were thirty, the probability is that they would still be crowded into the same space. During the hot weather, all well-behaved persons are allowed to sleep outside and around the guard-house. The building was evidently constructed to meet the wants of a two-company post, and as such, would fairly answer the purpose, but during the past two years it has been designated as a place of confinement for military prisoners throughout the Territory. It is totally unfitted for the purpose for which it has been set apart, and is always overcrowded.

The post-hospital is located on a line with and between the company quarters. It is a one-story building, 80 feet front by 35 feet deep. At one end is a ward, 30 by 29 feet; at the other end is another ward, 20 by 29 feet; between them, in front, is the dispensary, 22 by 16 feet, and in rear of it two rooms of equal size, the steward's room and a storeroom. The bath-room is a small wing resting chiefly against the rear of the large ward; its dimensions are 10 by 8 feet. It is provided with a bath-tub and wash-sink, has a good supply of water, but, like the hospital, is very much out of repair. A convenient dead-house, 10 by 8 feet, adjoins the rear of the smaller ward. These two rooms are really portions of the rear veranda, inclosed. The kitchen, a building 20 feet square, stands twenty feet in rear of the rear veranda of the hospital. The hospital sink is three hundred feet in rear of the building. Like the other sinks, it is a large covered trench, and serves the purpose of a water-closet and urinal. Patients unable to leave the ward make use of the close-stool and earth-closet.

The large ward contains ten beds, allowing an average air-space of 1,080 cubic feet to each. The small ward contains six beds, giving 1,200 cubic feet of air-space per bed. The wards are each warmed by a large fire-place, and lighted by two large windows in each of three sides. These windows extend from floor to ceiling; ample ventilation is effected by means of these fire-places and windows. Iron bedsteads of the new pattern, furnished with straw ticks, mattresses, and the usual bed-linen, one large table on which food is served to patients, chairs and bedside-tables, constitute the furniture.

Since its erection in 1854, very little has been done in the way of repairs; it is consequently, so far as general appearance is concerned, the most unsightly building at the post. Several square yards of plastering were blown down in 1869, and have never been renewed. The floor is nearly worn through; the window-frames and door-frames have become so warped by the climate, that a space of half an inch is left open everywhere; this latter defect is of little moment during the summer, but in cold weather when it becomes necessary to warm the wards, it is found impossible to do so by the fire-places, the only means of heating at the post. It is true, ventilation is thus provided, and it is, perhaps, better that the building should remain as it is until a proper system of ridge-ventilation can be established. The roof leaks badly, and during the heavy rain-storm of July, 1873, it was necessary to keep the patients and beds moving from one part of the ward to another, to prevent their being soaked.

The supply of water, both for drinking and culinary purposes, is abundant. It is obtained from the Colorado River, and forced by a steam-pump into a tank having a capacity of twenty-five hundred gallons. The tank is located on a knoll of the bluff, high enough to give a fall for the supply of every building at the garrison. Each set of officers' quarters is provided with a bath-room and bath-tub. Except during the high stage of the Gila, the water is always "soft" for washing purposes. It matters not how muddy it may be, no better water could be desired for bathing; when, however, the Gila is in force and commingles its waters with the Colorado, a difference is noted, it becomes brackish and "hard." Water for drinking and cooking is retained in "ollas," in which it settles rapidly, and is kept comparatively cool (at 70°) during the hottest day. The best "ollas" are made by the "Pimos," and are obtained from Tuscon; those made by the "Yumas" are of an inferior quality, and become impervious in a short time.

*Meteorological report, Fort Yuma, Cal., 1870–'74.*

| Months. | 1870–'71. Temperature. Mean. | Max. | Min. | Rain-fall in inches. | 1871–'72. Temperature. Mean. | Max. | Min. | Rain-fall in inches. | 1872–'73. Temperature. Mean. | Max. | Min. | Rain-fall in inches. | 1873–'74. Temperature. Mean. | Max. | Min. | Rain-fall in inches. |
|---|---|---|---|---|---|---|---|---|---|---|---|---|---|---|---|---|
| | ° | ° | ° | | ° | ° | ° | | ° | ° | ° | | ° | ° | ° | |
| July | 98.53 | 115 | 83 | 0.60 | 96.16 | 114 | 72* | 0.00 | 91.53 | 108* | 71* | 0.00 | 93.58 | 112* | 69* | 0.00 |
| August | 91.03 | 110 | 76 | 1.15 | 96.60 | 112 | 77* | 0.25 | 89.96 | 109* | 60* | 2.38 | 88.17 | 106* | 71* | 1.60 |
| September | 87.07 | 111 | 70 | 0.00 | 90.67 | 109 | 61* | 0.24 | 82.89 | 102* | 60* | 0.06 | 84.81 | 104* | 59* | 0.00 |
| October | 67.24 | 103 | 35 | 0.60 | 77.46 | 98 | 53* | 0.00 | 74.98 | 98* | 46* | 0.00 | 72.86 | 100* | 48* | 0.00 |
| November | 60.69 | 84 | 34 | 0.00 | 62.95 | 83 | 43* | 0.00 | 60.36 | 80* | 34* | 0.00 | 66.14 | 86* | 46* | 0.00 |
| December | 53.29 | 80 | 30* | 0.00 | 61.56 | 79 | 39* | 0.00 | 57.87 | 79* | 38* | 0.00 | 53.25 | 68* | 39* | 0.64 |
| January | 59.83 | 81 | 34* | 0.00 | 57.29 | 77 | 29* | 0.00 | 57.78 | 80* | 37* | 0.00 | 56.14 | 72* | 37* | 0.55 |
| February | 58.83 | 79 | 41* | 0.08 | 62.96 | 81 | 41* | 0.24 | 55.44 | 76* | 30* | 0.00 | 53.48 | 70* | 35* | 0.85 |
| March | 67.26 | 85 | 46* | 0.00 | 64.91 | 85* | 42* | 0.00 | 69.33 | 92* | 42* | 0.90 | 59.21 | 82* | 40* | 0.20 |
| April | 71.77 | 95 | 45* | 0.00 | 68.08 | 98* | 42* | 0.00 | 70.47 | 100* | 42* | 0.00 | 69.24 | 95* | 45* | 0.00 |
| May | 81.35 | 107 | 52‛ | 0.00 | 82.33 | 108* | 51* | 0.00 | 77.43 | 98* | 54* | 0.00 | 79.96 | 102* | 50* | 0.00 |
| June | 92.32 | 111 | 63* | 0.00 | 88.33 | 110* | 61* | 0.05 | 87.91 | 112* | 60* | 0.00 | 88.71 | 108* | 66* | 0.00 |
| For the year | 74.10 | 115 | 30* | 2.71 | 75.77 | 114 | 29* | 0.78 | 72.99 | 112* | 30* | 3.34 | 72.14 | 112* | 35* | 3.84 |

* These observations are made with self-registering thermometers. The mean is from the standard thermometer.

*Consolidated sick-report, Fort Yuma, Cal., 1870–'74.*

| Year | 1870–'71. | | 1871–'72. | | 1872–'73. | | 1873–'74. | |
|---|---|---|---|---|---|---|---|---|
| Mean strength. { Officers | 3 | | 4 | | 5 | | 5 | |
| { Enlisted men | 82 | | 68 | | 57 | | 112 | |
| Diseases. | Cases. | Deaths. | Cases. | Deaths. | Cases. | Deaths. | Cases. | Deaths. |
| GENERAL DISEASES, A. | | | | | | | | |
| Remittent fever | 1 | 1 | 2 | | 6 | | | |
| Intermittent fever | 9 | | 10 | | 9 | | 9 | |
| Diphtheria | 1 | | | | | | | |
| Other diseases of this group | | | 2 | | 3 | | 2 | |
| GENERAL DISEASES, B. | | | | | | | | |
| Rheumatism | 6 | | 4 | | 4 | | 11 | |
| Syphilis | 17 | | 15 | | 19 | | 14 | |
| Consumption | 1 | 1 | 2 | 1 | 3 | 1 | | |
| Other diseases of this group | | | 4 | | 1 | | | |
| LOCAL DISEASES. | | | | | | | | |
| Catarrh and bronchitis | 17 | | 8 | | 13 | | 28 | |
| Pneumonia | 1 | 1 | 1 | | | | | |
| Diarrhœa and dysentery | 15 | | 24 | | 24 | | 34 | |
| Gonorrhœa | 8 | | 6 | | 5 | | 10 | |
| Other local diseases | 72 | | 36 | 1 | 41 | | 52 | 2 |
| Alcoholism | 7 | | 7 | | 2 | | 10 | |
| Total disease | 155 | 3 | 121 | 2 | 130 | 1 | 170 | 2 |
| VIOLENT DISEASES AND DEATHS. | | | | | | | | |
| Gunshot wounds | 1 | | 2 | | 1 | | | 1 |
| Drowning | | | | | | | | 1 |
| Other accidents and injuries | 19 | | 29 | | 20 | | 14 | |
| Homicide | | | | | | 1 | | 1 |
| Total violence | 20 | | 31 | | 21 | 1 | 14 | 2 |

# INDEX OF POSTS DESCRIBED.

O

CIRCULAR No. 9.

WAR DEPARTMENT,
SURGEON GENERAL'S OFFICE,
WASHINGTON, MARCH 1, 1877.

A

# REPORT TO THE SURGEON GENERAL

ON THE

# TRANSPORT OF SICK AND WOUNDED

BY

# PACK ANIMALS.

BY GEORGE A. OTIS,
ASSISTANT SURGEON, U. S. ARMY.

WASHINGTON:
GOVERNMENT PRINTING OFFICE.
1877.

# CIRCULAR No. 9.

WAR DEPARTMENT,

Surgeon General's Office,

*Washington, March 1, 1877.*

With the approval of the Honorable Secretary of War, the following Report, upon the different modes of transporting sick and wounded men in localities inaccessible to wheeled vehicles, embodying the experience of many years and various campaigns, is published for the information of the Medical Officers of the Army.

JOSEPH K. BARNES,

*Surgeon General U. S. A.*

# INDICATION OF CONTENTS.

A

# REPORT TO THE SURGEON GENERAL

ON THE

# TRANSPORT OF SICK AND WOUNDED

BY

# PACK ANIMALS.

---

BY

**GEORGE A. OTIS,**
ASSISTANT SURGEON, U. S. ARMY.

---

GENERAL: The subject of the transport of sick and wounded by pack animals has latterly attracted much attention in the army. For several years, the contests with Indian savages in which the troops have engaged have been of unusual magnitude and difficulty; the expeditions have frequently penetrated into unexplored regions, and the engagements have taken place in situations altogether inaccessible to wheeled vehicles. The conditions of such warfare entail the necessity of modifying the arrangements for providing surgical assistance for the wounded or disabled. The ambulance equipment must be able to keep up with the troops, and not to interfere with their rapid movements; must provide the essentials of surgical aid far from a base of supply; and often improvise for the comfort of the wounded appliances that cannot possibly be transported. Under these circumstances, officers have recalled the expedients of the hardy explorers of the frontiers, and have endeavored to improve them or to adapt them to unexpected exigencies; and a number of interesting reports on the various devices employed have been transmitted to your office. In accordance with your instructions to collect and arrange these documents, and to combine them with such other information on the subject as may appear to be of interest, I have had the honor to prepare this report.

When it is recollected that it was not until the close of the last century that any systematic ambulance service was adopted in civilized armies, and only within twenty years that the completeness of organization now attained in some European armies has been acquired; and when consideration is given to the alterations that have taken place in these periods in the destructive power of fire-arms, the increased proportion of severe wounds, the celerity in movements and combination of troops, it seems not remarkable that frequent revision of ambulance *matériel* and administration should be required. There was never a time when more attention was paid than at present to the improvement of the destructive implements of war, and the most effective methods of employing

1

them,[1] and it is assuredly of pressing necessity that corresponding efforts should be made for the abridgment or mitigation of the sufferings and preservation of the lives of those exposed to such formidable means of aggression. For the interests of the sick and wounded are not alone involved in the efficiency with which the ambulance service is performed. The strategic plans of the commander are promoted or thwarted according as the work is done well or ill; and, above all, the spirit of the soldiers, their tone of feeling and confidence in time of danger, is much affected by their estimate of the provision made for their succor, should they be disabled in action. A veteran soldier, Marshal Bugeaud, after his African victories, declared that "the courage of the French troops would not perhaps have sufficed for the conquest of Algeria, if we had not been able to save the sick and wounded from the Arabs." It is not to be supposed that any neglect in providing for the comfort of sick and wounded men will be without depressing influence on the *morale* of troops of our army employed in Indian hostilities, and inspired with a traditional dread of the tortures that await them should they fall captives to their savage opponents.

The introduction of measures tending to the establishment of an ambulance system in the United States Army is of recent date;[2] yet it has been acknowledged by the most competent foreign authorities,[3] that toward the close of the late war our sanitary field service had attained a thorough organization; and, particularly, that the difficult problem of the speedy and comfortable transport of the wounded from the battle-fields had been dealt with creditably, in the face of great obstacles. It would be deplorable should the efficiency of our ambulance service even relatively retrograde; but it is not to be expected that it can be kept up to the standard attained by the great military powers without constant efforts to improve the equipment, both in providing against the causes of failure revealed by experience, and by devising expedients for unusual exigencies.

Fortunately, progress in the improvement of the equipment provided for the ambulance[4] service tends to simplicity rather than complexity. The costliness of maintaining, in time of peace, establishments required only in time of war, is an argument often urged against all branches of the military service, which, whatever its relevancy to armaments of war in general, has little validity as applied to the ambulance service. The greater part of its material can be utilized in time of peace; its necessary outfit need not be large or extravagantly expensive. But it is of the last importance, as long as the necessity of standing armies is accepted, that the sanitary appliances furnished should be the best of their kind, that, when an emergency arises, there may not be a lavish outlay for unserviceable material, nor avoidable suffering from the want of suitable equipment. The material required in a complete system of army hospital transport may be classified as: 1, stretchers or litters[5] carried by men; 2, litters wheeled by men; 3, conveyances borne by animals (litters, cacolets); 4, conveyances drawn by animals (ambulance wagons). Moreover, although its appliances need not be kept on hand, there should be a matured system for the transport of sick and wounded by railway and by water, defining all details, that, in view of an impending war, the requisite resources may be promptly accumulated. When more attention has been

---

[1] Although, in the late war, the troops were armed, for the most part, with muzzle-loading muskets and smooth-bore cannon, our present inferiority in ordnance is not willingly conceded; but it is held that, theoretically at least, our improvements in gunnery keep pace with those of other nations.

[2] During the war of the first French republic, in 1796, LARREY and PERCY introduced plans for providing primary surgical aid for those wounded in battle, styled by one *ambulance volante*, and by the other *chirurgie de bataille*. As M. LEGOUEST remarks (*Traité de Chir. d'Armée*, 1863, p. 979), they were the first organizers of the ambulance systems now employed, with the modifications suggested by time and experience, in all civilized armies. In the United States, while efficient measures of giving surgical help to the combatants were not altogether neglected in the War of 1812, and the campaigns in Florida and Mexico, the first attempt to introduce a regular ambulance system dates from the assembling of a Board convened October 18, 1859. In March, 1864, Congress enacted a bill for the uniform ambulance system for the armies then in the field.

[3] LONGMORE (T.) (*Encyc. Britan.*, 9th ed., 1875, Vol. I, p. 665): "In the armies of the United States during the late great civil war, the ambulance system attained a very complete organization." The two-horse "Wheeling" ambulance wagon may be regarded as a model on which most of the recent attempts to devise an improved form of ambulance vehicle have been based. The HALSTEAD folding stretcher has been pronounced by Professor GURLT, of Berlin, an almost ideal stretcher, "if it only had a head-rest." HARRIS's method of suspending litters by rubber rings; SMITH's and HODGEN's wire-suspension splints, and many minor appliances devised in this country for the improvement of the field sanitary service, have been commended and adopted abroad.

[4] Ambulance is a term first applied to the French "ambulance" (*hôpital ambulant*), derived from the Latin *ambulare*, to move from place to place. As defined by LITTRÉ (*Dict. de la Langue Française*, 1873, P. I, p. 125), they are "temporary hospital establishments, organized near the divisions of an army, to follow their movements and to assure early succor to the wounded." Surgeon-General LONGMORE remarks (*Encyc. Britan.*, 9th ed., 1875, T. I, p. 665) that "the term is not unfrequently misapplied in common speech in England to the *ambulance wagons* or other conveyances by which the wounded are carried from the field to the ambulances hospitals;" and this abuse of the term is almost universal in the United States.

[5] Litter, *Lectica* (from *lectus*, bed), according to REE's Cyclopædia, Vol. XXII, a kind of vehicle borne upon shafts, anciently esteemed the most easy and genteel way of carriage. PLINY calls the litter the traveller's chamber. It was much in use among the Romans, among whom it was borne by slaves kept for that purpose; as it still continues to be in the East, where it is called a *palanquin*. The invention of litters, according to CICERO, was owing to the kings of Bithynia. In the time of TIBERIUS they were become very frequent at Rome, as appears from SENECA. Horse-litters were much used in Europe prior to the introduction of coaches.

paid to the subject, it is not improbable that the hand-stretcher[1] (*brancard, Tragebahre*) may be so perfected as to serve as the uniform means of support in almost all military exigencies, for patients who require transport in a recumbent position. Eventually, it will probably be so constructed as to answer not only as a litter to be carried by men, but as the permanent couch for the soldier from the moment he is disabled until he reaches a fixed hospital, having such adjustments that it may be placed on wheels and drawn by men, or be carried by pack-animals,[2] or laid on springs or swung in special ambulance wagons, supply wagons, or other wheeled vehicles drawn by animals, or transported by rail or on water. The difficulty of adapting any appliance to various uses without sacrificing some things desirable in each, is obvious; but the importance, in army organization, of uniformity in equipment is so imperious that I cannot doubt that, ultimately, the hand-stretcher, so adjusted as to be readily combined with the various means of transport, will come to be regarded as an implement as essential in the sanitary outfit as the musket and spade in military operations. Notwithstanding the many improvements of late years, the hospital transport service is still generally esteemed the least perfected of any branch of the military organization for campaigning.[3] And it must be admitted that the imperfect state of the arrangements for this service becomes painfully apparent when troops are employed remote from railway or water transportation, and especially when they are serving in regions impracticable for wheeled vehicles, where the sick and wounded must be *carried*, either by men or quadrupeds.

Various beasts of burthen have been used for transporting disabled men, and, in a systematic disquisition on the subject, it would be proper to relate how each has been found useful under certain circumstances, and to describe the conveyances most appropriate for them to carry. But, in our army, mules and horses are exclusively employed as pack-animals;[4] and attention may be here restricted to the conveyance of disabled men by them. The special purpose of this report is to record recent observations of medical officers on the practical working of horse and mule litters over considerable distances in difficult country; but, incidentally, former experiences on the subject will be recalled, the methods practised in other armies adverted to, and such reference made, as space will admit, to the utilization of other quadrupeds for sick transport, to different plans of packing, and to other information having a practical bearing on the subject.

In the Revolutionary War, and in the war with the mother country in 1812–13, our armies were unprovided with any ambulance system.[5] During the hostilities against the Seminole Indians, in Florida, however, in 1835–38, it appears that the wounded were methodically transported for long distances, by special ambulance wagons or by horse-litters, and that the medical director of the troops, the now venerable Brigadier-General Richard S. Satterlee, organized the *personnel* as well as the *matériel* of the medical field-service as systematically and effectively as the desultory

---

[1] *Stretchers* appear to derive their name, as Professor LONGMORE remarks (*op. cit.*, p. 115) "from the fact of the sustaining canvas being stretched within a frame." *Brancard*, the French term, is derived from the two poles (*branches*) between which the supporting canvas is held. This is M. LITTRÉ's etymology; and Baron PERCY states that the word was formerly written *branchard*. *Tragebahre*, the German term, is derived from *tragen* (to carry), and *Bahre*, from the Anglo-Saxon *baer*, English *bier*.

[2] A plan by which patients supported on hand-stretchers were successfully carried on the backs of the trained mules the French took with them to Mexico, in 1864, will be hereafter described.

[3] M. L. LEGOUEST, professor of surgery at Val-de-Grace, in the edition of his classic *Traité de Chirurgie d'Armée*, published after his experience in the Franco-German War of 1870–71, concludes that: "the removal of the wounded from the battle-field and their transport to the ambulance stations is the most defective part of the army medical field service" (*op. cit.*, 6d. 1872, p. 779). Surgeon-General T. LONGMORE, professor of surgery at the army medical school at Netley, declares (*Treatise of the Transport of Sick and Wounded Troops*, 1869, p. 1) that "the established arrangements for this service are generally regarded . . . as the most defective part of military organization, as they are certainly of the medical departmental organization in armies."

[4] Horses, mules, asses, oxen, camels, llamas, and elephants have been used for transporting wounded. The experiment of using camels as a means of transport in the desert regions of Texas and New Mexico, introduced, I believe, through the efforts of the Egyptian traveller G. R. GLIDDON and of Colonel G. H. CROSMAN, Assistant Quartermaster General, was in a fair way of proving a valuable addition to the means of transport in our army. The animals thrived and multiplied, and rendered good service. At the outbreak of the late war the herds were dispersed. It has been stated, but I am unable to verify the report, that, about this time, most of these animals were sold to circus managers or farmers by persons responsible for public property. There were still one or two camels rendering good services at posts in Arizona as late as 1870. No attempt to renew the promising experiment of acclimating the camel and employing it for army transport has been made since the war.

[5] "The origin of the ambulance system which now prevails in all civilized armies, though variously modified among them in particular details, only dates from the last decade of the last century" (LONGMORE, *Encyc. Britan.*, 9th ed., 1875, Vol. I, p. 665). Before then, wounded soldiers were either carried to the rear by comrades, or were left exposed and unheeded until the fighting was over. Surgical assistance often reached the field only on the day after the battle or even later, when it was of no avail to a large proportion of the wounded. It was in 1796, during the Italian campaigns (*Lodi, Arcola, Rivoli*), that the illustrious LARREY organized his system of *ambulance volantes*, and PERCY soon afterward introduced a somewhat similar establishment, with a corps of *brancardiers* or stretcher-bearers (*Mém. de Chir. Mil. et Campagnes* de D. J. LARREY, 1812, T. I, p. 150). NAPOLEON I warmly sustained LARREY in his endeavors to perfect the new system of immediate aid to the wounded in battle. In like manner, during the late war in this country, General GRANT showed a keen solicitude in the safe transport of the wounded, always maintaining intimate relations with the medical officer directing that service, and promoting his plans. Before Petersburg he personally supervised experiments with the methods proposed by LANGER and others for fitting up the emptied carriages of the supply train for the comfortable removal of the sick and wounded.

nature of the campaign would allow.   In a report to the Surgeon General, dated Fort Brook, Tampa Bay, Florida, January 5, 1838, Dr. Satterlee described the measures taken for the aid of the wounded after the engagement at O-kee-cho-bee:[1]

"Sir: I have the honor to inform you that the brigade to which I am attached as Medical Director has had a very severe engagement with the Mickasuckie and Seminole Indians, about one hundred and fifty miles from this place, near a lake called O-kee-cho-bee; it took place on the twenty-fifth ultimo, and lasted nearly two hours, and resulted in the total defeat of the Indians, but with great loss to our troops in killed and wounded.[1]   Under the circumstances, as we had no permanent hospital nearer than this, and as the troops must, from the nature of the country, retire from it long before the wounded could recover, I deemed it proper to bring them immediately to this place.   I arrived with them last evening, and have now the satisfaction to say that they are in comfortable quarters.   I found the ambulances very serviceable, but as some of the wounded could not be transported in them on account of the roughness of the road, between thirty and forty of them were brought, a part of the way, on litters between two horses.   This is a very comfortable means of transportation, but difficult on account of the number of men and horses required.   I have requested the quartermaster to have twenty litters constructed here, except the poles, which I think can be obtained in the woods.   We were obliged to use blankets, and raw-hides of the cattle which we found on our way, but the length of time taken to construct them, together with the want of proper tools, and at a time when the medical officers with me (Assistant Surgeons McLaren and Simpson), as well as myself, were fully occupied night and day with the wounded, it was found very difficult to construct them; this is the reason why I wish them to be on hand and ready for any emergency that may occur.   *   *"

In the war with Mexico, the wounded were transported mainly in wheeled vehicles; but Colonel G. E. Cooper has informed me of one instance, at least, in which a two-horse litter was used for sick-transport for a long distance.[2]  This litter, and those used by Medical Director Satterlee are not specifically described; but were probably similar to that referred to and figured by Inspector General R. B. Marcy, in his instructive handbook for travellers on overland expeditions to the Pacific coast.[3]  This is a very ancient form of litter, often employed prior to the introduction of coaches, in the XVI century, for conveying people

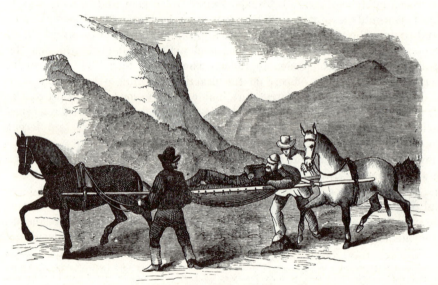

FIG. 1.—Two-horse litter.  [After Marcy.]

of consequence, or for the carriage of sick persons.   I take the liberty of copying his illustration of the mode of improvising this appliance and adapting it to the exigencies of frontier life.

"Should a party travelling with pack-animals, and without ambulances or wagons, have one of its members wounded or taken so sick as to be unable to walk or ride on horseback, a litter may be constructed by taking two poles about twenty feet in length, uniting them by two sticks three feet long lashed across the centre at six feet apart, and stretching a piece of stout canvas, a blanket, or hide between them to form the bed.   Two steady horses or mules are then selected, placed between the poles in the front and rear of the litter, and the ends of the poles made fast to the sides of the animals either by attachment to the stirrups or to the ends of straps secured over their backs.   The patient may then be placed upon the litter, and is ready for the march.   The elasticity of the long poles gives an easy motion to the conveyance and makes this method of locomotion much more comfortable than might be expected."—[The Prairie Traveler, p. 150.]

[1] After the engagement at O-kee-cho-bee, December 25, 1837, the commanding officer, Colonel ZACHARY TAYLOR, in his official report, referred "with the most pleasing and grateful recollections" to "the attention and ability displayed by Surgeon SATTERLEE, Medical Director," and his assistants, "in ministering to the wounded," as well as to "their uniform kindness to them on all occasions."

[2] "I have never seen a horse-litter used for transporting sick or wounded, save in one instance, which was in the case of an officer who was carried from the city of Mexico to Vera Cruz in one; and of this I have but little recollection, except that there were two horses—one in the front of the litter and the other behind it,—and that the litter was supported by shafts extending from the front and rear, to which the horses or mules were harnessed. The officer was, if my memory fails me not, Capt. WALKER, 6th U. S. Infantry.   Not having had anything to do with the getting up of the litter, and having seen it but once as it passed me on the road, I cannot give any reliable description of its construction."—Extract from a letter of Dr. COOPER dated Point San José, California, January 20, 1877.

[3] The Prairie Traveler, a Handbook for Overland Expeditions, etc.  By RANDOLPH B. MARCY, Captain, U. S. Army, New York, 1859, p. 150.

Dr. Satterlee's report from Florida is the earliest mention I have found of any scheme of ambulance administration and equipment in the field service of the United States Army.

During the Florida campaign, Captain H. L. Thistle, of the Louisiana volunteers, devised a single-litter horse conveyance, designed for the transport of wounded men through the narrowest defiles, or over the most encumbered and difficult ground. In August, 1836, the inventor proposed to the Quartermaster Department to furnish fifty sets of this appliance, the litter, saddle, and other appurtenances complete, at fifty dollars a set. In January, 1837, this contrivance was patented.[1] The adjacent wood-cut is copied from the drawing filed with the application of the patentee. The specifications are missing. Old officials at the War Department inform me that they remember seeing, in Washington, horses equipped

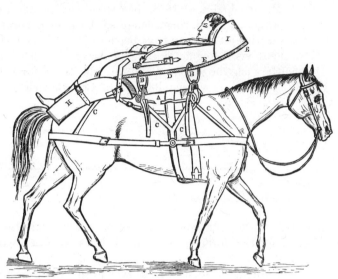

FIG. 2.—THISTLE'S single-litter for horse or mule.

with these litters under inspection; but to what extent, if any, they were issued to the troops, or how far they were tested in actual service, I have been unable to ascertain.[2]

In March, 1852, in an expedition from Fort Conrad, New Mexico, against the Apache Indians, Assistant Surgeon Lyman H. Stone, U. S. A., transported, for a considerable distance, several wounded men on two-horse litters. The question of suitable transport for the sick and wounded appears henceforward to have been a subject of solicitude in the army medical department. In 1858, various models of ambulance wheeled vehicles were constructed, and in October, 1859, a Board was convened to determine their relative merits.[3] The Board soon requested and received authority to examine the whole subject of hospital transport. Besides various recommendations regarding the kind of vehicles suitable for the conveyance of patients and of supplies, the Board advised that *two-horse litters* should be constructed and issued to the frontier posts. This recommendation was approved, and the specifications for the construction of such litters were incorporated in the Revised Regulations for the Army. The form of horse-litter recommended appears to have been derived from experiences in Florida and Mexico. It is illustrated in the next cut (FIG. 3). A supply of such litters were distributed to the western posts. The weight of the sample deposited

[1] Consult *Subject-matter Index of Patents for Inventions, issued by the United States Patent Office*, Washington, 1874, Vol. III, p. 1231, Patent No. 112.

[2] Several officers of distinction who served in the Florida campaign testify to the value of Captain THISTLE'S horse-litter. Major JOHN MOUNTFORT, U. S. Artillery, wrote from New Orleans June 18, 1836: "I have examined your single horse-litter and it affords me great pleasure to say that, for conveying wounded or sick men from the field, it certainly must be considered far superior to the two-horse litter generally used; and as it can always answer for a common pack-saddle, I regard it as all-important for our Indian campaigns, and hope the War Department will adopt it for our service." PERSIFER F. SMITH, in a letter dated June 20, 1836, states: "Captain H. THISTLE, who served the last campaign in Florida in the regiment of Louisiana volunteers, has invented a saddle or litter for sick or wounded men, which, as far as my experience permits me to say, is the best thing of the kind yet proposed. The want of such a conveyance for the wounded embarrasses the movement of all kinds of troops in that country, where there are no fortifications or depots at which they can be left; and the best plan of a campaign may fail of success from the unforeseen accumulation of sick or wounded without the means of their transportation, and in a warfare where they cannot be abandoned. This saddle of Captain THISTLE obviates the difficulty, for it may be adjusted to a pack-saddle tree and the animal be packed when not carrying any one." Dr. C. A. LUZENBERG, writing at the same place and date, took "pleasure in commending the ingenious saddle constructed by Captain THISTLE." He had "enjoyed ample opportunities of examining various contrivances for similar purposes in use in Europe; but none so well calculated to meet the exigencies that always accompanied Indian warfare as the one for which Captain Thistle claims originality."

[3] The Board was convened by S. O. 195, War Department, A. G. O., October 18, 1859. The order states that models of ambulance conveyances having been constructed according to the most approved plans, in accordance with General Order No. 1, A. G. O., 1859, Surgeons C. A. FINLEY, R. S. SATTERLEE, C. S. TRIPLER, J. M. CUYLER, and Assistant Surgeon R. H. COOLIDGE, will assemble at Washington, November 1, 1859, to examine and select the most suitable models, and to make such suggestions as it may deem practical and expedient, and also to perform any other duties connected with the subject that should be referred to it by the War Department. At the fifth meeting, November 5, 1859, the Boards after disapproving of all the model ambulance vehicles presented, submitted a statement to the Secretary of War, J. B. FLOYD, declaring that: "A complete ambulance *system* is very desirable and necessary for the hospital department in the field, and therefore asking that authority be given to the Board to consider and report on an ambulance *system* which will meet the exigencies of the service." At its fifteenth meeting, November 17, 1859, the Board decided that troops in the field should be furnished with ambulance transportation at the rate of forty men per thousand, provision to be made for twenty recumbent patients and twenty in the sitting posture. At the seventeenth meeting, November 19, 1859, the Board passed a resolution for the provision of two-horse litters, which was approved and adopted textually as paragraph 1292 of the Army Regulations (ed. of 1861), as cited above.

in the Army Medical Museum is eighty-eight pounds.[1]  I cannot learn that these litters were used during the late war; but in hostilities with Indians that have occurred since its termination, as in the Modoc campaign of 1873, they were sometimes carried into the field, and, in the last two years, improvised litters, constructed on the same general plan, have been extensively employed; and it is surprising that they have been regarded in some quarters as a novel device.[2]

In the Revised Regulations for the Army of the United States for 1861, Paragraph 1298 reads: "Horse-litters may be prepared and furnished to posts whence they may be required for service on ground not admitting the employment of two-wheeled carriages; said litters to be composed of a

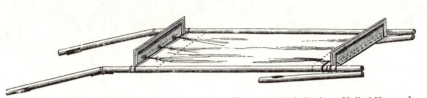

FIG. 3.—United States Army regulation two-horse-litter. [From a sample in the Army Medical Museum.]

canvas bed similar to the present stretcher, and of two poles each sixteen feet long, to be made in sections, with head and foot pieces constructed to act as stretchers to keep the poles apart."  Reports printed further on fully explain the mode of constructing extemporaneously and of using this form of two-horse litter;[3] but before introducing them it is proper, in chronological order, to allude to some other forms of sick-transport on pack-animals.

During the progress of the late war in this country, a number of persons, actuated by motives of patriotism, humanity, or interest, devised and brought to the notice of the War Department forms of conveyance for the sick and wounded, in localities impracticable for wheeled vehicles, that were represented as improvements upon existing patterns.  Several of these were apparently suggested by the descriptions of Delafield[4] and McClellan[5] of the horse litters and cacolets they had observed in the Crimea.  In October, 1861, W. C. H. Waddell forwarded to Secretary Cameron a proposal to construct cacolets and litters for army use, accompanied by drawings (FIGS. 7, 8), copied from Delafield's report, and suggested some trivial modifications.  In November, 1861, Mr. G. Kohler offered to furnish mule-litters and chairs of patterns imitated from those used in the Crimea.  In July, 1862, three hundred of these litters were purchased.  In April, 1862, Surgeon

[1] The litter deposited in the Army Medical Museum is numbered 2457, of Section I. (See *Catalogue of Surgical Section*, 1866, p. 625.) It weighs 88 pounds. The poles are of ash, cylindrical, and 2⅜ inches in diameter and 16 feet long, divided into sections, united by strong wrought-iron strap-hinges. The leading sections are 4½ feet; the middle, 8 feet; and the rear, 3½ feet in length. The side poles are kept apart by traverses of the same calibre, 25 inches in length, with ⅜-inch iron collars, 1¼ inch wide. Each traverse is supplied with 5 iron pins to which the sacking-bottom is corded, and is surmounted by a head- or foot-board of half-inch stuff, 8 inches high, and protected by an iron rim. The collars of the traverses rest against iron shoulders, 12 inches from either end of the middle sections. The strong canvas sacking-bottom is 6 feet by 2 feet 9 inches. The side poles are inserted through a wide hem. The end sections are furnished with heavy straps and girths.

[2] A palanquin, or two-horse litter, as used in the sixteenth century, is figured in a wood-cut in CHARLES KNIGHT'S *Old England*, compiled from

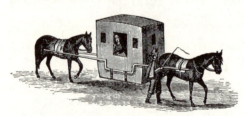

FIG. 4.—Two-horse litter of the XVI century.

several pictures in BRAUN'S *Civitates Orbis Terrarum*, 1584. In FIG. 4 the portion of the cut representing the horse-litter is copied. In *Shifts and Expedients of Camp Life*, by LORD and BAINES (London,1871, p. 687), there is a suggestion of an arrangement that "might, under favorable

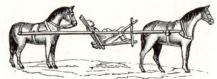

FIG. 5.—LORD and BAINES'S horse-litter.

circumstances, be made available for the carriage of a wounded man," with a cut (FIG. 5) of the appliance for suspending the patient either in a semi-recumbent or prone position. A conveyance much resembling this is used, according to Professor LONGMORE, in some parts of the East Indies, where it is called a "Tukta-rewan."

[3] Professor T. LONGMORE, in his excellent *Treatise on the Transport of Sick and Wounded Troops*, London, 1869, p. 292, thus refers to this form of litter: "It is necessary to notice another form of sick-transport litter issued for use in the early part of the late war in the United States, in which, instead of two litters being suspended across one horse or mule, one litter was suspended between two horses. This is a very ancient form of litter in Europe. Frequent notices of it occur, showing its common use on occasions of state and ceremony, as well as its employment for the carriage of sick persons, in the records of our own country prior to the introduction of coaches. It seems curious that its use should have been revived in modern times in America." In a note it is added: "This form of litter is referred to as late as the reign of CHARLES the 2d. A quotation introduced into the first volume of Knight's London, pp. 24 and 25, mentions that Major-General SKIPTON, coming in a horse-litter to London when wounded, as he passed by the brew-house near St. John street, a fierce mastiff flew at one of the horses and held him so fast that the horse grew mad as a mad dog; the soldiers were so amazed that none had the wit to shoot the mastiff; but the horse-litter, borne between the two horses, tossed the Major-General like a dog in a blanket."

[4] *Report of the Secretary of War, communicating the Report of Captain GEORGE B. McCLELLAN (First Regiment United States Cavalry), one of the Officers sent to the Seat of War in Europe in 1855 and 1856.* Washington, 1857.

[5] *Report on the Art of War in Europe in 1854, 1855, and 1856, by Major RICHARD DELAFIELD, Corps of Engineers, from his Notes and Observations made as a Member of a "Military Commission to the Theater of War in Europe" under the orders of the Hon. Jefferson Davis, Secretary of War.* Washington, 1860.

Glover Perin, U. S. A., and Assistant Surgeon Benjamin Howard, U. S. A., reported to Surgeon-General C. A. Finley the results of their inspection of cacolets and litters, devised by Mr. Charles Proal, of Louisville.[1]  Newspaper descriptions, almost textually quoted from Delafield's report, with figures of these appliances, were transmitted.  Mr. Proal claimed to have improved upon the French patterns by diminishing the weight and cost of construction.  Messrs. Lawrence, Bradley & Pardee, of New Haven, Connecticut, in 1861, applied for a patent for a cacolet, of cumbrous pattern, weighing 131 pounds. The chairs could not be detached from the saddle.  A sample, figured in the adjoining wood-cut (FIG. 6), was sent, in 1867, to the Army Medical Museum, and is numbered 824 in Section VI.  It combines in an unusual degree the undesirable qualities of weight, weakness, and inconvenience.  On September 25, 1862, a board of officers of the quartermaster department examined caco-lets submitted by Dr. Slade Davis, and reported[2] that, as compared with others that had been purchased for

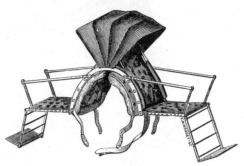

FIG. 6.—Cacolet of Lawrence, Bradley & Pardee. *Spec.* 824, SECT. VI, A. M. M.

the service, the only advantage of this form of cacolet was its lightness.  It was thought that those already on hand were as light as was consistent with the requisite degree of strength.  Mr. E. P. Woodcock,[3] of New York, in November, 1863, patented a pack-saddle with wooden outriggers from the pommel and cantle for the suspension of litters.  By securing litters to the projecting parts by straps, and protecting the side of the animal by pads, it was designed to carry two patients in the recumbent position.  This contrivance was exhibited by the United States Sanitary Commission at the Exposition in Paris in 1867, but met with no more approval abroad than at home.  Mr. J. Jones,[4] of New York, in December, 1862, proposed to the Surgeon General of the Army a mule-litter for carrying two persons either in a sitting or recumbent position, the litters being designed to serve also as efficient hand-stretchers or hospital-beds.  The "exceeding lightness, strength, and simplicity" of these conveyances were insisted on.  The saddle with two litters, girths, bridle, and other appurtenances weighed only 62 pounds, and could probably be reduced to 60 pounds.  In September, 1863, a board of medical officers was convened in Washington to examine into the merits of an "adjustable ambulance and pack-saddle," submitted by Spencer, Nichols & Co. Lightness, strength, simplicity, efficiency, adjustability, and cheapness were the merits claimed for this contrivance.[5]  Shortly afterward, December 1, 1863, another medical board assembled in Washington, to inspect and report on a mule-litter submitted by Messrs. Pomeroy & Co., which

[1] *Extract from a communication to Surgeon-General* C. A. FINLEY, *by Surgeon* G. PERIN *and Assistant Surgeon* B. HOWARD, dated Louisville, April 2, 1862: "The undersigned would respectfully state that Mr. Charles Proal, of this city, has submitted to our inspection a saddle-ambulance, which has been fairly tested by us in the open field.  Its chief excellencies, compared with other saddle-ambulances, are that it is lighter, is more easily adjusted, and combines both the litter and the chair, both of which can be packed away in a very small compass when the pack-saddle to which they belong is required for other purposes.  The weight of the entire ambulance, with saddle, etc., is about seventy-four pounds, that of the French being about one hundred and forty-two pounds.  The mode of adjustment is such that two litters, two chairs, or one chair and one litter, can be used at the same time, at discretion, each of which may be affixed to, or detached from, the saddle, while the patient remains undisturbed.  The harness appears to be very complete, the breeching and breast-band preventing motion backward or forward, while the surcingle, by being attached to the bottom of each chair or litter, prevents either undue oscillation, or shifting, which would be otherwise consequent upon any inequality in the weight of the two patients being carried.  *  *  The price of the ambulance and appurtenances completed is about fifty dollars."

[2] A Board of officers, consisting of Colonel D. H. RUCKER, Quartermaster, Captain J. J. DANA, A. Q. M., Captain E. E. CAMP, A. Q. M., was convened at Washington, September 25, 1862, to "examine a cacolet to be presented for inspection by Dr. SLADE DAVIS, and to report its opinion of the cacolet as compared with other patterns which have been purchased for the service."  The Board reported, that "in their opinion the cacolet presented by Dr. SLADE DAVIS possessed an advantage over those furnished by Mr. KOHLER (three hundred in number), all of which are now on hand, in light-ness only.  Those made by Mr. KOHLER are constructed in a strong and desirable manner, and are as light as is consistent with the requisite degree of strength.  No call has yet been made either for those first purchased or for those furnished by Mr. KOHLER, which cost $21,000.  We would not recom-mend the purchase of an additional number from any source."

[3] Compare LONGMORE (*Treatise on the Transport of Sick and Wounded, etc., op. cit.,* p. 290), *Subject-Matter Index of Patents for Inventions,* Washington, 1874, Vol. III, p. 1232, and SÉRURIER (*Conférences Internationales des Sociétés aux Blessés Militaires des Armées de Terre et de Mer tenues à Paris en 1867,* T. I, p. 47).

[4] MSS. Records of War Department for 1852.

[5] The Board, consisting of Surgeon T. H. BACHE, U. S. V., Surgeon C. ALLEN, U. S. V., and Assistant Surgeon W. MOSS, U. S. V., reported, September 16, 1863, 1. That the cacolets weighed 55½ lbs., and the saddle-girths and other equipment 38 lbs.  2. The saddle-tree was jointed, so that by turning screws it could be adapted to animals of different sizes.  3. As to simplicity, the saddle was provided with projecting crane-like supports of hickory covered with raw-hide, which were connected either with a flat framework of hickory, for packs, or with litters for patients.  4. As to strength, the saddle easily sustained two barrels of flour; but, when two soldiers, one of them a heavy man, mounted on the litters, there was "a slight yielding;" but the Board considered the litters "strong enough to bear any load that a horse or mule could carry."  Finally, the Board considered the pattern submitted as "comfortable as such a conveyance can be made."

was found to possess some good and some objectionable features.[1]  In addition to these essays in invention, cacolets and litters were submitted to the Quartermaster's Department, that purported

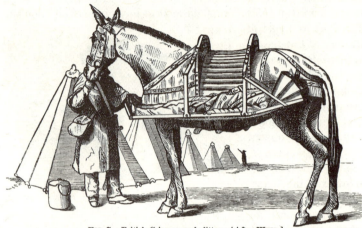

FIG. 7.—British Crimean mule-litter.  [After WEIR.]

to be constructed simply in accordance with drawings in General Delafield's report.[2]  August 20, 1861, Messrs. Lutz and Bridget, harness-makers, furnished twenty such sets with pack-saddles and harness.  These drawings, which are copied, of a reduced size, in FIGS. 7 and 8, though prepared by so distinguished an artist as Professor Weir, do not accurately represent the mechanical details of either the French or British Crimean litters and cacolets, and the ambulance equipments, made in imitation of them, did not prove

to be of utility.  Early in the war, however, probably as early as May, 1861, the Quartermaster's Department had purchased a number of cacolets and mule-litters of the patterns used in the

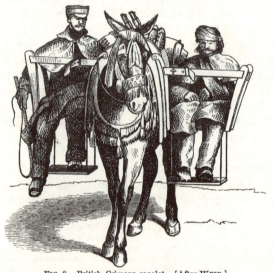

FIG. 8.—British Crimean cacolet.  [After WEIR.]

French army, and, in July, 1861, engaged Tiffany & Co., ot New York, to construct others, and employed a French agent to give instruction in the use of these cacolets and litters, and purchased animals specially adapted for their transport.  The Quartermaster General has remarked that these horses and mules were gradually appropriated as draft animals, and that the litters and cacolets were, for the most part, condemned as unserviceable.  The French litters and cacolets were what is known as the old pattern, such as the French used in Algeria and the Crimea.  They are figured in my surgical report in Circular 6, S. G. O., 1865, at page 82.  Surgeon-General Longmore correctly observes (op. cit., p. 291), that "the same drawings may also be seen in Chapter XX of M. Legouest's Traité de Chirurgie d'Armée, Paris, 1863, pp. 968–9.  I ventured to copy the drawings because they well represented the iden-

[1] The Board consisted of Medical Inspector J. M. CUYLER, U. S. A., Surgeon O. A. JUDSON, U. S. V., and Assistant Surgeon C. A. McCALL, U. S. A. The report is unaccompanied by a description or drawing of the conveyance, but states that it was simple in construction, with unusual capacity for providing for the comfortable carriage of two wounded men.  Some modifications were suggested, such as strengthening the attachments of the litters by substituting chains for straps; of supplying means for rendering their framework rigid so that they might be used temporarily as stretchers; of arranging that they might be detached from the saddle; of having rings and hooks for attaching necessary articles to the pack-saddle, and particularly a vessel for water.  The Board was unwilling to decisively approve of the conveyance until these alterations had been effected, and a trial in actual service had been successfully made.

[2] DELAFIELD (R.) (Report on the Art of War in Europe, 4to, Washington, 1860, p. 73) makes the following observations on mule-litters and cacolets: "The requisites for an ambulance should be such as to adapt it to the battle-field, among the dead, wounded, and dying; in plowed fields, on hill-tops, mountain slopes, in siege batteries and trenches, and a variety of places inaccessible to wheel carriages, of which woods, thick brush, and rocky ground are frequently the localities most obstinately defended, and where most soldiers are left for the care of the surgeons.  These difficulties were felt in a great degree by all the armies allied against Russia in the siege of Sebastopol, and the consequence was that the English, French, and Sardinian armies adopted finally, in part or altogether, pack-mules, carrying litters or chairs.  The careful and sure-footed mule can wind its way over any road or trail, among the dead, dying, and wounded, on any battle-field, as well as in the trench and siege battery.  It required but suitable arrangements to support the wounded from the mule's or horse's back to attain the desired object, and this the allied armies finally accomplished and put in practice. The merit of the plan renders it worthy our consideration, particularly so in our Rocky Mountain and other distant expeditions."  Further on he remarks: * * "I witnessed the transport of one hundred and ninety-six sick and wounded French soldiers, with their arms, accoutrements, and knapsacks, on the route from the Tchernaya to Kamiesch Bay, on these litters and chairs.  Fifty-two of them were on twenty-six mules in the horizontal litters, and one hundred and forty-four seated in chairs on seventy-two other mules.  A driver was provided for every two mules or four wounded men.  The appearances, with such an examination as I gave the whole equipment, were so favorable as to recommend it for trial in our service.  To make the system better understood, I annex two additional figures (FIGS. 7 and 8) showing the animal, the equipment, and position of the soldier, for which compilation and drawing I am indebted to Professor WEIR."

tical cacolets and litters issued in our army, and through an inadvertence which must be conceded to be unusual in me, I neglected to acknowledge my indebtedness to my honored friend and master. I trust this explanation will convince him and every one that I had no surreptitious design in using the cuts. In the mule-litters and cacolets now issued in the French army, there are improvements providing for making the sections of the litter rigid, so that it can be used temporarily as a hand-stretcher, for reduction in weight, and for greater compactness in packing.[1] The mule-chairs and litters now issued by the British Royal Carriage Department are lighter and more convenient than those used in the Crimea. I take the liberty of copying Surgeon-General Longmore's drawings of the cacolet (FIG. 9) and litter (FIG. 10) now employed in the British service.[2] The only reference I find of the actual employment in battle, during the late War in this country, of horse-litters or cacolets, is made by Professor F. H. Hamilton.[3] He mentions that, at the battle of Fair Oaks, May 31, 1862, when he was medical director of the Fourth Army Corps, eight pack-saddles, provided with a

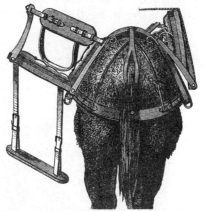

FIG. 9.—British mule-chair or cacolet, open for use and packed for traveling. [After LONGMORE.]

litter on one side and a cacolet on the other, were provided as a part of the ambulance outfit of that corps, and were used only on the first day of the battle, proving utterly unserviceable. Notes

are found in the War Department records of the transmission, August 26, 1861, of twelve of the mule-litters and cacolets made by Tiffany & Co., to the army in the Shenandoah valley, commanded by General Banks. A supply of litters and cacolets was provided for the advance of the Army of the Potomac from Yorktown toward Richmond in May, 1862. There were forty, at least, in store at White House,[4] but there were no trained animals to bear them. Moreover, the subordinate quartermasters and medical officers appear generally to have regarded the experiment with little favor. Medical Director Tripler, who, in 1859, in a report on the needs of the ambulance service, had urged the importance of supplying horse-litters to troops serving in regions impracticable for wheeled carriages, made several efforts to secure suitable equipment and proper animals[5] for this purpose, but without much success. His successor, also, Medical Director

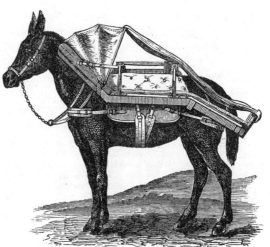

FIG. 10.—British army mule-litter attached to its pack-saddle. [After LONGMORE.]

Letterman, entertained similar views, in correspondence with the opinions of European authorities; and persevering, though ill-arranged, efforts were made to give the system a fair trial. In July, 1862,

---

[1] M. BOUDIN states (Système d'ambulances des armées française et Anglaise, 1855, p. 35) that the cacolet weighed something over 19 kilogrammes the pair. The pair in the Army Medical Museum weighs 40 pounds. Including the pack-saddle, Professor LONGMORE says a pair weighed in the Crimea was found to be 89 pounds and 12 ounces.

[2] The weight of a pair of English litters used in the Crimea was 138 pounds 12 ounces, without the pack-saddle. The present pattern weighs 84 pounds, without bedding or pack-saddle. With the paillasses and pack-saddle the weight is 167 pounds.

[3] HAMILTON (F. H.) (A Treatise on Military Surgery and Hygiene, 1865, p. 162): "Just before the battle of Fair Oaks, eight were sent to us for the use of the 4th Corps. They were only employed, however, on the first day of the battle. The horses were found to be impatient and restless under them, and six of the eight were soon broken and rendered unfit for use. Mules are better than horses for this purpose; they are not so high, and are less restive under the pressure of heavy weights upon their backs; but even mules require to be trained especially to this kind of service, before they can be rendered useful or safe."

[4] From a telegraphic order of May 27, 1862, recorded on the files of the War Department, and addressed from the Headquarters of the Army of the Potomac, by Lieutenant-Colonel J. A. HARDIE to Colonel S. VAN VLIET, Q. M., at White House, on the Pamunkey, it appears that a certain number of cacolets were at that depot prior to the battle of Fair Oaks. The dispatch reads: "The commanding General directs that you furnish the forty cacolets at the White House, belonging to the Medical Department, with horses, and report to the Medical Director here the moment they are ready." Doubtless the eight cacolets sent to the Fourth Corps were supplied from this source.

[5] March 13, 1862, on receiving the papers regarding Mr. Kohler's request for an examination of his litters and cacolets, Medical Director TRIPLER makes the endorsement that: "there are sufficient horse-litters for this army in the possession of the Quartermaster's Department. All we want now is horses or mules properly trained to carry them."

the Surgeon General requested the Quartermaster's Department to provide three hundred litters, and this number was purchased of Mr. G. Kohler.[1] Prior to the battle of Antietam, Medical Director Letterman asked for a supply of mules equipped with cacolets and litters. The Quartermaster's Department had an ample supply of the French patterns,

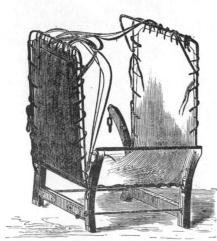

which were beyond all question the best that had been devised at that time. But there were no trained animals to bear them, and few, if any, available skilled packers. September 1, 1862, the Surgeon General requested that a hundred mule-litters should be sent to Medical Inspector R. H. Coolidge. A few weeks after the battle of Antietam a hundred and fifty mules were sent to the Army of the Potomac for ambulance service, but they were so unruly that it was

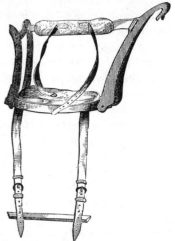

FIG. 11.—French litière folded. [After LEGOUEST.]

FIG. 12.—French cacolet unfolded. [After LEGOUEST.]

thought unwise to pack them with their equipment, and the litters and cacolets were sent along in wagons, and, as far as can be learned, never found their way to the backs of the mules.[2] Little could be anticipated from such essays. In November, 1862, the Surgeon General made another requisition for a hundred and fifty mules with drivers, with a view of having them drilled with cacolets in the field, by Dr. Slade Davis; but this, like previous experiments in this direction, proved abortive; and the ambulance material for transport by pack-animals, accumulated at no inconsiderable cost, was never really tested in the field.[3] There seems to have been a widespread distrust of the system on the part of officers of the Quartermaster's and the Medical Departments.

[1] June 17, 1862, Colonel RUCKER advises the Quartermaster General that he has advertised for proposals for mule-litters, and that the only proposal received is from Mr. G. KOHLER, and that the litter he proposes to furnish seems to be very high-priced; "it is intricate and cumbersome in construction, and, in my opinion, inferior to those now in Captain DANA's store-house" [the French cacolet and litière]. July 26, 1862, Surgeon-General HAMMOND states, in reply to a letter from the Quartermaster General concurring in Colonel RUCKER's opinion: * * "The litter presented by Mr. KOHLER has been examined by myself and a board of officers, who agree that it possesses sufficient merit to entitle it to trial in the field. I therefore request that *three hundred* of the mule-litters presented by Mr. KOHLER be purchased for-the use of the army." Quartermaster General MEIGS replies, July 29, 1862, that * * "inasmuch as the Surgeon General adopts and requests that these litters be constructed, though in the opinion of the Quartermaster's Department they are not as good as those already on hand, they will be contracted for under the proposal of Mr. KOHLER. The price bid is understood, as in other cases, to include the whole set, namely, head-stall, harness, saddle, and two litters for each mule." As early as December 9, 1861, this pattern of mule-litter had been reported on by a board convened by General McCLELLAN, consisting of Col. D. H. RUCKER, Surgeon C. H. LAUB, and Surgeon J. R. SMITH, it is presumed unfavorably, as further action was not had at the time.

[2] In October, 1862, the Surgeon General again made requisition on the Quartermaster's Department for one hundred and fifty mules provided with mule-litters, to be sent to Dr. JONATHAN LETTERMAN, Medical Director of the Army of the Potomac. In reference to delay in compliance with this requisition, Captain J. J. DANA, A. Q. M., reported, October 17, 1862, as follows: "The order was given by me, October 3d, immediately on its receipt, for one hundred and fifty mules and litters to be made ready for service. At that time we had no mules sufficiently well broken for the purpose. I directed fifty of the best to be taken from the ambulance train, the litters to be fitted upon them, and the mules drilled daily until they were fit to go into the field. On the 9th of October, fifty mules with litters upon them were started for Dr. LETTERMAN. Much difficulty was experienced in getting the mules forward, as they were, many of them, inclined to lie down and were otherwise unruly. Among a lot of mules received on the 10th instant, we found one hundred which were to some extent suitable for the purpose, and were sent forward on the 11th instant, the litters being sent by wagons in order to expedite the matter." October 3, 1862, Quartermaster-General MEIGS, in transmitting this report to Surgeon-General HAMMOND, stated: "I desire respectfully to call your attention to the fact mentioned in the report: that there are a large number of cacolets now in the possession of the Government which appear to have been overlooked by the officers of your department, and to suggest the expediency of directing their availing themselves of them as occasion may arise. General McCLELLAN issued orders, a year ago, for drill and practice of ambulance men, including, as I understand, the use of the mule-litters, of which, of French and American manufacture, there were then a considerable number provided by the Quartermaster's Department. Those lately purchased from Mr. KOHLER, on the requisition of the Surgeon General, cost $21,000, and are still in store."

[3] "From the papers laid before the Quartermaster General to-day, there appears an expenditure for purchase of cacolets and litters in 1861 and 1862 for the Army, partly upon reqnisions from the Surgeon General, partly from orders originating in this office, of over $20,000. To this, if the cost of animals and use of men, of forage, &c., supplied by this Department for the experiment of introducing these litters and cacolets, it would be found that not less than $100,000, and probably more has been expended in an experiment which was, so far as information in this office goes, entirely unsuccessful. There never was, to the knowledge of the Quartermaster General, a requisition from any military commander. All the requisitions came from the Surgeon General's office. It is not known to this office that these mule-litters ever were used in service, and the Quartermaster General believes that no wounded man was ever placed upon one of them. While the wheeled ambulances and hand-litters provided for the hospital equipments were in constant and useful use, the litters burdened the trains, and the mules were by the ordinary accidents of service taken for the ambulances and wagons. He believes that no better cacolet or mule-litter will be constructed than the French cacolet and litter, ordered at the beginning of the rebellion; and these, which though in his judgment inferior, were, at a later period, bought at the urgent requisition of the then Surgeon General. He is, therefore, of opinion that any further expenditure by this Department in this line of experiment will be a waste of public money, and he will not, therefore, unless under order of higher authority, expend money or make reports upon any models thus far submitted to him."—*Mem. of* QUARTERMASTER GENERAL, December 23, 1868.

In a letter of March 20, 1863, Surgeon George Suckley, U. S. V., Medical Director of the Eleventh Corps, wrote from the Army of the Potomac, near Fredericksburg, to Surgeon J. H. Brinton, U. S. V., at Washington:

"There are no cacolets in this Corps, and I want none. Three hundred and fifty pounds' weight is too much for a mule's back over rough ground, encumbered by bushes, stones, logs, and ditches. Among trees, cacolets will not answer at all; although used in European services and in Algeria, they have there been employed under some favorable circumstances, either on plains or on open ·rolling country. Here they would prove, I sincerely believe, only a troublesome and barbarous encumbrance, cruel alike to the wounded and the pack-animals."

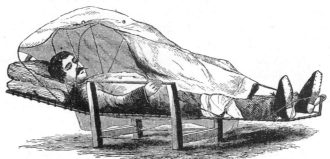

FIG. 13.—French litière unfolded. [After LEGOUEST.]

The French patterns, represented in FIGURES 11, 12, and 13, copied from M. Legouest's work, were, like the rest, considered unsuited to the requirements of field service in this country. Scarcely a word in favor of them is to be found in any reports of the medical directors[1] or field surgeons.

Surgeon John Moore, U. S. A., who long served as Medical Director in the Western armies, writes from San Antonio, January 24, 1877, in regard to the use of horse-litters and cacolets: "We had a few of these litters with the armies in the West, but they were very generally left in the depots of supply. I never knew of a single wounded man being carried on a horse-litter; for a man wounded in his arm or anywhere above the waist, was not so badly hurt as to prevent his riding a gentle horse, they are not needed; and for one so badly injured that he is unable to sit without being propped or supported, they are so uncomfortable as soon to become intolerable, and in all such cases where ambulance wagons or wheeled vehicles could not be had, hand-litters were improvised from slender poles cut in the woods and canvas or blankets fastened on them, upon which the wounded man was laid, and the litter either carried by men or by passing the ends of the poles through a kind of stirrup on each side of a horse or mule, an animal being at each end and the wounded man between them. In civilized warfare it rarely happens that men are wounded beyond the reach of our two-horse ambulance wagons, that horse-litters, at least such as I have seen, might well be excluded from the hospital equipment. There only remains, therefore, our Indian campaigns, in which the horse-litter may be utilized. But, unfortunately, the country where this kind of warfare takes place will usually be found so rocky and cut up by deep ravines as to make it impracticable to carry a badly wounded man in one of these horse-litters. Then the hand and horse-litter just referred to must be used, and nothing is better adapted to its construction than the Indian lodge-poles. There is usually little trouble in putting it together. Should it be necessary to carry a man for a long distance, the litter would be greatly improved by stretching over it, instead of canvas or blanket, the fresh hide of an ox, mule, or horse. If any of our litters have been found serviceable during the past year in the expeditions against the Sioux, I should be glad to know which; and also to learn the opinion of the men transported for two or three days in the Yellowstone region. The condition of the animal on which he was carried at the end of two or three days would not be without interest."

The absolute failure of the attempt to introduce, in our army, a system of sick-transport by cacolets and double litters[2] seems to have been due to defects, possibly insurmountable, in admin-

---

[1] Surgeon G. PERIN, Medical Director of the Army of the Cumberland, in a letter dated Fort Leavenworth, January 20, 1877, states: "In so far as I can now remember, this method of transporting sick or wounded was never used in any command with which I served. The hand-litter was all that was necessary to convey the wounded to points accessible by the ambulance trains. The only service where the cacolet or horse-litter would be found necessary, in my opinion, is that of scouting, where wagon transportation cannot be taken. I should prefer, for our Indian scouting, to take pieces of canvas about seven feet long by three feet wide, with eyelets six inches apart worked around the edges. These may be lashed over poles procured when needed. The poles can be fastened at one end to a pack-saddle and the other end allowed to drag upon the ground. This is the way the Indians transport their sick and wounded, and ordinarily answers well. In rough, stony grounds I have used litters mounted upon two pack-mules or horses, one being in front and one in rear, with a man to lead each animal." Dr. JOHN H. BRINTON, formerly Surgeon U. S. V., and Medical Director of the Middle Military Department, writes, January 13, 1877: "All that I can remember of the horse and mule-letters is the fact that a number of samples were inspected at the Surgeon General's office by a board appointed for the purpose, and my impression is that a limited number of the foreign models were issued to the brigade of regular cavalry then stationed near Washington. I subsequently enquired of many medical officers how this mode of transportation answered; and, to the best of my recollection, it was always condemned or spoken of as unsatisfactory, and unsuited to the American soldier. I imagine it will be found that very little, if any, real use was made of those horse-litters. As you know, I was present at many battle-fields, and witnessed the employment of almost every sort of transportation; but I am quite sure that I never saw one of these litters used." General J. M. CUYLER, who, as Medical Inspector General, had great opportunities for observation, writes from the headquarters of the Military Division of the Atlantic, January 10, 1877, that with the exception of the inspection at Carver Hospital [see note 1, p. 10, *ante*], in December, 1863, of the mule-litter submitted by Pomeroy & Co., he saw nothing of this mode of transport during the war. Colonel G. E. COOPER, Assistant Medical Purveyor, U. S. A., who was long at the head of the medical administration of the principal Western armies, writes, January 20, 1877, that: "I have never seen a horse-litter used for transporting sick or wounded, save in one instance." [The incident referred to, which occurred in the Mexican War, is noted at page 6, *supra*.] Surgeon JOSEPH B. BROWN, U. S. A., who was long intimately associated with the administration of the medical service of the Western armies, writes, January 19, 1877: "Concerning the use of horse-litters or cacolets in the Western Department, * * I have to state that I can recall no instances of my personal experience at all of the use of such transportation for wounded, for it has been my fortune to have been entirely unprovided with anything of the kind under circumstances and at times when they could have been used."

[2] Marshal LEROY DE SAINT-ARNAUD, in his *Rapport sur la réorganization des Equipages Militaires*, Paris, Février, 1852, says: "The use of the mule with a cacolet or litter was first adopted in Algeria. By means of these ingenious equipages, hundreds of wounded, amputated, and sick soldiers have been transported in safety to our base of operations."

istration, and not to demerits of the system. Without efficient animals and packers it was vain to anticipate useful results from the best-contrived appliances. Used with the greatest advantage in Algeria[1] and in the Crimea, the French cacolets and litters were adopted by the British army medical department with satisfactory results. In the Italian war of 1859, they were found serviceable in each of the different armies engaged. They were used, with what results I have not ascertained, in the armies of Spain and Portugal. The Italian Medical Inspector General, Dr. Cortese, reported most favorably of their utility in the rocky defiles and narrow wooded paths of the Tyrol (Fischer). Sent to India during the Sepoy rebellion, and to New Zealand during the Maori war, they proved altogether useless from lack of trained animals to bear them (Longmore). In the Franco-Austrian invasion of Mexico, the French contingent of the expeditionary army, carrying with them their train of pack-mules, used this mode of transport advantageously; whereas the Austrian contingent, relying on animals picked up in the country, derived little benefit from it.[2] On the whole, it may be asserted that the evidence of the value and importance of mule-litters and cacolets, as a part of the ambulance equipment, is conclusive. They can be packed compactly and easily carried on the march—the mules conveying supplies or doing other field service when not

---

[1] Marshal BUGEAUD, who served with great credit in his campaigns in the Spanish peninsula, from 1810 to 1814, and afterward commanded in Algeria, concluding in 1837 the treaty of Tafna with Abd-el-Kader, when recalled, in 1847, to command the army of Paris, was the warm advocate of supplying the army with means of transport by pack-animals, regarding the mule-litters and cacolets used in Africa as scarcely susceptible of improvement. He contrasted the efficiency of this mode of transport with what he had observed in Spain, where, for the want of transport suited to the field of operations, whole divisions had sometimes to abandon their wounded on the field. Such neglect, he argued, must produce a most depressing effect upon the troops. Marshal BUGEAUD recommended that the equipment for the transport of wounded of all the cavalry and infantry divisions of the French army should be exactly like that of the army of Africa, and that wheeled ambulance-wagons should be attached only to the reserves. Medical Inspector General HALL considered the merits of the French cacolets and litières,—their general applicability to the circumstances of warfare,—their admitting of the removal of sick and wounded from every description of ground and over every kind of ground where mules and horses can travel,—and the rapidity with which the removal could be effected over roads where wheeled carriages could not travel (*Parliamentary Report upon Hospitals of the British Army in the Crimea*, London, 1855). Colonel BLANE, Assistant Adjutant General for Lord RAGLAN, regarded "the cacolets and litières now in the French service as by far the most perfect system which has yet been devised for the transport of sick and wounded with an army in the field." See LONGMORE, *op. cit.*, p. 274.

[2] Dr. J. NEUDÖRFER, the chief medical officer of the Austrian expeditionary force in Mexico, in 1864-5, thus relates (*Handbuch der Kriegschirurgie*, Leipzig, 1867, p. 341) his experience of transport by mule-litters and cacolets: "Those who know these modes of transport only from descriptions and delineations, without personal experience, will be much prepossessed in their favor, as they appear simple, easy of conveyance, and practicable on every ground. We will show, however, that the system is not quite so simple as it appears. We had cacolets made of the French pattern, in the corps workshop at Puebla. The weight was 70 pounds, and could not, without risk to solidity and utility, be reduced to less than 60 pounds. Considering further the weight of the wounded man (with his full equipment, which is not allowed to be abandoned) as amounting to 150 pounds, and finally estimating the equipment of the mule leader, other traps of the wounded man, their victuals, and perhaps a little forage for the mule, as weighing 30 pounds, we have a round total of 400 pounds, to be transported by the mule. Four hundred pounds is a burden that cannot be borne continuously on the back of a horse. A horse may draw twice that amount, but cannot carry such a load. Mules, instead of horses, are selected for the transport of wounded by cacolets, because, as the cavalry say, mules have stronger backs than horses; besides, mules have the advantage of getting along better and more safely than horses in the mountains, although the Mexican horse (and probably every horse raised in the mountains) is not in any way inferior to the mule when it is necessary to surmount difficult passways. But even for the back of a mule 400 pounds is a burden that can only be carried by the largest and strongest mule. For this reason, the French in Mexico brought with them droves of large and strong mules. Such an outfit is directly very costly, and indirectly yet more expensive from the outlay for the care and feed of animals. But there was no alternative; for a sufficient number of strong capable mules could seldom be obtained in that country by requisition. The Austrian corps using the cacolets only as an auxiliary means for the transport of wounded, employed such mules as could be procured through requisition at the time and place, and it sometimes happened that these animals, although the largest and strongest of those on hand, would break down under their load, obliging the wounded to remain for hours lying on the roadway, until the mule could recover itself, or other means of transportation could be improvised. In accidents of this kind, we were quite satisfied if the wounded man did not sustain injury at the breaking down of the animal. Even the largest and strongest mules could not always be made immediately serviceable. In Mexico these animals live, as the horses, in wild droves on the fields. They are caught when wanted for sale, and then are unfit for service as pack-animals. They break and destroy everything that is packed on them. Several months elapse until they are tamed and can be employed to carry, and a mule, strong and tame as it must be for the purpose of carrying cacolets, costs at least 200 pesos (silver ounce). The cacolets as well as the litters have, besides the disadvantage that they afford to the sick or wounded man, little or no protection against the influences of the climate; yet such protection is as much needed as in Europe or Africa, for the sick man must be guarded against the tropical sun as well as against the tropical rain. But these do not exhaust the inconveniences of this means of transport. I have tried riding on a cacolet, and found that it depends on the gait and form of the animal as to what degree of discomfort the patient experiences. Some mules have such an unpleasant gait that the patient, either sitting or lying, feels as wretchedly as if subjected to the rolling motions of a small screw-steamer. Even with a well-gaited animal, the constant swinging motion is unpleasant. The upper part of the body of a man seated in a cacolet swings to and fro like a pendulum, pivoting at the level of the knee joints. Besides, the sitting posture, with the patient strapped to his seat, can only be borne by the slightly sick or wounded, and even these will be fatigued by the forced position and swinging motion in a transport of this kind. Finally, the cacolets and litters require so much room, that it is quite impossible to move them through narrow mountain passes, such as our wounded had to traverse repeatedly in the Sierra del Norte, in Mexico. In other cases, mountain roads passing a projecting rock made such abrupt curves that the mule burdened with two wounded men was obliged to keep close to the margin of the road, where one of the patients would be actually suspended over a yawning abyss, in constant danger of life. Moreover, from the method of packing, the centre of gravity is placed so high that, in the steep and abrupt descents to be passed, even the safe-going mule lost its balance. A mule carrying a mountain howitzer was precipitated down a ravine into a watercourse. It may be concluded that this mode of transport has neither the merit of simplicity nor of fulfilling its purpose, and can only be resorted to when no better means of transport can be had; moreover, that cacolets, at the present day, are to be considered as obsolete, and to be used only where they are still on hand, and that no more new cacolets or litters should be provided. We must, in fact, resort to entirely new measures for the transport of the wounded. We must consider not only the numerous wars carried on in late years in localities separated from the soldier's home by immeasurable oceans, in China, India, Mexico, and in the South American Republics, but the late European wars in Italy, in Schleswig-Holstein, and in Austria. There we shall see that already, with the field-sanitary regulations hitherto in use, the transport of wounded should be divided into two classes: 1, the transport of wounded and sick for short distances; 2, the transport of the same for greater distances. We need not repeat that transport by means of cacolets or litters, is adapted neither for short nor long distances. Moreover, in central Europe, the breeding of mules is less extensive than in Mexico. In Europe, there would be, for this reason, an insufficient number of suitable pack-animals."

required for sick-transport. They can be taken into broken and precipitous places where wheeled vehicles are utterly inadmissible; or can convey the wounded over distances far too great and tedious for the employment of hand-stretchers. Professor Longmore, after summing up these advantages, observes, with equal justice, that they are only attainable when, in the first instance, mules of sufficient strength and docility can be procured, with attendants capable of training and harnessing them properly, of placing patients on the conveyances in the best way, and taking care of them on the march. Without these adjuncts, in actual campaigning, the animals and appliances will be unserviceable (Longmore, *op. cit.*, p. 294).

In 1868, Mr. W. B. Rooker, of Prince George's county, Maryland, submitted to the Surgeon General and Quartermaster General a plan for "an attachment to a saddle for the use of a sick and wounded soldier," which he proposed should be made part of the cavalry equipment.[1] This proposal naturally met with little favor; but it was repeatedly brought to the attention of the War Department, and, in 1874, permission was granted that twelve of these contrivances might be made at Watervliet Arsenal. Subsequently a board examined[2] them, and reported that they might be serviceable at times, furnished in the proportion of two for each company, for cavalry expeditions in mountain regions. In the summer of 1875 the twelve experimental saddles were distributed to cavalry commands in Wyoming and Dakota, and pronounced valueless.[3] The form or arrangement of this apparatus is indicated in the adjoining wood-cuts (FIGS. 13, 14). Its alleged advantages were again brought before the military authorities, when, in August, 1876, General Sherman dismissed the

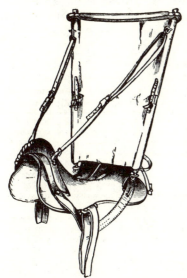

FIG. 13.—ROOKER'S saddle-attachment for the support of wounded men.

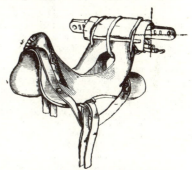

FIG. 14.—ROOKER'S saddle-attachment packed to a McClellan saddle.

---

[1] The following description of this contrivance was filed with the application for a patent: "This so-called ambulance saddle is an ordinary cavalry saddle, having an attachment consisting of two upright bars cut and hinged in the middle, a cross-bar at the top of the uprights to support the head, a canvas back, and two leather straps, with buckles, so arranged as to support the apparatus to be more or less inclined, to suit the rider. When the upright bars are placed in the canvas, they need not again be taken out, but may be folded at the hinges, and, with the straps inside, may be rolled into a compact bundle and attached by the coat-straps to the cantle. Its weight is four and six-sixteenths pounds, and probably this weight might be considerably diminished. When intended to be used it may be thus adjusted: Unstrap it from the cantle and place the sick or wounded man in the saddle; insert the iron keys in the lower ends of the uprights in the eye-bolts, especially attached to the saddle for this purpose, on each side, near the base of the cantle; put on the cross-bar and key it; hook the straps to the eyelets in the upper parts of the uprights, having first buckled the lower ends of the straps into the staples in front of the pommel; then by the middle buckles elevate or depress the head, as may be required." In a letter to the Secretary of War, dated January 5, 1874, * * "My invention is intended expressly for cavalry, but like any ambulance arrangement may be used for infantry if desired. It is so constructed that it may be taken apart, rolled in the piece of canvas forming the back, and strapped to the saddle like a valise or other bundle, its weight being under six pounds and its bulk inconsiderable. Each cavalryman may carry his own, and, in case of being wounded or taken sick on a long march, this apparatus may in the short space of five minutes be so adjusted as to afford him a comfortable conveyance. An umbrella may be readily attached, though not an essential part of the apparatus. I have had the pleasure of showing it to a number of army surgeons and other officers, who, I am happy to say, have expressed high approbation of the design, saying that numberless men by its use might be conveyed from the field who would otherwise be unavoidably left."

[2] The Board, consisting of Colonel F. D. CALLENDER, Ordnance Department, Assistant Surgeon J. S. BILLINGS, Medical Department, and Captain C. E. DUTTON, Ordnance Department, convened at Washington Arsenal in February, 1875, and gave the opinion that "The Board do not think it advisable to encumber the cavalry soldier with the carrying of this ambulance attachment, however light it may be made, as it is deemed important to his efficiency to diminish rather than increase the number of articles he is to carry, and to limit them to those of prime necessity. The Board are of the opinion that the use of the attachment in front of the saddle is of little or no value for the carrying of the sick or wounded soldiers; but, that altogether this ambulance saddle has sufficient merit to warrant its trial as an auxiliary to ambulances, stretchers, or other means in charge of the Medical Department for carrying the sick and wounded, and that the reports of officers who may use them in the field should furnish the basis of a final judgment upon their merits and usefulness. For a cavalry expedition or scouting party, which is not and cannot be provided with wheeled transportation, as in certain parts of Arizona and Utah and the Northwest, it is thought probable that if this apparatus were furnished in the proportion of about two to each company it would at times be of service. It would not do for the transportation of severely wounded men:" * * *

[3] The saddles were sent to Rock Island Arsenal April 10, 1875, subject to the order of the Lieutenant General, and from May 8th to July 6th, 1875, three were sent to Lieutenant-Colonel G. A. CUSTER'S command, two to Fort Laramie, two to Major E. M. BAKER'S command, three to Fort Leavenworth, one to Fort Brown, one to Colonel B. H. GRIERSON'S command. Two written reports respecting them were sent by the officers requested to test them. Captain J. MIX, 2d Cavalry, reported from Camp Brown, Wyoming, June 12, 1876: * * "The back is so arranged that the rider cannot lean back, and in going down steep places his position is painful in the extreme. I have never seen a place so destitute of resources that I could not improvise a more comfortable arrangement of carrying a sick or wounded man." Acting Assistant Surgeon T. G. MAGHEE reported, June 10, 1876, "I have examined and tested the new ambulance saddle, and for practical use consider it inferior to many, if not all, of the packs and litters commonly constructed to suit such occasions by every one serving in the mountains."

matter with the endorsement: "I have examined the Rooker ambulance-saddle and do not hesitate to pronounce it useless in war or peace." Assistant Surgeon S. S. Jessop, U. S. A., has communicated an instance in which an officer (Lieutenant F. B. Sherman, 15th Infantry), when disabled, was conveyed for some distance with the aid of a contrivance analogous to the Rooker saddle attachment. Mr. Sherman has had the goodness to furnish a statement, which is subjoined in a footnote,[1] of his recollection of this incident. In great exigencies, a wounded man may be carried off on horseback,[2] either tied on, suspended in a blanket,[3] or supported by a pad or pillion behind a comrade, to relieve him of exertion in guiding or holding on to the horse:[4][5][6]

In the operations against the Modoc Indians, in the lava-beds of California, extending from December, 1872, to May, 1873, the ordinary methods of transport were found unsuitable and a form of mule-litter, devised by Assistant Surgeon H. McElderry, U. S. A., proved serviceable and well adapted to the exigencies encountered. Dr. McElderry sent one of these litters to the Army Medical Museum, and in a letter dated Fort Klamath, March 3, 1874, described it as follows:

"I transmit a box containing a mule-litter, devised by me for use in the lava-beds about Rhett Lake, California, during the late Modoc campaign,—the ordinary form of litter drawn by two horses having been found entirely unfitted for service in such broken country, abounding in narrow and winding defiles. A harness gear, *aparejo*, and appliances, to be used with the litter, is also contained in the box. It is believed that this form of litter, besides being especially adapted to the character of country for which it was devised, will be found also of service in mountainous districts, and on the frontier generally; and it is

[1] Mr. SHERMAN'S note is dated Fort Union, New Mexico, January 25, 1877: * * "Dr. JESSOP has confounded two occasions. The only time I have been wounded my transportation was an army wagon, and I do not think a description of this mode of conveyance is needed, nor are my recollections of my twenty miles ride sufficiently pleasant to enable me to recommend such transport. But when out on a scout in Texas some years since, I was taken very ill and completely prostrated, so that I could not sit upon my horse. It was an absolute necessity for our party to get back to the fort, and I found myself an encumbrance. Some Tonkawa Indians, along with us, said they knew a way to carry me. I was placed in a saddle and a lean-back was made; a bent twig or sapling inclined at an angle of 50° was attached to the rings at the crupper of the saddle, and I was securely attached to it by a rope. My legs were stretched out along the side of the horse and also tied in some way to a small branch run along by them, and attached to the saddle. I was too sick to remember much about it, but know I felt secure. The back was made by running the ends of the sapling into the saddle-rings. My arms were tied to my body, but not closely. I think I have read of a similar method used in Europe, but much improved."

[2] PERCY (Art. *Despotats*, in *Dict. des Sci. Méd.*, T. VIII, p. 565) believed it historically established that the ancient Celts carried off their wounded in battle by laying them across the backs of horses. It is well known that under the reign of the Emperor LEO I, who obtained victories over the Huns, but was repulsed by GENSERIC in Africa, in the latter part of the Vth century, it was customary for ten or twelve mounted men, called *despotati* (their saddles provided with two stirrups on the near or left side of the horse), to follow each cohort, to pick up and transport wounded men. It is stated by ISENSEE and COHEN, in their history of medicine (Gröningen, 1843), that in the succeeding century the Emperor MAURITIUS ordered that each cavalry division of 400 men should be followed by 8 or 10 picked men of activity and determination, entrusted with the duty of aiding the wounded by giving restoratives, applying temporary dressings, and transporting them from the field of danger. FISCHER (*Lehrbuch der Kriegs.-Chir.*, 1806, p 208) adds that each received an honorarium for every wounded man he succored.

[3] In their most instructive work entitled *Shifts and Expedients of Camp Life*, Messrs W. B. LORD, Royal Artillery, and T. BAINES, F. R. C. S. (London, 1871, p. 687), suggest: "In a case of great emergency the ends of a blanket might be knotted together; and, two men being laid in the bights, the central part might be laid across the back of a horse, with one man hanging on each side, and secured with the best means available at the moment. Among civilized nations it would, perhaps, be better to leave the wounded to the mercy of a victorious enemy than to risk the extinction of life by such rough means; but in fighting savages, no living man ought, under any circumstances, to be left in their power, and a soldier had better die under the rough, though kindly, efforts of his comrades to remove him than become a prisoner—to be kept alive as long as he is capable of enduring torture."

[4] SCHMUCKER (J. L.) (*Chirurgische Wahrnehmungen*, Berlin, 1774, Theil I, p. 346) relates: "After the battle of Liegnitz, August 15, 1760, * * I ordered the severely wounded to be placed on pork-, provision-, or bread-wagons, and the slightly wounded to move along slowly without equipment. There yet remained five hundred men, mostly wounded in the upper extremities, for whom no means of transportation were provided. As it was necessary to follow the moving army, I quickly made up my mind as to the course to be pursued. I ordered the men to be put together in one place, and proceeded in person to the Adjutant General von Krusemarck. I informed him that these men were entirely unable to march; but if the General would give orders to unseat a regiment of dragoons, all might be carried along. My proposition was assented to; in the course of half an hour all the wounded were on horseback, and the dragoons marched alongside. In the evening we reached Parchwitz, where the army camped. The next day we marched in the same manner, until, on the third day, I reached Breslau with all the wounded."

[5] "After the abandonment of the siege of St. Joan d'Acre there was a total want of any kind of conveyance for the wounded, and Bonaparte directed that all the horses of mounted officers should be used for this purpose, an order he enforced by example, by marching on foot with the rest of his army. The wounded must otherwise have been abandoned in the desert to have their throats cut by the Arabs."—(LARREY, *Camp. d'Egypte*, p. 312.) In the Sepoy mutiny of 1857, in General LUGARD'S field force, on many occasions the number made helpless by wounds or sickness was greater than the regular means of transport would accommodate. To leave these disabled men would have exposed them to atrocities too horrible to contemplate. Yet an advance was imperative. Under such circumstances every available means of conveyance was adopted, and the disabled were taken to a place of safety under a strong cavalry escort, which promptly rejoined the main body and enabled the advance to be continued.—(GORDON (C. A.) *Army Hygiene*, London, 1866, p. 217.)

[6] Prof. A. BERTHERAND, Director of the School of Medicine of Algiers, remarks (*Campagnes de Kabylie*, Paris, 1862, p. 116): "Every one has heard of the sure and rapid means employed by the Arabs to transport from the field of battle the victims of shot-wounds. We have often seen from a distance, notably during the murderous expedition of 1840 and 1841, groups of the enemy assembled about a pack-animal or a stretcher hastily constructed of two branches, and carrying off at a run a precious burthen, revealed by a fluttering burnous or a pendant limb, or a dead or wounded soldier. But, at a distance, we could not discern how the patient was attached and supported on these improvised appliances. Thanks to Staff-Captain Dupin, who had occasion to make a nearer inspection of them, we are enabled better to appreciate their mechanism and adaptation to exigencies. The removal of the wounded on *traverses of wood* covered with moss, dry leaves, the cloaks or outer garments of the country (*burnous*, *haïk*), or sometimes by huge grain-sacks (their's), need not detain us. It is hammock system in its primitive rudeness, easily constructed of the first available materials, and far inferior to the perfected stretcher (brancard) of the French army. Transport on the back of mules or horses is of greater interest, responding to more important indications. The plan is this: On either side of the large pack-saddle with which the animal is equipped, at a level with its most projecting part, a large sack stuffed full of straw, leaves, or grass, is attached, in such position that the convexities of the two sacks and the upper surface of the saddle are all in the same horizontal plane. The surface is covered with a pallet of hay or straw or by some sort of mattress made of folded stuff, on which the patient is laid cross-wise to the animal, and in the line of the long axis of this couch. Afterward branches are arched over the litter to protect the patient, if need be, from the sun or rain."

respectfully suggested that a certain number of them be constructed and issued at frontier posts for trial. They should invariably be used with the *aparejo*, the back of the animal being first protected by two ordinary saddle-blankets properly folded. If this be done and the litter be properly secured in its place, the ordinary precautions being taken, the mule's back will never be made sore. As originally used, the litter was lashed with ropes to the *aparejo*. This is perhaps the more satisfactory way of fixing it in its place. As, however, a skilled packer may not always be on hand, it was thought advisable to secure it with a broad girth. This plan has been found to work well and satisfactorily. Owing to the want of the proper materials at the post, the litter forwarded could not be made exactly as was devised. For instance, all the hinges about it should be larger and stronger; the rings, through which the arm-straps pass, should be triangularly shaped; and all the rings that come in contact with the ropes or canvas should be made of galvanized iron, to prevent rusting. The litter forwarded was constructed for me by Hiram Field, quartermaster's employé at this post, and for many years past in the Government service. To him I am also indebted for several valuable suggestions in originally planning it."

An additional report on this subject, dated Washington Arsenal, January 17, 1877, was transmitted to the Surgeon General by Dr. McElderry, with drawings by Lieutenant J. P. Wisser, 1st Artillery, of the different parts of the apparatus.

"I have the honor to transmit for your consideration drawings of a mule-litter which I respectfully recommend for adoption in the army for use on the frontier in campaigns against hostile Indians. The following are some of the advantages of this form of litter. As was demonstrated by experience in the field during the Modoc campaign in the lava-beds in southern Oregon and northern California in 1873, the proposed style of litter is specially adapted for use in broken, rough, and mountainous country; along narrow and winding defiles, abounding in sudden and abrupt turns and angles; and in places and under circumstances generally where no other kind of litter could be employed. A wounded man can be transported on this litter with entire safety on the back of any steady pack-mule or horse, taken indiscriminately out of the pack-train; the animal not requiring any special training before he will pack it, otherwise than he has already received in the pack-train. Every officer of any practical experience in scouting on the frontier knows that, before the pack-mules or cavalry horses can be made to work satisfactorily in the double horse-litters now issued in the army, every such animal requires, in each case, a special and more or less prolonged system of training and daily drills in these litters. Several litters are usually broken to pieces before the animals can be made to work steadily. It is nearly always found impracticable to give the animals such special training, for the reason that on an Indian campaign transportation is always cut down to the minimum, and consequently no extra animals can be taken for use in the litter-train. It is seldom possible to obtain the quarter-

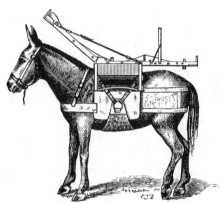

FIG. 15.—McELDERRY's single mule-litter.

master's pack-animals for such preparatory drills, as they are forced by the circumstances of the case to carry packs all day, and when camp is reached at night there is no time and the animals are in no condition for any such drills. The consequence is, that when the urgent necessity for the use of the litter-train actually arises, among all the animals turned over to the medical officer for such service there will not be more than one or two that can be used; the others all refuse to work in the litters, and ultimately some other means has to be resorted to for the transportation of the wounded. Only one animal is required for use

with this litter, and consequently there is no useless expenditure of labor, as when two horses are required for the transportation of one man. The litter can be folded compactly together, so as to permit a load of grain, provisions, etc., to be packed upon it. The animal having arrived at its destination, the load is removed, the litter is unfolded, and becomes available for the transportation of the wounded back to the base of supplies. By the use of the adjustable iron support, which raises up over the lower end of the litter, a wounded lower extremity can be suspended in the anterior or other splint, and the patient thus carried with much greater ease and comfort than when the wounded member is simply laid upon or fixed to the litter. Used upon the Mexican *aparejo*, which is now universally found in the pack-trains upon the Pacific coast and Texas frontiers, this litter, being well balanced, is easily and comfortably carried by the pack-animal, and consequently has no

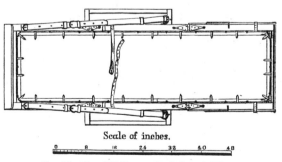

Scale of inches.

FIG. 16.—Plan of McELDERRY's single mule-litter.

tendency to make the animal's back sore. This is always found a source of serious trouble in packing the long poles of the double horse-litter now in use. They are so long that they have to be packed crosswise on the pack-saddle, and in consequence invariably cause so much wabbling of the saddle that, after they have been carried for a day or two, the pack-mule gets a sore back, and is henceforth unfit for use for some time during the campaign. As will be seen, the present form of litter is substantially the same as the one devised by me and constructed to meet the emergencies of the service in the Modoc campaign, and the model of which is now in the Army Medical Museum. Like that model it is intended to be constructed of strong wood braced with iron rods, with strong hinges to bear the rough usage of frontier field service, so as not to be easily broken or otherwise rendered unfit for service. Several modifications, suggested by experience and reflection, have been added, in order to cause the litter to fold up more compactly and to add to the comfort of the patient. The upper part of the heavy canvas which forms the bed is intended to be made of double thickness, to be left open above. Into the pocket thus formed, hay or prairie-grass is to be stuffed, and the upper edges of the canvas tied together with cords sewed on for the purpose. This forms the pillow. A canvas awning has been sketched on the plan, intended to be stretched from head to foot-board of the litter over the raised iron support, and tied in place by the cords attached to its edges. An *aparejo*, furnished with a good broad breast-strap and crupper, is first lashed to the animal's back with its girth in the usual way, and the litter, being then placed upon it, is firmly fixed in position by means of an extra-broad California horse-hair girth, as shown in the figure. It has been suggested to me that this litter might be constructed of iron, to render it lighter and more compact for transportation. It is possible that this might be done, and I intended to submit drawings for a model of this form of litter to be constructed of iron. Upon reflection, however, I am of the opinion that this could be much better done after due consultation and deliberation with some competent practical mechanic authorized to construct the litter of such material. It is believed that by the aid of the drawings herewith submitted, and the model already in the Army Medical Museum, and any required information that I should be able to furnish him, that a competent mechanic would have no difficulty in constructing two models, one of wood, braced with iron rods, and one entirely of iron. If the style of litter herewith submitted should receive the approbation of the Surgeon General and the construction of a number be authorized for use in the Army, I would respectfully suggest that two such model litters be made for inspection and comparison, when the one considered most suitable for the service may be selected as a model and guide for the construction of the others. The drawings herewith submitted were kindly made for me by Lieutenant J. P. Wisser, and I am greatly indebted to him for the artistic and accurate manner in which he has performed the work."

Dr. McElderry's litter weighs, without a mattress, fifty-four pounds. The *aparejo* and appurtenances weigh fifty-one pounds. Like the litter of Captain Thistle (*ante*, p. 5) and those exhibited by MM. Philippe and Locati,[1] at the Paris Exposition of 1867, it has the advantage that its width does not much exceed the outer limits of the flanks of the pack-animals; a condition adapting it to the passage of narrow defiles or cañons, or of roads encumbered by vehicles.

The following passage and illustrations are extracted from a report to the *Conseil de Santé* by M. Gouchet,[2] médecin-major, serving with the 1st Zouaves, in the French corps sent to Mexico, in 1864. Referring to a skirmish at *Espinosso del Diablo*, January 1, 1865, and describing the disposition made for the carriage of the slightly wounded, he remarks:

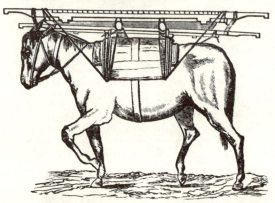

FIG. 17.—Single mule-litter used by the French in Mexico. [After GOUCHET.]

"It remained for us to provide for the transport over broken and difficult ground of four wounded men, who needed a recumbent position, and could not endure the cacolets, while we had no regulation mule-litters. On the pack-saddles of four strong and docile mules we applied two transverses, strongly bound to the front and rear ledges (pommel and cantle), to support two parallel bars arranged to support the side poles of the stretcher on which the wounded man was carried. The stretcher was securely attached on this framework by ropes fastened to the four handles of the stretcher and then knotted on rings of the pack-saddle. * * The patient's head, as he lay on the stretcher, was a little above and behind the mule's head * * with his feet stretched backwards. He experienced on the march little lateral oscillation, but only the longitudinal movement produced by the walk of the pack-animal. This was proportioned to the inclination of the roads, and when these were steep, the attendants were directed to support the stretcher during ascents and to press it down strongly when descending declivities. On commencing the march, the patient, laid on the stretcher, was placed on the pack-mule, and the handles of the stretcher were strongly secured, as already said, and the men of the train being at their posts, they moved off at a very gentle gait, to avoid jolting over the narrow and rugged paths. The patients on the stretchers bore the journey very well, and, after a little experience, preferred this mode of conveyance to the regulation litters, which have great lateral swaying, very fatiguing on such difficult roads. They only complained of feeling on their backs the pressure of the forward bow of the pack-saddle, which, after a while, much incommoded them. But the patients themselves remedied this inconvenience by shifting their positions, or by

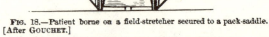

FIG. 18.—Patient borne on a field-stretcher secured to a pack-saddle. [After GOUCHET.]

stuffing in something to increase the thickness of the pallet at that part."

This adaptation of ordinary hand-stretchers to the purposes of a single-litter mule conveyance is admirable in principle; and if means can be devised to secure such stretchers on pack-animals without pitching them so high as to endanger the patient and encumber the animal, such arrangement would be the simplest and best.

[1] VAN DOMMELEN (G. F.), *Essai sur les moyens de Transport et des Secours en général aux Blessés et Malades en Temps de Guerre*, La Haye, 1870 pp. 12, 13, et Planche VI, Figs. 1, 2. See GROSSHEIM's comments on McELDERRY's litter, in *Deutsche Mil. Zeitschr.*, 1877, p. 68.

[2] *Recueil de Mémoires de Médecine de Chirurgie et de Pharmacie Militaires*, 3me série, 1865, T. XIV, p. 520.

A mode of transporting sick and wounded by conveyances that at one end rest on the ground, so that the patient is drawn, but only partially sustained, by the pack-animal, is mentioned by early travellers among the North American Indians. Parkman indicates[1] that in the war with Pontiac, in 1763, the colonists carried their wounded by this contrivance, and, in a later work,[2] refers to the *travail* used by the Oregon Indians; and Lewis and Clark[3] resorted to it in 1805, to carry a wounded hunter of their party. Latterly, this method of transport has received much attention from medical officers, as well adapted to the exigencies of frontier service. Surgeon C. R. Greenleaf, U. S. A., has remarked on this form of conveyance:

"I know of nothing better for scouting parties, than a litter made after the following plan, which is borrowed from a custom among the Indians, quite familiar to all officers who have seen any service on our frontiers. It consists of four ash poles, two for shafts and two for litter-poles—the former are 7 feet 6 inches long, 2 inches wide, 2¾ inches deep at the butt, and 1¾x1¼ inches at the point; the latter are 8 feet 6 inches long, 2 inches wide, and 2¾ inches deep, with rounded edges and corners. On one end of the litter-pole is riveted two wrought-iron (best Norway) bands ⅛ inch thick and 1½ inch wide. One of these collars is set 2 inches from the end of the litter-pole, and has a diameter of 4⅜ inches by 2 inches; the other is set 12 inches from the end of the poles, and has a diameter of 5⅜ inches by 2 inches. The opposite end of the litter-pole is shod with an iron thimble 1 foot long. Two cross-bars, 30 x 1½ x 2¼ inches, with a square collar of iron ⅛ inch thick by 1½ inch wide on each end, serve to keep the poles separated and steady; the collars should have a diameter of 2 x 2¾ inches, and the litter-pole must be square at its front end and 2¼ feet from the rear end for their reception. A canvas bed 6 feet by 32 inches, with strongly bound eyelets 8 inches apart on the upper end and upper three feet of the sides, and permanently fastened to the lower three feet of the

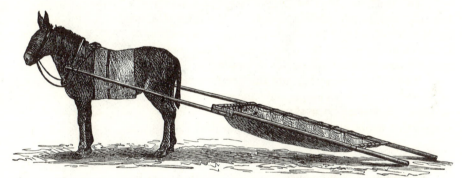

FIG. 19.—GREENLEAF'S combined hand and horse litter hitched to a mule. [From a drawing by Dr. GREENLEAF.]

sides, completes the affair. The litter is dragged by a horse or mule hitched into the shafts—the rear end of the litter-poles resting on the ground, the patient occupying the canvas bag in the middle. To put it together, the small end of the shaft is passed from behind forward, through the rear and largest collar on the front end of the litter-pole, thence through the smaller collar, and then "pulled home," until the butt of the shafts is tightly embraced by the collars; the cross-bars are then put into their respective places by slipping their collars over the front and rear ends of the litter-poles and pushing them securely home, the canvas bed lashed to the poles by rope passing through the side eyelets and around the poles, and through the end eyelets and around the cross-bars; the ropes at the head of the bed should be slack, to afford "bag" enough to the canvas to bring the head and shoulders of the patient nearly on a level with his feet. By the arrangement of splicing the shafts to the litter-poles through collars of unequal sizes, a constant tightening of the parts goes on by the force exerted by the animal in pulling the litter, and no opportunity for loosening occurs; while, as the greatest weight occurs at this point, additional strength is gained through the iron collar and the double thickness of pole. With a collar and harness, which could be carried without much trouble, the litter can be hitched to a mule by a chain attached to the harness, and having on its end a goose-neck pin to pierce the shaft from below, and be fastened above by a nut or linch-pin. To unship the litter, give a smart blow on the small end of the shaft, which will drive it back through the collars, when it can be taken out; remove the cross-bars, unfasten the ropes, and wrap the poles and cross-bars in the canvas, packing the whole thing like a tent on a pack-mule. For use as a hand-litter, it is only necessary to unship the shafts."[4]

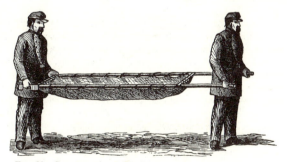

FIG. 20.—GREENLEAF'S combined hand and horse litter used as a hand-litter. [From a drawing by Dr. GREENLEAF.]

[1]PARKMAN (F., jr.), *History of the Conspiracy of Pontiac and the War of the North American Tribes*, Boston, 1855, p. 601. After the battle of Bushy Run, August 6, 1763, Colonel H. BOUQUET wrote to his excellency, Sir J. AMHERST, describing the litters constructed after the Indian fashion by the four companies under his command to carry off their wounded.

[2]PARKMAN (F., jr.), *California and Oregon Trail*, *being sketches of Prairie and Rocky Mountain Life*: 12 mo., New York, 1849, p. 165.

[3]*History of the Expedition under the command of Captains* LEWIS *and* CLARK *to the sources of the Missouri, thence across the Rocky Mountains and down the River Columbia to the Pacific Ocean, performed during the years 1804–5–6, by order of the Government of the United States.* By PAUL ALLEN, esquire, Philadelphia, 1814, Vol. II, p. 381.

[4]Extract from a Report made in compliance with Circular Orders No. 3, War Department. S. G. O., November 25, 1874, by Assistant Surgeon CHARLES R. GREENLEAF, U. S. A., dated Huntsville, Alabama, December 14, 1874. On October 27, 1876, Dr. GREENLEAF contributed to the Army Medical Museum a model of this combined hand- and horse-litter, which is numbered 804 in Section VI, A. M. M.

**Efforts were made by several other medical officers to systematize this mode of transport:**

In November, 1875, Assistant Surgeon P. J. A. Cleary, U. S. A., reported to the Surgeon General's Office his observations at Fort Sill and elsewhere, in the Indian Territory, on the facility with which the Indians transported their sick and aged or infirm on litters dragged by ponies, and suggested that analogous conveyances might be utilized for the transport of wounded in cavalry scouts, and in marches in difficult country where the use of wheeled vehicles was impracticable. April 15, 1876, Dr. Cleary sent to the Army Medical Museum a model and descriptive statement of a modification of this Indian litter that he would recommend as adapted to army use. This model is numbered **774**, Section VI, A. M. M., and is represented in the accompanying wood-cut (FIG. 21). Dr. Cleary writes: "In the process of constructing the model of a horse-litter which I send to the Museum by express, I have more than once altered the details of my original plan, and the model, although as near an approximation as I can make to my design, does not exactly carry out my ideas. The chief defects of the model

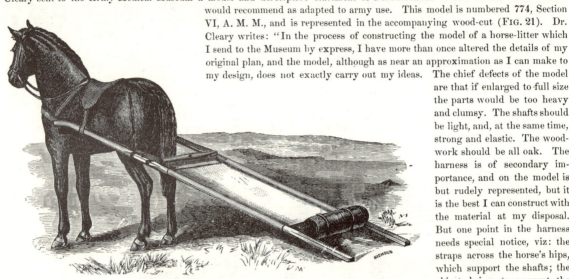

are that if enlarged to full size the parts would be too heavy and clumsy. The shafts should be light, and, at the same time, strong and elastic. The woodwork should be all oak. The harness is of secondary importance, and on the model is but rudely represented, but it is the best I can construct with the material at my disposal. But one point in the harness needs special notice, viz: the straps across the horse's hips, which support the shafts; the object being to prevent the horse, in case he rears up, from

FIG. 21.—Horse-litter proposed by Dr. CLEARY, U. S. A.

jumping out of the shafts, or kicking the patients; by this strap he *lifts* up the litter every time he attempts to kick, and so cannot reach the patient. However, a kicking horse is not the kind for the sick under any circumstances. As to the litter proper, it needs but little explanation. Each side-pole is jointed; by withdrawing a pin it comes apart, leaving the shafts in the harness, and the stretcher-frame disconnected. The length of the connected side-poles should be 17 feet, viz: 5 feet occupied by the horse, 3 feet from rear of horse to first traverse or cross-piece of litter, 7 feet for bed of litter, 2 feet from bed of litter to end, total 17 feet. I have a large one almost completed, and shall test it in a short time and report how it works. The advantages which the litter appears to me to possess are:

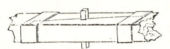

FIG. 22.—Splice of the shaft of the above litter.

1. Simplicity of construction. 2. Facility of transportation, as it can be easily rolled up and carried either in a wagon or strapped to a horse. 3. It can easily be drawn by one animal. 4. It requires but one man to work it, who can, by laying it on the ground, easily shift even a severely wounded man into it, and then lifting it can readily attach the litter proper to the part forming the shafts. It requires two or more persons to lift a wounded man into an ambulance wagon. 5. The facility with which a patient can be brought into a hospital—here, again, by detaching it at the joint it is converted into a hand-litter on which the patient can be conveyed by two men to the ward of the hospital. 6. Regularity of its motion; instead of jumping over irregularities of the road, as a wheeled vehicle, the poles, by dragging along, necessarily ascend and descend all irregularities of the ground by gradual motion. 7. Its general adaptability for any kind of ground—for instance in crossing cañons and deep gullies, the litter proper could be easily detached, and a man at either end carry it as a hand-litter over any obstruction and again attach it, and finally, for any slight obstruction, the driver, without detaching it, could lift the rear—the forward part being held in the harness—until the obstruction was passed; none of which can be done with an ambulance. Were it to be sent out with a cavalry command, and not required for actual use, it would occupy but a small space, and need not have even a horse sent with it—when, if required, the trooper's horse could be used to haul it. I should explain that the upper and lower straps [attached to the side poles but not represented in the drawing] are intended to pass under the patient's buttocks and over the thighs, fastening to the upper part of the litter—the upper one to pass under the arms and be similarly fastened; only one pair need be used at a time, this to counteract the tendency to slip, due to the incline of the litter.

**Assistant Surgeon Curtis E. Munn, U. S. A., in a report to the Medical Director of the Department of the Platte, dated April 12, 1876,[1] relates his experience in the use of horse-litters, or "travaux," in an expedition against hostile Indians on the Powder River:**

"The command left Fetterman on the morning of March 1st. I was supplied with four ambulance wagons and one supply wagon. * * Early on the morning of March 3d, at a camp on the south fork of the Cheyenne River, about thirty

---

[1] An expedition against hostile Indians, known as the "Big Horn Expedition," was organized at Fort Fetterman, Wyoming, in February, 1876. It consisted of five companies of the 2d Cavalry, five of the 3d Cavalry, and two of the 4th Infantry, under command of Colonel J. J. REYNOLDS, 3d Cavalry. Leaving Fort Fetterman March 1, 1876, the detachment reached Crazy Woman's Fork on March 7th, and there left the wagon-train and proceeded northward with a train of 350 pack-animals, and attacked an Indian village on Powder River March 17th. The troops resumed their stations March 27, 1876, having lost four killed and six wounded. The march was made in very inclement weather, the thermometer sometimes falling below 26° of the Fahrenheit scale.

miles north from Fetterman, a small party of Indians fired on two herders, who were on duty near the troops, and wounded one severely. During the next four days he was transported in an ambulance wagon eighty-four miles to camp on Crazy Woman's Fork, where he was left with the supply train, doing very well. On March 3d, at a camp on the Powder River, Indians fired into the groups standing by the camp-fires, and slightly wounded Private Slavey, Co. I, 4th Infantry. March 7th, at Crazy Woman's Fork, myself and assistants were occupied selecting stores to be carried on pack-mules, and generally preparing for cutting loose from the wagon train, which was to return to Old Fort Reno, and there camp until our return from the north. The two companies of Infantry were left for its protection. Here I left Acting Assistant Surgeon J. Ridgely, with instructions to establish a field-hospital, to be in readiness on our return, as it was highly probable there would be many wounded or sick. * * On the evening of the 7th, the Cavalry, accompanied by a 'pack-train' of about 360 mules, again started north, and marched all night. The medical supplies were carried on two pack-mules. They consisted of a valise of instruments and dressings, chloroform, etc. (a complete surgical outfit), a medicine pannier well stocked, and two blanket cases, each containing 12 blankets, a rubber bedcover, and several bottles of brandy. * * The march for days was over mountains, to, and then along the Tongue River, then across a divide in the direction of the Powder River. On March 16th, at two P. M., having marched 22 miles that day, the command was halted and divided; two battalions and the pack-train to remain, and three battalions, under Col. Reynolds, to follow a trail by night march. Medical stores were again divided, and, directing Acting Assistant Surgeon Stevens to remain with the train, I started, with the necessities indispensable for an engagement on the horses of myself and orderly. These comprised an amputating knife, ball-forceps, artery-forceps, and a pocket-case, two pots of beef-extract, a bottle of chloroform, one of brandy, oakum, rollers and lint, cigar-box covers and 'binders-boards.' My orderly had a field-medicine case complete. * * Up to this time, on our march over slippery roads, but one casualty had occurred of sufficient severity to incapacitate any one from horseback riding Corporal Moore, Co. D, 3d Cavalry, had been rendered helpless by a fall of his horse upon his body, and for several days he had been transported in the rear of his battalion

on a rude imitation of an Indian 'travail.' He was left, with several men suffering with inflammatory rheumatism, in care of Acting Assistant Surgeon C. R. Stevens. The idea of transport by the travail I took with me to the field, and it encouraged me to feel that my little outfit was adequate, and if to-morrow it should be found necessary, with poles from the woods and cavalry horses from the command, I would surely be able to transport the wounded with the column. On the morning of March 17th, after an exhausting night march, the command struck an Indian village on the Powder River and fought for several hours, the Indians making a brave defence. As soon as they were driven from their village, it was

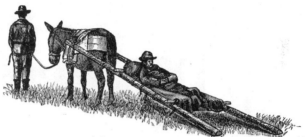

FIG. 23.—Wounded soldier on a "travail." [From a photograph.[1]]

easy to construct *travaux* from the lodge-poles, and upon one of these curious conveyances, which I constructed in fifteen minutes, Pt. Egan, of Co. K, 2d Cavalry, who received a penetrating wound of the abdomen, was brought about one hundred miles, over the roughest trails, to the ambulance station, which he reached in convalescing condition. I had never seen, or thought of, such a method of transportation for wounded before, and am naturally much pleased at the perfect success attending their use. We followed trails over mountains and ravines where it seemed impossible for a horse to go, and although the frequent exigencies of precipitous side-hills and deep gulches elicited much forcible and profane language, addressed to drivers

and mules, to secure safe conduction, no accident occurred. All, including two cases of acute rheumatism, were brought safely. To keep up with the column frequently necessitated the trot or gallop, and strangely enough the rheumatic cases seemed to improve while undergoing this harsh treatment. I would recommend the employment of this mode of transportation whenever troops are obliged to leave wagon-roads. A few well-seasoned poles about 16 feet long should be carefully prepared, and provided as part of the outfit. They can be dragged along in bundles behind two or three packed mules, until a drag should be

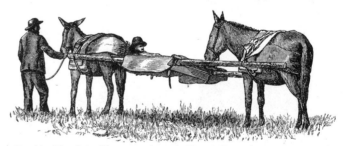

FIG. 24.—Wounded soldier conveyed on a double mule-litter. [From a photograph.[2]]

needed. Several of the animals in the train should be provided with collars and hames, with short chains and hooks to attach to rings in the poles. A common girth will support the poles over any saddle, and two lariats will make the cradle behind the mule or horse, and serve to bind the patient securely upon the apparatus. A patient can be more comfortably transported over a rough country in this way than by the best ambulance, but the poles must be well-seasoned and of elastic material, as ash, lance-wood, or hickory. * * The command reached the site of old Fort Reno on the evening of March 21st; a cold rain-storm during the afternoon completed a long sum total of discomfort. My notes say that we marched 10 hours, over the worst trails yet traversed. I had cheered my patients with repeated statements about the comforts prepared for them at camp at Reno. I found only the hospital tent pitched, its interior wet, no fire in or about it." * * *

---

[1] Dr. MUNN indicated, on the photographic print from which the cut is copied: "This is the picture of a poorly-contrived 'travail.' It should be drawn by two mules, and the poles should be elastic. When a stream is crossed, men take up the ends of the poles and carry them across."

[2] Assistant Surgeon MUNN, in transmitting the photograph copied above, remarks: "The litter with two mules, long in use, I believe to be inferior to the travail. When the animals move at an uneven pace, the result is disastrous to the harness and to the patient."

In connection with his report of sick and wounded for June, 1876, in relating the circumstances of an engagement with hostile Indians[1] at Rosebud Creek, Montana, June 17, 1876, Assistant Surgeon A. Hartsuff, U. S. A., made the following references to the conveyance of wounded by horse-litters and " travois":

"The fight commenced by a sharp attack from the hostile Indians, who evidently thought to surprise us. They were all well mounted and well armed, and seemed to have an abundance of ammunition. Their ponies carried them swiftly over ground that was difficult for us to get over at all, and they did all their firing from their horses, which we were unable to do. The attack was promptly met, both by our troops and our friendly Indians; and the Sioux were driven back, from hill to hill and crag to crag, the ground being a succession of sharp hills, crags, etc. Soon we discovered great numbers of the enemy on our flanks. Evidently they were trying to surround us, and to get to our rear, with a view of capturing our camp, transportation, stock, etc. For they presumed that we had a base; but, what was their surprise, when they got to the ground where they first found us, to find we had no rear! Our headquarters, base, and all, were in the saddle! Every officer and man was mounted, and all carried their rations and ammunition upon their persons, our only extra transportation being two pack-mules, one of which carried medical supplies, and the other tent-flies, shovels, picks, axes, etc. After the enemy, by great exertion of hard riding, had succeeded in finding our supposed base, and finding nothing, their next anxiety and hard work was to get back to their main column. Having no base, and being thus entirely surrounded, and the position of all the troops constantly changing, it was necessary that the medical officers of the command should be very active and vigilant to

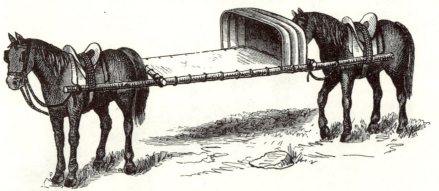

FIG. 25.—Extemporized horse-litter. [From a drawing by Dr. HARTSUFF.]

prevent any of our wounded falling into the hands of the enemy. The wounded were all collected together and their wounds hastily and rudely dressed, neither time nor circumstances allowing us to give them the necessary care and attention. Frequently, during the fight, we had to move the wounded to safer positions. Not a drop of water could be obtained during the day, for we were on the hills, and the nearest water, Rosebud, a miserable little stream, two miles away. At about one o'clock P. M. the firing had nearly all ceased, the Indians having retreated, through deep and narow cañons, down the Rosebud. It was about half-past six o'clock when the command reached the Rosebud River. Owing to the great heat of the day, no shelter, and no water, and very considerable loss of blood, many of the wounded were much exhausted. Their wounds were all dressed as speedily as possible, and all were made as comfortable as our limited means would allow; but our work then was not done, for the order was to return to the wagon train, and to march early in the morning; the time of marching to depend on time when the wounded could be moved. Mr. Moore and his packers gave

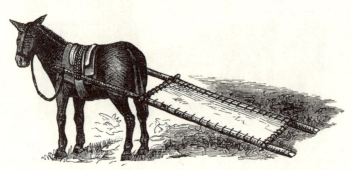

FIG. 26.—Extemporized Mule-"travois." [From a drawing by Dr. HARTSUFF.]

us the necessary assistance; and, by working the greater portion of the night, one horse-litter and five travois were made. Captain G. V. Henry, 3d Cavalry, was placed on the litter (FIG. 25), and five of the wounded soldiers were placed on the travois (FIG. 26); the remainder of the wounded [thirteen in number] rode their horses. At sunrise all was ready, and we at once moved out. I felt very considerable interest in this (to me) new mode of transportation of the wounded, and I carefully watched the behavior of the litter and travois. I soon discovered, however, that *the litter was much better in all respects than the travois, except, perhaps, over comparatively smooth ground;* much of our route was very rocky and broken, the hills were very steep and cañons deep. Occasionally a little stream and a narrow trail on steep mountain sides. Over such a country, the travois is very troublesome and uncomfortable; so much so did they prove to us, that at night, after the first march, we threw away all of them, and made litters in their stead. With these, we had no trouble; could move as fast as the columns could move over mountain sides, through cañons, over rocks, stones, and

[1] An expedition against hostile Sioux and other Indians, known as the "Big Horn and Yellowstone Expedition," started June 1, 1876, from Buffalo Wallow, Wyoming Territory, and reaching Rosebud Creek, in Montana, June 17th, was attacked by a force of Indians estimated at fifteen hundred in number. The detachments of United States troops consisted of ten companies of the 3d Cavalry, five of the 2d Cavalry, three of the 9th Infantry, and two of the 4th Infantry, twenty packers, and two hundred and fifty friendly Crow and Creek Indians, making an aggregate of twelve hundred and fifty men, commanded by Brigadier-General GEORGE CROOK. In the affair of the Rosebud the detachment lost nine killed and nineteen wounded.

even through deep rivers. We crossed the Tongue River, three or four feet deep, without trouble. The wounded occupants of the litters thought them very comfortable; and even when we reached the ambulance-train, some of the wounded did not want to give up their litters for the ambulance wagons. The horse-litter is quite as quickly and easily constructed as the travois; can be used wherever the travois can be used, and in many places where the latter is entirely useless. The travois are extensively used by all tribes of Indians of this country; but they have, I believe, no knowledge of the horse-litter. For the information of those who may not be familiar with the appearance and construction of the means of transportation to which I have referred, I insert the preceding sketches (FIGS. 25, 26). I also send a sketch of a splint much used by the Indians (FIG. 27): It is quickly made, of small willows, peeled, and woven or tied together by buckskin-strings. They may be of any length, are very pliable and easily fitted to any shape or condition. The splint is quickly applied, pressure is uniform, and, when wrapped around a fractured extremity and tied with strings or buckled with straps, it behaves better than any other form of dressing. Our killed were all buried on the field, and as the Indians did not get at their dead bodies, none of them were scalped or mutilated. Our Indians, Crows and Snakes, took thirteen Sioux scalps, and otherwise mutilated the bodies of the dead Sioux. Assistant Surgeon J. H. Patzki and Acting Assistant Surgeon C. R. Stephens were my assistants in the above-named engagements and on the field, *en route*, and at all times and places they were active and efficient in the discharge of their duties"

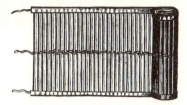

FIG. 27.—Splint of willow-twigs united by buckskin thongs. [From a drawing by Dr HARTSUFF.]

Assistant Surgeon J. W. Williams has supplemented his report of the killed and wounded at the disastrous engagement at the Little Big Horn,[1] June 25, 1876, with the following remarks on transport by horse-litters:

"The ordinary Teepe poles, with which the Indians pitch their tents when in villages, are also used in constructing the travois. The Dakota and Montana Sioux, who use mountain-pine or ash poles, select straight, well-proportioned saplings of those woods, trim them down to the proper size and taper, and then lay them aside to season. The dressed poles are about thirty feet long, two to two and a half inches at the butt, and one and a half inches at the other extremity. The oval couch rim is made exclusively of ash, bent into the desired shape while the wood is green. A network of raw-hide is afterward lashed to the rim and completes the bed. The bed is three and a half to four feet in its transverse, and two and a half to three feet in its conjugate diameter. When a travois is to be rigged, two or three Teepe poles, according to size and strength, are selected for each shaft and lashed together, butts to butts, with raw-hide. The system is then lashed to the pack-saddle with the same material, the small ends of the poles trailing on the ground. The Indians sometimes use a breaststrap as an additional stay. The bed, with the longer diameter laid transversely, is next secured to the shafts one foot in rear of the horse, about six inches of each end of the bed being allowed to overlap the shafts. A blanket, piece of canvas, or buffalo robe lashed to the lower half of the oval rim

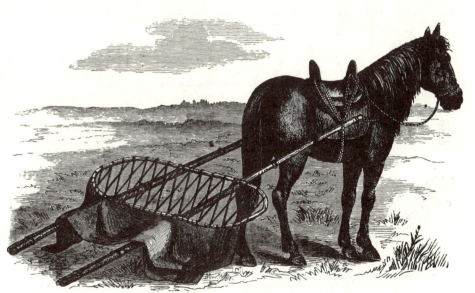

FIG. 28.—Dakota Indian litter. [From a drawing by Dr. J. W. WILLIAMS, U. S. A.]

of the bed completes the outfit. When a patient is to be carried, he is laid transversely on the bed, partly reclining on the side, with knees slightly drawn up, and head and shoulders bent forward and secured to the bed by drawing the blanket up over him and lashing it to the upper part of the rim. I made use of ten of these travoises to transport the wounded from the battle-field of the Little Big Horn, June 25 and 26, 1876, to the boat at the mouth of the Big Horn. The distance was thirty miles; time of march, night; the country to be traversed rough and broken; the Little Big Horn, which crossed our line of march in its windings toward the Big Horn, had to be forded six times—obstacles enough to test the merits of the travois as a carrier of wounded; yet, notwithstanding the difficulties in the way, the wounded were transported to the boat without accident or personal inconvenience and discomfort of any kind. I was particularly pleased with the results of this trial, and resolved to make

[1] Brigadier-General A. H. TERRY, with a force of cavalry and infantry numbering about fifteen hundred men, made an expedition into the Sioux country in June, 1876. On June 25th, the advance, consisting of eleven companies of the 7th Cavalry, under Lieutenant-Colonel G. A. CUSTER and Major M. A. RENO, encountered the Indians at the "Little Big Horn," and lost 15 officers, an acting assistant surgeon, and 232 men killed, and 59 men wounded.—See *Annual Report of the Surgeon General*, U. S. A., 1876, p. 13.

a more extended trial of the travois should future occasion offer. I am of the opinion that the travois is well adapted for transporting wounded over a rough country; that it is quite as safe and free from jar as the mule-litter, also resorted to on the same occasion; and that it is by far more economical than the latter in the number of attendants and animals which it requires.[1] In case of an Indian war, when villages are attacked and captured, there never will be any difficulty of obtaining material for building the travois; under different circumstances they will have to be prepared beforehand. My idea was to prepare twenty-five travoises and use them as part of the pack-train until needed for transporting wounded. It is well known that the Indians use the travois for carrying all sorts of baggage, and that it is no impediment to rapid marching, and that, further, in case of battle, their wounded are quite as speedily removed from the field by the same means."

Brigadier-General A. H. Terry is of opinion that the following memorandum, by Lieutenant G. C. Doane, 2d Cavalry, for the construction of two-horse litters, will "be of great value to at least every medical officer of the army":[2]

CAMP ON YELLOWSTONE RIVER, *July* 11, 1876. To the ASSISTANT ADJUTANT GENERAL, Department of Dakota. (*Through official channels.*) SIR: In compliance with a verbal request, I have the honor to submit the following memorandum of specifications for the construction of horse or mule litters for the transportation of wounded men in the field: Cut two poles sixteen feet long. These should be of green timber, three inches in diameter at small ends after being barked; four inches back from each end, cut a notch (FIG. 29) all around and tie in a loop of strong rope or raw-hide (FIG. 30); the loop to be about four inches aperture. Now lay the poles parallel and with the small end to the front, about three feet apart. For cross-bars take two pieces of pole, same size as above, and each about four feet long; cut notches about two-thirds of the way through one of them, three feet two inches apart, to fit down on the

FIG. 29.— Notched three-inch timber.

FIG. 30.—Notched timber with rope.

two poles at right angles; cut with a square shoulder to resist pressure inward (FIG. 31). Lay off from the small end of each parallel a distance of four feet four inches and mark, then tie in the notches downward firmly upon these points. Cut the other cross-bar in the same way, but have the notches three feet six inches apart. Lay off from the large ends of the parallel bars a distance of four feet eight inches, and tie down at these points the rear bar (FIG. 32) firmly as before; this gives a bed seven feet long, three feet two inches wide at one end and three feet six inches at the other, exclusive of thickness of parallel bars.

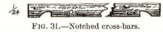

FIG. 31.—Notched cross-bars.

Now take a lariat or raw-hide thong and cord the bed-space in the following manner (FIG. 32): Tie one end at a corner over a lashing of a cross-bar notch, pass the rope over the opposite parallel bar nine inches advanced from where it is lashed to the cross-bar. The rope comes under the bar behind the first cord and back over it, making a similar turn over and under the other parallel bar eighteen inches from the point of starting; then back, gaining eighteen inches each time, until it reaches and passes over an intersection of the cross-bar at the other end of the bed; then pass the rope under both parallels and back over the opposite end of the bar, and cord back to the front end as before, dividing each space of eighteen inches, so that when finished the spaces will be nine inches between bearings approximately; the object of a second cording is to counterbalance the strain of the first, which would tend to throw one parallel forward and the other to the rear; draw the cords tightly. The bed is now complete. To fasten the litter on the mule, take for each end of the litter a lariat and *coil* it in loops long enough to reach over the saddle-seat and half way down on each side of the body of the animal. Fasten the ends in a tie around the middle of the coil; then slip the loops of the coiled lariat at end through the small loops tied at the end of the bars, and over the ends of the bars, slipping back into the notches; the ends of the bars will then hang in the ends of the lariat coil suspended. Now fasten into the small loop at each end of each bar a piece of rope about four feet long, and around each right-hand, or off-side notch, one end of another cord long enough for a belly-band for the mule. The litter is now complete. To put in the mules: lead up the front mule first, the smaller of the two; loose the lariat loops from one end of the shafts; back the mule between them, pass

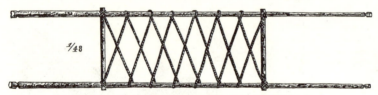

FIG. 32.—Litter of poles and raw-hide. [From Lieut. DOANE'S drawing.]

---

[1] Surgeon General T. LONGMORE remarks (*Op. cit., Treatise on Transport, etc.*, p. 293): "Two-horse litters seem to be conveyances of very doubtful expediency, if expedient at all, under any circumstances. It is a very unprofitable expenditure of labor for two horses to be devoted to the carriage of one sick man, when the same purpose can be more economically accomplished by other means. The comparatively little width of space occupied by such litters give them some advantage in moving along narrow ways through a partially cleared country, but they cannot travel along narrow tracks presenting short turns, such as winding paths with steep acclivities on one side, which are so frequently met with in hilly districts. The conveyance is too long and unyielding for such movement. Again, it is unsuited for any but tolerably level roads. It is destitute of any provision for preserving its level in case of the leading horse elevating the fore part of the long poles, while the hinder part is depressed, or *vice versa*, so that a road presenting either a steep ascent or descent would cause great inconvenience to any invalid in the litter during the act of transportation."

[2] "HEADQUARTERS DEPARTMENT OF DAKOTA, SAINT PAUL, MINNESOTA, *December* 7, 1876. To the ASSISTANT ADJUTANT GENERAL, Headquarters Military Division of the Missouri, Chicago, Illinois. Sir: After the action of the 25th of June last, the wounded men of the 7th Cavalry were carried to the Big Horn River in mule-litters constructed by 1st Lieutenant G. C. Doane, 2d Cavalry. These litters answered their purpose admirably, and I think that a knowledge of the manner in which they were constructed would be of great value to at least every medical officer of the army. At my request Lieutenant Doane has prepared a detailed report upon the method of construction used by him. I now have the honor to forward a copy of it, and I suggest that it be submitted to the Surgeon General of the Army. In this connection I desire to call the attention of the Lieutenant General commanding the division to the invaluable services rendered by Lieutenant Doane. I believe that I speak the sentiments of every officer and soldier who served under me in the field during the campaign of last summer, when I say that I feel the most hearty admiration for the zeal, skill, and energy displayed by this accomplished gentleman and soldier. I am, sir, very respectfully, your obedient servant, ADFRED H. TERRY, *Brigadier General*, commanding."—[*Forwarded by the Lieutenant General to the Adjutant General and referred by the latter to the Surgeon General.*]

the lariat loop over the seat of the saddle, lifting both shafts equally; slip the detached lariat loop to its place and drop the shafts so that they will hang equally; then tie each short rope at the side into the pommel-bars of the pack-saddle so as to keep the ends of the bars at an equal elevation. Tie the rope for the belly-band on the near side as on the opposite, and let the mule be led a short distance, with the litter dragging, to see if he is gentle. Put in the rear mule the same way except that he is led into the shafts, and the short ropes are tied into the cantle-bars of his saddle and his halter-strap fastened to the rear bar of the bed, short enough, so that he cannot get his head down under it. If the mules make trouble at all, it will be when first hitched up, and many which act badly at first will quiet down when they find they cannot break loose. They should be led around with the litter empty (care being taken to keep the front mule straight in the shafts) to accustom them to the work. To turn the litter, work the mules in *opposite* directions, the front one to the right, and the rear one to the left, or vice versa. To go down hill, hold back on the rear mule; to go up hill, whip up the rear mule; always start the rear mule first. On the road, a man should lead or ride each mule; also a man should walk or ride on each side of the litter to steady it or refasten ropes when required. Such litters will keep up with the cavalry column on the march if properly managed. The litter should be halted as seldom as possible. If one gets out of order it should be passed by the others if practicable, and closed up when fixed. The rear mule should always be unhitched first. Everything about the fastenings must be strong enough, so that if the mules pull in opposite directions they cannot break either the poles or the ropes. No brittle timber should be used that may weigh as much as one hundred and fifty pounds without detriment. The litters can be carried on cavalry horses with cavalry saddles as well as on mules, if the horses are gentle. I have had occasion to use these litters: one, after the Piegan affair in January, 1870; one, in the summer of 1875, to bring Colonel R. B. Marcy, Inspector General, U. S. A., from the Geysers to the Great Falls in the National Park;[1] and nineteen on June 27 to 30, 1876, transporting wounded men of General Custer's command, in the Little Big Horn Valley, Montana Territory. Very respectfully, your obedient servant, G. C. DOANE, 1st Lieut. 2d Cavalry.

A few weeks after these experiences in the command of General Terry,[2] Surgeon B. A. Clements, U. S. A., joined the co-operating column under General Crook, as Medical Director, and, in December, 1876, made an elaborate report on the operations of the medical department in the conjoined commands, a report[3] including many interesting observations on sick-transport, especially after the engagement at Slim Buttes, September 9, 1876. As it was hardly practicable to extract these remarks from the context without injustice to the narrative, at the request of Assistant

[1] In General W. E. STRONG's work, entitled *A Trip to the Yellowstone National Park*, 4to (illustrated), Washington, 1876, it is stated (p. 75) that General R. B. MARCY, accompanying the Secretary of War in a visit to the Geysers, fell ill August 3, 1875, and could not mount his horse, when Lieutenant GUSTAVUS C. DOANE, 2d Cavalry, constructed for him a litter to be carried by two pack-mules. The following day the General rode fifteen miles on the litter, and for five days subsequently occupied it occasionally when horseback riding was too fatiguing. General STRONG gives the following description of this litter: "Two poles, eighteen feet long and four inches in diameter, were lashed together in the centre, for the distance of seven feet, by weaving a network of pack-cord across, and forming a good, strong bed of sufficient width to admit a mule between the poles in front and one behind. The mules are to be fastened to this litter in precisely the same manner that a horse would be attached to the shafts of a buggy, the shafts of the litter being strongly fastened to pack-saddles by means of straps. Upon the bed of the litter a buffalo robe was spread, and upon this a mattress was placed, with plenty of blankets and a pillow. Two of the most gentle and surest-footed mules were selected and hitched in, with a reliable man on the back of each."

[2] Assistant Surgeon J. W. WILLIAMS, chief medical officer of General TERRY's command, furnished, January 9, 1877, the following memorandum of the arrangements made for the removal of the wounded after the lamentable affair of the Little Big Horn: "On the arrival of the infantry column under Colonel JOHN GIBBON, 7th Infantry, on June 26th, it was imperative that fifty-nine wounded men should be transported to the confluence of the Little Big Horn with the Big Horn, a distance of about thirty miles, where they could be placed on the transport steamer Far West. It was of urgency that they should be removed without delay from the immediate vicinity of the battle-field, made intolerable by the unburied bodies of men and horses. General GIBBON suggested transportation by hand-stretchers; Dr. WILLIAMS advised the construction of travois; Lieutenant G. A. DOANE advocated the use of two-mule litters. Specimens of the three varieties of conveyance were made the next day, June 27th, and were used in moving the wounded to a camp about five miles down, on the Little Big Horn. The hand-litters proved useless, for the men employed as bearers broke down, and sufficient relays could not be had. The travois worked well. The double-mule litters were ineffective, except for luggage, for the animals were so restive that the wounded feared to be placed on the litters. The next day, June 28th, new trials were made with the mule-litters and travois, selecting animals from General CUSTER's pack-train, in which the mules, recently subjected to long and fatiguing marches, were more docile and tractable. After these experiments, on June 29th, General GIBBON directed the construction of additional two-mule litters and travois, and, as fast as they were finished, the mules were exercised in marching with them. On June 30th, 19 of the more severely wounded were placed on the two-mule litters, 10 on travois, and 30 of the less severely wounded on horseback. Each mule-litter was attended by 4 men, one leading the forward mule, one the rear mule, while one walked on either side of the litter to steady the swaying movement of the side poles. Among the gravely wounded on the mule-litters was one amputated at the place of election in the leg, another with a shot perforation of the knee joint, and 4 with penetrating wounds of the chest or abdomen. On nearing the bank of the Big Horn, the leading mule of the litter bearing the amputated man knelt down and the patient rolled off, but was, fortunately, uninjured. Dr. WILLIAMS observed that much vigilance was requisite on the part of men leading the mules, to prevent serious accidents of this description. The travois, on which the wounded were carried transversely to the long side poles (see FIG. 28, p. 21), required the service of but a single attendant; the 10 less seriously wounded men carried on these conveyances all stated that they found this mode of transport easy and comfortable.

[3] The "Big Horn and Yellowstone Expedition," reinforced after the affair of the Rosebud, leaving its wagon-train and disabled men at Goose Creek, near the Big Horn Mountains, resumed the offensive, August 5, 1876, the command consisting of "about 1,500 cavalry, 450 infantry, 45 white volunteers, and 240 Snake and Ute Indians," an aggregate of 2,235 rank and file. A train of 240 pack-mules carried the supplies, 2 mules being assigned for medical and hospital stores and appliances. A medicine-chest, additional quantities of essential medicines, plaster, and surgical dressings, and 20 canvas sacking-bottoms for litters, were carried on the mules. There were six medical officers, and each carried instruments and dressings on his horse. On August 10th, a junction was effected with the troops under Brigadier General TERRY. The combined forces marched to the confluence of the Powder River with the Yellowstone, arriving August 17th. Here 34 disabled men were transferred to the steamer Far West. Marching northward, many of the men fell sick from the use of alkaline water and exposure to rain and hailstorms, and five of the men were transported on two-mule litters. After long and fatiguing marches, on September 9th an Indian village at Slim Buttes was attacked and captured. There were one man killed, an officer, and 15 men wounded, in this affair. Litters were constructed from the teepe poles, and the march was continued with 15 mule-litters in the ambulance-train. Approaching the Black Hills, the litter-mules struggled with difficulty through the tenacious mud, and some of them fell in crossing streams and ravines; but none of the occupants of the litters received injury. After a most exhausting march, the column reached the Belle Fourche and was joined by a wagon-train. Among the wounded who were carried for many days in mule-litters, in the most inclement weather, and over most difficult country, was one with a shot fracture of the femur put up in a plaster bandage, and an officer amputated at the place of election in the leg.

Surgeon-General C. H. Crane, U. S. A., Surgeon Clements forwarded from Fort Saunders, Wyoming, January 15, 1877, the following memorandum on the construction and management of horse or mule-litters:

"Litters drawn by mules or horses are not to be regarded as a last resort for the transportation of wounded men. On the contrary, they are superior to any other mode of land transportation for certain classes of wounds. These wounds are, especially, gunshot fractures of the bones of the lower extremity and, particularly, of the femur. Mules are preferable to horses, being smaller, more sure-footed, and having a shorter step. Ordinarily, and especially in Indian warfare, the mules will be selected from the pack-train; but in some cases it may be best to select them for this special purpose alone before leaving the supply depot. When not in actual use, the mules are left with the pack-train in charge of the packers. The packers in charge of the litter-mules assist in hitching up and unhitching, and instruct the men in the management of the mules, tying knots, etc., and accompany the litters on the march. The mules selected for each litter should have unequal steps, otherwise a swaying motion is given to the litter. The ordinary pack-saddle, as distinguished from the Mexican or Californian 'aparejo,' should be used. A litter consists of two poles about four inches in diameter and eighteen feet long; two stretcher-bars or poles, two and a half inches in diameter and three feet long; and a canvas bottom, five and a half feet long and two and a half feet broad, with eyelet-holes at sides and ends, which are to be lashed to the poles with rope. The 'travois' (so called) is similarly made; but the rear ends of the side-poles rest on the ground, and it is drawn by one mule. Raw-hide may be used in place of canvas, and it can be had, in case of a successful fight, by skinning dead horses or ponies. If the side-poles are less than eighteen feet long, the rear mule cannot see where he puts his feet, and his head will project over the body of the occupant of the litter, and may injure him; and for the same reason the rear mule is more apt to stumble or fall. The litter is best adapted for a rough country, and, for cases of fracture, the 'travois' (so called) will answer for a level or rolling country and for wounds other than fractures. Six to eight poles, and the same number of stretcher-bars, can be transported on one mule. Twenty-four canvas bottoms can be transported on one mule. The following number of men—mounted—is required: One private for each mule, one corporal for each set of two litters or four travois, one sergeant to each set of six litters or twelve travois, one or more line officers. The officers and men to be detailed from the same company—discipline and efficiency being better secured thereby. A medical officer has general charge of the litter-train, but confines himself to his professional duties and the general direction of the train on the march. A steward and nurses likewise accompany the train on the march. In hitching up and unloading, one man holds the horses of the men of each set of two litters or four travois. The front mule is always led; the rear mule will often move more evenly and more in harmony with the leading mule if left to himself. The rear mule of the empty litter may be detached, and the litter drawn as a travois until needed. The wounded man lies, preferably, facing to the rear. The loaded litters march in rear of the leading column of troops—preferably in rear of the Infantry—and start with the advance. The empty litters march in front of the rear guard, accompanied by a medical officer. Certain troops—preferably Infantry—are designated in orders to protect the litter-train in case of attack en route. The word 'travois' is used for convenience. I am in doubt as to its orthography, derivation, and true meaning. I have heard mentioned, incidentally, made that Parkman, in some one of his works on the Indian tribes, writes of their carrying their goods and children on 'travaux.'"

Assistant Surgeon J. H. Patzki, U. S. A., who was assigned to the charge of the wounded of the infantry detachment on this expedition, forwarded from Fort D. A. Russell, January 25, 1877, a report on sick-transport, from which the following extracts are made:

"In Indian warfare wagons and ambulances are usually pushed as far as the nature of the territory will permit, but when the column cuts loose from the train, accompanied only by pack-animals, there is, as a rule, nothing provided to carry the sick and wounded. The surgeon relies on the old, traditional travée, or on the mule-litter, which, ordinarily, can easily be extemporized by constructing a bed or seat of blankets, canvas, or raw-hide, between two stout but elastic saplings; the former fastened to one mule and dragged as a kind of sledge, the latter carried between two mules. I confess that the matter of transportation under these circumstances has always caused me much worry; there is nothing on hand except, occasionally, the canvas-bed, rarely the harness, but never, in my experience, the most important part, the poles, which, it is trusted, will be obtained from the timber along the river-banks, on which the hostile camps are usually met, or from the tepee-poles should a village be captured. In the latter case, abandoned travées, ready for use, are generally found. A load of barked and seasoned poles could be easily carried by a few mules; but, as a rule, no animals are set apart at the outset for transportation of sick and wounded. When the supplies are reduced by daily consumption, animals become available; but not to the extent one might suppose; as, in the course of the trip, they become progressively weaker, and their loads must be lightened. * * This want of ready transportation was felt during the engagements at the Rosebud, in June, 1876, when the command moved without even a pack-train; it was embarrassing in the extreme to shift the wounded, to secure for them shelter from the fire by mounting them on horses, on which some were supported by comrades mounted behind them, while others were carried in saddle-blankets supported by carbine-slings. * * Ready transportation, available at any moment, is a great desideratum in Indian warfare; it would expedite the movements of the troops, lessen suffering, and reduce the danger of the wounded and dead falling into the hands of the savages. I have no experience with Dr. McElderry's litter; but, in my opinion, the necessary material to quickly construct travées or two-mule-letters would meet all that can be desired. Both are excellent in their way; though I confess that I do not share the favorable opinion, amounting in some to enthusiasm, in regard to the travée as preferable to the litter. I think the popularity of the former is partly due to the fact that it is the most common conveyance, as saplings of sufficient length to construct mule-litters are not often found, and on account of the easier construction and the fewer animals required; partly to the opinion of the wounded, who glides along with less suffering than anticipated on a rude conveyance upon which he looked with dread; and, finally, to the relief felt by the surgeon when at last he sees his flock safely stretched on the travées and keeping pace with the troops. * * Its Indian origin also lends the travée, in the eye of the novice, a certain charm.

From personal experience, and from conversation with the wounded, I consider the travée decidedly inferior to the litter. The patients are comfortably carried in the latter, if properly constructed and provided with a hood; and, especially, if so arranged that the rear animal can see the ground and pick his way; and, if the animals are well selected as to gait and temper, and carefully led across the gulches and obstructions, to prevent the rear animal from jamming against the one in front. They have the additional advantage of allowing suspension of the fractured limbs and carrying some medicines and dressings in them, while streams of moderate depth are crossed with less difficulty than with travées. In deep snow, on account of the plunging and stumbling of the animals, hampered by the litter, and on account of the smooth gliding of the travée, I would prefer the latter. Perhaps, also, in the rare instance where the trail is abruptly winding the greater length of the litter may become a hindrance. The travée has the advantage, that its rear end can be lifted and carried over obstructions. I have found that wounds of the trunk, and even fractures of the thigh, if well dressed in plaster, are less painfully carried in travées than injuries of the head and fractures below the knee, as patients suffering with the last-named injuries are more distressed by the jarring and bumping, and by contact of the feet with the ground. If the poles are unduly slender and elastic, or the canvas too baggy, the patient is apt to have the greater part of the bed come in contact with the ground, especially if this be uneven or covered with brush. Weak, fainting patients are apt to collapse into a heap and to be dragged, or possibly dropped out, through the carelessness of nurses, as I have witnessed. In the litter, the patient can easily be secured by surcingles. Fractures of the upper extremities, well splinted or bandaged against the trunk, are best carried on horseback, as are all slighter injuries. Of course, where poles of sufficient length or the necessary number of animals cannot be obtained, then the travée, the simplest but rudest possible conveyance, is the last refuge; it enables the surgeon to drag his wounded along dead or alive, but the groans or set faces of the sufferers betray that they are not on a bed of roses. Some say that travées are more comfortable than even ambulances; this is not borne out by my experience; but, I think, the litters are; not, however, more so than ordinary hand-litters, or hammocks slung in wagons or ambulances. The travée, as I have seen it, constructed by our troops, is decidedly inferior to the Indian original. The latter is usually hooded with wicker-work; the poles are well-seasoned, longer, lighter, and more elastic; they converge at their lower extremity instead of diverging, thus preventing somewhat the sliding down of the patient; the seat or bed is of platted raw-hide covered with a robe, less baggy than blankets or canvas. In these, with their intimate knowledge of their territory, Indians carry their sick and wounded with comparative comfort over the short distances they ordinarily travel when changing camp for grass or game. I have noticed that they carry fractures of the leg on horseback, the limb dressed in their willow-splints,—similar but inferior to our co-aptation splints,—and suspended from the pommel of the saddle."

Acting Assistant Surgeon V. T. McGillycuddy, who immediately supervised the transport of the wounded carried on *travées* in this expedition, visited the Army Medical Museum November 15, 1876, and presented a miniature model of such an appliance attached to a horse. In this model, numbered 813 in Section VI, the ultimate limit of simplicity is aimed at. The draughtsman has tried to represent it in the adjacent wood-cut (FIG. 33). A sacking-bottom is lashed to two poles that are separated by traverses, and secured to the stirrup leathers of a cavalry horse equipped with the regulation saddle. The soldier's pack makes a pillow, and a blanket is thrown over him. Dr. McGillicuddy has communicated an account of the

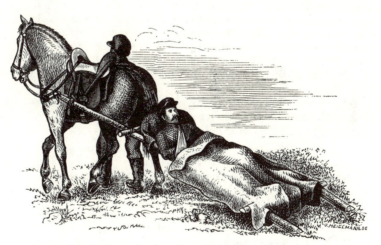

FIG. 33.—*Travée* or Indian horse-litter as figured by Dr. McGILLYCUDDY.

results of his observations on the utility of this form of drag, with comments on its merits when compared with the two-horse litter. Extracts are subjoined of such portions of this paper as has not been anticipated by previous reports. It is dated Camp Robinson, Nebraska, January 27, 1877:

* * "I have the honor to submit the following report on the comparative merits of the travois and two-horse litter as means of transportation for sick and wounded in service on the frontier. In reports heretofore rendered, more or less confusion has arisen from the indiscriminate application of the term horse-litter to both of these conveyances, whereas they are totally different, each having its own peculiar advantages and disadvantages. The horse-litter (properly speaking) is a two-animal arrangement, and is substantially the same as the ordinary hand-litter, or stretcher, in use in the army, either horses or mules being substituted for the men, who act as stretcher-bearers, one animal being harnessed between the poles before and the second between the poles behind; the patient being placed on a piece of canvas or other material, stretched between the poles in the intermediate space. The *travor, travoir, travois, traveau, travaise*, or *travail* (as it is variously spelled), is, on the contrary, not a litter or stretcher in the way it is used. * * The animal being hitched between the poles in front, the after ends of the poles rest on the ground and act as runners, the patient resting on canvas stretched between the poles in the rear

of the animal. In fact, the horse-litter is *carried* by the animals, while the travois is *drawn*. Sometimes two animals are used with the travois, harnessed in tandem; but, in my experience, I find one animal sufficient for the load for any ordinary march, even in a rough country. * * The travois may have been employed years ago by our medical officers on the frontier; but it certainly never was used so extensively nor brought before the public so prominently, as during the present Sioux war. I had good opportunities for observing the comparative advantages of the travois over the horse-litter while on the Big Horn expedition during the past summer, especially after the engagement at Slim Buttes, when I was placed in charge of the transport of the wounded by Surgeon Clements. For transportation I employed nine travois and three two-horse litters, and carried the wounded a distance of about eighty miles, from the field to the northern portion of the Black Hills, where wagons were procured. Our route was over a portion of country untravelled, and in some places very much broken and hilly, and, in other parts, very difficult on account of the numerous small streams, which made the ground very soft and almost impassable, even for cavalry. One objection to the two-horse litter is, that two animals are always required with two men to each animal, one to lead the other to drive. So, to transport one patient, two animals and four men are required. With a travois, but one animal and two men are necessary. With the two-horse litter, if the leading wishes to travel a little more rapidly than the after animal, one or other animal is apt to pull or be pulled out of the harness, and the litter come to the ground either by the foot or head, causing the animal that remains attached to be frightened, which results in more or less damage to the vehicle and patient; on the contrary, if the after animal hastens a little, then there is apt to be a collapse. If one of the animals stumbles and falls down, either the other has to come also or the conveyance is broken, and the person carried thrown out. There is another objection to the two-horse litter; if both animals keep step, the litter begins to vibrate, from the regularity of the motion, and increases to such a degree as to almost throw the patient out. It is for this reason that men employed as stretcher-bearers have to break step; if, on the other hand, the animals break step, the result is a kind of a compound joggling motion which is very unpleasant to the occupant of the litter. I find it necessary to carry long straps around the litter and patient, to prevent his being bounced out. If the animals become unmanageable, and the patient is by any means thrown out, or throws himself out, he has a long distance to fall, and is apt to sustain further injuries. In crossing soft swampy ground, should the animals get to floundering, they being both fastened to the same conveyance seriously interfere with each other, which renders them entirely unmanageable. Besides, owing to the peculiar manner in which the rear animal is fastened to the litter, it is impossible for him to regain his feet. The litter cutting off the sight of the ground from the rear animal, makes him particularly liable to stumble. In fact, in being forced to use two animals in the litter, the liability to accident and trouble is more than doubled, without a corresponding amount of benefit resulting. The travois, on the contrary, is easily constructed, requires but one animal and only one man to manage. Should the horse or mule for any reason become unmanageable, the patient has only to roll off, being but a few inches from the ground, and therefore runs very little risk of being injured. On moderately smooth ground I have frequently traveled with the travée at a trot, without inconveniencing the patient, a thing impossible to do with a two-horse litter. In view of these facts, I consider the travée in every way preferable to the horse-litter, and, unless over good roads, it is preferable to the ambulance-wagon. I have heard patients, after having been transferred to the wagons, wish themselves back to the travée. As I have before remarked, the travée is very easy of construction, and with a limited supply of tools, finding myself one day several miles in the rear of the column with a sick officer unable to travel on horseback, I succeeded in constructing a very comfortable travée in the course of an hour, using small pine trees for poles, and interlacing the lariats of the horses between the poles for the support of the patient; in this case the only tools available were our belt-knives."

**Assistant Surgeon J. R. Gibson, U. S. A., on returning from the Powder River expedition[1] against the Sioux in November and December, 1876, transmitted from Fort McPherson, Nebraska, January 24, 1877, the following observations:**

* * "The old traditional travois, with its rude construction and apparent imperfections, is, in reality, a great boon. It is open to objections; but, when the nature of the service, character of the country, and limited facilities are taken into consideration, the travois comes prominently forward as the means, *par excellence*, for the transport of the disabled. It is not equally well adapted to all the emergencies incident to Indian warfare; for, in many cases, doubless grave perplexities would arise, as, for instance, in shot fractures of the lower extremities; here its advantage is questionable. Yet, in the last campaign, two cases, one shot-fracture of the upper thigh and one involving the hip-joint, were carried for a distance of fifty or sixty miles, from battle-field to supply-camp, with the utmost comfort. These patients were in plaster of Paris dressings. In fact, on their subsequent transfer to ambulance wagons or to swinging litters in army wagons, their expressed preferences for the travois were most pronounced. * * The two-mule litter was not used in the Powder Run expedition. My experience with it is very limited, having seen it used in but one instance several years since. The objection to it consists in the difficulty of securing animals uniformly gaited, in the liability of the rear mule falling or being dragged by the lead mule; also in the varying deviations from a plane surface which the litter describes in traversing very abrupt country. It has also some advantages; for instance, in crossing fordable streams and swift currents the patient's position is far more secure and comfortable than on the travois, the latter necessitating the services of attendants to secure the free ends of the drag, and to wade the streams carrying their burden. The rate of travel attainable by mule-litter is much greater than by travois. The drag-litter is readily prepared from materials at hand; white-pine saplings are the poles, and canvas stretched on them forms the bed. The Indians use raw-hide or robes. Oftentimes the Indian litter is found ready for use in a captured village. * * The use of the modern expedients, with their elegant appliances, harness, gear, etc., seem to me to be excluded simply for the reason that, in such campaigns, the number of pack-animals is usually limited. If the number sufficient to transport medical supplies alone is furnished, the medical officer

---

[1] The "Powder River Expedition" against the Sioux, under the command of Brigadier General G. CROOK, commenced November 14, 1876, and terminated December 29, 1876. The expeditionary force consisted of eleven companies of cavalry, four of artillery, and eleven of infantry, an aggregate of 74 officers, 1,441 enlisted men, with 355 friendly Shoshone, Pawnee, and Arapahoe scouts. November 25, 1876, Colonel R. MACKENZIE, 4th Cavalry, attacked and captured a Cheyenne village on the north fork of the Powder River, on Bates Creek, and lost six killed and twenty-seven wounded.

may consider himself fortunate. A mule can be utilized in two ways: he goes out packed with commissary supplies, which, when consumed, make the animal, with his pack-saddle, available for emergencies,—he generally returns the bearer of a litter. Of course it would be desirable to have the means of transportation of sick and wounded entirely and solely under medical direction. The animals should be previously selected, accustomed to their harness and new duties; also, they should, from the start, be reserved for this service alone.[1] By this means the transportation of pack-saddles, harness, etc., is secured, otherwise it would prove a matter of no little difficulty and annoyance to have the gearing and poles of perhaps thirty to forty litters carried. For the above-cited reasons, chiefly, I consider the improvised litter preferable to more modern appliances."

**Assistant Surgeon D. L. Huntington, U. S. A., who has had much frontier experience, has kindly furnished the reporter, from Soldiers' Home, Washington, January 18, 1877, the following remarks on army sick-transport under conditions of exigency:**

"Such experience as I have had on the frontier and in the midst of hostile Indian tribes leads me to the conclusion that all the common forms of apparatus for transporting badly wounded men under circumstances where wheeled vehicles cannot be used are serviceable and useful; the circumstances and peculiarities of any given situation giving to each form of apparatus its particular value. Under the widely varying geographical diversity of our country, I doubt the possibility of determining upon any one apparatus which shall be equally serviceable in all places and under all conditions. The necessarily irregular and peculiar warfare waged with hostile Indians renders it impracticable, in many cases, to properly fit out a scout for an emergency with all that is desirable for the contingencies of action; and it often happens that, most unexpectedly, and in the most inopportune places, the ingenuity of a medical officer is taxed to the utmost to provide transportation for a man wounded in a sudden Indian attack, or injured by accident at a distance from camp or settlement. Even with expeditions fitted out for the express purpose of seeking and fighting Indians, the character of the country often presents such obstacles to the use of the ordinary conveyances for the wounded, that the medical officer is perplexed to know what material even can be taken, which may be serviceable in fitting up transport apparatus when needed. Again, it not unfrequently happens that in the hot pursuit of Indians who are seeking safety in almost inaccessible mountains and cañons, it is necessary to abandon, for a time, the pack-trains and follow the enemy in the lightest order. In such situations, the transport of an unfortunate wounded man to the base of supplies is a difficult and dangerous matter, and the medical officer is here required at once to suggest and practically carry out some plan that will ensure the safe removal of the man. Under such circumstances, I was once obliged to transport a soldier, wounded in the abdomen, a distance of twelve miles along the narrow bed of a creek filled with boulders and obstructions. I was fortunate enough to find two ash-saplings which, with a blanket stretched across, made an improvised litter, on which my patient was borne, by relays of men, with comparative ease and comfort. At another time, a man belonging to a small detachment sent out from a scouting party was wounded in the leg by the accidental discharge of a musket. Finding it impossible to place the man on horseback, and unsafe to detach a small party to seek the main command, his comrades carried him a distance of about three miles, by forming a seat with their hands and arms, similar to the chairs made by children in their games (FIG. 34). During the late war, I saw a soldier, who had been wounded at some distance from his command, conveyed to a place of safety by laying him prone across a saddle, the stirrup of one side being sufficiently lengthened to afford support for one foot. The horse with his burden was then led quite a distance. I am familiar with another instance, where a man, badly wounded, was conveyed about a three-days' journey in a cot or hammock formed by securing a blanket to two lariat ropes; the ends of the ropes were gathered and carried by his comrades on horseback. All military surgeons know of instances where wounded men have been carried rom the battle-field on muskets with an overcoat laid upon them for a bed. Under the urgent demands of necessity, the fruits of ingenuity are sure to come to the rescue. Of the

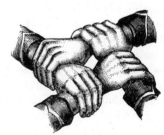

FIG. 34.—Seat made by clasping arms.

usual apparatus for conveying wounded, the ordinary hand-litter is the simplest and generally the most useful in the greater number of cases, particularly when the command is large and the distance to be travelled not excessive. It can be easily secured to a pack-saddle, and, with a little attention from the mule driver, it may be safely carried a long journey. If it becomes necessary to penetrate cañons or ravines, impracticable for the train, it can be carried on men's shoulders. If called into requisition for transport for long distances, it must, of course, be carried by relays of men. Over rough country, it is the easiest and most comfortable mode of conveyance for the wounded, although laborious and fatiguing to the command. The litter for two mules is a comfortable and easy mode of conveyance, provided the mules are quiet and have been trained to its use; otherwise, the unsteady motion and frequent jerks, cause much pain to the sufferer. It is inapplicable over very rough country, and in narrow-winding mountain trails or in densely-wooded and unbroken country. The travée is a common and familiar mode of conveyance, easily improvised, and not uncomfortable. The side-poles for its construction may be carried with any pack-train in the manner in which the Indians carry their lodge-poles. The most favorable condition for its use is over plain country. In rough country, and in mountains, it is dangerous. I have had no experience with the cacolet; but doubt if it would be of much service with the small mule so common in the West and over mountain trails. Judging from the description of such mounted litters for one mule as have been successfully employed on several occasions, I should think that probably future experience will succeed in perfecting it to such an extent as to make it a very desirable conveyance for general use. Even a limited experience in the Indian country will serve to bring out all the latent ingenuity of a medical officer in devising apparatus suitable to the end to be attained; and he will at once learn the value of such material as can be readily carried by man or beast, as rope, buckskin thongs, and blankets."

---

[1] The British *Military Train Manual* (1862, p. 37) remarks, in the directions for *Loading of Pack-Animals*, "Great judgment is required in loading pack-animals, and care should be taken that the animals are not over-weighted, that the load is well put on, that it is neither pitched too high upon the saddle, thereby causing it to roll upon the back, nor too low, which adds to the weight and encumbers the animal, but that the lower line of the load should be even with the shoulders."

Assistant Surgeon-General C. H. Crane, U. S. A., has noted a curious expedient by which, in the absence of any regular appliances, a wounded man was transported a long distance in the mountainous regions of Oregon:

"I believe that the nature of the country where troops are operating against Indians must determine the question as to the best way of transporting the wounded men; and that there will generally be found in the command sufficient ingenuity and means to successfully overcome all obstacles, and to devise and carry out the most appropriate methods of transport. I have had occasion, during several Indian campaigns in California and Oregon, to use litters for carrying wounded men over difficult mountain-trails; in one instance, for a distance of forty or fifty miles. This difficult and tedious undertaking was accomplished by hand-litters, constructed on the spot, from such material as happened to be available, generally by lashing canvas or thongs of raw-hide to poles cut in the woods. I have never used the so-called *travée* or traversine, or Indian litter; I have seen a wounded man safely carried by his comrades for a distance of over fifty miles, along bad mountain-trails, packed on an *aparejo* on a mule's back. He was placed in a semi-recumbent position facing the mule's tail, reclining in the frame of an old trunk, from which the lid and one end had been removed. His wound was from a rifle-bullet that had perforated the muscles of the upper third of the thigh without touching the femur. It was so painful that he could not be carried in the usual way, on horseback, as I have seen safely done in several other instances of shot wounds in the same location."

In an endorsement on the papers relating to the Rooker saddle attachment, General W. T. Sherman makes the following observations on the transport of wounded in cases of emergency:[1]

"When wagons are present or near they are, of course, the best possible, because the wounded man can be placed in a position for carriage by the surgeon in charge, according to the nature of the wound. When there are no wagons, the stretcher improvised on the spot out of blankets and poles is the best possible, carried by men or arranged to a horse, like the lodge-poles of the Sioux. These are better than this saddle. A wounded man, ninety-nine times out of the hundred, wants a recumbent position as soon as possible. If the occasion does not admit of this, then he must be carried on the back of a man, or on a horse, with a comrade behind him to support him and guide the horse. All sorts of saddles have been tried for carrying wounded men, but as a rule they are always left behind, and though I would not discourage the inventive genius and efforts of men humanely disposed, I would trust to the ingenuity of the officer and surgeon on the spot. Mr. Rooker's saddle seems to have been issued to General Custer and others competent to judge, and the only answers I find in this series of papers are that of Captain Mix, 2d Cavalry, and of Dr. Maghee, both of which are unfavorable. This matter, as well as others of a similar nature, may well be left to the ingenuity of the troops interested, who are fully qualified to take care of themselves in all the contingencies of war."

Notwithstanding the opinions of officers of distinction and of large practical experience, I am unable to convince myself that it is prudent or economical to confide the matter of sick-transport to the ingenuity of troops. Because there will generally be found in military commands sufficient ingenuity to construct a bridge, it is not considered expedient for the engineers to neglect the study of trestles and pontoons; and whatever aptitude the men may have for foraging, a regulated administration of commissary, quartermaster, and ordnance supplies is deemed essential. So, likewise, in the medical service of armies, if the difficult problems concerning the transport of sick and wounded men, with due care for the safety of their lives and alleviation of their sufferings, are not studied out in advance, there will be great detriment, on numerous occasions in campaigning, to the efficiency of the fighting force.[2] Experience having demonstrated that, in our army, some other mode of transport than by hand-litters and wheel-vehicles is imperatively necessary, it is

---

[1] Captain A. MOORE, 3d Cavalry, October 3, 1872, forwarded, from Fort McPherson, Nebraska, to the headquarters of the Department of the Platte, a memorandum in regard to the equipment necessary for the successful working of a pack-train to accompany expeditions against Indians, containing in substance the following practical hints: A thoroughly qualified chief packer should be engaged with two or four assistants, according to the duration of the proposed scout. He sees that the aparejos are properly fitted to the mules, which takes time and care. An aparejo fitted to a small mule, such as are used in Arizona and New Mexico, should not weigh over 18 pounds. In the Department of the Platte, where American mules are used, the weight of the aparejo should not exceed 22 pounds. The packer and his assistants should put on and off the aparejo, carefully attending to galls or sores on the pack-animal's back. He should forbid the blankets of the pack-animal from being used as bedding, and see that the dock or crupper is kept clean and well greased, as pack-mules in a mountainous country suffer more from lacerated tails than from any other injury. He should daily equalize the packs, favoring the weaker animals. The aparejos furnished in the Department of the Platte were not properly fitted to the mules. To procure competent packers Captain MOORE believed it to be necessary to send to Oregon, Idaho, Nevada, or Arizona, where the roughness of the country precludes the use of wagons. Captain MOORE states that he had used aparejos on Indian expeditions almost continuously since 1867, and was convinced of their superiority to other pack-saddles. In December, 1871, Captain MOORE turned over at Tucson a train of mules in perfect order, that had followed his company over 4,000 miles in less than a year, bearing packs on the aparejo. In forwarding the report of which the foregoing is a brief abstract, Brigadier-General E. O. C. ORD remarks that the "Mexican aparejo is much used throughout Mexico, California, and the mountains of Nevada, Arizona, and Utah, and that no intelligent packer will allow an old-style pack-saddle to gall his mules if he had means to make, buy, beg, borrow, or steal a decent aparejo." * * Lieutenant-General P. H. SHERIDAN, in transmitting the report, remarks: * * "There has been a great variety of opinions as to the relative value of pack-saddles. If a corps of Mexican packers are to be used, it is absolutely necessary to have aparejos, because that is the instrument which is their beau ideal, and there is no people so celebrated for beastly mule-cruelty as the Mexicans. When mules follow a scouting party which travels at a rapid gait, to keep their backs well is a difficult thing, and no odds how well adjusted the saddle may be when the mule starts out, in a few days, the fatigue and loss of flesh destroys the first adjustment of the saddle to the pack. I have packed extensively with skilful Mexican and American packers, with aparejos and pack-saddles, and have found the condition of the mules and the condition of their backs to depend very much upon the speed with which they were driven, and the roughness or smoothness of the country over which they travel."

[2] To such an extent that in several of the expeditions against Indians in 1876, four men and two animals were subtracted from the effective force for every man sick or wounded, a most unprofitable expenditure of labor.

important to determine the best method. Assuredly this cannot be the devotion of two animals and four soldiers to the carriage of one sick man. It is known that in countries varying in climate and geographical configuration as widely as Algeria, Russia, Italy, and Mexico,[1] it has been found possible to transport two wounded men by one mule, and that only one muleteer was needed for every two mules. The utility and economy of such an arrangement are so obvious, that, notwithstanding the expense and systematic care required to provide animals of sufficient strength and docility and men adequately instructed in the training of the animals and care of the wounded, it would be feasible and desirable to renew the attempt to secure its advantages, as has been successfully accomplished in other armies. It is probable that, with suitable pack-animals[2] and trained hospital men, the advantages in comfort and economy of perfected cacolets[3] and litters over rude improvisations,[4][5] however ingenious, would be recognized. In a shipwreck, one admires the ingenu-

---

[1] It has already been noticed (ante, p. 12) that the French invading force in Mexico, in 1865, took with them the ambulance-mules that had formerly served in Algeria, and had no difficulty in carrying two sick or wounded men on each; while the Austrians, provided with similar cacolets and litters, but without competent muleteers, or any animals but those procured in Mexico, failed wretchedly in their sick-transport. It would be presumptuous to propound a definite plan for sick-transport for our army for circumstances where wheeled-vehicles and water-transportation are unavailable, while the expressed opinions of experienced officers are so divergent, and old methods have repeatedly failed; but as steps in the right direction, it might be suggested that troops operating in frontier regions, and dependent on pack-trains for their supplies, should be accompanied not only by farriers, packers, and commissary and ordnance employés, but by hospital-men or infirmarians familiar with the handling of the sick and wounded, and capable of utilizing the means provided for their transport; and also by trained mules or ponies fit for ambulance-transport. Both men and animals could render other services until their special functions were called in requisition. Could even a small body of trained hospital men be distributed through the detachments of the army, they would serve as fuglemen, to drill two or more detailed men in each company in the duties requisite in emergencies for the care of the sick and wounded, and would constitute a corps of enlisted men from which competent hospital stewards could be recruited.

[2] The burden a mule can sustain continuously varies much, according to the breed or strain, as well as in individuals. "A good Spanish mule, of proper age, is said to be able to travel several months continuously with a weight of some six to eight hundred weight on its back; but only the best, full-sized, and well-limbed animals can accomplish this task. (LONGMORE, op. cit., p. 268). In the "Voyage of the Beagle," Mr. DARWIN mentions, with regard to South American mules, that it is the custom for each animal in a troop to carry a weight of 416 pounds when the ground is level; but that in a mountainous country the mule's load is only about 300 pounds. Dr. NEUDÖRFER (Handbuch der Kriegschir., 1867, B. I, p. 341) states, that the largest and strongest mules that could be obtained in Mexico by the Austrian expeditionary force in 1864–65, broke down under a weight of four hundred pounds. LORD and BAINES (Shifts and Expedients of Camp Life, London, 1871, p. 468) assert: "About 140 pounds is about as much as a mule of average power can travel well with from day to day," meaning probably the load in addition to the pack-saddle and accoutrement. They prefer animals of comparatively small size, and mare mules to horse mules as more tractable. "Baggage mules abound in some of the mountainous parts of Eastern India, but they cannot be turned to account for the carriage of European cacolets and litières with a couple of sick or wounded men upon them. They have not the requisite size or strength. They were tried for this purpose experimentally at Huzara, in 1854, by Captain HUGHES, commanding the Peshawur Mountain Battery, but were found to be quite incapable of sustaining such a load. These mules are thoroughly efficient for the tasks they have to perform, for carrying supplies over rocky and precipitous defiles, or in the interior of a country where there are no roads, because their loads are properly proportioned to their size and power of endurance; but only a mule that is capable of carrying without distress a weight of from four hundred pounds to five hundred pounds can do the work required in the European mode of sick-transport, and any attempt to get mules of less power to perform this service satisfactorily must always end in disappointment and loss."—LONGMORE, op. cit., p. 269. Pack, in commerce, denotes a quantity of goods made up in loads or bales for carriage (REES's Cyclopædia, Am. ed., Vol. XXVII). "A pack of wool is a horse's load, containing seventeen stone and two pounds, or two hundred and forty pounds weight." In the Report of G. B. MCCLELLAN it is stated (op. cit., p. 25) that in the Prussian service the normal load of a pack-animal was then (1855) estimated at two hundred and four pounds.

[3] The derivation of the term cacolet is doubtful. M. LITTRÉ (Dictionaire de la Langue Française, T. I, p. 449) says: "Mot usité dans les Pyrénées." It has been suggested, according to Professor LONGMORE (op. cit., p. 272), that the word may be derived from the resemblance in principle of the mule-chair to the arrangement for carrying milk in casks slung on a mule (câque au lait), employed by the peasantry in the south of France, where mule-litters and chairs were first provided, as a part of the ambulance outfit for the troops on their way to Algeria. It has also been supposed that "cacolet" is simply a corruption of "cabriolet," which originally denoted a sort of little arm-chair. It seems probable that the word was of local use in the Pyrenees to designate the burden of a pack-animal. The eminent Russian surgeon PIROGOFF commends the cacolet (Grundzüge der Allgemeinen Kriegschirurgie, 1864, p. 42): "In the Caucasus, I tested several times the Algerian transport saddle and chair. I conveyed in the same, on horses, through the narrow defiles of Dagestan, several wounded with compound fractures of the leg, after having secured the injured limb in paste bandages. The transported men found this mode very comfortable."

[4] An abstract from F. JAGON's Travels in the Philippines (London, Chapman & Hall, 1876) is given in Harper's New Monthly Magazine, for December, 1876 (Vol. LIV, p. 78), and contains, among its numerous illustrations, a drawing of a Pavava (FIG. 35), a conveyance drawn by a buffalo, and employed by the country people about Manila. The shafts, frame-work, and body are of bamboo; the collar and nose-band of the buffalo of chair cane, and the roof of pandanus leaves. This arrangement furnishes a hint for making travées more comfortable. Unhappily the bamboo, admirably suited to the construction of litters and stretchers, is not available in this country. RÖDLICH (Entwurf zu einer sowohl für den Frieden als Kriegszustand dauernd bleibenden Transportirungs-anstalt für Kranke und Verwundete, Aachen, 1815), has proposed to suspend a large litter for two or more wounded between two oxen, as in FIG. 36; but he considers this expedient unlikely to be of general application, since the movements of oxen are very slow, unfitting them for purposes of military transport.

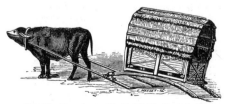

FIG. 35.—Pavava used in the Philippine Islands.

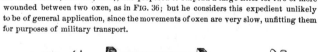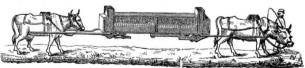

FIG. 36.—Bullock litter. [After H. FISCHER.]

[5] Early references to the Indian drag or litter use the word "travail" (plural travaux), a term possibly applied, by metonymy, to a labor-saving appliance. It seems more probable, however, that the early French voyageurs and missioners who visited the western wilderness gave to this contrivance the name of travée, with reference to the poles held apart by traverses. Travée, according to LITTRÈ (op. cit., T. IV, p. 2325), denotes two side-posts connected by cross-pieces. The various corruptions of the term, travois, etc., are probably Indian patois.

ity and intrepidity with which sailors construct a raft, yet does not hold the commander blameless if he has neglected the precaution of life-boats. It may be assumed that, to introduce in our army a system of sick-transport on pack-animals, it is requisite to provide suitable mules or ponies and men skilled in packing them. Opinions of officers charged with trains appear to incline in favor of the *aparejo* in preference to other forms of pack-saddle. Major-General Schofield, April 10, 1874, promulgated a set of instructions by the lamented Lieutenant Grant,[1] on the mode of pre-

---

[1] *Remarks on preparing and packing the aparejo.* By Lieutenant ALEXANDER GRANT, 1st Cavalry: "The most suitable size of the *aparejo* is four feet nine inches long by two feet wide. To set up an aparejo, prepare straight smooth sticks from one-half to one inch in diameter (wild-rose stems are the best, but any tough, elastic wood will answer), and the coarsest grass that can be obtained. The grass should be cut green, free from flower-stalks,

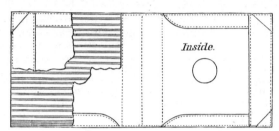

FIG. 37.—Interior view of aparejo.—[GRANT.]

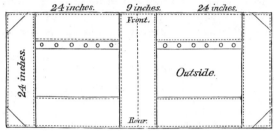

FIG. 38.—Exterior view of aparejo.—[GRANT.]

and dried slowly in the shade. Place the aparejo outside down, as in FIG. 37, shake the grass thoroughly, and place layer after layer on the sticks until the compartment is as full as it can be stuffed with the hand. Great care is necessary in order to insure an equal distribution of the grass in the compartment. The corners are stuffed as hard as possible, a sharp stick being used for the purpose. When stuffed the compartment should have uniform thickness, and when the aparejo is stuffed it should be put on the mule, and the crupper adjusted (FIG. 39). The aparejo-cinch (FIG. 41) is made of strong canvas, seventy-two inches long and twenty inches wide, folded so as to bring the edges in the centre of the cinch. The edges are stitched together, as shown in FIG. 41. A semicircular piece of strong leather, pierced with two holes, is stitched on one end, and two loops of strong leather on the other. A slider of hard wood, of the form shown in the figure, is placed in the loops, and a ring two inches in diameter is attached to the semicircular piece of leather by a thong. The latigo-strap is of strong bridle leather seventy-two inches long, an inch and a half wide on one end, and tapering to half an inch at the other. The wider end has holes punched in it, as shown in the figure. A saddle-blanket, of the pattern issued by the Quartermaster's Department, is first placed on the mule, and on this a corona or upper saddle-blanket, made of two or three folds of old blanket stitched together, with the mule's number stitched on it in colored cloth. Two men put the aparejo on the mule,—No. 1 placing it well back; No. 2 turning down the crupper, passing it under the tail, and then assisting No. 1 to push the aparejo forward as far as it will go. A hammer-cloth, made of matting or canvas of a size to exactly cover the aparejo, is now laid on. The hammer-cloth has two pieces of hard wood (see FIG. 40), twenty inches long, two inches wide, an inch and a half thick, flat on one side, beveled to an edge at the ends, with leather caps stitched over the ends. No. 1 passes the aparejo-cinch to the off-side until the slider-end will reach to the middle of the mule's belly; he then, assisted by No. 2, passes the latigo-strap from above over the slider, then from the outside through the ring, and again over the slider, drawing it tight. No. 2 now reaches over the mule's neck, seizing the front corners of the aparejo, drawing them forward and upward, No. 1 at the same time pulling on the latigo-strap. When the aparejo is set—that is, when the cinch is tight enough to prevent it slipping—No. 2 passes around to the near side of the mule. No. 1 places his left knee against the aparejo, his left hand as far down on the latigo-strap as possible, his right six inches from his left. No. 2, facing No. 1, places his right knee against the aparejo, his right hand between No. 1's hands and his left hand close to No. 1's right, and both draw on the latigo-strap, moving their hands forward as the cinch is tightened, when No. 1 passes a double of the latigo-strap through the loop on the cinch and draws it tight. The packers are provided with a sling-rope of half-inch hemp, sixteen feet long, and a lash-rope thirty-six feet long, one end spliced to a ring in the pack-cinch. This cinch is of strong canvas, thirty-three inches long by eleven inches wide, doubled so as to bring the selvages in the middle of the cinch, where they are stitched as in the aparejo-cinch. Two rectangular pieces of strong leather eight inches long by five and one-half inches wide are stitched on one end on either side. They are of the forms shown at *a, b,* FIG. 42. A piece of strong leather is cut

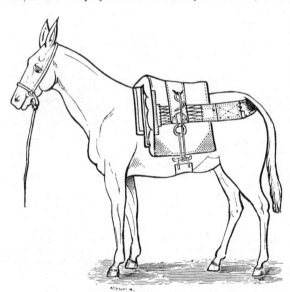

FIG. 39.—Aparejo, with crupper.—[GRANT.]

*Latigo Strap.*

*Hammer Cloth.*

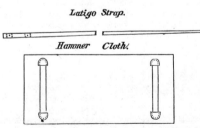

FIG. 40.—Hammer-cloth and Latigo-strap.—[GRANT.]

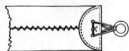

FIG. 41.—Mexican cinch (or synch).—[GRANT.]

of the form shown at *c,* FIG. 42, the circles being five and one-half inches in diameter. A ring three inches in diameter is placed between the circles, and these are folded on each other with the canvas cinch between them, and the whole firmly stitched together. The hook is made of hard wood of the form shown at *d,* FIG. 42. It is passed through the slit in the rectangular piece of leather, and firmly fastened with a leather thong. In putting on the pack No. 1 takes the sling-rope, doubles it, and passes the loop well over on the off-side; No. 2 raises the part of the load intended for his side of the pack and places it well up on the aparejo, holding it there with his left hand. With his right hand he then passes the loop of the sling-rope over the load to paring and packing this form of saddle, instructions so important that a condensed abstract of them, with illustrations, is placed in a foot-note. The cross-tree[1] and other patterns of pack-saddles have also their advocates. Ambulance-chairs and litters could probably be adjusted with almost equal facility to several varieties of pack-saddles; what is essential is that there should be trained mules or ponies[2] and skilled packers. Until these indispensable adjuncts are provided, the improved cacolets and litters found useful in European armies cannot be advantageously employed in our service, and medical officers will probably resort in emergencies to the Indian drag or travée,[3]

---

No. 1, who passes the ends of the sling-rope through the loop and draws them tight. No. 1 then places the part of the load intended for his side of the pack on the aparejo against that already there, and, holding it with his left hand, he passes one end of the sling-rope to No. 2, who carries it under either branch of the rope already round the pack on his side and hands it back to No. 1, who brings both ends of the sling-rope together, draws them tight, and ties them in a square knot. The two men then adjust the load to balance it equally and place the pack-cover, a hemmed piece of canvas five feet square, over the load. No. 1 then takes the lash-rope, coiled in his right hand, grasps it near the cinch with his left hand, and throws the rope to its full extent to his right. He passes the cinch under the mule, hook from him, and, without moving the cinch, he places the rope on the

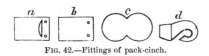

FIG. 42.—Fittings of pack-cinch.

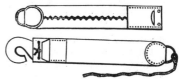

FIG. 43.—Outside and inside view of the pack-cinch.

centre of the pack lengthwise (FIG. 44). He then moves to the mule's shoulder and draws the rope forward two-thirds of its length, and, seizing it about six feet from the cinch, he passes it double to No. 2. No. 2 takes this double in his right hand and the hook of the cinch in his left; he

moves his hands until he can feel that it is tight, when he passes the rear branch of the rope from above into the hook and passes the slack back to No. 1. No. 1 draws this slack tight with his left hand, and passing his right hand under his left he seizes the rope in front of the pack and passes it to the rear; he then passes the part of the rope in his left hand under the standing branch from rear to front, and draws it well up on the pack; he then pushes the bight thus formed below the aparejo. No. 2, in the meantime, takes the end of the rope and passes it under the front standing branch on his side, from rear to front, pushing it to the top of the pack, and throwing the end in front of the pack on No. 1's side; he then seizes the front standing branch with both hands, well down, placing his left knee against the aparejo; he is now ready to pull. No. 1 seizes the front branch on his side, and places his left shoulder against the pack; he then says 'pull.' No. 2 pulls, and No. 1 takes in the slack; this is continued until No. 1 says

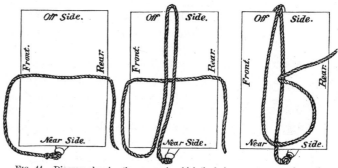

FIG. 44.—Diagram showing the manner in which the lash-rope passes round a pack.

'enough.' No. 2 leads the mule forward, while No. 1 sees that the pack is balanced. No. 1 passes to the rear, and pulls the branch under the aparejo tight. No. 2 passes to the rear, pulls the branch on his side tight, and passes it forward under the points of the aparejo. No. 1 goes to the mule's shoulder on his own side, takes the end of the rope, draws it tight, brings it down under the points of the aparejo and back to the centre of the pack, where he fastens it by drawing it under the standing branches, or, if it is too long, he passes it to No. 2, to be fastened in the same manner.

[1] Dr. D. L. HUNTINGTON, U. S. A., and other medical officers, who have served west of the Rocky Mountains, frequently advert to the so-called cross-tree saddle used by the traders and explorers of New Mexico and the Northwest, and the employés of the Hudson Bay Company, in transporting their stores and peltries. LORD and BAINES (op. cit., p. 465) give figures of two forms of this saddle: one (FIG. 45) the usual form; another (FIG. 46) made with natural forked branches. The girth used with this description of saddle is made in two parts, with eyelets at the end so that they may be laced together with a strip of hide. FIG. 47 represents a mule laden with a pack of this description. FRANCIS GALTON (Art of Travel, or Shifts and Expedients available in Wild Countries, London, 1855, p. 129), gives the following directions for improvised pack-saddles: "Cut four bent pieces of tough wood and two small planks, season them as well as you can and join them together, as in the drawing, using raw-hide in addition to nails or pegs. Stuffed cushions must be tied, or otherwise secured, inside the planks. The art of good packing is to balance the packs accurately, and to lash them very tightly to the saddle. The entire load is then secured to the animal's back by moderate girthing. It is going on a false principle to wind one long cord round the horse, saddle, and packs, making, as it were, a great faggot of them."

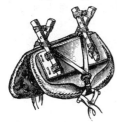

FIG. 45.—Hudson Bay cross-tree saddle. [After LORD & BAINES.]

FIG. 48.—Pack-saddle tree. (After GALTON.)

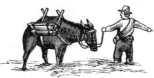

FIG. 47.—Mule laden with pack on cross-tree saddle.—[IBID.]

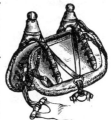

FIG. 46.—Modified cross-tree saddle.—[IBID.]

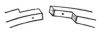

FIG. 49.—Joint of bent pieces. [After GALTON.]

[2] A pony is defined by COWPER: "a small horse; a horse less than fourteen hands high." S. JOHNSON says, "perhaps from puny;" but the ordinary significance of the term is the reverse of this,—stout-built, compact, and strong animals are often thus designated. Measuring at the fore-leg and shoulder, reckoning a hand at four inches, a horse under fifty-six inches in height is usually styled a pony; but this definition is not rigidly attended to in practice. G. B. McCLELLAN, in his Report on European Armies in 1855–56, states (op. cit., p. 248) that in the French service the average height of pack-horses was fixed at 14 hands 1½ inch to 15 hands 1 inch, and that of pack-mules at 13 hands 3 inches to 15 hands 1½ inch.

[3] In the Prairie Traveller, p. 153, General MARCY relates that: "The prairie Indians have a way of transporting their sick and children upon a litter very similar in construction to the one just described, excepting that one animal is used instead of two. One end of the litter is made fast to the sides of the animal, while the other end is left to trail upon the ground. A projection is raised for the feet to rest against and prevent the patient from sliding down. Instead of canvas, the Indians sometimes lash a large willow basket across the poles, in which they place the person to be transported. The animals harnessed to the litter must be carefully conducted upon the march, and caution used in passing over rough and broken ground.

or to the two-horse litter, conveyances that have been fully described in the preceding pages. As I close this report, the following communication is received from New Orleans, dated March, 1877, from Assistant Medical Purveyor E. Swift, U. S. A :

"During the Mexican war, Lieutenant Schuyler Hamilton, aide to General Scott, was severely wounded by a lance, two and a half inches wide, thrusted six and a half inches into the right lung from behind, at Mille Flores, a foundry where shot and shell were being manufactured for the Mexican army.  The lieutenant was conveyed a short distance to headquarters at Chalco, where a horse-litter was constructed of tent-cloth and two long canal-boat setting-poles—the extremities of the poles serving as shafts, to which were harnessed a horse or mule in front and rear of the patient; on this litter he travelled comfortably several days, with the army on its march to the city of Mexico.  Many sick and wounded were conveyed to the coast from the city of Mexico on litters provided with a covered frame-work for protection from the sun and rain.  Litters were frequently improvised and made temporarily by means of blankets knotted at the four corners to two muskets; also a blanket passing under the arm and knotted over the opposite shoulders of two men, forming a seat between them, on which the patient was conveyed in comparative ease and comfort.  Sometimes, wounded men were carried off the field on the backs of their comrades.  I have also known wounded to be carried upon the backs of men, in a kind of chair, after the manner of conveying travellers over mountains in South America.  The well-known Indian travois, rudely constructed of long poles and buffalo-hide—one end harnessed to a mule or horse while the other trails on the ground—almost equals the comfort presented in the first-described method, which I deem the best."

It was my design to treat somewhat more in detail of the different forms of cacolets and of double and single mule-litters used in foreign armies; but the limits allotted to this report are already attained if not exceeded.  For particulars regarding the conveyances of Hill, Shortell, and

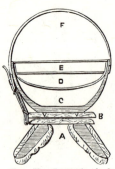

FIG. 50.—LOCATI'S single mule-litter. [After LONGMORE.]

Locati, I must refer to the admirable treatise on the transport of sick and wounded troops by Surgeon-General T. Longmore, my indebtedness to which I have repeatedly had occasion to acknowledge, and for descriptions of other European forms of cacolets and litters to the writings of MM. Legouest, Pirogoff, Gurlt, Van Dommelen, Grossheim, and others who have been cited in this report.  The single mule-litter of M. Locati, of Turin, designed for the passage of the narrowest defiles, avoiding as far as possible obstructions from tree-branches overhead or impediments on either side, is regarded in Europe as about the best appliance of this sort.  A cross-section of it is shown in the adjacent wood-cut.  Assistant Surgeon W. J. Wilson, U. S. A., who recently accompanied an incursion of the troops of the Khedive upon the Abyssinians, informs me that camels were there advantageously used for sick-transport by the Egyptian troops.  I had prepared wood-cuts of the camel-litters used by Larrey in the campaign in Syria, and the camel-kujawahs used in the Punjaub, devised by Surgeon W. B. Webb of the Bengal service, but have not space to introduce them, and must again refer to the exhaustive work of Professor Longmore, and to the memoirs and historical and surgical relation of the *Armée d'Orient* of the illustrious Larrey, for information on this means of sick-transport, apparently well adapted for army use in Texas, New Mexico, and Arizona.

Whatever incompleteness there may be in this report as a theoretical disquisition, the practical views and suggestions advanced by a considerable number of experienced medical officers cannot fail to receive your appreciation.

I am, General, very respectfully, your obedient servant,

GEORGE A. OTIS,
*Assistant Surgeon, U. S. A.*

Brigadier-General JOSEPH K. BARNES,
*Surgeon General U. S. A.*

paring and packing this form of saddle, instructions so important that a condensed abstract of them, with illustrations, is placed in a foot-note. The cross-tree[1] and other patterns of pack-saddles have also their advocates. Ambulance-chairs and litters could probably be adjusted with almost equal facility to several varieties of pack-saddles; what is essential is that there should be trained mules or ponies[2] and skilled packers. Until these indispensable adjuncts are provided, the improved cacolets and litters found useful in European armies cannot be advantageously employed in our service, and medical officers will probably resort in emergencies to the Indian drag or travée,[3]

---

No. 1, who passes the ends of the sling-rope through the loop and draws them tight. No. 1 then places the part of the load intended for his side of the pack on the aparejo against that already there, and, holding it with his left hand, he passes one end of the sling-rope to No. 2, who carries it under either branch of the rope already round the pack on his side and hands it back to No. 1, who brings both ends of the sling-rope together, draws them tight, and ties them in a square knot. The two men then adjust the load to balance it equally and place the pack-cover, a hemmed piece of canvas five feet square, over the load. No. 1 then takes the lash-rope, coiled in his right hand, grasps it near the cinch with his left hand, and throws the rope to its full extent to his right. He passes the cinch under the mule, hook from him, and, without moving the cinch, he places the rope on the

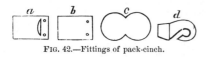

FIG. 42.—Fittings of pack-cinch.

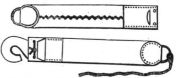

FIG. 43.—Outside and inside view of the pack-cinch.

centre of the pack lengthwise (FIG. 44). He then moves to the mule's shoulder and draws the rope forward two-thirds of its length, and, seizing it about six feet from the cinch, he passes it double to No. 2. No. 2 takes this double in his right hand and the hook of the cinch in his left; he moves his hands until he can feel that it is tight, when he passes the rear branch of the rope from above into the hook and passes the slack back to No. 1. No. 1 draws this slack tight with his left hand, and passing his right hand under his left he seizes the rope in front of the pack and passes it to the rear; he then passes the part of the rope in his left hand under the standing branch from rear to front, and draws it well up on the pack; he then pushes the bight thus formed below the aparejo. No. 2, in the meantime, takes the end of the rope and passes it under the front standing branch on his side, from rear to front, pushing it to the top of the pack, and throwing the end in front of the pack on No. 1's side; he then seizes the front standing branch with both hands, well down, placing his left knee against the aparejo; he is now ready to pull. No. 1 seizes the front branch on his side, and places his left shoulder against the pack; he then says 'pull.' No. 2 pulls, and No. 1 takes in the slack; this is continued until No. 1 says 'enough.' No. 2 leads the mule forward, while No. 1 sees that the pack is balanced. No. 1 passes to the rear, and pulls the branch under the aparejo tight. No. 2 passes to the rear, pulls the branch on his side tight, and passes it forward under the points of the aparejo. No. 1 goes to the mule's shoulder on his own side, takes the end of the rope, draws it tight, brings it down under the points of the aparejo and back to the centre of the pack, where he fastens it by drawing it under the standing branches, or, if it is too long, he passes it to No. 2, to be fastened in the same manner.

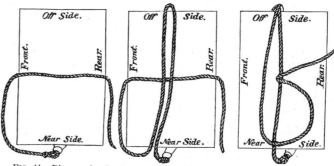

FIG. 44.—Diagram showing the manner in which the lash-rope passes round a pack.

[1] Dr. D. L. HUNTINGTON, U. S. A., and other medical officers, who have served west of the Rocky Mountains, frequently advert to the so-called cross-tree saddle used by the traders and explorers of New Mexico and the Northwest, and the employés of the Hudson Bay Company, in transporting their stores and peltries. LORD and BAINES (op. cit., p. 465) give figures of two forms of this saddle: one (FIG. 45) the usual form; another (FIG. 46) made with natural forked branches. The girth used with this description of saddle is made in two parts, with eyelets at the end so that they may be laced together with a strip of hide. FIG. 47 represents a mule laden with a pack of this description. FRANCIS GALTON (Art of Travel, or Shifts and Expedients available in Wild Countries, London, 1855, p. 129), gives the following directions for improvised pack-saddles: "Cut four bent pieces of tough wood and two small planks, season them as well as you can and join them together, as in the drawing, using raw-hide in addition to nails or pegs. Stuffed cushions must be tied, or otherwise secured, inside the planks. The art of good packing is to balance the packs accurately, and to lash them very tightly to the saddle. The entire load is then secured to the animal's back by moderate girthing. It is going on a false principle to wind one long cord round the horse, saddle, and packs, making, as it were, a great faggot of them."

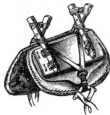

FIG. 45.—Hudson Bay cross-tree saddle. [After LORD & BAINES.]

FIG. 48.—Pack-saddle tree. (After GALTON.)

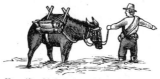

FIG. 47.—Mule laden with pack on cross-tree saddle.—[IBID.]

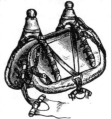

FIG. 46.—Modified cross-tree saddle.—[IBID.]

FIG. 49.—Joint of bent pieces. [After GALTON.]

[2] A pony is defined by COWPER: "a small horse; a horse less than fourteen hands high." S. JOHNSON says, "perhaps from puny;" but the ordinary significance of the term is the reverse of this,—stout-built, compact, and strong animals are often thus designated. Measuring at the fore-leg and shoulder, reckoning a hand at four inches, a horse under fifty-six inches in height is usually styled a pony; but this definition is not rigidly attended to in practice. G. B. McCLELLAN, in his Report on European Armies in 1855–56, states (op. cit., p. 248) that in the French service the average height of pack-horses was fixed at 14 hands 1½ inch to 15 hands 1 inch, and that of pack-mules at 13 hands 3 inches to 15 hands 1½ inch.

[3] In the Prairie Traveller, p. 153, General MARCY relates that: "The prairie Indians have a way of transporting their sick and children upon a litter very similar in construction to the one just described, excepting that one animal is used instead of two. One end of the litter is made fast to the sides of the animal, while the other end is left to trail upon the ground. A projection is raised for the feet to rest against and prevent the patient from sliding down. Instead of canvas, the Indians sometimes lash a large willow basket across the poles, in which they place the person to be transported. The animals harnessed to the litter must be carefully conducted upon the march, and caution used in passing over rough and broken ground."

or to the two-horse litter, conveyances that have been fully described in the preceding pages. As I close this report, the following communication is received from New Orleans, dated March, 1877, from Assistant Medical Purveyor E. Swift, U. S. A:

"During the Mexican war, Lieutenant Schuyler Hamilton, aide to General Scott, was severely wounded by a lance, two and a half inches wide, thrusted six and a half inches into the right lung from behind, at Mille Flores, a foundry where shot and shell were being manufactured for the Mexican army. The lieutenant was conveyed a short distance to headquarters at Chalco, where a horse-litter was constructed of tent-cloth and two long canal-boat setting-poles—the extremities of the poles serving as shafts, to which were harnessed a horse or mule in front and rear of the patient; on this litter he travelled comfortably several days, with the army on its march to the city of Mexico. Many sick and wounded were conveyed to the coast from the city of Mexico on litters provided with a covered frame-work for protection from the sun and rain. Litters were frequently improvised and made temporarily by means of blankets knotted at the four corners to two muskets; also a blanket passing under the arm and knotted over the opposite shoulders of two men, forming a seat between them, on which the patient was conveyed in comparative ease and comfort. Sometimes, wounded men were carried off the field on the backs of their comrades. I have also known wounded to be carried upon the backs of men, in a kind of chair, after the manner of conveying travellers over mountains in South America. The well-known Indian travois, rudely constructed of long poles and buffalo-hide—one end harnessed to a mule or horse while the other trails on the ground—almost equals the comfort presented in the first-described method, which I deem the best."

It was my design to treat somewhat more in detail of the different forms of cacolets and of double and single mule-litters used in foreign armies; but the limits allotted to this report are already attained if not exceeded. For particulars regarding the conveyances of Hill, Shortell, and

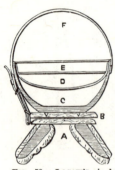

FIG. 50.—LOCATI'S single mule-litter. [After LONGMORE.]

Locati, I must refer to the admirable treatise on the transport of sick and wounded troops by Surgeon-General T. Longmore, my indebtedness to which I have repeatedly had occasion to acknowledge, and for descriptions of other European forms of cacolets and litters to the writings of MM. Legouest, Pirogoff, Gurlt, Van Dommelen, Grossheim, and others who have been cited in this report. The single mule-litter of M. Locati, of Turin, designed for the passage of the narrowest defiles, avoiding as far as possible obstructions from tree-branches overhead or impediments on either side, is regarded in Europe as about the best appliance of this sort. A cross-section of it is shown in the adjacent wood-cut. Assistant Surgeon W. J. Wilson, U. S. A., who recently accompanied an incursion of the troops of the Khedive upon the Abyssinians, informs me that camels were there advantageously used for sick-transport by the Egyptian troops. I had prepared wood-cuts of the camel-litters used by Larrey in the campaign in Syria, and the camel-kujawahs used in the Punjaub, devised by Surgeon W. B. Webb of the Bengal service, but have not space to introduce them, and must again refer to the exhaustive work of Professor Longmore, and to the memoirs and historical and surgical relation of the *Armée d'Orient* of the illustrious Larrey, for information on this means of sick-transport, apparently well adapted for army use in Texas, New Mexico, and Arizona.

Whatever incompleteness there may be in this report as a theoretical disquisition, the practical views and suggestions advanced by a considerable number of experienced medical officers cannot fail to receive your appreciation.

I am, General, very respectfully, your obedient servant,

GEORGE A. OTIS,
*Assistant Surgeon, U. S. A.*

Brigadier-General JOSEPH K. BARNES,
*Surgeon General U. S. A.*

O